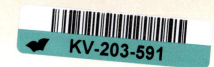

This book is dedicated to the men and women of the emergency medical services system, who are an integral part of the emergency medical team and have contributed to marked improvement in patient survival, especially in cardiac arrest and trauma—often while working under challenging conditions.

a **LANGE** medical book

DR S M BRUNDEN

CURRENT

Emergency Diagnosis & Treatment

Fourth Edition

Edited by

Charles E. Saunders, MD, FACEP, FACP
Associate Clinical Professor of Medicine
University of California School of Medicine
San Francisco and San Francisco General Hospital
Medical Director, Department of Health
Paramedic Division, City and County of San Francisco

Mary T. Ho, MD, MPH
Assistant Professor of Medicine
Emergency Medicine Service
University of Washington School of Medicine, Seattle
Co-Director, Center for Evaluation of Emergency
Medical Services, Seattle—King County Department of Public Health

with Associate Authors

 Prentice-Hall International Inc.

Copyright © 1992 by Appleton & Lange
Simon & Schuster Business and Professional Group
Copyright © 1990 by Appleton & Lange; copyright © 1985, 1983 by Lange Medical Publications

92 93 94 95 96 / 10 9 8 7 6 5 4 3 2 1

Prentice Hall International (UK) Limited, *London*
Prentice Hall of Australia Pty. Limited, *Sydney*
Prentice Hall Canada, Inc., *Toronto*
Prentice Hall Hispanoamericana, S.A., *Mexico*
Prentice Hall of India Private Limited, *New Delhi*
Prentice Hall of Japan, Inc., *Tokyo*
Simon & Schuster Asia Pte. Ltd., *Singapore*
Editora Prentice Hall do Brasil Ltda., *Rio de Janeiro*
Prentice Hall, *Englewood Cliffs, New Jersey*

ISBN: 0-8385-1306-9
ISSN: 0894-2293

Acquisitions Editor: Martin J. Wonsiewicz
Production Editor: Charles F. Evans

PRINTED IN THE UNITED STATES OF AMERICA

Table of Contents

Authors

Joseph A. Abbott, MD
Clinical Professor of Medicine (Cardiology and Clinical Electrophysiology) and Radiology (Cardiac Imaging), University of California School of Medicine, San Francisco.

David C. Aron, MD
Associate Professor of Medicine, Case Western Reserve University School of Medicine, Cleveland; Associate Chief, Medical Service, Veterans Administration Hospital, Cleveland.

Paul S. Auerbach, MD
Professor of Surgery and Chief, Division of EmergencyMedicine, Stanford University School of Medicine, Stanford, California.

Henry M. Bartkowski, MD, PhD
Clinical Associate Professor, Pediatric Neurosurgery, Children's Hospital, Ohio State University, Columbus, Ohio.

Charles E. Becker, MD
Professor of Medicine, University of California School of Medicine, San Francisco; Head, Division of Occupational/Environmental Medicine and Toxicology, San Francisco General Medical Center.

John P. Cello, MD
Professor of Medicine, University of California School of Medicine, San Francisco; Chief of Gastroenterology, San Francisco General Hospital.

Melvin D. Cheitlin, MD
Professor of Medicine, University of California School of Medicine, San Francisco; Associate Chief of Cardiology, San Francisco General Hospital.

Kevin Coulter, MD, FAAP
Assistant Clinical Professor, Pediatrics, University of California School of Medicine, San Francisco.

Richard A. Crass, MD
Professor of Surgery and Head, Division of General Surgery, The Oregon Health Sciences University, Portland, Oregon.

Roger L. Crumley, MD
Professor and Chief, Otolaryngology—Head and Neck Surgery, University of California, Irvine, California.

Steven A. Davis, MD
Associate Clinical Professor of Medicine, Division of Dermatology, University of Texas Health Science Center, San Antonio.

Ronald A. Dieckmann, MD, MPH, FAAP, FACEP
Associate Clinical Professor of Pediatrics and Medicine, University of California Medical Center, San Francisco; Director of Pediatric Emergency Medicine, San Francisco General Hospital.

Stephen H. Embury, MD
Professor of Medicine, University of California School of Medicine, San Francisco; Chief of Hematology, San Francisco General Hospital.

James E. George, MD, JD, FACEP
President, Emergency Physician Associates, and Partner, Law Firm of George & Korin, Woodbury, New Jersey.

Phillip J. Goldstein, MD
Obstetrician and Gynecologist-in-Chief, Sinai Hospital, Baltimore.

Phyllis A. Guze, MD
Professor of Clinical Medicine and Vice Chair, Department of Medicine, University of California School of Medicine, Los Angeles; Chief of Medicine, West Los Angeles Veterans Administration Medical Center (Wadsworth Division), Los Angeles.

Thomas Hearne, PhD
Emergency Medical Services Management Analyst, King County Emergency Medical Services Division, Seattle—King County Department of Public Health.

Mary T. Ho, MD, MPH
Assistant Professor of Medicine, Emergency Medicine Service, University of Washington School of Medicine, Seattle; Co-Director, Center for Evalua-

tion of Emergency Medical Services, Seattle—
King County Department of Public Health.

Michael H. Humphreys, MD
Professor of Medicine, University of California
School of Medicine, San Francisco; Chief of Ne-
phrology, San Francisco General Hospital.

John H. Karam, MD
Professor of Medicine and Director, Diabetes Clin-
ics, University of California School of Medicine,
San Francisco.

Eugene S. Kilgore, Jr., MD, FACS
Clinical Professor of Surgery and Emeritus Chief
of Hand Clinic, University of California School of
Medicine, San Francisco; Emeritus Chief of Hand
Clinics, Veterans Administration Medical Center,
San Francisco and Martinez, California.

David Knighton, MD, FACS
Associate Professor of Surgery, University of Minnesota Medical School, Minneapolis.

Charles A. Linker, MD
Associate Clinical Professor of Medicine, University of California School of Medicine, San Francisco.

Richard M. Locksley, MD
Associate Professor of Medicine and Chief, Division of Infectious Diseases, University of California School of Medicine, San Francisco.

John M. Luce, MD
Associate Professor of Medicine and Anesthesia,
University of California School of Medicine, San
Francisco; Associate Director, Medical-Surgical
Intensive Care Unit, San Francisco General Hospi-
tal.

W. Earle Matory, Jr., MD, FACS
Associate Professor of Surgery, Division of Plastic
and Reconstructive Surgery, University of Massachusetts Medical Center, Worcester, Massachusetts.

Jack W. McAninch, MD
Professor of Urology and Vice Chairman, Department of Urology, University of California School
of Medicine, San Francisco; Chief of Urology, San
Francisco General Hospital.

Sharron L. Mee, MD
Attending Urologist, Cedars-Sinai Medical Center,
Los Angeles.

Anthony A. Meyer, MD, PhD
Professor of Surgery, University of North Carolina, Chapel Hill, North Carolina.

John Mills, MD
Professor of Medicine and Microbiology, University of California School of Medicine, San Francisco; Professor of Clinical Pharmacy, University
of California School of Pharmacy, San Francisco;
Chief of Infectious Disease Unit, San Francisco
General Hospital.

Jerome A. Motto, MD
Professor of Psychiatry Emeritus and Associate
Director of Psychiatric Consultation/Liaison Ser-
vice, University of California School of Medicine,
San Francisco.

Pamela H. Nagami, MD
Clinical Associate Professor of Medicine, University of California School of Medicine, Los Angeles; Infectious Disease Section, Department of Internal Medicine, Southern California Permanente
Medical Group, Kaiser Medical Center, Woodland
Hills, California.

Julia Nathan, MD
Assistant Clinical Professor of Medicine, University of California School of Medicine, San Francisco; Attending Physician, Emergency Services,
San Francisco General Hospital.

William L. Newmeyer, MD
Associate Clinical Professor of Surgery, University of California School of Medicine, San Francisco.

Kent R. Olson, MD, FACEP
Associate Clinical Professor of Medicine and Lec-
turer in Pharmacy, University of California Medical Center, San Francisco; Medical Director, San
Francisco Bay Area Regional Poison Control Center.

Carol A. Raviola, MD
Clinical Assistant Professor of Surgery, University
of Pennsylvania; Vascular Surgery Division, Pennsylvania Hospital, Philadelphia.

Patricia R. Salber, MD, FACEP, FACP
Assistant Clinical Professor of Medicine, University of California School of Medicine, San Francisco; Staff Physician, Emergency Department,
Kaiser Permanente Medical Group, San Francisco.

Charles E. Saunders, MD, FACEP, FACP
Associate Clinical Professor of Medicine, University of California School of Medicine, San Francisco, and San Francisco General Hospital; Medi-

cal Director, Department of Health, Paramedic Division, City and County of San Francisco.

Roger P. Simon, MD
Professor of Neurology, University of California School of Medicine, San Francisco; Chief of Neurology, San Francisco General Hospital.

Khalid F. Tabbara, MD
Professor and Chairman, Department of Ophthalmology, College of Medicine, King Saud University, Riyadh, Saudi Arabia.

Thomas A. Tami, MD
Assistant Professor of Otolaryngology, University of California Medical Center, San Francisco; Chief, Department of Otolaryngology—Head and Neck Surgery, San Francisco General Hospital.

Peter G. Trafton, MD
Associate Professor of Orthopedic Surgery, Brown University; Surgeon-in-Charge, Division of Orthopedic Trauma, Rhode Island Hospital, Providence.

Donald D. Trunkey, MD
Professor and Chairman, Department of Surgery, The Oregon Health Sciences University, Portland, Oregon.

J. Blake Tyrrell, MD
Clinical Professor of Medicine, University of California School of Medicine, San Francisco.

Robert L. Walton, MD
Professor of Surgery, and Chairman, Division of Plastic and Reconstructive Surgery, University of Massachusetts Medical Center, Worcester, Massachusetts.

Preface

This fourth edition of *Current Emergency Diagnosis & Treatment* continues its problem-oriented approach to emergency management problems. It provides the emergency practitioner with ready information needed to both diagnose and treat life-threatening problems rapidly and also to organize the approach to the patient in the emergency setting.

OUTSTANDING FEATURES

Like all Lange medical books, *CEDT* provides a concise yet comprehensive source of current, clear, and correct information. As editors and practicing emergency physicians, we have tried to ensure that each chapter reflects the needs and realities of day-to-day practice.

Because of the book's practical orientation, basic science and pathophysiologic principles are emphasized only when they are germane to management. Likewise, discussion of management is generally limited to those measures customarily performed in the emergency department.

INTENDED AUDIENCE

This text is specifically designed for physicians, residents, and medical students who are providing emergency care. It will also be useful to emergency department nurses and emergency medical technicians.

ORGANIZATION

CEDT's organization is priority-based and problem-oriented. In actual emergency practice, the patient presents with a problem, and the diagnosis may, at first, be unknown. Because the emergency physician's evaluation and treatment is initially problem-oriented, this fact is reflected in the table of contents. Chapters are grouped in order of presenting clinical management problems, with the most life-threatening first. Next are traumatic emergencies, followed by nontraumatic emergencies. The book concludes with a comprehensive reference chapter of emergency problems.

NEW TO THIS EDITION

- A new chapter organization that emphasizes the priority-based, problem-oriented approach to emergency evaluation and management.
- Updates throughout.
- A completely new chapter on emergency airway management by Julia Nathan, MD, University of California School of Medicine, San Francisco.
- A completely new and expanded chapter on pediatric emergencies by Ronald A. Dieckmann, MD, and Kevin Coulter, MD, both from the University of California School of Medicine, San Francisco.

- A completely new chapter on multicasualty incidents and disaster management by Charles E. Saunders, MD, University of California School of Medicine, San Francisco.
- Expansion and division of cardiac emergencies into two chapters, Cardiac Emergencies by Melvin D. Cheitlin, MD, and Cardiac Arrhythmias by Joseph A. Abbott, MD, both from the University of California School of Medicine, San Francisco.
- Additions of several new procedures to the emergency procedures chapter.
- An expansion of the dermatology chapter.
- Updated coverage of AIDS throughout.

ACKNOWLEDGMENTS

We would like to thank the editorial staff of Appleton & Lange for their support and patience, and in particular, Nancy Evans, Carol Vartanian, and Rebecca Hainz-Baxter.

We welcome comments and criticisms regarding this text and ask that they be sent to Appleton & Lange.

July 1992

Charles E. Saunders, MD, FACEP, FACP
Mary T. Ho, MD, MPH

Section I.
Management of Common Emergency Problems

Basic & Advanced Cardiac Life Support

1

Mary T. Ho, MD, MPH, & John M. Luce, MD

The ABCs of CPR

After initial assessment, the steps of CPR may be remembered by using the mnemonic A–B–C:

$A = Airway$
$B = Breathing$
$C = Circulation$

Each step begins with an assessment phase.

BASIC LIFE SUPPORT

TECHNIQUE OF CARDIOPULMONARY RESUSCITATION (CPR)

Step 1: Verify Unconsciousness.

The physician confronted with a person in an apparently collapsed state who may require lifesaving resuscitation measures must first determine whether unconsciousness has occurred. Shake the victim gently, and shout, "Are you all right? Are you okay?" The victim may have fainted or may be just sleeping. Shouting and gentle shaking are usually enough to revive or awaken the victim in such cases. If there is no response, cardiac or respiratory arrest may be present, and the procedures listed below must be followed.

Step 2: Shout for Help.

Assistance is essential, since a single rescuer cannot perform CPR and call to activate the emergency medical services (EMS) system simultaneously. Even if no one is in sight, attempt to summon help by shouting, "Help, somebody, help." Whoever responds should be sent to activate the EMS system for out-of-hospital situations, or the advanced cardiac life support team for in-hospital cardiac arrests.

Step 3: Position the Patient.

The unconscious victim must be positioned to allow further assessment and management. Place the patient face up (extended supine position) on a firm, level surface. Be gentle while turning the patient, especially if signs of trauma are present, since fractures or internal injuries may be made worse by rough handling. If spinal cord injury is suspected, hold the patient's head in a neutral position and move it and the body as one unit (logroll).

Note: If a monitor-defibrillator and personnel trained in its use are immediately available, skip to step 7 and check for a palpable pulse. If the pulse is absent and the monitor or "quick-look" paddle rhythm shows ventricular fibrillation or tachycardia,

immediately defibrillate with 200 J. Repeat at 200–300 J and again at 360 J if rhythm or pulselessness persists.

If a defibrillator without monitor capability is immediately available, pulseless patients should be defibrillated as above.

If a defibrillator is not available and the arrest is witnessed, confirm pulselessness, and deliver a solitary precordial thump (see Fig 1–12).

If a defibrillator is not available or if defibrillation or precordial thump is not successful, proceed with CPR steps 4–9.

Step 4: Establish Airway.

Establish and maintain an open airway *immediately*. With unconsciousness, the tongue falls posteriorly and may obstruct the airway (Fig 1–1).

A. No Cervical Spine Injury: Opening and maintaining the airway is best achieved by the **head-tilt and chin-lift method.** Place one hand on the forehead and the other on the bony portion of the mandible (chin). Use the hand on the forehead to tilt the head backward and the fingers of the other hand to lift the chin forward (Fig 1–1B). The fingers must not press into the soft tissue under the chin, which might obstruct the airway. The thumb should not be used to lift the chin. The formerly recommended head-tilt and neck-lift method is less effective and should no longer be used.

B. Suspected Cervical Spine Injury: If a victim of respiratory arrest has a suspected or documented cervical spine injury—a rare combination—the ventilation technique must be modified to avoid further cervical spinal cord injury. The patient should be on a hard surface for CPR, as this factor alone provides some protection for the neck. Place sandbags, if available, on both sides of the neck and head to prevent lateral movement. Maintain the neck in a neutral position, and avoid extension and flexion. Open the airway with the **jaw-thrust maneuver.** Grasp the angles of the victim's lower jaw, and lift with both hands to displace the mandible forward (Fig 1–2). The rescuer should stand or kneel at the head of the patient and rest the elbows on the surface on either side of the patient's head. Two rescuers are generally needed to perform ventilation with the jaw-thrust technique—one to open the airway and the other to provide ventilation. If only one rescuer is available, the nostrils are occluded by the rescuer's cheek during mouth-to-mouth ventilation. A rubber nasal airway or plastic oropharyngeal airway may be helpful in keeping the tongue from occluding the upper airway.

Step 5: Check for Spontaneous Ventilation.
(See Fig 1–1D.)

Once the airway is open, check for signs of adequate respiratory exchange. Spontaneous ventilation

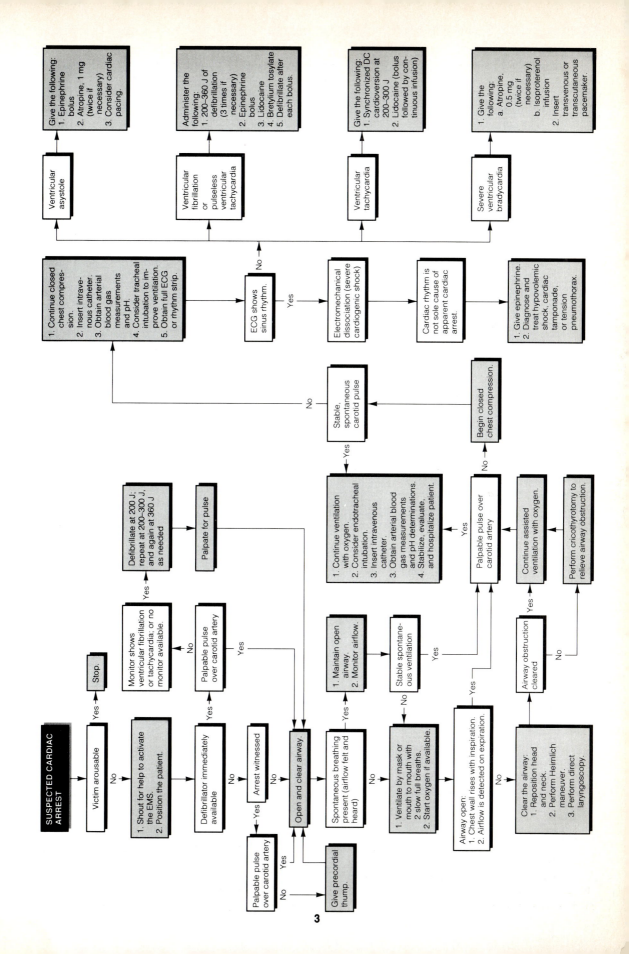

SUSPECTED CARDIAC ARREST

Victim arousable — Yes → Stop.

No ↓

1. Shout for help to activate the EMS.
2. Position the patient.

Defibrillator immediately available

No ↓ / Yes →

Palpable pulse over carotid artery — No / Yes

Give precordial thump.

Arrest witnessed — Yes → / No

Monitor shows ventricular fibrillation or tachycardia; or no monitor available.

Yes → Defibrillate at 200 J; repeat at 200–300 J, and again at 360 J as needed

No → Palpate for pulse

Open and clear airway.

Spontaneous breathing present (airflow felt and heard) — Yes →

1. Maintain open airway.
2. Monitor airflow.

No ↓

1. Ventilate by mask or mouth to mouth with 2 slow full breaths.
2. Start oxygen if available.

Airway open:
1. Chest wall rises with inspiration.
2. Airflow is detected on expiration.

Yes →

Clear the airway:
1. Reposition head and neck.
2. Perform Heimlich maneuver.
3. Perform direct laryngoscopy.

Airway obstruction cleared — Yes → Continue assisted ventilation with oxygen.

No → Perform cricothyrotomy to relieve airway obstruction.

Stable spontaneous ventilation — Yes →

Palpable pulse over carotid artery — Yes →

No → Begin closed chest compression.

1. Continue ventilation with oxygen.
2. Consider endotracheal intubation.
3. Insert intravenous catheter.
4. Obtain arterial blood gas measurements and pH determinations.
4. Stabilize, evaluate, and hospitalize patient.

Stable, spontaneous carotid pulse — Yes ↑ / No →

1. Continue closed chest compression.
2. Insert intravenous catheter.
3. Obtain arterial blood gas measurements and pH.
4. Consider tracheal intubation to improve ventilation.
5. Obtain full ECG or rhythm strip.

ECG shows sinus rhythm. — No ↑ / Yes →

Electromechanical dissociation (severe cardiogenic shock) →

Cardiac rhythm is not sole cause of apparent cardiac arrest. →

1. Give epinephrine
2. Diagnose and treat hypovolemic shock, cardiac tamponade, or tension pneumothorax.

Ventricular asystole →
Give the following:
1. Epinephrine bolus
2. Atropine, 1 mg (twice if necessary)
3. Consider cardiac pacing.

Ventricular fibrillation or pulseless ventricular tachycardia →
Administer the following:
1. 200–360 J of defibrillation (3 times if necessary)
2. Epinephrine bolus
3. Lidocaine
4. Bretylium tosylate
5. Defibrillate after each bolus.

Ventricular tachycardia →
Give the following:
1. Synchronized DC cardioversion at 200–300 J
2. Lidocaine (bolus followed by continuous infusion)

Severe ventricular bradycardia →
1. Give the following:
   a. Atropine, 0.5 mg (twice if necessary)
   b. isoproterenol infusion
2. Insert transvenous or transcutaneous pacemaker.

3

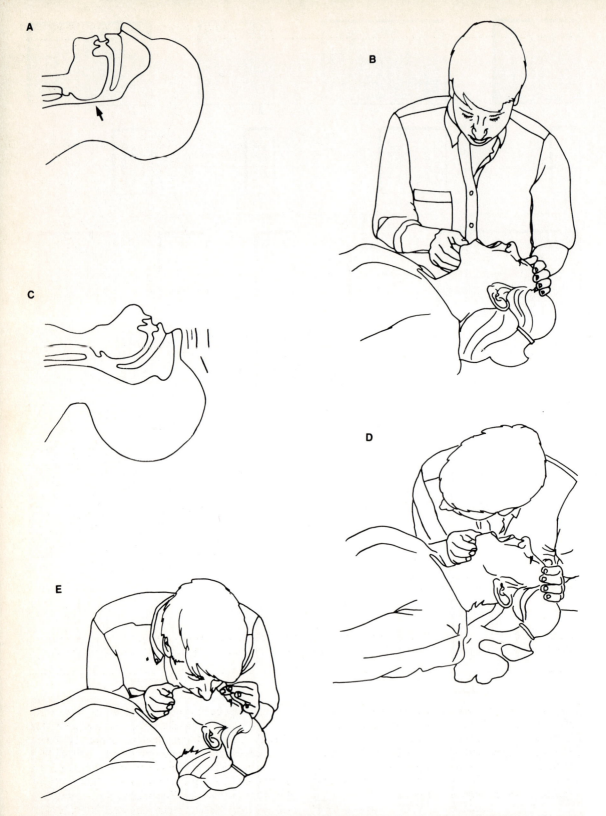

Figure 1–1. Opening the airway and providing ventilation. **A:** Obstruction of airway by posterior displacement of tongue (arrow) in resting, supine position. **B** and **C:** Relief of lingual airway obstruction in supine position by forward displacement of mandible (head-tilt and chin-lift method). **D:** Rescuer checks for spontaneous breathing by listening and feeling for exhaled air while looking for chest movement. **E:** Mouth-to-mouth ventilation. While maintaining head tilt and chin lift, the victim's nose is sealed shut by the rescuer's fingers; rescuer takes a deep breath, seals mouth over victim's mouth, and exhales, watching for chest movement. Look, listen, and feel for passive exhalation.

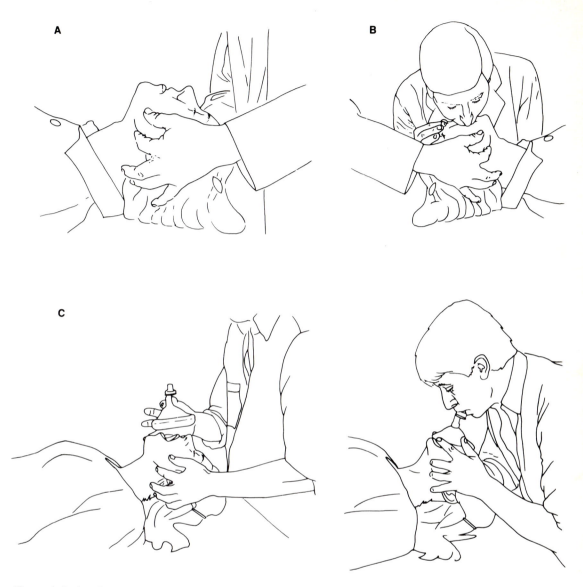

Figure 1–2. Jaw-thrust maneuver. **_A:_** If cervical spine injury is suspected, open airway by grasping and lifting angles of victim's lower jaw without tilting the head. **_B_** and **_C:_** Ventilation is best provided with the aid of a second rescuer or a pocket mask.

is accompanied by chest movement associated with airflow at the mouth. Put one ear close to the victim's mouth, and listen for breath sounds. Feel for exhaled air on your cheek, and look to see if the chest rises and falls. Spend 3–5 seconds checking for breathing before concluding that it is absent. If spontaneous ventilation is occurring, go to step 7.

Step 6: Begin Ventilation.
(See Figs 1–2 to 1–4.)

A. Technique: If there are no signs of breathing, begin ventilation immediately. To provide positive pressure ventilation through the mouth, the nasal air passage must be closed. Keep the airway open with the head-tilt and chin-lift maneuver, and pinch the victim's nostrils closed. Dentures should be left in place unless they are loose and obstruct access. Seal your mouth over the victim's mouth, and give 2 full breaths, each lasting 1–1½ seconds. Allow for exhalation between breaths. The breaths will average 0.8–1.2 L each. Deeper breaths delivered more rapidly may cause gastric distention. Watch the chest for movement, and listen and feel for exhalation (Fig 1–1). **_Note:_** The previously recommended initial ventilation with 4 quick successive breaths has been changed to 2 slow, full breaths to simplify training

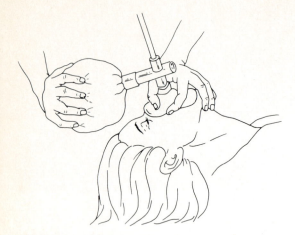

Figure 1–3. Ventilation technique using face mask and positive pressure ventilation (bag or valve). As in mouth-to-mouth ventilation, head must be tilted to keep airway open. Seal mask to face with one hand, with fingers under chin to maintain open airway. Use other hand to operate bag or valve.

and to lessen the chances of gastric distention, regurgitation, and aspiration.

If the victim's mouth is damaged or is too large to be covered by the rescuer's mouth, mouth-to-nose ventilation should be performed by blowing directly into the victim's nose with the victim's mouth closed. Open the victim's mouth to allow for passive exhalation. Mouth-to-nose ventilation may be an effective way to ventilate a victim with facial burns or one who has swallowed a caustic substance.

Mouth-to-mouth resuscitation must often be the initial step in active ventilatory support. Subsequently—or initially if equipment and well-trained, experienced personnel are available—use of a bag, valve, and mask system (eg, Ambu bag) can be used to provide a higher inspired oxygen concentration (Fig 1–3). A bag-valve mask or pocket mask should be used preferentially over mouth-to-mouth ventilation in patients with known or suspected communicable diseases to protect the provider.

B. Detection of Airway Obstruction: Airway obstruction may be detected in any of 4 ways: (**1**) The rescuer is unable to blow air into the victim's lungs, or doing so requires excessive expiratory effort; (**2**) the victim's chest does not rise with the ventilation as it should if the lungs are being inflated; (**3**) no airflow can be perceived on passive exhalation (Fig 1–1); or (**4**) auscultation of the chest by an assistant fails to disclose sounds of air exchange.

C. Relief of Airway Obstruction:

1. Reposition head–If attempts at ventilation are unsuccessful, reposition the head once again (Fig 1–1). *Note: Insufficient forward displacement of the mandible, causing obstruction of the airway by the tongue, is the commonest cause of airway obstruction during CPR.*

After the head is repositioned, attempt ventilation again. If the victim still cannot be ventilated, proceed with maneuvers to relieve airway obstruction, as follows:

2. Perform the Heimlich maneuver (subdiaphragmatic thrusts)–Kneel astride the victim's thighs, placing the heel of one hand midway between the navel and the xiphisternal notch in the midline, well away from the tip of the xiphoid. Place the second hand directly on top of the first. Taking care to deliver each as a separate and distinct thrust, deliver up to 10 upward thrusts as necessary to clear the airway (Fig 1–4A). The Heimlich maneuver has replaced back blows in all victims except infants under 1 year of age. **Chest thrusts** should be used instead of subdiaphragmatic thrusts in women in the advanced stages of pregnancy or in very obese people. Chest thrusts are accomplished by placing the hands in the position for closed chest compression (Fig 1–5) and delivering 6–10 distinct thrusts in rapid succession.

3. Use finger sweep–(See Fig 1–4C.) Check for a dislodged foreign body by using the finger sweep technique. Open the mouth by grasping the tongue and lower jaw together with one hand and lifting. Then sweep a curved index finger from the far side of the mouth along the cheek, deeply into the back of the throat, and then out the near side. Do not extend a finger straight into the center of the pharynx, since this may force a loose but not totally occluding foreign body deeper into the pharynx. Blind finger sweeps should be avoided in infants and young children for the same reason.

4. Reposition the head, and attempt ventilation again–If ventilation is unsuccessful, repeat the sequence of steps 1–3, above, in rapid succession.

5. Use further measures as necessary–If ventilation is still unsuccessful after several attempts, immediate cricothyrotomy (Chapter 46) is indicated. Alternatively, if equipment and expertise are available, visualization and extraction of the foreign body should be attempted by direct laryngoscopy (Chapter 46).

When the obstruction is removed, ventilate with 2 full breaths, and check for a pulse (step 7).

Step 7: Check Circulation.

Absence of a palpable pulse (associated with unresponsiveness) must be assumed to be due to cardiac arrest. Cardiac arrest may be due to ventricular fibrillation, cardiac asystole, severe tachyarrhythmias or bradyarrhythmias, or electrical depolarization with ineffective contraction (severe cardiogenic shock, also called "electromechanical dissociation"). In any case, immediate closed chest compression is necessary to ensure delivery of blood to vital organs.

Palpation of the carotid artery is the preferred

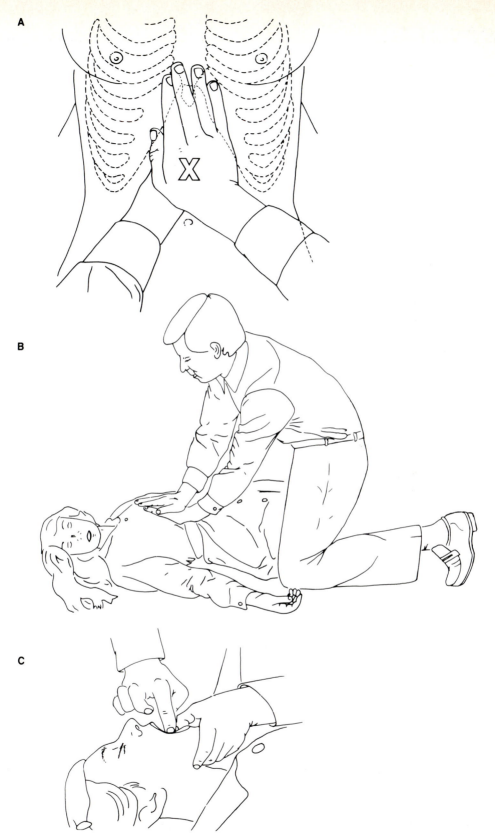

Figure 1–4. Clearing the obstructed airway. *A* and *B:* Supine Heimlich maneuver (subdiaphragmatic thrust). With victim level (or head down) and head turned to the side, rescuer kneels astride victim's thighs. Rescuer places heel of one hand midway between navel and xiphoid (well away from tip of xiphoid) and the other hand directly on top of the first. Deliver as many as 10 vigorous thrusts to victim's epigastrium. Proceed to next step. *C:* Finger sweep. Using a partially flexed index finger, sweep through far side of victim's mouth along cheek, deeply into back of the throat, and then out the near side.

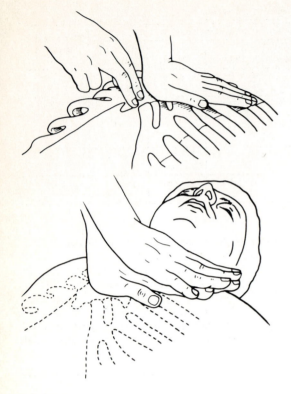

Figure 1–5. Hand placement for closed chest compression. Locate xiphoid, and place heel of one hand 2 fingerwidths cephalad to the xiphisternal notch. The other hand should be placed on top of first hand. Only the heel of the bottom hand should touch the chest wall—not the palm or fingers.

means of diagnosing cardiac arrest. Find the carotid artery by palpating the Adam's apple (larynx) and sliding the fingers laterally over the neck to the carotid groove, just anterior to the sternocleidomastoid muscle, where the pulse may be felt. Spend 5–10 seconds feeling for the carotid pulse before concluding that it is absent.

Other arteries should not be used to diagnose cardiac standstill for the following reasons: **(1)** The carotid is the largest and most central palpable artery; **(2)** peripheral arterial pulsations (eg, radial artery) may not be palpable if the patient is in shock; **(3)** atherosclerotic occlusion of the other arteries in older individuals is more common than occlusion of the carotid artery; **(4)** the carotid pulse is the easiest to reach in a fully clothed victim receiving artificial respiration; and **(5)** palpation of the carotid artery is less likely to be misinterpreted by bystanders than palpation of the femoral artery. *Note:* Listening for a heartbeat through the chest wall with a stethoscope is an insensitive and time-consuming method of diagnosing cardiac standstill and *should not be done*.

Keep the airway open while you are feeling the ca-

rotid pulse. If a pulse is present and the victim is not breathing, give one breath every 5 seconds (12 per minute), and monitor the pulse frequently. If there is a pulse and the victim is breathing, just keep the airway open, and frequently reassess the presence of breathing and pulse.

Step 8: Activate Emergency Medical Services (EMS) System.

Once the initial steps of CPR have been completed, the hospital or community EMS system must be activated to provide optimal emergency management. This may mean dialing 9–1–1 on a telephone in the USA where this service is available or calling the police, fire department, or an ambulance service. The function of the EMS system is to bring an advanced life support unit to the site to take over CPR.

Outside the hospital setting, the EMS system should be activated as soon as unconsciousness is established. In a setting where the rescuer and the victim are totally alone, the EMS system should be activated after 4 cycles of compression and ventilation (1 minute).

Step 9: Begin Closed Chest Compression.

Begin external closed chest compression combined with assisted ventilation if the patient is apneic and pulseless.

A. Position of Patient: The victim must be supine (face up) on a fixed, level, hard surface (ground, floor, or backboard).

B. Hand Placement: (See Fig 1–5.) Locate the lower (caudal) end of the rib cage with the middle finger, and slide the finger up the costal margin to the point where the ribs meet (xiphisternal notch). The heel of the other hand should be placed on the sternum 2 fingerwidths above the xiphisternal notch. It is best to use the hand nearest the victim's feet to find the landmark while the other hand is at rest on the victim's chest. Once the landmark is located and the heel of one hand is in the right position, place the other hand directly on top of the first. The fingers may be linked or extended but should not touch the chest; only the heel of the hand should be in contact with the sternum.

C. Compression Technique: (See Table 1–1.) The adult victim's sternum is compressed 4–5 cm (1½–2 in) at a rate of 80–100 compressions per minute. The proper rate can be determined by counting aloud and compressing at each count: "One-and-two-and-three-and. . . ." A single rescuer must stop after 15 compressions to deliver 2 full breaths (1–1½ seconds per breath with exhalation between breaths). The rescuer should then find the proper landmark and continue closed chest compressions.

The rescuer should be positioned with knees close to the victim's body, elbows held straight and locked, and shoulders above the hands (Fig 1–6). This posi-

Table 1–1. Summary of CPR techniques.

	Number of Rescuers	Ventilation		Cardiac Compression				Compression/Ventilation Ratio
		Rate	Switch Roles	Compressor	Rate	Depth	Switch Roles	
Adult or large child	1	10–14/min	After 2 breaths	2 hands	80–100/min	4–5 cm (1.5–2 in)	After 15 strokes	15:2
	2	16–20/min (after every 5 compressions)	None	2 hands	80–100/min	4–5 cm (1.5–2 in)	None	5:1
Small child	1	16–20/min	None	1 hand	80–100/min	2.5–4 cm (1–1.5 in)	None	5:1
Newborn or infant	1	20–30/min	None	2 fingers	At least 100/min	1.25–2.5 cm (0.5–1 in)	None	5–7:1

tion ensures that compressions are delivered with a piston-like motion from the shoulders (not the elbows) and that torso weight rather than the strength of forearms and shoulders is used. The compression maneuver should be smooth rather than abrupt or jerky, since it is not important for blood flow to be rapid. Compression and relaxation phases should be of the same duration to ensure optimal filling and emptying of the heart. The hands should not lose contact with the sternum even during the relaxation phase. The carotid pulse should be palpated after the first minute of CPR (4 compression-ventilation cycles) and every few minutes thereafter to determine if an effective heartbeat has returned.

D. Two-Rescuer CPR Technique: (See Fig 1–6.) In order to simplify training and improve skill

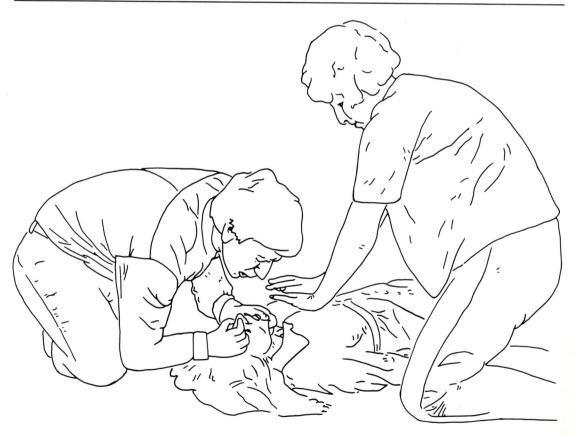

Figure 1–6. Positioning for 2-rescuer CPR. Ventilator and compressor should be on opposite sides of victim. Two-rescuer CPR should be performed only by professional rescuers.

retention, the American Heart Association in its 1986 Standards and Guidelines for Cardiopulmonary Resuscitation (CPR) and Emergency Cardiac Care (ECC) no longer recommends teaching of 2-rescuer CPR to the lay community. If a second person experienced in CPR comes to assist and is not a professional rescuer, he or she should activate the EMS system (if not already done) and perform one-person CPR when the first rescuer becomes fatigued. The first rescuer stops CPR after 2 ventilations. The second rescuer should check for a pulse for 5 seconds, and if it is absent, should give 2 full breaths and begin closed chest compression at the rate and compression-ventilation ratio for one-person CPR.

If both rescuers are health care professionals, they should perform 2-person CPR, since it is less fatiguing. One rescuer performs chest compression while the other maintains an open airway, provides ventilation, and monitors the carotid pulse. With 2 rescuers, the rate of compression should remain at 80–100/min. The compression-ventilation ratio is 5:1. The compressor should pause after the fifth compression to allow a full breath (1–1½ s) to be given. If a ventilation is omitted, one should be given after the next compression and the proper rhythm then resumed.

E. Changing Rescuer Roles: When the rescuer giving compressions becomes fatigued, the ventilator or another person able to help should take over. The tiring rescuer signals for a change by saying, "CHANGE and, *two* and, *three* and, *four* and, *five*" in synchrony with the compressions. On the fifth count the ventilator gives one breath and the 2 rescuers can then change positions, or a third rescuer can start performing the compressions. The new person performing ventilation should move to the head and check for breathing and pulse for 5 seconds. The new person performing compression should move to the chest, find the proper landmark on the sternum, and await the ventilator's instruction to begin compressions. If there is no pulse, the ventilator will give a breath and say, "Continue CPR." The compressor begins compressions at the rate of 80–100/min, and CPR continues.

PROBLEMS IN BASIC CPR

Complications

A. Gastric Distention: Gastric distention is a frequent complication of artificial ventilation (by mouth or mask) without esophageal balloon or endotracheal tube. Mild degrees of distention can be ignored; severe distention (gross abdominal distention with tympany) will elevate the diaphragm, interfere with ventilation and perfusion, and markedly increase the risk of vomiting or regurgitation, with subsequent aspiration. Gastric rupture may occur.

Gastric distention can be minimized by keeping the airway open and limiting inflation volumes as described earlier. Other methods that may prevent gastric distention include **(1)** mouth-to-nose ventilation, which decreases the pressure of gases reaching the pharynx; **(2)** slow inflation time during ventilation, which also produces less pressure and hence less tendency to open the esophagus; and **(3)** pressure on the cricoid cartilage against the cervical vertebrae to prevent regurgitation.

Severe distention can be corrected by turning the victim on the side, head down, and gently compressing the epigastrium. Belching indicates relief of distention. In the emergency department, the preferred technique is passage of a nasogastric tube.

Caution: Do not perform cardiac compression while also pressing on the epigastrium, since liver lacerations may occur.

B. Pneumothorax: Pneumothorax (often tension in type) may occur during CPR, and this complication should be considered in patients in whom correctly performed CPR fails to produce an adequate pulse or correct hypoxemia and acidosis. If pneumothorax is suspected, take corrective measures. If the patient is intubated and receiving assisted ventilation, thoracostomy will be both diagnostic and therapeutic: at the lateral fourth intercostal space just below the pectoralis major muscle, incise to the pleura with a scalpel, and puncture the pleura with a finger or Kelly clamp. In patients being ventilated without an endotracheal tube, needle thoracostomy (with a 16- to 14-gauge needle) may be safer. (See Chapter 46 for details on insertion of a thoracostomy tube.)

C. Skeletal Trauma: Rib fractures and costochondral separations occur commonly, even during perfectly executed CPR. These may then cause pneumothorax or any of the complications listed below.

D. Other Complications: Other complications are uncommon during correctly performed CPR but may occur when improper technique is used. These include sternal fractures, flail chest, hemothorax, coronary artery or myocardial contusion or laceration (with or without cardiac tamponade), liver lacerations, lung contusions, and fat emboli.

Common Mistakes

Most mistakes can be defined and prevented by repeated team CPR practice with a mannequin and evaluation of actual arrest situations after they have occurred. Videotapes of actual events are helpful as training materials.

A. Improper Positioning of Victim: Resuscitation attempts with the patient improperly positioned are ineffective. If the patient is not fully supine or is not on a firm surface, closed chest compression will not restore cardiac output. Laying the patient on the floor, ground, or a large (1 × 1 m [3 × 3 ft] or larger) backboard will ensure effective closed chest compression.

B. Inadequate Evaluation Techniques: Use of

outdated techniques for evaluation of the patient with potential cardiac arrest is a common cause of failure. Listening to the heart with a stethoscope and examining the pupils for evidence of constriction or dilatation are not useful in the early diagnosis or management of cardiac arrest. Only after stabilization of the victim is examination of the pupils indicated, and then only to determine the adequacy of brain perfusion. Cardiac auscultation is not indicated until an autonomous pulse with adequate blood pressure has been established. *The proper means of CPR evaluation is to feel the carotid pulse.*

C. Improper Closed Chest Compression: Other common mistakes include improper hand positioning during closed chest compression, rates of compression that are too fast or too slow, and repeated interruption of resuscitation to feel for the carotid pulse or to obtain or examine the ECG.

D. Delay and Fatigue: Other common errors include delays in resuscitation during transport or having an operator remain at one position too long, so that he or she becomes fatigued and ineffective.

MECHANISMS OF BLOOD FLOW DURING CLOSED CHEST COMPRESSION

The mechanism of blood flow during CPR has traditionally been assumed to be as follows: the heart is squeezed between the sternum and the spine during chest compression, causing raised pressure in the left ventricular chamber with resultant forward flow of blood across the aortic valve.

Recent studies have challenged this view with an alternative hypothesis called the "thoracic pump model." According to this hypothesis, chest compression raises the intrathoracic pressure, which results in an intrathoracic-extrathoracic pressure gradient. Blood flows along this gradient from the venous reservoir in the pulmonary vascular bed through the left atrium and ventricle, which act as a passive conduit. The cardiac valves serve to channel the direction of flow. During relaxation, blood returns to the pulmonary vascular bed through a passive right atrium and ventricle.

Consistent with this hypothesis is the observation that efforts to augment increases in intrathoracic pressure, such as simultaneous ventilation with chest compression, result in higher systemic blood pressures and greater cerebral blood flow. This model also predicts that CPR will fail to maintain adequate myocardial blood flow, since intrathoracic pressures are similar in both the aortic root and coronary sinus, with only a slight transmyocardial pressure gradient.

It is unknown to what extent either mechanism applies to the individual patient. Furthermore, simultaneous ventilation and chest compression CPR has not proved to be superior to conventional CPR in a recent trial. For these reasons, the methods described in this chapter should be followed.

DETERMINANTS OF CARDIAC ARREST SURVIVAL

Heart disease is the leading cause of death in adults in the USA, and in 1987 approximately 1.25 million persons suffered a heart attack. More than 500,000 people died, and of these, more than two-thirds died before reaching the hospital. Three-quarters of out-of-hospital cardiac arrests occurred in the victim's home.

Many factors have been identified that may affect outcome following cardiac arrest. Individual characteristics such as younger age, absence of prior heart disease, collapse that is witnessed, and presence of ventricular fibrillation or ventricular tachycardia when found are all associated with higher likelihood of survival. Bystander-initiated CPR and short time from collapse to defibrillation are the most important factors determining survival. In King County, Washington, 32% of cardiac arrest patients were discharged alive when CPR was initiated within 4 minutes of collapse compared with 17% when CPR was initiated later. In addition, when time to definitive care was less than 6 minutes, 37% were discharged alive versus 11% when care was delayed over 14 minutes. Greater involvement of the community in learning CPR, decreased response time of emergency personnel, and wider use of automated and semiautomated defibrillators by first responders are crucial to improving survival following cardiac arrest.

AIRWAY OBSTRUCTION IN THE CONSCIOUS VICTIM

Diagnosis
Airway obstruction in the conscious victim typically occurs in elderly persons, edentulous or with dentures, who have been drinking alcoholic beverages and eating foods that must be chewed before swallowing. *The victim suddenly becomes agitated but is unable to speak.* Cyanosis occurs, followed by unconsciousness. Whether deliberately or not, the victim often gives the universal signal of choking distress—fingers around the neck.

Treatment
A. Make Correct Diagnosis: Ask the victim to try to speak. If speech is possible even in a whisper, the problem is laryngospasm or partial rather than complete airway obstruction by a bolus of food. Offer to provide assistance if it is wanted. *Do not* perform the Heimlich maneuver, since there is no immediate threat to life.

B. Perform the Heimlich Maneuver (Sub-

diaphragmatic Thrusts): If the victim cannot speak, stand behind the victim (whether the victim is standing or sitting), and wrap your arms around the victim's waist. Place a fist thumb-side toward the abdomen, midway between the xiphisternal notch and navel, grasp the fist with the other hand, and compress the abdomen with pistonlike upward thrusts (Fig 1–7). Repeat until successful or until the victim loses consciousness.

If abdominal compression is not feasible (eg, victim is markedly obese or in the third trimester of pregnancy), use closed chest compression instead. Stand behind the victim, and encircle the victim's chest with your arms, placing the fist thumb-side toward the sternum on the middle of the sternum and avoiding the xiphoid. Place the other hand on top of the fist, and deliver backward thrusts to the sternum until the foreign body is dislodged or the victim loses consciousness.

C. Perform the Supine Heimlich Maneuver: If the above maneuver fails or the victim becomes unconscious, assist in positioning the victim supine on the floor. Open the airway, and attempt to ventilate the victim. If the airway is obstructed, call for help, and activate the EMS system. Then give 6–10 supine subdiaphragmatic thrusts (Fig 1–4A and 1–4B), followed by finger sweeps (Fig 1–4C). Attempt to ventilate the victim after each series of steps. Continue this sequence until the obstruction is relieved or until means to perform definitive resuscitative measures are available (see below). Complications of supine subdiaphragmatic compression include liver laceration, gastric rupture, vomiting and aspiration, rib fractures, and costochondral separations.

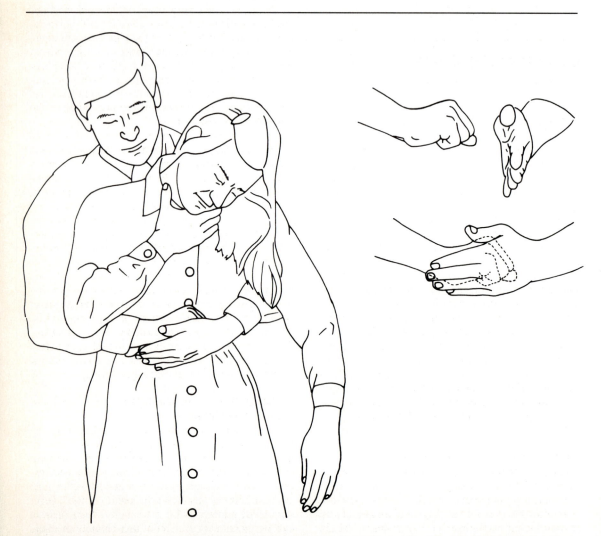

Figure 1–7. Clearing airway in conscious victim (Heimlich maneuver). Reach around the victim from the back, and deliver a sharp thrust to the epigastrium with the clenched fist, thumb-side toward the abdomen.

D. Perform Definitive Measures If Necessary: If the above maneuvers fail in an unconscious victim, perform cricothyrotomy (Chapter 46), or remove the obstruction under direct vision with a laryngoscope, depending on the resources available.

Disposition

Victims of airway obstruction in whom the obstruction was removed outside the hospital should be examined by direct or indirect laryngoscopy to be certain that no foreign material remains in the hypopharynx. If they are otherwise well, they may be discharged from the emergency department with written information on how airway obstruction may be prevented.

If complications have occurred as a result of airway obstruction (eg, cardiac arrest) or attempts to relieve obstruction (eg, vomiting and aspiration, cricothyrotomy), the patient should be hospitalized.

ADVANCED LIFE SUPPORT

ADVANCED VENTILATORY SUPPORT

Tracheal Intubation

The best way to maintain adequate ventilation and oxygenation and to protect the airway in an unconscious patient is to intubate the trachea under direct vision using a cuffed low-pressure endotracheal tube (Chapter 46). Intubation ensures that the airway remains patent while the victim is transported to the hospital. It also permits administration of positive pressure ventilation and increased oxygen concentration and markedly reduces the risk of aspiration. In addition, several drugs used in advanced life support (epinephrine, atropine, lidocaine) are effective when given endotracheally, providing a route for their administration until intravenous access is established. Tracheal intubation should only be attempted by skilled personnel using appropriate equipment. If neither appropriate equipment nor personnel are available, supplemental oxygen should be delivered either by nasal cannulas or by a bag, valve, and mask system.

Pharyngotracheal Lumen Airway

The pharyngotracheal lumen airway is an effective method of airway management that is increasingly being taught to emergency medical technicians. It is more effective than the esophageal obturator airway, has fewer complications, and is easy to learn. The airway consists of a long endotracheal type tube that is located within a shorter tube. Each tube has a low-pressure cuff at the distal end that is inflated after insertion. When inserted, the short tube opens at the level of the pharynx above the epiglottis. Whether the long tube was inserted into the trachea or the esophagus is determined by blowing into the short tube. If the long tube is in the esophagus, blowing into the short tube will inflate the lungs and cause the chest to rise, since the inflated cuff at the end of the long tube seals the esophagus and the inflated cuff at the end of the short tube prevents air escape from the mouth or nose. If the long tube is in the trachea, blowing into the short tube will not cause the chest to rise but blowing into the long tube will. Air or oxygen is delivered through the short tube if the long tube is in the esophagus, and through the long tube if it is in the trachea. Any leakage in the cuffs will decrease the effectiveness of the pharyngotracheal lumen airway.

Esophageal Obturator Airway

Emergency medical technicians in many parts of the USA utilize esophageal airways to deliver ventilation. A flexible tube is inserted in the esophagus, and a balloon is inflated to obstruct the esophagus. A face mask is fitted, and air delivered to the oropharynx is diverted to the lungs by the esophageal balloon. *Caution:* Be sure that the tube is in the esophagus and not in the trachea (breath sounds heard in the lungs but *not* in the stomach).

Controversy exists about the efficacy of the esophageal airway as a means of delivering assisted ventilation to a respiratory arrest victim. Some studies have shown that the esophageal airway is less effective than the bag-mask system, and it is far inferior to tracheal intubation. Furthermore, an esophageal airway produces some gastric distention, and if the esophageal balloon is removed *before* airway protection is provided, massive aspiration can occur. *Caution: Always perform endotracheal intubation before removing an esophageal airway in patients who are comatose or lethargic.* In the alert and awake patient, have a large-bore suction device ready (eg, tonsillar suction), and place the patient on one side (preferably also in the Trendelenburg position) before deflating the balloon and removing the esophageal airway. Regurgitation of gastric contents almost always occurs following removal of an esophageal airway.

Transtracheal (Translaryngeal) Catheter Ventilation

Percutaneous insertion of a transtracheal catheter (Chapter 46) is a rapid temporary method of gaining airway control until cricothyrotomy or tracheostomy can be performed in patients in whom endotracheal intubation is difficult or contraindicated (eg, severe cervical spine injury, massive maxillofacial injury, unrelieved upper airway obstruction). Transtracheal catheter ventilation requires a high-pressure or high-frequency high-flow oxygen source. A second catheter may need to be inserted to facilitate exhalation.

The exhalation catheter must be closed during inspiration. This technique of ventilation has not been adequately studied in children.

Cricothyrotomy

If ventilation cannot be achieved by mask-to-mouth or mouth-to-mouth breathing and if orotracheal or nasotracheal intubation cannot be performed, emergency cricothyrotomy is indicated (Chapter 46). Tracheostomy is much inferior to cricothyrotomy during cardiac arrest because of the time and experience needed to perform the procedure correctly in the acutely ill patient and the potential for serious complications and long-range adverse effects.

INTRAVENOUS ACCESS

An intravenous catheter should be inserted as soon as possible after adequate CPR has been established. The preferred and fastest method is to place large ($\geq$ 16-gauge) plastic cannulas in veins of the upper extremity, usually the basilic veins. If 3 or more people are available for the CPR effort, one person may be spared to try to pass a central venous cannula via a basilic vein either by venous cutdown or by use of a long needle-clad catheter (Chapter 46). This procedure is more time-consuming than insertion of a peripheral intravenous catheter, but it is preferable for monitoring and therapy. Access routes in patients without adequate upper extremity veins include the external and internal jugular veins (difficult to enter during active CPR, especially if the patient has not yet been intubated) and the subclavian vein (interruption of chest compression is necessary; technique requires personnel skilled in insertion). The femoral vein is the least desirable route of access. It is difficult to enter in obese patients; accidental arterial cannulation may be difficult to detect; and the catheter must extend above the diaphragm. Although central line insertion is associated with more complications than peripheral site insertion (eg, pneumothorax, bleeding, laceration of internal structures), it is preferable when perfusion is not rapidly restored. Drugs administered via the central line are more rapidly effective and have higher peak levels than those given through peripheral sites.

Caution: Internal jugular and subclavian venipunctures are relatively contraindicated in patients who have known bleeding disorders or are taking anticoagulants. Thrombolytic therapy is contraindicated in any patient in whom internal jugular or subclavian venipuncture has been attempted.

CORRECTION OF ACIDOSIS

Although correction of systemic acidosis by means of intravenous injection of sodium bicarbonate immediately after insertion of an intravenous catheter was once recommended, numerous studies suggest that bicarbonate produces a paradoxical cerebrospinal fluid and mixed venous acidosis through the generation of CO_2. It also induces hyperosmolarity and hypernatremia and fails to improve the outcome of CPR. It should therefore not be given empirically and probably should be reserved for patients with known (ie, by blood gas measurement) or suspected (ie, patients on dialysis for renal failure) severe acidosis with or without hyperkalemia. The dose for such patients is 1 meq/kg initially and no more than 0.5 meq/kg every 10 minutes thereafter, depending on the results of arterial blood pH and $PaCO_2$ measurements. Arterial blood pH should be maintained near physiologic levels ($\geq$ 7.2). Ideally, adequate ventilation will help correct acidosis in most individuals. If it does not, physicians should exercise their own judgment regarding bicarbonate.

DIAGNOSTIC TESTS

Only 2 diagnostic tests are essential: electrocardiography and arterial blood gas and pH analysis.

ECG & Rhythm Monitoring

Although a full 12-lead ECG is preferable, rhythm strips are adequate to make the diagnosis of ventricular fibrillation, ventricular tachycardia, severe bradyarrhythmia, or asystole. Tachyarrhythmias may require many leads for correct diagnosis but are uncommonly a cause of clinically evident cardiac arrest (except for ventricular tachycardia). A quick rhythm strip can be obtained by using a monitor defibrillator with paddle electrodes. *Note:* If the ECG shows asystole, double-check to make sure that all electrical leads are connected.

Arterial Blood Gases & pH

Measurement of arterial blood gases is useful chiefly as a means of judging the adequacy of ventilatory and cardiac compression efforts and as a guide for treating acidosis with bicarbonate. With optimum CPR, especially in a patient who has been intubated and is receiving supplemental oxygen, arterial PO_2 should be normal (or higher than normal); PCO_2 should be between 30 and 45 mm Hg; and pH should be near physiologic levels ($\geq$ 7.2). Cardiac performance and antiarrhythmic and inotropic drug effects are markedly impaired by hypoxemia and acidosis.

A. Hypoxemia: Severe hypoxemia ($PO_2 < 50$ mm Hg) despite a high FIO_2 may be due to (**1**) inadequate ventilation (pneumothorax, improper endotracheal tube placement), (**2**) grossly inadequate cardiac output (depressed myocardium, tamponade, etc), or (**3**) increased pulmonary shunt (atelectasis, congenital heart disease, pulmonary embolism).

B. Acidosis: Persistent acidosis (with a normal

or nearly normal PCO_2) indicates hypoperfusion; acidosis accompanying hypoxia may indicate either inadequate ventilation or inadequate perfusion.

C. Hypercapnia: CO_2 retention is always due to inadequate ventilation.

CORRECTION OF ARRHYTHMIAS

Drugs mentioned below are listed in Table 1–2 and discussed in more detail below in the section on intravenous infusion of essential drugs. In the management of cardiac arrest, all drugs are given intravenously if possible, unless otherwise specified. The doses given are for adults. If the patient is intubated before intravenous access is established, epinephrine, atropine, and lidocaine can be given through the endotracheal tube in the same doses, followed by one inflation of air or oxygen.

Ventricular Asystole

Cardiac arrest associated with electrical asystole is usually associated with extensive myocardial injury and has a poor prognosis. Occasionally, it results from high levels of parasympathetic tone, which cause a cessation of pacemaker activity. Because very fine ventricular fibrillation can mimic asystole,

it is important to check at least 2 different lead configurations to confirm the diagnosis.

A. Epinephrine: Establish intravenous access. Give a bolus of 0.5–1 mg (5–10 mL) of aqueous epinephrine solution (1:10,000). A higher dose of epinephrine, 200 μg/kg (15 mL for a 70-kg person) of 1:1000 solution given by bolus injection, may be more effective than the standard, much smaller Advanced Cardiac Life Support (ACLS)–recommended dose. However, whether a high dose improves survival has not yet been demonstrated in human trials. If this treatment does not induce cardiac electrical activity, give atropine.

B. Intubation: Intubate the patient when possible.

C. Atropine: Give atropine, 1-mg intravenous bolus, repeated in 5 minutes.

D. Repeat Epinephrine: If asystole persists, epinephrine injections should be repeated at 5-minute intervals.

E. Defibrillation: Since very fine ventricular fibrillation may appear as asystole on the ECG, defibrillation with an energy load of 360 J may be tried for asystole that persists in spite of the above measures.

F. Sodium Bicarbonate: Although not routinely recommended, use of sodium bicarbonate, 1

Table 1–2. Drugs for advanced life support: Doses for adults.

Drug and Dosage Form	Usual Adult Dosage and Route of Administration	Comments
Packaged in Prefilled Syringes Containing 1 Ampule Each		
Sodium bicarbonate 8.4% solution (50-meq ampule that contains 1 meq/mL)	Initial intravenous bolus of 1 meq/kg, then 0.5 meq/kg every 10–15 minutes, or amount based on results of arterial blood gas determinations.	Do not use in first 10 minutes of resuscitation. Do not put in intravenous line with catecholamines or calcium. Repeat as arterial blood gas measurements indicate. Stop when pH is ≥ 7.2.
Epinephrine 1:10,000 aqueous solution (1 mg in 10-mL ampule [0.1 mg/mL])	0.5–1 mg bolus (5–10 mL or ½–1 ampule).	Repeat every 5 minutes and as indicated. Also effective intratracheally.
Lidocaine 1% solution (50 mg in 5-mL ampule [10 mg/mL]; also comes in 2% solution) Also in bottles of 25 mg/mL and 40 mg/mL	Cardiac arrest: 1 mg/kg bolus, then 0.5 mg/kg every 5–10 minutes, until a maximum of 3 mg/kg has been given.	Repeat 50-mg bolus at 5- to 10-minute intervals. Also effective intratracheally.
	Noncardiac arrest: 1 mg/kg bolus, then 2–4 mg/min by continuous intravenous infusion.	
	For 4 mg/mL solution, add 1 g to 250 mL of 5% dextrose in water.	
Atropine 1 mg in 10-mL ampule (0.1 mg/mL)	0.5–1 mg (5–10 mL) intravenously.	Repeat every 5 minutes but not more than 2 mg total dose. Also effective intratracheally.
Calcium chloride 10% solution (1 g in 10-mL ampule [100 mg/mL])	0.5 g (½ ampule) intravenously over 1–2 minutes.	Do not put in intravenous line with bicarbonate solutions. To be used only for hyperkalemia, hypocalcemia, and toxicity due to calcium channel-blocking agents.

(continued)

Table 1–2. Drugs for advanced life support: Doses for adults. (continued)

Drug and Dosage Form	Usual Adult Dosage and Route of Administration	Comments
Packaged in Single-Use Glass Vials		
Epinephrine 1:1000 aqueous solution (30 mg in 30-mL vial [1 mg/mL])	Cardiac arrest: Higher dose of 200 μg/kg (15 mg for 70-kg person) may be more effective.	Repeat every 5 minutes and as indicated.
Isoproterenol 1 mg in 5-mL vial (0.2 mg/mL)	Add 1 vial (1 mg) to 500 mL of 5% dextrose in water (2 μg/mL). Give as intravenous infusion at a rate of 2–20 μg/min.	Now used only for hemodynamically unstable bradycardia refractory to atropine. *Do not use in cardiac arrest.*
Dopamine 200 mg in 5-mL vial (40 mg/mL)	Add 1 vial (200 mg) to 500 mL of 5% dextrose in water (400 μg/mL). Give as intravenous infusion at a rate of 2–20 μg/kg/min.	Useful for hypotension not due to hypovolemia; increases blood flow to viscera at low doses. Synergistic effects when used with dobutamine for cardiogenic shock. See text.
Dobutamine 250 mg in 20-mL vial (12.5 mg/mL)	Add 2 vials (500 mg) to 250 mL of 5% dextrose in water (2 mg/mL). Give as intravenous infusion at a rate of 2.5–20.0 μg/kg/min.	Drug of choice for cardiac inotropic effects in treatment of cardiogenic shock; reduces both preload and afterload. Synergistic effects when used with dopamine. *Do not use in cardiac arrest.*
Procainamide 1000 mg in 10-mL vial (100 mg/mL) **or** 1000 mg in 2-mL vials (500 mg/mL)	Give 1000-mg loading dose in 50- to 100-mg increments every 5 minutes, then 1–4 mg/min by continous intravenous infusion. For 2 mg/mL solution, add 500 mg to 250 mL of 5% dextrose in water.	Do not exceed rate of 20 mg/min. Stop if QRS complex becomes 50% wider than original measurement or if hypotension develops.
Bretylium tosylate 500 mg in 10-mL vial (50 mg/mL)	Ventricular fibrillation or pulseless ventricular tachycardia: 5 mg/kg (0.1 mL/kg) by bolus intravenous injection. Defibrillate. If arrhythmia persists, give 10 mg/kg (0.2 mL/kg) every 15–30 minutes until arrhythmia is halted or a total dose of 30 mg/kg is reached.	Antiarrhythmic agent with minimal negative inotropic effects. Enhances ability to convert ventricular fibrillation. Perform electrical defibrillation after each dose.
	Persistent recurring ventricular tachycardia: Dilute 500 mg (10 mL) to 50 mL, and give 5–10 mg/kg intravenously over 8–10 minutes, then 1–2 mg/min by continous intravenous infusion.	
	For 2 mg/mL solution, add 500 mg to 250 mL of 5% dextrose in water.	
Verpamil 5 mg in 2-mL vial (2.5 mg/mL)	5 mg intravenously. Give 10 mg after 15–30 minutes if supraventricular tachycardia persists.	Do not use in Wolff-Parkinson-White syndrome, Lown-Ganong-Levine syndrome, atrioventricular block, wide-complex atrial fibrillation, or chronic heart failure. Hypertension may be reversed with calcium chloride, 0.5–1 g intravenously.
Norepinephrine (levarterenol) 2% solution that contains 8 mg per vial	Add 1 vial to 500 mL of 5% dextrose in water (16 μg/mL). Give as intravenous infusion at an initial rate of 2–10 μ/min. Increase as needed.	Potent vasoconstrictor; visceral ischemia common. Use only if dopamine is not available. Phentolamine, 5–10 mg in 10–15 mL of saline, should be given subcutaneously and in the same intravenous catheter if norepinephrine extravasates. Contraindicated in patients receiving monoamine oxidase inhibitors.

meq/kg, can be considered at this point. If used, half the original dose should be given at 10-minute intervals for as many doses as needed, guided by arterial blood gas measurements when available (eg, initial dose 100 meq, additional doses 50 meq every 10 minutes).

G. Pacemaker: If these measures fail, transvenous, transthoracic, or transcutaneous electrical pacing may be tried. The immediate success rate is less than 10%, and the long-term survival rate is very low.

Ventricular Fibrillation & Pulseless Ventricular Tachycardia
(See Fig 1–8.)

Immediate defibrillation should be performed in all victims with ventricular fibrillation and pulseless ventricular tachycardia. This may be accomplished by a precordial thump in a victim with a witnessed arrest. However, if the precordial thump is unsuccessful or if the victim has had an unwitnessed arrest, immediate DC defibrillation should be used instead.

A. Defibrillation: Be sure to warn everyone in-

volved before applying the shock, so that no one is touching the victim or the bed without intervening electrical insulation. *Caution:* CPR effort should not be interrupted for more than a few seconds while defibrillation is being administered. Do not interrupt CPR while searching for a defibrillation machine, paddles, or saline pads or adjusting the instrument. All these tasks should be performed by others while closed chest compression continues.

1. For most adults, administer 200 J of DC countershock with one defibrillator paddle at the aortic position and the other at the cardiac apex (Fig 1–9). If there is no response, repeat immediately at 200–300 J, and then again at 360 J if there is still no response.

2. Children and small adults require lower maximum defibrillation levels of about 2–3 J/kg and, ideally, smaller defibrillation paddles. Anteroposterior paddle placement may be useful in these patients.

3. Very large or obese patients may require larger paddles, higher-voltage defibrillation machines, or anteroposterior paddle placement.

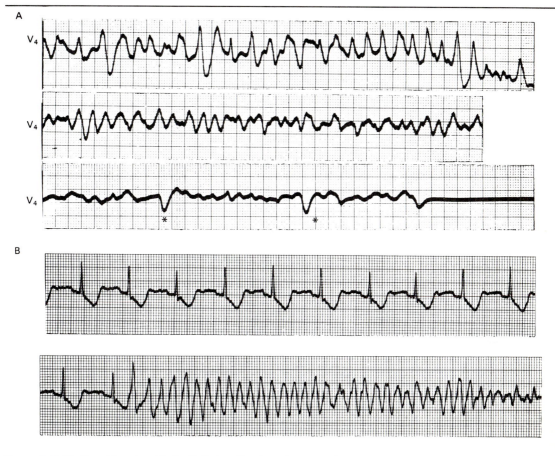

Figure 1–8. Rhythm strips of ventricular fibrillation. Note irregular rate and amplitude of fibrillating waves and CPR artifact in V$_4$(*) that can mimic wide-complex ventricular beats. **A:** Ventricular fibrillation recorded in precordial leads. **B:** Continuous rhythm strip showing sinus rhythm terminating abruptly in ventricular fibrillation. (The 2 strips are actually continuous.) (Reproduced, with permission, from Goldman MJ: *Principles of Clinical Electrocardiography,* 12th ed. Lange, 1986.)

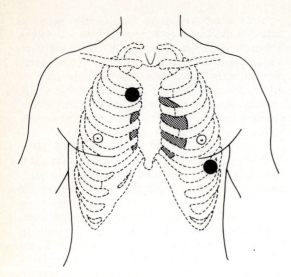

Figure 1–9. Contact points for defibrillation electrodes (solid circles). Place one paddle electrode to the right of the sternum in the second or third interspace; the other paddle should be at the cardiac apex. In children and thin adults, paddles may be placed directly over the heart in anteroposterior orientation.

B. Evaluation After Defibrillation: Return of normal cardiac action is detected by the presence of a carotid pulse and a more normal rhythm on the ECG. In the absence of a pulse, closed chest compression must be resumed immediately.

Refractory Ventricular Fibrillation & Tachycardia

Failure of ventricular fibrillation and tachycardia to revert to normal sinus rhythm after DC countershock (as opposed to conversion to sinus rhythm with subsequent deterioration to fibrillation; see below) may be due to severe hypoxemia, improper defibrillation, myocardial failure, or a combination of these causes. CPR should be continued while the following measures are undertaken:

A. Administer Epinephrine: Establish intravenous access, and give epinephrine, 0.5–1 mg (5–10 mL of 1:10,000 solution). Epinephrine, 200 μg/kg of 1:1000 solution (15 mL for a 70-kg person), may be more effective. Repeat bolus injections every 5 minutes if ventricular fibrillation or tachycardia persists.

B. Intubate: If possible, intubate the patient. Check arterial blood gases, and correct hypoxemia and hypercapnia if present.

C. Repeat Defibrillation: Repeat defibrillation at 360 J with close attention to paddle position, conducting medium (saline pads or paste), paddle pressure, and current energy. An anteroposterior paddle position should also be tried at least once.

D. Administer Other Drugs: If ventricular fi-

brillation or tachycardia continues, administration of one or more of the following may be useful:

1. Lidocaine–Bolus of 1 mg/kg, then 0.5 mg/kg bolus every 5–10 minutes to a total of 3 mg/kg. Repeat defibrillation at 360 J after each bolus injection, **followed by**—

2. Bretylium tosylate–Bolus of 5 mg/kg, followed by defibrillation; if unsuccessful, increase bolus to 10 mg/kg every 15–30 minutes to a maximum total dose of 30 mg/kg. Defibrillate after giving each bolus.

3. Sodium bicarbonate–1 meq/kg initially, then 0.5 meq/kg every 10 minutes, guided by arterial blood gas measurements. Sodium bicarbonate is not recommended in the initial 10 minutes of a resuscitation.

E. Defibrillate: Defibrillate at 360 J after giving each bolus of drug.

Unstable Sinus Rhythm

Ventricular fibrillation or tachycardia that converts to sinus rhythm after defibrillation but then deteriorates again may be due to acidosis, hypoxemia, or ventricular irritability (as may occur after myocardial infarction).

A. Correct Acidosis and Hypoxemia: See pp 14–15 for corrective measures.

B. Control Ventricular Irritability:

1. Lidocaine is the drug of choice. Give 1 mg/kg by intravenous bolus injection, followed by continuous infusion of 2–4 mg/min.

2. Other agents may be tried if instability persists. Give bretylium tosylate initially, followed by procainamide if the patient fails to respond (Table 1–2). *Caution:* Ventricular ectopy that does not degenerate into ventricular fibrillation should not be treated with large doses of antiarrhythmic drugs, since these medications depress cardiac output and may cause asystole.

Sustained Ventricular Tachycardia With a Pulse (See also Chapter 28.)

A. Hemodynamically Unstable: The presence of chest pain, dyspnea, altered mentation, hypotension, or congestive heart failure suggests hemodynamic compromise. Monitor the pulse closely, since its disappearance necessitates CPR and initiation of treatment discussed above under Ventricular Fibrillation & Pulseless Ventricular Tachycardia.

1. Administer oxygen, and establish intravenous access (consider sedation if the patient is awake and does not have hypotension or pulmonary edema).

2. Use cardioversion, 50 J. If there is no response, double the energy level and repeat at 100 J, 200 J, and 360 J until successful or until up to 360 J has been given. Synchronized cardioversion should be used unless the patient has hypotension or pulmonary edema, is unconscious, or has a rapid heart rate (QRS and T waves are indistinguishable).

3. If the above techniques are unsuccessful or if sustained ventricular tachycardia with a pulse recurs, administer lidocaine as a bolus of 1 mg/kg. Also, repeat cardioversion at the level that was previously successful or at a level of 360 J if cardioversion was previously unsuccessful.

4. Administer procainamide or bretylium tosylate. If the patient is still unresponsive, administer procainamide, 20 mg/min up to 100 mg, or bretylium tosylate, 5–10 mg/kg diluted to 50 mL infused over 8–10 minutes (follow with 1–2 mg/min given as a continuous infusion). Repeat cardioversion as described in step 3. If hypotension or pulmonary edema is present or if the patient is unconscious, give bretylium tosylate instead of procainamide. Otherwise, use procainamide and, if necessary, bretylium tosylate.

B. Hemodynamically Stable: Follow the treatment outlined above in ¶ A as soon as any signs of hemodynamic compromise appear.

1. Administer oxygen, and establish intravenous access.

2. Administer lidocaine, 1 mg/kg as an initial bolus. If ventricular tachycardia persists, give 0.5 mg/kg as a bolus every 8–10 minutes until tachycardia resolves or until a total dose of 3 mg/kg has been reached.

3. Administer procainamide if lidocaine is unsuccessful. Give 20 mg/min until ventricular tachycardia resolves or until 1000 mg has been given.

4. If still unsuccessful, use cardioversion as described in ¶ A, above.

Severe Bradyarrhythmias

Bradycardia requires treatment only if there are associated signs of hemodynamic compromise such as hypotension, congestive heart failure, chest pain, dyspnea, altered mental status, or premature ventricular contractions. If cardiac arrest occurs, guidelines for electromechanical dissociation should be followed.

A. Atropine: Give atropine, 0.5–1 mg intravenously, and repeat after 5 minutes if there is no response. The total dose should not exceed 2 mg.

B. Isoproterenol: Begin isoproterenol infusion at a rate of 2–4 µg/min; increase the dose up to 20 µg/min, depending on ventricular response. Isoproterenol is a temporizing measure and should be used only until a pacemaker can be inserted.

C. Transcutaneous or Transvenous Pacemaker: A transcutaneous pacemaker (Chapter 46) can be applied temporarily until a transvenous pacemaker can be inserted.

Electromechanical Dissociation

Electromechanical dissociation, also known as profound cardiogenic shock, is present when the ECG reveals relatively normal ventricular complexes occurring at a nearly normal rate, but there is no detectable arterial pulse. The prognosis for resuscitation is poor, since this condition usually signifies massive myocardial damage. However, it is important to remember that potentially reversible disorders may mimic electromechanical dissociation. Therefore, after intravenous access and, whenever possible, endotracheal intubation have been established, search for and correct the following conditions:

A. Myocardial Failure: Give 0.5–1 mg (5–10 mL) of epinephrine (1:10,000). Epinephrine, 200 µg/kg of 1:1000 solution (15 mL for a 70-kg person), may be more effective. Repeat every 5 minutes as needed.

B. Hypovolemia: Give a fluid bolus challenge (crystalloid solution, 500 mL as rapidly as possible). Look for an unsuspected site of bleeding. Cardiac arrest due to massive hemorrhage (eg, ruptured abdominal aortic aneurysm) may require emergency thoracotomy and aortic cross-clamping for control of bleeding.

C. Tension Pneumothorax: Perform needle thoracostomy by insertion of a 14-gauge needle in the fourth intercostal space at the anterior axillary line. If air rushes out of the needle, tube thoracostomy should be performed.

D. Cardiac Tamponade: Look for signs of tamponade (distended neck veins), and perform pericardiocentesis (Chapter 46) if tamponade is suspected. Cardiac arrest due to traumatic cardiac tamponade requires emergency thoracotomy to open the pericardium and to occlude or repair cardiac injuries (Chapters 18 and 46).

E. Severe Acidosis and Hypoxemia: Treat as discussed on pp 14–15.

F. Consider Open Chest Compression: If all else fails, open chest compression may be indicated (Chapters 18 and 46).

Supraventricular Tachyarrhythmias

Supraventricular tachyarrhythmias in themselves rarely cause cardiac arrest. For diagnosis and treatment, see Chapter 29.

Successful Resuscitation

Resuscitation is successful if arterial pulses are palpable without the need for chest compression.

A. Check Blood Pressure: As soon as a spontaneous pulse is detectable by palpation, try to obtain a blood pressure reading. If blood pressure is less than 60 mm Hg or if a pulse cannot be felt in the brachial artery, resume chest compressions.

B. Treat Arrhythmias: Treat any unstable rhythms that are incompatible with good cardiac output (see above and Chapter 29).

C. Correct Volume Depletion: If hypotension is due to hypovolemia, treat with intravenous crystalloid solution or blood products (Chapter 3).

D. Give Inotropic Agent: (See below and Table

1–2.) If systolic blood pressure is below 90 mm Hg, give dopamine as a continuous intravenous infusion at a rate of 2–20 µg/kg/min.

E. Transfer Patient: As soon as the patient's condition has stabilized, with systolic blood pressure higher than 90 mm Hg, transport the patient to an intensive care unit for further definitive therapy and management.

DRUGS USED IN ADVANCED LIFE SUPPORT
(See Table 1–2.)

Sodium Bicarbonate

As noted above, routine administration of bicarbonate during CPR is no longer recommended, and it should not be used during the first 10 minutes of resuscitation. If it is used at all, its administration should be guided by determination of pH through arterial blood gas analysis unless severe acidosis, with or without hyperkalemia, is suspected (ie, patient requiring dialysis for renal failure). The usual dose is 1 meq/kg, followed by 0.5 meq every 10 minutes as needed. It should not be given in the same intravenous line as any other medication.

Catecholamines

Most catecholamines have mixed sympathomimetic effects; an important exception is isoproterenol, which is a pure beta agonist. Alpha receptor stimulation results in peripheral vasoconstriction, which redistributes blood to the brain and other vital organs; β_1 receptor stimulation increases the vigor and rate of the cardiac contraction; and β_2 receptor stimulation causes vasodilation in some organs.

A. Epinephrine: Epinephrine has mixed alpha- and beta-stimulating effects. It increases cerebral blood flow and provides a high diastolic aortic root pressure that improves coronary perfusion. The dose for adults is 0.5–1 mg (5–10 mL of 1:10,000 solution or 1 mL of 1:1000 solution diluted appropriately) intravenously. Higher doses may be useful, as noted earlier. Epinephrine is also effective by intratracheal administration (use the same dose as for intravenous administration). The intramuscular and subcutaneous routes, although generally effective, should be avoided in cardiac arrest victims, because the drug is poorly absorbed.

B. Dopamine: Dopamine has variable effects, depending on the dose. Low doses (2–5 µg/kg/min) have a dopaminergic effect that dilates renal and mesenteric blood vessels. Higher doses (5–20 µg/kg/min) have dopaminergic and mixed adrenergic effects. Doses of more than 20 µg/kg/min have predominantly alpha-adrenergic effects. Generally speaking, dopamine is the vasopressor drug of choice in the treatment of shock after hypovolemia has been ruled out or treated. Fortunately, there is little decrease in

urinary output at higher dosage levels (up to 20 µg/kg/min). The drug should be administered by continuous intravenous infusion via an infusion pump.

C. Dobutamine: Dobutamine increases myocardial contractility with minimal increase in oxygen demand by stimulating myocardial β_1 and α receptors without inducing norepinephrine release. Its β_2 stimulation induces vasodilation, which decreases peripheral resistance. The combined positive inotropic effect and afterload reduction increases cardiac output with minimal tachycardia or change in blood pressure at lower doses. Dobutamine is the drug of choice in patients with cardiogenic shock or significant right ventricular infarction. When used in combination with dopamine, arterial blood pressure and cardiac output are maintained at lower doses of each drug than when either drug is used alone. The dosage of dobutamine for adults is 2.5–20 µg/kg/min given as a continuous intravenous infusion via an infusion pump.

Note: Dobutamine is not usually recommended for resuscitation from cardiac arrest because of its vasodilating effects.

D. Isoproterenol: Isoproterenol is a potent beta-stimulating drug whose principal usefulness is in the treatment of hemodynamically significant bradycardia unresponsive to atropine. The major disadvantages of isoproterenol are that it increases myocardial oxygen consumption and redistributes blood flow away from the brain to the periphery of the body. It is administered by continuous intravenous infusion at a rate of 2–20 µg/min. Occasionally, the magnitude of the heart block becomes less severe with isoproterenol infusion; more often, a slow ventricular pacemaker accelerates to a faster level that supports an adequate ventricular pulse and output.

E. Norepinephrine (Levarterenol): Norepinephrine is a potent alpha-adrenergic stimulator. The dose is 2–10 µg/min by continuous intravenous infusion. When norepinephrine is given to a patient in shock, there is usually a prompt rise in blood pressure, which increases myocardial and brain perfusion. The disadvantage of this medication is that it markedly decreases renal perfusion and urine output, and prolonged use may lead to acute tubular necrosis.

Antiarrhythmics

A. Lidocaine: Lidocaine is a potent antiarrhythmic drug that is effective in suppressing ventricular ectopy, especially premature ventricular contractions and ventricular tachycardia. A loading dose of 1 mg/kg is given by bolus injection, followed by continuous intravenous infusion at a rate of 2–4 mg/min (adult dose). If significant ventricular arrhythmia reappears after the loading dose, an additional 50-mg bolus may be given. In the setting of cardiac arrest, bolus therapy should be used. Following the initial bolus of 1 mg/kg, boluses of 0.5 mg/kg may be given every 8–10 minutes as needed, not exceeding a total of 3 mg/kg. The drug is also effective (temporarily) by intratracheal administration; the dose is the same as for the intravenous route.

Lidocaine causes few cardiac side effects and does not worsen atrioventricular conduction. The principal toxic effects of lidocaine are on the central nervous system, and these are more likely to occur in patients with shock, congestive heart failure, or severe liver disease. Failure to suppress ventricular ectopy after adequate doses of lidocaine may be an indication for administration of procainamide or bretylium tosylate.

B. Bretylium Tosylate: Bretylium tosylate is a quaternary ammonium compound useful in the treatment of ventricular fibrillation and ventricular tachycardia unresponsive to cardioversion and other antiarrhythmic agents. Its mechanism of action is unclear, but it accumulates in postganglionic adrenergic neurons and inhibits norepinephrine release. Antifibrillatory cardiac actions may be seen within minutes. The effects on ventricular arrhythmias (including ventricular tachycardia) may not be manifest for 20 minutes to 2 hours. Severe hypotension may occasionally occur.

To treat ventricular fibrillation and pulseless ventricular tachycardia, give undiluted bretylium solution, 5 mg/kg by intravenous bolus injection. If arrhythmia persists, increase to 10 mg/kg, and repeat at intervals of 15–30 minutes to a maximum total dose of 30 mg/kg. Electrical defibrillation should be performed after each bolus of bretylium. To treat persistently recurring ventricular tachycardia, dilute 500 mg (10 mL) to 50 mL, and give 5–10 mg/kg intravenously over 8–10 minutes, followed by continuous intravenous infusion at a rate of 1–2 mg/min.

C. Procainamide: Procainamide is effective in suppressing ventricular irritability. It is the second drug of choice after lidocaine for the treatment of ventricular premature beats and ventricular tachycardia with a pulse. It is given in intravenous boluses of 50–100 mg every 5 minutes until the arrhythmia is suppressed or until 1 g has been given. The boluses should be followed by a continuous intravenous infusion of 1–4 mg/min. Blood pressure and the ECG should be monitored closely during administration. The drug should be temporarily discontinued if hypotension or a widening of the QRS complex by 50% of its original width develops.

D. Atropine: Atropine is a potent vagolytic (parasympatholytic) drug useful in accelerating the heart rate and raising the blood pressure in patients with severe bradycardia due to vagotonic states such as may be seen in acute inferior myocardial infarction. The dose is 0.5–1 mg by bolus injection, but no more than 2 mg should be administered over 2 hours. Atropine is also effective when administered intratracheally; the dose is the same as that for the intravenous route. Atropine may induce ventricular irritability or increase the magnitude of myocardial infarction by inordinately accelerating the sinus rate.

Atropine also has central nervous system, visual, and genitourinary toxicity and should therefore be used only for *symptomatic* bradyarrhythmia. Infants younger than 6 months of age with a heart rate of less than 80/min should also be treated.

Calcium Chloride

Calcium has traditionally been used during CPR for its inotropic effects. The use of calcium in conditions such as ventricular fibrillation and electromechanical dissociation is not supported by experimental studies, however. Investigators have demonstrated that severe hypercalcemia may result from calcium administration and that high intracellular concentrations of calcium may be harmful. Furthermore, calcium channel–blocking agents may aid resuscitation. Calcium should therefore be given only to patients with known hyperkalemia, hypocalcemia, or toxicity due to calcium channel-blocking agents. Both the chloride and gluconate salts of calcium are effective, but the chloride form is preferred because it is substantially cheaper. The dose is 5 mL of 10% solution given intravenously.

ADVANCED PERFUSION SUPPORT

Open Chest Cardiac Compression

Open chest cardiac compression (Chapters 4 and 46) is indicated in patients whose chest wall cavities are too large, stiff, or deformed to permit effective closed chest compression. The best indicators of inadequate external massage are a feeble or absent carotid pulse and refractory acidosis and hypoxemia. Open chest compression is also indicated in patients who have had (or need to have) emergency thoracostomy as a result of a chest wound, hypovolemic shock, tension pneumothorax, air embolism, or cardiac tamponade (see below and Chapter 18).

Chest Compressors

A number of mechanical devices are available for performing closed chest compression. They are effective and safe substitutes for manual compression only in experienced hands. They can be extremely useful, however, when CPR must be performed for a prolonged period, in a confined space, or during transport of the patient over difficult terrain. Sternal fracture is a common complication, but major complications occurring with properly placed and monitored mechanical devices are probably no more frequent than with manual compression. All the problems that may occur during manual compression can also occur with mechanical devices. Additional considerations are availability, maneuverability, and expense.

STABILIZATION OF PATIENTS

It is recommended that patients with cardiac arrest be adequately stabilized in the emergency department or at the scene of arrest by the advanced life support unit rather than being transported prematurely, because attempts at CPR during transport (hallway, stairs, elevator, etc) may be ineffective. Victims have a better chance of survival if their condition is stabilized at the scene or in the emergency department before they are transported to a hospital or intensive care area that may be some distance away.

CEREBRAL RESUSCITATION

Ideally, properly performed basic and advanced cardiac life support provides an adequate amount of oxygenated blood for the brain. Additional therapies to help resuscitate the central nervous system during and after CPR are being investigated. Animal studies suggest that barbiturates, such as thiopental, and calcium channel blockers, such as lidoflazine, might be effective in reducing the ischemic and hypoxic damage that results from cardiac and respiratory arrest. However, thiopental loading within 30 minutes of arrest did not improve outcome in an international clinical trial, and calcium channel blockers also were not successful. As a result, these agents cannot be generally recommended.

CPR IN INFANTS & CHILDREN

BASIC LIFE SUPPORT

Basic CPR techniques in infants and children are similar to those used in adults. Some differences are discussed below. As a guideline, infants are younger than 1 year, and children are between the ages of 1 and 8 years. For children 8 years of age and older, the techniques are the same as those used in adults.

Diagnosis of Cardiac Arrest

Absence of cardiac output is more easily diagnosed in infants by palpating the brachial artery than by palpating the carotid artery. Palpation of the precordial impulse is no longer recommended.

Airway

Marked extension of the neck may occlude the airway in infants; hence, a more neutral position is recommended. See Table 1–3 for guidelines on the size of endotracheal tubes to be used.

Position

In infants, the head and back can be braced with one palm, the head-tilt position maintained by the weight of the head, and closed chest compression performed with the index and middle fingers of the other hand while the rescuer's mouth seals both the mouth and the nose of the infant during respiratory maneuvers (Fig 1–10A). Children too large to be supported by one hand should be placed supine on a hard surface and the airway opened with the head-tilt and chin-lift method described for adults.

Inflation Rate & Volume

The inflation rate for children should be faster than that for adults (16–20 breaths per minute), and small puffs rather than large volumes of air should be blown into the child's lungs to prevent pneumothorax (Table 1–1). In the newborn, only cheek pressure (mouth air) should be used to inflate the lungs. In general, use just enough air and force to cause the chest to rise.

Airway Obstruction

If the airway of an infant (< 1 year of age) is occluded, hold the infant straddled face down over one arm with the head lower than the trunk and the head and neck supported by the hand (Fig 1–11). Deliver 4 sharp blows between the scapulas with the heel of the hand. Immediately turn the infant face up on the thigh, with the head lower than the trunk. Deliver 4 chest thrusts with 2 fingers in the mid sternum.

An infant too large to hold in one arm should be placed horizontally over the thighs, with its head lower than the trunk. The chest thrust can be performed with the infant lying on the floor.

In children over 1 year of age, the Heimlich maneuver should be performed to relieve airway obstruction, as described above for adults.

Table 1–3. Guidelines for endotracheal tube selection.[1]

Age	Orotracheal Tube[2]	Nasotracheal Tube
Premature	Uncuffed ≤ 2.5	Not applicable
Term	Uncuffed 3.0	Not applicable
3–12 months	Uncuffed 3.0–3.5	Not applicable
1–3 years	Uncuffed 4.0–4.5	Not applicable
3–5 years	Uncuffed 5.0–5.5	6–7
5–7 years	Uncuffed 5.5–6.0	7–8
8–13 years	Cuffed 6.5–7.0	8–9
Over 13 years		
Female	Cuffed 7.5–8.0	8–10
Male	Cuffed 8.0–9.0	9–12

[1] In children over 1 year of age, the following formula may be used: Age (in years) + 16 ÷ 4.
[2] Internal diameter in mm.

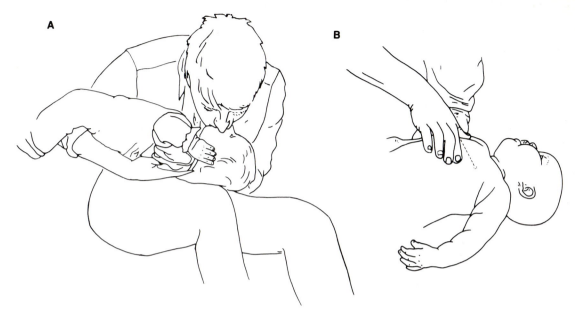

Figure 1–10. CPR in infants (< 1 year of age). **A:** To ventilate, rescuer's mouth occludes both mouth and nose of victim during inspiratory phase. In small infants, air expelled from rescuer's mouth and cheeks is sufficient to provide adequate ventilation. Avoid overextension of infant's head. **B:** Closed chest compression is achieved with the rescuer's index and middle fingers placed one fingerwidth below an imaginary line connecting the nipples. Head tilt can be maintained by bracing the back with one palm.

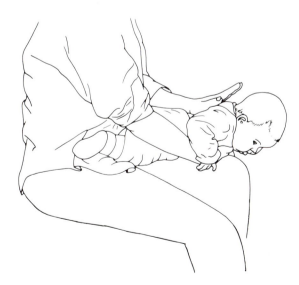

Figure 1–11. Clearing airway in infant. Place infant in prone position, head down. With heel of hand, deliver 4 sharp blows between the scapulas. Immediately turn the infant face up, and deliver 4 chest thrusts with 2 fingers in the sternum, one fingerwidth below an imaginary line connecting the nipples (Fig 1–10B).

Closed Chest Compression

The heart is more centrally placed in the chest in newborns and infants, so that the correct position for closed chest compression is on the sternum, one fingerwidth below an imaginary line connecting the nipples (Fig 1–10B). *Note:* This is lower than was previously recommended. In infants, chest compression is achieved with 2–3 fingers compressing the sternum to a depth of 1.25–2.5 cm (½–1 in) at a rate of at least 100/min (counting: "One, two, three. . ." at a normal rate). In children, adequate chest compression can be performed with the heel of one hand in the same position as for adults, to a depth of 2.5–4 cm (1–1½ in) at a rate of 80–100/min (counting: "One-and-two-and-three. . ."). Pause after every 5 compressions to give one breath. In infants and children, the 5:1 compression-ventilation ratio is used for both single and 2-rescuer CPR. As for adults, 2-rescuer CPR should be performed only by health care professionals. Reassess the victim for the presence of spontaneous respiration and pulse after 10 cycles of ventilation and compression and every few minutes thereafter.

ADVANCED LIFE SUPPORT

Intravenous Access

In addition to the basilic and femoral veins, cannulation of the external jugular and saphenous veins may also be tried in infants. The scalp may also be cannulated, using a rubber band around the forehead as a tourniquet. Intraosseous administration of fluids and drugs by means of the tibial bone marrow may be tried if venous access cannot be achieved (Chapter 46). The efficacy of this route during CPR has not been determined.

Dosage of Drugs for CPR

Drugs used for the treatment of arrhythmias in infants and children are similar to those used in adults; however, the dosages and frequency of administration may differ, as shown in Table 1–4.

Defibrillation

Because ventricular fibrillation is uncommon in children, unmonitored defibrillation should not be attempted in infants and children. When defibrillation is indicated, use the largest size electrode paddle that makes maximal chest wall contact. Paddle position is the same as that for adults. Administer 2 J/kg initially, and if unsuccessful, double the energy and repeat twice. Severe acidosis and hypoxemia must be corrected for successful defibrillation and maintenance of normal sinus rhythm.

SPECIAL PROBLEMS & SITUATIONS

PRECORDIAL THUMP

Precordial thump is indicated for adult patients with *witnessed* or *monitored* cardiac arrest or bradycardiac arrest that can be paced by chest thump. Chest thump defibrillation may be especially useful in victims of high-voltage electrocution.

The thump is administered sharply as a blow that uses the ulnar aspect of the clenched fist (Fig 1–12) and is delivered from a point 25–30 cm (10–12 in) above the chest. The fist should strike the center of the sternum with a single brisk motion. This delivers a low-energy wave (approximately 4 J) to the myocardium, and occasionally this carries sufficient energy to convert ventricular fibrillation of less than 1–2 minutes' duration to normal rhythm.

Caution: The precordial thump should not be used in children. In adults, the precordial thump should be attempted only in patients whose arrest is witnessed or monitored and when a defibrillator is not immediately available, because (theoretically) the thump may actually induce ventricular fibrillation rather than convert it. In patients with marked bradycardia, any energy delivered to the heart during the down-

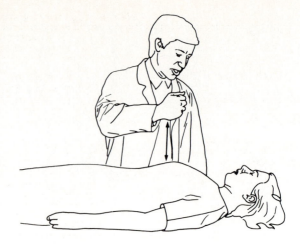

Figure 1–12. Precordial thump for witnessed cardiac arrest. Deliver a sharp blow to the center of the sternum with a clenched fist, initiating the blow from a point *no more* than 25–30 cm (10–12 in) above the sternum.

stroke of the T wave (so-called vulnerable period) may induce sustained ventricular arrhythmia.

TRAUMATIC CARDIAC ARREST

Cardiac arrest occurring in victims of trauma is usually the result of tension pneumothorax, severe hypovolemia, or cardiac tamponade rather than primary arrhythmias or myocardial failure. The ABCs of basic life support must still be followed. If cervical spine injury is suspected, the jaw-thrust technique (with the cervical spine appropriately immobilized) should be used to open the airway. Endotracheal intubation should be established as soon as possible. Tension pneumothorax (deviated trachea, distended neck veins, unilateral increased tympany, or absent breath sounds) must be searched for and treated immediately by tube thoracostomy (Chapter 46), preferably, or by insertion of a 14-gauge needle in the fourth intercostal space at the anterior axillary line. Emergency thoracotomy should be performed (Chapter 46) if tension pneumothorax is absent or if decompression does not achieve return of the pulse. Exposure of the chest cavity allows for (**1**) treatment of cardiac tamponade, (**2**) direct cardiac compression (closed chest compression is ineffective in severe hypovolemia), (**3**) control of bleeding from the myocardium and great vessels, and (**4**) cross-clamping of the aorta to control massive bleeding below the diaphragm and increase cardiac output to the brain and myocardium. Insert several large-bore (≥ 16-gauge) intravenous catheters for rapid crystalloid infusion. If thoracotomy cannot be done, perform pericardiocentesis to search for and temporarily treat cardiac tamponade. Apply a MAST (military antishock trou-

Table 1–4. Drugs for life support: Dose for infants and children.

Drug and Dosage Form	Usual Dosage and Route of Administration	Comments
Sodium bicarbonate 8.4% solution that contains 1 meq/mL **or** 7.5% solution that contains 0.9 meq/L	Initial intravenous bolus of 1 meq/kg, then 0.5 meq/kg every 10 minutes or 0.3 × weight (kg) × base deficit (meq/L).	Use only for prolonged cardiac arrest or documented metabolic acidosis. Do not put in intravenous line with catecholamines or calcium. Repeat dosage as arterial blood gas measurements indicate. Stop when pH is ≥ 7.2. In infants, dilute 1:1 with 5% dextrose in water.
Epinephrine 1:10,000 aqueous solution (0.1 mg/mL) **or** 1:1000 aqueous solution (1.0 mg/mL) for older children	Cardiac arrest: 0.1 mL/kg intravenously. 0.2 mg/kg bolus injection may be more effective. Repeat every 5 minutes as needed.	Effective intratracheally.
	Hypotension: 0.1 µg/kg/min by continuous intravenous infusion. Increase by 0.1 µg/kg/min up to a maximum of 1 µg/kg/min as needed.	
Atropine Prefilled syringe of 0.1 mg/mL **or** Vials of 1 mg/mL, 0.5 mg/mL, 0.4 mg/mL	0.02 mg/kg intravenously, with a minimum dose of 0.1 mg and a maximum dose of 1 mg. May be repeated every 5 minutes for a total dose of up to 1 mg in children and 2 mg in adolescents.	May be given endotracheally using the same dose as for the intravenous route.
Calcium chloride Prefilled syringe of 10% solution (1 g in 10 mL [100 mg/mL])	0.2 mL/kg intravenously over 5 minutes.	Recommended only for hypocalcemia, hyperkalemia, hypermagnesemia, and toxicity due to calcium channel–blocking agents. Never mix with bicarbonate solutions.
Dextrose 50% dextrose in water	Dilute 50% dextrose in water 1:1 with water to make 25% dextrose in water, and give 2 mL/kg intravenously.	
Naloxone 0.4 mg/mL **or** 0.02 mg/mL	0.01 mg/kg intravenously.	Repeat at 2- to 3-minute intervals as indicated.
Dopamine 200 mg in 5-mL vials (40 mg/mL)	Mix 6 mg/kg in 100 mL of 5% dextrose in water so that 1 µg/kg/min = 1 mL/h. Give by continuous intravenous infusion at a rate of 2–20 µg/kg/min.	Increase concentration for infants and newborns depending on volume needs.
Isoproterenol 1 mg in 5-mL vial (0.2 mg/mL)	Mix 0.6 mg/kg in 100 mL of 5% dextrose in water so that 0.1 µg/kg/min = 1 mL/h. Give by continuous intravenous infusion at a rate of 0.1 µg/kg/min, and increase by 0.1 µg/kg/min as indicated.	Use only for hemodynamically unstable bradycardia resistant to atropine. Not recommended in asystole.
Lidocaine 1% solution (50 mg in 5-mL vial [10 mg/mL]) **or** 2% solution (20 mg/mL)	Initial bolus of 1 mg/kg, then 20–50 µg/kg/min by continuous intravenous infusion (120 mg in 100 mL of 5% dextrose in water infused at a rate of 1–2.5 mL/kg/h).	Reduce infusion rate to 1 mL/kg/h in presence of shock, chronic heart failure, or cardiac arrest.
Bretylium tosylate 500 mg in 10-mL vial (50 mg/mL)	Ventricular fibrillation or pulseless ventricular tachycardia: intravenous bolus of 5 mg/kg; if arrhythmia persists, give 10 mg/kg every 15–30 minutes as needed, for a maximum total dose of 30 mg/kg.	Defibrillate after each bolus. Second-line drug: use if arrhythmia is refractory to lidocaine.
	Ventricular tachycardia: Dilute to 10 mg/kg, and give 5 mg/kg over 6–8 minutes.	

sers) suit (Chapter 46) and, if resuscitation is successful or still possible, transport the patient to a facility with cardiothoracic surgical capability.

Traumatic cardiac arrest following blunt trauma has a dismal prognosis. Emergency thoracotomy is unlikely to be of benefit except in selected cases (signs of life during the prehospital phase or cardiothoracic operation immediately available). In contrast, cardiac arrest resulting from penetrating trauma may be associated with survival rates as high as 30–40% if emergency thoracotomy is performed.

HYPOVOLEMIA
(Massive Bleeding)

Massive bleeding (gastrointestinal tract; ruptured abdominal aneurysm or aortic dissection) may not be apparent initially to emergency department personnel. However, severe volume depletion can lead to cardiovascular collapse mimicking cardiac arrest. Hypovolemia should not be overlooked, especially if there is no other explanation for the collapsed state. Appropriate diagnostic procedures and tests such as hematocrit, aspiration of stomach contents, abdominal or thoracic paracentesis, examination of feces for blood, and central venous pressure measurements usually suggest the proper diagnosis. Therapy should be directed initially at volume replacement and identification of the bleeding source and rate of blood loss before definitive therapy is selected (Chapter 3).

AORTIC DISSECTION

Dissection of the aorta is an emergency that may require medical rather than surgical therapy. (See Chapter 32 for further discussion.) The therapeutic approach varies depending on the size and progression of the lesion. Patients with dissection often present with pain that frequently mimics myocardial infarction or even renal colic. The patient may be in shock, and physical examination may reveal new murmurs of aortic insufficiency, absent pulses, pulsatile abdominal masses, or an enlarged aorta on chest or abdominal x-rays. Since diagnosis and therapy usually depend on the site of the initial tear and its extension, emergency angiography or CT scan is required.

DROWNING

Although mouth-to-mouth resuscitation may be successfully performed in the water, the drowning victim should always be moved to land, to a boat, or to some other hard surface before chest compression is attempted. Standard CPR measures should be started even though the victim has been submerged

for many minutes, since hypothermia induced by immersion and the diving reflex that redistributes blood flow to vital organs may protect the brain from hypoxic damage during cardiac arrest. This is especially true in children. (See Chapter 38 for further discussion.)

ACCIDENTAL ELECTRIC SHOCK

Cardiac arrhythmias, especially ventricular fibrillation, may develop if the voltage the victim is exposed to is high ($\geq$ 1000 V). The continuous 50- to 60-cycle current from household electrical outlets may span the "vulnerable" period of many ECG waves and thus cause ventricular fibrillation. If the current passes through the head, apnea may result that is particularly responsive to CPR. The death rate from high-voltage electrocution is high, but resuscitation should always be initiated as soon as the victim is safely removed from the energy source. Defibrillation with DC countershock is indicated (Chapter 38).

CARDIAC TAMPONADE

Traumatic wounds of the chest cavity may not be apparent on initial examination. Such a victim may arrive in the emergency department pulseless, unconscious, and unresponsive as a result of cardiac tamponade. This diagnosis should be considered if closed chest compression fails to produce adequate cardiac output, particularly if there is marked jugular venous distention. CPR itself, especially if improperly performed, can cause cardiac tamponade.

Cardiac tamponade must be relieved immediately. For obvious chest wounds, this is best accomplished by limited thoracotomy and direct pericardiotomy in the emergency department (Chapter 4). Repeated attempts to treat this problem with transthoracic needle pericardiocentesis should be performed *only* until the surgeon who is to perform the thoracotomy or laparotomy arrives. Needle aspiration is useful for both diagnosis and therapy in patients who do not have obvious chest wounds (Chapter 46).

CRITERIA FOR
TERMINATING CPR

Absence of spontaneous respirations or palpable pulse after 30 minutes of effective CPR (good pulses with closed chest compression, relatively normal arterial blood gas measurements) in a patient whose core temperature is 32 °C (90 °F) or higher usually indicates cerebral death and can be taken to mean that further resuscitative efforts will be futile. Inability to maintain independent mechanical systole despite adequate ventilation and intravascular volume, an arterial blood pH greater than 7.2, and absence of cardiac tamponade or tension pneumothorax are indications that the heart is functionally dead. Resuscitation can be withheld from a patient who is obviously dead for other reasons (decapitation, rigor mortis, evidence of tissue decomposition). Other factors that may justify termination or withholding of resuscitative efforts include team exhaustion or a prior written agreement with the patient and family not to resuscitate (eg, in chronic incurable illness).

ROLE OF EMERGENCY DEPARTMENT STAFF IN CPR

The staff of every emergency department must be able to deliver basic resuscitation and to initiate advanced resuscitative maneuvers as required. This is best achieved by designating a CPR team leader for each shift who assigns specific roles to individuals. The role of the team leader is to make certain that resuscitative techniques are initiated promptly, to guide resuscitative efforts, and to decide if CPR should be terminated. The leader maintains a high standard of performance in resuscitation by reviewing every case and by developing and maintaining a system for ongoing training. Medical personnel who have been poorly trained or are unfamiliar with the dynamics of the team may interfere with delivery of optimal resuscitation. An ongoing, approved training program with annual recertification in CPR is essential to maintain proficiency. The American Heart Association and the American National Red Cross teach CPR techniques both to lay persons and to medical and paramedical professionals. CPR certification of physicians is now required for maintenance of hospital staff privileges in many areas.

REFERENCES

Advanced Cardiac Life Support (ACLS) Task Force on Early Defibrillation: Automated external defibrillation. In: *Textbook of Advanced Cardiac Life Support.* American Heart Association, 1990.

American Heart Association: *Textbook of Advanced Cardiac Life Support.* American Heart Association, 1987.

Barton C, Callaham ML: High-dose epinephrine improves the return of spontaneous circulation rates in human victims of cardiac arrest. Ann Emerg Med 1991;20:722.

Bedell SE et al: Survival after cardiopulmonary resuscitation in the hospital. N Engl J Med 1983;309:569.

Bircher N, Safar P: Manual open-chest cardiopulmonary resuscitation. Ann Emerg Med 1984;13:770.

Bjork RJ et al: Medical complications of cardiopulmonary arrest. Arch Intern Med 1982;142:500.

Callaham ML: High-dose epinephrine therapy and other advances in treating cardiac arrest. West J Med 1990; 152:697.

Dronen SC: Antifibrillatory drugs: The case for bretylium tosylate. Ann Emerg Med 1984;13:805.

Eisenberg MS, Hallstrom A, Bergner L: Long-term survival after out-of-hospital cardiac arrest. N Engl J Med 1982;306:1340.

Eisenberg MS et al: Cardiac arrest and resuscitation: A tale of 29 cities. Ann Emerg Med 1990;19:179.

Eisenberg MS, Cummins RO, Ho MT (editors): *Code Blue: Cardiac Arrest and Resuscitation.* Saunders, 1987.

Goetting MG, Paradis NA: High-dose epinephrine improves outcome from pediatric cardiac arrest. Ann Emerg Med 1991;20:22.

Guzy PM: Emergency cardiac pacing. Emerg Med Clin North Am 1986;4:745.

Hedges JR et al: Central versus peripheral intravenous routes in cardiopulmonary resuscitation. Am J Emerg Med 1984;2:385.

Hoffman JR: Treatment of foreign body obstruction of the upper airway. West J Med 1982;136:11.

Koster RW, Dunning AJ: Intramuscular lidocaine for prevention of lethal arrhythmias in prehospitalization phase of acute myocardial infarction. N Engl J Med 1985; 313:1105.

Krischer JP et al: Comparison of prehospital conventional and simultaneous compression-ventilation cardiopulmonary resuscitation. Crit Care Med 1989;17:1263.

Longstreth WT Jr et al: Neurologic recovery after out-of-hospital cardiac arrest. Ann Intern Med 1983;98:588.

Martin GB et al: Verapamil in the treatment of asystolic and pulseless idioventricular rhythm cardiopulmonary arrest: A preliminary report. Ann Emerg Med 1984;13:221.

Michael JR et al: Mechanisms by which epinephrine augments cerebral and myocardial perfusion during cardiopulmonary resuscitation in dogs. Circulation 1984;69: 822.

Murphy DJ et al: Outcomes of cardiopulmonary resuscitation in the elderly. Ann Intern Med 1989;111:199.

Nayler WG: The role of calcium in the ischemic myocardium. Am J Pathol 1981;102:262.

Niemann JT: Differences in cerebral and myocardial perfusion during closed-chest resuscitation. Ann Emerg Med 1984;13:849.

Neimann JT, Rosborough JP: Effects of acidemia and sodium bicarbonate therapy in advanced cardiac life support. Ann Emerg Med 1984;13:781.

Olson DW et al: A randomized comparison study of bretylium tosylate and lidocaine in resuscitation of patients from out-of-hospital ventricular fibrillation in a paramedic system. Ann Emerg Med 1984;13:807.

Otto CW, Yakaitis RW: The role of epinephrine in CPR: A reappraisal. Ann Emerg Med 1984;13:840.

Ralston SH, Voorhees WD, Babbs CF: Intrapulmonary epinephrine during prolonged cardiopulmonary resuscitation: Improved regional blood flow and resuscitation in dogs. Ann Emerg Med 1984;13:79.

Roberts D et al: Early predictors of mortality for hospital patients suffering cardiopulmonary arrest. Chest 1990; 97:413.

Standards and guidelines for cardiopulmonary resuscitation (CPR) and emergency cardiac care (ECC). JAMA 1986;255:2905.

Stueven HA et al: The effectiveness of calcium chloride in refractory electromechanical dissociation. Ann Emerg Med 1985;14:626.

Stueven HA et al: Lack of effectiveness of calcium chloride in refractory asystole. Ann Emerg Med 1985;14:630.

Weaver WD et al: Use of the automatic external defibrillator in the management of out-of-hospital cardiac arrest. N Engl J Med 1988;319:661.

Weil MH et al: Difference in acid-base state between venous and arterial blood during cardiopulmonary resuscitation. N Engl J Med 1986;315:153.

Compromised Airway

2

Julia Nathan, MD

IMMEDIATE MANAGEMENT OF THE COMPROMISED AIRWAY (See algorithm.)

Securing the airway and assuring adequate ventilation are the first priorities in the resuscitation of any acutely ill or injured patient. Without a patent airway and adequate gas exchange, other resuscitative measures will usually be futile. Thus, attention to the airway must precede or occur simultaneously with any other type of management. The exception is the initial defibrillation in cardiac arrest due to ventricular fibrillation, if defibrillation can be performed immediately.

Assess the Airway

A. Determine the patient's level of consciousness, and note the presence of any respiratory effort. In patients with known or suspected cervical spine injury, all assessments and maneuvers should be undertaken with the cervical spine immobilized in a neutral position to prevent cord injury.

B. In an apneic, unconscious patient—

1. Open the airway with a chin-lift or jaw-thrust maneuver. If the cervical spine is not injured, place the head in the "sniffing" position (see Chapter 1 and Fig 2–1).

2. Clear the airway of obstructions, using a rigid suction catheter to remove any blood, vomitus, or se-

cretions from the oropharynx. Remove any large obstructing foreign bodies from the oropharynx manually or with Magill forceps (Chapter 1).

3. If the patient remains apneic, assist ventilation using a bag-valve-mask device (eg, Ambu bag) device or mouth-to-mouth breathing (Chapter 1). If adequate personnel and equipment are available, immediately perform endotracheal intubation. Administer high-flow oxygen.

C. In a patient with respiratory effort—

1. Administer high-flow oxygen.

2. Clear and position the airway as described above.

3. Identify evidence of upper airway obstruction. Prolapse of the tongue and accumulation of secretions, blood, or vomitus are common causes of obstruction. Signs may include wheezing, sonorous respirations, stridor, cough, and dysphonia. Upper airway obstruction should be removed if present. Back blows or the Heimlich maneuver may clear the obstruction. If not, use suction or direct visualization and a Magill forceps or finger. Blind sweep is contraindicated. Obstructions that recur or persist require endotracheal intubation, either orotracheally or via cricothyroidotomy, tracheostomy, or percutaneous transtracheal jet ventilation (Chapters 1 and 42).

4. Evaluate the effectiveness of the patient's respiratory effort. Helpful signs include respiratory rate, tidal volume, accessory muscle use, level of consciousness, skin color, upper airway sounds, and auscultated lung sounds. Further assessment may include pulse oximetry, arterial blood gas measurement, and chest radiography.

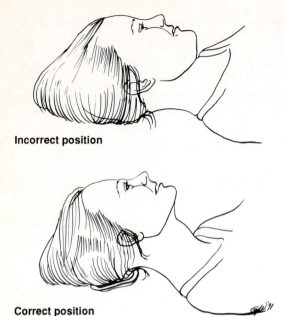

Incorrect position

Correct position

Figure 2–1. In the sniffing position, the head is slightly extended and the neck is flexed on the shoulders. This aligns the axis of the airway with the mouth and pharynx, facilitating direct visualization of the cords during intubation. It is particularly important in young children and infants, in whom the larynx is considerably more anterior. A pad beneath the occiput improves flexion of the neck. This position cannot be used when there is cervical spine injury.

5. If intubation is indicated (Table 2–1), continue high-flow oxygen and assist ventilation as needed. Assemble all items necessary for the appropriate method of intubation (Tables 2–2 and 2–3). Check for equipment malfunction. If the patient is alert, inform him or her of your plan.

Table 2–1. Indications for intubation.

Respiratory insufficiency
Apnea
Hypoxia
Hypoventilation
Airway obstruction
Foreign body
Fixed mass
Traumatic deformity
Continued bleeding, secretions, or emesis
Inability to protect airway
Altered mental status
Loss of normal airway reflexes
Need for hyperventilation
Head injury
Metabolic acidosis in critically ill or injured patient
Anticipated or impending airway compromise
Shock
Multiple trauma
Need for sedation or paralysis

Table 2–2. Essential airway management equipment.

Oxygen
Nasal cannula
Nonrebreathing masks of various sizes
Suction—rigid pharyngeal, flexible
Oral airways—range of sizes
Nasal airways—range of sizes
Bag-valve-mask units—adult and pediatric sizes
Water-soluble lubricant
Vasoconstrictive topicals
Anesthetic topicals (jelly and spray)
Laryngoscope handles
Laryngoscope blades—range of sizes (curved or straight based on operator preference)
Low-pressure cuff endotracheal tubes of varying sizes
Stylets
Intravenous access (advised)

Prepare for Intubation

A. High-Flow Oxygen: All patients with airway or ventilatory compromise require high-flow oxygen. A nasal cannula at flow rates up to 6 L/min provides a patient with 20–40% inspired oxygen concentration. A variety of masks are available that can accept oxygen flow rates of 5–15 L/min. Masks equipped with reservoirs and nonrebreathing valves can deliver oxygen concentrations close to 100% at flow rates of 10 L/min if an adequate seal can be maintained between the mask and face.

Before attempting intubation, preoxygenate the patient with 100% oxygen for 2–3 minutes. In a ventilating patient, this provides 6–7 minutes of protection against hypoxia should the patient become apneic. In an apneic patient, preoxygenation with a bag-valve-mask unit provides 2–3 minutes of protection against hypoxia. Unsuccessful attempts at intubation should be stopped at 30 seconds so that the patient may be reoxygenated.

B. Suction: A rigid tipped suction catheter should be available at all times to keep the airway

Table 2–3. Optional equipment for difficult intubations.

Alternative laryngoscope blades and handles
Flexible-tipped stylets
Lighted stylets
Flexible-tipped endotracheal tubes
Fiberoptic laryngoscope or bronchoscope
Kit for retrograde intubation[1]
Kit for percutaneous transtracheal ventilation[1]
Kit for cricothyroidotomy[1]

[1]Either commercially available or preassembled in a sterile tray.

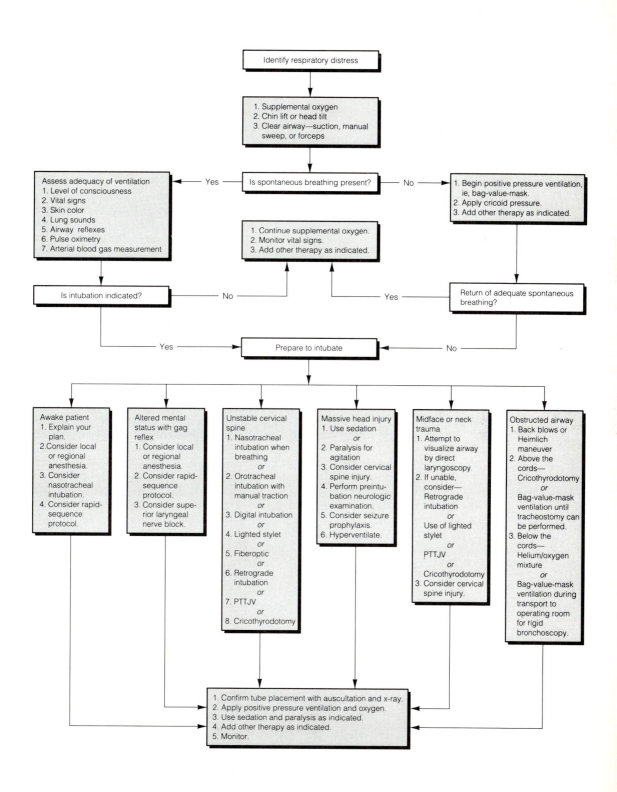

Identify respiratory distress

1. Supplemental oxygen
2. Chin lift or head tilt
3. Clear airway—suction, manual sweep, or forceps

Is spontaneous breathing present?

Yes →

No →

Assess adequacy of ventilation
1. Level of consciousness
2. Vital signs
3. Skin color
4. Lung sounds
5. Airway reflexes
6. Pulse oximetry
7. Arterial blood gas measurement

1. Begin positive pressure ventilation, ie, bag-value-mask.
2. Apply cricoid pressure.
3. Add other therapy as indicated.

1. Continue supplemental oxygen.
2. Monitor vital signs.
3. Add other therapy as indicated.

Is intubation indicated? —— No ——

—— Yes —— Return of adequate spontaneous breathing?

Yes → Prepare to intubate ← No

Awake patient
1. Explain your plan.
2. Consider local or regional anesthesia.
3. Consider nasotracheal intubation.
4. Consider rapid-sequence protocol.

Altered mental status with gag reflex
1. Consider local or regional anesthesia.
2. Consider rapid-sequence protocol.
3. Consider superior laryngeal nerve block.

Unstable cervical spine
1. Nasotracheal intubation when breathing
   or
2. Orotracheal intubation with manual traction
   or
3. Digital intubation
   or
4. Lighted stylet
   or
5. Fiberoptic
   or
6. Retrograde intubation
   or
7. PTTJV
   or
8. Cricothyrodotomy

Massive head injury
1. Use sedation
   or
2. Paralysis for agitation
3. Consider cervical spine injury.
4. Perform preintubation neurologic examination.
5. Consider seizure prophylaxis.
6. Hyperventilate.

Midface or neck trauma
1. Attempt to visualize airway by direct laryngoscopy.
2. If unable, consider—
   Retrograde intubation
   or
   Use of lighted stylet
   or
   PTTJV
   or
   Cricothyrodotomy
3. Consider cervical spine injury.

Obstructed airway
1. Back blows or Heimlich maneuver
2. Above the cords—Cricothyrodotomy
   or
   Bag-value-mask ventilation until tracheostomy can be performed.
3. Below the cords—Helium/oxygen mixture
   or
   Bag-value-mask ventilation during transport to operating room for rigid bronchoscopy.

1. Confirm tube placement with auscultation and x-ray.
2. Apply positive pressure ventilation and oxygen.
3. Use sedation and paralysis as indicated.
4. Add other therapy as indicated.
5. Monitor.

clear of blood and secretions. The suction device should be set at 120 mm Hg. After intubation, suction the tracheobronchial tree with a sterile, flexible catheter as described below, under Care of the Intubated Patient—Pulmonary Toilet.

C. Oral and Nasal Airways: When the jaw thrust or chin lift is ineffective in airway opening, a nasal or oral airway may support collapsed oropharyngeal tissues and permit adequate ventilation. A range of sizes should be readily available in all areas of the emergency department (Fig 2–2).

1. The oral airway is best used in an obtunded patient. It may be inserted over a tongue-blade or positioned backward as it enters the mouth and rotated after the tongue is cleared. Positioned correctly, it retracts the tongue upward and anteriorly. Care must be taken not to push the tongue backward into the pharynx, worsening the obstruction. An overly long oral airway can push the epiglottis over the larynx, causing complete obstruction.

2. The soft, rubber, noncuffed nasopharyngeal tube tends to be better tolerated in a semi-obtunded patient. Lubricate the tube with anesthetic jelly before insertion. Insert it through the least obstructed nostril, advancing it posteriorly along the floor of the nostril until it bypasses the tongue. If it is too long, it

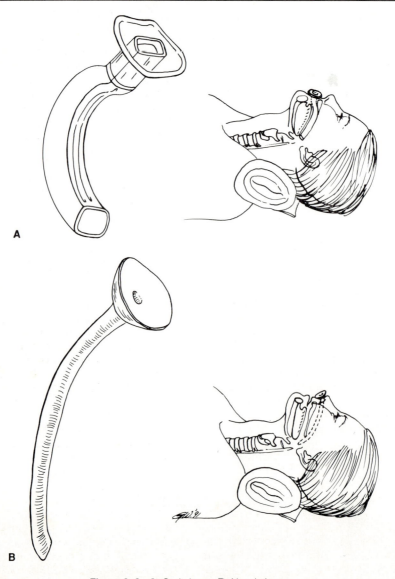

Figure 2–2. A: Oral airway. **B:** Nasal airway.

may enter the esophagus, resulting in ineffective positive pressure ventilation and gastric distention. Epistaxis may occur during insertion, and suction should be available.

3. In patients with intact airway reflexes, placement of either device may cause emesis, gagging, or laryngospasm. During and after placement, head position should be maintained to optimize airway patency. Where indicated, spinal precautions must be maintained. Evaluate breath sounds after placement of either device to ensure that obstruction has not occurred. Care must be taken to avoid trauma during placement.

D. Positive Pressure Ventilation: Following airway opening, positive pressure ventilation may be used to preoxygenate a patient before intubation. Occasionally it may be the only form of ventilation in an apneic patient when an airway cannot be secured, or when a patient responds rapidly to other therapy. In general, however, it is not recommended for prolonged ventilation owing to gastric dilatation and technical difficulty.

1. The bag-valve-mask (BVM) unit is the most common device used to provide positive pressure ventilation in the emergency department. The bag-valve-mask unit has a self-inflating bag that accepts 15-L/min oxygen flows. A nonrebreathing valve permits reservoir air to enter through a separate port from expired air. At these flow rates, inspired air will approach 100% oxygen. The self-filling bag permits use with spontaneously breathing patients. The unit can usually be attached to an endotracheal tube after intubation for manual bag-assisted tracheal ventilation.

2. The procedure for using the bag-valve-mask unit is described in Chapter 46. Use of this device is difficult in the hands of a single operator because effective bag-valve-mask ventilation depends on a tight seal between the mask and face. Often this requires 2 hands and a second operator to compress the bag. Many circumstances of anatomic variation or maxillofacial trauma make a tight seal impossible. During bag-valve-mask ventilation, proper head positioning must be maintained to preserve airway patency. Monitor the effectiveness of ventilation closely by frequent assessments of chest wall movement, lung sounds, and gastric dilatation.

3. The positive pressure generated by bag-valve-mask ventilation leads to gastric dilatation and abdominal distention. This results in decreased lung compliance and significant risk of emesis and aspiration. A clear mask is recommended to reveal emesis. Suction equipment must be available. In patients with unprotected airways, cricoid pressure (the Sellick maneuver) is recommended. To perform the Sellick maneuver, apply firm, direct pressure on the circumferential cricoid cartilage. This will compress the esophagus posteriorly, decreasing gastric dilatation and reflux. If emesis occurs, release pressure on the

cricoid to prevent esophageal rupture. Fracture of the cricoid has been reported. If bag-valve-mask ventilation must be prolonged for any reason, place a nasogastric tube to reduce gastric dilatation and its consequences (Fig 2–3).

4. Because of operational difficulties and risks of aspiration, the bag-valve-mask is a temporizing measure under most circumstances. Patients who require bag-assisted ventilation should generally be intubated as soon as it can be accomplished safely and practically.

5. The mouth-to-mask technique is another method of providing positive pressure ventilation. This method may be easier for a single operator, since both hands can be used to seat the mask. Supplemental oxygen is provided via a port in the mask or via a nasal cannula worn by the operator. Several devices of this type are on the market or in testing. Manually triggered oxygen-powered devices also are available for use with face masks or endotracheal tubes.

E. Esophageal Obturators and Related Devices: An esophageal obturator airway (EOA) or similar device may be placed in the prehospital setting. The emergency physician must be familiar with those devices used in his or her area of practice. Because of a high rate of complications and uneven efficacy, their use in the prehospital setting is controversial, especially since endotracheal intubation has been shown to be safe and successful in many prehospital systems. There are no indications for the esophageal obturator airway in the emergency department.

These tubes are designed to provide airway protection and ventilation. The esophageal obturator airway is a 34-cm, semirigid plastic tube fitted at the distal end with an inflatable cuff and at the proximal end with a face mask. The proximal portion of the tube is hollow with multiple side ports. The distal end is solid. It is passed blindly into the esophagus with the balloon positioned distal to the tracheal bifurcation. The balloon is then inflated, obstructing the esophagus. Ventilation through the mask provides air to the region of the trachea (Fig 2–4).

Since introduction of this device, several modifications have been made. The esophageal gastric tube (EGT) airway has a hollow esophageal tube that permits passage of a nasogastric tube for gastric decompression. The esophageal tracheal combitube (ETC) may be used as an endotracheal tube if blind insertion results in tracheal placement. Similarly, the pharyngeal tracheal lumen airway (PTLA) may be ventilated through either a long or short tube depending on tube position after placement.

Because these tubes are placed blindly, they require less expertise to place and may present less hazard of cord injury in patients with cervical spine injury. They are contraindicated in awake and semi-obtunded patients and in infants, children, and patients less than 120 cm in height. Do not use them

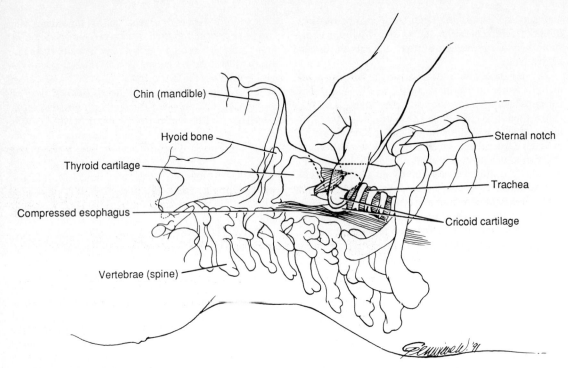

Figure 2–3. The Sellick maneuver. Firm pressure on the cricoid cartilage compresses the esophagus, preventing aspiration of gastric contents when airway reflexes are absent.

when there is known esophageal injury or ingestion of caustic substances. Complications are listed in Table 2–4. The true complication rate is unknown owing to lack of autopsy follow-up and confounding factors such as concomitant cardiopulmonary resuscitation. Because of reports of esophageal trauma, some authors recommend Gastrografin swallow or endoscopy after use of an esophageal obturator airway–like device (Table 2–4).

Patients intubated with an esophageal obturator airway in the field will need endotracheal intubation upon arrival in the emergency department unless they are awake or the trachea is intubated with the esophageal tracheal combitube or pharyngeal tracheal lumen airway. Disconnect the mask, suction the oropharynx, and intubate the trachea before deflating the esophageal balloon and removing the esophageal obturator airway. If endotracheal intubation is difficult, try partially deflating the esophageal balloon, or apply downward pressure on the cricoid cartilage to shift

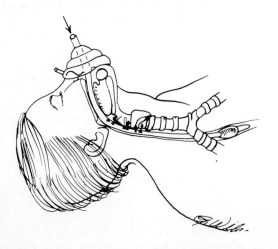

Figure 2–4. The esophageal obturator airway in position.

Table 2–4. Complications of esophageal airways.

Unrecognized endotracheal intubation

Incorrect positioning in pharynx

Inadequate mask-to-face seal

Esophageal or pharyngeal trauma due to placement, cardiopulmonary resuscitation, or retching

Tracheal compression due to incorrect balloon position

Balloon rupture or leakage

Anterior displacement of larynx

Emesis on removal

Gastric rupture

the larynx more posteriorly. If the patient is awake and ventilating adequately, suction fully and remove the esophageal obturator airway with the head turned to the side.

PRINCIPLES OF INTUBATION

These principles of preintubation management apply to all methods of airway management described in this chapter. Airway positioning, suction, and administration of 100% oxygen must precede any attempt at advanced airway control. Keep protective gear with the airway equipment, and use it routinely.

Choice of Method

Most patients can be intubated orally by direct laryngoscopic visualization of the cords. This is the method of choice, since the best assurance of correct tube placement is seeing the tube pass through the cords into the trachea. When direct visualization is not possible (Table 2–5), airway control can be achieved using a wide variety of special equipment and alternative methods described below (Table 2–6).

Choice of a blind or surgical technique depends on the patient's condition, availability of equipment, and operator experience. Advantages, indications, and problems associated with each technique are summarized below. Most alternative procedures require some training and expertise. Become comfortable with several alternative techniques, and be sure that the emergency department stocks the appropriate equipment.

Intubation by any method carries risks of hypoxia, aspiration, laryngospasm, unrecognized esophageal intubation, bleeding, airway trauma, cord trauma, right or left main-stem intubation, arrythmia, and death. Delayed complications include soft tissue infection, mediastinitis, tracheal stenosis, and dysphonia.

Table 2–5. Relative contraindications for orotracheal intubation.

On-going bleeding in the hypopharynx

Excessive secretion or vomitus in the hypopharynx

Mechanical obstruction in the hypopharynx or at the cords

Craniofacial or neck trauma

Need for cervical spine immobilization

Unusual anatomic features

Presence of wiring due to jaw fracture

Greater advantage for nasotracheal intubation or tracheal airway

Table 2–6. Alternative methods of intubation.

Blind Techniques
 Nasal intubation
 Digital intubation
 Use of lighted stylet
 Use of fiberoptic endoscope
Surgical Techniques
 Retrograde intubation
 Percutaneous transtracheal jet ventilation (PTTJV)
 Cricothyroidotomy
 Tracheostomy

Any blind technique (nasal, digital, lighted stylet) carries increased risk of unrecognized esophageal tube placement and trauma to the hypopharynx and airway. These methods should be used only when direct visualization is dangerous or cannot be successfully completed.

Surgical and needle techniques are generally rapid but in inexperienced hands may lead to massive bleeding or trauma that makes control of the airway impossible. They share the relative contraindications of coagulopathy, goiter, overlying tumor, or overlying skin infection. There are no absolute contraindications other than the ability to obtain an airway by less invasive means. Although each invasive method of airway control has unique complications, as a group they share an increased risk of bleeding, extratracheal tube placement, and trauma to the airway and surrounding tissues over less invasive routes. Loss of integrity of the tissues of the neck may result in barotrauma and significant soft tissue infection. Delayed complications include hoarseness and subglottic stenosis.

Universal Precautions

Airway management presents many opportunities for exposure to patient secretions. Wear adequate protective clothing, including a gown, gloves, mask, and either a face shield or goggles, any time the airway is manipulated. When the intubator's fingers are in the patient's mouth (eg, digital intubation, lighted stylet), care must be taken to prevent bite wounds. Place a bite block or dental prod before initiating intubation. Alternatively, place several layers of gauze between the intubator's hand and the patient's teeth. Remove dentures before airway manipulation.

Laryngoscopy & Oral & Nasal Intubation

See Chapter 46.

Postintubation

After intubation, assess tube position by observing the chest wall for expansion. Auscultate both lung fields and the abdomen while ventilating. Inaudible lung sounds or the presence of abdominal sounds suggest esophageal placement. If breath sounds are louder on the right than the left, suspect right mainstem intubation. Withdraw the tube 1–2 cm, and reauscultate. Confirm tube position by chest x-ray.

NONSURGICAL ALTERNATIVES FOR MANAGING THE DIFFICULT AIRWAY

Digital Intubation

This method has been used successfully when the cords cannot be visualized because of anatomic features or copious secretions. In the hands of experienced clinicians, it is rapid and can be achieved with little movement of the cervical spine. There are no absolute contraindications to this method, but it is a blind method and should not be used when direct visualization of the cords can be safely done. Because of the risk of being bitten, select this method only in deeply comatose patients.

If necessary, one person can perform digital intubation unaided. No special equipment is necessary beyond an oxygen delivery system, suction, and an appropriately sized endotracheal tube with stylet. Lubrication may aid passage of the tube. Take precautions against the accidental or reflex bite. Place a stylet into the lubricated tube as far as the side hole, and bend the tube into a gentle hook at the end.

To perform digital intubation, stand at the patient's right shoulder. Insert the index and middle fingers into the patient's mouth, and advance along the midline of the tongue until the epiglottis is palpated. Pass the endotracheal tube along the fingers until the tip reaches the epiglottis. Move the 2 fingers posteriorly, and advance the tube past the epiglottis while exerting gentle anterior pressure to guide the tip of the tube into the trachea. Once past the cords, remove the stylet before further advancement to prevent damage to the anterior trachea. After removing the stylet, adjust the final tube position, secure the tube, and verify its placement in the usual way. Never advance the tube against resistance. Cricoid pressure may be used until the endotracheal cuff is inflated.

Complications are similar to those described for other methods of blind intubation.

Variations on Basic Equipment

Several variations on the basic equipment have been developed for managing the difficult intubation. Use of these devices may be helpful under some circumstances, but few data are available on emergency department use.

A. Flexible-tipped endotracheal tubes (Endotrol,

others) have a built-in thread that extends from the distal tip to the proximal end, where it attaches to a plastic ring. Traction on the ring flexes the tip of the tube, directing the tube more anteriorly, simulating the function of a flexible stylet.

B. Flexible lumen finders (Flexiguide, others) are modified stylets with a design similar to that described above. In this case, the lumen finder protrudes beyond the endotracheal tube and can be maneuvered with traction on a thumb ring at the proximal end. When the end of the finder is threaded into the glottis, the endotracheal tube can be advanced over the finder into final position.

C. Specialized laryngoscope blades and handles are also available. A shortened laryngoscope handle may assist in intubation of individuals whose chest anteroposterior diameter is increased. One type has an adjustable angle laryngoscope handle. The Bainton blade is designed to encircle the endotracheal tube to prevent collapse of edematous or redundant pharyngeal tissues. The Siker blade has a mirrorlike surface to improve visibility, and the Huffman modification is a prism that fits on a standard laryngoscope to improve visibility.

Fiberoptic Techniques

A. Lighted Stylet: Lighted stylet and light wand (eg, Tube-stat, Flexi-lum) devices have been developed to aid in blind intubation. This method can be used when blood, secretions, or vomitus fill the hypopharynx. Because laryngoscopy need not be used, lighted stylets may be advantageous when the cervical spine must remain immobilized. Blind intubation with a lighted stylet is most suitable for deeply comatose or apneic patients when there is little risk of stimulating protective reflexes or biting of the intubator's hand. Use a bite block or dental prod for protection. A lighted stylet can also be combined with direct laryngoscopy. Although there are no absolute contraindications to this technique, ambient lighting must be low to maximize its benefit. Obesity may diminish the intensity of transillumination. As for other blind techniques, avoid this method when direct laryngoscopy can be performed.

1. If necessary, one person can perform this technique unaided. These devices have a battery-powered light source at the top of a semiflexible stylet. A longer, floppy stylet is available for nasal intubations. The stylet is threaded into an endotracheal tube. Aside from the lighted stylet, no special equipment is required.

2. Form the assembly of stylet and endotracheal tube into a hook of slightly greater than 90 degrees. The patient may be approached from the head if laryngoscopy is used. Otherwise, approach the patient from the right shoulder. While placing gentle traction on the tongue, pass the assembly into the mouth. When the epiglottis is reached, use a scooping or ladling motion to place the tip into the glottis. The appearance of transillumination at the neck indicates the position of the tube. Tracheal placement results in a bright, well-circumscribed area of transillumination at the cricothyroid membrane. The endotracheal tube can then be advanced over the stylet into the trachea. Transillumination lateral to the midline indicates piriform sinus placement and need for repositioning. Esophageal placement causes little or no transillumination. The procedure is essentially the same for nasal intubation with a lighted stylet.

3. This procedure shares the same complications of inadvertent malpositioning of the tube, hypoxia, and tissue damage as other blind techniques.

B. Fiberoptic Bronchoscope: Fiberoptic bronchoscopes may be used to locate the opening of the glottis when direct laryngoscopy cannot be used or is unsuccessful. The endotracheal tube can then be advanced over the endoscope into the trachea. Although this procedure can be carried out without movement of the cervical spine, it requires skill and practice. It may be time consuming when the hypopharynx is filled with blood or secretions. In addition, the equipment is expensive and easily damaged.

NEEDLE CRICOTHYROIDOTOMY

Cricothyroidotomy is the standard approach to creating an emergent surgical airway. Two methods using needle penetration of the cricothyroid membrane are described below. They are acceptable alternatives to cricothyroidotomy in selected case and may be easier and less invasive than emergent cricothyroidotomy for inexperienced operators.

Identification of the cricothyroid membrane is critical to performing either needle or surgical cricothyroidotomy (Fig 2–5). Palpation of the tracheal midline will identify the hyoid bone superiorly. Below this, the thyrohyoid space leads to the laryngeal prominence of the thyroid cartilage. The vocal cords lie behind the thyroid cartilage. The cricothyroid membrane is about 1.5 fingerwidths below the prominence and is bounded caudally by the cricoid cartilage. It is approximately 10 mm high and 22 mm wide. Each landmark must be clearly identified by palpation in both the caudal and the cephalad direction to prevent incision of the thyrohyoid space with entry into the hypopharynx, above the cords. Penetration of the cricothyroid membrane will enter the trachea about 1 cm below the vocal cords. Penetrate the cricothyroid membrane in the lower third of the membrane to avoid the superior cricothyroid vessels that run transversely across the upper third of the cricothyroid membrane. When subcutaneous air, trauma, or body habitus obscure the usual landmarks,

the approximate position of the cricothyroid membrane may be determined by placing the small finger of the right hand in the sternal notch while the hand is held in neutral position. The cricothyroid membrane will lie approximately 4 fingerwidths above the sternal notch. If time allows, prepare the skin with an iodine skin disinfectant, and raise a wheal of local anesthetic over the cricothyroid membrane before inserting the needle.

Percutaneous Transtracheal Jet Ventilation (See also Chapter 46.)

Percutaneous transtracheal jet ventilation (PTTJV) is an alternative technique for oxygenating and ventilating a patient who cannot be intubated in a more standard fashion. It is unique in that positive pressure is generated by high-pressure oxygen delivered as an intermittent jet through high-pressure tubing and a percutaneously placed large-bore tracheal catheter. No bag reservoir or nonrebreathing valve is employed. This technique must be distinguished from high-frequency jet ventilation, which is used for other purposes. PTTJV is less invasive than cricothyroidotomy and less time consuming than retrograde intubation (see below). It is relatively easily learned. With attention to detail, there are few complications. It can be used in awake or obtunded patients. Other advantages include presumed protection of the cervical spine and possible expulsion of a pharyngeal foreign body by expired air. Although it has been reported to be safe and effective in the recovery room setting for 24–48 hours, in the emergency department it is regarded as a temporizing measure while radiographic cervical spine clearance is being obtained or other methods of airway control can be established. Indications for PTTJV are the same as for cricothyroidotomy. Use in the pediatric population is under study.

Disadvantages include the need for either makeshift or commercially available special equipment. With prolonged use, CO_2 retention may develop. Contraindications are not yet well defined. They include anterior neck trauma, where high delivered pressures may lead to severe tissue disruption, and complete airway obstruction, where expired air cannot escape through the glottis. PTTJV shares the relative contraindications mentioned above for all invasive methods of airway control. Prior unsuccessful attempts at catheter placement may lead to air leak or subcutaneous emphysema after a second, successful attempt.

The materials required for PTTJV are listed in Table 2–7. The system may be built out of items normally stocked in the emergency department and operating room. Several companies now produce specialized delivery systems and cannulas for PTTJV. The components of the system must be immediately available to be useful in emergency department airway management.

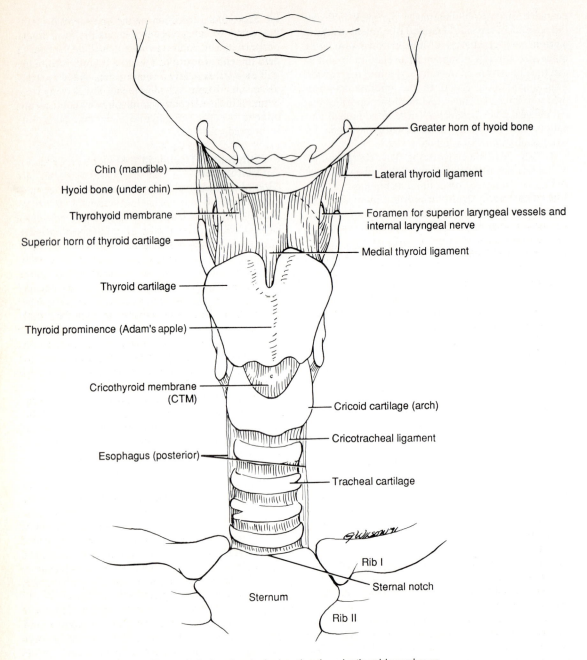

Figure 2–5. Landmarks for locating the cricothyroid membrane.

To obtain the 50 psi of pressure necessary to generate adequate volume to expand the patient's chest, the high-pressure tubing must be attached to the oxygen tank through a step-down regulator (or demand valve). A wall O_2 outlet or the flush valve of the anesthesia machine are also potential sources of high-pressure O_2. A bag-valve-mask unit cannot generate adequate pressure to ventilate a patient with this system.

The high-pressure tubing is fitted with an interrupt valve along its length. If an interrupt valve is not available, a Y connector or side port in the oxygen tubing can be used as an alternate port. It is then attached directly to the tracheal catheter via a Luer-Lok adapter. If necessary, an adapter can be constructed using the male end from intravenous tubing, a 3-way stopcock, or the barrel of a 3-mL syringe. All connections should be reinforced with plastic ties to prevent separation under pressure (Chapter 46).

The over-the-needle catheter must be kink-resistant and meet the specifications noted in Table 2–7.

Table 2–7. Equipment required for percutaneous transtracheal ventilation (PTTJV).

Oxygen source capable of delivering 50 psi line pressure
Stryker valve to access high-pressure oxygen
High pressure tubing
Cut-off or interrupt valve for tubing
Luer-Lok adaptor at the catheter end of the tubing
5- to 8-cm over-the-needle, 12- to 14-g catheter
10-mL syringe for needle placement

The commercially available catheters have distal side holes that diffuse the jet of air entering the trachea, preventing focal trauma. They also have a proximal flange for securing the catheter to the neck.

Significant deviations from recommended equipment may lead to inadequate ventilatory volumes, hypoxia, and hypercapnia.

To place the catheter, prepare the neck and locate the cricothyroid membrane as described above. Insert the over-the-needle catheter and needle into the lower third of the cricothyroid membrane in a caudal direction at an angle of 30–45 degrees. Aspiration of air should confirm catheter position. Advance the catheter, and remove the needle. In its final position, the tip of the catheter should be near the carina. Secure the catheter at the neck, attach the O_2 delivery system to the catheter, and begin ventilation.

When the alternate port is covered with a finger, O_2 is delivered to the patient, generating about 20 cm H_2O pressure in the airway. Much of the 50-psi pressure is lost through the glottis during O_2 delivery. When the alternate port is released, there is a period of passive exhalation while the patient's chest wall and diaphragm recoil. Recommended ventilatory rates vary from 12 to 20 cycles per minute with an inspiratory to expiratory ratio of 1:2 (eg, 1 second with the alternate port covered leading to ventilation, 2 seconds with the alternate port opened allowing passive exhalation). During ventilation, the chest wall will rise and a significant volume of O_2 will be expelled out the glottis. This produces a spray of blood and secretions through the patient's mouth and nose, creating potential for hazardous exposure. During passive exhalation, the chest wall muscles recoil, expelling (less forcefully) some of the volume, and the chest wall should fall. If passive exhalation is inadequate, some authors recommend a 20-gauge needle adjacent to the first for venting. There are few data on this method. The rise and fall of the chest wall must be monitored closely, because without chest wall recoil and passive exhalation, hypercapnia, acidosis, and barotrauma may develop quickly.

Complications include all those noted above for needle placement. Needle misplacement may cause perforation of the trachea or esophagus, leading to tissue disruption and emphysema of the deep tissues

or mediastinitis owing to the high pressures of ventilation. Local subcutaneous emphysema is common. Inadequate monitoring may lead to hypoxia, hypercapnia, and acidosis as noted above. The awake patient may experience cough during the procedure. Even with good technique, prolonged ventilation using PTTJV will result in respiratory acidosis and hypoxia.

Retrograde Intubation

Retrograde intubation (RI) is indicated when oral or nasal intubation is contraindicated or technically impossible owing to anatomic, pathologic, or traumatic abnormalities. The advantages of this technique include maintenance of the cervical spine in a neutral position and the benefits of any blind technique. In addition, it requires less skill than fiberoptic intubation. Disadvantages include its time-consuming nature and the need to have the patient ventilating adequately throughout. This method is contraindicated when the airway is obstructed at or above the level of the cords. If the patient is unable to open the mouth, the retrograde wire must be passed out the nose for nasal intubation, which can be difficult and suboptimal in some settings. Contraindications include apnea and those described above, under Choice of Methods.

Retrograde intubation can be performed by one operator, although an assistant is extremely helpful. Special equipment includes a needle large enough to accept a catheter or guide wire and a wire or catheter, approximately 70 cm in length. Local anesthetic is recommended. A small clamp is useful.

The principle of retrograde intubation involves entering the trachea at the cricothyroid membrane with a guide wire that is threaded out the mouth or nose and used as a guide for blind oral or nasal intubation. After appropriate preparation of the neck, identify the cricothyroid membrane and surrounding landmarks. Pass a needle through the skin, and puncture the inferior third of the cricothyroid membrane with the needle directed about 30 degrees caudad. Aspiration of air confirms tracheal placement. Rotate the needle to about 30 degrees cephalad, and reaspirate to confirm tracheal position. Introduce the catheter or wire through the needle. As the catheter is threaded through the needle, it often exits spontaneously through the mouth. Occasionally, however, it must be retrieved with fingers or forceps. Guiding the wire out through the nares is more difficult. When the wire is in hand at the lips or nares, the needle is removed. Fix the wire at the cricothyroid membrane with fingers or a small clamp. Thread the proximal end of the wire into the endotracheal tube through the side hole (Murphy's eye). It should pass up through the lumen of the tube, exiting at its proximal end. Advance the lubricated tube along the wire until resistance is met, indicating that the tube is in the trachea, below the cords, pulled tight against the fixed wire. Release the wire at the skin, and pull it out through the proximal end of the tube. Advance the tube to the appropriate position, and confirm in the usual manner.

Only a small number of cases of retrograde intubation have been described. Few serious complications have been reported. In addition to the risks that accompany any surgical intubation, broken needles have been reported.

SURGICAL AIRWAYS

Cricothyroidotomy

When there is complete upper airway obstruction or massive facial trauma that prohibits intubation from above, immediate access to the trachea can be obtained with cricothyroidotomy. In experienced hands, it is a rapid technique that maintains immobilization of the cervical spine. It is a radical procedure with risk of significant short- and long-term negative outcomes. It is contraindicated whenever the airway can be secured by less invasive means. In children, cricothyroidotomy becomes technically more difficult as the landmarks become smaller. Patient age less than 10 years is a relative contraindication for inexperienced practitioners. In children under 5 years, PTTJV or a tracheostomy is preferable if possible. Other relative contraindications include preexisting laryngeal disease, coagulopathy, anatomic deformities of the neck due to trauma or other causes, and lack of familiarity with the procedure.

The equipment and technique for cricothyroidotomy are described in Chapter 46. The clinician preparing for this eventuality should be aware that new products are continually becoming available to facilitate placement of an emergent surgical airway. Kits are available that use over-the-wire techniques, progressive dilatation, and trochar placement.

Early and delayed complications of cricothyroidotomy are shared with other invasive techniques (see above).

Tracheostomy

Tracheostomy has little indication in emergency department management of the airway. Its only true indication is severe blunt trauma to the neck with fracture of the thyroid or cricoid cartilage preventing access to the cricothyroid membrane. Tracheostomy is the preferred method of surgical airway management in the very small child when PTTJV is not possible. Because of the close location of vascular, nerve, and visceral tissue, the risk of negative sequelae is high. A thorough knowledge of anatomy and careful surgical technique are critical to success.

It should be performed only by surgeons experienced with the procedure.

USE OF DRUGS TO ASSIST IN INTUBATION

Many patients in the emergency department can be intubated without the use of pharmacologic intervention other than oxygen. However, when pharmacologic adjuncts are indicated, their use may dramatically reduce the difficulty of intubation and speed control of the airway. The overall condition of the patient and the goal of intubation determine the choice of agent.

Awake oral or nasal intubations are best carried out under local, topical, or regional anesthesia. Occasionally, sedation alone may be useful in preparing for intubation. For a semi-obtunded or combative patient, use of neuromuscular blockade with sedation, usually in a rapid-sequence induction protocol, provides rapid control of the airway while protecting against aspiration of gastric contents.

Drugs that induce apnea must be used by or under the direct supervision of experienced clinicians prepared to obtain a surgical airway in the event of failed intubation. Equipment necessary for intubation and surgical airway must be prepared in advance and be available at the bedside before the patient is sedated or anesthetized.

Topical Anesthesia

A. General Considerations: Awake intubation presumes a patient with enough ventilatory effort to allow time to anesthetize the airway. The patient must be able to cooperate with, or at least tolerate, the noxious process of passing an endotracheal tube. Anesthesia of the airway causes loss of the normal protective airway reflexes, with concomitant risk of aspiration. Absorption of topical agents occurs more readily from tracheal tissues than from oral or nasal mucosa, increasing the risk of systemic toxicity if excessive doses are used.

B. Choice of Agent: The most common choices for topical anesthesia of the airway are lidocaine, tetracaine, and cocaine (Table 2–8). Agents such as procaine and mepivacaine are too poorly absorbed to be effective topically. All local anesthetics have central nervous system toxicities including confusion, coma, and seizures. All local anesthetics also have cardiovascular effects including slowed conduction, myocardial depression, arrhythmogenesis, and peripheral vasodilation. Hypotension and cardiac arrest may occur.

1. Topical lidocaine may be administered as a

Table 2–8. Properties of local anesthetics.

	Lidocaine	Tetracaine	Cocaine
Available concentration	2–4%	1–2%	4–11%
Common routes	Gargle, spray, or atomizer	Saturated packing or spray	Saturated swabs or packing
Time to onset	3–5 minutes	3–8 minutes	5–10 minutes
Duration	30–45 minutes	30–60 minutes	30–90 minutes
Toxic doses	> 4–5 mg/kg or 200–250 mg in adults	> 80 mg	> 3–4 mg/kg (toxicity has been reported with therapeutic doses)
Toxicities	Seizure, coma, contusion, respiratory arrest, cardiovascular depression	Similar to those of lidocaine	Tachycardia, cardiac arrhythmias, stroke, cardiac arrest, elevated blood pressure

gargle of 10-mL aliquot repeated 3 times. The drug must be spit out, not swallowed, between each dose to avoid toxic systemic levels. To aerosolize, 4 mL of a 4% solution may be administered through a standard nebulizer at 8 L/min with either a mouth piece or face mask. Alternatively, tetracaine and lidocaine are available in a commercial spray.

2. Topical cocaine combines anesthetic and vasoconstrictive properties. A local vasoconstrictor is unnecessary with cocaine and can be dangerous. Owing to risks associated with cocaine, its use is generally limited to anesthesia of the nares prior to nasal intubation. Saturate several cotton-tipped applicators in a commercially available solution of 4% cocaine, and place the applicators in the nares. Wait 5–10 minutes for adequate anesthesia before attempting intubation (Table 2–8).

C. Topical Vasoconstrictors: If nasal intubation is planned, addition of a local vasoconstrictor is necessary to decrease the risk of epistaxis. The best drugs for this purpose are phenylephrine, 0.005–0.15%, or ephedrine, 1%. Topical epinephrine is ineffective. Do not use a topical vasoconstrictor in combination with cocaine.

D. Topical Laryngeal Anesthesia: After nasal and oropharyngeal anesthesia is induced, the posterior pharynx and larynx may require additional local anesthesia. Gentle direct laryngoscopy will permit local anesthesia of more distal tissues with a spray. Tracheal anesthesia can also be obtained by direct injection of 2–3 mL of 1–2% lidocaine through the cricothyroid membrane.

Superior Laryngeal Nerve Block

Sensory innervation of the larynx, epiglottis, and lower pharynx is supplied by the internal branch of the superior laryngeal nerve that branches from the vagus bilaterally. It pierces the thyrohyoid membrane between the thyroid cartilage and the hyoid bone below the greater horn of the hyoid, and runs in the submucosa of the piriform fossa. It may be blocked in the sitting patient by inserting the needle laterally just above the thyroid cartilage below the greater horn and injecting 2–3 mL of 2% lidocaine. The injection is then repeated on the other side. A median approach

with the needle directed laterally and upward toward the greater horn on either side also will be effective (Fig 2–6).

Rapid-Sequence Intubation

A. General Considerations: Use of sedation alone to intubate a patient in the emergency department can be difficult and risky. Titration of a narcotic or sedative to an intubating dose is time consuming. Delays in airway control can delay other care. Unwanted central nervous system or cardiovascular side effects can persist, complicating the patient's postintubation course. Hypoventilation often occurs before the patient is adequately relaxed for intubation, and prolonged bag-valve-mask ventilation may be required. Many emergency department patients present with a full stomach. This, combined with gastric distention due to bag-valve-mask ventilation, depressed airway reflexes, and the emetic effects of sedatives, raises the risk of aspiration.

The rapid-sequence induction protocol diminishes these difficulties in the awake patient who is agitated or who has altered mental status and requires oral intubation. A rapid-acting neuromuscular blocker is given to paralyze the patient. A short-acting sedative may be added to decrease agitation and the noxious sensations associated with paralysis and intubation. The patient is intubated immediately after paralysis. Further sedation or paralysis may then be effected as indicated.

During the short period when the patient is paralyzed and not intubated, the airway must be protected from aspiration with cricoid pressure.

The rapid-sequence protocol is unnecessary in a completely obtunded, relaxed patient. Contraindications include contraindications to the specific drugs that will be used. Do not induce apnea if there are contraindications to oral intubation or evidence that it is not likely to be successful. The rapid-sequence protocol will obscure the neurologic examination and physical manifestations of status epilepticus, so alternative plans to follow the neurologic condition of the patient must be made before inducing paralysis.

B. Equipment and Personnel Required: At least 2 individuals must be available to safely initiate

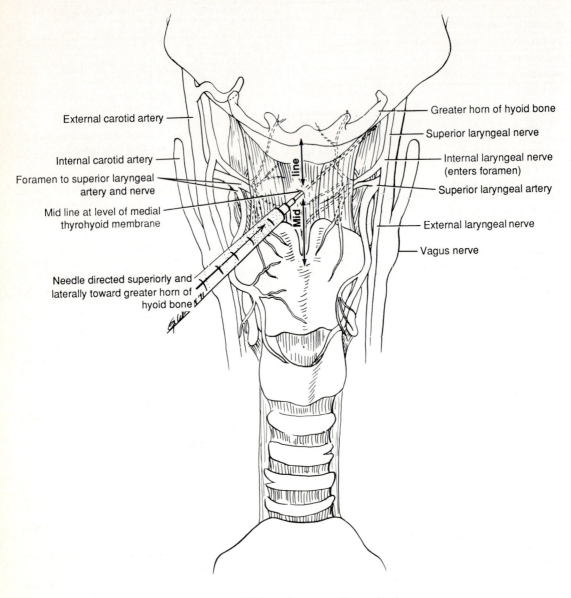

External carotid artery

Internal carotid artery

Foramen to superior laryngeal artery and nerve

Mid line at level of medial thyrohyoid membrane

Needle directed superiorly and laterally toward greater horn of hyoid bone

Greater horn of hyoid bone

Superior laryngeal nerve

Internal laryngeal nerve (enters foramen)

Superior laryngeal artery

External laryngeal nerve

Vagus nerve

Mid line

Figure 2–6. The superior laryngeal nerve block.

the rapid-sequence protocol. Other than the drugs, no special equipment is required to induce neuromuscular blockade. Before giving any sedative or neuromuscular blocking agent, review the checklist in Table 2–9. The choice of sedative or anesthetic and neuromuscular blocking agent depends on the indication for intubation, patient condition, and user familiarity.

C. Procedure: Table 2–10 outlines the steps of the rapid-sequence protocol. The characteristics of the recommended drugs are mentioned below, under Drugs Used During Intubation.

D. Additional Drugs: Several agents may be added to the rapid-sequence protocol under specific circumstances.

1. Vecuronium—Vecuronium, 0.01 mg/kg given 3–5 minutes before succinylcholine, will abolish fasciculations. Fasciculations may cause muscle pain, increased intragastric pressure, increased intraocular pressure, and increased intracranial pressure and may displace bony fractures. Although vecuronium can attenuate these effects, many physicians use fasciculation as an indicator that paralysis is being initiated and intubate immediately upon cessation of fasciculation.

Table 2–9. Checklist for initiation of anesthesia.

Baseline neurological exam is completed.

All materials for intubation are assembled.

Materials for surgical airways are immediately available.

Suction is working and available.

The patient is preoxygenated.

2. Atropine–Atropine, 0.01–0.02 mg/kg given immediately before the sedative, attenuates the vagal bradycardia associated with succinylcholine. Children, who tend to be more sensitive to the bradycardiac and hypotensive effects of succinylcholine, benefit from pretreatment with atropine. Pretreat adults with bradycardia and those receiving a second dose of succinylcholine.

3. Lidocaine–Lidocaine, 1.5 mg/kg given 1 minute before intubation, may attenuate elevations in intracranial pressure associated with succinylcholine and intubation. It may have some protective effect against laryngeal spasm and ventricular arrhythmias during intubation.

4. Analgesics–If pain control is part of the management plan, a narcotic such as morphine sulfate, 2–4 mg intravenously, or other analgesic should be added after intubation, since barbiturates have little analgesic effect and neuromuscular blockers have none.

5. Antiseizure agents–If status epilepticus is present before intubation, load the patient with antiseizure medications such as phenytoin, 15 mg/kg, after intubation. The drugs used in the rapid-sequence protocol mask, but do not stop, central nervous system seizure activity.

Table 2–10. Rapid-sequence induction protocol.

Preoxygenate with 100% oxygen.
  (Use bag-valve-mask ventilatory assistance only as needed.)

Give rapid intravenous injection of thiopental, 1–4 mg/kg, followed immediately by

Rapid intravenous injection of succinylcholine, 1–2 mg/kg.

Initiate cricoid pressure, and stop bag-valve-mask ventilation.

Observe for fasciculations followed by apnea.

Immediately intubate upon onset of apnea.

Confirm tube position clinically.

Begin ventilation.

Inflate endotracheal tube cuff, and release cricoid pressure.

Secure tube.

Provide additional sedation and paralysis as indicated.

  Alternative sedative drugs
    Methohexital, 0.5–1 mg/kg
    Midazolam, 0.1–0.3 mg/kg
    Fentanyl, 1–5 μg/kg
    Ketamine, 1–2 mg/kg

  Alternative neuromuscular blocker
    Vecuronium, 0.1–0.25 mg/kg
    (Use only when succinylcholine is contraindicated.)

Drugs Used During Intubation

A. Succinylcholine: A depolarizing neuromuscular blocking agent.

1. Dose–1–1.5 mg/kg in adults, 1.5–2 mg/kg in children.

2. Onset–60 seconds to complete relaxation.

3. Duration–5–10 minutes.

4. Metabolism–Degraded by pseudocholinesterase.

5. Indications and advantages–

a. Drug of choice for the rapid-sequence protocol under most circumstances owing to rapid onset, complete muscular relaxation, and short duration.

b. Single dose in emergency department setting usually well tolerated if appropriate precautions are taken (see below).

6. Contraindications–

a. Risk factors for hyperkalemia (see ¶ 7, below).

b. Hereditary pseudocholinesterase deficiency (1/2800 patients).

c. Penetrating ocular trauma or glaucoma.

d. Known family or personal history of malignant hyperthermia.

e. Hypersensitivity to succinylcholine.

7. Adverse effects and precautions–

a. Cardiovascular effects include bradycardia and hypotension, ventricular arrhythmias, and tachycardia or hypertension. Use with care in setting of irritable myocardium.

b. Fasciculation (see above for sequelae).

c. Hyperkalemia occurs in settings of subacute burns, subacute crush injuries, upper and lower motor neuron disease, and tetanus. Levels in excess of 9 meq/L have been reported, and cardiac arrest may occur.

d. Pseudocholinesterase inhibition may occur in pregnancy, in renal or hepatic insufficiency, and with a variety of drugs.

e. Malignant hyperthermia occurs in 1/50,000 patients.

f. Histamine release may cause bronchospasm or anaphylactoid reaction.

g. Intraocular pressure is elevated during fasciculations.

h. Intracranial pressure may increase.

i. Intragastric pressure may increase; use cricoid pressure until endotracheal tube cuff is inflated.

j. Always use sedation with alert patients; succinylcholine has no intrinsic analgesic or sedative effect.

B. Vecuronium: A nondepolarizing neuromuscular blocking agent.

1. Dose–Standard dose is 0.1 mg/kg. To achieve rapid intubating conditions, 0.25 mg/kg may be used.

2. Onset–Dose dependent; standard doses achieve paralysis in 3–5 minutes, larger doses in 1–1.5 min.

3. Duration–Dose dependent; standard doses

last 20–40 minutes, and larger doses may prolong paralysis 2–3 times the usual duration.

4. Metabolism–Hepatic metabolism, renal excretion; no dose changes recommended in patients with congestive heart failure or hepatic or renal insufficiency.

5. Indications and advantages–

a. Drug of choice for the rapid-sequence protocol when succinylcholine cannot be utilized.

b. Short duration allows neurologic reevaluation and provides satisfactory paralysis for procedures such as CT scan in emergent setting.

c. Minimal cardiovascular effects at usual doses.

d. Reversible after partial recovery (evidence of head lift, respiratory effort, or muscle twitch response) with neostigmine, 0.04 mg/kg intravenously. Atropine, 0.02 mg/kg intravenously, must also be administered to prevent muscarinic side effects.

e. Does not cause fasciculations or elevate intracranial pressure.

6. Contraindication–Known hypersensitivity to vecuronium.

7. Adverse effects and precautions–

a. Reduce dosage in myasthenia gravis to avoid prolonged blockade.

b. Use cricoid pressure before inflation of endotracheal tube cuff.

c. Must use sedation/anesthesia in awake patients.

d. Block is prolonged by aminoglycosides, lithium, quinidine, lidocaine, and propranolol and in hypermagnesemia, hyperkalemia, dehydration, hypothermia, and respiratory acidosis.

e. Use during pregnancy only if clearly indicated.

C. Pancuronium: A longer acting nondepolarizing neuromuscular blocking agent.

1. Dose–0.05–0.2 mg/kg.

2. Onset–1–3 minutes.

3. Duration–Dose dependent, averaging 60–90 minutes.

4. Metabolism–Hepatic metabolism, renal excretion. Dosage adjustments are indicated.

5. Indications and advantages–

a. Main use is prolonged blockade after intubation is complete.

b. Does not promote bronchospasm.

c. Reversible after partial recovery (see vecuronium).

d. No elevated intracranial pressure or fasciculation.

6. Contraindications–

a. Known hypersensitivity to pancuronium.

b. Cardiovascular instability or history of congestive heart failure.

7. Adverse effects and precautions–

a. History of myasthenia gravis (see vecuronium).

b. Cardiovascular effects include increased heart rate, increased afterload, and ventricular arrhythmias.

Use with caution in the setting of irritable myocardium.

c. Blockade is prolonged by multiple drugs (see vecuronium).

d. Onset and duration profile are not optimal for use with the rapid-sequence protocol.

e. Use cricoid pressure before inflation of endotracheal tube cuff.

f. Always use sedation or anesthesia in awake patients.

g. Use in pregnancy only if clearly indicated.

D. Thiopental: A short-acting, highly lipid soluble barbiturate sedative.

1. Dose–1–4 mg/kg. A test dose of 25–75 mg is recommended and may be sufficient alone.

2. Onset–60 seconds.

3. Duration–5–20 minutes.

4. Metabolism–Hepatic.

5. Indications and advantages–

a. Barbiturate drug of choice for the rapid-sequence protocol owing to rapid onset and short duration.

b. Decreases intracranial pressure and cerebral O_2 consumption.

c. Produces amnesia.

6. Contraindications–

a. Known sensitivity to barbiturates.

b. Lack of intravenous access.

c. Variegate or acute intermittent porphyria.

7. Adverse effects and precautions–

a. Respiratory depression and apnea.

b. Cardiovascular effects include myocardial depression, dilation of veins, tachycardia, and hypotension. Dehydrated patients are at greatest risk for hypotension. Use with care in cardiovascular disease and shock and in hypotensive patients.

c. Cough, laryngospasm, bronchospasm, and hiccups. Consider an alternative drug for status asthmaticus.

d. Nausea and vomiting.

e. Pain on injection and local necrosis with extravasation.

f. Anaphylactoid reactions.

g. Effect prolonged or intensified by other sedatives, narcotics, probenecid, advanced age, Addison's disease, renal or hepatic insufficiency, myasthenia gravis, and anemia.

h. Effect antagonized by aminophylline.

i. Consider an alternative drug in pregnancy.

E. Methohexital: A rapid ultra-short-acting barbiturate anesthetic.

1. Dose–0.5–1.5 mg/kg.

2. Onset–Less than 60 seconds.

3. Duration–5–7 minutes.

4. Metabolism–Hepatic metabolism, renal excretion.

5. Indications and advantages–

a. Slightly shorter acting alternative to thiopental in the rapid-sequence protocol.

b. See thiopental.

6. Contraindications–See thiopental.

7. Adverse effects and precautions–See thiopental.

F. Midazolam: A short-acting benzodiazepine central nervous system depressant.

1. Dose–1–2.5 mg, recommended to be given at 1 mg over 2 minutes.

2. Onset–1–5 minutes, depending on rate of injection when given intravenously.

3. Duration–10–90 minutes.

4. Metabolism–Hepatic metabolism with delayed elimination in congestive heart failure, renal insufficiency, and old age.

5. Indications and advantages–

a. Alternative induction agent for sedation in the rapid-sequence protocol (may have prolonged sedative effect).

b. Minimal cardiovascular effects.

c. May produce amnesia for several hours.

d. Blunt intracranial pressure responses at high doses.

6. Contraindications–

a. Known sensitivity to midazolam or benzodiazepines.

b. Acute narrow-angle glaucoma.

7. Adverse effects and precautions–

a. Respiratory depression or arrest.

b. Cardiovascular effects usually minimal with bigeminy, premature ventricular contractions, and nodal rhythms.

c. Laryngospasm and bronchospasm, cough, hives.

d. Local irritation at injection site.

e. Nausea and vomiting.

f. Potentiated by other central nervous system depressants; dose modifications recommended.

g. Dose modifications recommended in chronic obstructive pulmonary disease and congestive heart failure and in elderly patients and patients with renal failure.

h. Possible increase in fetal malformations with pregnancy.

G. Fentanyl: A short-acting narcotic anesthetic.

1. Dose–1–5 mg/kg intravenously.

2. Onset–60 seconds.

3. Duration–30–60 minutes.

4. Metabolism–Hepatic.

5. Indications and advantages–

a. Alternative drug for sedation in the rapid-sequence protocol (sedation may be prolonged with thiopental).

b. Both analgesic and sedative effects.

c. No histamine release.

d. Blunts intracranial pressure response to intubation.

e. Reversible with naloxone, 1–4 mg intravenously.

6. Contraindications–Known sensitivity to fentanyl.

7. Adverse effects and precautions–

a. Respiratory depression and apnea. Respiratory depression may persist beyond analgesic and sedative effects.

b. Muscle rigidity, which may occur with rapid injection of high doses.

c. Bradycardia or cardiovascular depression.

d. Nausea and vomiting.

e. Effects potentiated by other central nervous system or respiratory depressants.

f. Dose modifications recommended in chronic obstructive pulmonary disease and congestive heart failure and in elderly patients and patients with renal failure.

g. Possible increase in fetal malformations. Consider alternative drugs in pregnancy.

H. Ketamine: A dissociative anesthetic agent.

1. Dose–1–2 mg/kg.

2. Onset–60 seconds.

3. Duration–5–10 minutes.

4. Metabolism–Hepatic.

5. Indications and advantages–

a. Alternative drug for sedation and analgesia during the rapid-sequence protocol, particularly in hypotension.

b. May cause bronchodilation.

c. Airway reflexes are usually maintained. Respiratory depression is usually minimal and transient.

d. Myocardial depression is uncommon.

e. Prominent analgesic effects.

6. Contraindications–

a. Hypersensitivity.

b. Head injury.

c. Severe hypertension.

7. Adverse effects and precautions–

a. Elevated blood pressure and pulse rate are the most common cardiovascular effects. Hypotension, bradycardia, and arrhythmias have been reported. Use with caution with irritable myocardium or where hypertension would adversely affect patient course.

b. Respiratory stimulation and maintained airway most common but apnea, respiratory arrest, and laryngospasm also have been reported.

c. Dysphoric emergence reactions.

d. Nausea and vomiting.

e. Local irritation at injection site.

f. Increased intracranial pressure.

g. Intraocular pressure may be increased.

h. Muscle rigidity or myoclonus.

i. Increased secretions. Consider pretreatment with atropine.

j. Possible prolonged recovery when used concurrently with narcotics or barbiturates.

k. Consider alternative drug in pregnancy and for patients below 2 years of age.

SPECIAL CASES

Management of the Pediatric Airway

Basic principles of airway management are similar for all age groups. However, anatomic and physiologic differences affect the emergency physician's equipment needs and management decisions when confronted with a pediatric airway emergency.

A. Unique Features:

1. In infants, the head is relatively larger in proportion to the body.

2. The neck is more supple owing to a greater proportion of cartilaginous support tissue.

3. The airway is smaller, resulting in increased resistance and susceptibility to obstruction due to edema, blood, or secretions.

4. The mucosa is looser, permitting obstruction due to positioning and greater, faster distention from blood or edema.

5. The adenoidal and tonsillar lymphatic tissues are larger and more friable than those of adults.

6. The larynx is more cephalad and anterior.

7. The epiglottis is larger and more floppy and protrudes into the airway more prominently.

8. The narrowest portion of the airway in children less than 5 years of age is the cricoid cartilage rather than the larynx, as in adults.

9. The cricothyroid membrane is very small and does not lend itself to surgical manipulation.

10. The carina branches symmetrically at 45 degrees.

11. The chest wall is thinner, and both airway and gastric sounds radiate easily, making auscultation less reliable.

12. The chest wall is more pliable, and ventilation depends significantly on diaphragmatic movement.

13. Oxygen consumption is 6–8 mL/kg/min in children, whereas adults usually consume about 3–4 mL/kg/min. Hypoxemia can occur more rapidly and is tolerated less well.

14. Apnea occurs suddenly during a wide range of illnesses and injuries.

15. Normal vital signs vary for different age groups (Table 2–11).

B. Equipment Required:

1. All essential equipment (O_2 delivery systems, face masks, bag-valve-mask units, oral and nasal airways, laryngoscope blades, endotracheal tubes, stylets, and suction devices) should be stocked in a variety of sizes to accommodate the anticipated population served by the facility (Table 2–11).

2. Oxygen should be humidified and warmed to prevent drying of secretions and subsequent airway obstruction.

3. Endotracheal tubes for children less than 8 years of age should be noncuffed to prevent damage to the cricoid ring. Correct tube size may be obtained from a table or gauged based on one of the 3 following methods.

a. The tube size should closely approximate the size of the child's small finger at the distal interphalangeal joint.

b. The tube size should closely approximate the size of the child's nares.

c. The tube size in millimeters is equal to 16 + patient's age in years ÷ 4.

4. For patients under the age of 4 years, a straight blade is preferred owing to the tendency of the epiglottis to protrude and cover the airway.

5. In emergency departments where pediatric resuscitation is rare, precalculate the doses of commonly needed drugs, based on weights, and post them clearly in the resuscitation area.

C. Decisions and Techniques:

1. Evaluate for respiratory distress by assessing vital signs, skin signs, overall patient condition, use of accessory muscles, retractions, nasal flaring, and arterial blood gases or pulse oximetry.

2. Supplemental O_2 must be given. Children often cannot tolerate a face mask. Adequate oxygen supplementation can frequently be achieved by directing a stream of humidified 100% O_2 across the patient's face.

3. Airway positioning is essential. The alert patient will often choose the position of greatest airway patency and should not be forced to lie down. The infant and the obtunded patient must be placed in the sniffing position (Fig 2–1) unless cervical spine in-

Table 2–11. Pediatric vital signs and airway equipment sizes.

Age	Premature	Neonate	1 mo	6 mo	1 yr	3 yr	5 yr	7 yr	> 10 yr
Weight (kg)	1	2–3	4	7	10	12–14	16–18	20–26	> 30
Heart rate	145	125	120	130	125	115	100	100	75
Respiratory rate	30–40	30–40	25–35		20–30		12–25		12–18
Endotracheal tube size (inner diameter in mm)	2.5–3.0 Uncuffed - - - -	3	3.5	3.5	4	4.5	5–6	6–6.5 - - - Cuffed	7
Length at teeth (cm)	8	10	12		12	16	16	18	20–22
Laryngoscope blade size	0	0–1	1	1	1–2	1–2	2	2–3	3
		- - - - - - - - - Straight - - - - - - - - -						- - - Curved - - -	
Suction catheter size (Fr)	5	6	6–8	6–8	8	8–10	10	10–12	12

jury is suspected or present. In this position, the neck is flexed slightly, and the head is extended on the neck. The jaw thrust or chin lift is then used to lift the soft tissues out of the airway.

4. Obstruction should be cleared.

5. Oral and nasal airways are less useful in children because they frequently stimulate laryngospasm or emesis when reflexes are intact. In addition, placement may traumatize the adenoidal or tonsillar soft tissues, resulting in significant bleeding, which can be difficult to control and further complicate airway management.

6. In an obtunded or paralyzed child, cricoid pressure should be used during positive pressure ventilation until intubation is confirmed.

7. Bag-valve-mask ventilation is a better option for emergent oxygenation and ventilation in children because of the ease of attaining a seal and the smaller size of the chest cavity. Adequacy of ventilation is best assessed by observing chest wall motion; auscultation is less reliable. Nasogastric tube placement should accompany bag-valve-mask ventilation where safe to decrease the risk of emesis and aspiration. Care should be taken to coordinate breaths with the bag-valve-mask unit with spontaneous ventilations, when present.

8. When prolonged airway control or hyperventilation is indicated, endotracheal intubation should be undertaken. The optimal method is orotracheal intubation. Blind nasal intubation may be tried if the oral route is contraindicated but is technically more difficult. The increased adenoidal tissue is at risk for bleeding, and the anterior position of the larynx with the overlying epiglottis makes nasal tube placement more difficult.

9. When possible, children should be premedicated with atropine, 0.02 mg/kg, to prevent bradycardia with intubation.

10. Since auscultation is not reliable, tube placement should be confirmed by observation of chest wall movement, skin color, and radiographs.

11. When a cervical fracture is suspected and immediate airway control is essential, options include either nasotracheal intubation or PTTJV. The rapid-sequence protocol may be used with in-line traction if necessary. Otherwise, temporize with bag-valve-mask ventilation during clinical and radiographic clearance.

12. PTTJV has been shown to be effective in the pediatric model. Perform needle cricothyroidotomy as described for adults. The smaller size of the airways should be taken into account. The possibility of obstruction at the cricoid cartilage must be considered, since ventilation at the level of the cricothyroid membrane would be ineffective in that situation. The use of retrograde, fiberoptic, and digital techniques has not been well studied in children.

13. Surgical airways in young children and infants are extremely difficult. They should be performed only as a last resort by surgeons with experience in pediatric head and neck surgery. There are high failure and complication rates. Most airways will be adequately managed by bag-valve-mask or oral intubation techniques.

D. Epiglottitis and Croup: These illnesses may cause severe airway edema and sudden obstruction. Diagnosis is based on clinical features and, where necessary, anteroposterior and lateral neck soft tissue views.

1. Croup–Croup progresses more slowly than epiglottitis, causing subglottic swelling and a barking cough, and it is often accompanied by signs of viral upper respiratory infection. Croup rarely requires intubation. Treatment includes intravenous fluids, humidified air, racemic epinephrine, and occasionally steroids.

2. Epiglottitis–Epiglottitis progresses rapidly with a toxic-appearing, drooling child sitting in the upright position with the neck hyperextended. Abrupt, complete airway obstruction can occur with minimal stimulation of the patient. When suspicion is high for epiglottitis, supplemental O_2 should be supplied and the patient transported with minimal disturbance to the operating room, where the epiglottis can be directly visualized. More than half of patients with epiglottitis will require intubation, which is best done in the operating room by the most experienced intubator before airway obstruction occurs. If intubation fails, an emergent tracheostomy must be performed, preferably by a pediatric ear, nose, and throat specialist. Treatment includes antibiotics and intravenous fluids after the airway is secured (Chapter 42).

Management of Foreign Bodies in the Airway

Management of foreign bodies in the airway is dictated by the location of the object and the age and condition of the patient. Most airway obstruction due to foreign bodies occurs between the ages of 1 and 5 years. More than 3000 deaths annually are due to this disorder.

Assessment begins with observation for tachypnea, air movement, stridor, retractions, agitation or lethargy, and cyanosis. Auscultation and chest x-ray may be helpful. Examination of the oropharynx may reveal the foreign body.

If the foreign body is visible, the airway may be cleared with a manual sweep. Blind sweep is not recommended. If the patient is coughing, do not interfere; the normal reflexes often clear the airway. O_2 should be administered to all patients with foreign body aspiration. A 70% helium/30% oxygen mixture may decrease airway turbulence, and O_2 delivery may be enhanced while definitive management is being arranged.

If there is total obstruction, the Heimlich maneuver should be attempted in patients older than 1 year; in younger children, back blows and chest thrusts are recommended. If these methods are unsuccessful, position the airway to optimize patency. Attempt to remove the object under direct observation with a laryngoscope. If this is unsuccessful, a surgical airway is necessary. Subglottic obstructions may not be relieved by cricothyroidotomy or tracheostomy. Removal in the operating room with rigid bronchoscope may be the only option.

Management of the partially obstructed airway must be individualized. Bronchial obstructions often do not require intubation, and compromise may be subacute. If there is air movement and the object cannot be visualized on direct observation, the safest method for removal is under general anesthesia with the rigid bronchoscope. Take care not to cause complete obstruction while inserting the laryngoscope or bronchoscope.

Management of Airway in Status Asthmaticus

The asthmatic patient requires intubation when clinical evidence of fatigue is accompanied by increasing respiratory acidosis due to CO_2 retention and increasing hypoxia in the face of aggressive therapy. Intubation is dangerous for the asthmatic. These patients are susceptible to barotrauma while intubated, and intubation does not ensure bronchodilation or adequate ventilation and oxygenation. Because of the difficulties of bag-valve-mask ventilation in status asthmaticus, many practitioners prefer awake nasal intubations with topical anesthetic. The asthmatic's active respiratory effort helps tube placement through the cords, but agitation often complicates this procedure. If the rapid-sequence protocol is used, succinylcholine is relatively contraindicated owing to histamine-induced bronchospasm. Similarly, thiopental may worsen the condition. Better choices include vecuronium, midazolam, fentanyl, and ketamine. Ketamine has bronchodilating effects. After intubation, halothane may be administered to provide strong bronchodilating effects as well as anesthesia.

Management of Airway in Trauma Patients

A. Patients with Unstable Cervical Spines or Facial Injuries: The optimal route of intubation for patients with known or suspected cervical spinal injuries is controversial. When possible, the cervical spine should be cleared radiologically and clinically prior to intubation. When airway control must precede definitive stabilization of the spine, options include orotracheal intubation with manual in-line stabilization, blind techniques such as nasal or digital intubation, use of lighted accessories, and transtracheal methods. No method is fully supported by the literature, and many of these techniques are not widely used at present. Most large series report no bad neurologic outcomes with any carefully done technique. Although nasal intubation is most commonly recommended in this setting, the decision must be individualized based on the patient's level of consciousness, injuries, the urgency of the need for airway control, and the intubator's skill with various techniques.

When severe facial, mandibular, and upper neck trauma occur, the best option is needle cricothyroidotomy followed by endotracheal tube placement or later tracheostomy. Blunt laryngeal trauma may render cricothyroidotomy very difficult, requiring bag-assisted ventilation and urgent tracheostomy in the operating room. A technique for blind localization of the cricothyroid membrane in the setting of massive neck swelling has been devised by Simon. It is based on the fact that the distance from the mentum to the hyoid is one-half the distance from the angle of the jaw to the mentum. A needle placed into the midline of the neck at the appropriate measured site should locate the hyoid. A skin hook hooked under the hyoid can be used to stabilize and retract the trachea forward. A midline incision inferiorly from the hyoid will locate the cricothyroid membrane for cricothyroidotomy. This technique has not been widely used. It may be considered a last resort when all landmarks are lost.

B. Patients with Head Trauma: Intubation of patients with severe head trauma is indicated to treat hypoventilation and hypoxia and to protect and control the airway in patients who are unstable or combative and agitated enough to require paralysis for necessary studies and procedures. Additionally, it is the only way to hyperventilate the patient to a low PCO_2 as part of the treatment for elevated intracranial pressure. Approach to the airway must take into consideration other potential traumatic injuries to the mid face, cervical spine, soft tissues of neck, and respiratory tract. When nasotracheal intubation is contraindicated, oral intubation with the rapid-sequence protocol often is recommended. If the rapid-sequence protocol is used, lidocaine, 1–5 mg/kg intravenously, may attenuate the rise in intracranial pressure. Although succinylcholine is reported to raise intracranial pressure, it remains the recommended agent for neuromuscular blockade in the setting of head trauma because of the ability to rapidly control the airway and begin treatment. Digital intubation or light-assisted or surgical airways may be used as indicated if oral intubation is unsuccessful.

CARE OF THE INTUBATED PATIENT

Adjunctive Drugs

Intubated patients often require sedation to prevent coughing or "bucking" the endotracheal tube and to reduce agitation. Prolonged paralysis may be indicated during procedures or during early stages of management. In any awake patient, neuromuscular blockade should be accompanied by sedation to blunt the noxious sensation of paralysis. Paralysis may mask the manifestations of status epilepticus. All these patients must have full anticonvulsant loading before, during, or immediately after paralysis. If the patient remains paralyzed, control of seizures must be demonstrated with electroencephalographic recording.

Pulmonary Toilet

After the endotracheal tube position is confirmed by clinical evaluation and x-ray, it is secured by taping about the head or neck to prevent accidental extubation. All intubated patients require regular suctioning. The frequency of suctioning depends on the amount of secretion produced. Indicators of the need to suction may include visible secretions welling up in the endotracheal tube, hypoxia, agitation, and increased difficulty with bagging. In the emergency department, most patients will be manually ventilated with a bag-valve-mask unit, at least initially. If on a mechanical ventilator, a patient should be preoxygenated with several minutes of bag-valve ventilation at 100% O_2 to ensure against hypoxia during suctioning. Disposable, sterile, narrow-gauge, flexible suction catheters are available for suctioning the endotracheal tube. The diameter of the catheter should be less than half the internal diameter of the endotracheal tube. Insert the catheter with the side port open. When the catheter is in the trachea, apply suction by covering the side port. Rotate the catheter several times to suction both right and left main stem. Continue suction and rotary movement during catheter removal. The patient is then reoxygenated. No single suctioning episode should last longer than 10–15 seconds. Preoxygenate for 30–60 seconds before reinserting the catheter. Suctioning may be aided by administering 1–2 mL of sterile normal saline down the tube to moisten secretions. Complications of suctioning include hypoxia, arrhythmias, hypotension, mucosal trauma, and pulmonary collapse. There is also a surge in intracranial pressure during suctioning, which may be blunted by the use of tracheal or intravenous lidocaine. Occasionally the oropharynx must be suctioned with the rigid, tipped catheter to control oral secretion or blood.

Endotracheal Medication

Medications that are safe and probably effective when given endotracheally include epinephrine, atropine, lidocaine, diazepam, naloxone, and oxygen. Doses are the same as those for intravenous use. Delivery is enhanced if the drugs are diluted in 10 mL of normal saline before administration and aerosolized during administration by rapid injection through a pediatric feeding tube positioned in the trachea.

Monitoring

A. Observation: Any patient intubated in the emergency department requires close observation. A respiratory technician, nurse, or physician should be present at all times. In addition to adding critical clinical observations to the data obtained by monitoring devices, they may note complications of intubation and positive pressure ventilation and address them before they compromise the patient.

Complications that may occur while a patient is intubated include barotrauma with tension pneumothorax, atelectasis, and obstructions or disconnections in the ventilatory circuit. In critically ill patients, continuous observation for changes in the patient's hemodynamic or mental status is the standard of care.

B. Pulse Oximetry: A pulse oximetry sensor can be clipped over the tip of a digit or an earlobe to detect the oxygen saturation of arterial blood. Oximetry reflects trends in oxygenation before, during, and after intubation. At oxygen saturations over 70%, the 95% confidence limits are ± 4%. When the PaO_2 is greater than 60–80 mm Hg, a large change in PaO_2 may result in only a small change in O_2 saturation measured by the pulse oximeter. Oxygenation can also be maintained to some degree by hyperventilation (PCO_2 declines); however, pulse oximetry provides no information about the adequacy of ventilation. Consequently, the pulse oximeter cannot substitute for arterial blood gas determinations in many clinical settings. The presence of nail polish, skin pigmentation, methemoglobin, carboxyhemoglobin, intravascular dye, hypothermia, and hypoperfusion all may reduce the accuracy of the pulse oximeter.

C. Capnography: Capnometers may be attached to the expired air circuit to monitor the end tidal carbon dioxide tension ($P_{et}CO_2$). In healthy patients, the plateau $P_{et}CO_2$ is usually 1 mm Hg less than the PCO_2. Numerous clinical conditions and manipulations can change the $P_{et}CO_2$, and its role as a monitoring device remains to be determined. Since the absence of $P_{et}CO_2$ indicates esophageal intubation, disposable devices may be helpful to indicate successful endotracheal tube placement.

D. Arterial Blood Gases: The measured pH, $PaCO_2$, and PaO_2 remain the standard for monitoring respiratory status. The method for obtaining a sample is described in Chapter 46. The main disadvantage of using the arterial blood gas measurement is the discontinuous nature of the data. Transient changes and trends may be missed. Overall, however, it remains the best indicator of gas exchange and acid-base balance.

E. Cardiac Monitoring: Most intubated patients require continuous cardiac monitoring and frequent checks of blood pressure and heart rate. Hypoxia and other complications of intubation are often reflected early in changes in vital signs.

F. Other Monitoring Methods: Several other devices may assist in monitoring an intubated patient.

Some are useful only in specific settings and others when intubated patients must be held for prolonged periods in the emergency department while awaiting a bed in an intensive care unit. Transcutaneous PO_2 devices are available for neonates in whom $P_{tc}O_2$ correlates well with PaO_2. Arterial lines and pulmonary artery catheters allow intra-arterial measurement of PaO_2 and measurement of mixed venous O_2 saturation. Pulmonary functions may be monitored, particularly in patients who are likely to be extubated in the emergency department.

General Care

Paralyzed patients are unable to shift their weight from pressure points at will. Consequently, they must be turned every hour and must have particular pressure points padded. If they are in a cool environment, they must be adequately covered. Lubricate and tape the eyes to prevent corneal ulceration.

Mechanical Ventilation

If mechanical ventilation is used in the emergency department, the choice of ventilator and ventilator settings must be individualized to the patient's condition. In many circumstances, a tidal volume of 15 mL/kg, a rate of 12, and the "assist control" mode are reasonable settings. For hyperventilation, start with a rate of 20 and check an arterial blood gas measurement for confirmation. The use of a ventilator does not obviate the need for close observation of the patient's condition by a physician or qualified nurse.

Extubation

In several circumstances, a patient may require extubation in the emergency department. Before electing to extubate, be certain that the patient has spontaneous ventilation and is able to generate a vital capacity of 15 mL/kg. The indication for intubation must be resolved, and airway reflexes should be intact. Optimally the patient should be able to follow commands and understand the planned procedure. If possible, decompress the stomach with nasogastric suction. Assemble equipment for suctioning and reintubation. Suction the oropharynx and tracheobronchial tree, manually oxygenate with 100% O_2, release the cuff, and withdraw the tube at the end of inspiration. Ventilate with a mask, and observe for laryngospasm or respiratory insufficiency. If laryngospasm occurs, continue bag-valve-mask ventilation with 100% O_2. Consider racemic epinephrine, 0.5 mL of 2.25% in 4 mL of normal saline via nebulizer. If these methods fail, reintubation or a surgical airway may be necessary.

REFERENCES

American College of Surgeons Committee on Trauma: *Student Manual for Advanced Trauma Life Support Course for Physicians.* American College of Surgeons, 1988.

American Heart Association: *Textbook of Advanced Cardiac Life Support.* American Heart Association, 1987.

Ampel L et al: An approach to airway management in the acutely head injured patient. J Emerg Med 1988;6:1.

Anton W et al: A disposable end-tidal CO_2 detector to verify endotracheal intubation. Ann Emerg Med 1991;20:271.

Barkin R: Pediatric airway management. Emerg Med Clin North Am 1988;6:687.

Batlan D, Zaid G, Johnston W: Neuromuscular blockade in the emergency department. J Emerg Med 1987;5:225.

Bergman K, Harris B: Airway management in pediatric trauma. Emerg Care Q 1991;7:58.

Chameides L: *Textbook for Pediatric Advanced Life Support.* American Heart Association, 1988.

De Garmo BH, Dronen S: Pharmacology and clinical use of neuromuscular blocking agents. Ann Emerg Med 1983;12:48.

Hardwick W, Bluhm D: Digital intubation. J Emerg Med 1984;1:317.

Hawkins M: The esophageal obturator airway and related devices. Emerg Care Q 1991;7:13.

Holley J, Jorden R: Airway management in patients with unstable cervical spine fractures. Ann Emerg Med 1989;18:1237.

Jorden R: Airway management. Emerg Med Clin North Am 1988;6:671.

Jorden R: Percutaneous transtracheal ventilation. Emerg Med Clin North Am 1988;6:745.

McNamara RL: Retrograde intubation of the trachea. Ann Emerg Med 1987;16:680.

Mizrahi S et al: Major airway obstruction relieved by helium/oxygen breathing. Crit Care Med 1986;14:986.

Odom J, Boyd C: Airway management and cervical spine fractures. Emerg Care Q 1991;7:51.

Piotrowski J, Moore E: Emergency department tracheostomy. Emerg Clin North Am 1988;6:737.

Redan J et al: The value of intubating and paralyzing patients with suspected head injury in the emergency department. J Trauma 1991;31:371.

Roberts D, Clinton J, Ruiz E: Neuromuscular blockade for critical patients in the emergency department. Ann Emerg Med 1986;15:152.

Sanders A: Capnography in emergency medicine. Ann Emerg Med 1989;18:1287.

Sellick BA: Cricoid pressure to control regurgitation of stomach contents during induction of anesthesia. Lancet 1961;2:404.

Shock 3

Donald D. Trunkey, MD, Patricia R. Salber, MD, FACEP, FACP, & John Mills, MD

IMMEDIATE MANAGEMENT OF SHOCK
(See algorithm.)

Shock is a state of circulatory failure characterized by inadequate tissue perfusion. Blood flow is insufficient to provide the nutritional requirements of cells and remove the waste products of metabolism. This insufficiency leads to cellular dysfunction and, ultimately, death. Table 3–1 sets forth some of the different causes of the shock syndrome. Correct management of patients in shock involves treating both the underlying cause of shock and the physiologic abnormalities associated with the shock state.

See also Chapter 42 for treatment of shock in infants and children.

Classification
(See Table 3–1.)

The causes of shock can be classified on the basis of 4 major pathophysiologic mechanisms involved.

A. Hypovolemic Shock: The chief abnormality in hypovolemic shock is decreased intravascular volume, which may occur as a result of loss of blood or plasma or of fluid and electrolytes. These losses may be exogenous (eg, gastrointestinal tract bleeding, diarrhea) or endogenous ("third-spacing," hematomas).

B. Cardiogenic Shock: The chief abnormality in cardiogenic shock is abnormal cardiac function due to arrhythmia, "pump failure," or valvular dysfunction.

C. Obstructive Shock: The chief abnormality in obstructive shock is an impediment to filling of the right or left ventricle (decreased preload). If decreased filling is sufficiently severe, the resulting fall in cardiac output causes shock. Obstruction may occur in the systemic circulation (eg, obstruction of the vena cava) or pulmonary circulation (eg, massive pulmonary embolus) or may be due to pericardial disease (eg, cardiac tamponade) or cardiac disease (eg, atrial myxoma).

D. Distributive Shock: The chief abnormality in distributive shock is abnormal distribution of vascular volume due to changes in vascular resistance or permeability. The end result is a decrease in ventricular filling that leads to inadequate cardiac output. The derangement of vascular volume characterizing distributive shock may occur as a result of sepsis, anaphylaxis, or neurogenic shock.

Diagnosis
A. Suspect Shock If the Following Signs Are Present:

1. Hypotension–Systolic blood pressures of 90 mm Hg or less in adults or proportionately lower in children usually signify hypotension. (The normal systolic blood pressure in children can be estimated

Table 3–1. Classification of shock by mechanism and common causes.

Hypovolemic shock
 Loss of blood (hemorrhagic shock)
  External hemorrhage
   Trauma
   Gastrointestinal tract bleeding
  Internal hemorrhage
   Hematoma
   Hemothorax or hemoperitoneum
 Loss of plasma
  Burns
  Exfoliative dermatitis
 Loss of fluid and electrolytes
  External
   Vomiting
   Diarrhea
   Excessive sweating
   Hyperosmolar states (diabetic ketoacidosis, hyperos-
    molar nonketotic coma)
  Internal ("third-spacing")
   Pancreatitis
   Ascites
   Bowel obstruction

Cardiogenic shock
 Dysrhythmia
  Tachyarrhythmia
  Bradyarrhythmia
 "Pump failure" (secondary to myocardial infarction or other
  cardiomyopathy)
 Acute valvular dysfunction (especially regurgitant lesions)
 Rupture of ventricular septum or free ventricular wall

Obstructive shock
 Tension pneumothorax
 Pericardial disease (tamponade, constriction)
 Disease of pulmonary vasculature (massive pulmonary
  emboli, pulmonary hypertension)
 Cardiac tumor (atrial myxoma)
 Left atrial mural thrombus
 Obstructive valvular disease (aortic or mitral stenosis)

Distributive shock
 Septic shock
 Anaphylactic shock
 Neurogenic shock
 Vasodilator drugs
 Acute adrenal insufficiency

by adding 80 to twice the child's age in years, eg, for a 10-year-old, $80 + [2 \times 10] = 100$.) Some healthy adults may have systolic blood pressures that are normally this low; conversely, patients with preexisting hypertension may develop shock at blood pressure levels within the normal range. Orthostatic vital signs should be measured if equivocal blood pressure readings are found and no spinal injury exists.

2. Orthostatic change in vital signs–Orthostatic vital signs should be measured in patients who are not clearly hypotensive in the supine position. Both blood pressure and pulse are measured in the supine and then in the sitting (legs dangling over the side of the bed) position. If no change occurs in the sitting position, repeat the determinations with the patient standing. Wait about 3–5 minutes between measurements to allow pulse and blood pressure to stabilize. Although there is a wide varia-

tion in both blood pressure and pulse response to standing in euvolemic patients, in general a drop in systolic blood pressure of 20 mm Hg or more associated with an increase in pulse rate of more than 20 beats/min suggests depletion of intravascular volume. An increased heart rate with no change in blood pressure in the seated or erect position may be seen in some patients with mild hypovolemia. On the other hand, normovolemic patients with autonomic neuropathies or those taking certain medications (eg, some antihypertensive drugs) may demonstrate an orthostatic fall in blood pressure, usually without an associated increase in pulse rate.

3. Tachycardia–Tachycardia, although a nonspecific finding, is usually present in mild to moderate shock. An orthostatic fall in blood pressure will help confirm shock as the cause of tachycardia.

4. Adrenergic responses–Restlessness, anxiety, and diaphoresis may accompany the shock state.

5. Peripheral hypoperfusion–Cool or mottled extremities (livedo reticularis) and weak or impalpable peripheral pulses are signs of peripheral hypoperfusion.

6. Altered mental status–Patients in shock may demonstrate normal mental status or may be restless, agitated, confused, lethargic, or comatose as a result of inadequate perfusion of the brain.

B. Determine Severity of Shock: (See Table 3–2.)

1. Mild shock–Mild shock is defined as decreased perfusion of nonvital organs and tissue only, eg, skin, fat, skeletal muscle, and bone. These tissues

Table 3–2. Clinical classification of shock.[1]

	Pathophysiology	Clinical Manifestations
Mild (< 20% of blood volume lost)	Decreased peripheral perfusion only of organs able to withstand prolonged ischemia (skin, fat, muscle, and bone). Arterial pH normal.	Patient complains of feeling cold. Postural hypotension and tachycardia. Cool, pale, moist skin; collapsed neck veins; concentrated urine.
Moderate (20–40% of blood volume lost)	Decreased central perfusion of organs able to tolerate only brief ischemia (liver, gut, kidneys). Metabolic acidosis present.	Thirst. Supine hypotension and tachycardia (variable). Oliguria or anuria.
Severe (> 40% of blood volume lost)	Decreased perfusion of heart and brain. Metabolic acidosis is severe. Respiratory acidosis may also be present.	Agitation, confusion, or obtundation. Supine hypotension and tachycardia are invariably present. Rapid, deep respiration.

[1] These clinical findings are most consistently observed in hemorrhagic shock but apply to other types of shock as well.

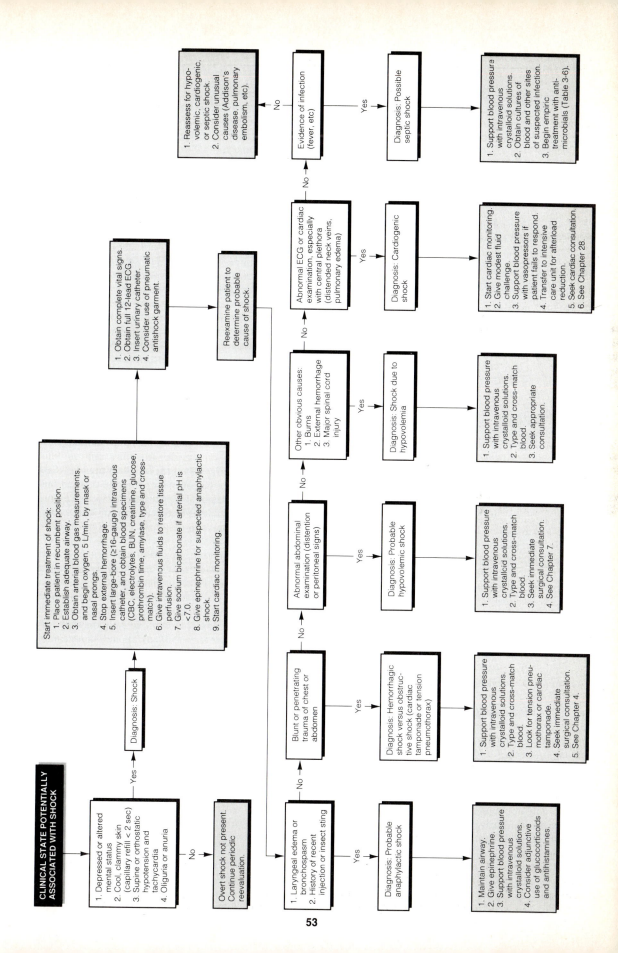

CLINICAL STATE POTENTIALLY ASSOCIATED WITH SHOCK

1. Depressed or altered mental status
2. Cool, clammy skin (capillary refill < 2 sec)
3. Supine or orthostatic hypotension and tachycardia
4. Oliguria or anuria

→ No → Overt shock not present. Continue periodic reevaluation.

→ Yes → Diagnosis: Shock

Start immediate treatment of shock:
1. Place patient in recumbent position.
2. Establish adequate airway.
3. Obtain arterial blood gas measurements, and begin oxygen, 5 L/min, by mask or nasal prongs.
4. Stop external hemorrhage.
5. Insert large-bore (≥16-gauge) intravenous catheter, and obtain blood specimens (CBC, electrolytes, BUN, creatinine, glucose, prothrombin time, amylase, type and cross-match).
6. Give intravenous fluids to restore tissue perfusion.
7. Give sodium bicarbonate if arterial pH is <7.0.
8. Give epinephrine for suspected anaphylactic shock.
9. Start cardiac monitoring.

1. Obtain complete vital signs.
2. Obtain full 12-lead ECG.
3. Insert urinary catheter.
4. Consider use of pneumatic antishock garment.

Reexamine patient to determine probable cause of shock.

Laryngeal edema or bronchospasm / History of recent injection or insect sting

→ Yes → Diagnosis: Probable anaphylactic shock →
1. Maintain airway.
2. Give epinephrine.
3. Support blood pressure with intravenous crystalloid solutions.
4. Consider adjunctive use of glucocorticoids and antihistamines.

→ No → Blunt or penetrating trauma of chest or abdomen

→ Yes → Diagnosis: Hemorrhagic shock versus obstructive shock (cardiac tamponade or tension pneumothorax) →
1. Support blood pressure with intravenous crystalloid solutions.
2. Type and cross-match blood.
3. Look for tension pneumothorax or cardiac tamponade.
4. Seek immediate surgical consultation.
5. See Chapter 4.

→ No → Abnormal abdominal examination (distention or peritoneal signs)

→ Yes → Diagnosis: Probable hypovolemic shock →
1. Support blood pressure with intravenous crystalloid solutions.
2. Type and cross-match blood.
3. Seek immediate surgical consultation.
4. See Chapter 7.

→ No → Other obvious causes:
1. Burns
2. External hemorrhage
3. Major spinal cord injury

→ Yes → Diagnosis: Shock due to hypovolemia →
1. Support blood pressure with intravenous crystalloid solutions.
2. Type and cross-match blood.
3. Seek appropriate consultation.

→ No → Abnormal ECG or cardiac examination, especially with central plethora (distended neck veins, pulmonary edema)

→ Yes → Diagnosis: Cardiogenic shock →
1. Start cardiac monitoring.
2. Give modest fluid challenge.
3. Support blood pressure with vasopressors if patient fails to respond.
4. Transfer to intensive care unit for afterload reduction.
5. Seek cardiac consultation.
6. See Chapter 28.

→ No → Evidence of infection (fever, etc)

→ Yes → Diagnosis: Possible septic shock →
1. Support blood pressure with intravenous crystalloid solutions.
2. Obtain cultures of blood and other sites of suspected infection.
3. Begin empiric treatment with antimicrobials (Table 3-6).

→ No →
1. Reassess for hypovolemic, cardiogenic, or septic shock.
2. Consider unusual causes (Addison's disease, pulmonary embolism, etc).

can survive relatively long periods of decreased perfusion without undergoing irreversible changes. Mentation is unimpaired, urine output is normal or only slightly decreased, and metabolic acidosis is absent or mild.

2. Moderate shock–Moderate shock is defined as decreased perfusion of vital organs other than heart and brain (liver, gut, kidneys, and others). These organs do not tolerate hypoperfusion as long as fat, skin, and muscle do. Oliguria (urine output < 0.5 mL/kg/h in adults, < 1 mL/kg/h in children, or < 2 mL/kg/h in infants) and metabolic acidosis are present, but the sensorium is relatively intact.

3. Severe shock–Severe shock is defined as inadequate perfusion of the heart or brain. The compensatory mechanisms of shock act to preserve blood flow to these 2 vital organs at the expense of all others. Thus, in advanced shock there is constriction of all other vascular beds. In addition to severe oliguria and acidosis, altered mentation and signs of cardiac hypoxia (abnormal ECG, decreased cardiac output) occur.

Initial Treatment:
General Measures

A. Position the Patient: Place the patient supine and level to maximize blood flow to the brain. (Remember to prevent unnecessary heat loss with a blanket when the patient is not being examined.)

B. Establish Adequate Oxygenation: Open or maintain the airway. Support inadequate ventilation with a bag-mask combination or endotracheal tube. Obtain arterial blood gas measurements as a guide both to the adequacy of oxygenation and to the severity of hypoperfusion, as indicated by the presence or absence of metabolic acidosis. Pending the results of blood gas measurements, give oxygen, 5–10 L/min, by mask or nasal prongs.

C. Stop Obvious External Hemorrhage: Use direct manual compression. Blind clamping of vessels should be avoided, since it causes further injury. Tourniquets are rarely indicated except in traumatic amputation.

D. Gain Intravenous Access: The type and number of venous access sites, as well as the type and size of the intravenous catheters used, depend in part on the type of shock suspected.

1. Suspected hypovolemic shock–In patients with apparent hypovolemic shock, insert 2 large-bore (≥ 16-gauge in adults or the largest possible in children) peripheral venous catheters. If necessary, a large-bore catheter may be inserted percutaneously into the common femoral vein just below the level of the inguinal ligament. Alternatively, perform a venous cutdown in the saphenous vein at the ankle or in the basilic vein in the antecubital fossa (Chapter 46). In infants and young children, rapid access for fluid administration can be gained by the intraosseous route. Percutaneous catheterization of the subclavian

or internal jugular veins may be difficult in hypovolemic shock owing to vessel collapse. In addition, central venous catheters offer more resistance to fluid flow owing to their longer length. Obtain a sample of venous blood for CBC, electrolyte studies, renal function tests, and typing and cross-matching. In the presence of severe shock or massive blood loss, multiple simultaneous venous cutdowns may be performed if a sufficient number of trained personnel are available.

2. Cardiogenic shock–In a patient with suspected cardiogenic shock—especially if shock is mild and pulmonary edema is present—an 18- to 20-gauge percutaneous catheter may suffice for administration of appropriate drugs, although more than one intravenous access site may be necessary if critical illness requires rapid administration of incompatible medications (eg, sodium bicarbonate and catecholamines). Obtain a sample of venous blood for CBC, electrolyte studies, renal function tests, and cardiac enzyme determinations.

3. Shock of unknown cause–If the cause of shock is unknown, insert a large-bore percutaneous catheter (≥ 16-gauge), and obtain a sample of venous blood for CBC, electrolyte studies, and renal function tests.

E. Administer Appropriate Intravenous Fluids: Give appropriate intravenous fluids at once to restore adequate tissue perfusion. The type of fluid and rate of administration depend on the severity and cause of shock. Specific recommendations for fluid therapy are discussed under Emergency Treatment of Specific Causes of Shock, below.

F. Correct Metabolic Acidosis: The best way to correct the metabolic acidosis associated with shock is to restore tissue perfusion. If acidosis is profound (pH < 7.0), give sodium bicarbonate, 0.5–1 meq/kg intravenously over 5–10 minutes, with administration of additional doses being guided by the results of repeated arterial blood gas measurements.

G. Monitor Cardiac Rhythm and Obtain 12-Lead ECG: Although cardiac monitoring is especially important in cardiogenic shock, shock of any cause may result in myocardial ischemia due to hypoperfusion, and arrhythmias due to electrolyte and acid-base disturbances.

H. Insert Urinary Catheter: Insert an indwelling urinary catheter (eg, Foley) for urinalysis and monitoring of urine output.

I. Use Pneumatic Antishock Garment: In the past, an antishock garment (eg, military antishock trousers, or MAST) has been used as a temporizing measure in patients in whom venous access is difficult or impossible to obtain. However, its use has not been shown to increase survival in large clinical trials, and complications have occurred (eg, compartment syndrome).

Correct application and inflation of antishock garments are described in Chapter 46.

SEEK CAUSE OF SHOCK IN ORDER TO PROVIDE SPECIFIC THERAPY

Perform a rapid assessment of the most likely cause of shock in order to provide more specific and definitive therapy. Obtain a brief history from the patient, family, friends, bystanders, police, or ambulance attendants. Pay careful attention to clues available from physical examination (eg, obvious trauma, melena, fever, diarrhea).

HISTORY OF TRAUMA
(See also Chapter 4.)

Is There Obvious External Blood Loss or Penetrating Injury?

Turn the patient to examine the back (logroll the patient to maintain axial orientation if cervical spine injury is suspected).

Has There Been Chest Trauma?

Chest trauma may be due to obvious penetrating injury or to blunt trauma causing hemothorax, tension pneumothorax, cardiac tamponade or rupture, or myocardial contusion.

Has There Been Abdominal Trauma?

Intra-abdominal or retroperitoneal bleeding may result from visceral or vascular injuries. *Note: Intra-abdominal or retroperitoneal bleeding must be assumed to be present in any injured patient with severe shock, a normal chest x-ray, and no signs of significant external bleeding. Early surgical exploration is required.* In a more stable patient, peritoneal lavage (Chapter 46), abdominal CT scan (if obtainable without delay), or both may be useful for diagnosing intra-abdominal bleeding.

Has There Been Deceleration Injury?

Deceleration injury may be associated with lacerations of the aorta, especially in the region of the isthmus. A widened mediastinum may be visible on chest x-ray, but aortic angiography is required for definitive diagnosis.

Have There Been Pelvic or Thigh Injuries?

Injuries to the pelvis or thigh may be associated with a large volume of concealed blood loss.

Is There Evidence of Significant Spinal Cord Injury?

Neurogenic shock may occur after traumatic quad-riplegia or paraplegia. However, severe shock with the patient in the supine position is usually due to other concomitant causes of shock, such as blood loss.

Did a Preexisting Medical Condition Cause Trauma?

An example of a preexisting condition that results in trauma is an acute myocardial infarction that causes a motor vehicle accident.

NO HISTORY OF TRAUMA

Is This Hemorrhagic Shock?

Blood loss may be difficult to recognize if there is preexisting anemia or if not enough time has elapsed for compensatory mechanisms to cause hemodilution. Serial hematocrit measurements are needed to rule out hemorrhagic causes of shock.

A. Seek Evidence of Gastrointestinal Tract Blood Loss: (See Chapter 8.) Ask about prior hematemesis, melena, or abdominal pain. Perform a test for occult blood on a sample of feces, and insert a nasogastric tube to search for blood loss in the gastrointestinal tract.

B. Seek Evidence of Aortic Dissection or Ruptured Abdominal Aortic Aneurysm: (See Chapter 32.) The sudden onset of severe back or abdominal pain in a patient with a history of hypertension should suggest contained aortic dissection. Hematuria, neurologic deficit, or diminished peripheral pulses may be present. Abdominal pain with a palpable abdominal mass or abdominal tenderness and distention suggests rupture of an abdominal aortic aneurysm. *Note: Severe hemorrhagic shock in a patient without an obvious source of blood loss should be considered to be caused by ruptured abdominal aortic aneurysm, and exploratory laparotomy should be performed immediately.* Patients with aneurysms that have been repaired with aortoiliac grafts may occasionally present with massive gastrointestinal tract bleeding resulting from rupture at the suture site into the colon or duodenum.

C. Seek Evidence of Ectopic Pregnancy: Consider ruptured ectopic pregnancy in a woman of childbearing age who presents in shock, especially if there is a history of pelvic pain, vaginal bleeding, or amenorrhea. Culdocentesis (Chapter 30) often reveals free blood in the pelvis.

Is This Nonhemorrhagic Hypovolemic Shock?

Fluid or fluid and electrolyte loss may be the cause of hypovolemic shock in a patient with no evidence of external hemorrhage in whom serial hematocrit measurements remain stable (Table 3-1).

Is There a Cardiac Cause of Shock?

Cardiac causes of shock include arrhythmias, acute valvular dysfunction, rupture of the ventricular septum or free ventricular wall, or "pump failure" (cardiogenic shock). Ask about a history of hypertension, chest pain, or cardiac disease. Perform a careful physical examination, and pay special attention to the presence of distended neck veins, rales, and abnormal cardiac sounds (S_3 gallop, murmurs, rubs). An ECG may show arrhythmias or ischemic changes such as ST segment abnormalities.

Is There Evidence of Pericardial Disease?

Cardiac tamponade may occur in the patient with aortic dissection, pericarditis, uremia, or recent myocardial infarction. Occasionally, patients with constrictive pericarditis may present in shock. Assess the patient for pulsus paradoxus, Kussmaul's sign, or distended neck veins without evidence of pump failure (clear lung fields on chest x-ray, no S_3 gallop). If the patient is stable, obtain an echocardiogram to confirm the presence of pericardial fluid and to assist in pericardiocentesis. *Note: If the patient is in severe shock, immediate percutaneous pericardiocentesis may be lifesaving* (Chapter 46).

Is There Evidence of Sepsis?

Fever or hypothermia, rigors, leukocytosis, or petechiae suggest septic shock. Infants, the elderly, and immunocompromised or severely leukopenic patients may lack symptoms that localize the site of infection. Consider the possibility of **toxic shock syndrome** in young women, especially if there is a history of tampon use or recent menses.

Does the History Suggest Anaphylactic Shock?

A history of a bee or wasp sting, recent administration of drugs, or ingestion of certain foodstuffs should raise a suspicion of anaphylactic shock. Urticaria, laryngeal edema, and bronchospasm often (but not invariably) accompany anaphylaxis. Since most cases of anaphylaxis are due to parenteral administration of medications and occur within minutes of exposure to the inciting agent, the diagnosis usually is readily apparent.

Is This Obstructive Shock?

Tension pneumothorax, an obstructive cause of shock, should be considered in a setting of chest or upper abdominal trauma when diminished breath sounds are present unilaterally with tracheal deviation. Other causes of obstructive shock, resulting from obstruction to filling of the right or left ventricle, are difficult to diagnose rapidly in the emergency department. Obstructive shock may be due to such diverse conditions as massive pulmonary embolus, mural thrombus, or atrial myxoma. (Although diseases of the pericardium such as tamponade and constriction are also obstructive disorders, symptoms and signs often permit early specific diagnosis.) Pulmonary embolus should be suspected in the patient who presents in shock with signs of right heart failure (distended neck veins, right-sided S_3 gallop), refractory hypoxemia (especially if there is evidence of decreased pulmonary compliance as manifested by difficulty in ventilating the patient with a bag-mask combination), and an ECG that shows evidence of right heart strain (large R wave in lead V_1, right axis deviation, or incomplete right bundle branch block).

Are There Other Causes of Shock?

Unusual and infrequently encountered causes of shock include pheochromocytoma, addisonian crisis, and severe hypothyroidism (Chapter 35). Drug or toxin may also produce shock through a variety of mechanisms, including vasodilatation (eg, phenothiazines) and direct cardiac effects (eg, tricyclic antidepressants).

EMERGENCY TREATMENT OF SPECIFIC CAUSES OF SHOCK

HYPOVOLEMIC SHOCK

Hypovolemic shock may result from loss of whole blood, plasma, or fluid and electrolytes (Table 3–1).

In many patients with hypovolemic shock who are seen in the emergency department, the cause of shock will be immediately apparent, eg, obvious bleeding or history of severe diarrhea. Common causes that may not be readily apparent include ruptured abdominal aortic aneurysm, aortic dissection, splenic rupture (which may occur after seemingly inconsequential trauma), intestinal obstruction, and peritonitis.

Diagnosis

The clinical features of shock are present. In addition, there may be signs suggesting hypovolemia as the cause, eg, obvious hemorrhage or clinical features associated with volume loss due to burns, peritonitis, bowel obstruction, or ruptured abdominal aneurysm. Central venous pressure is low, and both venous and arterial pressures improve rapidly with intravascular volume replacement.

Treatment

See also Initial Treatment: General Measures, above.

A. Place the patient in a recumbent position.

B. Give oxygen by nasal prongs or mask.

C. Gain intravascular access. The number of intravenous cannulas required depends on the severity of shock. For adults, catheters inserted either by venous cutdown or by percutaneous methods should be 16-gauge or larger; size 5F or 10F pediatric feeding tubes should be used if shock is profound. During insertion of the intravenous line, blood may be conveniently obtained for CBC, electrolytes, BUN and creatinine, and prothrombin time. If hemorrhage is suspected, a clot should be sent for blood typing and cross-matching.

1. Long saphenous vein–The safest site for a venous cutdown is the long saphenous vein at the ankle (Chapter 46). If shock is not severe and the vein is not collapsed, insert a 16-gauge percutaneous catheter.

2. Basilic vein–The basilic vein in the antecubital fossa is also a good site for a large-gauge percutaneous catheter or venous cutdown. It can be used to achieve central venous pressure monitoring (Chapter 46).

3. Femoral vein–If an individual is attempting resuscitation without assistants, a temporary percutaneous catheter inserted in the femoral vein may permit rapid access to the circulation without major complications (Chapter 46).

4. Central veins–*Avoid* percutaneous catheterization of the subclavian or jugular veins for treatment of hypovolemic shock, since the great veins are usually collapsed, and the chances of complications such as hemothorax and pneumothorax are greatly increased. (For a patient in hypovolemic shock, the additional physiologic insult of hemothorax or tension pneumothorax may be rapidly fatal.)

5. Intraosseous infusion–In infants and young children, rapid access for fluid administration can be gained through intraosseous infusion (Chapter 46).

D. Administer intravenous fluids at once to restore adequate intravascular volume. The goal is normal cardiac output and tissue perfusion.

1. Types of fluids–Table 3–3 lists various solutions used in resuscitation of patients in shock. These solutions may be divided into 2 main types: crystalloids and colloids.

a. Crystalloids–(See Inside Back Cover.) Crystalloid solutions include isotonic (0.9%, or normal) saline and balanced salt solutions (lactated Ringer's injection, Plasma-Lyte, Isolyte, etc). Balanced salt solutions contain varying amounts of acetate or lactate (or both) that are metabolized to bicarbonate when there is adequate perfusion of the liver. Crystalloids have the advantages of being readily available and relatively inexpensive.

Hypertonic sodium chloride (7.5%) has been em-

Table 3–3. Fluids used for resuscitation of the patient in shock.

Crystalloids (See Inside Back Cover)
Isotonic sodium chloride (normal saline)
Hypertonic sodium chloride
Balanced salt solutions
Lactated Ringer's injection
Acetated Ringer's injection
Normosol, Plasma-Lyte, etc
Colloids
Blood
Low-titer O-negative (universal donor)
Type-specific
Typed and cross-matched
Washed red cells
Fresh warm blood
Plasma and its components
Plasma (fresh-frozen)
Albumin
Plasmanate
Plasma substitutes
High-molecular-weight dextran (MW 70,000)
Low-molecular-weight dextran (MW 40,000)
Hetastarch

ployed experimentally for hypovolemic shock due to hemorrhage (some preparations also include 6% dextran). These fluids osmotically draw water from extravascular spaces and can quickly expand blood volume. However, their safety has not yet been established, and there is growing concern over the value of rapidly expanding intravascular volume before hemorrhage is controlled surgically. Otherwise, hemorrhage may actually increase, accompanied by progressive hemodilution.

b. Colloids–Colloid solutions contain high-molecular-weight substances that do not easily diffuse across normal capillary membranes. This property may enable these fluids to be retained longer in the intravascular space. Colloid solutions also cause an increase in plasma oncotic pressure which, in accordance with Starling's law, should draw fluid from the interstitial space into the intravascular space to cause additional volume expansion. Both of these properties should prevent accumulation of pulmonary interstitial fluid that would hinder oxygen diffusion. Capillary membranes are often damaged in the patient in shock, however, so that larger molecules (from the high-molecular-weight substances) may leak from the intravascular space into the interstitium, where they could theoretically have an adverse effect on pulmonary function. Common colloid solutions include the following:

(1) Blood–Blood is most commonly available as packed red blood cells or whole blood. In patients in mild hemorrhagic shock, especially if blood pressure can be maintained with asanguineous fluids, typed and cross-matched packed red blood cells are preferred. Because it may take 45 minutes or longer to type and cross-match blood, patients with moderate or severe hemorrhagic shock may require type-specific, Rh-negative blood or universal donor blood (O-negative blood with low antibody titers to erythrocyte antigens) if shock persists after administration of more than 2–3 L of crystalloid solutions in adults or 20–40 mL/kg in children. Whole blood should be used as soon as possible in patients with moderate to severe hemorrhagic shock. Because hypothermia is a frequent side effect of transfusion of large amounts of blood stored at 4 °C, blood should be administered through blood warmers. (See also Principles of Transfusion Therapy in Chapter 33.) Blood *should not* be given to patients with other types of hypovolemic shock in whom the hematocrit is higher than 30–35%.

(2) Plasma or albumin solutions–Plasma or albumin solutions are effective volume expanders; however, they are expensive and, as noted above, may be harmful if they enter the pulmonary interstitium as a result of capillary leakage. They may also transmit infectious agents. The authors feel, therefore, that plasma and plasma products should not be used until capillary integrity has been regained (about 24 hours after correction of the initial insult).

(3) Plasma substitutes–Plasma substitutes such as dextrans have been used for initial volume replacement in hypovolemic shock, but their use is not recommended. Both low- and high-molecular-weight dextran may interfere with reticuloendothelial function. High-molecular-weight dextran coats red cells and makes typing and cross-matching difficult. Low-molecular-weight dextran coats platelets and can create a bleeding diathesis. Hetastarch (Hespan), a branched polymer of glucose, also affects coagulation and may cause bleeding.

2. Choice of fluids– The choice of fluid for resuscitation depends on the type of hypovolemic shock present (hemorrhagic versus nonhemorrhagic) and on the severity of shock.

a. Mild shock–Normal saline, lactated or acetated Ringer's injection, and plasma or other blood products are equally effective in treating patients in mild shock. Crystalloid solutions are strongly preferred because of their low cost, lack of adverse effects, and ready availability.

b. Moderate to severe shock–Considerable controversy exists regarding the correct fluid to use in patients in moderate to severe shock. Some authorities feel that colloids are associated with fewer adverse pulmonary effects than crystalloids in patients in severe shock, whereas other authorities feel that colloids are potentially more harmful than crystalloids (see above). A review suggests that crystalloids and colloids probably have equivalent effects if the amounts given achieve the same hemodynamic end points. The authors generally recommend crystalloids because of their low cost and lack of adverse effects.

c. Hemorrhagic shock–Isotonic saline or one of the balanced salt solutions should be used for ini-

tial resuscitation, because these substances are cheap and readily available, and they effectively restore vascular volume for short periods. As much as 2–3 L of crystalloid solution (adult dose; in children, 20–40 mL/kg) may be given to maintain adequate blood pressure for the 30–40 minutes required for definitive cross-matching of blood. As noted above, patients in mild hemorrhagic shock can be treated with cross-matched packed red cells, whereas patients in moderate to severe shock should receive whole blood and may require the use of type-specific or universal donor blood (see above). Patients with severe, persistent hemorrhagic shock due to hemothorax are candidates for autotransfusion (reinfusion of blood collected from chest tube drainage; see Chapters 4 and 46).

d. Nonhemorrhagic hypovolemic shock–Hypovolemic shock due to dehydration or third-spacing should be managed with crystalloid solutions alone.

E. Evaluate the Effectiveness of Resuscitation:

1. Monitor indices of resuscitation–(See Table 3–4.) The best indicators of successful resuscitation are improved atrial filling pressures and improved urine output. Additional guidelines include improved state of consciousness and peripheral perfusion (as measured by clinical criteria, including arterial blood pH). In an intensive care unit setting, measurements of cardiac output are also useful.

a. Atrial filling pressure– The only estimate of atrial filling pressure available in most emergency departments is the central venous (right atrial) pressure. It is generally a good measure of intravascular volume but may be unreliable in patients with cardiac or pulmonary disease or in those who require mechanical ventilatory support. Such patients require measurement of pulmonary capillary wedge pressure, a procedure that should be performed only in an intensive care unit.

Atrial filling pressure should be kept at or near normal levels (3–8 cm water), especially if there is severe shock associated with pulmonary capillary leakage. Filling pressure higher than 3–8 cm water may cause or exacerbate pulmonary edema.

b. Urine output–Urine output is a good index of visceral blood flow (specifically, renal blood flow) and should be maintained at more than 0.5 mL/kg/h in adults, 1 mL/kg/h in children, and more than 2

Table 3–4. Indices of successful resuscitation.

Atrial filling pressures (left or right) at or near normal (central venous pressure 3–8 mm water)
Urine output > 0.5 mL/kg/h or improving (in children, > 1 mL/kg/h; in infants, > 2 mL/kg/h)
Level of consciousness improving
Peripheral perfusion improving
Cardiac output increasing (normal ≥ 3.5 L/min in adults)

mL/kg/h in infants. This measurement is unreliable in patients with preexisting serious renal damage or when renal damage has occurred as a result of prolonged shock (eg, acute tubular necrosis).

2. Record progress of resuscitation–Documentation, preferably entered on an emergency department critical care flow sheet such as the one shown in Fig 3–1, is essential both for emergency department management and for later management once the patient has been transferred to an intensive care unit or operating room. The following information should be systematically recorded:

a. Vital signs–Record blood pressure, pulse, and respiration rate every 5–15 minutes.

b. Fluids–Note the quantity and type of fluid administered.

c. Central venous pressure–If central venous access has been obtained, measure and record central venous pressure every 30–60 minutes or as dictated by the progress of resuscitation.

d. Urine output–Measure urine output (with an indwelling catheter), and record every 30–60 minutes.

e. Other factors–Obtain and record serial hematocrits, arterial blood gas determinations, electrolyte measurements, and renal function tests as indicated.

F. Aggressively Search for the Cause of Persistent Shock: Persistent shock or recurrence of shock in a patient who initially responded to treatment suggests ongoing, often occult hemorrhage. Obtain serial hematocrit measurements, give whole blood, and search for hidden sources of blood loss. Patients with severe, refractory shock may require immediate surgery (eg, left thoracotomy to cross-clamp the aorta; exploratory laparotomy). Possible sources of blood loss include the following:

1. Thorax–Each hemithorax may contain up to 2 L of blood; therefore, a quick upright or lateral decubitus chest x-ray should always be obtained before surgery is considered.

2. Abdomen–Hidden blood loss in the abdomen is common. Distention is a late and unreliable sign. Intra-abdominal hemorrhage must be assumed to be present in any patient in shock who has a normal chest x-ray and no external signs of significant bleeding. Diagnostic peritoneal lavage (Chapter 46) may be helpful if gross blood is found or if a hematocrit of 2% or more is noted on the lavage sample. Absence of these signs does not exclude the possibility of intra-abdominal bleeding. A CT scan may demonstrate intraperitoneal fluid and help identify injury to specific solid organs. Its use should be restricted to patients who are relatively stable and for whom it can be obtained rapidly.

3. Retroperitoneum–Bleeding in the retroperitoneum cannot be diagnosed with routine studies. A CT scan is a helpful diagnostic aid if the patient's condition is stable enough to permit this delay.

4. Pelvis–The pelvis may conceal a large amount of blood; hemorrhagic shock is a common sequela of pelvic fracture.

5. Thigh–The thigh may contain 3–4 L of blood after a major fracture or crush injury.

G. Consider a Pneumatic Antishock Garment: A pneumatic antishock garment (eg, MAST) is a useful device for temporarily controlling hemorrhage below the level of the diaphragm. It is primarily indicated for patients with suspected pelvic hemorrhage in whom definitive control of bleeding must be delayed. However, studies to date have not shown a benefit on survival by the use of MAST, and complications (eg, compartment syndrome) have been noted. Thus, its routine use for patients in hemorrhagic shock cannot be recommended. If the patient arrives in the emergency department with a MAST already in place, *do not remove the suit until secure access to the circulation has been achieved and the patient has been stabilized hemodynamically. The MAST should then be deflated little by little, with close monitoring of the blood pressure.* In patients in hemorrhagic shock, the MAST is generally best removed in the operating room. The correct application and deflation of an antishock garment are described in Chapter 46.

Disposition

All patients in hypovolemic shock must be hospitalized.

CARDIOGENIC SHOCK

Broadly defined, the term cardiogenic shock denotes a shock syndrome resulting from some abnormal cardiac function, such as arrhythmias, valvular disease or pericardial disease (eg, cardiac tamponade), as well as shock resulting from severe myocardial dysfunction ("pump failure"). This section will consider mainly "pump failure." Shock due to pericardial disease or cardiac tumors is discussed under Obstructive Shock, below. Further discussion of the diagnosis and treatment of arrhythmias, valvular disease, and pericardial disease may be found in Chapters 28 and 29.

Cardiogenic shock due to "pump failure" is usually associated with acute myocardial infarction but may also result from end-stage cardiac disease of any cause, including valvular heart disease or cardiomyopathy. Cardiogenic shock is a complication of acute myocardial infarction in about 10% of patients and carries a grave prognosis (mortality rate > 50%) even with appropriate therapy. Potentially correctable myocardial—and nonmyocardial—factors may contribute to, or be the sole cause of, shock in a patient with myocardial infarction (Table 3–5). These factors must be sought and treated vigorously.

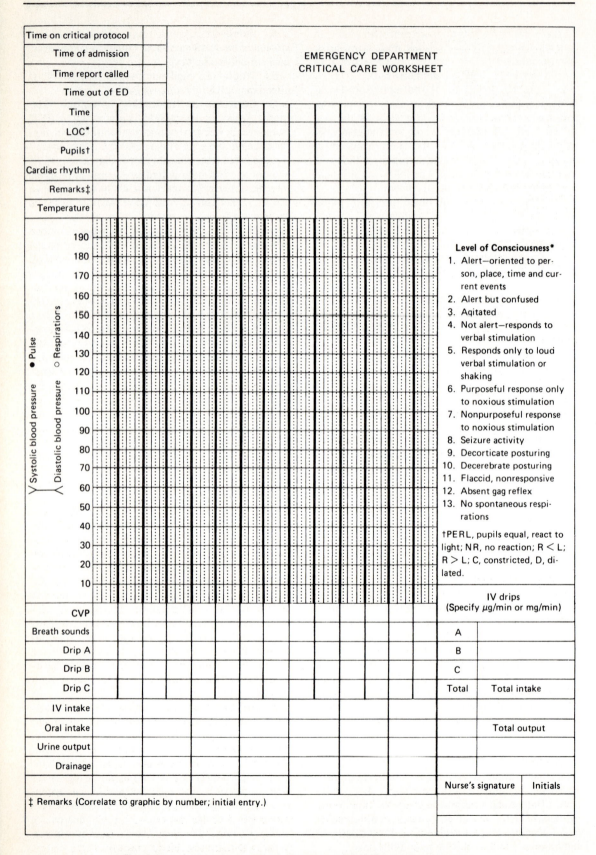

Time on critical protocol		
Time of admission		
Time report called		
Time out of ED		

EMERGENCY DEPARTMENT
CRITICAL CARE WORKSHEET

Time											
LOC*											
Pupils†											
Cardiac rhythm											
Remarks‡											
Temperature											

Level of Consciousness*
1. Alert—oriented to person, place, time and current events
2. Alert but confused
3. Agitated
4. Not alert—responds to verbal stimulation
5. Responds only to loud verbal stimulation or shaking
6. Purposeful response only to noxious stimulation
7. Nonpurposeful response to noxious stimulation
8. Seizure activity
9. Decorticate posturing
10. Decerebrate posturing
11. Flaccid, nonresponsive
12. Absent gag reflex
13. No spontaneous respirations

†PERL, pupils equal, react to light; NR, no reaction; R < L; R > L; C, constricted, D, dilated.

Pulse ● Respirations ○
Systolic blood pressure ∨
Diastolic blood pressure ∧

190
180
170
160
150
140
130
120
110
100
90
80
70
60
50
40
30
20
10

IV drips (Specify µg/min or mg/min)	
CVP	

Breath sounds									A	
Drip A									B	
Drip B									C	
Drip C									Total	Total intake
IV intake										
Oral intake									Total output	
Urine output										
Drainage										
									Nurse's signature	Initials

‡ Remarks (Correlate to graphic by number; initial entry.)

Figure 3–1. Critical care flow sheet. (Courtesy of Kaiser Foundation Hospitals.)

Table 3–5. Potential correctable causes
of cardiogenic shock.

Cardiac
  Mitral regurgitation from papillary muscle dysfunction or rupture; rupture of chordae tendineae
  Acute aortic regurgitation
  Rupture of interventricular septum
  Ventricular aneurysm
  Rupture of free ventricular wall
  Severe valvular or infravalvular stenosis
  Arrhythmias
Pericardial
  Cardiac tamponade
  Pericardial constriction
Noncardiac
  Hypoxemia
  Acidosis
  Hypovolemia
  Pulmonary embolus
  Tension pneumothorax
  Hemothorax
  Drugs
  Sepsis

Diagnosis

The hallmark of cardiogenic shock is hypotension (systolic blood pressure usually < 90 mm Hg, though it may be higher) accompanied by clinical signs of increased peripheral vascular resistance (weak, thready pulse; cool, clammy skin) and inadequate organ perfusion (altered mental status, decreased urine output). The patient also shows signs of acute myocardial infarction or preexisting severe cardiac disease.

A. Early Signs: Tachycardia and decreased pulse pressure (due to elevated systemic vascular resistance) are early signs of decreased cardiac output and should alert the physician to potential problems even if systolic blood pressure is normal. Diaphoresis or other signs of an increase in circulating catecholamines may be present. Restlessness, agitation, or confusion is an early manifestation of decreased cerebral blood flow. A fall in urinary sodium concentration to 20 meq/L or less or an increase in the ratio of urine osmolality to serum osmolality greater than 1.2–1 may occur before urine output falls significantly.

B. Central Venous Pressure: Central venous pressure (assessed by examination of the patient's neck veins) varies in cardiogenic shock depending on intravascular volume and the degree of associated right ventricular failure; central venous pressure is not a reliable means of diagnosing severe left ventricular failure.

Treatment

Although initial treatment of cardiogenic shock should be started in the emergency department, definitive therapy often requires hemodynamic monitoring using pulmonary and other systemic pressure catheters. Therefore, the patient should be transferred to an intensive care unit as quickly as possible.

A. Using arterial blood gas measurements as guidelines, establish adequate ventilation and oxygenation. Give supplemental oxygen, 2–5 L/min, by nasal prongs, pending the results of blood gas determinations; adjust oxygen supplementation to maintain arterial PO_2 at 60 mm Hg or higher. Pulse oximetry may also be used to maintain oxygen saturation ≥ 90%. If hypercapnia and acidosis are present, tracheal intubation may be necessary (Chapter 46).

B. Place the patient supine or supine with the legs elevated if systolic blood pressure is less than 70–80 mm Hg. Conversely, a patient with pulmonary edema and a normal or low normal blood pressure should be seated upright.

C. If hypotension is profound (systolic blood pressure < 70 mm Hg) and there is no evidence of pulmonary edema, gain intravenous access and infuse a crystalloid solution (normal saline or lactated Ringer's injection); if pulmonary edema is present, use 5% dextrose in water at a minimal rate sufficient to maintain an open vein.

D. Draw a sample of venous blood for CBC, electrolyte measurements, renal function tests, cardiac enzymes (CK and LDH isoenzymes); coagulation studies (prothrombin and partial thromboplastin times and platelet count) are essential if invasive monitoring or placement of a central venous catheter is anticipated.

E. Obtain a 12-lead ECG, and begin continuous cardiac monitoring.

F. Monitor urine output hourly. Bladder catheterization may be necessary.

G. Search for and treat nonmyocardial factors that may be causing or contributing to shock.

1. Acidosis–(See Chapter 36.) Respiratory acidosis (low arterial blood pH, high PCO_2) indicates hypoventilation, which should be corrected by bag-mask ventilation or, preferably, tracheal intubation (Chapter 46). Metabolic acidosis (low pH, normal or low PCO_2) in cardiogenic shock is due to hypoperfusion, with production of lactic acid. In addition to measures to improve cardiac output, give sodium bicarbonate if arterial blood pH is less than 7.0. Give 0.5–1 meq/kg over 5–10 minutes, and repeat as needed, using arterial blood gas determinations as a guideline. *Caution:* Do not administer sodium bicarbonate through the same intravenous line as catecholamines.

2. Arrhythmias–(See Chapter 29.) Cardioversion is the treatment of choice for tachyarrhythmias causing hypotension. Initial treatment for bradyarrhythmias causing hypotension is atropine, 0.5 mg intravenously every 5 minutes up to a total dose of 2 mg for adults; in children, give 0.02 mg/kg, with a minimum single dose of 0.1 mg and a maximum total dose of 1 mg. If the patient fails to respond, infuse isoproterenol (2 mg in 500 mL of 5% dextrose in water) at a rate that maintains an adequate heart rate (> 60 beats/min) and blood pressure. If the patient still fails to respond, a transvenous or transcutaneous pacemaker should be used.

3. Hypovolemia–In the patient with acute myocardial infarction, recent use of diuretics, excessive sweating, vomiting, or diarrhea may cause hypovolemia. In the patient without supine hypotension, measurement of orthostatic vital signs may provide a valuable clue to possible depletion of intravascular volume. Cautious administration of intravenous fluid should be attempted in patients who have no evidence of pulmonary edema. Give intravenous fluids in 50- to 100-mL increments over 5–10 minutes, and watch closely for signs of improvement (decreased heart rate, increased blood pressure) or deterioration (increased dyspnea or decreased arterial PO_2).

4. Tamponade–Rupture of the free ventricular wall or pericarditis with effusion may result in cardiac tamponade and may be confused with cardiogenic shock of myocardial origin. Perform a careful physical examination, and look for evidence of cardiac tamponade (elevated neck veins with clear lung fields on chest x-ray, pulsus paradoxus, pericardial friction rub, low voltage on the ECG). Immediate pericardiocentesis may be lifesaving (see also Obstructive Shock, below).

5. Acute valvular disease or ventricular septal rupture–Listen carefully for characteristic murmurs. Definitive diagnosis may require cardiac catheterization or echocardiography. Treatment with intra-aortic balloon pumping or drugs that reduce afterload may gain time to prepare the patient for lifesaving surgery (see also Chapter 28).

H. If the patient fails to respond to intravenous fluids, give dopamine, 200 mg in 250 mL of 5% dextrose in water (800 μg/mL) at the lowest rate that maintains adequate blood pressure (usually between 4 and 15 μg/kg/min). Norepinephrine (starting at a rate of 2–8 μg/min) may be tried if the patient fails to respond to high doses of dopamine.

Dobutamine is not useful for emergency department treatment of cardiogenic shock, because it has only minimal effects on the peripheral (alpha) receptors that mediate vasoconstriction and, hence, little effect on blood pressure. *Stabilization* in the emergency department may require maintaining blood pressure by means of such vasoconstriction while the patient is awaiting transfer to the intensive care unit.

Digitalis glycosides have no role in the initial treatment of cardiogenic shock.

I. Assess the need for urgent transfer of the patient to an intensive care unit. A patient with frank pulmonary edema and hypotension is difficult to manage in the emergency department, and every effort should be made to transfer the patient as rapidly as possible to an intensive care unit for hemodynamic monitoring and drug therapy.

J. Treat pulmonary edema. If the patient's blood pressure is only slightly decreased and the major clinical findings suggest pulmonary edema (elevated neck veins, rales, and decreased oxygenation) rather than decreased tissue perfusion (hypotension, clammy skin, etc), small doses of intravenous furosemide (20–40 mg in adults; in children, 0.5–1 mg/kg) or a preload reducing agent (nitroglycerin ointment, 1.5–2 cm [½–1 in] under an occlusive dressing) may be tried. Pay close attention to the effect of these drugs on blood pressure and clinical signs of tissue perfusion.

Disposition

All patients in cardiogenic shock should be hospitalized in an intensive care unit.

OBSTRUCTIVE SHOCK

Obstructive shock results from impaired filling of the ventricles (decreased preload) (Table 3–1) that is severe enough to cause a significant fall in cardiac output. With the exception of acute cardiac tamponade and tension pneumothorax, obstructive disorders are difficult to diagnose and even more difficult to treat in the emergency department. Knowledge of the patient's medical history can be crucial in management. Clues to the specific cause of shock are discussed below.

Cardiac Tamponade
(See also Chapter 28.)

A history of cancer, uremia, or infectious illness should suggest the possibility of pericardial effusion; distended neck veins without evidence of "pump failure" (clear lung fields on chest x-ray, absent S_3 gallop) suggest cardiac tamponade. Pulsus paradoxus, a fall in systolic blood pressure of 12 mm Hg or more during inspiration, occurs in almost every case of cardiac tamponade. A pericardial friction rub may or may not be present. Distant heart sounds, an enlarged cardiac silhouette on chest x-ray, and low voltage on the ECG are additional (but insensitive) clues to the presence of pericardial effusion. Sudden onset of shock in a patient with recent myocardial infarction may be due to rupture of the free ventricular wall that causes cardiac tamponade. If the patient's condition permits, obtain an echocardiogram to confirm the diagnosis and to guide pericardiocentesis. In the desperately ill patient, blind pericardiocentesis (Chapter 46) may be lifesaving. See Chapters 4 and 28 for a more complete discussion of the diagnosis and treatment of cardiac tamponade.

Massive Pulmonary Embolism
(See also Chapter 27.)

Ask about a history of thrombophlebitis, pulmonary emboli, or hypercoagulable state (use of oral contraceptives, pregnancy, family history of thromboembolic disease, cancer). Search for evidence of lower extremity deep venous thrombosis or for some other predisposing factor (lower extremity injury; recent prolonged immobility). Pleuritic chest pain, dyspnea, apprehension, or cough occurs frequently in patients with massive pulmonary embolism; hemoptysis or syncope occurs less commonly. Accentuation of the pulmonary closure sound (P_2) may occur. Massive pulmonary embolism with acute pulmonary hypertension may result in signs of right ventricular overload, eg, jugular venous distention and a right-sided S_3 gallop. The ECG may show evidence of acute right heart strain, eg, R > S in lead V_1, S1Q3T3 pattern (large S wave in lead I, Q wave in lead III, inverted T wave in lead III). Patients with massive pulmonary embolism typically are hypoxemic, and it is difficult to increase the PO_2 even with the administration of 100% oxygen. Attempt to maintain blood pressure with intravenous fluids (an initial bolus of 500–1000 mL of normal saline should be infused rapidly); if the patient fails to respond, give vasopressors as described above. Administration of thrombolytic agents such as streptokinase or tissue plasminogen activator may be tried; however, the prognosis in patients with massive pulmonary embolism is poor. See Chapter 27 for further discussion. Emergency surgery (eg, Trendelenburg procedure) is rarely successful.

Atrial myxoma, mitral thrombus, coarctation of the aorta, obstructive valvular disease, and pulmonary hypertension are rare causes of shock in patients presenting to the emergency department. Tension pneumothorax is discussed in Chapters 6 and 18. Supportive treatment with fluids, vasopressors, and oxygenation should be started as described under Initial Treatment: General Measures, above. Echocardiography and right heart catheterization may help to establish the diagnosis.

DISTRIBUTIVE SHOCK

Distributive shock occurs when distribution of intravascular volume is markedly abnormal as a result of decreased vascular resistance (as occurs in fainting, when blood pools in the venous rather than the arterial portion of the circulation). Cardiac output may be increased, normal, or low in patients with this type of shock. The causes of distributive shock are diverse and include septic shock, anaphylactic shock, and neurogenic shock, which will be discussed below; acute adrenal insufficiency is discussed in Chapter 35. Some drugs and toxins may produce vasodilation and may also result in distributive shock. See Chapter 39 for a discussion of drug overdose and poisoning.

1. SEPTIC SHOCK
(See also Chapter 34.)

Septic shock is usually caused by gram-negative bacteria that invade the bloodstream ("endotoxic shock"), although other bacteria and some fungi may produce a similar syndrome. Septic shock may occur without frank bacteremia if there is extensive local infection (eg, intra-abdominal abscess). Shock also occurs in toxic shock syndrome as a result of absorption of a staphylococcal toxin.

Factors predisposing to development of septic shock include trauma, diabetes, leukemia, severe granulocytopenia, disease of the genitourinary tract, radiation treatment, and treatment with corticosteroids or immunosuppressive agents. Immediate precipitating causes may include surgical or other manipulation of the urinary, biliary, or gynecologic tracts.

Relative hypovolemia develops as a result of pooling of blood in the microcirculation and loss of fluid from the intravascular space because of a generalized increase in capillary permeability. Cardiac function may also be depressed. Peripheral resistance is usually decreased owing to the opening of arteriovenous shunts, and the result is a further decrease in arterial blood pressure.

Diagnosis
Clinical features of shock and infection are present.

A. Systemic Signs: Rigors, fever (hypothermia is noted in 5–10% of patients), petechiae, leukocytosis, or leukopenia with a shift to the left may be noted.

B. Localized Signs: Abdominal tenderness, perirectal abscess, and extensive pneumonia may be present. Localizing symptoms and signs may be absent, however, especially if the patient is immunocompromised, very young, or very old. Typical sites of occult infection include the urinary tract, biliary system, pelvis, retroperitoneum, and perirectal area.

C. Other Signs: Hyperventilation with hypocapnia is common. The presence of infection should be confirmed by microscopic examination, culture, or other definitive test. Samples of body fluids and tissues that may harbor infection should be submitted for culture, including 2 or 3 blood cultures.

In **toxic shock syndrome,** toxins from localized staphylococcal colonization or infection cause severe hypotension or shock associated with a diffuse red rash (which later desquamates) and other symptoms and signs (nausea and vomiting, diarrhea, thrombocytopenia). The majority of cases have occurred within 5 days of onset of a menstrual period in women using tampons; however, any type of staphylococcal infection may produce this syndrome. The clinical diagnosis is supported by recovery of *Staphylococcus aureus* from the vagina, wounds, or elsewhere. Blood cultures are rarely positive. See Chapter 34 for details of treatment.

Treatment

A. Medical Measures:

1. Volume replacement–As in hypovolemic shock, a balanced salt solution should be used for initial fluid replacement. Colloids should not be used, because capillary endothelial permeability is increased in the shock state, which allows colloid solutions to pass into the interstitial space, thus worsening interstitial edema. The amount of fluid administered follows the same guidelines governing fluid replacement in severe hypovolemic shock (see above). In general, 1–2 L given over 30–60 minutes (adult dose; in children, 10–20 mL/kg) will improve blood pressure and urine output; further administration of fluid depends on clinical response (urine output, blood pressure, and pulse) and measurements of atrial filling pressure (central venous pressure or, preferably, pulmonary arterial wedge pressure).

2. Inotropic agents–Give dopamine (3–15 μg/kg/min) if the patient fails to respond to measures that raise central venous or pulmonary capillary wedge pressure to normal levels. Follow the dosage guidelines given in the table on the inside front cover.

3. Antibiotic therapy–Antibiotic treatment should be specific for the causative organism, but the etiologic agent may not be known at the onset of shock. Prompt empirical treatment with antibiotics, using the recommendations in Table 3–6, should be started as soon as cultures of blood and other materials have been obtained.

B. Surgical Measures: Antibiotics and fluid replacement are much less effective if an abscess or other localized source of infection is left undrained. It is therefore critical to identify any source of sepsis as soon as possible, eg, intra-abdominal abscess, biliary obstruction with cholangitis, or any other disorder requiring surgery.

C. Special Measures:

1. Corticosteroids–Recent studies have shown conclusively that administration of pharmacologic doses of glucocorticoids has no beneficial effect in patients with septic shock and may even be harmful. Therefore, high-dose corticosteroids should not be used as adjunctive therapy in septic shock.

2. Heparin–Disseminated intravascular coagulation (Chapter 33) may occur in septic shock. If treatment of septic shock is successful, consumption of coagulation factors usually ceases and rapid regeneration of these factors occurs. If coagulation studies

Table 3–6. Suggested empiric antibiotics in septic shock.

Suspected Site of Infection or Predisposing Factor	Common Pathogens	Suggested Antibiotics[1]
Genitourinary tract	Aerobic gram-negative bacilli (*Escherichia coli, Klebsiella, Proteus, Pseudomonas*); group D streptococci	Ampicillin[2] plus aminoglycoside.[3]
Respiratory tract	*Streptococcus pneumoniae; Staphylococcus aureus;* aerobic gram-negative bacilli; anaerobes	Penicillin G[4] or clindamycin,[5] plus aminoglycoside.[3] Cefoxitin[2] or cefazolin[6] may be substituted for penicillin.
Below the diaphragm Intra-abdominal abscess; decubitus ulcers; pelvic or perirectal abscess	Aerobic gram-negative bacilli; anaerobes (including *Bacteroides fragilis*)	Clindamycin[5] plus aminoglycoside.[3]
Biliary tree	Aerobic gram-negative bacilli; group D streptococci; anaerobes	Ampicillin[2] plus aminoglycoside[3]. (Clindamycin[5] may be added.)
Skin, bone, or joint	*S aureus;* streptococci; aerobic gram-negative bacilli; *Clostridium* or other anaerobes	Nafcillin, oxacillin, or methicillin;[7] aminoglycoside[3] or clindamycin[5] may be added.
Immunocompromised host (immunosuppressive drugs; corticosteroids; cancer)	Usual pathogens as well as higher incidence of aerobic gram-negative bacilli (including *Pseudomonas*); staphylococci; yeasts (especially *Candida albicans*)	Ticarcillin[8] plus aminoglycoside.[3] (Cefotaxime[9] may be added.)
Unknown	*S pneumoniae; S aureus; Neisseria meningitidis,* aerobic gram-negative rods	Ampicillin[3] plus aminoglycoside.[3] (Nafcillin[7] may be added.)

[1]Doses are for patients with normal renal and hepatic function.
[2]Ampicillin: give 150–200 mg/kg/d intravenously in 4 divided doses.
[3]Gentamicin or tobramycin: give 5–6 mg/kg/d intravenously in 3 divided doses.
[4]Penicillin G: give 20–24 million units intravenously in 6 divided doses.
[5]Clindamycin: give 30–40 mg/kg/d intravenously in 3 divided doses.
[6]Cefazolin: give 100 mg/kg/d intravenously in 3 divided doses.
[7]Nafcillin, oxacillin, or methicillin: give 150 mg/kg/d intravenously in 4 divided doses.
[8]Ticarcillin, piperacillin, or mezlocillin: give 250 mg/kg/d intravenously in 4 divided doses.
[9]Cefotaxime: give 200 mg/kg/d (up to 12 g) intravenously in 4 divided doses.

confirm the presence of persistent intravascular coagulation (prolonged prothrombin and partial thromboplastin times, decreased number of platelets, depressed fibrinogen levels, and the presence of fibrin degradation products) *and if there is significant bleeding,* give heparin, 100 units/kg intravenously to start, followed by 10–40 units/kg/h by continuous intravenous administration (infusion pump preferred). Response to heparin is indicated by slowing of bleeding and a rise within 12 hours of the levels of fibrinogen and factors V and VII. Platelet counts may rise at a slower rate. Discontinue heparin therapy when the cause of disseminated intravascular coagulation has been corrected and coagulation factors have been restored to hemostatic levels.

3. Naloxone–Preliminary animal and clinical trials have shown that administration of narcotic antagonists such as naloxone (Narcan, others) may reverse the hypotension associated with septic shock. Confirmatory studies are pending, and the use of naloxone in septic shock is considered investigational. No adverse effects have been reported. One recommended dosage schedule is 1 mg/kg as an intravenous bolus, followed by 0.7 mg/kg/h by continuous intravenous infusion if the patient responds to the initial dose (increased blood pressure, etc).

Disposition

All patients should be hospitalized, preferably in an intensive care unit.

2. ANAPHYLACTIC SHOCK

Anaphylactic shock is a catastrophic and frequently fatal type of allergic reaction that occurs within minutes after parenteral (rarely oral) administration of drugs or nonhuman proteins, including foods, sera, or venoms. In cases obviously caused by injections of drugs or sera, there is seldom any reason for delayed treatment.

Diagnosis

Symptoms and signs include marked apprehension, generalized urticaria or edema, back pain, a choking sensation, cough, bronchospasm, or laryngeal edema. In severe cases, hypotension, loss of consciousness, dilatation of the pupils, incontinence, and convulsions may be present; sudden death may occur.

Three modes of presentation of anaphylaxis (based on the most conspicuous presenting features) are recognized; however, any combination of these may occur: **(1)** urticaria or angioedema that may be associated with upper airway obstruction and laryngeal edema, **(2)** bronchospasm, or **(3)** vascular collapse (ie, severe hypotension).

Treatment

Begin treatment as soon as anaphylaxis is suspected; *do not wait until it is fully developed.*

A. Position: Place the conscious patient in a comfortable position, and ensure unimpeded ventilation. The unconscious patient should be placed supine, in a level or slightly head-down position (do this as quickly as possible).

B. Airway: Keep the airway open (Chapter 1), and give supplemental oxygen by mask or nasal prongs at a rate of 5–10 L/min. If the patient is not breathing, assist ventilation with a bag-mask until endotracheal intubation can be performed (Chapters 1 and 46). If equipment for insertion of an endotracheal tube is not available or if intubation is unsuccessful because of airway obstruction by laryngeal edema, cricothyrotomy (Chapter 46) may be necessary.

C. Intravenous Access: Insert an intravenous catheter, and begin infusion of a balanced salt solution or normal saline, 0.5–1 L over 30 minutes (adult dose; in children, 5–15 mL/kg), with further administration governed by blood pressure and urine output.

D. Drugs: Epinephrine is the drug of choice for emergency use and should be given as soon as anaphylactic shock is suspected or diagnosed. It may be necessary to supplement epinephrine with antihistaminic drugs or corticosteroids and—in intense bronchospasm—with intravenous aminophylline.

1. Aqueous epinephrine–For mild anaphylaxis, give epinephrine, 0.3–0.5 mg (0.3–0.5 mL of 1:1000 solution) intramuscularly (adult dose; for children, give 0.01 mL/kg/dose up to a maximum of 0.4 mL/dose). An additional 0.2–0.3 mL of 1:1000 solution can be infiltrated around the sting or injection site (with or without a tourniquet proximally) to delay absorption of antigen. For severe anaphylaxis, epinephrine should be administered intravenously or via an endotracheal tube; give 1–5 mL of 1:10,000 solution. Repeat every 10 minutes if symptoms continue or recur. A continuous infusion may be necessary in some patients. Add 1 mg of a 1:1000 solution of epinephrine to 250 mL of 5% dextrose in water (4 μg/mL); begin the infusion at a rate of 1 μg/min (0.1 μg/kg/min in children), and increase up to 4 μg/min as needed.

2. Diphenhydramine–Give diphenhydramine (Benadryl, many others), 50 mg intravenously (2 mg/kg for children) or intramuscularly, early in treatment.

3. Glucocorticoid–A soluble glucocorticoid preparation should be given as an adjunct to epinephrine. Give hydrocortisone sodium succinate, 100–250 mg intravenously; or methylprednisolone sodium succinate, 50–100 mg intravenously. The total dose depends on the severity of anaphylaxis; the drug may be repeated at intervals of 1–4 hours as indicated by the patient's clinical condition.

4. Beta-agonist aerosol–If bronchospasm is present, give metaproterenol or other beta-agonist inhalant solutions, 0.1–0.5 mL in 3–5 mL of sterile saline, by nebulizer every 30–60 minutes.

5. Aminophylline–For severe bronchospasm, aminophylline may also be of limited benefit; give 6 mg/kg as a loading dose in 50–100 mL of saline by intravenous infusion over 30 minutes. Follow with a maintenance infusion (Chapter 27).

Prevention

Inquire carefully about any history of drug allergy before giving drugs. In drunk, unconscious, or obtunded patients, search for a card, bracelet, or necklace specifying drug allergies or medical conditions (eg, diabetes) requiring special attention. Be cautious when administering parenteral medications to patients with a history of drug allergy. If there is a history of previous reaction to the agent to be injected, use an alternative drug whenever possible. Give intravenous injections slowly, and observe individuals who have received parenteral medication for at least 30 minutes after injection. Patients with a history of anaphylactic reactions to insect venoms or other environmental agents that cannot be easily avoided should be prescribed a kit with epinephrine for self-administration and should be advised to carry it at times of high risk of exposure.

Disposition

Recurrent episodes of anaphylaxis may occur 12–24 hours after the initial episode; therefore, patients who have experienced life-threatening anaphylaxis should be hospitalized for observation and treatment. Patients who have shown only mild manifestations of anaphylaxis (eg, urticaria) that have resolved with treatment may be discharged from the emergency department after treatment (Chapter 40); follow-up should follow the principles outlined in Chapter 40.

3. NEUROGENIC SHOCK

Neurogenic shock is due to failure of vasomotor regulation that results in pooling of blood in dilated capacitance vessels and a subsequent fall in blood pressure. True neurogenic shock should be distinguished from vasovagal syncope (Chapter 11). Although the mechanism of hypotension is similar in both conditions—sudden failure of vasomotor regulation—the condition is not prolonged enough in vasovagal syncope to produce diffuse tissue ischemia and clinical features of shock.

Neurogenic shock is rare. It is most commonly due to traumatic quadriplegia or paraplegia ("spinal shock"), although a similar syndrome can be induced by high spinal anesthesia and is occasionally seen in severe Guillain-Barré syndrome and other neuropathies. In patients with traumatic spine injuries, it is important to remember that *hypovolemic shock* (due to associated injuries) is still the most common cause of shock and must be presumed to be present until proved otherwise.

Diagnosis

The symptoms and signs of neurogenic shock are similar to those of hypovolemic shock. Signs of neurologic disease often associated with neurogenic shock are also present (eg, traumatic quadriplegia or paraplegia).

Treatment

Place the patient supine, and give oxygen. If blood pressure and peripheral perfusion are not rapidly restored, begin other measures.

The treatment of choice is volume replacement with crystalloid solution to "fill up" the dilated capacitance vessels. For adults, give 1 L (for children, 10–20 mL/kg) of crystalloid solution intravenously over 20–40 minutes (depending on the severity of shock). An intravenous vasopressor agent with alpha-agonist activity, such as dopamine in high doses (> 10–20 µg/kg/min) or phenylephrine (10 mg in 250 mL of normal saline at a rate of 10 µg/min [25 mL/min]) may be started to restore the tone of capacitance vessels. Phenylephrine should be given only to patients who have no other disorder, such as a ruptured spleen, that would contraindicate the use of pressor agents.

Disposition

All patients should be hospitalized, preferably in an intensive care unit.

REFERENCES

Barach EM et al: Epinephrine for treatment of anaphylactic shock. JAMA 1984;251:2118.

Doyle WP, O'Rourke RA: Pathophysiology and management of cardiogenic shock. Curr Probl Cardiol 1983;7:6.

Greenfield RH, Bessen HA, Henneman PL: Effect of crystalloid infusion on hematocrit and intravascular volume in healthy, non-bleeding subjects. Ann Emerg Med 1989;18:51.

Gross D et al: Is hypertonic saline resuscitation "safe" in uncontrolled hemorrhagic shock? J Trauma 1988;28:751.

Hodge D III, Fleisher G: Pediatric catheter flow rates. Am J Emerg Med 1985;3:403.

Kabeck KR, Sanders AB, Meislin HW: MAST suit update. JAMA 1984;252:2598.

Mattox KL et al: Prospective MAST study in 911 patients. J Trauma 1989;29:1104.

Mazzoni MC et al: The efficacy of iso- and hyperosmotic fluids as volume expanders in fixed-volume and uncontrolled hemorrhage. Ann Emerg Med 1990;19:350.

McCabe WR, Olans RN: Shock in gram-negative bacteremia: Predisposing factors, pathophysiology, and treatment. Page 121 in: *Current Clinical Topics in Infectious Disease.* Remington JS, Swartz MN (editors). McGraw-Hill, 1980.

Parker MM, Parrillo JE: Septic shock: Hemodynamics and pathogenesis. JAMA 1983;250:3324.

Parrish GA, Turkewitz D, Skiendzielewski JJ: Intraosseous infusions in the emergency department. Am J Emerg Med 1986;4:59.

Rackow EC et al: Fluid resuscitation in circulatory shock: A comparison of the cardiorespiratory effects of albumin, hetastarch, and saline solutions in patients with hypovolemic and septic shock. Crit Care Med 1983;11:839.

Rock P et al: Efficacy and safety of naloxone in septic shock. Crit Care Med 1985;13:28.

Sheffer AL: Anaphylaxis. J Allergy Clin Immunol 1985;75:227.

Todd JK et al: Corticosteroid therapy for patients with toxic shock syndrome. JAMA 1984;252:3399.

Tranbaugh RF, Lewis FR: Crystalloid versus colloid for fluid resuscitation of hypovolemic patients. Adv Shock Res 1983;9:203.

Trauma management: State of the art. Proceedings of the 1986 American College of Emergency Physicians Winter Symposium, March 17–20, 1986, Orlando, Florida. Ann Emerg Med 1986;15:1381. [Entire issue.]

Wayne MA, Macdonald SC: Clinical evaluation of the antishock trouser: Retrospective analysis of five years of experience. Ann Emerg Med 1983;12:342.

4

The Multiply Injured Patient

Donald D. Trunkey, MD

IMMEDIATE MANAGEMENT OF LIFE-THREATENING PROBLEMS (See algorithm.)

PREPARE FOR PATIENT'S ARRIVAL

Obtain Information About Patient's Status

If radio contact with the emergency transport technicians is available, learn as much as possible about the circumstances of the accident and the patient's status. This information will indicate whether major trauma is present and will guide preparations for the patient's arrival. Circumstances of the accident that suggest major trauma include information such as

motor vehicle accident at a speed of more than 50 mph, a fall of more than 15 feet, ejection from the vehicle, prolonged extrication time, or associated deaths. Important facts about the patient's status include such information as blood pressure below 100 mm Hg; inadequate or labored respirations; multiple fractures; penetrating injuries to the head, neck, or torso; depressed sensorium; burns over more than 25% of the body surface area; or impending loss of a limb.

Injury-scoring instruments, such as the Glasgow Coma Score, Trauma Score, or Revised Trauma Score (similar to the Trauma Score but without capillary refill and respiratory expansion), may be used to objectively quantify the degree of injury (Fig 4–1). The threshold for major trauma is lower in pediatric, geriatric, and obstetric patients.

If it becomes apparent that your emergency depart-

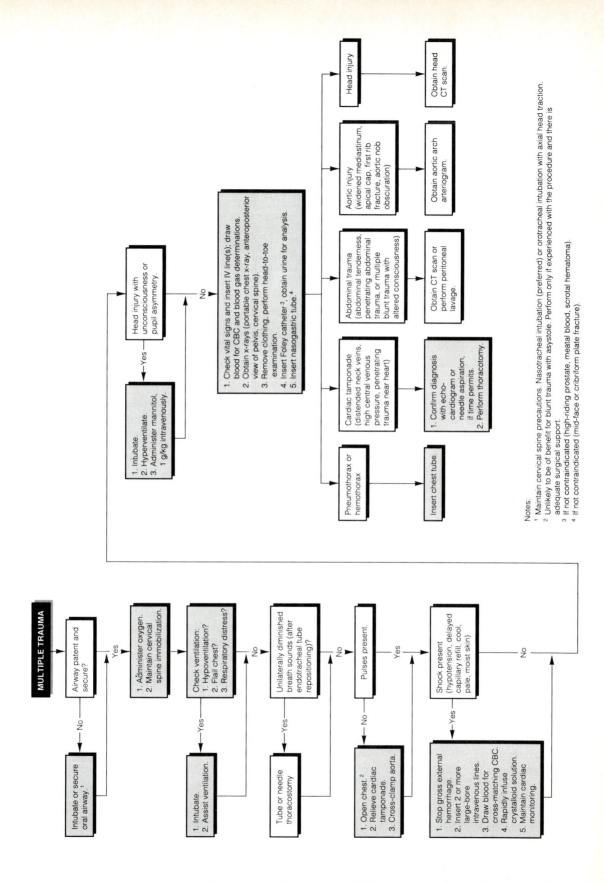

MULTIPLE TRAUMA

Airway patent and secure?

Intubate or secure oral airway. [1]

1. Administer oxygen.
2. Maintain cervical spine immobilization.

Check ventilation:
1. Hypoventilation?
2. Flail chest?
3. Respiratory distress?

1. Intubate.
2. Assist ventilation.

Unilaterally diminished breath sounds (after endotracheal tube repositioning)?

Tube or needle thoracostomy

Pulses present.

1. Open chest. [2]
2. Relieve cardiac tamponade.
3. Cross-clamp aorta.

Shock present (hypotension, delayed capillary refill, cool, pale, moist skin)

1. Stop gross external hemorrhage.
2. Insert 2 or more large-bore intravenous lines.
3. Draw blood for cross-matching CBC.
4. Rapidly infuse crystalloid solution.
5. Maintain cardiac monitoring.

Head injury with unconsciousness or pupil asymmetry.

1. Intubate.
2. Hyperventilate.
3. Administer mannitol, 1 g/kg intravenously.

1. Check vital signs and insert IV line(s); draw blood for CBC and blood gas determinations.
2. Obtain x-rays (portable chest x-ray, anteroposterior view of pelvis, cervical spine).
3. Remove clothing, perform head-to-toe examination.
4. Insert Foley catheter [3], obtain urine for analysis.
5. Insert nasogastric tube. [4]

Pneumothorax or hemothorax

Insert chest tube.

Cardiac tamponade (distended neck veins, high central venous pressure, penetrating trauma near heart)

1. Confirm diagnosis with echo-cardiogram or needle aspiration, if time permits.
2. Perform thoracotomy.

Abdominal trauma (abdominal tenderness, penetrating abdominal trauma, or multiple blunt trauma with altered consciousness)

Obtain CT scan or perform peritoneal lavage.

Aortic injury (widened mediastinum, apical cap, first rib fracture, aortic nob obscuration)

Obtain aortic arch arteriogram.

Head injury

Obtain head CT scan.

Notes:

[1] Maintain cervical spine precautions. Nasotracheal intubation (preferred) or orotracheal intubation with axial head traction.

[2] Unlikely to be of benefit for blunt trauma with asystole. Perform only if experienced with the procedure and there is adequate surgical support.

[3] If not contraindicated (high-riding prostate, meatal blood, scrotal hematoma).

[4] If not contraindicated (mid-face or cribriform plate fracture).

A Glasgow Coma Scale

Eye opening	Spontaneous	4
	To verbal command	3
	To pain	2
	None	1
Verbal responsiveness	Oriented	5
	Confused	4
	Inappropriate words	3
	Incomprehensible sounds	2
	None	1
Motor response	Obeys	6
	Localizes	5
	Withdraws	4
	Abnormal flexion	3
	Abnormal extension	2
	None	1

Total: _____

B Trauma Score

Glasgow Coma Scale total	14–15	5
	11–13	4
	8–10	3
	5–7	2
	3–4	1
Respiration rate (breaths/min)	> 35	2
	25–35	3
	10–24	4
	1–9	1
	None	0
Respiratory expansion	Normal	1
	Shallow	0
	Retracts or absent	0
Blood pressure	> 89	4
	70–89	3
	50–69	2
	0–49	1
	No pulse	0
Capillary refill	< 2 seconds	2
	> 2 seconds	1
	None	0

Total: _____

Figure 4–1. Trauma score used to quantify degree of injury. **A.** Determine total on Glasgow Coma Scale. **B.** Convert Glasgow Coma Scale total to trauma score points and determine trauma score total.

ment is not equipped to provide adequate care for a patient, instruct the emergency transport technicians to go to a trauma center if one is available in the area.

Organize Staff & Equipment

Instruct the nursing staff to prepare the resuscitation room (eg, have chest tubes and surgical supplies available; make sure intravenous solutions are prepared, warmed, and ready for administration; set up and turn on suctioning equipment and oxygen delivery systems [eg, Ambu bag]; have a long spine board in place). Activate the trauma team or contact medical personnel and ask them to come to the emergency department (eg, surgeons, anesthesiologists, respiratory therapists, x-ray or CT scan technicians). Ask them to prepare the necessary equipment (eg, bring a portable x-ray machine and film cassettes for anteroposterior chest and pelvic views and a lateral cervical spine view; turn on CT scanner). Inform the operating room staff or intensive care staff that a trauma patient is expected so that they can call for additional personnel, if necessary.

Assign specific tasks to the emergency department resuscitation team so that the resuscitation can proceed smoothly. Designate one person to be the team leader, another to provide intravenous access, and another to perform other procedures. In some emergency departments, there is a preestablished "trauma protocol."

Proceed in Organized Manner When Patient Arrives

Maintain order, and keep noise to a minimum so that a clear report can be obtained from the emergency transport technicians. This report should include a brief history of the events; extent of damage to the vehicle; whether or not a seat belt was in place; whether loss of consciousness occurred; caliber of the weapon; and physical assessment, most recent status, and vital signs of the patient.

Transfer the patient from the ambulance stretcher to the emergency department stretcher, taking care to maintain cervical spine and back immobilization (in the case of multiple blunt injuries). Secure the patient to a long spine board with neck rolls and tape. Proceed with the initial survey of the patient's status at the same time as other medical personnel are performing their assigned tasks. Placing a chest x-ray cassette on the trauma gurney before the patient arrives will help integrate chest radiography into the early stages of care.

ESTABLISH AIRWAY

Clear Oropharynx

Turn the head to the side unless there is concern for a cervical spine injury, in which case axial orientation should be maintained (logroll the patient).

In the *unconscious* victim, insert a gloved finger into the mouth, and sweep out all clots, debris, and any fragments of bone, teeth, or vomitus in the upper airway. In the *conscious* victim, use a tonsil sucker to clear most of the obvious debris.

Open the Airway
(See also Chapter 1.)

Opening of the airway is best accomplished by lifting the chin and tilting the head (see Fig 1–1). If cervical spine injury is suspected, keep the neck immobilized, and open the airway by placing the fingers behind the angle of the jaw and displacing the mandible forward (chin lift). Occasionally, it may be necessary to apply a towel clip to the tongue and draw it forward in order to establish the airway. Oropharyngeal or nasopharyngeal tubes may be useful to maintain a patent airway; however, they should only be used in *unconscious* victims, since they can induce vomiting in the conscious patient.

Maneuvers to open the airway may be all that is required to ensure adequate ventilation in a conscious, spontaneously breathing patient, although supplemental oxygen, 2–10 L/min by nasal prongs or mask, may be used until adequacy of ventilation is confirmed by arterial blood gas measurements.

If the patient is not breathing or if respiratory efforts are inadequate or the airway is unprotected by a gag reflex (eg, central nervous system depression, flail chest), maintain ventilation with oxygen delivered by a bag-mask combination at a high flow rate (10 L/min) until tracheal intubation can be performed. In patients with suspected cervical spine injuries who are breathing spontaneously, it is safer to perform nasotracheal intubation, since the neck need not be extended for this procedure (Chapter 46). If nasotracheal intubation is not possible, orotracheal intubation may be performed with the neck carefully stabilized (rigid cervical collar, tape, neck rolls, and an assistant to provide axial head traction), although this method carries the risk of spinal cord injury in the presence of an unstable cervical spine. Cricothyrotomy alternatively produces no neck extension but may be difficult for an inexperienced person to perform (Chapter 46). If there are laryngeal fractures or severe maxillofacial injuries, cricothyrotomy may be the only method of airway control possible.

Newer methods of airway control have also been used successfully, including nasotracheal intubation over a fiberoptic laryngoscope, "blind" orotracheal intubation using a ligated stylet (transillumination appears at the anterior neck when the tube tip passes the glottis), and retrograde intubation (which involves passing the endotracheal tube along a guide wire inserted through the cricothyroid membrane and directed cephalad through the oropharynx). If the airway is lacerated and exposed in the neck, intubate directly at the site of injury.

Establish Adequacy of Ventilation

The adequacy of ventilation should be confirmed by inspecting the chest wall for adequate expansion; noting labored breathing, flail segments, sucking wounds, etc; and auscultating for the presence of symmetric breath sounds.

If breath sounds are unilaterally diminished and the patient is intubated, withdraw the endotracheal tube 2–3 cm in case the tip is residing in a main stem bronchus, and recheck the breath sounds. Persistent diminished breath sounds imply pneumothorax. If the patient is hypotensive, in shock, or laboring to breathe, perform a tube thoracostomy immediately. Should a delay exist before this can occur, decompress the chest with a 14-gauge Angiocath or other catheter-clad needle inserted in the fourth intercostal space at the anterior axial line. A patient with diminished breath sounds who is stable may await a chest x-ray for confirmation first.

Treat a sucking chest wound by sealing the wound with an occlusive dressing (eg, petrolatum-impregnated dressing) at 3 points and then performing a tube thoracostomy (not through the chest wall defect). Adequacy of ventilation can be confirmed with arterial blood gas determinations.

CHECK CARDIAC ACTIVITY
(Feel for Pulse)

Pulse Absent

If spontaneous cardiac activity is not detected by palpation of the carotid artery, perform immediate thoracotomy, and assist circulation by direct cardiac massage (see Cardiac Tamponade, below). In the multiply injured patient without a detectable pulse, there is a high probability of severe hypovolemia, cardiac tamponade, or tension pneumothorax. Closed chest compression cannot produce effective cardiac output in the presence of hypovolemia or cardiac tamponade. Emergency thoracotomy also allows access to the pericardium for relief of tamponade and to the descending aorta, which can be cross-clamped with a vascular clamp or with the hand. Aortic cross-clamping controls massive hemorrhage below the diaphragm and preserves perfusion of the 2 most critical organs: the heart and the brain. In contrast to patients who have suffered penetrating trauma, the prognosis for victims of blunt chest trauma without detectable cardiac activity is extremely poor. Emergency thoracotomy is *not* indicated if there is obvious brain injury.

Pulse Present

If pulses are present, proceed to examine the patient for shock.

STOP OBVIOUS
EXTERNAL HEMORRHAGE

Obvious external hemorrhage should be stopped by gentle compression with sterile dressings. Bleeding vessels should not be indiscriminately clamped. Rarely, exsanguinating arterial hemorrhage from an extremity will not abate with compression. A blood pressure cuff inflated proximal to the wound will serve as an effective tourniquet temporarily until surgical control of the bleeding can be achieved. However, except as a last resort, tourniquets should be avoided.

EXAMINE FOR SHOCK

Shock is defined as inadequate perfusion of tissue and is further classified as mild, moderate, or severe, based primarily on clinical criteria (see Table 3–2).

Cool, pale skin; diaphoresis; delayed capillary re fill (>2 seconds return from thenar eminence blanch); and tachycardia are reliable indicators of shock. Cerebral insufficiency, hypotension, and oliguria are presumed to be due to shock until proved otherwise. The physician should not assume that perfusion is good on the basis of supine pulse and blood pressure alone, because these 2 signs may change only late in shock, particularly in healthy young adults—who are the most common victims of multiple trauma.

PERFORM BRIEF
NEUROLOGIC ASSESSMENT

Quickly assess the level of responsiveness to determine if the patient is **awake and alert;** responds to **verbal stimuli** with eye opening or following of commands; responds to **painful stimuli** (eg, sternal rub, muscle or tendon squeeze) by appropriate movement, localization, or posturing; or is **unresponsive.**

Assess the pupils for symmetry, size, and reactivity. An asymmetrically enlarged pupil in an unresponsive patient may imply transtentorial herniation and should be treated with endotracheal intubation, hyperventilation, and other measures to reduce intracranial pressure (Chapter 16).

TREATMENT OF THE INJURED
PATIENT WITH SHOCK
(See also Chapter 3.)

Evaluation and treatment must proceed rapidly and simultaneously. Shock in the traumatized patient is usually due to hypovolemia from hemorrhage; cardiac tamponade, tension pneumothorax, and brain injury may contribute to shock or (rarely) may cause shock without concurrent volume loss.

Establish Secure
Intravenous Access
(See Chapter 46.)

Multiple large-bore catheters should be inserted in patients with profound shock. Ideally, one line should monitor central venous pressure.

A. Percutaneous Approach: Insert a large-bore catheter ($\geq$ 16-gauge) into a femoral or antecubital vein. *Caution:* Avoid subclavian and internal jugular lines initially, since the subclavian and jugular veins are flaccid in the shock state. Insertion of the lines is therefore difficult, and there is increased risk of pneumothorax and laceration of the subclavian or carotid artery.

B. Cutdown Approach: Either the saphenous vein in the ankle or the antecubital vein in the arm can be used. A large-bore catheter (eg, pediatric feeding tube or intravenous tubing) should be inserted into the vein.

Take Specimens
for Laboratory Tests

Obtain blood specimens for hematocrit or CBC, typing and cross-matching for at least 4 units of whole blood, electrolyte measurements, and renal function tests. If the history suggests possible substance abuse (alcohol, opiates, etc), samples of blood and urine should be submitted for toxicology studies.

Administer Fluids

Begin intravenous infusion of crystalloid solution (balanced salt solution). Up to 2 L of crystalloid solution should be given to support intravascular volume before blood is given. Only rarely is blood that is type-specific but not cross-matched required initially (eg, patient with preexisting severe anemia or very rapid hemorrhage). In such an event, administer O blood initially until type-specific or cross-matched blood is available. Patients in profound shock should receive fluids administered by infusion pump or pressure bag.

Further Management

A. *Keep the neck immobilized if cervical injury is suspected* (Chapter 21). Portable cervical spine x-rays can be obtained once the patient is stable.

B. Remove all of the patient's clothing immediately, and examine the entire body on all sides for injuries. Logroll the patient (ie, roll the patient from side to side, keeping the head and entire trunk aligned as one unit) if cervical spine injury is suspected.

C. Obtain arterial blood gas samples. Arterial blood pH and bicarbonate values are good indicators of the degree of hypoperfusion; PO_2 and PCO_2 monitor the adequacy of ventilation and pulmonary parenchymal function. Continuously monitor oxygen saturation by pulse oximetry, if available.

D. Obtain an ECG, and maintain cardiac monitoring.

E. Insert a urinary catheter (Chapter 46) in all patients with shock. Measurement of urinary output aids in the diagnosis of shock and monitors the effectiveness of resuscitation. Urinary output below 0.5 mL/kg/h indicates significant hypovolemia. Urinalysis is essential for evaluation of renal trauma. A urine sample can be tested for the presence of hemoglobin with a urine test reagent strip. False-positive results may occur, however, because of the sensitivity of the reagent and the cross-reactivity with iodine-containing cleaning solutions. Therefore, a microscopic evaluation for hematuria is essential. *Caution:* Do not insert a urethral catheter if there is obvious injury to the external genitalia, obvious urethral bleeding, scrotal hematomas, a malpositioned or high-riding prostate on rectal examination, or difficulty in passing the catheter (Chapter 20).

F. Seek the underlying cause of shock while performing the procedures discussed above. In the multiply injured patient, hemorrhage is the commonest cause of shock. Cardiac tamponade, tension pneumothorax, or head injury may worsen hemorrhagic shock, but head injury alone rarely causes shock.

G. Insert a nasogastric tube. (If a cribriform plate fracture is suspected, or if there are massive maxillofacial fractures, insert the tube via the orogastric route.)

H. Obtain surgical consultation as soon as possible.

Persistent or Worsening Shock

Persistent shock or shock that worsens despite administration of fluids indicates either continuing occult hemorrhage or another cause of shock.

A. Obtain a chest x-ray to diagnose or rule out tension pneumothorax and hemothorax. Treat these conditions if present.

B. If renal trauma is suspected, perform emergency urography. Give 90 mL (adult dose) of water-soluble urographic contrast medium intravenously over about 5 minutes. Obtain a supine abdominal x-ray 5–20 minutes after injection; several films during this interval are preferable if the patient's condition permits.

C. Consider cardiac tamponade as a potential cause of persistent shock if there is penetrating trauma near the heart or blunt trauma to the anterior chest. If tamponade is probable, treat with pericardiocentesis or, preferably, thoracotomy.

D. Perform an immediate laparotomy to control intra-abdominal hemorrhage.

E. Consider application of a pneumatic antishock garment (eg, MAST; see Chapters 3 and 46) if laparotomy cannot be performed immediately or if transfer is necessary and no contraindication exists. MAST may effectively control hemorrhage below the diaphragm, but its use has not been shown to improve survival and complications have been reported (eg, compartment syndrome). If a patient arrives with

MAST in place, it should be deflated slowly and only after the patient has been stabilized hemodynamically. Otherwise, sudden deterioration may occur.

TREATMENT OF THE INJURED PATIENT WITHOUT SHOCK

If the patient arrives in the emergency department with shock that resolves with administration of fluids, or if the patient arrives in stable condition, the situation is less urgent and a more thorough evaluation can be performed. The evaluation should proceed in an orderly fashion so that nothing is overlooked.

Immediate Measures

A. Check vital signs, including (whenever possible) pulse and blood pressure with the patient sitting and standing if readings with the patient supine are normal and there is no back or neck injury.

B. Insert a large-bore percutaneous intravenous catheter ($\geq$ 16-gauge). Avoid inserting a catheter into an extremity that is obviously injured.

C. Send blood for CBC and typing and cross-matching to reserve blood in the blood bank. Reserve samples of blood and urine for toxicology screening, if indicated.

D. Obtain portable cervical spine x-rays before moving a patient with suspected cervical spine injury.

Examine the Patient

A. Remove all of the patient's clothing.

B. Logroll the patient from side to side and look for injury on all sides. (Logrolling is not a guarantee that the spine will maintain axial alignment. Studies on cadavers with unstable spinal injuries have demonstrated considerable subluxation during the logroll. Extreme caution should be exercised if a spinal injury is suspected.)

C. Examine the patient thoroughly. Be sure to examine scalp, perineum, gluteal folds, and all bones and joints. Perform a rectal examination to evaluate the tone of the anal sphincter, look for a high-riding prostate gland, and assess the possibility of occult gastrointestinal tract bleeding.

Laboratory Tests & Special Examinations

A. Urinalysis is mandatory. Try to obtain urine without bladder catheterization. Test the urine for blood using a test strip; if positive, send a specimen for microscopic analysis. In the setting of trauma, even microscopic hematuria may indicate significant genitourinary tract trauma (Chapter 20). Serum electrolyte and blood glucose determinations, renal function tests, and arterial blood gas measurements are often helpful.

B. X-rays are obtained as indicated on the basis of physical examination and history. A chest x-ray should be obtained on every patient. In most cases, an anteroposterior view of the pelvis and complete cervical spine films are routinely obtained as well.

C. CT scans and arteriography are also useful in evaluating the trauma patient. Table 4–1 lists the indications for arteriography. CT scanning is particularly useful in evaluating the abdomen for intra-abdominal or retroperitoneal bleeding, for the head, for areas of the vertebral column and spine, and for facial bones.

EMERGENCY TREATMENT OF SPECIFIC DISORDERS

FLAIL CHEST
(See also Chapters 5 and 18.)

Diagnosis
Flail chest is easily diagnosed by the paradoxical motion of a portion of the rib cage (inward with inhalation and outward with exhalation).

Treatment
Assist ventilation with a bag-mask combination; endotracheal intubation need not be performed immediately if arterial blood gas levels are satisfactory ($PO_2 > 65$ mm Hg, $PCO_2 < 44$ mm Hg, $O_2 \geq 90\%$) (Chapter 18). Give oxygen as indicated.

Disposition
Hospitalize the patient immediately. If arterial blood gas abnormalities are present or if the flail segment is large, hospitalize the patient in an intensive care unit.

Table 4–1. Indications for arteriography following trauma.

Neck injuries—zones I and III (see Fig 32–3 and Chapter 32 for details)
Chest injuries
    Obscuring of aortic shadow or aortopulmonary window
    Widening of mediastinum
    Fracture of first rib
    Deviation of trachea to the right
    Apical cap
Abdominal injuries
    Nonvisualizing kidney on urography
    Pelvic fractures requiring more than 8 units of blood
All penetrating wounds of extremities near major vessels
Knee dislocation
All fractures associated with abnormal pulses

TENSION PNEUMOTHORAX

Tension pneumothorax interferes with venous return to the heart and thus decreases cardiac output and perfusion. Oxygenation is also impaired; the combination is quickly lethal.

Diagnosis
Tension pneumothorax is manifested by respiratory distress, distended neck veins, contralateral shift of the trachea, and asymmetry of breath sounds and percussion tympany. Chest x-ray confirms the diagnosis or detects more subtle and unsuspected cases.

Profound shock and cardiac arrest may be refractory to usual treatment unless tension pneumothorax is relieved.

Treatment
Tension pneumothorax may be treated on a temporary basis by inserting a 14-gauge needle into the fourth intercostal space of the involved hemithorax (anterior axillary line). A rush of air confirms the diagnosis. If tension pneumothorax is due to an open wound, open the wound with a finger or clamp to release trapped air, and then cover it with petrolatum-impregnated gauze. Definitive treatment is tube thoracostomy performed as quickly as possible (Chapter 46).

Disposition
All patients should be hospitalized.

CARDIAC TAMPONADE
(See also Chapters 18 and 28.)

Cardiac tamponade interferes with diastolic filling of the heart and causes inadequate cardiac output and perfusion. It may progress rapidly.

Diagnosis
The key to diagnosis is the combination of shock and distended neck veins. The neck veins may not be distended initially if tamponade is accompanied by untreated hemorrhagic shock.

A. Penetrating Injury: Suspect cardiac tamponade in any patient with penetrating trauma to one of the hemithoraces. However, remember that with penetrating trauma (and especially with gunshot injuries), injury to the heart may occur even with remote wounds.

B. Blunt Trauma: Blunt anterior chest trauma occasionally causes tamponade, particularly in steering wheel injuries. Clinical findings may be delayed, and associated myocardial contusion is common.

Treatment
A. For the Patient Not at Point of Death: If cardiac tamponade is suspected before the patient is

at the point of death, an emergency echocardiogram can be useful to confirm the diagnosis and guide pericardiocentesis. Pericardiocentesis (Chapter 46) may be helpful in temporarily treating the patient, but it is not definitive treatment for posttraumatic tamponade.

B. For the Patient at Point of Death: If shock is rapidly progressive despite therapy or if cardiac arrest occurs from tamponade, perform immediate emergency thoracotomy (Chapter 46) with minimal preparation of the chest in order to decompress the pericardium.

Disposition

Immediate hospitalization and surgery are required.

MASSIVE HEMORRHAGE

Diagnosis

A. Obvious Sources of Blood Loss: External sources of hemorrhage are usually obvious. *Be sure to examine the patient's back.* Serial hematocrit readings are useful to determine the extent of blood loss.

B. Hidden Sources of Blood Loss: In most cases, serial hematocrit determinations must be obtained to document persistent internal bleeding. Rising serial white blood cell counts may be due to peritoneal irritation caused by blood in the abdomen. Possible internal sources of blood loss are as follows:

1. Thorax–Each hemithorax may contain up to 2 L of blood. For this reason, a quick upright or lateral decubitus chest x-ray should always be obtained before surgery is performed. For patients who are at the point of death, a supine film will suffice.

2. Abdomen–The abdomen is another common area of hidden blood loss. Distention is a late and unreliable sign. Intra-abdominal hemorrhage must be assumed to be present in any patient in shock who has a normal chest x-ray and no external signs of significant bleeding. Diagnostic peritoneal lavage (Chapter 46) may be helpful if positive; a negative test does not exclude the possibility of intra-abdominal bleeding.

3. Retroperitoneum–Bleeding in the retroperitoneum cannot be diagnosed with routine studies and is usually discovered at laparotomy. CT scan is helpful diagnostically if the patient's condition is stable enough to permit this delay.

4. Pelvis–The pelvis can conceal a large amount of blood, and hemorrhagic shock is a common sequela of pelvic fracture.

5. Thigh–The thigh may contain 3–4 L of blood after a major fracture or crush injury.

Treatment

A. Direct Pressure: Obvious external bleeding can usually be controlled with direct pressure. Tourniquets are rarely indicated except in the case of traumatic amputation.

B. Pneumatic Antishock Garment: A pneumatic antishock (eg, MAST) garment may be a useful method of temporarily controlling hemorrhage below the diaphragm; however, its use is controversial and has not been shown to improve survival in large series. It may be considered for patients with suspected intra-abdominal, pelvic, or lower extremity hemorrhage in whom definitive control of bleeding must be delayed. It is contraindicated if pulmonary edema is present.

If the patient arrives in the emergency department with a MAST already in place, *do not remove the suit until there is access to the circulation and the surgeon is ready to treat the specific injury.* In general, the MAST is best removed in the operating room with the patient prepared for or already under anesthesia.

C. Supportive Measures: Guidelines for volume restoration indicating successful resuscitation are set forth in Table 3-4.

1. Crystalloid solution–In general, 2 L of crystalloid solution can be safely infused in the hypovolemic patient before it is necessary to give whole blood.

2. Blood–The amount of blood administered depends on the clinical situation and the amount and kind of other intravenous fluid replacement. (Ideally, in the severely traumatized patient, the hematocrit should be kept at or about 30%). Older patients require a hematocrit of 35–40%, especially if preexisting cardiopulmonary disease is present.

3. Autotransfusion–Autotransfusion is a useful and occasionally lifesaving practice that makes it possible for patients to receive autologous blood with minimal delay. Because of the risk of infection, only blood from the thoracic cavity (ie, hemothorax) should be used. The simplest method of autotransfusion involves collection of blood from chest tube drainage into receptacles containing citrate anticoagulant (10 mL of sodium citrate per 100 mL of blood); this mixture should be continually agitated and can then be infused directly into the recipient through a blood filter. Commercial autotransfusion devices are available (Chapter 46).

4. Warming of blood–Hypothermia is a frequent side effect of transfusion of blood stored at 4 °C. Therefore, blood should be administered through blood warmers or specially designed heat exchangers.

Disposition

Hospitalize for emergency surgery or observation as indicated.

HEAD TRAUMA
(See also Chapter 16.)

Diagnosis

Suspect significant head trauma in any traumatized patient with cranial hematomas or lacerations or with altered sensorium with or without focal neurologic findings.

A. Examine the scalp carefully for evidence of trauma.

B. Any clear fluid in the ear canal or coming from the nares must be assumed to be cerebrospinal fluid. If the fluid is cerebrospinal fluid, a dipstick glucose test will usually be positive, since cerebrospinal fluid contains glucose and mucus does not. False-negative results may occur in patients with hypoglycemia.

C. Blood behind the eardrum, a postauricular hematoma (Battle's sign), or bilateral circumorbital hematomas ("raccoon eyes") suggest basilar skull fracture.

D. The form of the neurologic examination should be standardized and the results carefully recorded (Fig 4–1), so that changes noted on subsequent examinations may be readily detected. Pay particular attention to the following:

1. Level of consciousness.

2. Ocular movements, pupillary and corneal reflexes, decorticate or decerebrate posturing, doll's eye sign (dissociation between the movements of the eyes and those of the head), or response to caloric stimulation.

3. General motor function and pain response (truncal and all 4 extremities).

4. Deep tendon and plantar reflexes.

E. CT scan should be performed if the patient's condition is not deteriorating so rapidly (worsening noticeably every 10–20 minutes or less) that emergency surgery is mandatory.

Treatment

Obtain emergency neurosurgical consultation. Rapidly progressive neurologic abnormalities are an indication for emergency decompressive craniotomy. In the unusual case of extremely rapid deterioration, burr holes may be drilled in the skull in the emergency department.

Disposition

Hospitalize for observation or surgery as indicated.

INJURIES TO NECK REGION
(See also Chapter 21.)

Diagnosis

A. Cervical Spine: See Chapter 21.

B. Upper Airway (Larynx, Trachea, Bronchi): Injury to the upper airway is characterized by hoarseness or aphonia, apnea or respiratory distress, stridor, and subcutaneous emphysema. The airway may be lacerated in massive neck injury.

C. Esophagus: (See Chapter 18.) Injury to the esophagus is uncommon even in penetrating trauma. Difficulty in swallowing and neck pain are common, but clinical findings may not be present initially. Confirm the diagnosis by esophagography or esophagoscopy.

D. Vascular Injury: Clinical findings are variable and depend on the type of injury. Also, they maybe inapparent initially; for this reason, arteriography or surgical exploration of the neck is recommended for most penetrating injuries deep to the platysma and for most cases of severe blunt trauma.

Treatment

A. Cervical Spine: Maintain axial orientation of the head and neck with lateral neck rolls or traction if cervical spine injury is suspected. (See Chapter 21.)

B. Upper Airway (Larynx, Trachea, Bronchi): If the airway is exposed, intubate directly; otherwise, intubate orally under direct vision with a laryngoscope. If an endotracheal tube cannot be inserted, perform cricothyrotomy (Chapter 46) pending tracheostomy. If subcutaneous emphysema is present, assume that fracture of the trachea or main stem bronchus has occurred, and intubate the airway (preferably under bronchoscopic guidance) distal to the break or in the contralateral bronchus if the lacerated bronchus is inaccessible.

C. Esophagus: Suction the pharynx, and insert a nasogastric tube. Give penicillin, 200,000 units/kg/d intravenously in 6 divided doses (about 12 million units/d for an adult). Obtain surgical consultation.

D. Vascular Injury: Prepare to treat hemorrhagic shock (Chapter 3). Obtain surgical consultation to determine whether arteriography or surgical exploration is indicated (Chapter 32).

Disposition

All patients with injury to neck structures require hospitalization. The only exceptions are patients with minor blunt or penetrating trauma (eg, whiplash injuries, superficial lacerations).

MYOCARDIAL CONTUSION
(See also Chapter 18.)

Diagnosis

Suspect myocardial contusion in any patient who has sustained high-velocity blunt chest trauma. The diagnosis can be confirmed by ECG, serial CK-MB enzymes, and 2-dimensional echocardiography. The most lethal manifestations are arrhythmias, which usually occur in the first hour following injury. There is increasing evidence that myocardial contusion without hemodynamic instability, heart failure, or sustained arrhythmias has a benign course.

Treatment

Treat arrhythmias as indicated (Chapter 29). Obtain serial ECGs, and send blood samples to the laboratory for analysis of serum CK and MB fraction isoenzymes.

Disposition

Hospitalize in a monitored bed for further tests, continuous cardiac monitoring, and observation.

PULMONARY CONTUSION
(See also Chapter 18.)

Diagnosis

The diagnosis of pulmonary contusion is based on chest x-ray findings of abnormal opacities after chest trauma when there is no other explanation. These findings may be delayed for 24 hours or more.

Treatment

Administer supplemental oxygen as needed. Intubation and ventilatory support may be required in patients with extensive pulmonary contusion.

Disposition

Hospitalize for observation.

AORTIC RUPTURE OR ANEURYSM
(See also Chapter 32.)

Diagnosis

The possibility of aortic injury must be considered in patients with blunt chest trauma.

A. Blood pressure higher in the arms than in the legs, appearance of new murmurs, or diminution of lower extremity pulses all suggest aortic injury. However, physical findings are often absent.

B. Chest x-ray may show mediastinal widening or blurring of the aortic outline. The diagnosis is confirmed by aortography.

Treatment & Disposition

Patients with significant blunt chest trauma and possible aortic rupture should be hospitalized for surgical consultation, diagnostic studies, and immediate surgery if indicated. Until surgery is performed, support blood pressure with intravenous fluids (crystalloid solution and blood), and maintain the hematocrit at more than 30%. Since rupture may occur into the pleural space, autotransfusion from tube thoracostomy drainage may be utilized (Chapter 46).

SPINAL TRAUMA
(See also Chapter 21.)

Immobilize the neck and spine until x-rays are interpreted. Consider the use of skeletal traction (Chapter 21). If the patient must be moved, cautiously use the logroll technique.

Diagnosis

A. Conscious Patient: Suspect spinal trauma if the patient reports pain overlying the spine. Neurologic deficits may or may not be present. X-rays confirm the diagnosis.

B. Unconscious Patient: The type and site of injury may suggest spinal injury. X-ray all suspected areas.

Treatment & Disposition

The patient with suspected spinal trauma must be immobilized and hospitalized for neurosurgical or orthopedic consultation and care as indicated.

FRACTURES
(See also Chapter 22.)

Diagnosis

Examine all bones and joints, and x-ray suspected areas if the patient's condition is stable.

Treatment

Splint fractures (Chapter 22) as soon as possible after initial resuscitation to prevent further blood loss and neurovascular damage, to relieve pain, and to prevent continued microembolization. Wrap open fractures in clean dressings in preparation for irrigation and debridement in the operating room, and administer antibiotics (eg, cefazolin, 1 g intravenously). Obtain orthopedic consultation.

Disposition

Hospitalize the patient for observation or surgery as indicated.

CRUSH INJURY

Diagnosis

Crush injuries are characterized by massive swelling and skin and soft tissue ecchymosis; concomitant degloving injuries are common. Absent pulses are also common. Fractures may or may not be present. Urinalysis may demonstrate hemoglobinuria or myoglobinuria.

Treatment

Treat shock with intravenous crystalloid solution. Whole blood may be necessary in some cases. Search for and treat myoglobinuria (Chapter 12).

Disposition

Hospitalize the patient, and obtain immediate surgical consultation for operative decompression and debridement.

ABDOMINAL TRAUMA
(See also Chapter 19.)

Diagnosis

Repeated physical examination is the most useful means of evaluating blunt abdominal trauma.

A. Peritoneal Lavage: (See Chapter 46.) Peritoneal lavage is useful in evaluating some patients with blunt abdominal trauma, particularly those who are unconscious or unable to cooperate. Obtain surgical consultation.

B. Radiologic Studies: CT scans and arteriography may be warranted. Plain films of the abdomen are helpful in about one-third of cases.

Treatment

Treat shock and blood loss as required.

Disposition

Hospitalize the patient for observation and surgery as required.

GENITOURINARY TRAUMA
(See also Chapter 20.)

Diagnosis

In patients with gross urethral bleeding, a urethrogram should be performed before a urinary (Foley) catheter is inserted. When a urinary (Foley) catheter is inserted and bloody urine is recovered, a biplane cystogram should be obtained. If this is negative, excretory urography is indicated.

Treatment

Treat shock if present.

Disposition

Hospitalize as required. Obtain urgent urologic consultation.

REFERENCES

American College of Surgeons Committee on Trauma: Hospital and prehospital resources for optimal care of the injured patient. Bull Am Coll Surg (Oct) 1986;71:4.

American College of Surgeons Committee on Trauma: *Student Manual for Advanced Trauma Life Support Course for Physicians.* American College of Surgeons, 1984.

Baxt WG et al: The failure of prehospital trauma prediction rules to classify trauma patients accurately. Ann Emerg Med 1989;18:1.

Baxter BT et al: Emergency department thoracotomy following injury: Critical determinants for patient salvage. World J Surg 1988;12:671.

Cayten CG (editor): Multiple trauma. (Symposium.) Emerg Med Clin North Am 1984;2:1. [Entire issue.]

Daum GS et al: Dipstick evaluation of hematuria in abdominal trauma. Am J Clin Pathol 1988;89:538.

Greenfield RH, Bessen HA, Henneman PL: Effect of crystalloid infusion on hematocrit and intravascular volume in healthy, non-bleeding subjects. Ann Emerg Med 1989;18:51.

Kearney PA et al: Computed tomography and diagnostic peritoneal lavage in blunt abdominal trauma: Their combined role. Arch Surg 1989;124:344.

Mattox KL et al: Prospective MAST study in 911 patients. J Trauma 1989;29:1104.

McGill J, Clinton JE, Ruiz E: Cricothyrotomy in the emergency department. Ann Emerg Med 1982;11:361.

Moore EE, Eiseman B, van Way CW: *Critical Decisions in Trauma.* Mosby, 1983.

Odling-Smee W, Crockard A: *Trauma Care.* Grune & Stratton, 1981.

Shires GT: *Principles of Trauma Care,* 3rd ed. McGraw-Hill, 1984.

Trunkey D (editor): Symposium on trauma. Surg Clin North Am 1982;62:1. [Entire issue.]

Dyspnea, Respiratory Distress, & Respiratory Failure

5

John Mills, MD, & John M. Luce, MD

IMMEDIATE MANAGEMENT OF LIFE-THREATENING PROBLEMS
(See algorithm.)

Assess Severity & Give Immediate Necessary Care

The first step in the evaluation of the patient with suspected respiratory disease is to quickly assess the severity by noting the patient's general appearance and heart and respiratory rate. Rapidly examine the heart and chest. If severe respiratory distress is present (eg, too short of breath for speech)—and especially if it has developed over a short period of time (minutes to hours)—proceed rapidly with simultaneous evaluation and therapy (see algorithm). As in all life-threatening conditions, providing and maintaining an adequate airway is the first consideration.

Perform Arterial Blood Gas Analysis

If time and the clinical situation permit, arterial blood gas analysis should be performed as quickly as possible to determine the presence or absence of respiratory failure. The diagnosis is made if (1) the oxygen tension (PO_2) in arterial blood is less than 50 mm Hg (hypoxemic respiratory failure) while the patient is breathing room air, or (2) the arterial carbon dioxide tension (PCO_2) is greater than 50 mm Hg (hypercapnic respiratory failure). The acuteness of the respiratory failure is reflected in arterial blood pH, which will fall from a normal level of 7.4 to 7.3 or lower if the $PaCO_2$ rises acutely by 10 mm Hg or more. Chronic respiratory failure, in which the pH is near normal owing to compensatory processes, usually reflects severe pathophysiologic disturbances but is not an immediate threat to life. On the other hand, acute respiratory failure generally demands prompt intervention. Only with arterial blood gas analysis can respiratory failure be diagnosed and its degree of acuity assessed. Such analysis also helps to direct supplemental oxygen therapy and may be essential in making decisions regarding intubation and mechanical ventilation.

Pulse oximetry, which measures the saturation of hemoglobin by oxygen, provides a guide to the oxygenation of arterial blood. However, because hyperventilation can raise the PO_2, a normal saturation may be observed despite an abnormal elevated alveolar to arterial oxygen gradient. In addition, pulse oximetry provides no information about PCO_2 tension or the adequacy of ventilation, and it is inaccurate when carbon monoxide is present in the blood. Thus, patients with severe hypoxemia (eg, saturation below 90%) or ventilatory insufficiency should also have arterial blood gas determinations. Pulse oximetry is most helpful when the saturation is normal or near normal; it cannot be used to diagnose respiratory failure.

CARDIAC ARREST

Diagnosis

In patients who are unresponsive, check for patency of the airway, and position the head and jaw properly (Chapter 1). Quickly begin ventilating the lungs and palpate the carotid artery to see if the heart is beating. Terminal gasping respirations may simulate respiratory distress—and, conversely, conditions that produce severe respiratory distress may lead to hypoxic cardiac arrest.

Treatment & Disposition

Start CPR at once if the carotid pulse is not palpable (Chapter 1).

Hospitalization is always required for these severely ill patients if they survive initial resuscitation attempts.

SEVERE UPPER AIRWAY OBSTRUCTION

Diagnosis

Listen for inspiratory and expiratory stridor. Look for ineffective inspiratory efforts characterized by suprasternal, supraclavicular, and intercostal retractions, often coupled with cyanosis, which indicate gross upper airway obstruction. The diagnosis may be confirmed by asking the patient to speak; patients with complete upper airway obstruction are unable to speak even in a whisper.

Treatment

A. Away From Hospital: (See also Chapter 1.) Remove possible obstructing foreign bodies by performing the Heimlich maneuver repeatedly until successful. If the victim loses consciousness, call for help to activate the Emergency Medical Services system, and perform 6–10 supine subdiaphragmatic thrusts (supine Heimlich), followed by a finger sweep and attempt to ventilate. Repeat this series of steps until the obstruction is cleared or until help arrives. If the victim is markedly obese or in the third trimester of pregnancy, use closed chest compression instead of the Heimlich maneuver. A foreign body may be removed by trained rescue personnel under direct visualization using a laryngoscope and suction device or forceps. Rarely, cricothyrotomy may be necessary, but it should be performed *by rescuers trained in the technique.*

B. In a Hospital Emergency Department:

1. Laryngoscopy– Immediate direct laryngoscopy is indicated if the obstruction cannot be quickly

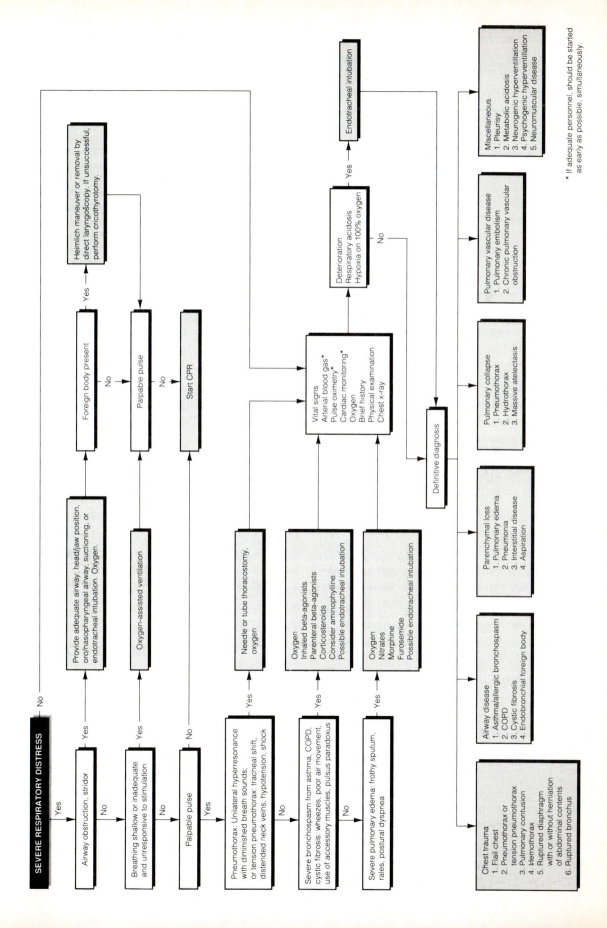

SEVERE RESPIRATORY DISTRESS

Airway obstruction, stridor
— Yes → Provide adequate airway: head/jaw position, oro/nasopharyngeal airway, suctioning, or endotracheal intubation. Oxygen. → Foreign body present
— Yes → Heimlich maneuver or removal by direct laryngoscopy. If unsuccessful, perform cricothyrotomy.
— No

Breathing shallow or inadequate and unresponsive to stimulation
— Yes → Oxygen-assisted ventilation → Palpable pulse
— Yes → (Vital signs...)
— No → Start CPR

Palpable pulse
— Yes
— No → Start CPR

Vital signs
Arterial blood gas*
Pulse oximetry*
Cardiac monitoring*
Oxygen
Brief history
Physical examination
Chest x-ray

→ Deterioration
Respiratory acidosis
Hypoxia on 100% oxygen
— Yes → Endotracheal intubation
— No → Definitive diagnosis

Pneumothorax: Unilateral hyperresonance with diminished breath sounds; or tension pneumothorax: tracheal shift, distended neck veins, hypotension, shock
— Yes → Needle or tube thoracostomy, oxygen
— No

Severe bronchospasm from asthma, COPD, cystic fibrosis: wheezes, poor air movement, use of accessory muscles, pulsus paradoxus
— Yes → Oxygen
Inhaled beta-agonists
Parenteral beta-agonists
Corticosteroids
Consider aminophylline
Possible endotracheal intubation
— No

Severe pulmonary edema: frothy sputum, rales, postural dyspnea
— Yes → Oxygen
Nitrates
Morphine
Furosemide
Possible endotracheal intubation

Definitive diagnosis:

Chest trauma
1. Flail chest
2. Pneumothorax or tension pneumothorax
3. Pulmonary contusion
4. Hemothorax
5. Ruptured diaphragm with or without herniation of abdominal contents
6. Ruptured bronchus

Airway disease
1. Asthma/allergic bronchospasm
2. COPD
3. Cystic fibrosis
4. Endobronchial foreign body

Parenchymal loss
1. Pulmonary edema
2. Pneumonia
3. Interstitial disease
4. Aspiration

Pulmonary collapse
1. Pneumothorax
2. Hydrothorax
3. Massive atelectasis

Pulmonary vascular disease
1. Pulmonary embolism
2. Chronic pulmonary vascular obstruction

Miscellaneous
1. Pleurisy
2. Metabolic acidosis
3. Neurogenic hyperventilation
4. Psychogenic hyperventilation
5. Neuromuscular disease

* If adequate personnel, should be started as early as possible, simultaneously.

removed. This may be the first step in emergency department treatment. Foreign bodies may be removed under direct vision using forceps. Obstruction caused by soft tissue swelling or local edema (as in anaphylaxis) may be relieved by passage of an endotracheal tube. Anaphylaxis requires specific treatment (p 65). Epiglottitis may cause upper airway obstruction in either children or adults; if this condition is suspected, obtain a lateral soft-tissue radiograph of the neck (Chapter 26).

2. Surgery– If the upper airway obstruction cannot be bypassed with an endotracheal tube or cannot be physically removed, cricothyrotomy or tracheostomy is required (Chapter 46).

Disposition

Patients who are asymptomatic after uncomplicated and easy removal of an obstructing foreign body may be sent home with instructions to eat more slowly, chew more thoroughly, and swallow more carefully. Alcohol intoxication is often contributory. Patients who lost consciousness but otherwise appear well should be examined and observed in the emergency department. Patients who required intubation or surgery or who remain symptomatic should be hospitalized for treatment and observation.

STUPOR OR COMA WITH SHALLOW BREATHING

Diagnosis

Stupor or coma in a patient with obvious respiratory distress is commonly due to CO_2 retention or profound tissue hypoxia. Alternatively, the patient may be stuporous or breathing shallowly without signs of distress. If the patient's condition is stable enough to permit brief evaluation, either the absence of a gag reflex (unprotected airway) or an arterial blood gas sample showing severe hypercapnia or hypoxemia (ie, respiratory failure) supports the necessity for endotracheal intubation in the emergency department. When possible, the arterial blood gas sample should be obtained before respiratory support or supplementary oxygen is provided.

Treatment

Ventilatory support (bag-mask or mouth-to-mouth) should be given until endotracheal intubation can be accomplished. Provide supplemental oxygen, 10 L/min, by mask (nonrebreathing, if available), nasal prongs, or Ambu bag.

As soon as oxygenation and CO_2 exchange have been partially corrected by assisted ventilation, the patient should be intubated. This will protect the airway (preventing aspiration) and make possible effective respiratory support.

If there is doubt about the need for intubation, err on the side of intubation.

Disposition

Hospitalize for further diagnosis and treatment.

TENSION PNEUMOTHORAX (See also p 86.)

Diagnosis

Severe respiratory distress associated with tension pneumothorax occurs usually (though not exclusively) following blunt or penetrating chest trauma (including chest compressions during CPR), and it may rarely occur spontaneously in patients prone to spontaneous pneumothorax. Tracheal shift, hyperresonant hemithorax with markedly decreased breath sounds, hypotension, and distended neck veins are classical signs, although not invariably present. If time permits, the clinical diagnosis may be confirmed by chest x-ray (a simple anteroposterior view is sufficient).

Treatment

A. Give oxygen at once (10 L/min, by mask or nasal prongs).

B. Perform tube thoracostomy (Chapter 46). For immediate relief, perform needle thoracostomy with a large-bore (14- to 16-gauge) needle if delay is anticipated in obtaining equipment for chest tube insertion. The risk of needle or tube thoracostomy without x-ray confirmation of tension pneumothorax must be weighed against the severity of respiratory distress or hemodynamic compromise and the certainty of the clinical diagnosis. If the procedure is properly performed, the risks of tube thoracostomy are minimal even in a patient without pneumothorax.

Disposition

Hospitalize immediately.

MASSIVE ASPIRATION (See also p 88.)

Diagnosis

If the patient with severe respiratory distress has vomitus with particulate matter in the oropharynx, significant aspiration has probably occurred.

Treatment

A. Clear the airway with a large-bore suction device (eg, tonsil sucker). Endotracheal intubation is often required because of depressed consciousness with hypercapnia and severe hypoxemia.

B. Begin oxygen, 5–10 L/min, by mask or nasal prongs.

C. Antibiotics and corticosteroids have been suggested by some authorities because of the risk of pneumonia. However, there is evidence that antibiotics are ineffective in this situation, since the initial infiltrate appearing on chest x-ray is due to a chemical pneumonitis. Corticosteroids have also not been shown to be effective in decreasing the death rate from aspiration pneumonitis. In addition, pneumonia due to gram-negative organisms is more likely to develop in patients who have received corticosteroids than in those who have not.

Disposition

Hospitalize immediately for definitive treatment and follow-up.

SEVERE PULMONARY EDEMA
(See also Chapters 27 and 28.)

Diagnosis

Patients with severe pulmonary edema are extremely dyspneic, especially in the supine position, and may also cough up frothy, pink material. Rales (crackles) are present, and the chest x-ray almost always reveals bilateral infiltrates. Fever is uncommon. In cardiogenic pulmonary edema, other manifestations of heart failure are usually present: tachycardia, distended neck veins or hepatojugular reflux, peripheral edema, cardiomegaly, or a ventricular (S_3) gallop. Wheezing may also be present (so-called "cardiac asthma," probably caused by reflex bronchospasm). Patients with cardiogenic pulmonary edema often give a history of heart disease and have had pulmonary edema before.

The physical findings of cardiogenic pulmonary edema are usually absent in noncardiogenic pulmonary edema, as is a history of heart disease; nevertheless, some patients with cardiogenic pulmonary edema may have some component of noncardiogenic pulmonary edema, and vice versa. Noncardiac pulmonary edema has many causes, including drug overdose (especially heroin and other narcotics), septic shock, pulmonary contusion, pancreatitis, and fat embolism. These conditions are collectively known as adult respiratory distress syndrome (ARDS).

Treatment

A. All patients with severe pulmonary edema should receive supplemental oxygen, 10–15 L/min, by mask or nasal prongs. Endotracheal intubation with mechanical ventilation may be required if distress is severe and not easily relieved, and especially if respiratory failure (hypercapnia) is present.

B. Morphine, 5–10 mg intravenously and/or nitrates given sublingually (0.4 mg), cutaneously (1–2 inches of nitroglycerin ointment), or by intravenous infusion (begin at 10 µg/min, and titrate to desired effect), cause peripheral venous pooling; and furosemide, 40–80 mg intravenously, will often improve respiratory function in patients with both cardiogenic and noncardiogenic pulmonary edema, at least temporarily.

C. Additional treatment depends on whether the edema is cardiogenic or noncardiogenic (Chapters 27 and 28). Placement of a pulmonary artery catheter for measurement of pulmonary artery wedge pressure is essential to the differentiation of these conditions. This procedure is usually not performed in the emergency department.

Disposition

Hospitalize immediately.

SEVERE ASTHMA, CHRONIC OBSTRUCTIVE PULMONARY DISEASE, OR CYSTIC FIBROSIS
(See also Chapter 31.)

Diagnosis

Patients with asthma, chronic obstructive pulmonary disease, or cystic fibrosis may present with severe dyspnea and respiratory distress similar to those of patients with pulmonary edema. However, dyspnea in the former group of patients is less likely to be much worse when they are supine, and they usually have a history of previous acute respiratory failure—if they are able to give a history at all. Cough is common to the obstructive disorders, but sputum may be scanty. Most important, patients with asthma, chronic obstructive pulmonary disease, or cystic fibrosis usually have wheezing on auscultation of the chest, although some patients may not have sufficient tidal volumes to produce audible wheezing. In such patients, the principal physical findings are tachypnea, tachycardia, cyanosis, chest hyperexpansion, and markedly diminished breath sounds. In severe episodes, a pulsus paradoxus may be present. The use of the sternocleidomastoid muscles during inspiration is common, and intercostal retractions and nasal flaring are often visible. Chest x-ray shows only hyperexpanded lung fields unless another pathologic process such as bacterial pneumonia is present. These patients usually do not have pneumonia; rather, viral or (rarely) bacterial tracheobronchitis or exposure to an allergen has exacerbated their chronic underlying disease. Objective measures of airflow, such as the peak expiratory flow rate (PEFR) or forced expiratory volume in 1 second (FEV_1), may be measured in the emergency department. They are often useful in following improvement and comparing the degree of obstruction to a known baseline for a given patient.

Treatment

The measures outlined below may be used safely in the emergency department even in the absence of precise diagnosis. Further management of patients with these disorders is discussed in Chapter 27.

A. Oxygen: Give oxygen, 1–3 L/min by mask or nasal prongs, in an attempt to raise arterial saturation to $\geq 90\%$ or PO_2 to between 60 and 80 mm Hg without causing respiratory depression and a marked increase in arterial PCO_2. Arterial blood gas analysis is vital in directing therapy. Tracheal intubation and mechanical ventilation should be avoided but may be necessary if a patient is comatose or is in acute respiratory failure (hypercapnia with respiratory acidosis).

B. Beta-Adrenergic Sympathomimetic Bronchodilators: In adults, beta-adrenergic sympathomimetic bronchodilators should be given in aerosol form if possible; otherwise, they may be given parenterally. A typical regimen is metaproterenol, 0.2–0.3 mL in 3 mL normal saline, delivered by nebulizer over 5 minutes every 30–60 minutes; or albuterol, 0.2–0.3 mL in 3 mL normal saline, delivered by nebulizer over 5 minutes every 30–60 minutes. Parenteral therapy includes epinephrine, 0.2–0.3 mL (1:1000 dilution) every 20–30 minutes subcutaneously, or terbutaline, 0.25 mg subcutaneously every 2–4 hours. Parenteral therapy is occasionally of value in severe exacerbation, or when the patient is unable to cooperate with drug administration by nebulizer (eg, a small child). However, parenteral administration of sympathomimetics can produce marked tachycardia and may occasionally induce myocardial ischemia, especially in elderly patients or those with preexisting coronary artery disease. Therefore, they should be used cautiously in this group and be withheld if chest pain or extreme tachycardia develops.

C. Corticosteroids: Corticosteroids should be given early in the course of treatment of patients who fail to respond adequately to nebulized or parenteral beta-adrenergic agents alone. The recommended regimen is methylprednisolone, 125 mg intravenously initially, followed by 30–60 mg intravenously 4 times daily if the patient is hospitalized.

D. Magnesium Sulfate: Magnesium sulfate ($MgSO_4$) has a bronchodilating effect that may be of benefit in asthma, and it has been safely administered to preeclamptic women for years. Although it should still be considered experimental and its role in acute asthma is currently being investigated, it is being used clinically by some. If used, it should be reserved for life-threatening bronchospasm that fails to respond to sympathomimetic bronchodilators. In adults, 1 g of $MgSO_4$ in 50 mL of normal saline or 5% dextrose in water is infused over 30 minutes. If necessary, an infusion of 1 g/h may be maintained. The effects are short-lived and abate after the infusion is discontinued. Blood pressure should be monitored and the infusion stopped if hypotension occurs. Deep tendon reflexes will be lost once serum magnesium concentration reaches 7–10 meq/L (normal concentration is 1.5–2 meq/L); the infusion should be stopped if reflexes are lost. At magnesium concentrations of 10–15 meq/L, respiratory depression occurs, and at 30 meq/L, cardiac arrest may occur. However, the dose used for asthma is low (approximately one-fourth the dose used in preeclampsia).

E. Theophyllines: Theophyllines exert an inotropic effect on respiratory muscles, although they are less effective bronchodilators than the beta-adrenergics and have much greater toxicity. Randomized trials of theophyllines in the emergency department treatment of acute asthma exacerbations have failed to show a benefit, and many emergency physicians no longer use them in this setting. However, there may be a benefit over the longer term or in hospitalized patients. If using this class of drugs, give a loading dose of aminophylline, 5–6 mg/kg intravenously, to patients not already receiving theophylline on a regular basis; in other patients, reduce or eliminate the loading dose. The maintenance dose of aminophylline is 0.5–0.9 mg/kg/h; dosage should be adjusted so that serum theophylline levels are between 10 and 20 mg/dL.

F. Hydration: Hydration can be achieved using oral or intravenous fluids. Overhydration should be avoided, since it may precipitate pulmonary edema.

Disposition

Hospitalize patients with life-threatening bronchospasm that does not respond immediately to treatment, or those with moderate bronchospasm who fail to improve after 4–6 hours of treatment.

FURTHER DIAGNOSTIC EVALUATION

Diagnostic Information

A. Data Base: After supplemental oxygen has been started and life-threatening problems have been corrected, proceed as follows to construct an *emergency cardiopulmonary data base:*

1. Brief history directed toward cardiopulmonary disease, with emphasis on the duration of this attack of dyspnea.

2. Complete list of prescribed and unprescribed medications (current and recent past), including most recent dosage history.

3. Examination of the heart, lungs, abdomen, and other areas as indicated.

4. CBC, urinalysis, serum creatinine or blood urea nitrogen, serum electrolytes, and glucose.

5. Arterial blood gas and pH analysis if not already obtained.

6. Chest x-ray and ECG.

B. Interpretation of Diagnostic Data: Information from this data base usually will allow the emergency physician to identify the cause of dyspnea as shown below and in Table 5–1. The basis of this categorization is discussed below and in greater detail in Chapter 27.

Table 5–1. Essentials of diagnosis of diseases causing dyspnea and respiratory distress.[1]

Disorder	Specific Condition	Onset History	Symptoms Other Than Dyspnea	Signs	Chest X-Ray	Comment
Chest wall defect	Flail chest.	Trauma.	Pain with respiration.	Paradoxical motion of chest wall.	Rib fractures.	Coexistent pneumothorax common.
	Muscular weakness.	Gradual onset.	Weakness of other muscles.	Weakness of non-respiratory muscles.	Normal.	Dimished inspiratory force.
Pulmonary collapse	Pneumothorax.	Sudden onset; occasionally trauma.	Cough and chest pain common.	Tympany and decreased breath sounds; decreased blood pressure and tracheal shift if tension.	Lung collapse; mediastinal shift if tension.	
	Hydrothorax.	Gradual onset.		Dullness and decreased breath sounds.	Pleural effusion (decubitus views)	
	Atelectasis.	Variable onset.		Variable.	Signs of atelectasis.	
Loss of functional lung parenchyma	Plumonary edema.	Usually abrupt onset (hours to days).	Cough common.	Bibasilar rales (occasional wheezing).	Bilateral alveolar infiltrates, often symmetric.	Most common cause is cardiogenic, in which case will have associated signs of heart failure.
	Pneumonia.	Usually abrupt onset (hours to days).	Cough, pleurisy common.	Rales with or without dullness over affected areas; fever.	Patchy alveolar infiltrates, usually asymmetric.	Leukocytes and often bacteria in sputum.
	Diffuse interstitial disease.	Previous dyspnea common.	Cough.	Often dry rales.	Interstitial disease (or negative).	Patient often aware of diagnosis.
	Aspiration.	Abrupt onset; history of vomiting.	Cough.	Vomitus in oropharynx.	Normal or infiltrate.	Usually associated with coma or obtundation.
Airway disease	Upper airway obstruction.	Often sudden onset.	Hoarseness or aphonia.	Inspiratory stridor.	Normal.	Soft tissue x-rays of neck may be helpful.
	Asthma.	Usually previous attacks; onset variable.	Wheezing.	Wheezing; hyperinflation and decreased breath sounds in status asthmaticus.	Hyperinflation.	Patient usually aware of diagnosis.
	Chronic obstructive lung disease and cystic fibrosis.	Previous dyspnea common; onset variable.	Cough, wheezing.	Wheezing; hyperinflation and decreased breath sounds.	Hyperinflation; occasional pneumonitis.	Clubbing with cystic fibrosis; patient usually aware of diagnosis.
Pulmonary vascular disease	Acute pulmonary embolism.	Abrupt onset.	Cough, pleurisy, hemoptysis.	Tachycardia; occasionally signs of acute cor pulmonale.	Usually normal; occasionally infiltrates, atelectasis, elevaed hemidiaphragm.	Lung scan or pulmonary arteriogram for diagnosis.
	Repeated small pulmonary emboli.	Gradual onset.	Rarely, pleurisy or chest pain.	Occasionally signs of cor pulmonale.	Rarely helpful.	May require formal pulmonary function tests for diagnosis.
Miscellaneous	Pleurisy.	Often abrupt onset.	Pleurisy.	Rub (about 80%).	Normal.	Rule out pulmonary embolism.
	Metabolic acidosis.	Gradual onset.	Often not dyspneic.	Hyperventilation.	Normal.	Low arterial blood pH and bicarbonate.
	Neurogenic.		Usually not dyspneic.	Signs of cardiac or neurologic disease.	Normal.	Stroke, heart failure are usual causes.
	Psychogenic.	Previous attacks common; abrupt onset with stress.	Circumoral and acral tingling.	Tetany.	Normal.	Reliet obtained with rebreathing system (eg, paper bag).

[1] The most helpful tests or findings are shaded.

Disposition
(See also specific conditions, below.)

If the emergency data base suggests a significant acute abnormality but an exact diagnosis cannot be made that would permit specific therapy to be started, the patient should be hospitalized even if the clinical status would not otherwise warrant hospitalization. It is not uncommon for more than one abnormality to be present in the same patient (eg, acute exacerbation of chronic bronchitis and pneumonia).

EMERGENCY TREATMENT OF SPECIFIC DISORDERS

CHEST WALL DEFECTS

1. FLAIL CHEST

Diagnosis

Posttraumatic flail chest is usually apparent on physical examination as painful paradoxical motion of the rib cage or sternum (inward with inhalation and outward with exhalation).

Treatment

A. Provide supplemental oxygen. Use a bag-mask to support ventilation of patients with obvious hypoventilation.

B. Intubation for respiratory support need not be performed immediately if saturation is > 90% or arterial blood gas levels are satisfactory (PO_2 > 65 mm Hg, PCO_2 < 44 mm Hg) (Chapter 18). Give oxygen as indicated.

C. Provide analgesia (morphine, 1–4 mg intravenously), and watch carefully for signs of respiratory depression. Do not use if respiratory failure is imminent.

Disposition

All patients with flail chest injuries require immediate hospitalization.

2. NEUROMUSCULAR DISEASES

Diagnosis

Patients with dyspnea or respiratory distress associated with progressive neuromuscular disease usually have hypoventilation (arterial blood gases showing hypoxemia and hypercapnia) and objective weakness of other muscle groups, though the latter is not always present. Among many possible causes are Guillain-Barré syndrome, myasthenia gravis, periodic paralysis, botulism, and tick paralysis.

Treatment & Disposition

Believe the patient's complaints of dyspnea, and evaluate respiratory status using arterial blood gas analysis and pulmonary function tests (eg, vital capacity and maximal inspiratory force). Intubation may be postponed if initial blood gas levels are satisfactory. Specific therapy should focus on the neuromuscular disease (Chapter 12). Immediate hospitalization is mandatory.

PULMONARY COLLAPSE

Moderate degrees of pulmonary collapse that do not cause severe respiratory distress or obvious physical findings are apparent on chest x-ray. Treatment depends on the specific cause as discussed below.

1. PNEUMOTHORAX

Diagnosis

The patient often has both chest pain and severe respiratory distress, with tympany elicited by chest percussion of the affected side. The degree of dyspnea or respiratory distress depends on the amount of collapse and on the degree of pressure (in tension pneumothorax). The involved side is hyperresonant and tympanitic, with decreased breath sounds. Chest x-ray shows collapse of lung and air in the pleural space. Small amounts of fluid may also be present in the pleural space. Tension pneumothorax presents in a similar manner and is often (not always) associated with shift of the mediastinum away from the side of the involvement; distended neck veins, hypotension, and shock may be present.

Treatment

Immediate thoracostomy is indicated for bilateral pneumothoraces or unilateral tension pneumothorax, even if the patient appears stable, since sudden deterioration is always a possibility. Patients with unilateral large, simple (nontension) pneumothoraces are also best treated by thoracostomy tube in the emergency department before hospitalization. Patients with other types of pneumothoraces may be treated with a chest tube or, if the pneumothorax is simple and uncomplicated, by catheter aspiration and observation in the emergency department with the catheter connected to a Heimlich valve for 6 hours. If a follow-up chest x-ray demonstrates persistent reexpansion, the patient may be discharged with instructions to return if symptoms reappear.

Disposition

A. Hospitalization is indicated for patients who

have received tube thoracostomy, including all patients who present with tension pneumothorax or bilateral pneumothoraces of any type or who fail to maintain lung reexpansion after catheter aspiration.

B. Patients with small to moderate-sized unilateral simple pneumothoraces of recent onset may be observed for a few days in the hospital without a chest tube to see if the condition is stable or improving.

C. Patients with stable small spontaneous unilateral pneumothoraces with no symptoms may be referred for follow-up on an outpatient basis. They should be seen within 1–2 days.

2. HYDROTHORAX & HEMOTHORAX (Pleural Fluid or Blood)

Diagnosis

Fluid in the pleural space results in pulmonary collapse. Small amounts of air may be present as well. The patient shows moderate dyspnea or respiratory distress and has dullness with chest percussion of the affected side. Chest x-ray is diagnostic.

Treatment

A. Hydrothorax: If dyspnea of acute onset is thought to be secondary to hydrothorax, immediate drainage in the emergency department is indicated; a needle or small-gauge catheter should be used if the fluid is watery; viscous effusions may require tube thoracostomy. No more than 1–2 L should be removed at any one time because of the risk of expansion injury to the lung. The fluid should be sent for analysis (pH, specific gravity, cell count, glucose, protein, lactate dehydrogenase, and amylase), culture (for *Mycobacterium tuberculosis* and other bacteria), and cytologic studies.

B. Hemothorax: In hemothorax due to penetrating trauma, autotransfusion may be indicated (Chapter 46). Otherwise, thoracentesis or tube thoracostomy (or both) should be done, followed by investigation into the source of bleeding (eg, aortic angiography, exploration) as indicated (Chapter 18).

Disposition

Hospitalization is required for all patients except those with chronic recurrent pleural effusions of known cause.

3. MASSIVE ATELECTASIS

Diagnosis

Atelectasis is alveolar collapse that is not due to pneumothorax or hydrothorax (Chapter 27). Decrease in chest motion on the affected side, dullness to percussion, and decreased to absent breath sounds are noted. Dyspnea, tachycardia, and cyanosis may

be present. The disorder is evident radiologically as an increase in density of the collapsed lung, with reduced volume of the involved hemithorax (narrowed rib interspaces, elevated hemidiaphragm, and mediastinal shift to the side of involvement).

Treatment

In the rare patient with respiratory failure, respiratory support (administration of oxygen and usually also assisted ventilation) should be initiated in the emergency department. Otherwise, no emergency therapy is indicated, although administration of oxygen (5 L/min by nasal prongs) is wise pending results of blood gas analysis.

Disposition

Hospitalization is required unless the process is known to be chronic and nonprogressive.

LOSS OF FUNCTIONAL LUNG PARENCHYMA

A number of conditions can produce acute or chronic dyspnea through loss of functional pulmonary parenchyma.

The hallmarks of diseases causing loss of functional lung parenchyma are inspiratory rales (crackles) on physical examination, dullness to percussion, auscultatory pitch changes (eg, egobronchophony, bronchophony, and bronchial breath sounds), and one or more infiltrates on chest x-rays.

These disorders may be divided into those associated with (**1**) pulmonary edema, (**2**) pneumonia (including aspiration "pneumonia"), and (**3**) interstitial disease. Pulmonary contusion following blunt chest trauma is covered in Chapter 18.

In patients with dyspnea, several processes may be occurring simultaneously. For example, aspiration pneumonia may be a combination of chemical pulmonary edema and bacterial pneumonia, with varying degrees of airway obstruction; viral pneumonias are often interstitial in their early phases; and cardiogenic pulmonary edema starts as interstitial edema before progressing to the alveolar filling stage. Additionally, it may be difficult to differentiate these conditions in the emergency department (eg, pneumonia from pulmonary edema).

1. PULMONARY EDEMA (See also p 81.)

Diagnosis

The clinical presentation of less severe pulmonary edema is similar to that associated with the more severe form discussed above. Patients generally are less dyspneic and have a history of such symptoms and signs as paroxysmal nocturnal dyspnea, gradually increasing peripheral edema, and intermittent chest pain if the pulmonary edema is cardiogenic. Noncardiogenic edema usually begins more abruptly and is more severe than the cardiogenic form.

Treatment

A. Give oxygen as needed.

B. Additional treatment depends on whether the diagnosis is cardiogenic or noncardiogenic pulmonary edema (Chapters 27 and 28). Endotracheal intubation may be required if hypoxemia cannot be corrected with high-flow oxygen by mask.

Disposition

Many patients with dyspnea from acute pulmonary edema require hospitalization. Some patients with chronic or recurrent pulmonary edema (usually cardiogenic) can be managed on an ambulatory basis.

2. PNEUMONIA
(See also Chapter 34.)

Diagnosis

Patients with pneumonia generally give a history of fever and cough; dyspnea is a secondary or late symptom. Production of purulent sputum and pleuritic chest pain are common.

Physical examination usually shows a febrile patient with localized rales and dullness, often associated with signs of consolidation (egobronchophony, bronchial breath, and vocal sounds). In children, fever and cough are the only constant symptoms.

Chest x-ray shows one or more infiltrates, an exception being patients with early pneumonia or concomitant dehydration, in whom observation and rehydration over 4–6 hours generally will make the infiltrates visible on x-ray. Patients with severe leukopenia or acquired immunodeficiency syndrome (AIDS) may also have pneumonia without infiltrates.

Patients with AIDS may develop pneumonia due to *Pneumocystis carinii*. Despite cough, fever, dyspnea, and hypoxemia (or an elevated alveolar to arterial oxygen gradient calculated from arterial blood gas data), their clinical findings may be few and x-ray findings extremely subtle or normal. However, typical x-ray findings, if present, are a diffuse heterogeneous alveolar or "interstitial" infiltrate.

Treatment

Begin antibiotics based on the clinical situation and the results (if available) of a Gram-stained smear of sputum. If the patient is to be hospitalized but is not desperately ill, antibiotic therapy should be deferred until the attending physician has had an opportunity to evaluate the patient. (See Chapter 34 for a more extensive discussion of evaluation and treatment of patients with pneumonia, including those with AIDS.)

Disposition

Hospitalization is warranted for all seriously ill patients; for very young or very old patients; for patients with significant concurrent illnesses; for unreliable patients; and for patients with pneumonia of unknown cause. Patients with pneumocystis pneumonia should be admitted.

Adolescents and young adults with mild viral, mycoplasmal, or pneumococcal pneumonia usually can be managed on an outpatient basis (Chapter 34).

3. DIFFUSE INTERSTITIAL PULMONARY DISEASE (See also Chapter 27.)

Diagnosis

Most patients with interstitial pulmonary disease have a history of chronic dyspnea, are aware of their diagnosis, and come to the emergency department because of recent worsening of symptoms. If the patient has not sought medical attention previously, interstitial pulmonary disease should be suspected if the physical examination shows diffuse "dry" rales, the chest x-ray shows interstitial infiltrates, and arterial PCO_2 and PO_2 are low.

Treatment

Supportive care is the only treatment recommended in the emergency department.

Disposition

Hospitalization should be considered for all newly diagnosed patients and for patients with known interstitial disease with significant recent increase in dyspnea or hypoxemia.

4. ASPIRATION

Diagnosis

Aspiration may present clinically as pneumonia *without* obvious prior aspiration or as respiratory distress *with* obvious aspiration (vomitus in mouth and on clothing and elsewhere). This latter presentation is more common in obtunded patients.

Treatment

Supportive care should be given immediately in all cases. If obvious aspiration has occurred, clearing the airway is the most important emergency measure. This is best accomplished with a large-bore suction device (eg, tonsil sucker). Endotracheal intubation for better airway control and toilet should be considered, as should emergency bronchoscopy. Although glucocorticoids have been recommended in the past, they are not beneficial and may increase the risk of bacterial superinfection.

Disposition

Hospitalize all patients. The patient's initial status is not a reliable guide to the need for hospitalization, because pulmonary function may worsen progressively for 24–72 hours after aspiration.

AIRWAY DISEASE

Obstruction to airflow (airway obstruction) is a principal manifestation of all types of airway disease.

1. UPPER AIRWAY OBSTRUCTION

Lesions of the oropharynx, larynx, or trachea may occlude the airway sufficiently to cause dyspnea.

Diagnosis

Upper airway obstruction usually causes pronounced stridor (obstruction of inspiratory airflow equal to or greater than expiratory airflow), which may be accentuated by forced ventilatory efforts. The stridor may be accompanied by intercostal, suprasternal, or supraclavicular retractions or other signs of increased respiratory effort. The diagnosis can be made with lateral soft-tissue x-rays of the neck. In some cases, fiberoptic laryngoscopy is necessary.

Causes of upper airway obstruction include foreign bodies, tonsillar hypertrophy, croup, epiglottitis, anaphylaxis with laryngeal edema, retropharyngeal abscess, and tumors. If epiglottitis is suspected, obtain a lateral neck x-ray before attempting to visualize the upper airway directly (Chapter 26). Small children may aspirate small objects (eg, pearl, raisin, peanut) that lodge in the trachea or mainstem bronchus. Wheezing may be mistaken for bronchospastic disease. A chest x-ray is diagnostic, showing unilateral hyperexpansion on the affected side due to the ball-valve effect of the obstructing object (which may not be visible).

Treatment

A. A foreign body should be removed if present.

B. Anaphylaxis with laryngeal edema requires immediate intramuscular injection of epinephrine, 0.5–1 mg (0.5–1 mL of 1:1000 solution). Alternatively, give 0.1–0.2 mg (1–2 mL of 1:10,000 solution) intravenously. Repeat in 3–10 minutes as needed (Chapter 3). Additionally, administration of diphenhydramine, 25–50 mg intramuscularly or intravenously, will block further histamine release. Discharged patients should receive diphenhydramine, 25 mg orally, every 6 hours for 24–48 hours to prevent recurrence. Surgical cricothyrotomy may be emergently required if obstruction progresses. Occasionally, patients with hereditary angioedema (due to C1q esterase inhibitor deficiency) will present with signs and symptoms similar to those of allergic anaphylaxis. These patients are affected little by epinephrine and require C1q esterase inhibitor replacement (or fresh-frozen plasma if C1q esterase inhibitor is unavailable).

C. Children with epiglottitis (Chapter 42) should not receive direct or indirect laryngoscopy in the emergency department, since laryngeal spasm may precipitate complete obstruction. They should be carefully intubated in the operating room with surgeons present who can perform an emergency tracheostomy if needed. Adults with epiglottitis are less prone to sudden airway obstruction but should be admitted and monitored closely. Both children and adults should receive intravenous antibiotics.

D. Other disorders should be treated specifically to the extent possible.

Disposition

Patients with dyspnea from documented or suspected upper airway obstruction require hospitalization unless the problem is chronic, mild, and nonprogressive or is due to a foreign body that can be removed in the emergency department. Successfully treated upper airway obstruction due to anaphylaxis may recur when epinephrine wears off. Therefore, a 4- to 6-hour period of observation (or hospitalization) is advisable.

2. ASTHMA, CHRONIC OBSTRUCTIVE PULMONARY DISEASE, & CYSTIC FIBROSIS (See also Chapter 27.)

In these disorders, expiratory airflow tends to be reduced proportionately more than inspiratory flow. Patients with dyspnea caused by these types of airway disease usually have a history of respiratory symptoms and are aware of their diagnosis.

Diagnosis

Cough is commonly a feature, although sputum production is variable. Most of these patients have wheezing on auscultation, accentuated during forced expiration. Other findings are similar to those discussed on p 83.

Treatment

The therapy discussed under treatment of severe forms of these disorders can be modified.

Disposition

Hospitalization is indicated for patients with severe or rapidly worsening dyspnea that does not respond to a few hours of treatment in the emergency department.

PULMONARY VASCULAR DISEASE

Dyspnea from pulmonary vascular disease may be one of the most difficult diagnostic problems confronting the emergency physician. The manifestations of pulmonary vascular disease are extremely varied in character and severity, and there is a significant risk of labeling patients with these illnesses as hysterical personalities or malingerers.

1. ACUTE PULMONARY EMBOLISM (See also Chapter 27.)

Diagnosis

Patients with acute pulmonary embolism and infarction usually have dyspnea, tachypnea, pleuritic chest pain, tachycardia, hypoxemia, and hypocapnia. Low-grade fever, cough, hemoptysis, and wheezing may also be present. Pulmonary infiltrates, occasionally with effusion, may be seen on x-ray.

Patients with embolization without infarction have similar manifestations but often without pulmonary infiltrates, fever, and hemoptysis.

In massive pulmonary embolization, crushing anterior chest pain, dyspnea, severe hypoxemia, syncope, and shock are common.

Patients with right-sided endocarditis and other causes of septic pulmonary embolization usually have high fever and rigors associated with symptoms of embolization; the chest x-ray often shows multiple scattered infiltrates that frequently cavitate after several days of illness.

Confirm the diagnosis by ventilation-perfusion lung scanning (or a perfusion scan alone), followed by pulmonary angiography if indicated. A completely normal ventilation-perfusion lung scan excludes the diagnosis of pulmonary embolism, but an abnormal scan is not specific for pulmonary emboli (see Chronic Pulmonary Vascular Obstruction, below).

Treatment

A. Give oxygen.

B. Give morphine as necessary for pain.

C. Treat shock if present.

D. Heparin should be started (unless contraindicated) if embolization is strongly suspected. *Do not* give heparin in cases of suspected *septic* embolization. For adults, give a bolus of 10,000 units intravenously, followed by continuous infusion of about 1000 units per hour, adjusting the rate to maintain the prothrombin time at 1.5–2 times control values. This treatment may be started in the emergency department and continued in the hospital. Thrombolytic therapy (Chapter 27) should rarely be started in the emergency department.

Disposition

Patients with suspected or documented pulmonary embolization require hospitalization.

2. CHRONIC PULMONARY VASCULAR OBSTRUCTION (Repeated Small Pulmonary Emboli)

A much more difficult problem is presented by patients with repeated small pulmonary emboli without infarction or with progressive pulmonary vascular occlusion from other causes (intravenous drug abuse, sickle cell anemia, vasculitis).

Diagnosis

These patients usually complain of dyspnea yet may have no abnormal findings in the emergency cardiorespiratory data base. Although significant hypoxemia and hypocapnia are often present, blood gas values are occasionally normal at rest. Evidence of pulmonary hypertension and right ventricular overload is found infrequently, and then only in patients with advanced illness. A normal perfusion lung scan virtually excludes pulmonary emboli and is evidence against other types of pulmonary vascular disease. On the other hand, abnormal lung scans can be produced by practically any type of pulmonary disease: asthma, bronchitis, and emphysema are the most common offenders in patients with normal chest x-rays.

Treatment & Disposition

Obtain an arterial blood gas sample for determination of PO_2, PCO_2, and pH before starting treatment. Start low-flow oxygen (2 L/min by mask or nasal prongs, or 24% by Ventimask), and adjust the flow based on results of arterial blood gas analysis.

Hospitalization is indicated for patients with respiratory failure or if symptoms are worsening rapidly. Dyspneic patients with unexplained hypoxemia should not be discharged home without arranging for an evaluation to exclude pulmonary vascular disease (screening pulmonary function tests with diffusing capacity, measurement of alveolar-arterial PO_2 gradient during rest and exercise, perfusion lung scan, pulmonary arteriography, etc). Furthermore, if a patient comes to the emergency department on 2 or 3 occasions with dyspnea and no abnormalities are noted in the cardiopulmonary data base, referral to a chest physician is warranted for evaluation and complete pulmonary function testing.

MISCELLANEOUS CONDITIONS

1. PLEURISY

Diagnosis

Pleurisy and pleuritic pain from any cause may produce a sensation of dyspnea. Even conditions such as rib fractures that produce pleuritic pain in the absence of significant underlying pulmonary parenchymal abnormalities may cause splinting and atelectasis sufficient to produce hypoxemia. When pleural fluid forms, the pain and friction rub may lessen or disappear. Pleurisy is often part of a viral syndrome (which may occasionally be accompanied by pericarditis). Fever, myalgias, headache, nasal congestion, or influenzalike symptoms may be present. A chest x-ray is required to exclude underlying lung disease, pleural effusion, or pneumothorax.

Treatment

Other than measures for relief of pain, therapy must be directed toward the underlying lesion.

Disposition

Hospitalization is required if the patient is severely hypoxemic (arterial $PO_2 \leq 60$ mm Hg as a new finding), if parenteral analgesia is required for pain relief, or if the underlying disease requires hospital treatment.

2. METABOLIC ACIDOSIS

Diagnosis

Metabolic acidosis (diabetic ketoacidosis, salicylate overdose, etc) can produce secondary hyperventilation that may be mistaken for dyspnea or respiratory distress. Arterial blood gas analyses usually show a normal or high PO_2, marked hypocapnia (PCO_2 10–20 mm Hg), and metabolic acidosis (low serum bicarbonate concentration).

Treatment & Disposition

Treatment depends on the underlying condition.

These patients almost always require hospitalization for management of the underlying cause of metabolic acidosis (Chapter 36).

3. ANEMIA, PREGNANCY, & THYROTOXICOSIS

These 3 conditions may at times have accompanying dyspnea, and therapy for the underlying condition is all that is required.

4. NEUROGENIC HYPERVENTILATION

Primary central nervous system disease can produce a variety of abnormal breathing patterns, including central hyperventilation and Cheyne-Stokes respiration, any of which could be mistaken for respiratory distress. Cheyne-Stokes respiration may

also occur when the circulation is slowed, as in heart failure.

Diagnosis

The diagnosis is based on finding obvious neurologic or cardiac disease consistent with the respiratory pattern. The arterial PO_2 is usually normal; PCO_2 may be low or high.

Treatment

No treatment of the respiratory condition is required.

Disposition

Disposition depends on the underlying disease.

5. PSYCHOGENIC HYPERVENTILATION & PULMONARY NEUROSIS

Diagnosis

Patients with psychogenic hyperventilation usually present with a history of acute dyspnea and anxiety, often precipitated by personal or environmental factors. Hyperventilation to the point of tetany is diagnostic. Lightheadedness (due to cerebral vasoconstriction) and circumoral or limb paresthesias are often present. Another helpful feature is that the dyspnea often improves with exercise. Patients can be calmed enough to speak, whereas in organic dyspnea, patients are not capable of speech. There are usually no abnormalities on the screening data base other than a low arterial PCO_2, normal or high arterial PO_2, and elevated pH. Most of these patients can be diagnosed in the emergency department as having neuroses, but the possibility of pulmonary vascular disease must be considered.

Patients with pulmonary neurosis or cardiac neurasthenia have complaints of chronic dyspnea with or without fatigue, often with vague or nonspecific chest pains. Results of arterial blood gas analyses are often normal.

Treatment

There is no specific treatment. Reassurance is usually helpful. Patients with symptomatic hypocapnia (circumoral tingling, carpopedal spasm, tetany) or marked respiratory alkalosis (pH > 7.55) should breathe into an airtight bag for several minutes to relieve hypocapnia.

Disposition

The patient should be referred to a pulmonary clinic or internist for complete evaluation and reassurance.

REFERENCES

Albert RK, Martin TR, Lewis SW: Controlled clinical trial of methylprednisolone in patients with chronic bronchitis and acute respiratory insufficiency. Ann Intern Med 1980;92:753.

Bell RC et al: Multiple organ system failure and infection in adult respiratory distress syndrome. Ann Intern Med 1983;99:293.

Benatar SR: Fatal asthma. N Engl J Med 1986;314:423.

Dorinsky PM, Gadek JE: Mechanism of multiple non-pulmonary organ failure in ARDS. Chest 1989;96:885.

Fowler AA et al: Adult respiratory distress syndrome: Risk with common predispositions. Ann Intern Med 1983; 98:593.

Jones J et al: Continuous emergency department monitoring of arterial saturation in adult patients with respiratory distress. Ann Emerg Med 1988;17:463.

Karpel JP et al: A comparison of atropine sulfate and metaproterenol sulfate in the emergency treatment of asthma. Am Rev Respir Dis 1986;133:727.

Littenberg B, Gluck EH: A controlled trial of methylprednisolone in the emergency treatment of acute asthma. N Engl J Med 1986;314:150.

Maunder RJ, Pierson DJ, Hudson LD: Subcutaneous and mediastinal emphysema: Pathophysiology, diagnosis, and management. Arch Intern Med 1984;144:1447.

Mayo-Smith MF et al: Acute epiglottitis in adults: An eight-year experience in the state of Rhode Island. N Engl J Med 1986;314:1133.

McNamara RM et al: Intravenous magnesium sulfate in the management of acute respiratory failure complication asthma. Ann Emerg Med 1989;18:197.

Moser KM: Venous thromboembolism. Am Rev Respir Dis 1990;141:235.

Natanson C, Shelhamer JH, Parrillo JE: Intubation of the trachea in the critical care setting. JAMA 1985;253:1160.

Pepe PE et al: Clinical predictors of the adult respiratory distress syndrome. Am J Surg 1982;144:124.

Siegel D et al: Aminophylline increases the toxicity but not the efficacy of an inhaled beta-adrenergic agonist in the treatment of acute exacerbations of asthma. Am Rev Respir Dis 1985;132:283.

Stein LM, Cole RP: Early administration of corticosteroids in emergency room treatment of acute asthma. Ann Intern Med 1990;112:882.

Vallee P et al: Sequential treatment of a simple pneumothorax. Ann Emerg Med 1988;17:936.

Vathener AS et al: High-dose inhaled albuterol in severe chronic airflow limitation. Am Rev Respir Dis 1988;138:850.

Chest Pain*

6

Mary T. Ho, MD, MPH, & John Mills, MD

---

*Chest pain due to trauma is discussed in Chapter 18.

I. IMMEDIATE MANAGEMENT OF LIFE-THREATENING PROBLEMS (See algorithm.)

INITIAL MANAGEMENT

Begin Supplemental Oxygen

Give oxygen, 5 L/min, by nasal prongs or face mask, pending further evaluation.

Begin Continuous Cardiac Monitoring

Begin cardiac monitoring, and treat life-threatening arrhythmias (Chapters 1 and 29).

Obtain Vital Signs

If blood pressure and pulse are normal in the supine position, obtain blood pressure and pulse in the sitting and then the standing positions (unless contraindicated) to detect more subtle hypovolemia.

Look for Markedly Abnormal Hemodynamics

1. Look for signs of shock. Arterial hypotension and poor peripheral perfusion cause altered sensorium; pale, clammy skin; oliguria; and, frequently, respiratory distress.

2. Look for central plethora. Central venous hypervolemia is manifested initially by distended superficial veins (best seen in the neck); later, pulmonary edema (causing cough, dyspnea, rales, and frothy sputum) or peripheral edema may be seen, although peripheral edema is usually absent in conditions of acute onset.

Central plethora may be caused by conditions obstructing venous return (eg, tension pneumothorax, pulmonary embolization) or by cardiac disease (eg, infarction, tamponade). Pulmonary edema is usually not seen in conditions causing only interference with venous return.

MANAGEMENT OF THE PATIENT WITH CHEST PAIN & ABNORMAL HEMODYNAMICS

Diagnosis

The patient is in obvious distress, and signs of abnormal hemodynamics are obvious on examination.

Treatment & Disposition

A. Immediate Measures:

1. Insert 2 large-bore (≥ 16-gauge) intravenous catheters.

a. Draw blood for CBC, serum electrolyte measurements, glucose, and tests for renal function; reserve 2 tubes of clotted whole blood for other studies that may be needed.

b. Begin administration of intravenous fluids based on estimate of intravascular fluid volume.

(1) No central plethora; hypotension or shock present—Begin intravenous infusion of crystalloid solutions (eg, normal saline or lactated or acetated Ringer's injection), about 300–500 mL in 20 minutes. Monitor the response (blood pressure, urine output, sensorium).

(2) Central plethora (with or without shock or hypotension)—Pending more precise diagnosis, infuse 5% dextrose in water solely to keep the intravenous catheter patent.

2. Briefly examine the pulmonary and cardiovascular systems, and palpate the abdomen for presence of a pulsatile mass.

3. Obtain a 12-lead ECG.

4. Obtain arterial blood for blood gas and pH determinations. Avoid unnecessary arterial punctures if the patient is a candidate for thrombolytic therapy for acute myocardial infarction.

5. Arrange for a portable chest x-ray as soon as possible.

6. Insert a urinary catheter.

B. Life-Threatening Abnormalities:

1. **No central plethora; hypotension or shock present**—Hypovolemia is manifested by collapsed neck veins, clear lung fields on physical examination or chest x-ray, and absence of peripheral edema. The central venous and pulmonary capillary wedge pressures are low. The differentiating features of the 3 most important conditions causing chest pain with hypotension but without central plethora are set forth in Table 6–1.

If the diagnosis is uncertain, treatment should be oriented primarily toward aortic dissection (Chapter 32).

a. Type and cross-match for 10 units of whole blood.

b. Expand intravascular volume with administration of intravenous crystalloid solution. Consider inserting a central line. For severe hypovolemia with shock, up to 3 L of crystalloid solution may be given rapidly (over 30–60 minutes) to restore normal hemodynamics until whole blood is available. Rarely, type-specific or universal donor blood (O-negative, low antibody titer to erythrocyte antigens) may be needed (Chapter 33). Maintain blood pressure with continued infusion of blood and crystalloid solution. Blood should be given to keep the hematocrit above 30%.

c. Obtain emergency vascular or thoracic surgical consultation.

d. Reexamine the patient for pulse deficits or an abdominal mass, and check urine for occult blood; these findings indicate aortic aneurysm or dissection. Obtain chest and abdominal x-rays.

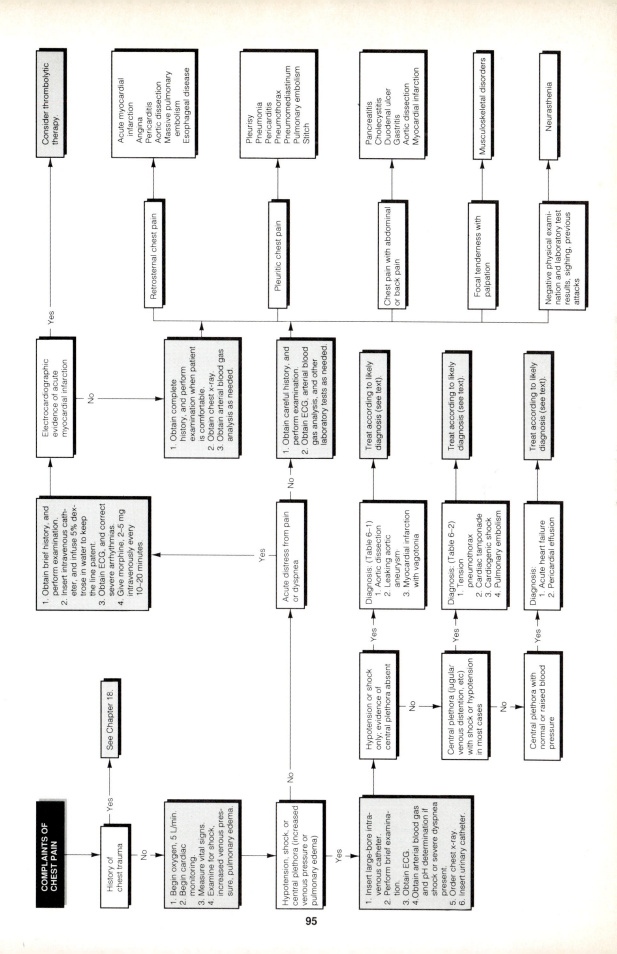

COMPLAINTS OF CHEST PAIN

History of chest trauma

Yes → See Chapter 18.

No →

1. Begin oxygen, 5 L/min.
2. Begin cardiac monitoring.
3. Measure vital signs.
4. Examine for shock, increased venous pressure, pulmonary edema.

Hypotension, shock, or central plethora (increased venous pressure or pulmonary edema)

Yes →

1. Insert large-bore intravenous catheter.
2. Perform brief examination.
3. Obtain ECG.
4. Obtain arterial blood gas and pH determination if shock or severe dyspnea present.
5. Order chest x-ray.
6. Insert urinary catheter.

Hypotension or shock only; evidence of central plethora absent

Yes → Diagnosis: (Table 6–1)
1. Aortic dissection
2. Leaking aortic aneurysm
3. Myocardial infarction with vagotonia

Treat according to likely diagnosis (see text).

No →

Central plethora (jugular venous distention, etc) with shock or hypotension in most cases

Yes → Diagnosis: (Table 6–2)
1. Tension pneumothorax
2. Cardiac tamponade
3. Cardiogenic shock
4. Pulmonary embolism

Treat according to likely diagnosis (see text).

No →

Central plethora with normal or raised blood pressure

Yes → Diagnosis:
1. Acute heart failure
2. Pericardial effusion

Treat according to likely diagnosis (see text).

No →

Acute distress from pain or dyspnea

Yes →

1. Obtain brief history, and perform examination.
2. Insert intravenous catheter, and infuse 5% dextrose in water to keep the line patent.
3. Obtain ECG, and correct severe arrhythmias.
4. Give morphine, 2–5 mg intravenously every 10–20 minutes.

Electrocardiographic evidence of acute myocardial infarction

Yes → Consider thrombolytic therapy.

No →

1. Obtain complete history, and perform examination when patient is comfortable.
2. Obtain chest x-ray.
3. Obtain arterial blood gas analysis as needed.

No →

1. Obtain careful history, and perform examination.
2. Obtain ECG, arterial blood gas analysis, and other laboratory tests as needed.

Retrosternal chest pain →
Acute myocardial infarction
Angina
Pericarditis
Aortic dissection
Massive pulmonary embolism
Esophageal disease

Pleuritic chest pain →
Pleurisy
Pneumonia
Pericarditis
Pneumothorax
Pneumomediastinum
Pulmonary embolism
Stitch

Chest pain with abdominal or back pain →
Pancreatitis
Cholecystitis
Duodenal ulcer
Gastritis
Aortic dissection
Myocardial infarction

Focal tenderness with palpation →
Musculoskeletal disorders

Negative physical examination and laboratory test results, sighing, previous attacks →
Neurasthenia

95

Table 6–1. Differentiating features of conditions causing chest pain with hypovolemia but without central plethora.

Diagnosis	Findings			
	History	Examination	ECG	X-Rays
Myocardial infarction with vagotonia	Crushing chest pain; nausea and vomiting	Bradycardia; stable hypotension	Acute infarction pattern and bradycardia	Nonspecific.
Aortic dissection	Tearing chest pain; back pain; often history of hypertension	Tachycardia; pulse deficits; progressive hypotension	Nonspecific or may show ischemia or infarction pattern	Widened mediastinum; pleural fluid. CT scan is more sensitive than x-ray.
Leaking upper abdominal aortic aneurysm	Chest and epigastric pain	Tachycardia; pulsatile epigastric mass	Nonspecific	Abdominal aneurysm. Sonogram is more sensitive than x-rays.

e. Hospitalize the patient in an intensive care setting immediately for further evaluation and treatment.

2. Central plethora with hypotension or shock–Superficial veins (especially neck veins) are distended; pulmonary and peripheral edema may be present as well. See Table 6–2 for guidelines to differential diagnosis. **Tension pneumothorax** should be considered immediately, since this condition may be quickly and reliably differentiated from the others and is easy to treat. Look for marked respiratory distress, a laterally deviated trachea away from the affected side, and a hyperresonant hemithorax with markedly decreased or absent breath sounds on the affected side. Chest x-ray confirms the diagnosis, but treatment should not be unduly delayed to obtain a chest x-ray, since many patients require definitive treatment quickly.

Table 6–2. Distinguishing features of conditions causing chest pain, hypotension, or shock in association with distended neck veins (central plethora).

Diagnosis	Helpful Distinguishing Features
Tension pneumothorax	Hyperresonant hemithorax with decreased breath sounds; chest x-rays diagnostic.
Cardiac tamponade	Faint heart sounds; ECG with diffuse low voltage or electrical alternans. Pulmonary edema rare. Echocardiography diagnostic.
Cardiogenic shock (arrhythmogenic)	ECG or cardiac monitor shows severe bradycardia (ventricular rate < 50 beats/min, usually < 40 beats/min) or tachycardia (rate > 160 beats/min, usually > 180 beats/min). Signs of myocardial ischemia may also be present.
Cardiogenic shock (myocardial)	Pulmonary edema almost always present. ECG almost always shows pattern diagnostic of infarction.
Pulmonary embolism (massive)	Physical examination, ECG, and chest x-ray show signs of right heart strain. Chest x-ray may show infiltrates, effusions, or truncation of pulmonary vasculature. Confirm diagnosis by ventilation-perfusion scanning or pulmonary arteriography.

Cardiac tamponade should also be diagnosed early, since treatment is reasonably effective but differs markedly from that for cardiogenic shock, heart failure, or pulmonary embolism. Look for faint heart sounds and low voltage on all leads of the ECG, electrical alternans, or diffuse ST segment elevation typical of pericarditis. A narrow pulse pressure and pulsus paradoxus may also be present. Pulmonary edema is rare. Chest x-ray is not helpful, because acute tamponade does not cause a detectable increase in heart size. Definitive diagnosis by noninvasive methods is best done by echocardiography, but tamponade may be confirmed (and treated) by pericardiocentesis alone in desperate cases.

a. **Tension pneumothorax**–(See Chapter 18.) Insert a thoracostomy tube if one is readily available (Chapter 46). Otherwise, a 16-gauge needle inserted in the second intercostal space lateral to the sternum or in the fourth intercostal space at the anterior axillary line relieves tension in the chest until a thoracostomy tube can be inserted. Hospitalize the patient for further care.

b. **Cardiac tamponade**–(See Chapter 28.) Attempt volume expansion with intravenous administration of 300–500 mL of crystalloid solution over 20–30 minutes if the diagnosis is confirmed (this therapy is disastrous for cardiogenic shock). If the initial trial succeeds in raising the blood pressure, volume expansion may be repeated once in a patient whose systolic pressure subsequently drops to less than 90 mm Hg.

If time permits, obtain emergency cardiothoracic consultation for therapeutic pericardiocentesis, which should be performed in the operating room or under echocardiographic or fluoroscopic guidance. Otherwise, perform immediate pericardiocentesis (Chapter 46) if rapid, progressive hypotension develops and the patient fails to respond to volume expansion. Hospitalize the patient at once in an intensive care unit.

c. **Cardiogenic shock (arrhythmogenic)**–See Chapter 29 for further details on the diagnosis and treatment of cardiac arrhythmias.

(1) Severe bradyarrhythmia (heart rate usually < 40 beats/min)–Give atropine, 0.5 mg intravenously; if necessary, repeat every 5–10 minutes up to a total dose of 2 mg. An external transcutaneous pacemaker (Chapter 46) may be applied to increase the heart rate until a percutaneous transvenous pacemaker can be inserted. Isoproterenol may be given temporarily until a pacemaker becomes available. Give 2–4 µg/min initially by continuous intravenous infusion, and increase as needed up to 20 µg/min. Isoproterenol must be used with extreme caution and only with continuous electrocardiographic monitoring and frequent blood pressure readings, because it may cause arrhythmias. Because of the vasodilator (β_2-adrenergic) effect of isoproterenol, blood pressure may fall if the heart rate does not increase.

Dopamine can be used instead of isoproterenol to support blood pressure by increasing myocardial contractility (Inside Front Cover). Mix 200 mg of dopamine in 250 mL of 5% dextrose in water for a solution of 800 µg/mL. Give at a rate of 2–12 µg/kg/min by continuous intravenous infusion, and observe the response. The dosage may be increased as needed but should not exceed 20 µg/kg/min.

In the occasional patient with hypotension or shock due to severe bradyarrhythmia *without central plethora,* fluid challenge may be given as described in the section on cardiac tamponade. If there is no response to the above measures or if the patient develops left heart failure with fluid challenge, a percutaneous transvenous pacemaker should be inserted. This is the treatment of choice. Hospitalize all patients in an intensive care unit.

(2) Severe tachyarrhythmia (heart rate usually > 180 beats/min)–Immediate cardioversion is the treatment of choice. Intubate the patient to protect the airway, and use intravenous anesthesia (supervised by an anesthesiologist, if possible). Deliver 50–100 J of synchronized DC countershock initially, and increase the shock by 50- to 100-J increments if there is no response.

d. Cardiogenic shock (myocardial infarction)–(See also Chapter 3.)

(1) In patients with no evidence of pulmonary edema, give intravenous crystalloid solution, 100–300 mL over 30 minutes. If blood pressure improves, maintain the infusion at a rate of 100–200 mL/h.

(2) Give dobutamine, dopamine, or a combination of both if no change in blood pressure occurs or if severe shock or pulmonary edema is present initially. Mix 500 mg (2 vials) of dobutamine in 250 mL of 5% dextrose in water for a 2 mg/mL solution, and give at a rate of 2.5–20 µg/kg/min by continuous intravenous infusion. Begin at the lower dose, and increase as needed, guided by clinical response. Dobutamine is the drug of choice for treatment of cardiogenic shock due to pump failure. *Caution:* Observe for signs of arrhythmia.

(3) Give morphine, 2–4 mg intravenously every 5–20 minutes, until pain and dyspnea are controlled. Carefully monitor the patient's respiratory status.

Avoid unnecessary arterial punctures in patients who may be candidates for thrombolytic therapy.

(4) Nitroglycerin ointment, 1.25–2.5 cm (½–1 in) applied under an occlusive dressing, can be used for additional preload reduction. If the patient's condition worsens because of the effect of the ointment, it can be discontinued by simply wiping it off.

(5) Notify the cardiology consultant immediately if an acute infarction pattern is evident on the 12-lead ECG. Ideally, patients eligible for thrombolytic therapy (Chapter 28) should have treatment begun in the emergency department by the emergency physician, avoiding the delay necessitated by obtaining cardiologic consultation or transporting the patient to the coronary care unit. Emergency reperfusion therapy with thrombolytic agents or percutaneous transluminal coronary angioplasty (PTCA) has been shown to be of benefit in decreasing the mortality rate and the size of the infarct.

(6) Hospitalize the patient immediately in a coronary care or intensive care unit, and insert a pulmonary artery (Swan-Ganz) catheter and an arterial line as soon as possible to monitor blood pressure.

e. Massive pulmonary embolism–(See Chapter 27.) Because massive pulmonary embolism is an uncommon diagnosis and difficult to confirm rapidly, every attempt should be made to exclude other causes of chest pain with shock (Table 6–2).

Attempt volume expansion with administration of 300–500 mL of normal saline over 20–30 minutes to raise systolic blood pressure. The dose may be repeated if the trial is successful and if heart failure does not develop. In the rare patient with hypotension without central plethora, a fluid challenge should also be given, but a larger dose (500–1000 mL of normal saline instead of 300–500 mL) may be administered.

Give dopamine (see above and Inside Front Cover). If clinical signs strongly suggest pulmonary embolism, begin heparin (see Pulmonary Embolism, below, for dosages). Obtain pulmonary consultation, and consider surgical consultation and thrombolytic therapy.

3. Central plethora with normal or raised blood pressure–Superficial veins (especially neck veins) are distended. Pulmonary and peripheral edema is common. Blood pressure is normal or (more commonly) elevated.

Acute congestive heart failure is the commonest cause. It most frequently results from acute myocardial infarction (acute cardiogenic pulmonary edema), although acute myopericarditis or pericardial effusion without frank tamponade may be present occasionally.

a. Give furosemide, 20–40 mg by bolus intravenous injection. The initial effect of rapid preload reduction is of immediate benefit; diuresis occurs later.

b. Give morphine, 2–4 mg intravenously, and repeat every 5–10 minutes until pain and dyspnea are relieved.

c. Give nitroglycerin, 0.4 mg sublingually, or use nitroglycerin ointment, 1.25–2.5 cm (½–1 in) applied under an occlusive dressing. Nitroglycerin by intravenous infusion, beginning with a rate of 10 μg/min and increasing by 5–10 μg/min every 3–5 minutes as needed, can be started in the emergency department. Monitor the blood pressure closely, and if hypotension develops, place the patient in the Trendelenburg position and decrease the infusion rate.

d. Give aspirin, 160–325 mg, chewed if not contraindicated.

e. Hospitalize the patient immediately in an intensive care setting, and monitor hemodynamic status with a pulmonary artery catheter and arterial catheter as needed.

MANAGEMENT OF THE PATIENT WITH SEVERE CHEST PAIN & NORMAL HEMODYNAMICS

Diagnosis

The patient is in acute distress because of chest pain but is neither hypotensive nor in shock. There is no readily apparent central plethora.

Treatment

A. Give oxygen, 3–5 L/min, by nasal prongs or mask.

B. Begin continuous electrocardiographic monitoring.

C. Insert an intravenous catheter (18-gauge is satisfactory), and begin an infusion of 5% dextrose in water as slowly as necessary to keep the catheter open.

D. Obtain a 12-lead ECG as soon as possible. If the ECG reveals evidence of acute myocardial infarction, evaluate the patient for possible thrombolytic therapy (Chapter 28).

E. Give morphine, 2–5 mg slowly intravenously; or nitroglycerin, 0.4 mg sublingually. Morphine may be repeated every 10–20 minutes until the patient is more comfortable; sublingual nitroglycerin may be repeated twice with 5 minutes between doses. If pain continues despite morphine and sublingual nitroglycerin and if acute myocardial infarction is suspected, begin nitroglycerin by intravenous infusion (see above).

F. Give aspirin, 160–325 mg, chewed if the patient has no aspirin allergy or other contraindications.

G. Send blood samples to the laboratory for CBC, renal function tests, and serum electrolyte, glucose, and amylase determinations. Send blood samples for cardiac enzyme measurements (CK with MB isoenzymes and LDH isoenzymes) if myocardial infarction is suspected and the patient is to be hospitalized.

H. Obtain arterial blood for blood gas and pH measurements if thrombolytic therapy is not antici-

pated and the patient is dyspneic or pneumothorax or pulmonary embolism is a possibility.

I. Correct any significant cardiac arrhythmias (Chapter 29). Ventricular premature contractions are the most common arrhythmia and should be treated with lidocaine. A loading dose of 1 mg/kg by bolus intravenous infusion is followed by 1–4 mg/min by continuous intravenous infusion. A second bolus of 0.5 mg/kg can be given after 15 minutes.

J. Take a thorough medical history with emphasis on the location, quality, and duration of chest pain, and perform a complete physical examination (see below).

K. Obtain a chest x-ray. An anteroposterior view with portable equipment is satisfactory if the patient is too sick to tolerate a better examination.

L. Obtain additional tests as indicated on the basis of the history, physical examination, and results of laboratory tests obtained above.

Disposition

Patients with chest pain severe enough to cause objective distress should be hospitalized for evaluation unless a condition not requiring hospitalization is diagnosed with certainty or they have a documented history of malingering.

II. FURTHER EVALUATION OF THE PATIENT WITH CHEST PAIN

Differential Diagnosis by Location & Quality of Pain

Evaluation of patients who complain of chest pain but are not in severe distress should proceed in a systematic fashion. The single most useful means of evaluation is the carefully elicited history supplemented by examination of the heart, lungs, abdomen, and peripheral vessels in conjunction with electrocardiography, chest x-ray, and arterial blood gas measurements. Consider most of the diagnostic possibilities at least briefly in every patient who presents with chest pain (Table 6–3).

A. Retrosternal Discomfort: Retrosternal discomfort, especially if it is a tightness, pressure, or "squeezing" pain, should suggest serious underlying disease, eg, **(1)** myocardial infarction, **(2)** angina due to atherosclerosis or valvular heart disease, **(3)** pericarditis, **(4)** dissection of the aorta, or **(5)** pulmonary embolism. When the above diagnoses are excluded, esophageal disease (eg, spasm, esophagitis) is the most common cause of retrosternal distress (see below). Because esophageal disease is relatively benign and rarely requires hospitalization, the more serious causes of retrosternal discomfort must be excluded with a high degree of certainty before concluding that the pain is of esophageal origin.

Hospitalize all patients with oppressive retrosternal pain for observation unless a condition not requiring hospitalization is diagnosed with certainty.

B. Pleuritic Pain: Pain that is markedly worse on inspiration should suggest pleurisy associated with pneumonia, pulmonary embolism, or isolated pleuritis. The pain of pneumothorax, pneumomediastinum, ruptured esophagus, and pericarditis frequently has a pleuritic component. The fleeting pain of a "stitch in the side" is often pleuritic in nature as well. Infrequently, chest pain due to myocardial infarction may have a pleuritic component.

Patients with pleurisy who have normal chest x-rays, ECGs, and arterial blood gas levels can be discharged unless there are other symptoms sufficiently suggestive of pulmonary embolism to warrant performing a ventilation-perfusion lung scan or pulmonary arteriogram. Disposition of patients with pleurisy who have abnormal laboratory tests should be guided by the most likely diagnosis, or if unknown, these patients should be hospitalized for evaluation.

C. Back or Abdominal Pain With Chest Pain: Abdominal pain that is inferior to the xiphoid process and associated with chest pain should suggest intra-abdominal disease or dissecting aortic aneurysm. These patients should usually be hospitalized unless a condition not requiring hospitalization is diagnosed with certainty.

D. Musculoskeletal Discomfort: Musculoskeletal disease with chest pain (Tietze's syndrome, rib fracture) is usually associated with marked tenderness localized over the affected site. Patients with chest pain referred from intrathoracic structures may also have some associated tenderness of superficial structures, however. Most patients with chest pain from musculoskeletal disorders can be treated in the emergency department and discharged for outpatient follow-up care.

E. Neurasthenic Pain: Neurasthenic pain is often bizarre, may be fleeting or constant, and is customarily described as being over the cardiac apex. Patients report fatigue but not true dyspnea. Sighing is a common sign. The results of physical and laboratory examination are normal. Neurasthenia is a diagnosis of exclusion that should be considered only after thorough evaluation. Generally, the diagnosis can be made with certainty only after repeated observation.

If life-threatening disease is suspected on the basis of history and physical examination alone, the patient should be hospitalized *even if laboratory test results are normal.* It is better to hospitalize a few patients with neurasthenia than to discharge inadvertently even one patient with myocardial infarction.

III. MANAGEMENT OF SPECIFIC DISORDERS CAUSING CHEST PAIN

CARDIOVASCULAR DISORDERS

ANGINA
(See Chapter 28.)

MYOCARDIAL INFARCTION
(See Chapter 28.)

MITRAL VALVE PROLAPSE

Diagnosis

Mitral valve prolapse should be considered in any patient with a mitral regurgitant murmur or clicks (without other known heart disease or other cause of chest pain) who presents with recurring atypical chest pains. The ECG may show nonspecific T wave abnormalities. Echocardiography is required for definitive diagnosis.

Treatment

No specific emergency therapy is required. Although life-threatening arrhythmias may occur, they are rare. Beta-blocker therapy (eg, metoprolol, 50 mg orally twice daily) may be offered to patients who are uncomfortably symptomatic.

Disposition

The patient should be referred to a cardiologist or primary-care physician for definitive evaluation and management.

AORTIC STENOSIS & INSUFFICIENCY

Diagnosis

Chest pain in patients with severe aortic stenosis or insufficiency is clinically similar to that of angina and is probably the result of a similar mechanism, ie, relative myocardial ischemia secondary to diminished coronary blood flow.

Anginal pain in a patient with aortic valve disease may signify that hemodynamically significant abnormalities of the valve are present, with a higher risk of impending sudden death. Murmurs of aortic stenosis or insufficiency are present on physical examination,

Table 6-3. Diagnostic clues to cause of chest pair.[1]

Cause	Previous Attacks of Similar Pain	History — Pain — Location	History — Pain — Character	History — Pain — Onset	History — Duration	Common Associated Findings	Signs	Other Abnormalities	Other Comments
Angina	Usually.	Retrosternal, radiating to left arm.	Squeezing, oppressive.	With stress or exercise.	2–10 minutes up to 20–30 minutes.	Occasionally dyspnea. Dizziness and syncope rare.	Often none. S₄ occasionally.	ECG often normal between attacks.	Relieved by nitroglycerin.
Acute myocardial infarction	In some cases.	Retrosternal, radiating to left arm, neck. Rarely in back.	Squeezing, oppressive, increases with time.	No precipitating factor necessary.	> 30 minutes.	Nausea and vomiting, diaphoresis, dyspnea.	Heart failure, restlessness, shock; cardiac examination often normal.	ECG may be diagnostic or normal.	Elevated CK, LDH, or CK-MB isoenzymes. Normal isoenzyme levels on one determination do not exclude diagnosis.
Mitral valve prolapse	Usually.	Variable.	Variable.	Variable.	Variable; usually hours.	Dyspnea, dizziness common; syncope in some.	Mdsystolic click or murmur in most cases.	ECG may show inverted T waves on leads II, III, and aVF. Echocardiogram is diagnostic.	Arrhythmia or sudden death may occur. Usually seen in young women. High-arched palate or chest or spine deformities may be present.
Aortic stenosis	May have occurred.	Like angina.	Like angina.	Like angina.	Like angina.	Syncope, dyspnea.	Systolic ejection murmur transmitted tc carotid arteries; delayed carotid pulse.	ECG usually shows left ventricular hypertrophy. Echocardiography and angiocardiography are diagnostic.	More common in older men.
Aortic insufficiency	May have occurred.	Like angina.	Like angina.	Like angina.	May be prolonged.	Dyspnea.	Ciastolic murmur transmitted to carotid arteries. Waterhammer and Quincke's pulse. Wide arterial pulse pressure.	ECG may be normal or may show left ventricular hypertrophy. Echocardiography and angiocardiography are diagnostic.	History of rheumatic heart disease, connective tissue disease, or syphilis.
Pericarditis	May have occurred.	Retrosternal.	Variable; often pleuritic and relieved by sitting.	Variable.	Hours to days.	Variable.	Pericardial friction rub in many.	ECG may be diagnostic, nonspecific, or normal. Echocardiography often shows fluid.	
Aortic dissection	No.	Retrosternal and back.	Tearing, maximal at onset.	Sudden.	Variable.	Myocardial infarction, stroke, limb ischemia, syncope.	Stroke, absent pulses, hematuria, shock.	Chest x-ray shows widened mediastinum. ECG may show acute myocardial infarction. Pulsatile abdominal mass.	Angiography or CT scan is definitive. Hypertension or connective tissue disease may be present.
Pleurisy	In some cases.	Variable; usually lateral thorax.	Pleuritic.	Usually sudden.	Variable.	Subjective dyspnea.	Often none. Occasionally friction rub, low-grade fever.	Occasionally pleural effusion.	Negative lung scan or pulmonary angiogram.

Disorder									
Pneumothorax	May have occurred.	Variable.	Variable; often pleuritic.	Usually sudden.	Variable.	Dyspnea and cough; shock if tension pneumothorax is present.	Tachycardia, lung collapse with or without mediastinal shift.	Chest x-ray is diagnostic but needs careful examination. Expiratory views may be helpful.	Consider esophageal perforation as cause.
Pneumomediastinum	No.	Retrosternal.	Variable; often pleuritic.	Usually sudden.	Variable.	Dyspnea.	Mediastinal crunch.	Chest x-ray is diagnostic. Pneumothorax common.	
Pulmonary hypertension	Usually.	Retrosternal.	Like angina.	Like angina.	Variable.	Dyspnea, fatigue, exercise syncope.	Loud P_2, right ventricular lift.	ECG shows right heart strain. Chest x-ray shows signs of pulmonary hypertension.	
Pulmonary embolism	May have occurred.	Variable; usually lateral thorax.	Usually strong pleuritic component.	Usually sudden.	Minutes to hours.	Dyspnea, cough, and tachypnea; Hemoptysis sometimes.	Friction rub or splinting in some.	Hypoxemia and hypocapnia. Chest x-ray usually abnormal, but findings are not specific.	Abnormal ventilation-perfusion radionuclide lung scan or pulmonary angiogram.
Pneumonia	Rare.	Over affected lobe.	Pleuritic.	Variable.	Variable.	Fever and chills, cough, dyspnea, sputum production.	Fever, rales with or without consolidation, friction rub.	Infiltrates on chest x-ray; purulent sputum.	
Esophagitis Esophageal spasm Hiatal hernia	Usually.	Retrosternal or epigastrium.	Changes with eating.	Usually gradual.	Variable.	Gastrointestinal symptoms.	None.	Positive barium swallow and Bernstein (acid perfusion) test.	Relieved by antacids or topical anesthesia.
Perforated esophagus	No.	Retrosternal.	Severe.	Usually sudden.	Variable.	Variable.	Subcutaneous emphysema, mediastinal crunch.	Chest x-ray usually shows pneumomediastinum, pneumothorax, or pleural effusion. Esophagogram is diagnostic.	History of severe retching or vomiting or esophageal trauma or instrumentation.
Perforated duodenal ulcer	No, or milder pain of ulcer.	Retrosternal to epigastrium.	Severe.	Variable.	Variable.	Variable.	Epigastric pain. May have prominent findings of peritoneal irritation.	Free air in peritoneum; elevated amylase.	Rare as cause of chest pain.
Pancreatitis	May have occurred.	Retrosternal to epigastrium.	Variable.	Variable.	Hours to days.	Vomiting, anorexia.	Epigastric or upper quadrant tenderness.	Markedly elevated urine or serum amylase.	Rare as cause of chest pain.
Cholecystitis	Usually.	Right upper quadrant; occasionally epigastrium or retrosternal.	Variable.	Usually sudden.	Hours to days.	Vomiting, anorexia.	Epigastric or right upper quadrant tenderness.	Abnormal liver function tests. Sonography is often diagnostic.	Rare as cause of chest pain.
Musculoskeletal disorder (Tietze's syndrome, stitch, etc), rib fracture	Variable.	Costochondral junctions; retrosternal and lateral.	Pleuritic ache, "sticking" sensation.	Gradual to sudden.	Variable: fleeting for stitch.	Splinting.	Tender (or, rarely, swollen) costosternal junctions, especially first and second ribs. Point tenderness over affected ribs.	None.	Relieved by lidocaine-corticosteroid injection.

¹ The shaded areas are the most helpful diagnostically.

101

often with adjunctive findings indicating severe valvular disease (eg, thrill over the carotid artery, wide pulse pressure, etc [Table 6–3]).

Treatment

Provide symptomatic treatment pending further evaluation for definitive treatment. Begin oxygen, 3–5 L/min, by mask or nasal prongs, and obtain an ECG. Insert an intravenous catheter (18- to 20-gauge), and begin an infusion of 5% dextrose in water to keep the catheter open. Give nitroglycerin, 0.3–0.4 mg sublingually, for pain. If nitroglycerin is not effective, give morphine, 2–4 mg intravenously.

Disposition

Hospitalization is warranted because of the imminent risk of infection or sudden death. The patient should be evaluated for valve replacement with or without coronary bypass.

PERICARDITIS
(See Chapter 28.)

AORTIC DISSECTION
(See Chapter 32.)

PULMONARY DISORDERS

PLEURISY & PLEURODYNIA
(See also Chapter 27.)

Diagnosis

Patients with idiopathic pleurisy or pleurodynia are generally young, and the onset of illness is acute, with severe pleuritic chest pain. Apart from low-grade fever in some patients and possible friction rub, other findings on physical examination are usually normal. Chest x-ray may show a small pleural effusion, with or without a small pulmonary infiltrate. Viruses (especially enteroviruses) are the usual causative agents.

An accurate diagnosis of pleurisy is important because its symptoms are similar to those of pulmonary embolism. Pleurisy is often a diagnosis of exclusion after a normal perfusion lung scan.

Treatment

Pleurisy and pleurodynia are benign, self-limited diseases, and only symptomatic measures are necessary. Although aspirin is sufficient for most patients, indomethacin, 25–50 mg orally 3 times daily, is reported to be more effective.

Disposition

Hospitalization is rarely indicated, and then only for relief of severe pain. Patients should be referred to an outpatient clinic for tuberculin testing and repeat chest x-ray.

SPONTANEOUS PNEUMOTHORAX
(See Chapter 27.)

TRAUMATIC PNEUMOTHORAX
(See Chapter 18.)

PNEUMOMEDIASTINUM
(See also Chapter 27.)

Diagnosis

Pneumomediastinum is frequently associated with pneumothorax. It is characterized by severe boring pain located retrosternally or in adjacent areas; the pain sometimes radiates to the back. Chills, fever, and shock may be present, especially if there is concurrent mediastinitis. A mediastinal "crunch" on auscultation or air in the mediastinum on chest x-ray is diagnostic.

Treatment

A. Give oxygen, 3–5 L/min, by nasal cannula or mask.

B. Insert an intravenous line ($\geq$ 16-gauge), and keep it open with 5% dextrose in water.

C. Give morphine, 2–4 mg intravenously, for pain; the dose may be repeated.

D. Treat pneumothorax with tube thoracostomy as indicated.

E. Evaluate the patient thoroughly to rule out serious underlying disease, ruptured bronchus, or a ruptured esophagus. Rupture of the esophagus is invariably associated with mediastinitis.

Disposition

Hospitalize the patient for observation and examination to rule out serious precipitating factors such as rupture of the trachea, bronchus, or esophagus. Patients with chronic or recurrent pneumomediastinum should be referred for outpatient care.

PULMONARY HYPERTENSION
(See also Chapter 28.)

Diagnosis

Severe or sudden onset of significant pulmonary hypertension may cause an oppressive retrosternal sensation or frank angina associated with dyspnea on exertion. A history of easy fatigability, weakness, syncope on exertion, and hemoptysis may be elicited.

A loud P_2 and right ventricular lift on physical examination suggest pulmonary hypertension. The ECG may reveal strain in the right side of the heart or cor pulmonale (right axis deviation; depressed ST segment and inverted T waves in leads II, III, aVF, and V_{1-5}; and tall, peaked P waves in leads II, III, and aVF). A large right ventricle or large pulmonary vessels on chest x-ray are diagnostic.

Treatment

No specific treatment is available for pulmonary hypertension. Administer oxygen for hypoxemia and treat other abnormalities (bronchopulmonary infection, recurrent pulmonary emboli, heart failure) that may be exacerbating the pulmonary hypertension.

Disposition

Hospitalization is indicated for severe pain, marked hypoxemia, or severe heart failure. Refer the patient to a cardiologist for complete evaluation and examination to rule out reparable lesions.

PULMONARY EMBOLISM
(See Chapter 27.)

PNEUMONIA
(See Chapter 34.)

GASTROINTESTINAL DISORDERS

ESOPHAGEAL DISORDERS

Diagnosis

Esophageal disorders such as esophagitis, spasm, motility disorders, and gastroesophageal reflux frequently cause retrosternal chest pain that can be difficult to differentiate from pain due to cardiac causes. When cardiac disease is excluded, esophageal disorder is the most common cause of chest pain. Characteristic features of chest pain of esophageal origin include pain that is burning in nature, often radiates along the sternum, is made worse by lying down and relieved by sitting, may be induced by swallowing, and often persists for hours after a shorter episode of more intense pain. Rest, sublingual nitroglycerin, and calcium channel blockers can relieve pain of both cardiac and esophageal origin and should not be used as diagnostic aids. Because cardiac disease is more life threatening, cardiac causes of chest pain must be excluded with a high degree of certainty before esophageal disorder is diagnosed as the cause of pain.

Diagnostic tests include barium swallow, endoscopy, manometry, use of provocative agents, pH monitoring, acid infusion (Bernstein test), and scintiscanning. Definitive emergency diagnosis of the esophageal disorder is seldom warranted.

Treatment

General symptomatic treatment can be offered to patients who are in discomfort, since the specific esophageal disorder is not usually known at the time of the emergency visit. A trial of viscous lidocaine, 15 mL mixed with 15 mL of an antacid given orally, can be tried for acute relief. Other measures include eating frequent small meals, using antacids, avoiding food before sleep, and using bed blocks (10–15 cm [4–6 in] high) under the head of the bed. If gastroesophageal reflux is suspected, H_2-receptor blocker therapy may be tried. The patient should be reassured that the chest pain was not of cardiac origin but should not be made to feel foolish for seeking emergency care.

Disposition

If esophageal disorder is diagnosed as the cause of chest pain and cardiac disease or other life-threatening conditions can be confidently excluded, the patient should be referred for outpatient care within 1–2 weeks.

PERFORATED ESOPHAGUS
(See also Chapter 18.)

Diagnosis

Esophageal perforation is marked by agonizing retrosternal chest pain associated with pneumomediastinum, pneumothorax, pneumonia, or purulent pleural effusion. A recent history of severe retching, vomiting, or endoscopy is often present. The diagnosis is confirmed by an esophagogram using water-soluble contrast medium.

Treatment

See Chapter 18.

Disposition

Hospitalize the patient for evaluation for possible surgery.

PERFORATED STOMACH OR DUODENUM
(See also Chapter 7.)

Diagnosis

Perforation distal to the esophagus is characterized by sudden onset of severe pain that is usually epigastric but may be retrosternal and may radiate to the back. There is often a history of chronic epigastric pain or ulcer disease. Epigastric tenderness and diminished or absent bowel sounds may be found. If peritonitis has supervened, rebound tenderness and a rigid abdomen are present. Air under the diaphragm may be seen on an x-ray. Serum amylase levels may be elevated as a result of posterior perforation into the pancreas. Leukocytosis with a shift to the left is often present.

Treatment

A. Insert a large-bore (≥ 16-gauge) intravenous catheter, and give crystalloid solutions intravenously to support blood pressure.

B. Give morphine, 2–4 mg intravenously, for pain; the dose may be repeated.

C. Insert a nasogastric tube, and begin continuous suction.

D. Obtain urgent surgical consultation.

E. Begin prophylactic intravenous antibiotics (penicillin 200,000 units/kg/d, and cefoxitin, 150 mg/kg/d; see also Table 7–1).

Disposition

Hospitalize the patient at once for emergency surgery.

PANCREATITIS
(See Chapter 7.)

CHOLECYSTITIS
(See Chapter 7.)

MUSCULOSKELETAL DISORDERS

COSTOCHONDRAL SEPARATION, RIB FRACTURES, & INTERCOSTAL MUSCLE STRAIN
(See also Chapter 18.)

Diagnosis

In this group of musculoskeletal disorders, pain is usually worse with movement and breathing. There is often a history of minor trauma, strenuous exercise, or severe coughing. Pain is localized and elicited by palpation. Chest x-ray may be normal or may show rib fractures if they are present.

Treatment

Oral analgesics and nonsteroidal anti-inflammatory agents (eg, aspirin or indomethacin) are effective for analgesia. Local heat alone may provide relief. In rib fractures, splinting is generally not recommended,

since it may impair respiratory function and promote atelectasis or pneumonia.

Disposition

Refer the patient for outpatient follow-up if pain is severe or persistent.

DISK DISEASE
(Cervical & Thoracic)

Diagnosis

Disk disease may cause paroxysmal pain radiating from the back of the neck into the arms and fingers. The pain is aggravated by coughing, sneezing, and straining. Movement of the neck is restricted by cervical muscle spasm. The patient may have paresthesias and pain in the fingers, weakness of hand and forearm muscles, and decreased biceps and triceps reflexes. Narrowing of the vertebral interspace is seen on a plain film, and a CT scan or myelogram confirms the diagnosis.

Treatment

Treatment consists of bed rest and cervical halter traction. Local heat may be of value. In mild cases, a light cervical collar during the day may be helpful.

Disposition

Severe cases require hospitalization. Mild cases can be treated on an outpatient basis.

TIETZE'S SYNDROME
(Costochondritis)

Diagnosis

Tietze's syndrome affects the costochondral or chondrosternal junctions, with visible swelling and erythema of the overlying skin and localized tenderness.

Treatment

Pain is relieved by salicylates, indomethacin, or other oral analgesics. Injection of lidocaine-corticosteroid preparations into the joints also relieves pain.

Disposition

Refer the patient for outpatient follow-up if pain is severe or persistent.

MUSCLE SPASM & FIBROSITIS
("Stitch")

Diagnosis

The patient complains of aching pain, usually in localized areas but sometimes more generalized. Pain often increases with movement and palpation. There may be a history of minor trauma or strenuous exercise.

Treatment

Massage, heat, and other local treatments are effective. Aspirin or other nonsteroidal anti-inflammatory agents are useful.

Disposition

Refer the patient for outpatient follow-up as needed. A search for more serious illnesses (myositis, arteritides, Pancoast's tumor, etc) may be necessary in recurrent or persistent cases that have no obvious cause.

MISCELLANEOUS DISORDERS

INTRATHORACIC NEOPLASM

Diagnosis

Intrathoracic neoplasm is suggested by a mass seen on chest x-ray with no other explanation for the chest pain.

Treatment

Give analgesics and other supportive measures as required.

Disposition

Depending on their general condition, patients with intrathoracic neoplasms should be either hospitalized or referred for evaluation.

ZOSTER
(See also Chapter 40.)

Diagnosis

In the preeruptive stage of zoster, pain felt on the skin surface in dermatomal distribution may occur several days before the characteristic skin lesions (clusters of clear, fluid-filled vesicles in a dermatomal distribution) appear. Pain is typically unilateral and does not cross the midline. Hypoesthesia in dermatomal distribution may also be present.

The appearance of the skin lesions confirms the diagnosis. Rarely, zoster may present with pain as the only manifestation of the disease; in such patients, a rise in antibody titer is diagnostic.

Treatment

Give analgesics as necessary; narcotics may be required for relief. Acyclovir, 800 mg orally 5 times daily for 7–10 days, if given within a few days of onset may alleviate symptoms, shorten the duration of illness, and reduce the incidence of postherpetic neuralgia, a special concern in elderly patients. Local nerve block with long-acting anesthetics (eg, bupivacaine [Marcaine, Sensorcaine]) is effective and obviates the need for narcotics and their associated side effects. It may also decrease the incidence and severity of postherpetic neuralgia. Prednisone, 60 mg orally daily (tapered over 2 weeks), may also decrease the incidence and severity of postherpetic neuralgia in elderly patients.

Disposition

Severe cases (extensive localized disease, dissemination) may require hospitalization for pain control and possible treatment with intravenous acyclovir. Other patients may be referred for outpatient evaluation and continued treatment (analgesia).

REFERENCES

American College of Emergency Physicians: *Clinical Policy for Management of Adult Patients Presenting with a Chief Complaint of Chest Pain, with No History of Trauma.* American College of Emergency Physicians, 1990.

Brundage BH: A sensible approach to chest pain. Postgrad Med (March) 1981;69:120.

Chambers CE, Leaman DM: Management of acute chest pain syndrome. Crit Care Clin 1989;5:415.

Goldman L et al: A computer protocol to predict myocardial infarction in emergency department patients with chest pain. N Engl J Med 1988;318:797.

Gruppo Italiano per lo Studio della Streptochinasi nell'Infarto Miocardico (GISSI): Effectiveness of intravenous thrombolytic treatment in acute myocardial infarction. Lancet 1986;1:397.

Lee HE et al: Acute chest pain in the emergency room: Identification and examination of low-risk patients. Arch Intern Med 1985;145:65.

Levine HJ: Difficult problems in the diagnosis of chest pain. Am Heart J 1980;100:108.

Loeser JD: Herpes zoster and postherpetic neuralgia. Pain 1986;25:149.

Nowakowski JF: Use of cardiac enzymes in the evaluation of acute chest pain. Ann Emerg Med 1986;15:354.

Pozen MW et al: A predictive instrument to improve coronary-care unit admission practices in acute ischemic heart disease. N Engl J Med 1984;310:1273.

Rusnak RA et al: Litigation against the emergency physician: Common features in cases of missed myocardial infarction. Ann Emerg Med 1989;18:1029.

Rustgi AK, Chopra S: Chest pain of esophageal origin. J Gen Intern Med 1989;4:151.

Second International Study of Infarct Survival (ISIS-2) Collaborative Group: Randomized trial of intravenous streptokinase, oral aspirin, both, or neither among 17,187 cases of suspected acute myocardial infarction. Lancet 1988;2:349.

Wears RL et al: How many myocardial infarctions should we rule out? Ann Emerg Med 1989;18:953.

Abdominal Pain

7

Richard A. Crass, MD, & Donald D. Trunkey, MD

IMMEDIATE MANAGEMENT OF LIFE-THREATENING PROBLEMS (See algorithm.)

Perform Brief Examination

Record complete vital signs, including blood pressure and pulse with the patient in the sitting (or standing) position if blood pressure is normal in the supine position. Assess peripheral perfusion (alertness; skin and extremity temperature). Gently examine the abdomen to find an obvious aortic aneurysm or the presence of an "acute" abdomen, ie, boardlike (involuntary) guarding. Perform a rectal examination, and check the stool for blood. A brief history may often be obtained simultaneously. (If there has been abdominal trauma, proceed as outlined in Chapter 19.)

Caution: Patients with acute myocardial infarction, especially involving the inferior or posterior wall, may present with epigastric or upper abdominal pain. A carefully elicited history and an ECG should be obtained, especially if no abdominal disorder is clearly identified.

Identify Candidates for Urgent Surgery

If hypotension (supine or postural) without gastrointestinal bleeding, an aneurysm, or a rigid abdomen is present in the patient with abdominal pain, there is a strong possibility of underlying life-threatening disease requiring early surgical correction. The surgeon on call and operating room personnel should be notified.

Treat Shock

Note: Persistent shock despite fluid resuscitation in the patient with acute abdominal pain requires urgent laparotomy.

Treat hypotension or frank shock (Chapter 3). To reiterate—

A. Insert 2 large-bore ($\geq$ 16-gauge) intravenous catheters in an upper extremity. If possible, one of the catheters should be a central venous pressure line.

B. Obtain blood for CBC with differential, serum electrolyte measurements, amylase determination, and renal function tests. Send a tube of clotted blood for typing and cross-matching.

C. Immediately begin rapid infusion of crystalloid solution (eg, a balanced salt solution). Adjust the rate of infusion based on blood pressure; initially, give 1 L over 10–20 minutes (adult dose).

D. Administer oxygen, 5–10 L/min, by nasal cannula or mask.

E. Insert a urinary catheter to monitor urine output, which is a sensitive indicator of visceral blood flow. Send a urine sample for analysis.

F. Obtain arterial blood gas and pH measurements, since they are a useful guide to the patient's overall physiologic condition.

G. Insert a nasogastric tube if the patient shows evidence of peritonitis, severe ileus, intestinal obstruction, or gastrointestinal bleeding. The tube should be inserted before other diagnostic measures are undertaken. (See p 126 for further management.)

H. Obtain a 12-lead ECG, and begin continuous cardiac monitoring.

I. If bacterial peritonitis is suspected, begin antibiotics (Table 7–1).

FURTHER EVALUATION OF THE PATIENT WITH ABDOMINAL PAIN

When vital functions have been normalized, reassess the patient as described below unless immediate surgery is required (Table 7–2).

Pain is usually present in acute intra-abdominal disorders. Diagnosis depends upon meticulous history taking and physical examination. The history is usually the most important diagnostic aid, though physical examination and laboratory and x-ray studies provide important confirmatory data. In general, 85–90% of diagnoses may be based on history alone, whereas laboratory examination alone or physical examination alone accounts only for an additional 5–8% each. The physician's time should be allocated accordingly.

Table 7–1. Antimicrobials for prevention of infection after suspected fecal soilage.

Drug	Dose
Cefoxitin	150 mg/kg/d intravenously in 4–6 divided doses.
Clindamycin[1] **plus**	40 mg/kg/d intravenously in 3 divided doses.
Tobramycin[2] **or**	5 mg/kg/d intravenously in 3 divided doses.
Gentamicin	5 mg/kg/d intravenously in 3 divided doses.
Penicillin (may be added to any of the above regimens for activity against enterococci)	200,000 units/kg/d intravenously in 4–6 divided doses.

[1] Metronidazole may be substituted for clindamycin. Give 15 mg/kg over 1 hour (loading dose), then 10 mg/kg every 8 hours. *Note:* Penicillin (as above) must be combined with this regimen.

[2] A second- or third-generation cephalosporin (eg, cefuroxime, 75 mg/kg/d in 4 divided doses) may be substituted for the aminoglycoside.

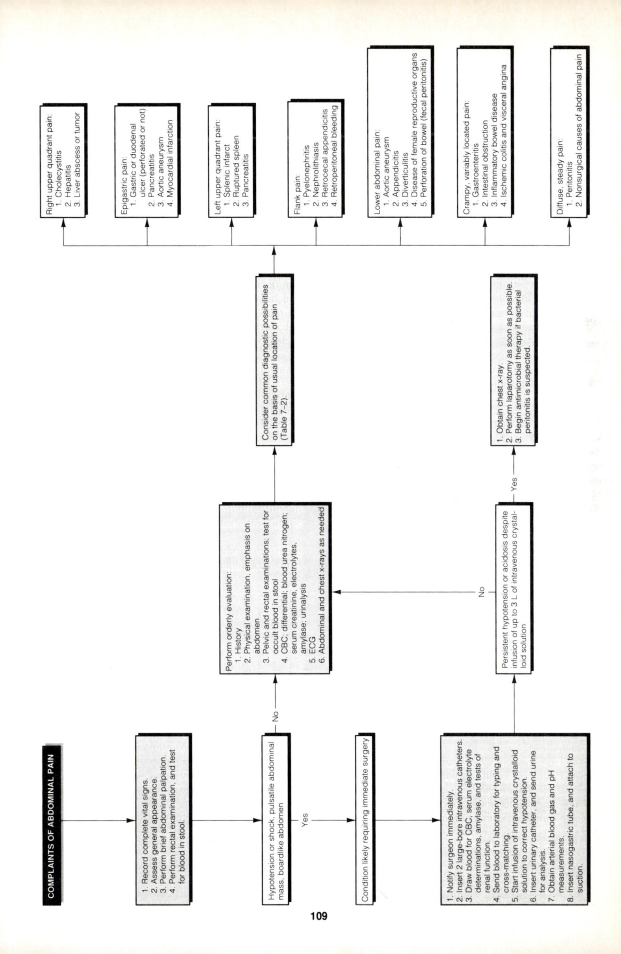

COMPLAINTS OF ABDOMINAL PAIN

1. Record complete vital signs.
2. Assess general appearance.
3. Perform brief abdominal palpation.
4. Perform rectal examination, and test for blood in stool.

Hypotension or shock, pulsatile abdominal mass, boardlike abdomen

— Yes → Condition likely requiring immediate surgery

— No →

Perform orderly evaluation:
1. History
2. Physical examination, emphasis on abdomen
3. Pelvic and rectal examinations; test for occult blood in stool
4. CBC; differential; blood urea nitrogen; serum creatinine, electrolytes, amylase; urinalysis
5. ECG
6. Abdominal and chest x-rays as needed

Consider common diagnostic possibilities on the basis of usual location of pain (Table 7–2).

Right upper quadrant pain:
1. Cholecystitis
2. Hepatitis
3. Liver abscess or tumor

Epigastric pain:
1. Gastric or duodenal ulcer (perforated or not)
2. Pancreatitis
3. Aortic aneurysm
4. Myocardial infarction

Left upper quadrant pain:
1. Splenic infarct
2. Ruptured spleen
3. Pancreatitis

Flank pain:
1. Pyelonephritis
2. Nephrolithiasis
3. Retrocecal appendicitis
4. Retroperitoneal bleeding

Lower abdominal pain:
1. Aortic aneurysm
2. Appendicitis
3. Diverticulitis
4. Disease of female reproductive organs
5. Perforation of bowel (fecal peritonitis)

Crampy, variably located pain:
1. Gastroenteritis
2. Intestinal obstruction
3. Inflammatory bowel disease
4. Ischemic colitis and visceral angina

Diffuse, steady pain:
1. Peritonitis
2. Nonsurgical causes of abdominal pain

1. Notify surgeon immediately.
2. Insert 2 large-bore intravenous catheters.
3. Draw blood for CBC, serum electrolyte determinations, amylase, and tests of renal function.
4. Send blood to laboratory for typing and cross-matching.
5. Start infusion of intravenous crystalloid solution to correct hypotension.
6. Insert urinary catheter, and send urine for analysis.
7. Obtain arterial blood gas and pH measurements.
8. Insert nasogastric tube, and attach to suction.

Persistent hypotension or acidosis despite infusion of up to 3 L of intravenous crystalloid solution

— No →

— Yes →

1. Obtain chest x-ray.
2. Perform laparotomy as soon as possible.
3. Begin antimicrobial therapy if bacterial peritonitis is suspected.

109

Table 7–2. Differential diagnosis of the common causes of acute abdominal pain.

Disease	Location of Pain and Prior Attacks	Mode of Onset and Type of Pain	Assosciated Gastro-intestinal Symptoms	Physical Examination	Helpful Tests and Examinations
Acute appendicitis	Periumbilical or localized generally to right lower abdominal quadrant.	Insidious to acute and persistent.	Anorexia common; nausea and vomiting in some.	Low-grade fever. Epigastric tenderness initially; later, right lower quadrant.	Slight leukocytosis. Ultrasound of the appendix may be helpful if diagnosis is uncertain.
Intestinal obstruction	Diffuse.	Sudden onset. Crampy.	Vomiting common.	Abdominal distention; high-pitched rushes.	Dilated, fluid-filled loops of bowel on abdominal x-ray.
Perforated duodenal ulcer	Epigastric. History of ulcer in many.	Abrupt onset. Steady.	Anorexia; nausea and vomiting.	Epigastric tenderness. Involuntary guarding.	Upright abdominal x-ray shows air under diaphragm. Water-soluble contrast study shows perforation.
Diverticulitis	Left lower quadrant. History of previous attacks.	Gradual onset. Steady or crampy.	Mild diarrhea common.	Fever common. Mass and tenderness in left lower quadrant.	Barium enema shows diverticulitis. CT scan shows inflammatory mass.
Inflammatory bowel disease	Diffuse; primarily in lower abdomen. Prior attacks common.	Gradual onset. Often crampy.	Diarrhea common, often with blood and mucus.	Fever. Diffuse abdominal tenderness.	Blood and leukocytes in stool. Abnormal results on proctosigmoidoscopy or barium enema.
Acute cholecystitis	Epigastric or right upper quadrant; may be referred to right shoulder.	Insidious to acute.	Anorexia; nausea and vomiting.	Right upper quadrant tenderness.	Right upper quadrant sonography shows gallstones. Radionuclide scan shows nonvisualization of gallbladder.
Biliary colic	Intermittent right upper quadrant. Prior attacks common.	Often abrupt onset. Dull to sharp.	Anorexia; nausea and vomiting common.	Right upper quadrant tenderness.	Sonography shows gallstones; oral cholecystogram shows stones or nonvisualization on repeat dose.
Ischemic colitis	Epigastric; diffuse. Prior attacks common.	Often abrupt. Crampy.	Diarrhea, commonly bloody.	Diffuse abdominal tenderness. Vascular disease elsewhere.	Barium enema shows "thumbprinting" of mucosa. Visceral angiography shows vascular obstruction.
Ruptured abdominal aortic aneurysm	Epigastrium and back.	Abrupt. Sharp and severe.	Variable; may be none.	Hypotension or shock. Abdominal aneurysm.	Lateral abdominal x-ray shows calcification in aneurysm. Sonography, CT scan, or angiography shows aneurysm.
Rupture of spleen	Left upper quadrant or diffuse. May be referred to left shoulder. History of trauma common.	Abrupt. Severe.	Usually none.	Hypotension or shock. Peritonitis. Left upper quadrant tenderness; fractured left ribs in some.	CT scan or liver-spleen scan shows rupture. Peritoneal lavage reveals blood.
Renal colic	Costovertebral or along course of ureter.	Sudden. Severe and sharp.	Frequently nausea and vomiting.	Flank tenderness.	Hematuria. Abnormal excretory urogram(obstruction, hydronephrosis).
Acute pancreatitis	Epigastric penetrating to back.	Acute. Persistent, dull, severe.	Anorexia; nausea and vomiting common.	Epigastric tenderness.	Elevated serum amylase. CT scan shows pancreatic inflammation.
Acute salpingitis	Bilateral adnexal; later, may be generalized.	Gradually becomes worse.	Nausea and vomiting may be present.	Cervical motion elicits tenderness. Mass if tubo-ovarian abscess is present.	Culdocentesis reveals purulent material.
Ectopic pregnancy	Unilateral early; may have shoulder pain after rupture.	Sudden or intermittently vague to sharp.	Frequently none.	Adnexal mass. Tenderness.	Culdocentesis shows blood. Pelvic ultrasound reveals adnexal mass or blood. Positive serum pregnancy test. (Urine pregnancy test may be negative.)

Often it is impossible to diagnose abdominal pain definitively in the emergency department. If pain is significant, it is prudent to hospitalize the patient for observation and further diagnostic procedures.

HISTORY

If there is a history of abdominal trauma, the diagnostic approach differs from that for spontaneous abdominal pain and is discussed in Chapter 19. Pelvic pain in women is discussed in Chapter 30.

Mode of Onset
of Abdominal Pain
(See Fig 7–1 and Table 7–2.)
A. Abrupt Onset:

1. If the patient was well one moment and seized with agonizing (explosive) pain in the next, the most probable diagnosis is rupture of a hollow viscus or a vascular accident (eg, ruptured aortic aneurysm). In these instances, the pain is maximal or nearly maximal at time of onset. Renal or biliary colic may be very sudden in onset but is less likely to cause severe and prostrating pain.

2. Pain that begins abruptly, is only moderately severe at first, and worsens rapidly suggests acute pancreatitis, mesenteric thrombosis, or small bowel strangulation. If pelvic pain is present, consider a possible ruptured ectopic pregnancy or ovarian follicle cyst (Chapter 30).

B. Gradual Onset: Gradual onset of slowly worsening pain is characteristic of peritoneal infection or inflammation. Appendicitis and diverticulitis often present in this way.

Character of Pain
(See Fig 7–1.)
A. Excruciating Pain: Excruciating pain not relieved by ordinary doses of narcotics usually indicates a vascular lesion such as coronary occlusion, rupture of an abdominal aneurysm, or a ruptured viscus. Biliary or renal colic occasionally produces similar excruciating pain.

B. Severe Pain: Severe pain that is readily controlled by medication is typical of acute pancreatitis or peritonitis associated with ischemic bowel (as from strangulation or vascular thrombosis).

C. Dull Pain: Pain that is dull, vague, and poorly localized and does not require analgesia is also likely to have been gradual in onset. Such findings strongly suggest an inflammatory process or a low-grade infection. Appendicitis and diverticulitis present in this way.

D. Intermittent Pain With Cramps and Rushes: This picture is common in gastroenteritis. However, if the pain comes in regular cycles, rises in crescendo fashion, and then subsides to a pain-free interval, the most likely diagnosis is mechanical small bowel obstruction. Occasionally, this type of pain occurs in early subacute pancreatitis or in renal colic. If auscultation reveals intermittent peristaltic

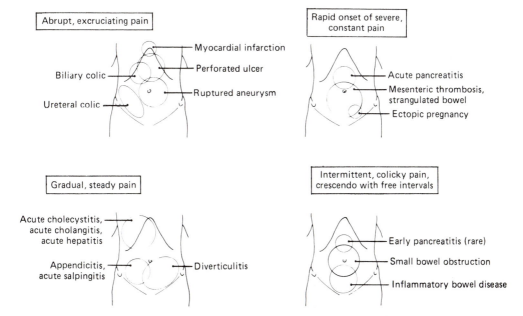

Figure 7–1. Correlation between nature of abdominal pain and underlying condition. (Reproduced, with permission, from Way LW [editor]: *Current Surgical Diagnosis & Treatment,* 9th ed. Lange, 1991.)

rushes that rise in a crescendo and are synchronous with the pain, small bowel obstruction is likely. In the colic of gastroenteritis, on the other hand, peristaltic rushes have little or no relation to abdominal cramps.

E. Absence of Pain: Occasionally, a patient presents with no abdominal pain but rather a sense of fullness and a feeling that a bowel movement would bring relief. A bowel movement, whether it is spontaneous or due to administration of cathartics or an enema, usually fails to relieve discomfort, however. This so-called "gas stoppage sign" is characteristic of retrocecal appendicitis but may be present when any inflammatory lesion is walled off from the free peritoneal cavity.

Location of Pain

Generally, pain fibers within the abdominal cavity are confined to the visceral peritoneum, parietal peritoneum, and blood vessels. The parietal peritoneum is innervated by somatic nerve fibers and will therefore localize pain. Pain due to visceral peritoneal involvement alone is poorly localized. In conditions that do not involve the parietal peritoneum, the most common sources of pain are distention of a hollow viscus and visceral ischemia. These general principles are a useful guide to a systematic evaluation of the cause of abdominal pain.

A. Localized Abdominal Pain: (See Table 7–2.) In general, when abdominal pain becomes localized, it does so over or near the involved viscus, eg, epigastric or right upper quadrant pain of acute cholecystitis, or right lower quadrant pain of appendicitis. However, the physician must remember anatomic variants (eg, an inflamed retrocecal appendix produces flank pain or nonlocalizing abdominal pain) and must consider all structures that might cause pain (eg, vascular disease).

B. Radiation of Pain or Shift in Localization: Radiation of pain or shift in localization of pain has particular diagnostic significance.

1. Shoulder pain may be due to ipsilateral diaphragmatic irritation from air, blood, or infection in the peritoneal cavity. For example, cholecystitis may be associated with referred right shoulder pain or even epigastric and left shoulder pain mimicking angina.

2. Diffuse periumbilical and epigastric pain gradually localizing to the right lower quadrant is a classic sign of appendicitis. With early appendicitis, only the visceral peritoneum surrounding the appendix is involved in the inflammatory process, and localization is therefore poor. As inflammation spreads and involves the parietal peritoneum, pain then localizes to the right lower quadrant. If the appendix is retrocecal, however, as it is in 15% of cases, the parietal peritoneum is not involved, and the pain remains poorly localized.

3. Pain radiating from the flank to the groin or genitalia usually signifies ureteral colic, as seen in urolithiasis.

Anorexia; Nausea & Vomiting

Anorexia and nausea and vomiting occur more commonly in disease of the upper abdomen; however, advanced intra-abdominal disease may be present without any of these symptoms. If the peritoneum is well protected from infection or inflammation, as in retrocecal appendicitis or when the appendix is completely isolated by omentum, the patient may retain a normal appetite.

If nausea and vomiting *precede* the onset of pain, an acute abdominal emergency requiring operation is unlikely. The most likely diagnoses are gastroenteritis and food poisoning, acute gastritis, acute pancreatitis, and (much less frequently) common duct stone and high intestinal obstruction. In most acute surgical emergencies, nausea and vomiting are not dominant or early symptoms, although they may be present by the time the patient seeks medical attention.

Severe vomiting with retching—particularly after a dietary indiscretion or an alcoholic bout—followed by abdominal pain with or without hematemesis should immediately suggest mucosal laceration of the gastroesophageal junction (Mallory-Weiss syndrome) or an esophageal perforation (Boerhaave's syndrome). Massive hematemesis or severe pain radiating into the chest and left shoulder in association with severe vomiting and retching are classic symptoms of Boerhaave's syndrome. The presence of pleural fluid on chest x-ray further supports the diagnosis.

Fever & Rigors

Fever is common with most causes of acute abdominal pain. In appendicitis, the temperature is usually not high, and rigors (shaking chills) are uncommon. High fever or rigors in suspected appendicitis strongly suggest diffuse peritonitis from perforation of a viscus, pylephlebitis (septic thrombophlebitis of the portal vein), or another disorder entirely (eg, pyelonephritis). Very high fever with peritoneal signs in a female patient with no apparent general systemic illness is characteristic of acute salpingitis with pelvic peritonitis. Repeated shaking chills and fever are most common in infections of the biliary or urinary tract. Acute cholangitis and acute pyelonephritis usually present with intermittent rigors and fever. Chills, fever, rigors, jaundice, and hypotension suggest suppurative cholangitis, which is a surgical emergency.

Diarrhea, Constipation, & Obstipation

Diarrhea, constipation, and obstipation may occur in acute abdomen but are not often major symptoms in acute intra-abdominal disease requiring surgery. Colitis (vascular or some other kind) usually is associated with early and severe diarrhea. Occasionally, patients with diverticulitis, appendicitis, or salpingitis may also experience diarrhea.

PHYSICAL EXAMINATION

The basic steps of the physical examination of the acute abdomen are outlined in Table 7–3. Remember that physical findings may be subtle in elderly or immunocompromised patients.

Inspection

The physician should first inspect the abdomen and look for such striking features as the scaphoid, contracted abdomen of an early perforated viscus; the visible peristalsis and distention of mechanical obstruction; or the soft, doughy distention of early ileus.

Auscultation

A. A silent abdomen, with complete absence of audible peristalsis, usually signifies diffuse peritonitis; however, peristalsis may persist in the face of established peritonitis. Other manifestations of diffuse peritonitis such as rigidity and distention are usually also present. It may be necessary to listen for as long as 2–3 minutes to establish absence of peristalsis, since peristalsis diminishes if the patient has not eaten.

B. Intermittent crescendo peristaltic rushes with the onset of pain and with periods of silence at regular intervals are diagnostic of acute small bowel obstruction. For reasons that are not entirely clear, the only other lesion that produces peristalsis of this type is early acute pancreatitis, in which the dilated sentinel loop seen on x-ray appears to undergo cyclic peristaltic contractions simulating those of acute mechanical obstruction.

C. In gastroenteritis, dysentery, and active ulcerative colitis, there may be abnormal high-pitched peristalsis with rushes that are not synchronous with the episodes of pain.

Palpation

A. Examine Hernial Rings and Male Genitalia: Examine the inguinal and femoral canals in both sexes and the genitalia in the male, and look for incarcerated hernias that may be causing intestinal obstruction. This must be done by asking the patient to

cough, but should be done gently so as to cause as little discomfort as possible.

B. Elicit Cough Tenderness: In most acute inflammatory conditions arising within the abdomen, coughing elicits pain in the involved area. Directing the patient to point one finger to the area of pain provides objective localization of the lesion. With this information, the examiner can proceed to examine the abdomen and deliberately examine last the area now known to be most tender.

C. Feel for Spasm of Rectus Abdominis Muscle: The next step is to establish the presence or absence of true muscle spasm by placing a hand gently over the rectus abdominis muscle and depressing it slightly and gently without causing pain. Properly performed, this maneuver is comforting to the patient. The patient is asked to take a long, slow breath. If the spasm is voluntary, the muscle will immediately relax underneath the gentle pressure of the palpating hand. If there is true spasm, however, the muscle will remain taut and rigid through the respiratory cycle. This maneuver alone may be sufficient to establish the presence of peritonitis.

Except for rare neurologic disorders, renal colic, or rectus muscle injury, only peritoneal inflammation produces abdominal muscle rigidity (for reasons not understood). In renal colic, the spasm is confined to the entire rectus muscle on the involved side. The distinction is important, because marked rigidity of the entire length of one rectus muscle with relaxation of the opposite rectus cannot occur in peritonitis, since the peritoneal cavity is not compartmentalized. It is possible to have segmental spasm of a rectus muscle involving only the upper or lower portion of one side, or to have segmental spasm of both rectus muscles in upper or lower abdominal peritonitis. In generalized peritonitis, however, both muscles are usually involved to the same degree.

D. Perform One-Finger Palpation: Abdominal tenderness must be assessed with one finger, since it is impossible to localize peritoneal inflammation accurately if palpation for tenderness is done with the entire hand. Careful one-finger palpation, beginning as far away as possible from the area of tenderness elicited by coughing and gradually working toward it, will usually enable the examiner to delineate the area of abdominal tenderness precisely. In early acute appendicitis, this area is often no larger than 3 cm (1³⁄₁₆ in) in diameter and sometimes smaller. Diffuse abdominal tenderness *without* associated involuntary rigidity of the muscles suggests gastroenteritis or some other inflammatory process of the intestines without peritonitis.

Do not test for peritoneal inflammation by looking for classic "rebound" tenderness (deep palpation of the abdomen with abrupt release). This maneuver yields no additional information and is so painful in patients with significant abdominal tenderness that further examination may be impossible.

Table 7–3. Routine for physical examination of acute abdomen.

Inspection
Auscultation
Palpation
    Examination of hernial rings and male genitalia
    Cough tenderness
    Rectus muscle spasm
    One-finger palpation
    Costovertebral angle tenderness
    Deep palpation
Percussion
Special signs (iliopsoas and obturator signs, etc)
Pelvic and rectal examinations

E. Look for Costovertebral Angle Tenderness: Palpation should be followed by gentle percussion of the costovertebral angles. This will cause pain in individuals with pyelonephritis, retroperitoneal abscesses, and retrocecal appendix. Excessively vigorous percussion should be avoided, since it is not helpful in localizing tenderness and the pain it causes will make further examination difficult.

F. Perform Deep Palpation: Having established the presence or absence of muscular rigidity and localized the area of tenderness, the examiner now palpates more deeply for the presence of abdominal masses. Among the more common lesions identifiable by careful palpation in patients with acute abdominal pain are the distended, tender gallbladder found in acute cholecystitis, the right lower quadrant tender mass of appendicitis with early abscess formation, the left lower quadrant mass of sigmoid diverticulitis, and the midline pulsatile mass indicating a leaking abdominal aneurysm.

Percussion

In free perforation of a hollow viscus with air under the diaphragm, there may be diminished or absent liver dullness. Tympany located laterally in the midaxillary line, 5 cm (2 in) or more above the costal margin, is due to free air; tympany located anteriorly over the liver may be due to air in distended loops of bowel.

Special Signs

Several maneuvers in physical examination may help localize an acute abdominal lesion:

A. Iliopsoas Sign: (See Fig 7–2.) The patient flexes the thigh against the resistance of the examiner's hand. A painful response indicates an inflammatory process involving the psoas muscle.

B. Obturator Sign: (See Fig 7–3.) The patient's thigh is flexed to a right angle and gently rotated, first

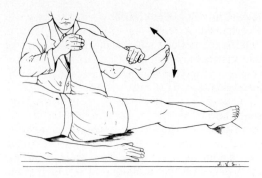

Figure 7–3. Performing the obturator test. (Reproduced, with permission, from Way LW [editor]: *Current Surgical Diagnosis & Treatment,* 6th ed. Lange, 1983.)

internally and then externally. If pain is elicited, there is an inflammatory lesion involving the obturator internus muscle (pelvic appendicitis, diverticulitis, pelvic inflammatory disease).

C. Fist Percussion Sign: Gentle percussion with the fist over the anterior chest wall elicits sharp pain if there is acute inflammation involving the space between the diaphragm and liver on the right and the stomach or spleen on the left.

D. Inspiratory Arrest (Murphy's Sign): The patient is asked to take a slow, deep breath as the examiner gently palpates the right upper quadrant. With descent of the diaphragm with the liver and gallbladder, an acutely inflamed gallbladder comes in contact with the examining fingers, causing pain, and the patient stops inspiration in an attempt to avoid the pain.

Pelvic & Rectal Examination

The importance of pelvic and rectal examination cannot be overstressed. In men a rectal examination plus simultaneous lower abdominal palpation with the other hand often reveals masses or localized pain not disclosed by abdominal examination alone. Likewise, pelvic examination in women provides essential information not revealed by other maneuvers. Evaluation of lower abdominal pain in women is discussed further in Chapter 30.

Examination of stool for occult blood must be performed in every patient with abdominal pain. Occult blood may result from intestinal tumors (possibly causing intestinal obstruction), inflammatory bowel disease, and ischemic bowel disease.

LABORATORY EXAMINATION

CBC with differential, amylase measurements, and urinalysis are called for in all cases. Electrolyte determinations and tests of renal function should be obtained if there is vomiting, diarrhea, hypotension, or

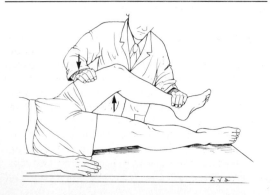

Figure 7–2. Performing the iliopsoas test. (Reproduced, with permission, from Way LW [editor]: *Current Surgical Diagnosis & Treatment,* 6th ed. Lange, 1983.)

shock or if there is a strong chance that surgery will be performed. A pregnancy test, preferably serum, should be obtained in women of child-bearing age with intact pelvic organs.

Blood Count

The hematocrit reflects changes both in plasma volume and in red cell volume. It is most useful diagnostically if it is markedly elevated (indicating dehydration) or depressed (indicating anemia). Additionally, the hematocrit should be corrected toward normal values (between 30% and 45% is usually satisfactory) in preparation for surgery.

The white cell count may be helpful if it is significantly elevated. However, normal or even low counts can occur in established peritonitis or sepsis (although usually with a marked shift to the left), and elevated counts may occur in gastroenteritis. A normal or low white count, particularly with lymphocytosis, may suggest viral infection. A progressively rising white count is of considerable diagnostic value and usually indicates progression of an inflammatory or septic process. A shift to the left on a blood smear may be a clue to an inflammatory reaction in the presence of a normal or only moderately elevated white count.

Serum Amylase

Serum amylase levels require cautious evaluation. Patients with abdominal pain and elevated serum amylase usually have acute pancreatitis. However, some patients with severe hemorrhagic pancreatitis have normal or low serum amylase, and patients with persistent or chronic pancreatitis often have normal serum amylase levels. In the presence of pancreatic pseudocysts, however, serum amylase often remains elevated.

Serum amylase may be elevated in mesenteric arterial thrombosis, intestinal obstruction, or perforated duodenal ulcer and occasionally in other conditions. It is also elevated in macroamylasemia, a common benign condition in which urinary amylase clearance is markedly reduced as a result of complex formation with other serum proteins.

Urine

Urinalysis (including microscopic examination of the sediment) is critical in ruling out urinary tract infection, urolithiasis, and diabetes. Hematuria strongly suggests urolithiasis. Rarely, however, urolithiasis with complete obstruction of the ureter may be associated with normal results on urinalysis. Low urine specific gravity associated with severe vomiting may be the earliest clue to renal disease.

Serum Electrolytes & Tests of Renal Function

Serum electrolyte determinations and a test of renal function (blood urea nitrogen, serum creatinine, or both) are required to document the nature and ex-

tent of fluid losses if vomiting or diarrhea has been significant or if the illness has lasted for more than 48 hours with diminished oral intake. Abnormalities should be corrected as much as possible in preparation for surgery (Chapter 36).

Pregnancy Test

A pregnancy test (preferably serum) should be obtained in all women of child-bearing age unless pregnancy is physically impossible (eg, complete hysterectomy, bilateral oophorectomy). Women with a history of pelvic infection, current intrauterine device use, prior ectopic pregnancy, and failed tubal ligation are at increased risk for ectopic pregnancy. A negative urine pregnancy test does not exclude the possibility of ectopic pregnancy.

Electrocardiogram

A 12-lead ECG should be obtained in patients with epigastric or upper abdominal pain in whom no clear cause of the pain is identified and cardiac ischemia is a possibility.

Peritoneal Fluid

If the diagnosis is obscure but a critical condition requiring surgery is suspected, examination of the peritoneal fluid for blood and pus may be required. This is particularly true in elderly, obtunded patients in whom peritonitis cannot be excluded because of scanty history and physical findings that are unreliable or difficult to interpret. It may be best to tap a single quadrant of the abdomen. In other cases, particularly if intraperitoneal bleeding is suspected, insertion of a peritoneal dialysis catheter with peritoneal lavage is more reliable (Chapter 46).

RADIOLOGIC EXAMINATION

Radiologic examination may provide important evidence for diagnosis of acute abdominal disease. Close cooperation between the radiologist and the physician caring for the patient is essential.

Suggested Studies

In most cases of acute abdominal disease and in all cases in which the diagnosis is obscure, obtain supine and upright anteroposterior and lateral abdominal x-rays. A left lateral decubitus (right side up rather than upright) view of the abdomen can be performed in patients unable to stand. The patient in whom perforation is suspected should be in the upright or left lateral decubitus position for 5–10 minutes before the x-ray to make certain that free air, if present, accumulates under the diaphragm or over the liver.

Interpretation

When these films are reviewed, the following questions should be asked: **(1)** Are the outlines of the liver, spleen, kidneys, and psoas muscles clearly defined? (**2**) Are the peritoneal fat lines identifiable? (**3**) Is the gas pattern in the stomach, small bowel, and colon within normal limits? (**4**) Is there evidence of air outside the bowel or beneath the diaphragm? (**5**) Is there air in the biliary ducts and ductules? (**6**) Are there abnormal opaque shadows such as gallstones, ureteral stones, fecaliths, or calcification in lymph nodes, pancreas, aorta, or other soft tissue masses?

On the basis of these observations, the following important pieces of evidence may be obtained:

A. Psoas Shadow: Obliteration of the psoas shadow may indicate a retroperitoneal hematoma or abscess (Fig 7–4).

B. Kidney Shadow: An enlarged or displaced kidney shadow may indicate a urologic lesion simulating an acute abdominal process.

C. Splenic Shadow: Enlargement of the splenic shadow with displacement of stomach or colon may suggest blood clot due to delayed rupture of the spleen.

D. Gas Patterns: Gas patterns are of particular importance. Proper interpretation requires prior passage of a nasogastric tube and an empty stomach before x-ray.

1. Residual gas and fluid within the stomach suggest pyloric obstruction.

2. Dilated loops of small bowel with air-fluid levels and no gas in the colon are indicative of small bowel obstruction (Fig 7–5).

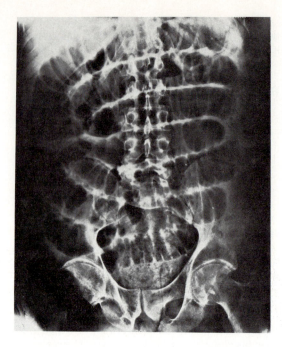

Figure 7–5. Upright abdominal x-ray showing dilated loops of small bowel with air-fluid levels and no gas in the colon. Patient had small bowel obstruction. (Reproduced, with permission, from Way WL [editor]: *Current Surgical Diagnosis & Treatment,* 9th ed. Lange, 1991.)

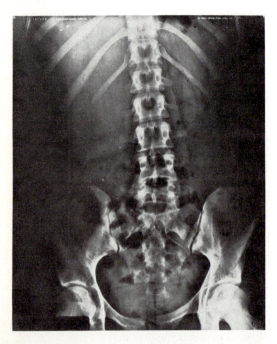

Figure 7–4. Obliteration of the psoas shadow on the right by a subhepatic abscess. (Reproduced, with permission, from Way LW [editor]: *Current Surgical Diagnosis & Treatment,* 6th ed. Lange, 1983.)

E. Cecum:

1. The position of the cecum may be a clue to appendicitis in an unusual location.

2. Marked dilatation and rotation of the cecum or sigmoid are typical of volvulus.

F. Dilatations:

1. Marked dilatation of the entire colon suggests colonic obstruction.

2. Massive dilatation of the colon in acute colitis indicates toxic megacolon.

3. Distention of both the small and the large bowel is characteristic of ileus, peritonitis, and pseudo-obstruction of the bowel (Fig 7–6). The differentiation between distended small and large bowel may at times be difficult. In advanced cases, the clinical signs may be more reliable than x-rays in the differentiation between intestinal obstruction and peritonitis.

G. Air in Abnormal Locations:

1. Except following laparotomy, free air under the diaphragm usually indicates a perforated viscus, most commonly seen in perforated duodenal or gastric ulcer (Fig 7–7).

2. Massive amounts of air beneath the diaphragm suggest colonic perforation.

3. An encapsulated air shadow outside the contours of small or large bowel may indicate localized perforation of the intestine.

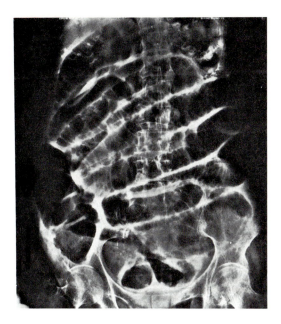

Figure 7–6. Abdominal x-ray showing dilated loops of small and large bowel without air-fluid levels, typical of diffuse peritonitis. (Reproduced, with permission, from Way LW [editor]: *Current Surgical Diagnosis & Treatment,* 6th ed. Lange, 1983.)

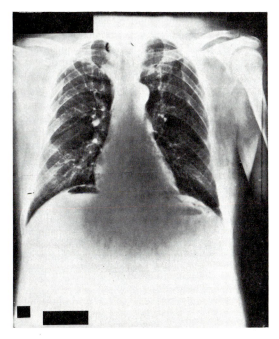

Figure 7–7. Upright film of the abdomen showing free air under the diaphragm—in this case, from a perforated duodenal ulcer. (Reproduced, with permission, from Way LW [editor]: *Current Surgical Diagnosis & Treatment,* 6th ed. Lange, 1983.)

4. Air in the biliary tract is diagnostic of a free communication between some portion of the gastrointestinal tract and the biliary tree. If there is evidence of intestinal obstruction, this pattern is characteristic of gallstone ileus.

5. Air in the portal venous system indicates pylephlebitis with a gas-forming organism but also occurs in pneumatosis cystoides intestinalis and has been described following the introduction of hydrogen peroxide into the rectum.

6. Rarely, free air in the peritoneum may be seen in asymptomatic or minimally symptomatic women with no signs of apparent underlying disease. The free air has presumably entered the peritoneum from the genital tract.

H. Calcifications and Opacities: X-rays of the abdomen may establish the presence of gallstones, ureteral stones, pancreatic calcification, retroperitoneal calcification, and vascular calcification. Such findings must be carefully correlated with the history and physical examination to establish their significance.

Special Studies
(See Table 7–4.)

Special x-ray contrast studies, ultrasonography, or CT scans may be helpful.

A. Contrast Media Swallow: Rarely, a swallow of diatrizoate meglumine (Gastrografin) or other water-soluble contrast medium may be necessary to confirm or exclude a diagnosis of high intestinal obstruction or perforation of the stomach or duodenum.

B. Barium Enema: Avoid barium enema if possible in the presence of acute abdominal disease and peritonitis. In rare cases, a water-soluble contrast enema is necessary to establish a diagnosis of diverticulitis, retrocecal appendicitis, sigmoid volvulus, or a low, partial colonic obstruction due to carcinoma.

C. Ultrasonography: Ultrasonography is a useful technique for evaluating the gallbladder, biliary ducts, pancreas, appendix, and kidneys. It is probably the best single diagnostic test for evaluating patients with right upper quadrant pain (Table 7–4).

D. CT Scan: CT scan is often the diagnostic procedure of choice for evaluating enigmatic abdominal pain or masses. It is useful for evaluating solid organs (liver, spleen, pancreas, etc) and the retroperitoneum, but rarely provides useful information about the gastrointestinal tract. Its utility is limited by its expense and the time required to perform the procedure.

E. Angiograms: Angiograms are being used less frequently than before in trauma, since CT scan has been found to be more useful in cases of rupture of a solid viscus such as the spleen or kidney. Mesenteric angiography is the best way to identify the site of bleeding in massive lower gastrointestinal tract hemorrhage, although radionuclide blood pool scans are more sensitive in intermittent or less severe hemorrhage (Chapter 8).

Table 7–4. Definitive diagnosis of conditions causing acute abdominal pain.

Usual Location of Pain	Condition	Most Sensitive and Specific Signs and Diagnostic Tests
Right upper quadrant	Cholecystitis	Right upper quadrant sonogram; radionuclide scan
	Biliary colic	Right upper quadrant sonogram; oral cholecystogram
	Cholangitis	Right upper quadrant sonogram
	Hepatitis	Liver function tests, especially transaminases
	Liver abscess or tumor	Right upper quadrant sonogram; CT scan; radionuclide liver scan
	Right lower lobe pneumonia	Chest x-ray
Epigastrium or midline	Peritonitis	Smear and culture of peritoneal fluid; laparoscopy or laparotomy
	Pancreatitis	Serum amylase; CT scan
	Duodenal perforation	Upright or left decubitus flat plate of abdomen; upper gastrointestinal series with water-soluble contrast media; CT scan with oral contrast media
	Abdominal aortic aneurysm	Sonogram; lateral abdominal x-ray; CT scan
	Myocardial infarction	ECG; CK isoenzymes
Left upper quadrant	Rupture of spleen	Peritoneal lavage; CT scan of abdomen
	Splenic infarct	CT scan
Flank	Pyelonephritis	Urinalysis and Gram's stain of urine; urine culture
	Renal colic	Urinalysis; excretory urogram
	Renal infarct	Urinalysis; renal scan or angiography
Lower abdomen	Appendicitis	History and examination; sonogram; laparoscopy or laparotomy
	Diverticulitis	History and examination; barium enema
	Ectopic pregnancy	Culdocentesis; pelvic sonogram; laparoscopy or laparotomy; positive serum pregnancy test
	Salpingitis	History and examination; pelvic sonogram; culdocentesis
	Ruptured ovarian follicle cyst	(Chapter 23.)
Diffuse or variable	Gastroenteritis	History and examination; stool smear and culture (Chapter 13)
	Intestinal obstruction	History and examination; supine and upright abdominal x-ray
	Volvulus and intestinal strangulation	Supine and upright abdominal x-ray
	Intestinal perforation	Supine and upright abdominal x-ray; upper gastrointestinal series with water-soluble contrast media
	Ischemic colitis	Barium enema; visceral angiography
	Idiopathic inflammatory bowel disease	Proctosigmoidoscopy; barium enema
	Mesenteric thrombosis	History and examination; visceral angiography; laparotomy
	Retroperitoneal hemorrhage	CT scan; flat plate x-ray
	Porphyria	History; hirsutism; elevated urinary porphobilinogens
	Addison's disease	Low serum sodium and high serum potassium; low serum cortisol level
	Poisoning	Toxicology screen (lead, arsenic, iron)
	Familial Mediterranean fever	History—patient and family
	Diabetes mellitus	Severe diabetes with neuropathy; previous attacks
	Tertiary syphillis	Presence of syphilis; previous attacks
	Preeruptive zoster	Unilateral dermatomal distribution

ADDITIONAL MEASURES FOR THE MANAGEMENT OF ACUTE ABDOMEN

Repeated Examination

When the diagnosis is in doubt and the patient is not critically ill, a period of active observation is in order. Frequent inquiries about progression or alteration of symptoms combined with repeated, gentle examinations of the abdomen and, occasionally, repeat laboratory tests will avoid many unnecessary operations without risking dangerous delays. If the physician feels that a diagnosis cannot be made within 6–12 hours, the patient should be hospitalized for observation. Observation in the emergency department for more than 4–6 hours is unwarranted for reasons of patient comfort, quality of care, and cost. Even in the absence of a tentative diagnosis, hospitalization is indicated for patients with severe pain and abdominal tenderness or peritoneal signs and for those with laboratory test abnormalities suggesting significant disease.

Relief of Pain

Parenteral narcotic analgesics should be given at once to relieve severe pain. Evaluation of acute abdominal disease can be performed more accurately after severe pain is relieved and the patient can cooperate. What at first appears to be diffuse tenderness may become better localized. Abdominal masses not palpable initially often become obvious after moderate sedation and relief of pain.

Antimicrobials

Antimicrobial agents should be withheld until the diagnosis is at least tentatively established, except in the presence of obvious signs of systemic infection (high fever, rigors, hypotension). In obscure cases, antibiotic therapy may mask progression of disease and lead to serious complications with increased illness (eg, appendicitis).

Surgical Consultation

Early surgical consultation is helpful for both the patient and the surgeon. Since the surgeon, like the emergency physician, must rely on repeated examinations for diagnosis, the earlier observation begins, the faster a definitive diagnosis can be made. Furthermore, delays in consultation may allow worsening of the condition, with possible disastrous sequelae.

MANAGEMENT OF SPECIFIC DISORDERS CAUSING ABDOMINAL PAIN

INTESTINAL DISORDERS

1. APPENDICITIS

Diagnosis

The initial symptom is poorly localized abdominal pain around the umbilicus or epigastrium, rarely in the right lower quadrant over McBurney's point. Later, the pain shifts to the periumbilical region and finally to the right lower quadrant. Anorexia and nausea and vomiting usually accompany the illness. Localized abdominal tenderness and guarding are noted on physical examination. Fever is low-grade, and the white count is moderately elevated. Variations from the classic clinical picture are common, especially in retrocecal appendicitis, where the pain commonly remains poorly localized. Ultrasonography of the appendix may be helpful if the diagnosis is uncertain.

Treatment & Disposition

The patient should be hospitalized and prepared for surgery within a few hours. Begin nasogastric suction; administer intravenous crystalloid solution to replace any volume deficits. Antimicrobial therapy is generally not used until the decision is made to operate.

2. INTESTINAL OBSTRUCTION

Diagnosis

The patient usually complains of intermittent colicky abdominal pain of sudden onset that rises to a peak and then subsides. Bowel habits may be altered. Vomiting may occur and will be feculent if obstruction is distal and long-standing. The abdomen is distended and tender, and peristaltic rushes as well as high-pitched tinkling may be heard. Dilated loops of bowel with air-fluid levels on abdominal x-ray confirm the diagnosis (Fig 7–5). Occasionally, x-ray findings are absent, and the diagnosis is based on clinical suspicion or abdominal CT scan with contrast.

Treatment & Disposition

Nasogastric suction and intravenous hydration should be initiated and the patient hospitalized for evaluation and possible surgery. Some cases resolve without surgery.

3. PERFORATED PEPTIC ULCER

Diagnosis

Perforation of a duodenal ulcer usually causes sudden severe upper abdominal pain. The pain of perforation subsides when gastric contents are diluted by peritoneal secretions but reappears later, with progressive worsening. Shoulder pain may occur owing to diaphragmatic irritation. The patient is usually in severe distress, with shallow breathing and knees drawn up to the chest in an effort to minimize pain. Upper abdominal tenderness is accompanied by boardlike rigidity of the abdomen. Percussion over the liver may reveal tympany resulting from escaped air, and sounds of peristalsis are reduced or absent. X-ray with the patient upright may show air under the diaphragm.

Treatment & Disposition

Insert a nasogastric tube for drainage of gastric acid. Administer crystalloid solution intravenously to correct volume depletion. Immediate hospitalization for surgery is necessary.

4. PERFORATION OF THE BOWEL

Diagnosis

Perforation of the bowel is accompanied by sudden or explosive onset of severe, agonizing mid or lower abdominal pain. Shock may be present and can be profound. Nausea and vomiting are common. The abdomen is rigid and tender. The temperature may be high and is accompanied by leukocytosis. A history of diverticulitis can often be elicited.

Treatment & Disposition

A. Treat shock with intravenous crystalloid solution.

B. Insert nasogastric tube for continuous gastric suction.

C. Obtain blood and urine cultures.

D. Begin antimicrobials (Table 7–1).

E. Hospitalize the patient, and prepare for surgery within 1–2 hours.

5. DIVERTICULITIS

Diagnosis

Diverticulitis is associated with lower abdominal pain which is usually gradual in onset and localized, predominantly in the left lower quadrant, but which may be midabdominal or in the right lower quadrant. There may be a history of diverticulosis. Fever is low-grade, accompanied by slight leukocytosis. Other findings may include abdominal tenderness, a palpable abdominal mass, and alterations in bowel function (either constipation or frequent defecation).

Treatment & Disposition

The patient should be hospitalized for administration of intravenous fluids and antimicrobial drugs (Table 7–1) and further observation.

6. INTESTINAL STRANGULATION

Diagnosis

Intestinal strangulation occurs most frequently in volvulus or femoral hernia and occasionally in inguinal hernia. Onset of pain is usually rapid. Pain increases in severity and may be intermittent and colicky. The patient may complain of an urge to defecate. The abdomen is distended, rigid, and diffusely tender. Exquisite tenderness is present in the region of strangulation. Shock appears early. Other findings include nausea and vomiting, high fever, and leukocytosis. In the case of volvulus, findings on abdominal x-ray may be diagnostic.

Treatment & Disposition

The patient should be hospitalized and prepared for surgery within an hour.

7. GASTROENTERITIS
   (See also Chapter 9.)

Diagnosis

The patient complains of mild to severe cramping and pain that may have come on gradually or abruptly. There may be nausea and vomiting, retching, and diarrhea, in any combination. These symptoms usually precede the onset of pain, in contrast to conditions requiring surgery, in which pain is usually the first symptom. Abdominal examination reveals generalized discomfort. In contrast to situations requiring surgery, involuntary guarding, localized tenderness, and peritoneal signs (eg, cough tenderness) are absent. Fever and leukocytosis are generally absent or mild, although patients with shigellosis typically have high fever and rigors. The patient may be dehydrated. Stool should be tested for blood, examined microscopically for leukocytes, and sent for culture if the patient has prolonged or severe diarrhea associated with fever.

Treatment & Disposition

Severely ill or dehydrated patients should be hospitalized. Mild to moderately ill patients can be sent home with instructions for rehydration. If symptoms persist or worsen, patients should receive follow-up evaluation. Bismuth subsalicylate (Pepto-Bismol, many others) may be used for symptomatic relief. Opiate-containing antidiarrheal agents (diphenoxylate with atropine [Lomotil, many others]) should be used, with caution, only in patients with mild diarrhea without evidence of dysentery. See Chapter 9 for details.

8. IDIOPATHIC INFLAMMATORY BOWEL DISEASE

Diagnosis
The patient complains of abdominal cramps and intermittent bloody diarrhea and usually gives a history of previous episodes of the same symptoms. There may be a long history of colitis. Weight loss, fever, and anemia may be present. Cramps may come on gradually or suddenly. The abdomen is slightly tender. Infectious causes of colitis (eg, *Shigella, Clostridium difficile, Campylobacter, Entamoeba histolytica*) should be systematically ruled out.

Treatment & Disposition
A. For the Seriously Ill Patient or for Uncertain Diagnosis:
1. Treat hypotension or shock with administration of intravenous crystalloid solution.
2. Give nothing by mouth; nasogastric suction may be helpful if the patient is vomiting.
3. Hospitalize the patient for definitive diagnosis and treatment. Indications for hospitalization are uncertain diagnosis, shock, fever, toxic megacolon, anemia, or gross blood in the stool.
B. For the Ambulatory Patient With Certain Diagnosis:
1. Begin sulfasalazine (Azaline, Azulfidine, Azulfidine EN-tabs, S.A.S.-500), 1 g orally 4 times a day.
2. Prescribe hydrocortisone enemas, 100 mg each night.
3. Refer the patient to an internist or gastroenterologist within 4–5 days.

HEPATOBILIARY DISORDERS

1. BILIARY COLIC

Diagnosis
Biliary colic is due to intermittent obstruction of the biliary tree by stones, usually at the cystic duct. The pain occurs in discrete episodes (frequently after ingestion of food), which usually begin abruptly and subside gradually. During an attack, there is steady upper abdominal pain that extends all the way across the abdomen but is more severe on the right. Pain may be referred to the scapula. A careful history often reveals prior attacks of similar pain. Abdominal examination shows right upper quadrant tenderness and, occasionally, a palpable gallbladder. A right upper quadrant sonogram is diagnostic and shows gallstones or a dilated gallbladder and cystic duct. An

oral cholecystogram may be nonvisualizing or may show gallstones.

Treatment
In the absence of acute cholecystitis or ascending cholangitis, no specific emergency treatment is necessary. Provide adequate analgesia.

Disposition
Refer the patient for possible elective cholecystectomy.

2. ACUTE CHOLECYSTITIS

Diagnosis
Acute cholecystitis is characterized by acute right upper quadrant pain and tenderness that may be referred to the right scapula. There may be a history of similar episodes. The discomfort may be moderate to severe and prostrating. Anorexia and nausea and vomiting usually occur also. There is low-grade fever and leukocytosis. In some cases, the gallbladder is palpable.

Ultrasonography of the abdomen demonstrating gallstones, dilatation of the intra- or extrahepatic bile ducts or thickening of the gallbladder wall confirms the diagnosis. Ultrasonography is the preferred diagnostic technique, since it is sensitive, specific, rapid, inexpensive, and without adverse effects. Nonvisualization on nuclear imaging (DISIDA) of the biliary tract is also diagnostic.

Treatment
A. Give pentazocine, 30–60 mg intramuscularly; if pentazocine is not available or does not relieve pain, give meperidine, 50–100 mg intramuscularly.
B. Insert a nasogastric tube, and attach it to continuous suction.
C. Give crystalloid solution (lactated Ringer's injection or equivalent) intravenously if the patient is dehydrated.
D. Give nothing by mouth.

Disposition
Hospitalize patients with cholecystitis, and obtain immediate surgical consultation. Patients with suspected cholelithiasis who are not acutely ill should receive surgical consultation and undergo elective gallbladder surgery; an appointment within a few days is satisfactory. Confirmatory diagnostic studies (ultrasonography of the abdomen or oral cholecystogram) should be scheduled in the meantime.

3. ACUTE SUPPURATIVE CHOLANGITIS

Diagnosis
Acute suppurative cholangitis is a surgical emergency commonly accompanied by bacteremia and

septic shock. Symptoms are abdominal pain, jaundice, fever and chills, mental confusion, and shock. Because of the overwhelming suppurative process, the biliary obstruction may not be apparent, and the actual diagnosis is therefore sometimes missed. Right upper quadrant sonography is the diagnostic procedure of choice and shows dilated, obstructed intrahepatic biliary ducts.

Treatment

A. Treat shock with infusion of intravenous crystalloid solution.

B. Insert a nasogastric tube, and connect it to a continuous suction device.

C. Insert a Foley catheter to monitor urine output.

D. Administer antimicrobials: ampicillin, 200 mg/kg/d intravenously (in 4–6 divided doses); plus tobramycin, 1.7 mg/kg every 8 hours intravenously.

Disposition

Hospitalize the patient, and prepare for surgery or endoscopic papillotomy within 1–2 hours.

4. HEPATIC ABSCESS

Diagnosis

When liver abscess results from other intra-abdominal infections, increasing toxicity, high fever, jaundice, and a deteriorating clinical picture are seen. Right upper quadrant pain may be present. In primary liver abscess (eg, caused by *Entamoeba histolytica*), the onset is insidious, and it may be several weeks before the disease becomes fulminant. High fever and leukocytosis often accompany the abscess, and rigors occur in approximately one-fourth of patients. The liver becomes enlarged and is often tender. Right upper quadrant sonography, CT scan, or liver scan is diagnostic. Obtain blood for culture and amebic serologic tests. Many patients with amebic liver abscesses do not have intestinal amebiasis; hence, stool examination for parasites is not helpful.

Treatment & Disposition

Hospitalize immediately for evaluation and treatment. Empiric antimicrobial therapy must be active against amebas, anaerobes, and coliform bacteria; metronidazole (750 mg 3 times a day intravenously or orally) plus a cephalosporin (eg, cefamandole, 2 g intravenously every 6 hours) is a satisfactory combination.

5. HEPATITIS

Diagnosis

Hepatitis is manifested by anorexia, nausea and vomiting, malaise, symptoms of upper respiratory tract infection or flulike syndrome, and bilirubinuria. Fever, jaundice, and an enlarged, tender liver are usually present. The white cell count is low or normal, and liver function tests show elevated bilirubin and hepatic enzymes (AST [SGOT], ALT [SGPT], and alkaline phosphatase).

The commonest causes are viral infection (hepatitis viruses, yellow fever, cytomegalovirus, Epstein-Barr virus) and alcohol. Alcoholic hepatitis can often be distinguished from viral hepatitis by the history and physical examination (evidence of alcohol abuse) and by AST and ALT levels (usually < 1000 IU/L in alcoholic hepatitis). In alcoholic hepatitis, AST (SGOT) levels are the same as or higher than ALT (SGPT) levels; in viral hepatitis, the situation is reversed.

Treatment & Disposition

Severely ill patients with persistent vomiting, dehydration, hepatic encephalopathy, or significant coagulopathy (prothrombin time > 15 seconds) should be hospitalized. Other patients can be referred to a primary-care physician and treated at home. The patient should be instructed to maintain hydration and strict hygiene and to avoid potential hepatotoxins (alcohol). Patients with viral hepatitis must avoid handling food that will be consumed by others. Tests that help in specific diagnosis (eg, HBsAg and hepatitis A IgM antibody) can be obtained in the emergency department if the physician so chooses. Close family contacts should be advised regarding appropriate immunizations if hepatitis viruses are suspected.

VASCULAR DISORDERS

1. RUPTURED AORTIC ANEURYSM

Diagnosis

Rupture of an abdominal aneurysm is accompanied by severe abdominal pain of sudden onset that may radiate into the back. In some patients, pain is confined to the flank, low back, or groin. Faintness or syncope may occur as a result of blood loss. After the first hemorrhage, pain may lessen and faintness may disappear, but these symptoms recur and progress further until shock finally supervenes. While dissection is occurring, a discrete pulsatile mass can be palpated in the abdomen. If rupture occurs in the retroperitoneum, a poorly defined midabdominal fullness can be felt, and shock becomes profound. A lateral abdominal x-ray and abdominal sonogram are useful for confirming the diagnosis. A chest x-ray should also be obtained in order to evaluate the thoracic aorta.

Treatment
(See also Chapter 32.)

A. Insert at least 2 large-bore (≥ 16-gauge) percutaneous catheters for vascular access. Consider a venous cutdown.

B. Draw blood for CBC, electrolytes, and tests of renal function. Type and cross-match for 8 units of whole blood.

C. Treat shock with intravenous crystalloid solution followed by whole blood as soon as available. In patients who are exsanguinating, type-specific or universal donor blood may be used until cross-matched blood is available (Chapter 33).

D. Obtain immediate vascular or general surgical consultation.

E. Prepare the patient for surgery as rapidly as possible.

Disposition

All patients must be hospitalized; the mortality rate is virtually 100% without surgical treatment.

2. ISCHEMIC COLITIS

Diagnosis

Patients with ischemic colitis are usually elderly and have evidence of vascular disease elsewhere in the body. There is often a history of similar attacks, abrupt in onset and of varying degrees of severity. The pain may be localized anywhere in the abdomen or may be diffuse. Severe colitis is usually accompanied by bloody diarrhea. Ischemic areas may progress to gangrene if the ischemia is sufficiently severe; if ischemia is milder, the areas may heal, often with strictures. Routine laboratory tests do not show specific abnormalities, although hemoconcentration and azotemia are common. Tests that confirm the diagnosis of ischemic colitis include sigmoidoscopy or colonoscopy, barium enema, and visceral angiography.

Treatment

A. Treat shock and hemoconcentration with intravenous crystalloid solution.

B. Administer antimicrobials (Table 7–1).

Disposition

All patients with suspected or documented ischemic colitis should be hospitalized for further diagnostic tests and possible surgery.

3. MESENTERIC THROMBOSIS

Diagnosis

The patient usually complains of the sudden onset of severe, diffuse abdominal pain in the mid or lower abdomen. The pain is poorly localized and very severe, often not relieved by narcotics. It is constant rather than crampy. There may be nausea and vomiting and diarrhea, with gross or occult blood in the stool. There are no physical findings initially. As the condition progresses, abdominal distention and tenderness appear and shock supervenes. Marked leuko-cytosis, hemoconcentration, azotemia, and acidosis are commonly associated with mesenteric thrombosis.

Treatment & Disposition

Treat shock and hemoconcentration with intravenous crystalloid solutions, and administer antimicrobials (Table 7–1). Hospitalize the patient and prepare for emergency surgery. Visceral angiography may be used to confirm the diagnosis.

4. RUPTURE OF THE SPLEEN
(See also Chapter 19.)

Diagnosis

Rupture of the spleen is usually caused by trauma to the lower left rib cage that is often associated with rib fractures. Occasionally, the spleen may rupture after trivial or overlooked injury, usually when pathologic enlargement has occurred (eg, infectious mononucleosis, AIDS, leukemia). Actual splenic rupture may occur several days after initial injury. Blood leaking into the peritoneal cavity causes abdominal pain and tenderness that may radiate to the left side of the neck or left shoulder. Tachycardia, hypotension, and falling hematocrit are present, and shock may develop. Occasionally, patients present with syncope, hypotension, or shock without abdominal symptoms. Palpation of the left upper quadrant may reveal tenderness, mild spasm, and distention. Tenderness over the ninth and tenth ribs on the left is a diagnostic clue. CT scan and peritoneal lavage showing gross blood are helpful in unclear cases but should not be performed routinely.

Treatment

A. Insert at least 2 large-bore ($\geq$ 16-gauge) percutaneous intravenous lines.

B. Obtain a CBC; type and cross-match for 6 units of whole blood.

C. Treat shock initially with intravenous infusion of crystalloid solution. Administer whole blood as soon as available, using hematocrit and blood pressure as guides to dosage.

Disposition

All patients with suspected splenic rupture should be hospitalized, and most will require emergency surgery.

5. SPLENIC INFARCT

Diagnosis

Infarction of the spleen usually occurs in patients with abnormal spleens due to hematologic disease (eg, sickling hemoglobinopathies). Rarely, it occurs as a result of arterial embolization, eg, in patients with endocarditis. There is left upper quadrant pain of variable degree, occasionally referred to the shoulder. Left upper quadrant tenderness is usually present as well. CT scan is helpful in confirming the diagnosis.

Treatment

No specific treatment is necessary. Symptomatic measures (eg, relief of pain) and treatment of the underlying disease may be necessary.

Disposition

Hospitalization is advisable until the diagnosis is confirmed. Likewise, hospitalization may be required for pain relief or treatment of the underlying disease.

URINARY DISORDERS

1. RENAL COLIC
(See also Chapter 31.)

Diagnosis

Sudden, severe flank pain followed by hematuria is characteristic of renal colic. There may be a history of passage of stones. Examination reveals costovertebral angle tenderness on the side of the stone, with the pain shifting anteriorly and inferiorly as the stone progresses down the ureter toward the bladder. The stone can usually be visualized on x-ray. Excretory urography confirms the diagnosis by demonstrating obstruction to urinary flow. Urinary tract infection may coexist, and urinalysis should be performed in every case along with culture of the urine for organisms if infection is suspected.

Treatment & Disposition

Large stones and a severe clinical picture require hospitalization for administration of parenteral analgesia and maintenance of hydration. The patient with small stones can be treated on an ambulatory basis with appropriate oral analgesia, hydration, and follow-up care with a primary care physician or urologist. Treat coexisting urinary tract infections.

2. PYELONEPHRITIS
(See also Chapter 34.)

Diagnosis

Patients with pyelonephritis typically have dysuria, urinary urgency and frequency, fever, and sometimes rigors. Pain, if present, is usually over the costovertebral angle or occasionally the abdomen. The pain is dull and usually gradual in onset. Malaise and nausea and vomiting are commonly present as well. Many bacteria and leukocytes are seen on stained smears of the urinary sediment.

Treatment & Disposition

A patient who is severely ill (vomiting, high fever, rigors), pregnant, very young or very old, or immunocompromised, or who has known anatomic abnormalities of the genitourinary tract requires hospitalization for intravenous hydration and parenteral antibiotics. For other patients (ie, those not requiring hospitalization), urine culture and administration of oral antibiotics on an empiric basis are acceptable.

3. RENAL INFARCT

Diagnosis

Infarction of the kidney usually occurs because of arterial embolization (eg, from endocarditis or atrial fibrillation). In addition to flank pain and tenderness, hematuria is usually present. The diagnosis may be confirmed by CT scan, renal scan, or angiography.

Treatment

No specific treatment is required for renal infarct. However, anticoagulation or other measures may be required to treat the underlying disease.

Disposition

Hospitalization is advisable for definitive diagnosis, administration of appropriate analgesia, treatment of underlying disease, and rapid anticoagulation measures if indicated.

PANCREATIC DISORDERS

1. ACUTE PANCREATITIS

Diagnosis

Acute pancreatitis is characterized by abrupt onset of severe, unrelenting epigastric pain radiating to the back, often accompanied by vomiting and retching. In severe cases, the patient may be in shock. A predisposing condition (alcoholism, glucocorticoid administration, diabetes mellitus) may be present. Abdominal examination reveals decreased or absent bowel sounds and tenderness usually localized to the epigastrium. Rarely, an abdominal mass is palpated in the epigastrium. Elevated serum amylase and lipase levels, mild fever, and leukocytosis are often present. If there is uncertainty about the diagnosis, abdominal CT scan can often demonstrate changes pathognomonic of pancreatitis. Patients may have a history of recurrent pancreatitis; alcohol abuse is a common predisposing factor.

Treatment

A. Send blood for CBC and serum electrolyte, glucose, calcium, and amylase measurements and renal function tests.

B. Insert an intravenous catheter ($\geq$ 18-gauge), and begin an infusion of crystalloid solution (change the composition of the fluid depending on the results of serum electrolyte determinations).

C. Give morphine, 2–4 mg intravenously, for pain; the dose may be repeated. For patients who are not vomiting and are less severely ill, oral analgesics (eg, codeine compounds, meperidine, or pentazocine) may be sufficient.

D. Insert a nasogastric tube attached to a suction device if the patient is vomiting or if the abdomen is distended, especially if ileus is present.

E. Give nothing by mouth to patients who are more severely ill.

Disposition

Patients with severe pain or persistent vomiting should be hospitalized for analgesia, intravenous hydration, and correction of electrolyte abnormalities. Even if they are not acutely ill, patients with no history of pancreatitis should be hospitalized for evaluation and treatment. Patients with chronic and recurrent pancreatitis may not require hospitalization if they can take fluids by mouth and do not require parenteral analgesics. Patients with recurrent acute pancreatitis due to alcohol abuse may be treated with oral analgesics and hydration on an outpatient basis if they are not severely ill.

GYNECOLOGIC DISORDERS
(See also Chapter 30.)

1. ECTOPIC PREGNANCY WITH RUPTURE

Diagnosis

In ectopic pregnancy with rupture, the patient experiences sudden, severe unilateral abdominal or pelvic pain that may be referred to the shoulder. Prior to rupture, pain may be vague or intermittent. There may be occasional nausea and vomiting but usually no fever. Irregular menses or other symptoms of pregnancy may be present as well. Postural hypotension or shock may be found on initial examination. Pelvic examination often reveals a unilateral doughy mass and tenderness on movement of the cervix. There is nonclotting blood in the cul-de-sac on culdocentesis. Pelvic sonography reveals free blood and an adnexal mass. A serum pregnancy test is positive, but urine pregnancy tests may be negative in about one-fourth of patients.

Treatment & Disposition

Treat shock or hypotension with intravenous crystalloid solution and whole blood if necessary. Hospitalize the patient at once for emergency surgery, or laparoscopy if the diagnosis is in doubt (Chapter 30).

2. ACUTE SALPINGITIS
(See also Chapter 34.)

Diagnosis

The patient with salpingitis experiences gradual onset of pelvic and lower abdominal pain that slowly increases in severity. There may be headache and lassitude with high fever and tachycardia. Nausea and vomiting may be present. The patient shows exquisite tenderness to vaginal examination and particularly to movement of the cervix. Adnexal fullness or mass (tubo-ovarian abscess) may be present.

Treatment & Disposition

Most patients should be hospitalized, treated with parenteral antibiotics, and kept under observation to decrease the risk of subsequent infertility. Surgery may be necessary if abdominal symptoms persist or if the patient's condition deteriorates.

3. RUPTURED OVARIAN FOLLICLE CYST

Diagnosis

Patients with ruptured ovarian follicle cyst experience sudden, moderately severe pelvic or lower abdominal pain. There usually are no gastrointestinal symptoms, and the patient is afebrile without leukocytosis. Tenderness may be elicited over the affected ovary. There should be no masses on pelvic examination, and the serum pregnancy test should be negative.

Treatment & Disposition

The patient should be kept under observation in the hospital until the diagnosis is confirmed. Operation is not necessary.

4. TORSION OF OVARIAN TUMOR

Diagnosis

Torsion of an ovarian tumor is characterized by sudden unilateral lower abdominal or pelvic pain precipitated by a change in position. There are no menstrual disorders and no gastrointestinal symptoms.

Treatment & Disposition

The patient should be hospitalized for observation and possible surgery.

5. ENDOMETRIOSIS

Diagnosis

Patients with endometriosis usually have a history of infertility, dysmenorrhea, and previous cyclic attacks of cramps and pains in the lower abdomen and possibly in the flank. Pain is worse with menses.

Onset of symptoms may be gradual or sudden if there is associated bleeding. Painful defecation and dyspareunia are present. Aching pelvic discomfort and general tenderness on pelvic examination suggest endometriosis. Acquired secondary dysmenorrhea should be attributed to endometriosis until proved otherwise.

Treatment & Disposition

If symptoms are mild, the patient should be given analgesics and referred to the obstetrics and gynecology department for follow-up. If pain is severe, the patient should be hospitalized for evaluation and possible surgery.

PERITONEAL DISORDERS

1. PRIMARY PERITONITIS

Diagnosis

Primary peritonitis occurs almost exclusively in patients with preexisting ascites, especially those with cirrhosis or nephrotic syndrome. (Peritonitis secondary to traumatic fecal soilage is discussed in Chapter 19.) The symptoms and signs vary, but fever and abdominal pain and tenderness are common. The most helpful tests are blood culture and abdominal paracentesis for Gram-stained smear, cell count, and culture. Most cases of primary bacterial peritonitis demonstrate positive blood cultures, peritoneal fluid leukocyte counts over 1000/μL (with a predominance of PMNs), and bacteria on Gram-stained smears or culture. Occasionally, all of these findings are present except that peritoneal fluid smears and cultures are negative. Familial Mediterranean fever produces sterile peritonitis that is difficult to distinguish from bacterial peritonitis.

Treatment

A. Culture blood and peritoneal fluid (include a culture for *Mycobacterium tuberculosis*).

B. Treat shock, if present, with intravenous crystalloid solution.

C. Begin parenteral antimicrobials; a cephalosporin in full doses (eg, cefazolin, 100 mg/kg/d intravenously in 3 divided doses) is satisfactory pending results of cultures.

Disposition

All patients with suspected or confirmed acute peritonitis should be hospitalized for diagnostic evaluation and treatment.

RETROPERITONEAL DISORDERS

1. RETROPERITONEAL HEMORRHAGE

Diagnosis

Retroperitoneal hemorrhage is a rare condition that may occur secondary to minor trauma in individuals with defective clotting factors resulting from medication or disease. Back pain and abdominal pain are present, and the psoas sign is often positive. Abdominal CT scan localizes the bleeding in most cases.

Treatment

A. Treat shock with intravenous crystalloid solution, followed by cross-matched whole blood as soon as available.

B. Correct coagulation defects by administering platelets or clotting factors as needed.

Disposition

Patients with copious hemorrhage, active bleeding, severe clotting abnormalities, or severe pain should be hospitalized.

CONDITIONS CAUSING ACUTE ABDOMINAL PAIN THAT ARE NOT AMENABLE TO SURGERY

A variety of conditions not amenable to surgery may cause abdominal pain. Aside from common conditions such as pyelonephritis, salpingitis, myocardial infarction, and lobar pneumonia, a number of rare conditions are capable of mimicking abdominal disorders requiring surgery. Most of these conditions simulate acute diffuse peritonitis. Helpful differential diagnostic tests are listed in Table 7–4.

REFERENCES

Beal JM, Raffinsperger JG: *Diagnosis of Acute Abdominal Pain.* Lea & Febiger, 1979.

Botsford TW, Wilson RE: *The Acute Abdomen,* 2nd ed. Saunders, 1977.

Brewer RJ et al: Abdominal pain: Analysis of 1000 consecutive cases in a university hospital emergency room. Am J Surg 1976;131:219.

Eisenberg RL et al: Evaluation of plain abdominal radiographs in the diagnosis of abdominal pain. Ann Intern Med 1982;97:257.

Graff L, Radford MJ, Werne C: Probability of appendicitis before and after observation. Ann Emerg Med 1991;20:503.

Jess P et al: Prognosis of acute nonspecific abdominal pain: A prospective study. Am J Surg 1982;144:338.

Lewis FR et al: Appendicitis: A critical review of diagnosis and treatment in 1000 cases. Arch Surg 1975;110:677.

Nauta RJ, Magnant C: Observation versus operation for abdominal pain in the right lower quadrant: Roles of the clinical examination and the leukocyte count. Am J Surg 1986;151:746.

Ranson JH: Acute pancreatitis. Curr Probl Surg (Nov) 1979;16:1. [Entire issue.]

Silen W: *Cope's Early Diagnosis of the Acute Abdomen,* 16th ed. Oxford, 1983.

Steinheber FV: Medical conditions mimicking the acute surgical abdomen. Med Clin North Am 1973;57:1559.

Szlabick RE et al: Hepatobiliary scanning in the diagnosis of acute cholecystitis. Arch Surg 1980;115:540.

Thomson HG, Jones PF: Active observation in acute abdominal pain. Am J Surg 1986;152:522.

Way LW (editor): *Current Surgical Diagnosis & Treatment,* 9th ed. Appleton & Lange, 1991.

Welch CE, Malt RA: Abdominal surgery (3 parts). N Engl J Med 1983;308:624, 685, 753.

8   Gastrointestinal Tract Bleeding

Richard A. Crass, MD, John P. Cello, MD, & Donald D. Trunkey, MD

Most patients with gastrointestinal tract bleeding present with obvious symptoms of hemorrhage, such as hematemesis (vomiting of blood), melena (passage of stool made black by large amounts of altered blood), and hematochezia (passage of bright red stools). Rarely, patients with brisk gastrointestinal tract hemorrhage do not demonstrate these findings and present with shock of unknown cause. For this reason, any patient in shock without an obvious cause must be rapidly evaluated by gastric lavage and rectal examination for blood or melena (Chapter 3) to assess the possibility of gastrointestinal tract bleeding. The physician must quickly estimate the severity and rapidity of blood loss, so that appropriate diagnostic and therapeutic measures can be started.

IMMEDIATE MANAGEMENT OF LIFE-THREATENING BLEEDING (See algorithm.)

Assess Rate & Volume of Bleeding

Patients who have active hematemesis or hematochezia on arrival in the emergency department are in danger of exsanguinating, and volume replacement must be started at once. Proceed immediately to treat exsanguinating gastrointestinal tract hemorrhage, as described below.

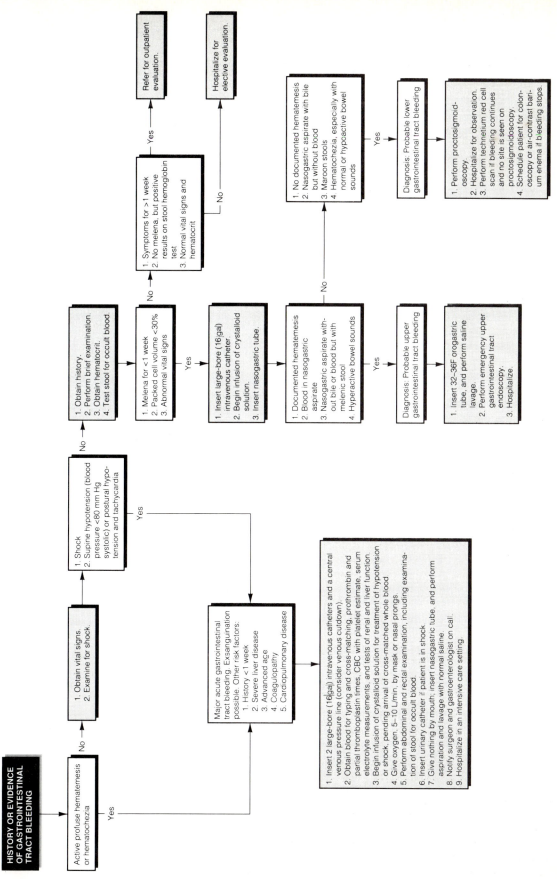

HISTORY OR EVIDENCE OF GASTROINTESTINAL TRACT BLEEDING

Active profuse hematemesis or hematochezia

No →

1. Obtain vital signs.
2. Examine for shock.

Yes →

1. Shock
2. Supine hypotension (blood pressure <80 mm Hg systolic) or postural hypotension and tachycardia

No →

1. Obtain history.
2. Perform brief examination.
3. Obtain hematocrit.
4. Test stool for occult blood.

Yes →

Major acute gastrointestinal tract bleeding. Exsanguination possible. Other risk factors:
1. History <1 week
2. Severe liver disease
3. Advanced age
4. Coagulopathy
5. Cardiopulmonary disease

1. Insert 2 large-bore (16 ga) intravenous catheters and a central venous pressure line (consider venous cutdown).
2. Obtain blood for typing and cross-matching, CBC with platelet estimate, serum electrolyte measurements, and tests of renal and liver function.
3. Begin infusion of crystalloid solution for treatment of hypotension or shock, pending arrival of cross-matched whole blood.
4. Give oxygen, 5–10 L/min, by mask or nasal prongs.
5. Perform abdominal and rectal examination, including examination of stool for occult blood.
6. Insert urinary catheter if patient is in shock.
7. Give nothing by mouth; insert nasogastric tube, and perform aspiration and lavage with normal saline.
8. Notify surgeon and gastroenterologist on call.
9. Hospitalize in an intensive care setting.

1. Melena for <1 week
2. Packed cell volume <30%
3. Abnormal vital signs

No →

1. Symptoms for >1 week
2. No melena, but positive results on stool hemoglobin test
3. Normal vital signs and hematocrit

Yes → Refer for outpatient evaluation.

No → Hospitalize for elective evaluation.

Yes →

1. Insert large-bore (16 ga) intravenous catheter.
2. Begin infusion of crystalloid solution.
3. Insert nasogastric tube.

1. Documented hematemesis
2. Blood in nasogastric aspirate
3. Nasogastric aspirate without bile or blood but with melenic stool
4. Hyperactive bowel sounds

Yes →

Diagnosis: Probable upper gastrointestinal tract bleeding

1. Insert 32–36F orogastric tube, and perform saline lavage.
2. Perform emergency upper gastrointestinal tract endoscopy.
3. Hospitalize.

No →

1. No documented hematemesis
2. Nasogastric aspirate with bile but without blood
3. Maroon stools
4. Hematochezia, especially with normal or hypoactive bowel sounds

Yes →

Diagnosis: Probable lower gastrointestinal tract bleeding

1. Perform proctosigmoidoscopy.
2. Hospitalize for observation.
3. Perform technetium red cell scan if bleeding continues and no site is seen on proctosigmoidoscopy.
4. Schedule patient for colonoscopy or air-contrast barium enema if bleeding stops.

If active blood loss is not obvious in a patient in whom gastrointestinal tract bleeding is suspected, proceed as follows:

Obtain Vital Signs

Check blood pressure and pulse with the patient in the supine position; if normal (blood pressure > 110 mm Hg systolic and pulse < 100 beats/min for adults), determine vital signs also with the patient sitting and, if still normal, in the standing position.

Recognize Possible Exsanguinating Hemorrhage

Factors that may indicate exsanguinating hemorrhage are as follows:

A. Profuse hematemesis or hematochezia.

B. Supine hypotension or shock (Table 8–1).

C. Postural hypotension or tachycardia.

D. Possible aortoduodenal fistula (history of aortic aneurysm, previous aortic operation [especially if graft is in place], or palpable abdominal aortic aneurysm).

E. Known or suspected varices.

Treat Exsanguinating Gastrointestinal Tract Hemorrhage

A. Gain Venous Access: Insert a large-bore intravenous catheter. In an adult, this should be 16-gauge or larger. If shock is present, a second intravenous catheter should be inserted as well (Chapters 3 and 46).

B. Perform Laboratory Studies: Obtain blood for immediate hematocrit. Type and cross-match blood, and order 6 units of packed red blood cells.

Measure the platelet count, prothrombin time, and partial thromboplastin time in order to discover any bleeding abnormality. Send blood for renal and liver function tests and measurement of serum electrolytes. Arterial blood gas and pH measurements may be helpful in determining the adequacy of perfusion. (Metabolic acidosis is indicative of poor perfusion.)

C. Begin Rapid Infusion of Crystalloid Solution: Give balanced salt solution or normal saline to restore intravascular volume and blood pressure until compatible blood becomes available for transfusion.

D. Begin Blood Transfusion: Infuse cross-matched packed red blood cells as soon as possible. Give 2 or more units (depending on vital signs and hematocrit) at a rate of 250–500 mL/h. Gastrointestinal tract bleeding is seldom rapid enough to justify transfusion of unmatched (eg, type-specific) blood.

E. Administer Oxygen: If the patient shows signs of shock (Table 8–1), give oxygen, 5–10 L/min, by mask or nasal prongs.

F. Perform Rectal Examination: Perform rectal examination, and obtain stool for occult blood testing.

G. Perform Abdominal Examination: Examine the abdomen to detect tenderness (perhaps indicating active ulcer or bowel infarction) or an aortic aneurysm (with possible aortoduodenal fistula), which might make urgent surgery necessary.

H. Perform Bladder Catheterization: Insert a urinary catheter to monitor urine output of patients in shock or with unstable cardiac or renal function.

I. Insert Nasogastric or Orogastric Tube:

1. If hematemesis has not been documented, insert a 16–18F nasogastric tube, and perform gastric lavage with at least 500 mL of normal saline (the temperature is not critical). Brisk, persistent bleeding during lavage indicates possible life-threatening upper gastrointestinal tract bleeding.

2. If hematemesis has been documented, insert a 32–36F Ewald or Edlich orogastric tube for lavage with saline (temperature is not critical) until all clots and food are removed. With the patient in the left lateral decubitus position to avoid aspiration, begin brisk lavage with normal saline until the return is no longer bloody (continued brisk bleeding generally indicates a need for urgent therapy). The large tube may then be replaced with a 16–18F nasogastric tube, which should then be connected to standard low-pressure suction, so that further blood loss can be monitored.

J. Withhold Foods and Antacids: Since most patients who are bleeding vigorously will require endoscopy, neither antacids nor foods should be administered by mouth or nasogastric tube. They will coat the upper gastrointestinal tract and impair endoscopic visualization and therapy of lesions.

K. Seek Early Consultation: Notify the surgeon and gastroenterologist on call as soon as a diagnosis of life-threatening hemorrhage has been made.

Table 8–1. Clinical classification of shock.[1]

Degree of Shock	Pathophysiology	Clinical Manifestations
Mild (< 20% of blood volume lost)	Decreased peripheral perfusion only of organs able to withstand prolonged ischemia (skin, fat, muscle, bone). Arterial pH normal.	Patient complains of feeling cold. Postural hypotension and tachycardia. Cool, pale, moist skin; collapsed neck veins; and concentrated urine.
Moderate (20–40% of blood volume lost)	Decreased central perfusion of organs able to tolerate only brief ischemia (liver, gut, kidneys). Metabolic acidosis present.	Thirst. Supine hypotension and tachycardia (variable). Oliguria or anuria.
Severe (> 40% of blood volume lost)	Decreased perfusion of heart and brain. Metabolic acidosis severe. Respiratory acidosis may also be present.	Agitation, confusion, or obtundation. Supine hypotension and tachycardia invariably present. Rapid, deep respiration.

[1] These clinical findings are most consistently observed in hemorrhagic shock but apply to other types of shock as well.

Disposition

Hospitalize patients with active blood loss in an intensive care unit, and monitor vital signs and blood loss. Continued bleeding, persistent supine hypotension or tachycardia, postural hypotension, and decreased peripheral perfusion all indicate inadequate volume replacement or persistent blood loss. Most of these unstable patients should have a central venous or pulmonary artery wedge (Swan-Ganz) pressure line inserted to serve as a guide to blood replacement. An arterial line should also be strongly considered.

DETERMINE SITE OF BLEEDING

Once vital signs and the hematocrit have returned toward normal, an attempt should be made to localize the site of bleeding if it is not already apparent. About 90% of patients presenting to the emergency department with gastrointestinal tract bleeding have upper gastrointestinal tract lesions, ie, located in or proximal to the duodenum (Table 8–2); only about 10% have lower gastrointestinal tract lesions. Furthermore, in about three-fourths of patients with lower gastrointestinal tract bleeding, the bleeding stops shortly after arrival at the emergency department or hospital.

Diagnostic Characteristics of Upper Gastrointestinal Tract Bleeding (See Fig 8–1.)

A. Hematemesis:

1. Hematemesis (exclude hemoptysis or epistaxis with subsequent vomiting of swallowed blood) is observed.

2. Frank blood or material in the nasogastric lavage contents that is positive for blood by the guaiac test is observed.

3. In about 10% of patients with gastrointestinal tract bleeding originating in the duodenum, frank blood is not found in the nasogastric aspirate, because the nasogastric tube does not reach the duodenum and blood has not refluxed into the stomach.

If the nasogastric lavage contents reveal bile but not blood, active upper gastrointestinal tract bleeding at the time of nasogastric sampling can be excluded with confidence.

If there is neither blood nor bile in the lavage material (inconclusive lavage), a postpyloric upper gastrointestinal tract bleeding lesion cannot be definitively ruled out. Patients who report recent unwitnessed hematemesis and in whom results of gastric lavage have been inconclusive should therefore be hospitalized for evaluation.

B. Melena: (Liquid, tarry, foul-smelling black stools.) Melena usually is due to bleeding from the

Table 8–2. Cause and severity of upper gastrointestinal tract hemorrhage in all patients undergoing diagnostic endoscopy at the San Francisco General Hospital over 3 years.

Source of Hemorrhage	Severity of Hemorrhage (%)	
	Mild-Moderate (n = 246 patients)	Severe (n = 140 patients)
Esophagus		
Esophagitis	12	7
Ulcer	2	2
Mallory-Weiss tear	5	19
Esophageal varices	5	31
Total, esophagus	24	59
Stomach		
Gastric ulcer	15	14
Prepyloric ulcer	2	4
Pyloric channel ulcer	4	2
Gastric erosions	2	0
Gastritis	7	0
Varices	1	2
Portal-hypertensive gastropathy	2	
Gastric cancer	2	
Polyp	0	2
Dieulafoy's lesion	0	
Total, stomach	35	24
Duodenum		
Ulcer	31	15
Duodenitis	8	
Aortoenteric fistula	2	
Pancreatic pseudocyst		2
Total, duodenum	41	17
	100	100

upper gastrointestinal tract and indicates that more than 500 mL of blood has been lost over a 24-hour period. Seemingly melenic stool should always be tested for occult blood, since many substances (bismuth, iron, spinach, etc) may cause dark stools.

The extent to which red blood is converted to melena is proportionate to the time the red blood is within the intestinal lumen; therefore, *slow* lower gastrointestinal tract bleeding rarely produces melena. Thus, melena may occur occasionally in lower gastrointestinal tract bleeding from the distal small bowel or proximal colon when intestinal transit is slow.

Diagnostic Characteristics of Lower Gastrointestinal Tract Bleeding (See Fig 8–2.)

A. Hematochezia: (Bright-red blood passed per rectum.) Hematochezia is usually associated with lower gastrointestinal tract (primarily colonic) bleeding. Hematochezia may occur with extremely brisk upper gastrointestinal tract bleeding. When from an

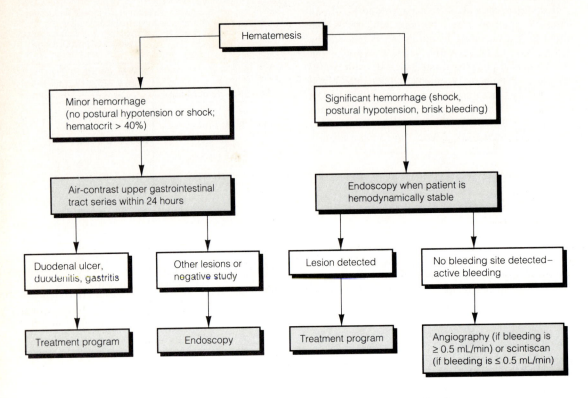

Figure 8–1. Diagnostic schema for upper gastrointestinal tract bleeding.

upper gastrointestinal source, hematochezia is invariably associated with severe intravascular volume depletion and hyperactive bowel sounds. Posterior duodenal bulbar ulcer and aortoduodenal fistulas are the upper gastrointestinal tract lesions most commonly associated with hematochezia.

B. Maroon Stools: (Gross blood with melena.) Bleeding distal to the duodenum is the usual cause of maroon stools. Brisk upper gastrointestinal tract bleeding is occasionally associated with maroon stools.

C. Melena: True melena (black, tarry stools) is rarely associated with lower gastrointestinal tract bleeding.

D. Absence of Bleeding: If nasogastric lavage contents reveal bile but not blood, a diagnosis of upper gastrointestinal tract bleeding is excluded.

FURTHER EVALUATION OF GASTROINTESTINAL TRACT BLEEDING

For the seriously ill patient, the following more thorough evaluation should be started as soon as the patient's hemodynamic status becomes relatively

normal and the site of bleeding has been tentatively identified. For the patient not at risk of acute exsanguination, this evaluation may be performed initially.

History

A. Inquire about bleeding diathesis, peptic ulcer disease, use of alcohol or nonsteroidal anti-inflammatory drugs, recent weight loss, altered bowel habits, pain suggesting duodenal ulcer or gastritis, gastric surgery, documented cirrhosis, and other documented episodes of gastrointestinal tract bleeding.

B. A history of recent vigorous retching or emesis before an episode of hematemesis or melena suggests Mallory-Weiss tear of the gastroesophageal junction.

C. Inquire about possible rectal trauma (rectal intercourse, dildos, etc).

D. In AIDS or other immune deficiencies, bleeding may be related to Kaposi's sarcoma or lymphoma or to cytomegalovirus ulcerations. Visceral Kaposi's sarcoma is usually associated with cutaneous lesions with their classical dusky violaceous nodules.

Physical Examination

A. Vital Signs: Assess cardiovascular status by checking blood pressure and pulse every 15 minutes,

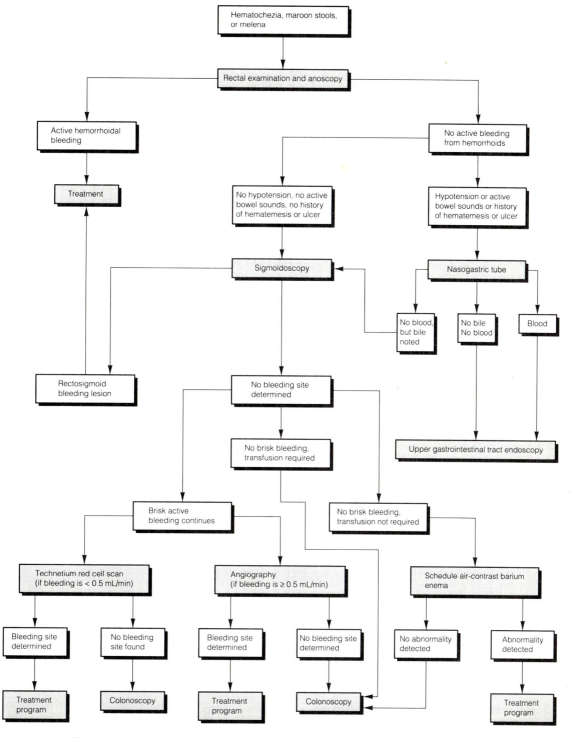

Figure 8–2. Diagnostic schema for evaluating apparent lower gastrointestinal tract bleeding.

with the patient in the supine and upright positions if possible.

B. Liver Disease: Look for signs of chronic liver disease (hepatosplenomegaly, ascites, spider angiomas, enlarged abdominal veins, jaundice, asterixis, palmar erythema). *Caution:* The mere presence of liver disease does not itself warrant attributing upper gastrointestinal tract bleeding to esophageal varices. Up to half of patients with cirrhosis and upper gastrointestinal tract hemorrhage have bleeding from sites other than varices.

C. Osler-Weber-Rendu Disease (Hereditary Hemorrhagic Telangiectasia): Look for telangiectasias of skin (particularly digits) and lips that may possibly indicate the presence of this disease, in which bleeding occurs from gastrointestinal tract vascular malformations.

D. Surgical Scars: Note surgical scars that may represent previous procedures for peptic ulcer disease or vascular disease with placement of graft.

E. Hyperactive Bowel Sounds: Auscultation of the abdomen may provide an indication of the briskness of bleeding, since severe upper gastrointestinal tract hemorrhage is usually associated with hyperactive bowel sounds owing to the strong laxative effect of intraluminal blood.

F. Pain and Tenderness: (See also Chapter 7.) Abdominal pain and tenderness are common in gastritis and peptic ulcers but rare in patients with Mallory-Weiss tears, cancer, or hemorrhage from varices. A tender abdomen without bowel sounds in a hypotensive patient with melena should suggest bowel infarction (a surgical emergency).

G. Rectal Examination: Obtain stool for visual inspection and testing for occult blood. The appearance of the stool can help determine the briskness of bleeding and differentiate upper from lower gastrointestinal tract bleeding sites (see above).

Special Examinations

A. Upper Gastrointestinal Tract Bleeding: (See Fig 8–1.)

1. Endoscopy–Endoscopy is the most rapid and accurate means of identifying the site of upper gastrointestinal tract hemorrhage. Once the condition of patients with upper gastrointestinal tract bleeding has stabilized, endoscopy should be the first test performed for those with evidence of marked active blood loss. In addition to being a highly reliable diagnostic tool, endoscopy allows for several therapeutic options such as sclerotherapy of varices and coagulation of bleeding vessels.

2. Upper gastrointestinal series–Upper gastrointestinal tract x-rays are a useful first test for the patient with minimal or no active bleeding who stabilizes quickly, has Hct $\geq 40\%$, and does not require transfusions. In most instances, radiography should be performed using the "double-contrast" or "air-contrast" technique rather than the single-contrast

method. Single-contrast barium upper gastrointestinal radiography has a sensitivity of less than 30% in patients with acute hemorrhage compared to 80% sensitivity when double-contrast techniques are used. Active bleeding, inability to cooperate, recent ingestion of food, or use of antacids will prevent effective coating of the mucosa by the barium and will decrease the test's sensitivity.

3. Angiography–Angiography is rarely employed in upper gastrointestinal tract hemorrhage. However, angiography should be considered in patients with continuing melena in whom results of endoscopy have been negative, particularly if the bleeding is judged to be faster than 0.5 mL/min. For patients with negative findings on endoscopy and bleeding at a rate of less than 0.5 mL/min, a technetium red blood cell scan should be performed first.

B. Lower Gastrointestinal Tract Bleeding: (See Fig 8–2.)

1. Anoscopy and sigmoidoscopy–Anoscopy and sigmoidoscopy should be performed as soon as the patient's hemodynamic status has normalized. This procedure will detect hemorrhoidal bleeding and exclude ulcerative colitis, distal sigmoid colon or rectal neoplasms, rectal lacerations, and distal ischemia.

Be especially careful to examine the anorectal junction for hemorrhoidal bleeding. Remember also that retrograde passage of blood from the rectum to the proximal colon may occur. On sigmoidoscopy, blood—even fresh blood—that seems to come from above the level of insertion of the sigmoidoscope may not necessarily originate there. If there is a large amount of stool or clotted blood in the rectum, a gentle enema performed with 1 L of tap water often clears the visual field. Flexible fiberoptic sigmoidoscopy enhances visualization of the distal bowel and is more acceptable to patients; however, it requires more thorough preparation of the bowel than rigid sigmoidoscopy, since the suction channels have small lumens and are easily clogged by feces and blood clots.

2. Barium enema–Patients with hemodynamically critical lower gastrointestinal tract hemorrhage whose bleeding stops shortly after admission to the emergency department or hospital, who are not anemic, and who do not require transfusions should undergo a barium enema with air-contrast study *following a 24-hour observation period during which bleeding does not recur.* Barium in the colon will interfere with visceral angiography, should it become necessary.

3. Colonoscopy–Because large amounts of blood clots and fecal material are present, colonoscopy is not technically feasible in most patients with brisk bleeding. In patients who are actively bleeding but not massively so, colonoscopy may be performed after careful preparation of the bowel. The best preparation for emergency colonoscopy uses a balanced solute solution in which the major ingredients are nonabsorbable sulfate salts and polyethylene glycol (Golytely Colyte, or equivalent). Give 3–4 L (adult dose) orally or by nasogastric tube over 2–3 hours; watery diarrhea will ensue, and adequate preparation of the colon will have occurred within a few hours.

4. Angiography–If brisk bleeding recurs during the observation period, emergency angiography may be performed.

a. Diagnose bleeding site–Selective mesenteric angiography is indicated to determine the site of bleeding in patients who continue to bleed massively or have substantial recurrence of bleeding after entering the hospital.

b. Control bleeding–Vasoconstrictor drugs (vasopressin), autogenous clot, metal coils, or Gelfoam infused selectively into the vessels feeding the bleeding segments often stops the bleeding.

5. Technetium red cell scintigraphy–In a patient with active hematochezia whose blood loss is less than 0.5 mL/min, a technetium red cell scan may localize the bleeding site. A portion of the patient's own red cells are labeled with technetium-99m and reinfused, and scanning with a gamma camera is started. If no bleeding is detected, scanning is repeated frequently over the next 18 hours. Bleeding into the gastrointestinal tract can be detected and localized by the scanner. Since both anterograde and retrograde passage of blood may occur, apparent bleeding sites identified by scanning must be interpreted with caution if many hours have passed between scans.

Monitoring for Rebleeding

A. Gastric Lavage: Perform lavage through the nasogastric tube frequently, and record the volume and appearance of the material aspirated from the stomach. Continued presence of bright red blood is an indication for consultation with a surgeon and gastroenterologist. In patients with hemodynamically significant upper gastrointestinal tract hemorrhage, a nasogastric tube should be in place for 24 hours to assist in identifying any rebleeding.

B. Stool: Record the frequency, color, and approximate amount of stool passed by the patient. In briskly bleeding patients, frequent defecation is the rule, since blood is an excellent cathartic. Continued frequent passage of bright red or melenic stools usually indicates persistent or recurrent bleeding and the need for continued monitoring and treatment (eg, further transfusions).

C. Hematocrit: Although they are not helpful in exsanguinating patients, frequent hematocrit checks are essential in patients with active gastrointestinal tract bleeding. Changes in the hematocrit will not occur until endogenous or exogenous fluids cause hemodilution. In patients with recent or active bleeding, the hematocrit must be checked at least every hour until there is no further decrease.

EMERGENCY TREATMENT OF SPECIFIC DISORDERS CAUSING UPPER GASTROINTESTINAL TRACT BLEEDING
(See Fig 8–1.)

Possible sites of upper gastrointestinal bleeding are shown in Table 8–2. An approach to identification of the site of hemorrhage in patients with upper gastrointestinal tract hemorrhage is shown in Fig 8–1. Endoscopy is the diagnostic procedure of choice in the patient with acute hemorrhage, whereas an upper gastrointestinal series is satisfactory for the patient who is not bleeding or who has stable, low-grade blood loss. Since emergency management does vary slightly depending upon the underlying cause, specific conditions are discussed below.

PEPTIC ULCER DISEASE; GASTRIC OR DUODENAL ULCERS

Peptic ulcer disease is responsible for almost half of all episodes of upper gastrointestinal tract bleeding (Table 8–2).

Diagnosis

The classic symptoms of peptic disease are epigastric distress and nocturnal pain promptly relieved by food or antacids. In many instances, patients have had dyspeptic complaints for years. However, ulcer pain may not be present prior to bleeding in up to 40% of patients bleeding from ulcers.

Clinical presentation varies according to the rapidity of bleeding.

(1) Acute: Sudden and massive bleeding, with shock on presentation.

(2) Chronic: Weakness, chronic anemia, and occult blood in stools due to slow blood loss may be the only findings, particularly among elderly patients with gastric ulcers.

Treatment

A. Provide emergency management as outlined on p 128.

B. Cimetidine (300 mg orally before meals and at bedtime) or sucralfate (1 g orally before meals and at bedtime) may be given to patients with gastric or duodenal ulcers. Three additional H_2 receptor antagonists are also available: ranitidine or nizatidine (150 mg twice daily) and famotidine (20 mg twice daily). These may be substituted for cimetidine. During the first few days in the hospital, continuous intravenous H_2 receptor antagonists may be used for ulcer patients (eg, cimetidine, 37.5 mg/hr).

C. Patients must be instructed not to smoke, since cigarette smoking is associated with high rates of failure for all peptic ulcer treatment programs. No special dietary restrictions are needed; however, alcohol and nonsteroidal anti-inflammatory drugs (including aspirin and phenylbutazone) should be avoided.

D. Recurrent or persistent hemorrhage requires evaluation for possible surgery.

Disposition

Patients with active bleeding should be hospitalized for observation and evaluation. Patients with normal hematocrits, normal vital signs, and bleeding that has stopped may be discharged with a prescription for one of the medications listed above and should be referred for further evaluation within 1 week.

GASTRITIS (Esophagitis or Duodenitis)

Gastritis has been recognized more frequently since the introduction of fiberoptic endoscopy in the diagnosis of acute upper gastrointestinal tract bleeding. Ingestion of large amounts of alcohol or of other injurious agents such as salicylates or other nonsteroidal anti-inflammatory agents is an important causative factor. Esophagitis or duodenitis may coexist or occur as isolated findings, with similar pathogenesis. The presence of esophagitis implies an incompetent lower esophageal sphincter with free gastroesophageal reflux.

Diagnosis

Gastritis is often asymptomatic. Some patients may experience anorexia, nausea, dyspepsia, and immediate postprandial emesis. There are no other distinguishing features. Endoscopy is the best diagnostic test, since upper gastrointestinal tract x-rays are insensitive. Occasionally, especially in patients with portal hypertension or coagulopathies, bleeding due to gastritis may be massive.

Treatment

A. Provide emergency management as outlined above.

B. Continue nasogastric suction until brisk bleeding has stopped. (Rarely, bleeding will not stop, in which case surgery must be considered.)

C. Give antacids hourly or every 2 hours to maintain a pH greater than 4.0. Sucralfate may be used in-

stead of antacids; give 1 g orally $\frac{1}{2}$–1 hour before meals and at bedtime.

D. Give cimetidine or another H_2 receptor antagonist as described above under ulcer disease.

E. For those patients requiring nonsteroidal anti-inflammatory drugs for severe arthritis, misoprostol (a prostaglandin cytoprotective agent), 200 μg, may be given twice a day.

Disposition

Patients with active bleeding (eg, continued appearance of fresh blood in nasogastric aspirate) should be hospitalized for treatment and observation. Surgery is rarely required to stop bleeding.

Patients with documented gastritis in whom bleeding is mild or has stopped and who have normal vital signs in the upright position and hematocrits of 30% or better may be treated with antacids and referred for outpatient follow-up (within 1–3 days).

MALLORY-WEISS SYNDROME

Tears of the gastroesophageal junction due to vigorous retching or emesis are responsible for about 10% of cases of acute upper gastrointestinal tract hemorrhage. Patients usually have one or more longitudinal tears 1–4 cm ($\frac{3}{8}$–$1\frac{1}{2}$ in) long in the mucosa near the gastroesophageal junction. The disruption extends through the mucosa into the submucosa but usually not into the muscularis.

Diagnosis

This disorder most commonly follows a bout of forceful retching and vomiting, although cases have been reported following closed chest compression, coughing, sneezing, or even straining at stool. Some cases have no identifiable predisposing factors.

Most patients are alcoholics.

Esophagogastroscopy is the only definitive diagnostic test.

Treatment

A. Provide emergency management as outlined above.

B. Gastric lavage with normal saline may help control the hemorrhage. Control forceful vomiting with antiemetics.

C. For patients with persistent bleeding not controlled by saline lavage, endoscopic coagulation, using a heater probe or multiple pole probe, endoscopic epinephrine injection, or angiographic embolization of the bleeding vessel may control the bleeding. If these procedures fail or are unavailable, surgery may be necessary.

Disposition

Hospitalize for observation, diagnosis, and treatment. Late rebleeding is unusual.

ESOPHAGEAL VARICES

Massive gastrointestinal tract bleeding secondary to esophageal or gastric varices carries a mortality rate of about 50%. The poor outcome is due to the poor general condition of many of these patients as well as to the severity of hemorrhage.

Diagnosis

Variceal hemorrhage does not occur unless significant portal hypertension *and* large-sized varices are present. In the USA, this usually is secondary to alcoholic cirrhosis. Elsewhere in the world, it may be due to other types of cirrhosis or portal hypertension resulting from parasitic infestations (eg, schistosomiasis).

Bleeding from varices cannot be diagnosed on clinical grounds alone even if previous endoscopy or upper gastrointestinal tract radiography has established the presence of varices, since alcoholic patients with varices have an increased incidence of peptic ulcer disease, gastritis, and Mallory-Weiss tears.

However, massive upper gastrointestinal tract hemorrhage in the patient with known or suspected cirrhosis is likely to be due to esophageal varices.

Treatment

A. Emergency Measures: Provide emergency management as outlined above.

B. Monitor Cardiovascular Status: Central venous pressure monitoring through a 16-gauge catheter is a useful measure of intravascular volume in most patients. A pulmonary artery line to measure pulmonary wedge pressure is also satisfactory.

C. Infuse Intravenous Fluids: Replace volume carefully to keep central pressures relatively low (central venous pressure ≤ 10 cm water and pulmonary capillary wedge pressure ≤ 8 mm Hg) while maintaining systolic blood pressure above 110 mm Hg. *Caution:* Overzealous hydration will elevate portal pressure and can exacerbate or cause a recurrence of variceal bleeding.

D. Give Vasopressin: Continuous peripheral intravenous vasopressin infusion (0.1–0.4 unit/min) may be started in an attempt to slow the hemorrhage. Cardiographic monitoring should be maintained while vasopressin is administered. *Caution: This drug must be given by a peripheral vein, not by central venous line or by Swan-Ganz line, since severe coronary vasospasm may result.* Vasopressin is contraindicated in patients with known coronary artery disease.

E. Perform Emergency Endoscopic Sclerotherapy: In patients with vigorous hemorrhage and known or suspected variceal hemorrhage, emergency endoscopy is strongly indicated both for diagnosis of variceal hemorrhage and for treatment with endoscopic variceal sclerosis (sclerotherapy). By directly injecting bleeding varices with various sclerosants, immediate control of hemorrhage is achieved in over 90% of patients.

F. Perform Balloon Tamponade: In rare instances (eg, in the exsanguinating patient), it may be necessary to insert the Sengstaken-Blakemore (SB) tube or one of its variations (eg, Minnesota tube) in the emergency department to control hemorrhage prior to endoscopic confirmation (Chapter 46). The patient must have airway protection by intubation prior to balloon tamponade in order to prevent massive aspiration.

Disposition

Once a balloon tamponade tube is inserted, the patient must be admitted to the intensive care unit for special monitoring and observation. The gastric balloon must not be deflated while the esophageal balloon is still inflated, since migration of the esophageal balloon can cause upper airway obstruction.

Active variceal bleeding not requiring balloon tamponade is also an indication for hospitalization in most cases.

Rarely, patients with advanced cirrhosis will have chronic low-grade gastrointestinal tract bleeding (occult blood in stools) with stable (but not necessarily normal) vital signs and hematocrit; these patients may be referred to their regular physician (within 1–3 days).

HEMOBILIA

Rarely, hepatic trauma (often several weeks before), hepatic tumors, gallstones, and parasites *(Ascaris)* may cause bleeding into the biliary tract (hemobilia) with resulting gastrointestinal tract hemorrhage.

Diagnosis

Hemobilia presents as gastrointestinal tract bleeding. Biliary colic and jaundice are usually present as well and may occupy most of the clinician's attention, since bleeding is often mild. Hepatic angiography is the diagnostic study of choice.

Treatment & Disposition

Hospitalize for evaluation. Embolization with autogenous clot or metal coils or infusion of Gelfoam into the site of bleeding during hepatic angiography can often be therapeutic. Support blood pressure with intravenous infusion of crystalloid solutions and whole blood as needed.

AORTIC ANEURYSM
(Aortoduodenal Fistula)
(See also Chapter 32.)

Diagnosis

Upper gastrointestinal tract bleeding in the presence of an abdominal aortic aneurysm (or graft) should be assumed to be secondary to aortoduodenal fistula until proved otherwise.

Upper gastrointestinal tract bleeding may be only moderate initially, but exsanguinating hemorrhage will occur eventually in most cases unless proper treatment is given. Inquire about previous abdominal vascular surgery, and palpate the abdomen carefully for an aneurysm. Neither endoscopy nor angiography can definitely exclude the diagnosis of aortic aneurysm, although both may be helpful in suggesting this condition. A cross-table lateral abdominal x-ray or abdominal ultrasound examination may help establish the presence and size of an aneurysm. Abdominal CT scans are the most useful for detecting disruption or infection of a graft or aneurysm.

Treatment

Treat for exsanguinating hemorrhage (p 130), and obtain emergency surgical consultation. Angiography should be done to confirm that the diagnosis of the patient's hemodynamic condition is stable.

Disposition

All patients with aortic aneurysm or aortic grafts and gastrointestinal tract bleeding must be hospitalized for careful evaluation.

EMERGENCY TREATMENT OF SPECIFIC DISORDERS CAUSING LOWER GASTROINTESTINAL TRACT BLEEDING
(See Fig 8–2.)

Extensive hemorrhaging from the colon in adults is usually caused by diverticular disease, angiodysplasia (vascular ectasias), or colitis (Table 8–3). Benign or malignant neoplasms and ischemic colitis rarely cause massive bleeding.

The site of bleeding in the colon can be identified in 90% of patients using the diagnostic schema shown in Fig 8–2. Massive bleeding originates in the right colon as often as in the left. Although diverticulosis is preponderantly left-sided, bleeding diverticula and vascular ectasias (angiodysplasias) are predominantly in the right colon.

Accurate identification of the bleeding site allows selective colonic resection if surgery becomes necessary.

Table 8–3. Cause of hematochezia in 72 hospitalized patients undergoing colonoscopy (and endoscopy if colonoscopy negative) at the San Francisco General Hospital.

Source of Hemorrhage	Percentage
Colonic cancer	7
Colonic polyps	11
Diverticula	23
Colitis	11
Vascular ectasia	1
Large hemorrhoids only	12
Ulcer/tear (rectum)	10
Upper gastorintestinal or small bowel source	10
No site identified	15
Total	100

DIVERTICULOSIS

Diagnosis

Diverticulosis is often asymptomatic. There may be a remote history of cramping, lower abdominal pain, and mild left lower quadrant tenderness. A history of alternating constipation and diarrhea also may be elicited.

Bleeding may be massive and usually occurs without any symptoms or signs of diverticulitis (eg, fever, left lower quadrant mass, or abdominal tenderness).

Treatment & Disposition

See above for general emergency management. Surgery must be considered in patients with massive bleeding. Localization of the bleeding site by technetium scintigraphy or angiography is needed. Hospitalize for observation, diagnosis, and, if indicated, surgery. Long-term treatment with dietary bulk and bulk additives (bran and bulk cathartics such as psyllium hydrophilic mucilloid) is appropriate.

ANGIODYSPLASIA
(Vascular Ectasias of Bowel)

Diagnosis

Angiodysplasia is characterized by painless bleeding, which may be mild to massive in amount (with signs ranging from occult blood in stools or iron deficiency anemia to brisk hematochezia). Many patients are elderly, with a history of cardiac disease (especially aortic stenosis) or renal disease.

When brisk hemorrhage is occurring, radionuclide scintigraphy (preferable) or angiography should be performed to identify the site of hemorrhage.

Colonoscopy in a patient in whom brisk bleeding is not occurring may show classic spider angioma–like lesions. These lesions are most common in the right colon but may be seen throughout the bowel. There are usually no accompanying skin or mucous membrane changes, in contrast to those seen in Osler-Weber-Rendu syndrome.

Treatment

A. Emergency Measures: General emergency measures are outlined above.

B. Medical Management: Brisk colonic hemorrhage may respond to peripheral intravenous vasopressin (0.1–0.4 units/min). In high-risk patients, selective arterial catheterization should be performed either for local infusion of vasopressin or for deliberate embolization to control hemorrhage. Most cases stop spontaneously.

C. Surgical Measures: If brisk bleeding continues despite medical measures, subtotal colectomy is indicated. Colonoscopic electrocoagulation or argon laser therapy is being used as an alternative to colectomy in many centers with excellent results.

Disposition

Hospitalize the patient for careful monitoring in the intensive care unit. Surgical and gastroenterologic consultation should be sought early.

HEMORRHOIDS

Diagnosis

Bleeding is usually the first symptom of internal hemorrhoids. There may be a history of straining on defecation, and the patient will present with frank hematochezia often mixed with well-formed, normal-appearing stools. Occasionally, recurrent bleeding can result in marked anemia. Exsanguinating hemorrhage is rare unless portal hypertension is present. The diagnosis should be confirmed by proctoscopy in the emergency department. Careful anoscopy must be done to fully visualize hemorrhoids. If a flexible fiberoptic sigmoidoscope is being used, retroflexion of the insertion tube (bending the section back to examine the rectum from above) is necessary to ensure good visualization of the anorectal junction.

Treatment

A. Medical Measures: Most early cases can be managed with high-roughage diet, local measures (sitz baths, suppositories for hemorrhoids [Anusol, many others]), and stool softeners (psyllium [Meta-

mucil, many others], dioctyl sodium sulfosuccinate [Colace, many others]).

B. Surgical Measures: Operation is required in occasional cases to arrest hemorrhage not controlled by medical measures.

Disposition

Hospitalize the patient for surgery to arrest persistent brisk bleeding. It is prudent to hospitalize patients with portal hypertension as well. Otherwise, refer the patient to an outpatient clinic for follow-up.

COLONIC POLYPS

Diagnosis

Painless rectal bleeding and discovery of a polyp on sigmoidoscopy, colonoscopy, or barium enema confirm the diagnosis of colonic polyposis.

Treatment

For significant bleeding, see p 128. If bleeding persists, the polyps should be removed immediately. If bleeding has stopped, the patient can be referred for elective colonoscopic polypectomy.

Disposition

Hospitalization is necessary if bleeding persists; otherwise, refer the patient for outpatient colonoscopic polypectomy.

COLITIS

Diagnosis

The chief findings are abdominal cramps, diarrheal stools containing blood and mucopurulent material, fever, weight loss, and anemia. On sigmoidoscopy, the rectal mucosa is eroded and friable. Infectious causes of colitis (particularly *Shigella, Campylobacter, Entamoeba histolytica,* and *Salmonella*) must be ruled out (Chapter 9).

Occasionally, particularly in elderly patients, ischemic colitis can present with brisk hematochezia. Differentiation from idiopathic or infectious colitis is often possible on sigmoidoscopy. Ischemic colitis rarely, if ever, involves the rectum, while other forms of colitis almost always involve the rectum.

Treatment

See above for emergency management of severe bleeding. Medical measures can usually control most symptoms in mild to moderate cases. Surgery is reserved for severe problems.

Disposition

Severe cases are medical emergencies requiring immediate hospitalization. Mild cases can be referred to the proper clinic for further evaluation and treatment after stool samples have been collected for evaluation for enteric pathogens.

CROHN'S DISEASE

Diagnosis

Frank blood is seen in about one-third of patients with Crohn's disease, but massive bleeding is unusual. Patients have abdominal pain and tenderness; diarrhea occurs but is rarely a prominent symptom. There may be fever and sepsis.

Fistula formation, fissures, and hemorrhoids are common. However, Crohn's disease may not involve the rectum or sigmoid. A normal proctosigmoidoscopic examination does not exclude Crohn's disease.

Treatment

The patient should be managed medically. Surgery is indicated only rarely, when massive bleeding is not controlled by medical measures. Amebic disease must be excluded before corticosteroids are used.

Disposition

Patients with severe bleeding or systemic symptoms (eg, fever, weight loss) must be hospitalized for observation and treatment. Patients with mild Crohn's disease can be referred for outpatient follow-up.

SOLITARY RECTAL ULCER

Diagnosis

Rectal ulcer is an unusual lesion associated with rectal prolapse. It may result from straining at stool. The patient passes blood and mucus per rectum. Many patients are elderly with chronic constipation.

Treatment & Disposition

General measures to aid defecation should be offered (eg, hydration, stool softeners). Surgery should be avoided. Refer the patient to the appropriate clinic for evaluation and follow-up.

MECKEL'S DIVERTICULUM

Diagnosis

About 25% of patients with Meckel's diverticulum become symptomatic, and 25% of these have lower gastrointestinal tract bleeding. This disorder usually occurs before age 2 years and rarely after age 10. Symptoms may mimic acute appendicitis. Meckel's diverticulum may be diagnosed by technetium pertechnetate scintigraphy or angiography.

Treatment & Disposition

Hospitalize all patients for observation, since surgery may be required for severe bleeding.

REFERENCES

Allison DJ, Hemingway AP, Cunningham DA: Angiography in gastrointestinal bleeding. Lancet 1982;2:30.

Athanasoulis CA: Therapeutic applications of angiography. (2 parts.) N Engl J Med 1980;302:1117, 1174.

Cello JP: Gastrointestinal hemorrhage. In: Wyngaarden JB, Smith LH, and Bennett JC (editors): *Cecil Textbook of Medicine,* 19th ed. Saunders, 1992.

Cello JP, Thoeni RF: Gastrointestinal hemorrhage: Comparative values of double-contrast upper gastrointestinal radiology and endoscopy. JAMA 1980;243:685.

Cello JP et al: Management of the patient with hemorrhagic esophageal varices. JAMA 1986;256:1480.

Fleischer D: Etiology and prevalence of severe persistent upper gastrointestinal bleeding. Gastroenterology 1983; 84:538.

Jensen DM, Machicado GA: Diagnosis and treatment of severe hematochezia: The role of urgent colonoscopy after purge. Gastroenterology 1988;95:1569.

Laine L: Multipolar electrocoagulation in the treatment of

active upper gastrointestinal tract hemorrhage: A prospective controlled trial. N Engl J Med 1987;316: 1613.

Markisz JA et al: An evaluation of 99mm Tc-labelled red blood cell scintigraphy for the detection and localization of gastrointestinal bleeding sites. Gastroenterology 1982;83:394.

Rex DK et al: Flexible sigmoidoscopy plus air contrast barium enema versus colonoscopy for suspected lower gastrointestinal bleeding. Gastroenterology 1990;98:855.

Storey DW et al: Endoscopic prediction of recurrent bleeding in peptic ulcers. N Engl J Med 1981;305:915.

Tedesco FJ et al: Colonoscopic evaluation of rectal bleeding: A study of 304 patients. Ann Intern Med 1978;89: 907.

Tedesco FJ et al: Role of colonoscopy in patients with unexplained melena: Analysis of 53 patients. Gastrointest Endosc 1981;27:221.

Diarrhea & Vomiting

9

John Mills, MD

IMMEDIATE MANAGEMENT OF LIFE-THREATENING PROBLEMS
(See algorithm.)

HYPOTENSION OR SHOCK

Diagnosis

Obtain vital signs, and look for signs of shock (cool, pale skin; abnormal mentation, etc) (Chapter 3). Hypotension (systolic pressure < 90 mm Hg) seen in the recumbent position or when upright posture is assumed indicates significant hypovolemia.

Treatment

Insert a large-bore intravenous catheter (≥ 16-gauge), and draw blood for CBC, electrolyte determinations, renal function tests, serum amylase and—if blood loss is suspected—typing and cross-matching. Begin intravenous fluid replacement with crystalloid solution, 200–1000 mL/h (the rate depending on the severity of dehydration, patient's size, and cardiac and renal status) until hypotension is corrected. Replacement therapy should be guided by the results of serum electrolyte determinations as soon as they are available (Chapters 3 and 36).

Disposition

Hospitalize the patient for observation and supportive treatment.

NEUROLOGIC ABNORMALITIES

Diagnosis

Botulism or neurotoxic seafood poisoning produces mild gastrointestinal symptoms with neurologic symptoms, eg, paresthesias, weakness, or diplopia. Because weakness may result in fatal respiratory insufficiency, rapid recognition and treatment of these disorders are required.

Treatment & Disposition

Maintain airway and ventilation. Obtain arterial blood gas samples to determine adequacy of respiratory exchange. Further evaluation and treatment are discussed in Chapter 12.

Hospitalization is required if neurologic signs are present.

PERITONEAL INFLAMMATION

Diagnosis

Search for the conditions listed in Table 9–1 which cause peritoneal inflammation in association with vomiting or diarrhea and which may mimic gastroenteritis.

Suspect abdominal or pelvic disease in the presence of the following: focal abdominal tenderness or peritoneal signs; continuous pain that is localized or precedes the vomiting or diarrhea; or protracted vomiting with nonspecific abdominal pain, as seen in partial small bowel obstruction. If obstruction is a possibility, include an upright or left lateral decubitus abdominal x-ray in evaluation.

Table 9–1. Conditions that may cause peritoneal inflammation ("surgical abdomen") in association with vomiting or diarrhea.

Pancreatitis
Cholecystitis
Appendicitis
Diverticulitis
Hepatitis
Peptic ulcer disease
Salpingitis (pelvic inflammatory disease)
Pyelonephritis
Generalized peritonitis
Intestinal obstruction (including intussusception)

Treatment & Disposition

Obtain complete vital signs, and examine the patient for shock and postural hypotension. Give nothing by mouth. Insert an intravenous catheter (≥ 16-gauge), and draw blood for CBC, electrolyte determinations, renal and liver function tests, and serum amylase. Reserve one tube of clotted blood for possible typing and cross-matching. Start intravenous infusion of crystalloid solution to restore or maintain intravascular volume. Insert a nasogastric tube, and connect it to intermittent suction. See Chapter 7 for evaluation of the acute abdomen.

Hospitalization for observation is indicated if there are objective signs of peritoneal inflammation. Obtain early surgical consultation.

OTHER ACUTE ABDOMINAL EMERGENCIES

1. ISCHEMIC COLITIS

Diagnosis

Ischemic colitis may present with abdominal pain and diarrhea. Although abdominal pain and tenderness are present, peritoneal signs are usually absent. Diarrhea contains occult or gross blood and leukocytes. Ischemic colitis should be suspected in older patients with other evidence of atherosclerosis or low cardiac output states. Although ischemic colitis is not as catastrophic as acute mesenteric ischemia, these patients may progress to sepsis or perforation.

Treatment & Disposition

Obtain complete vital signs, and treat shock and postural hypotension with intravenous crystalloid solution, being careful not to overload if congestive heart failure is present. Draw blood for CBC electrolyte determinations, renal and liver function tests, and serum amylase, and reserve one tube for possible blood typing and cross-matching.

Hospitalize the patient for observation, and obtain early surgical consultation.

2. INTUSSUSCEPTION

Diagnosis

Intussusception occurs mainly in infants and is characterized by abdominal pain, vomiting, and bloody diarrhea, which often has a "currant jelly" appearance. The abdomen is typically tender and may be distended; in some cases, a sausage-shaped mass can be palpated on the right. The blood leukocyte count is usually elevated, and abdominal x-rays (lateral decubitus view) show signs of obstruction.

Treatment & Disposition

See Treatment & Disposition under Peritoneal Inflammation, above. Obtain pediatric surgical consultation as soon as possible. Barium enema is diagnostic and may spontaneously reduce the intussusception.

See also Chapter 42.

FURTHER MANAGEMENT OF VOMITING & DIARRHEA

Once-life-threatening conditions have been treated and improvement is established, proceed with efforts to make a specific diagnosis, and begin further supportive and specific therapy as outlined below.

Diagnosis
(See Table 9–2.)

A. History:

1. Toxic substances–Evaluation should focus on toxic substances as a likely cause of illness if there is a history of exposure to or ingestion of antimicrobials, nonabsorbable sugars (eg, mannitol, sorbitol), wild mushrooms, drugs, heavy metals, or radiation.

2. Food poisoning–If symptoms suggest food poisoning, obtain a history of foods consumed during the preceding 24 hours. Particularly suspect are seafoods or foods containing protein that have been cooked and stored (chicken or potato salads, stews, meat pies, filled pastries, custards, etc). "Poisoned" foods rarely have a bad odor or taste.

3. Travel or residence in developing countries–A history of recent travel or residence in developing countries suggests that diarrhea may be due to infectious agents. Although enteric infection may be acquired anywhere (eg, within the USA), the risk is greater in developing nations.

4. Antibiotic use–Recent antibiotic use increases the likelihood of diarrhea due to *Clostridium difficile.*

5. Sexual transmission–Amebiasis, giardiasis, campylobacteriosis, salmonellosis, and shigellosis

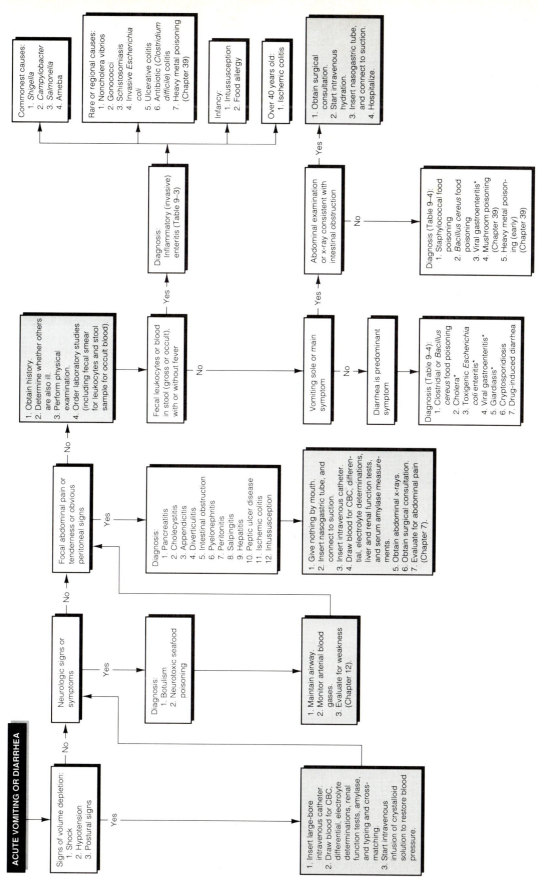

ACUTE VOMITING OR DIARRHEA

Signs of volume depletion:
1. Shock
2. Hypotension
3. Postural signs

— Yes →
1. Insert large-bore intravenous catheter.
2. Draw blood for CBC, differential, electrolyte determinations, renal function tests, amylase, and typing and cross-matching.
3. Start intravenous infusion of crystalloid solution to restore blood pressure.

— No →

Neurologic signs or symptoms

— Yes →

Diagnosis:
1. Botulism
2. Neurotoxic seafood poisoning

→
1. Maintain airway.
2. Monitor arterial blood gases.
3. Evaluate for weakness (Chapter 12).

— No →

Focal abdominal pain or tenderness or obvious peritoneal signs

— Yes →

Diagnosis:
1. Pancreatitis
2. Cholecystitis
3. Appendicitis
4. Diverticulitis
5. Intestinal obstruction
6. Pyelonephritis
7. Peritonitis
8. Salpingitis
9. Hepatitis
10. Peptic ulcer disease
11. Ischemic colitis
12. Intussusception

→
1. Give nothing by mouth.
2. Insert nasogastric tube, and connect to suction.
3. Insert intravenous catheter.
4. Draw blood for CBC, differential, electrolyte determinations, liver and renal function tests, and serum amylase measurements.
5. Obtain abdominal x-rays.
6. Obtain surgical consultation.
7. Evaluate for abdominal pain (Chapter 7).

— No →

1. Obtain history.
2. Determine whether others are also ill.
3. Perform physical examination.
4. Order laboratory studies (including fecal smear for leukocytes and stool sample for occult blood).

→

Fecal leukocytes or blood in stool (gross or occult), with or without fever

— Yes →

Diagnosis: Inflammatory (invasive) enteritis (Table 9–3)

→

Commonest causes:
1. *Shigella*
2. *Campylobacter*
3. *Salmonella*
4. Ameba

Rare or regional causes:
1. Noncholera vibrios
2. Gonococci
3. Schistosomiasis
4. Invasive *Escherichia coli*
5. Ulcerative colitis
6. Antibiotic (*Clostridium difficile*) colitis
7. Heavy metal poisoning (Chapter 39)

Infancy:
1. Intussusception
2. Food allergy

Over 40 years old:
1. Ischemic colitis

— No →

Vomiting sole or main symptom

— Yes →

Abdominal examination or x-ray consistent with intestinal obstruction

— Yes →
1. Obtain surgical consultation.
2. Start intravenous hydration.
3. Insert nasogastric tube, and connect to suction.
4. Hospitalize.

— No →

Diagnosis (Table 9–4):
1. Staphylococcal food poisoning
2. *Bacillus cereus* food poisoning
3. Viral gastroenteritis*
4. Mushroom poisoning (Chapter 39)
5. Heavy metal poisoning (early) (Chapter 39)

— No →

Diarrhea is predominant symptom

→

Diagnosis (Table 9–4):
1. Clostridial or *Bacillus cereus* food poisoning
2. Cholera*
3. Toxigenic *Escherichia coli* enteritis*
4. Viral gastroenteritis*
5. Giardiasis*
6. Cryptosporidiosis
7. Drug-induced diarrhea

*Patient may be febrile.

143

Table 9–2. Evaluation of acute gastroenteritis.

History
    Ingestion of wild mushrooms, seafood, drugs, heavy metals,
        nonabsorbable sugars (eg, mannitol), antimicrobials
    Radiation therapy
    Travel
    Current or recent antibiotic use
    Present illness: time of onset, initial symptoms, other symp-
        toms (sore throat, coryza, fever, chills, vomiting, abdom-
        inal pain, diarrhea)
    Illness among acquaintances
    Food history for preceding 24 hours if food poisoning is
        suspected
Physical examination
    General appearance
    Temperature
    Blood pressure and pulse: lying and standing or sitting
    Weight
    Abdominal examination
    Rectal examination
Laboratory tests and other procedures
    Usually required:
        Stool for gross or occult blood
        Stool microscopy (after staining)
        Stool culture for *Shigella, Salmonella,* and *Campylobacter*
    Occasionally required:
        Stool for ova and parasites (including *Cryptosporidium*)
        Stool culture for *Neisseria, Vibrio,* herpes simplex virus
        Stool for culture and toxin testing for *Clostridium difficile*
        CBC and differential
        Blood cultures
        Abdominal x-rays
        Sigmoidoscopy
        Abdominal ultrasound
    Rarely required:
        Amebic serology
        Duodenal aspirate or biopsy (for *Giardia*)
        Toxicology screen
        Barium enema

are common among homosexual males and may be transmitted by heterosexual contact as well. If receptive rectal intercourse has occurred, ask about symptoms of proctitis (constipation, anorectal pain, tenesmus and anorectal discharge), and consider *Chlamydia trachomatis,* herpes simplex, and *Neisseria gonorrhoeae* as possible causative agents. Watery diarrhea in homosexually active men may also be due to *Cryptosporidium,* cytomegalovirus, and *Mycobacterium avium-intracellulare.*

6. Features of the present illness–See Tables 9–3 and 9–4 for differential diagnostic features of common types of acute gastroenteritis. Important features of the present illness include time of onset, nature of symptoms (both initially and later), and duration of illness. Inquire about vomiting, abdominal pain, and diarrhea; note the character of vomitus (bloody or bilious) and stool (color, odor, and presence of blood or mucus). Confirm the presence of fever, chills, sore throat, and coryza. Note any genitourinary and gynecologic symptoms.

7. Similar illness in others–If others have been sick with a similar illness, the incubation period and

clinical features of the illness can be better defined, and a vector (food or water) may be identified.

B. Physical Examination: Physical examination is needed mainly to rule out "surgical abdomen" and to determine the need for hospitalization.

1. General appearance–The patient may appear "toxic" or severely ill, suggesting the need for hospitalization.

2. Fever–Invasive bacterial and parasitic infections of the intestinal tract almost always cause fever, which is often accompanied by rigors. Viral gastroenteritis is accompanied by fever in about half of cases, but the patient's temperature rarely exceeds 38.8 °C (101.8 °F). The presence of fever virtually rules out chemicals or toxins (eg, food poisoning) as the cause of illness.

3. Blood pressure and pulse rate–If the patient is not obviously dehydrated or hypotensive or in shock, take a blood pressure reading with the patient supine, sitting, and standing to detect more subtle degrees of volume depletion (systolic pressure drop ≥ 10 mm Hg and pulse rise ≥ 15 beats/min).

4. Weight–Weigh the patient so that subsequent changes in hydration can be documented (imperative in infants and children).

5. Abdominal examination–Significant abdominal tenderness is rare in enteritis, although subjective crampy pain is common. If abdominal examination elicits pain and especially if the pain is localized or peritoneal signs are found, seek surgical consultation after appropriate laboratory studies (see below).

6. Rectal examination–Perform rectal examination to detect fecal impaction, melena, or hematochezia. Anoscopy may be helpful to detect proctitis. In homosexually active men, proctitis may be due to *Chlamydia,* gonococcus, or herpes simplex.

C. Laboratory Studies:

1. Usually required–The following laboratory studies are usually required:

a. Stool sample–Obtain stool to check for gross or occult blood.

b. Stool smear–In patients with acute diarrhea, microscopic examination of a stool smear stained with Gram's stain or methylene blue for cells is the most helpful initial laboratory procedure (Table 9–5).

(1) PMNs–Patients with invasive infectious dysentery or ulcerative colitis (acute inflammatory bowel disease) usually demonstrate abundant PMNs in the stool smear. Amebiasis is an important exception; patients with amebiasis have erythrocytes in the stool but only a few PMNs. Fecal leukocytes may also occur in patients with pseudomembranous (antibiotic-associated) colitis, ischemic colitis, and diverticulitis. Erythrocytes are usually found in these conditions also. Patients with *Campylobacter* dysentery may have recognizable organisms on Gram-stained stool smear ("gull wing" appearance of

Table 9–3. Differential diagnostic features of common types of dysentery.[1]

	Mode of Transmission	Clinical Features						Definitive Diagnostic Procedures	Comments	Specific Treatment (in Addition to Supportive Measures)
		Incubation Period	Onset	Nausea and Vomiting	Abdominal Pain or Cramps	Diarrhea	Other			
Heavy metal poisoning	Variable—often food.	1–2 hours.	Abrupt.	+	+	+	Hepatic and renal failure; central nervous system signs.	Toxicology: blood, urine, tissue.	May be accidental or deliberate.	Chelating agents (Chapter 39).
Shigellosis	Water. Contact.[2]	1–7 days.	Abrupt.	Occasionally.	+	+	Fever, rigors common; seizures or coma, especially in children. Odorless stool with blood.	Culture of stool or rectal mucosal swab for enteric pathogens.	Symptomatic disease seen primarily in children; colonic infection.	Trimethoprim-sulfamethoxazole, 5 mg trimethoprim/kg/d orally (2 divided doses) for 5 days; or ciprofloxacin, 500 mg twice a day (adult dose) for 3–5 days.
Campylobacter dysentery	Contact. Animals. Water.	? 1–2 days.	Variable; often abrupt.	Occasionally.	+	+	Illness similar to shigellosis.	Stool culture—must specifically request *Campylobacter* culture.	As common as shigellosis.	Ciprofloxacin, 500 mg twice a day (adult dose) for 5–7 days.
Salmonella gastroenteritis	Water. Foods. Contact.[2] Animals.	12–72 hours.	Variable.	Occasionally.	±	+	Foul-smelling, pea soup stools, rarely bloody; fever common, rigors rare.	Routine stool culture.	Most strains are non-human-adapted (ie, primarily animal-associated); small bowel infection.	Antimicrobials prolong disease and secretion of salmonellae and are contraindicated, unless bacteremia is suspected.
Invasive *Escherichia coli*	Water. ? Other.	12–72 hours.	Abrupt.	Occasionally.	+	+	Similar to shigellosis, but milder.	None currently available for clinical use; bioassay for invasiveness.	Exact prevalence not yet defined; colonic infection.	None proved. Try trimethoprim-sulfamethoxazole as for shigellosis.
Amebiasis	Water. Contact.[2]	1–8 weeks.	Usually gradual.	Rare.	+	+	Bloody stool with little pus; fever, tenesmus uncommon.	Stool microscopy for amebas; stool for ova and parasites.	Illness usually associated with travel or living in developing countries; colonic infection.	Metronidazole, 750 mg 3 times a day for 5–10 days; or tetracycline, 250 mg orally 4 times a day for 10 days. See text.
Vibrio parahaemolyticus	Shellfish. ? Water.	8–30 hours.	Abrupt.	Occasionally.	+	+	Diarrhea, occasionally bloody; can mimic shigellosis.	Stool culture—must specifically request culture for vibrios.	Rare in USA; common in Japan.	None proved. Try tetracycline, 250 mg orally 4 times a day for 7 days.
Gonococcal proctocolitis	Sexual contact.	?	Variable.	Rare.	+	+	Variable.	Gram's stain and culture of stool (special media).	Rare; usually associated with rectal intercourse.	See Chapter 34.
Idiopathic inflammatory bowel disease (colitis)	Not applicable.	Not applicable.	Variable.	Rare.	+	+	Fever, bloody stools common; may have arthritis, skin lesions.	Sigmoidoscopy; barium enema; diagnosis of exclusion.	Relatively rare; patient usually is known to have colitis or has had recurrent diarrhea in past.	Hospitalize. Intravenous ampicillin, 150 mg/kg/d in 6 divided doses.
Antibiotic-associated (*Clostridium difficile*) colitis	Not applicable.	Not applicable.	Variable.	Rare.	+	+	Fever, fecal leukocytes common; blood occasionally.	Sigmoidoscopy; stool specimen of *Clostridium difficile* toxin assay.	Associated with administration of antimicrobials in most cases.	Vancomycin, 125 mg orally 4 times a day for 10 days; or metronidazole, 500 mg orally 3 times a day for 100 days.
Ischemic colitis	Not applicable.	Not applicable.	Variable.	Occasionally.	+	+	Variable.	Barium enema and angiography.	Patients usually > 40 years; vascular disease elsewhere.	Hospitalize for diagnosis and possible surgery.

[1] Dysentery: Diarrheal disease associated with evidence of mucosal destruction, eg, fecal blood or leukocytes, fever.
[2] Contact: direct human-human, or human-animal transmission.

145

Table 9–4. Differential diagnostic features of common types of nondysenteric gastroenteritis.

	Mode of Transmission	Incubation Period	Onset	Clinical Features: Nausea and Vomiting	Abdominal Pain or Cramps	Diarrhea	Other	Definitive Diagnostic Procedures	Comments	Specific Treatment (in Addition to Supportive Measures)
Staphylococcal food poisoning	Prepared protein-containing foods.	1–6 hours.	Abrupt.	+	+	±	Afebrile.	Gram's stain and culture of food and stomach contents (notify Health Dept.).	Common; protein toxin produced in food only, not in patient. Infected food handler is source.	Antiemetics are of limited value.
Clostridial food poisoning	Cooked meats.	8–24 hours.	Abrupt.	Occasionally.	+	+	Afebrile.	Gram's stain and culture of food and stool (notify Health Dept.).	Common; protein toxin produced both in food and in patient.	None.
Bacillus cereus food poisoning	Food (especially fried rice).	1–6 hours.	Abrupt.	+	+	Occasionally.	Usually afebrile.	Culture of food (notify Health Dept.).	Exact incidence uncertain.	None.
Scombroid fish poisoning	Scombroid fish (tuna, mackerel, etc).	1–2 hours.	Abrupt.	+	+	+	Afebrile. Skin rash and pruritus common.	Culture of fish for *Proteus* or assay for amines (notify Health Dept.).	Exact incidence uncertain.	Antihistamines (eg, diphenhydramine, 25–50 mg intravenously or intramuscularly) may alleviate symptoms.
Neurotoxic seafood poisoning	Various fish and shellfish.	1–8 hours.	Abrupt.	+	+	Occasionally.	Afebrile; paresthesias or paralysis may be dominant symptoms.	Bioassay of seafood (notify Health Dept.).	Probably rare, but small epidemics do occur.	May require ventilatory support as well; hospitalization mandatory.
Botulism	Canned food.	12–36 hours.	Abrupt.	+	+	+	Gastroenteritis is followed by paralytic symptoms.	Bioassay of serum and food (notify Health Dept.).	Very rare; gastroenteritis may be very mild.	Support ventilation; hospitalization mandatory. See Chapter 12.
Toxigenic *Escherichia coli* diarrhea	Water. ? Contact.	12–72 hours.	Usually abrupt.	+	+	+	Infants may be febrile; adult "turista" usually afebrile.	Serotyping of fecal *E coli* (unreliable); bioassay for toxin production (notify Health Dept.).	Common cause of gastroenteritis in adults, acquired while traveling ("turista").	Trimethoprim-sulfamethoxazole, 5 mg trimethoprim/kg/d (2 divided doses) orally for 5 days.
Cholera	Water. Contact.	12–72 hours.	Abrupt.	+	+	+	Fever common. Death from dehydration in 4–12 hours if untreated.	Gram's stain and culture of stool (special media or laboratory notification required in USA).	Not acquired in USA (except Gulf Coast).	Tetracycline, 250 mg orally 4 times a day for 3–5 days, or trimethoprim-sulfamethoxazole as for toxigenic *E coli.*
Giardiasis	Water. Contact.	1–4 weeks.	Variable.	+	+	+	Stools may be malabsorptive; often chronic; fever occasionally.	Stool for parasites; duodenal aspiration or biopsy. Therapeutic trial with quinacrine.	Patients with IgA deficiency more susceptible.	Metronidazole, 500 mg orally 3 times a day for 7–10 days. Alternative is quinacrine, 100 mg orally 3 times a day for 7 days.
Viral gastroenteritis	Contact. ? Water.	12–48 hours.	Abrupt.	+	+	+	Low-grade fever, malaise; blood in stool (rare).	Immunoassay of stool for rotaviruses. None available for other causative organisms.	Common; occasional epidemics, especially in infants and small children.	None.

Table 9–5. Evaluation of stained stool smears in patients with diarrheal disease.[1]

Predominant Cell Type	Implication and Diagnosis
PMN	Bacterial dysentery (eg, shigellosis) Idiopathic ulcerative colitis Antibiotic-associated colitis Diverticulitis (occasionally) Ischemic colitis (occasionally)
Mononuclear leukocyte	Viral gastroenteritis (occasionally) Allergic gastroenteritis (occasionally) Typhoid fever Giardiasis (occasionally)
No Inflammatory cells (may have epithelial cells)	Food poisoning Toxigenic diarrhea (eg, cholera) Viral and parasitic gastroenteritis

[1] Stained with methylene blue or Gram's stain.

Campylobacter jejuni), and a darkfield examination of a fecal wet preparation may show the characteristic morphology and motility of these bacteria.

(2) Mononuclear leukocytes–Mononuclear inflammatory cells may be seen with typhoidal (bacteremic) *Salmonella* infections and occasionally with viral and parasitic infections.

(3) Lack of leukocytes–Patients with food poisoning or toxigenic bacterial diarrhea do not have fecal leukocytes, because intestinal inflammation is absent. Despite an inflammatory response in the intestinal mucosa, patients with viral or parasitic infections usually do not have inflammatory cells in the stool.

2. Occasionally required–The following laboratory studies are occasionally required:

a. Stool culture–Stool culture should be performed for all patients with moderate or severe diarrheal disease who have fecal leukocytes or blood in the stool. Either fresh stool or a rectal swab may be submitted for culture. A rectal mucosal swab that avoids gross fecal contamination is the best way of obtaining material for culture of gonococci and probably also of *Shigella* and *Campylobacter.* A stool culture for "enteric pathogens" in most North American laboratories will detect *Salmonella, Shigella, C jejuni,* and staphylococci. *N gonorrhoeae, Vibrio,* and *C difficile* are not detected by routine culture in most laboratories, and such tests must be specially requested.

b. Stool for ova and parasites–If parasitic infection is suspected, fresh stool should be examined for ova and parasites. (Most acute diarrheas do not require ova and parasite examination.) Stool preserved with polyvinyl alcohol may be used if fresh stool cannot be obtained.

c. Stool for detection of *C difficile*–Stool for detection of *C difficile* toxin in addition to culture should be obtained in patients with suspected antibiotic-associated colitis.

d. Blood cultures–Blood cultures should be obtained if the patient has fever or rigors, but cultures are seldom positive.

e. Electrolyte determinations–Electrolyte determinations and tests of renal function should be obtained in patients with severe or protracted diarrhea or vomiting, especially if signs of intravascular volume depletion are present, or in elderly individuals, especially those taking digoxin.

f. CBC–White blood cell count and differential may be helpful in detecting gastrointestinal disease requiring surgery (eg, appendicitis, diverticulitis).

3. Rarely required–The following laboratory studies are rarely required: duodenal aspiration or biopsy for *Giardia lamblia,* toxicologic studies, barium enema, and rectal culture for herpes simplex virus or *Chlamydia trachomatis.*

D. Other Diagnostic Procedures: X-rays of the abdomen should be obtained if "surgical abdomen" is suspected. Abdominal ultrasound may be useful for diagnosing gallstones and pancreatic pseudocysts. Sigmoidoscopy is seldom warranted during initial evaluation but may be helpful if unexplained bloody diarrhea persists. Initial sigmoidoscopy may be indicated if gonococcal proctitis or ulcerative, pseudomembranous, or ischemic colitis is suspected.

E. Diagnostic Tests for AIDS-Related Diarrhea: Tests that should be obtained initially in AIDS patients who have diarrhea include stool culture for enteric pathogens, gonococcus, and *Campylobacter;* stool ova and parasite examination on 3 separate days; stool stain for protozoa; and 2 blood cultures. If results of these tests are nondiagnostic and the patient continues to have diarrhea despite symptomatic treatment, consider repeating the above tests and obtain esophagogastroduodenoscopy with biopsy and colonoscopy with biopsy.

F. Differentiation of Dysenteric and Nondysenteric Illness:

1. Dysenteric–The presence of either blood or leukocytes in the feces is evidence of mucosal inflammation or destruction and signifies dysenteric diarrheal illness. Fever is a helpful confirmatory sign. Clinical features of the common causes of dysentery are shown in Table 9–3.

2. Nondysenteric–Nondysenteric illnesses have neither leukocytes nor blood in the feces. Clinical features of the common causes of nondysenteric gastroenteritis are shown in Table 9–4.

Treatment

A. Replacement of Fluid and Electrolytes: Replacing lost fluid and electrolytes is the most important therapeutic measure in acute vomiting or diarrhea. In many cases, this is the only treatment required. Adequacy of replacement can be monitored by postural blood pressure and pulse measurements and serial body weights supplemented by measurements of urine output, serum electrolytes, and hematocrit.

1. Intravenous replacement–Fluids and electrolytes should be replaced intravenously in severely dehydrated patients, in those with hypovolemic shock, and in those with severe vomiting. Replacement of electrolyte and water loss should be guided by laboratory tests, but the intravenous fluid replacement solution recommended by WHO (Table 9–6) may be used satisfactorily until the results of serum electrolyte determinations are available.

2. Oral replacement–Since intestinal absorption is normal in most types of acute diarrheal disease, oral replacement is satisfactory if the patient is not vomiting and is not profoundly dehydrated. Sugar (glucose or fructose) should be included with the electrolyte solutions to provide calories and enhance absorption (Tables 9–6 and 9–7).

a. Mild diarrhea–Fruit juices, bouillon, and decarbonated cola beverages are satisfactory for mild cases of diarrhea (Table 9–7).

Table 9–6. Solutions for fluid replacement in diarrheal disease.[1]

Formula for fluid replacement solution.

Ingredient	Concentration (meq/l water)
Na^+	90–100
K^-	10–25
Cl^-	70–80
HCO_3^-	25–40
Glucose[2]	120 (mmol/L)
Citrate (optional)	20

For oral use, a rehydration solution may be conveniently made up by dissolving the following in 1 L of boiled water.

Ingredient	Metric Amount	Approximate Household Amount
NaCl (table salt)[3]	3.5 g	¾ tsp
NaHCO₃ (baking soda)	2.5 g	½ tsp
KCl	1.5 g	
or		
Potassium bitartrate (cream of tartar)		4 tsp
Glucose	20 g	
or		
Sucrose	40 g	
or		
Corn syrup		1 tbsp

[1] Modified and reproduced, with permission, from Sack RB et al: The use of oral replacement solution in the treatment of cholera. *Bull WHO* 1970;**43**:351.

[2] Sucrose, 240 mmol/L may be substituted for glucose.

[3] Lower sodium concentrations can be used safely in mildly ill patients and may be preferred in children.

Table 9–7. Electrolyte content (in meq/L) of commonly used replacement solutions for diarrhea.

	Na^+	K^+	Cl^-
Gatorade	22	2.5	. . .
Coca-Cola	0.4	13	. . .
Ginger ale	3	0.2	. . .
Pedialyte	30	20	30

b. Severe diarrhea–The solution recommended by WHO for oral use may be utilized in conjunction with measurement of serum electrolytes (Table 9–6).

B. Antiemetics: Vomiting may be treated with atropinic drugs, antihistamines, or phenothiazines.

1. Prochlorperazine–Prochlorperazine (Compazine), administered as a suppository, 5 mg 3 times a day in older children or 25 mg twice daily in adults; or by injection, 5–10 mg intramuscularly every 3–4 hours, appears most effective, although it also has the highest frequency of side effects. Dystonic reactions may occur.

2. Hydroxyzine pamoate–Hydroxyzine pamoate (Vistaril, many others), 25–50 mg intramuscularly every 4–6 hours for adults, may be effective.

3. Promethazine–Promethazine (Phenergan, many others), 12.5–25 mg (for adults) by suppository or intramuscular injection every 4–6 hours, may be effective.

C. Abdominal Cramps: Anticholinergic-antispasmodic drugs (eg, Donnatal, which contains scopolamine, atropine, hyoscyamine, and phenobarbital) may also be useful for relief of abdominal cramps. However, abdominal disorders other than hypermotility must be excluded. Opiates are also effective (see below).

D. Diarrhea: Treat diarrhea with bismuth compounds, loperamide, or opiate constipating agents such as diphenoxylate with atropine (Lomotil, many others).

1. Bismuth subsalicylate suspension–Bismuth subsalicylate suspension (Pepto-Bismol, many others), 2–4 tbsp every 30 minutes in adults until diarrhea resolves or an 8-oz bottle has been consumed, has been effective in various diarrheal illnesses. The exact mechanism of action is unknown but may involve binding of bacterial toxins by the bismuth as well as topical anti-inflammatory activity of the salicylate. It should not be used by persons allergic to or otherwise intolerant of aspirin.

2. Loperamide–Loperamide (Imodium), 2–4 mg orally after each unformed stool in adults (1–2 mg 3 times daily in children), may be effective. Daily dose should not exceed 16 mg. Loperamide is now available without a prescription.

3. Opiates–*Caution:* Although opiates are quite effective for relieving cramps and diarrhea, these drugs may prolong systemic symptoms or actually induce bacteremia in patients with salmonellosis or shigellosis. In patients with ulcerative or antibiotic-associated colitis, opiates may precipitate toxic megacolon. Therefore, use opiates only in patients with mild diarrheal disease without evidence of dysentery who are in situations (eg, traveling) where the presence of diarrhea itself may be incapacitating.

a. Diphenoxylate with atropine (Lomotil, many others)–Give one tablet after each loose stool but no more than 10–12 in 24 hours for adults.

b. Codeine–Codeine may be useful if diphenoxylate with atropine is unavailable. Give 30 mg orally every 4 hours as needed.

4. Kaolin-pectin suspension–Kaolin-pectin suspension (Kaopectate, many others) has not been helpful in clinical experiences with adults.

Specific Chemotherapy
(See also Tables 9–3 and 9–4.)

A. Bacterial Dysentery: If stool is negative for amebas on initial examination or if illness occurs in a setting where amebic dysentery is unlikely, common causes of bacterial dysentery that must be considered are *Shigella, Campylobacter,* invasive *Escherichia coli,* and *Salmonella.* Many cases of bacterial dysentery are self-limited and require no antibiotics. Patients with severe diarrhea, systemic toxicity, or prolonged symptoms (> 48–72 hours) should probably be treated. Because culture results are usually unavailable at the time of evaluation, the decision to treat should be empirical, based on the clinical setting and guided by knowledge of the common bacterial isolates from diarrhea specimens in the area (the hospital microbiology laboratory should be able to provide this information). The broadest-spectrum agent is ciprofloxacin, 500 mg orally twice daily for 5–7 days. This is effective for *Shigella, Campylobacter,* and probably invasive *Salmonella* infections. Trimethoprim-sulfamethoxazole (Bactrim, Septra), 5 mg/kg/d of trimethoprim divided into 2 doses for 5 days, is also effective, although it is not active against *Campylobacter.* If infection with *Campylobacter* is a possibility, give norfloxacin (Noroxin), 400 mg orally twice daily (or other quinolones) for 7–10 days. Erythromycin, previously recommended for *Campylobacter,* is effective in achieving bacteriologic cure but may not decrease duration or severity of symptoms.

B. Amebic Dysentery: In acute cases, give either metronidazole or tetracycline. The relapse rate is lower with metronidazole.

1. Metronidazole–Give metronidazole, 750 mg orally or intravenously (adult dose) 3 times daily for 5–10 days. Metronidazole should not be used in pregnant women.

2. Tetracycline–Give tetracycline, 250 mg orally 4 times daily for 10 days. Tetracycline should not be used in pregnancy or in children under 8 years of age.

3. Paromomycin–Give paromomycin (Humatin), 25–30 mg/kg/d orally in 3 divided doses (about 750 mg 3 times daily for adults) for 7 days. There are no contraindications to use of this drug.

4. Additional drugs–One of the following drugs should also be given in combination with or following metronidazole or tetracycline (but not paromomycin) in order to eliminate residual luminal cysts:

a. Diloxanide furoate, 500 mg 3 times a day for 10 days, is strongly preferred.

b. Diiodohydroxyquin, 650 mg 3 times a day for 3 weeks, may be used if diloxanide furoate is unavailable.

C. Watery Diarrhea: Viruses are also common causes of watery diarrhea (Tables 9–3 and 9–4).

1. If cholera or infection with toxigenic *E coli* is suspected and the patient is severely ill, give one of the following:

a. Tetracycline, 250 mg 4 times daily for 5 days (resistance to tetracycline is common). Many strains of *V cholerae* are now resistant to tetracycline.

b. Trimethoprim-sulfamethoxazole, (trimethoprim, 5 mg/kg/d) in 2 divided doses for 5 days. (Some strains are also resistant to trimethoprim.)

2. If *Giardia* is suspected, give one of the following:

a. Metronidazole, 500 mg orally 3 times daily for 7–10 days. (Lower doses are associated with a higher incidence of relapse.) Use with caution in pregnancy, and avoid the concurrent use of alcohol to prevent the disulfiramlike reaction.

b. Quinacrine, 100 mg orally 3 times daily for 7 days.

Disposition

Hospitalization is rarely required for vomiting or diarrhea due to food poisoning or viral gastroenteritis. Although severe, the vomiting or diarrhea rarely lasts long enough to require parenteral hydration. Patients with moderate to severe dehydration with persistent vomiting or diarrhea may require short-term hospitalization (12–36 hours) for investigation of more serious causes of vomiting such as small bowel obstruction.

Hospitalization is required for the following conditions:

(1) Extremes in age of patient. Newborns, infants, and the very old tolerate fluid depletion poorly.

(2) Systemic toxemia, as indicated by high fever and rigors.

(3) Mushroom or heavy metal poisoning.

(4) Preexisting dehydration.

(5) Massive diarrhea (> 0.5 L/h in an adult).

(6) Severe vomiting (preventing oral replenishment) with diarrhea.

(7) Possible "surgical abdomen."

(8) Poor home environment where required support cannot be provided.

REFERENCES

Avery ME, Snyder JD: Oral therapy for acute diarrhea. N Engl J Med 1990;323:891.

Blacklow NR, Greenberg HB: Viral gastroenteritis. N Engl J Med 1991;325:252.

DuPont HL: Bismuth subsalicylate in the treatment and prevention of diarrheal disease. Drug Intell Clin Pharm 1987;21:687.

DuPont HL: Subacute diarrhea: To treat or to wait? Hosp Pract (March 30) 1989;24:111.

DuPont HL, Ericsson CD, Johnson PC: Chemotherapy and chemoprophylaxis of travelers' diarrhea. Ann Intern Med 1985;102:260.

DuPont HL, Jong EC, Zanick DC: When a patient wants travel advice. Patient Care (July 15) 1991;25:51.

Ericsson CD et al: Ciprofloxacin or trimethoprim-sulfamethoxazole as initial therapy for travelers' diarrhea: A placebo-controlled randomized trial. Ann Intern Med 1987;106:216.

Ericsson CD et al: Treatment of traveler's diarrhea with sulfamethoxazole and trimethoprim and loperamide. JAMA 1990;263:257.

Gerding DN: Disease associated with *Clostridium difficile*. Ann Intern Med 1989;110:255.

Gerding DN et al: *Clostridium difficile*–associated diarrhea and colitis in adults. Arch Intern Med 1986;146:95.

Gorbach SL: Bacterial diarrhea and its treatment. Lancet 1987;2:1378.

Hill DR, Pearson RD: Health advice for international travel. Ann Intern Med 1988;108:839.

Hughes JM, Merson MH: Fish and shellfish poisoning. N Engl J Med 1976;295:1117.

Johanson JF, Sonnenberg A: Efficient management of diarrhea in the acquired immunodeficiency syndrome (AIDS): A medical decision analysis. Ann Intern Med 1990;112:942.

Plotkin GR, Kluge RM, Waldman RH: Gastroenteritis: Etiology, pathophysiology, and clinical manifestations. Medicine 1979;58:95.

Skirrow MB: *Campylobacter*. Lancet 1990;336:921.

Stoll BJ et al: Value of stool examination in patients with diarrhoea. Br Med J 1983;286:2037.

Todd E: Epidemiology of foodborne illness: North America. Lancet 1990;336:788.

Watson B et al: A comparison of the clinicopathological features with stool pathogens in patients hospitalised with the symptom of diarrhoea. Scand J Infect Dis 1986;18:553.

Coma

10

Roger P. Simon, MD

IMMEDIATE MANAGEMENT OF LIFE-THREATENING PROBLEMS (See Algorithm.)

For coma in victims of trauma, see Chapters 4 and 16.

Confirm Unconscious State

Attempt to arouse the patient by vigorous shaking or shouting to rule out sleep or a simple faint.

Secure Airway

Determine airway patency, and establish an adequate airway as necessary by tilting the head, lifting the chin, inserting an oral or nasal airway, or performing endotracheal intubation. Give supplemental oxygen (Chapter 1).

Establish Adequacy of Ventilation

If respirations are shallow or diminished, begin assisted ventilation (Chapter 1).

Establish Adequacy of Circulation

Assess pulses. If the carotid pulse is absent, begin

CPR (Chapter 1). Obtain vital signs, and treat shock, if present (Chapter 3).

Insert Intravenous Cannula into Upper Extremity

Insert a large-bore (≥ 18-gauge) intravenous catheter into an upper extremity, or use a large-bore needle if a catheter is not available. Secure it in place for later use.

Draw Blood

Obtain sufficient blood samples for the following determinations: blood glucose, CBC, hepatic and renal function tests, and measurements of serum electrolytes, calcium, and magnesium. A carboxyhemoglobin level should be obtained if carbon monoxide poisoning is suspected. Reserve 10 mL of blood for other tests requiring blood drawn before treatment is started, such as a toxicology screen.

Treat Immediately Reversible Causes of Coma

A. Hypoglycemia: Give glucose, 50 mL of a 50% solution (25 g of glucose) intravenously over 3–4 minutes. Hypoglycemic coma is a medical emergency that cannot tolerate the delay involved in obtaining blood glucose determinations before emergency treatment must be started.

B. Wernicke's Encephalopathy: Give thiamine, 100 mg by intravenous injection.

C. Opiate Overdose: Give naloxone (Narcan, others), 2 mg bolus intravenously; give 4 mg or more if propoxyphene (Darvon, others) ingestion is suspected.

Obtain Arterial Blood Gas Measurements

Arterial blood gas levels help to assess the adequacy of ventilation (by PCO_2 and PO_2), and blood pH is a useful clue to some drug intoxications (eg, salicylates) or metabolic encephalopathies (Table 10–1).

Perform Brief Evaluation

A. Obtain History From Relatives, Friends, or Others: Obtain a description of the onset of coma and a history of any chronic illnesses, eg, diabetes, hypertension, drug abuse, persistent headaches.

B. Obtain Complete Vital Signs: Include core body temperature in measurement of vital signs. If hypothermia is suspected, use a thermometer capable of measuring temperatures less than 33.3 °C (92 °F).

C. Perform a Rapid Physical Examination: Look for major abnormalities, especially traumatic injury (including injury of the back), cardiopulmonary disease, and meningismus.

D. Monitor Cardiac Rhythm: Rule out or treat life-threatening arrhythmias. Obtain an ECG as soon as possible.

Table 10–1. Differential diagnosis of metabolic coma by acid-base abnormalities.[1]

Respiratory alkalosis
  Hepatic encephalopathy
  Psychogenic coma
  Salicylate intoxication (early)
  Sepsis (very early)
Respiratory acidosis
  Respiratory depressant drugs (eg, bromides, ethanol, barbiturates, or other sedative-hypnotic drugs)
  Acute or chronic pulmonary failure
Metabolic acidosis
  Hyperosmolar coma
  Diabetic ketoacidosis
  Uremic encephalopathy
  Lactic acidosis
  Salicylate ingestion (late)
  Paraldehyde ingestion
  Methanol (wood alcohol) ingestion
  Ethylene glycol (antifreeze) ingestion
  Isoniazid ingestion
  Sepsis (late)
Metabolic alkalosis
  Coma (rare)

[1] Adapted and reproduced, with permission, from Plum F, Posner JB: *The Diagnosis of Stupor and Coma*, 3rd ed. Davis, 1980.

Continue Treatment of Specific Disorders

A. Hypoglycemia: The intravenous glucose already given should produce prompt lessening of hypoglycemic coma unless irreversible brain damage has occurred. *Note:* Beware of rebound hypoglycemia from long-acting insulin and oral hypoglycemic agents. A repeat dose of glucose or a glucose infusion may be necessary.

B. Wernicke's Encephalopathy: The intravenous thiamine already given usually protects against Wernicke's disease and will reverse the abnormalities over hours to days. Repeat daily until the patient starts a normal diet.

C. Opiate Overdose: Abnormalities should be reversed by the naloxone already given. *Note:* Symptoms of opiate intoxication may recur, particularly if the patient has taken a long-acting drug (eg, methadone), since naloxone has a short half-life. Repeat as necessary.

D. Hypoxemia or Hypercapnia: Severe hypoxemia or hypercapnia may present as coma. Generally, PCO_2 must rise acutely to > 80 mm Hg and PO_2 must fall to < 40 mm Hg before coma occurs. Give assisted ventilation with supplemental oxygen at once if blood gas abnormalities are life-threatening (PCO_2 > 60 mm Hg, PO_2 < 60 mm Hg); marked elevation in PCO_2 levels that are chronic (ie, near-normal pH) *should not* be rapidly corrected. (See Chapter 27 for further details.)

E. Active Seizures: Give diazepam, 5- to 10-mg bolus (or lorazepam, 2–4 mg) intravenously over 2–3 minutes, followed by phenytoin, 50 mg/min (in normal saline only) to a total dose of about 15–18 mg/kg

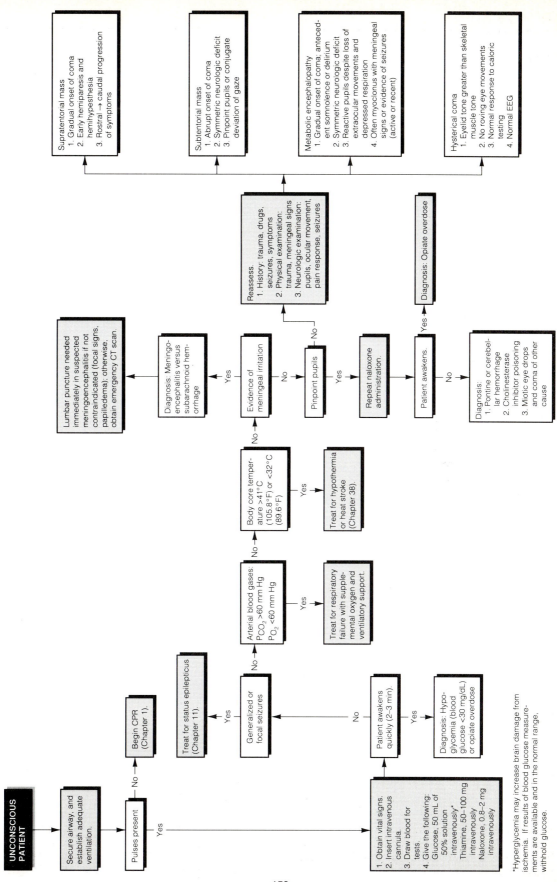

*Hyperglycemia may increase brain damage from ischemia. If results of blood glucose measurements are available and in the normal range, withhold glucose.

(1 g for normal-sized adult), since this is the treatment of choice for status epilepticus. Give diazepam only if seizures are actually occurring or if seizures recur and the patient fails to regain consciousness in between. When associated with coma, recurrent or continual focal motor activity such as repetitive movements of a single limb, hand, or one side of the face signifies status epilepticus. See Chapter 11 for detailed management of seizures.

F. Hypothermia or Hyperthermia: (See Chapter 38.) Body temperatures above 41–42 °C (105.8–107.6 °F) or below 32 °C (89.6 °F) may cause coma. *Hyperthermia in particular may cause rapid, irreversible brain injury and requires immediate corrective action.* If body temperature is 41 °C (105.8 °F) or higher, strip the patient, and sponge with cool water while directing air on the patient with a fan.

Hypothermia is generally much better tolerated than hyperthermia, and the physician may start corrective measures at a more deliberate pace.

Assess Meningeal Irritation

If meningismus is present (nuchal rigidity or Kernig's or Brudzinski's signs), perform lumbar puncture immediately to determine whether or not meningitis or subarachnoid hemorrhage is present.

Lumbar puncture is *contraindicated* (before CT scan or equivalent diagnostic procedure) in the following situations:

(1) If there is significant papilledema.

(2) If there are prominent lateralizing signs (eg, hemiparesis).

(3) If a brain abscess or other focal central nervous system lesion is *strongly* suspected for other reasons besides meningismus or lateralizing signs.

If both meningismus and a contraindication to lumbar puncture are present, emergency CT scan is the fastest means of ruling out an intracranial mass lesion and thereby permitting safe lumbar puncture. Under these circumstances, begin antimicrobial therapy (see Table 34–3) if there will be a delay of more than 1 hour in obtaining the CT scan.

See Chapters 13 and 34 for further comments on the management of meningitis and Chapter 46 for the technique of lumbar puncture and evaluation of the cerebrospinal fluid.

Look for Pinpoint Pupils

A. Opiate Overdose: Repeat administration of a narcotic antagonist (naloxone, 0.8–2 mg intravenously), particularly if the history and physical examination are suggestive of intravenous drug abuse (eg, sclerosed veins).

B. Cholinesterase Inhibitor Poisoning: Consider cholinesterase inhibitor poisoning if there is a history of exposure to insecticides or nerve gas and if paralysis, salivation, bronchorrhea, sweating, spontaneous defecation, or muscle fasciculations are present.

If cholinesterase inhibitor poisoning is suspected, give atropine, 1–2 mg (adult dose) intravenously, at once. Repeat every 2–5 minutes until signs of atropine effect (dilated pupils, flushed face, tachycardia) occur. See Chapter 39 for further evaluation and treatment.

C. Pontine or Cerebellar Hemorrhage: Pinpoint pupils, coma, and hypertension suggest pontine or cerebellar hemorrhage. If either condition is suspected, obtain immediate neurologic or neurosurgical consultation, since decompressive surgery may be lifesaving in the latter instance.

D. Factitious Pinpoint Pupils: Occasionally, pinpoint pupils are due to miotic eye drops used by the patient, and some other condition has caused the coma. This finding can be seriously misleading unless the use of miotic eye drops is considered and excluded (primarily on the basis of history).

FURTHER EVALUATION OF THE COMATOSE PATIENT

History

A history may be obtained from friends and family (at the hospital or by telephone), police, or ambulance technicians. Crucial points include the following:

A. Recent head trauma, even though seemingly trivial.

B. Drug use (including alcohol), recent or past (ask for pill containers).

C. History of seizures, diabetes, hypertension, cirrhosis, or previous neurologic disease that might explain the comatose state.

D. Precomatose activity and behavior (eg, headache, confusion preceding coma; sudden versus gradual onset of coma).

E. Multiple patients with coma or confusion suggest carbon monoxide poisoning or exposure to some other common-source toxin.

Physical Examination

Physical examination should include the following:

A. Obtain complete vital signs and rectal or tympanic temperature, and observe the respiratory pattern.

B. Search carefully for signs of head trauma. (Evidence of trauma elsewhere on the body is presumptive evidence of head trauma.)

C. Examine for signs of meningeal irritation (nuchal rigidity, Brudzinski's sign).

Neurologic Examination

It is essential to record the results of this simple neurologic examination accurately, since treatment decisions may depend on whether subsequent examinations show improvement or deterioration in the patient's condition. Evaluation of the following assists in determining involvement of the central nervous system:

A. Respiratory pattern.

B. Pupillary size, equality, and response to light. Examine the fundi (papilledema, subhyaloid hemorrhage), and check for corneal reflex.

C. Extraocular movements stimulated by the doll's eye maneuver (rotation of the head by the examiner) or, if no movement occurs, stimulated by ice-water lavage (caloric test) of the external ear canal (30–50 mL of ice water gently instilled against the tympanic membrane with the patient's head at a 30-degree angle from the horizontal). In hysterical unconsciousness, rapid nystagmus occurs. If the patient is unconscious because of an organic or metabolic cause, the eyes remain in mid position or deviate for several minutes to the side of the irrigation.

D. Motor response to pain, both centrally (elicited by pressure on the supraorbital ridge) and peripherally (elicited by pressure on the nail beds of the hands and feet). In coma, the response to pain is markedly blunted (eg, grunting) or grossly inappropriate or abnormal (eg, decorticate or decerebrate posturing). A satisfactory way to produce deep pain is to press on the nail beds or supraorbital ridge; these maneuvers produce no bruises that might be mistaken (by later examiners) as evidence of trauma.

E. Any repetitive, spontaneous movements that might indicate status epilepticus.

F. Say to the patient, "Open your eyes and look up at my finger," even though the patient appears comatose. Compliance suggests the "locked-in" syndrome (see below).

G. Deep tendon reflexes and Babinski's sign should be elicited to check for asymmetry.

Laboratory Tests

A. Blood Chemistry: The results of sodium, potassium, calcium, and glucose determinations and renal function tests previously obtained should now be available for evaluation.

B. Arterial Blood Gases and pH: Arterial blood PCO_2 and PO_2 should be determined to rule out abnormal respiratory function as a cause of coma and to determine the need for respiratory support. The pH abnormalities noted in arterial blood gas measurements are also used to differentiate among the metabolic causes of coma (Table 10–1).

C. Urinalysis: The bladder should be catheterized, a urine sample submitted for analysis, and a specimen reserved for culture and toxicologic studies, if needed.

D. Radiologic Examination: CT scan or magnetic resonance imaging (MRI) of the head (or, if unavailable, skull x-rays) should be obtained in all patients with a potential structural cause of coma.

EMERGENCY TREATMENT OF SPECIFIC DISORDERS

SUPRATENTORIAL MASS LESIONS

Diagnosis

In supratentorial mass lesions, symptoms and signs of unilateral hemispheric dysfunction are usually present before onset of coma and persist into the early stages of coma. Neurologic deficits follow a characteristic progression from rostral to caudal (cerebral hemisphere to medulla) involvement. Results on neurologic examination are consistent with the anatomic level of involvement of the brain (Fig 10–1). The lesion can usually be demonstrated by CT scan or angiography.

A. Cerebral Hemispheres: Patients are generally alert. Hemiparesis and hemihypesthesia are commonly present. Aphasia may also be present with involvement of the dominant hemisphere, or agnosia (denial of the deficit) with nondominant involvement.

B. Diencephalon: Somnolence and eventually coma occur because of bilateral cortical involvement or diencephalic compression. Asymmetric motor and sensory abnormalities usually persist because of prior involvement of the cortex. Surgical removal of the mass when involvement does not exceed the level of the diencephalon generally results in recovery of consciousness.

C. Midbrain:

1. Early stage–Herniation of the medial portion of the temporal lobe (the uncus) across the cerebellar tentorium produces midbrain signs, including unilateral pupillary dilation and impaired medial rectus muscle (oculomotor nerve) function which may occur prior to loss of consciousness.

Results on the remainder of the neurologic examination may be normal. It is critical to recognize that these findings represent early involvement at the midbrain level and carry the same serious prognosis as the more classic midbrain state resulting from transtentorial herniation (Fig 10–1).

2. Midbrain stage (fully developed)–Progressive uncal herniation causes loss of consciousness, and the fully developed midbrain stage appears rapidly. Marked ipsilateral pupillary dilatation and loss of reactivity to light are noted, and caloric testing (irrigation of the contralateral ear with ice water) fails to produce medial deviation of the eye ipsilateral to the

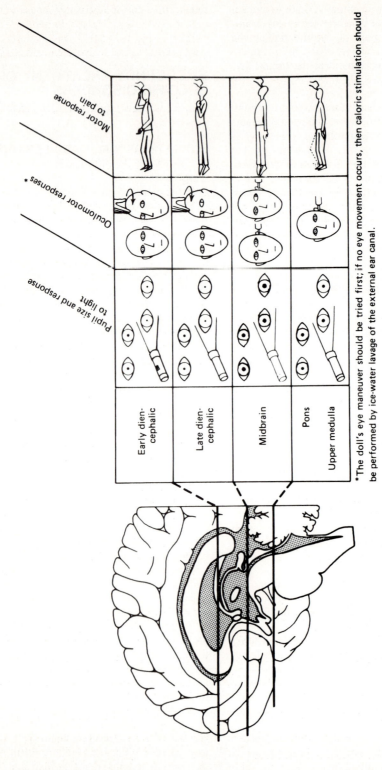

Figure 10–1. Symptoms at various levels of anatomic involvement of the brain. (Adapted and reproduced, with permission, from Plum F, Posner JB: *The Diagnosis of Stupor and Coma*, 3rd ed. Davis, 1980.)

*The doll's eye maneuver should be tried first; if no eye movement occurs, then caloric stimulation should be performed by ice-water lavage of the external ear canal.

156

lesion. Painful stimuli elicit decerebrate (extensor) posturing. If the patient's condition progresses to full midbrain dysfunction (absent oculocephalogyric reflexes), the chances of survival without severe neurologic impairment decrease rapidly, especially in adults.

D. Pons: Pupils remain in mid position and are unreactive to light. Extraocular movements (in response to the doll's eye maneuver and caloric testing) are absent. (Barbiturates and other drugs also abolish oculomotor reflexes.) Death is inevitable once the supratentorial mass lesion produces pontine-level dysfunction.

Focal pontine lesions (eg, pontine or cerebellar hemorrhage or infarction) as distinct from transtentorial herniation to the pontine level produce pinpoint pupils that react to light when viewed with a magnifying glass. (Pinpoint pupils induced by opiates and pilocarpine must be excluded.) Extraocular movements are not inducible.

Treatment

A. Immediate Measures: If a delay in surgery is unavoidable and the patient's neurologic status is worsening, hyperventilation to an arterial PCO_2 of 25–30 mm Hg and administration of mannitol and the most rapidly acting intravenous glucocorticoids to reduce cerebral edema (Table 10–2) may delay progression of the neurologic deficit.

B. Immediate Palliative Surgery: If the patient's neurologic status is worsening rapidly (eg, from cerebral hemispheric to midbrain level in less than 1 or 2 hours), immediate exploratory/decompressive craniotomy may be indicated, even if it must be done in the emergency department and even if the available personnel are not fully trained in neurosurgery.

C. Definitive Surgery for Removal of Mass: If a supratentorial mass lesion is suspected, emergency neurosurgical consultation is mandatory. Hematomas, tumors, and abscesses are the most common lesions causing supratentorial compression, and all may be amenable to surgery.

If neurologic signs and symptoms are stable and the lesion is at the diencephalic level or above, a CT scan or MRI should be done. If the routine CT scan is normal, contrast media should be used and the scan repeated. Angiography and radionuclide brain scanning are also valuable diagnostic aids if CT scanning or MRI is unavailable.

Disposition

Immediate hospitalization is mandatory in all patients.

1. SUBDURAL HEMATOMA

Diagnosis

The possibility of subdural hematoma must be considered in any comatose patient. Trauma is the most common cause, but in about 25% of cases, there is no history or evidence of trauma. Symptoms and signs are notoriously nonspecific, nonlocalizing, or absent (Table 10–3) and may be either stable or rapidly progressive. The frequency of bilateral hematomas makes localization of the lesion even more difficult, as does the coexistence of associated cerebral contusion. Hemiparesis, when present, is contralateral to the lesion in approximately 60% of cases, and ipsilateral pupillary dilatation occurs in approximately 75% of cases. Seizures may occur. Diagnosis is confirmed by CT scan (preferably) or cerebral angiography. Skull x-rays are not helpful.

Note: Lumbar puncture is contraindicated. Cerebrospinal fluid abnormalities are nonspecific and cannot differentiate subdural hematomas from cerebral contusion without hematoma.

Treatment & Disposition

Immediate hospitalization and emergency neurosurgical consultation are mandatory in all cases.

A. Stable patients or those with slowly worsening mild neurologic dysfunction should have radiologic confirmation of the diagnosis.

B. Unstable patients with rapidly worsening (min-

Table 10–2. Drug therapy for cerebral edema.

Drug	Dose	Route	Indications/Comments
Glucocorticoids			
Dexamethasone	10 mg, then 4 mg 4 times a day	Intravenous or oral	Dexamethasone preferred for the least mineralocorticoid effect; effective after 6–12 hours; concomitant antacid or H_2 blocker treatment probably indicated.
Prednisone	60 mg, then 25 mg 4 times a day	Oral	
Methylprednisolone	60 mg, then 25 mg 4 times a day	Intravenous or oral	
Hydrocortisone	300 mg, then 130 mg 4 times a day	Intravenous or oral	
Dehydration agents			
Mannitol	1.5–2 g/kg over 30 minutes to 1 hour	20% Intravenous solution	Effective immediately; major dehydrating effect is on normal tissue; osmotic effect is short-lived, and more than 2 intravenous doses are rarely effective; cause osmotic diuresis and electrolyte imbalance.
Urea	1–5 g/kg	Intravenous	
Glycerin (glycerol)	1.5–4 g/kg/d	Oral	Effective orally. Nausea and vomiting common.

Table 10–3. Common findings in patients with subdural hematomas.[1]

Clinical Findings	Acute[2] (82 Cases) (%)	Subacute[3] (91 Cases) (%)	Chronic[4] (216 Cases) (%)
Symptoms			
Headache	11	44	81
Confusion	12	41	37
Vomiting	24	31	30
Paresis	20	19	22
Seizures	6	3	9
Visual symptoms	0	0	12
Speech disturbance	6	8	6
Vertigo	0	4	5
Signs			
Depressed consciousness	100	88	59
Motor asymmetry	44	37	41
Pupillary inequality	57	27	20
Confusion/memory loss	17	21	27
Papilledema	1	15	22
Drysphasia	6	12	11
Hemianopia	0	4	3
Facial weakness	0	3	3

[1] After McKissock W: *Lancet* 1960;1:1365.
[2] Within 3 days of trauma.
[3] Within 4–20 days of trauma.
[4] More than 20 days after trauma.

utes to hours) neurologic deficit thought to be due to an expanding subdural hematoma may require emergency exploratory craniotomy without benefit of preoperative radiologic diagnosis.

Hyperventilation, mannitol, and glucocorticoids (Table 10–2) may be used to minimize cerebral damage while the patient is awaiting surgery.

2. HYPERTENSIVE INTRACEREBRAL HEMORRHAGE

Diagnosis

Intracerebral hemorrhage nearly always begins when the patient is awake. There are no prodromal features. Obtundation is unremitting and worsens steadily over minutes to hours, most often progressing to stupor or coma. Almost all patients are hypertensive (blood pressure ≥ 170/90 mm Hg) when seen, and high blood pressure persists even into the late stages of transtentorial herniation.

The ocular fundi may show hemorrhages secondary to the acute increase in intracranial pressure. Conjugate deviation of the eyes is common, with gaze directed toward the side of supratentorial (or away from the subtentorial) hemorrhage.

Headache occurs in 30–50% of patients and may be moderately severe; it overlies the location of the lesion. Vomiting and nuchal rigidity may also occur. Hemiplegia (contralateral to the hemorrhage) is a common early sign, because the site of hemorrhage (basal ganglia, 50% of cases; thalamus, 10%) abuts the internal capsule in most cases. Seizures are rare. CT scan provides the definitive diagnosis. The cerebrospinal fluid is grossly bloody in 90% of cases, and the pressure usually is above 200 mm water and often greater than 600 mm water. The total protein content is as high as 300–1200 mg/dL. The cerebrospinal fluid glucose level is normal initially but may fall later. The cerebrospinal fluid red blood cell count may be as high as 1 million/μL, and white cells are present in proportion (one white cell per thousand red cells). Peripheral blood leukocytosis (15,000–20,000/μL) is often present.

Treatment

Methods of treatment are frustratingly limited, especially because the hemorrhage occurs over a brief period and then stops. Bleeding probably does not recur, but the patient's condition worsens because of secondary cerebral edema. On the other hand, survivors of intracerebral hemorrhage may recover with minimal neurologic deficit as the clot resolves over a period of months.

Elevated intracranial pressure may respond temporarily to mannitol (Table 10–2). Glucocorticoids are not efficacious.

Surgical Measures: For hemorrhages originating deep within the brain (basal ganglia, thalamus), surgical attempts to evacuate the clot are as disappointing as supportive care alone. Surgery may be lifesaving, however, for hemorrhage into cortical white matter (lobar hemorrhage).

Disposition

Immediate hospitalization is required, primarily for supportive care.

3. BRAIN ABSCESS

Diagnosis

Brain abscess accounts for only 2% of intracranial masses. The presenting symptoms and signs are shown in Table 10–4. Progression to stupor and coma may be rapid, occurring over days or, rarely, hours. Often, the usual signs of infection are absent. The temperature is normal in half of patients, and the white blood cell count is below 10,000/μL in over one-fourth of patients. Brain abscess should be considered in patients with AIDS who develop changes in mentation (may be caused by *Toxoplasma gondii*).

Table 10–4. Principal presenting features in 88 cases of brain abscess.[1]

Headache	70%
Lethargy	48%
Hemiparesis	38%
Seizures	32%
Nuchal rigidity	25%
Nausea and vomiting	24%
Papilledema	23%
Dysphasia	11%
Ataxia or nystagmus	11%
Stupor	10%
Pupils unequal or ocular muscle palsy	10%
Visual field defect	7%

[1] Modified and reproduced, with permission, from Morgan H, Wood MW, Murphy F: Experience with 88 consecutive cases of brain abscess. *J Neurosurg* 1973;**33**:698.

Lumbar puncture is contraindicated. The results are nondiagnostic, varying between normal findings and those suggestive of meningitis. CT scan, radionuclide brain scan, or MRI will demonstrate the lesions in over 90% of cases. Antibiotics should be initiated immediately without awaiting the results of a CT scan in possible meningitis. Begin intravenous therapy with nafcillin (2 g intravenously every 4 hours), plus cefotaxime (150–200 mg/kg intravenously in 4 divided doses), plus metronidazole (30 mg/kg/d intravenously in 4 divided doses) (Chapter 34).

Treatment & Disposition

Neurologic and neurosurgical consultation are necessary. Hospitalize the patient for definitive diagnosis and treatment.

4. BRAIN TUMOR

Diagnosis

Coma is seldom the presenting symptom in primary or metastatic tumors of the central nervous system, although coma may result from seizures induced by the tumors. The patient typically has a history of days to weeks of headache, focal weakness, and altered or depressed consciousness. Papilledema is present in 25% of cases.

The chest x-ray is a useful screening test for brain tumors, because lung cancer that has metastasized to the brain is the most common intracranial tumor. Other common central nervous system metastases often involve the lung before they affect the brain.

Treatment & Disposition

Treatment with glucocorticoids (Table 10–2) is often dramatically effective in reducing surrounding edema and improving the neurologic deficit.

Hospitalize the patient for diagnosis and treatment.

5. CEREBRAL INFARCTION (Stroke) (See also Chapter 12.)

Diagnosis

The brain swelling of cerebral edema following massive hemispheric infarction can produce contralateral hemispheric compression or transtentorial herniation that will result in coma. Such cerebral swelling becomes maximal 48–72 hours after the infarct. The principal clinical findings are hemiparesis or hemisensory loss (and aphasia if the dominant hemisphere is involved). Evolving transtentorial herniation progresses slowly over many hours or several days to stupor and coma. Absence of blood in the cerebrospinal fluid or on CT scan of the brain rules out cerebral hemorrhage.

Treatment

Glucocorticoids and dehydrating agents can be tried (Table 10–2), but clear benefit from their use has not been demonstrated.

Antihypertensive drugs should be used with caution during the acute stage, because of the dangers of hypoperfusion of the ischemic hemisphere.

Disposition

Hospitalization is indicated for all patients.

SUBTENTORIAL MASS LESIONS

Diagnosis

Clinical findings depend on the anatomic level of involvement of the brain. Generally, there is coma of sudden onset without antecedent hemispheric signs (eg, hemiparesis or hemihypesthesia). With conjugate gaze deviation, the eyes are directed away from the side of the lesion and toward the hemiparesis. Disconjugate eye movements—especially internuclear ophthalmoplegia (lateral deviation of one eye on oculovestibular [doll's eye maneuver] or caloric testing without concomitant medial deviation of the contralateral eye)—strongly suggest a subtentorial lesion. Motor responses are not helpful in differentiating subtentorial from supratentorial lesions, because decerebrate or flaccid responses to painful stimulation occur with supratentorial lesions that progress to involve subtentorial structures. Respiration may be ataxic, gasping, or agonal. Differentiating a primary subtentorial process from transtentorial herniation in the late stage may be impossible except by extrapolating from the history.

In pontine or cerebellar hemorrhage or infarction, tiny (pinpoint) pupils are often present. (Remember that intoxication with cholinesterase inhibitors or opiates also produces pinpoint pupils.)

Treatment

Emergency neurosurgical consultation is mandatory. If surgery must be delayed and neurologic abnormalities are progressive, use glucocorticoids, mannitol, and hyperventilation (reduce PCO_2 to 25–30 mm Hg) to try to control swelling of the brain (Table 10–2).

Disposition

Immediate hospitalization is required in all cases.

1. BASILAR ARTERY THROMBOSIS OR EMBOLIC OCCLUSION

Diagnosis

Basilar artery thrombosis and embolic occlusion are relatively common vascular syndromes that cause coma because of direct involvement of the penetrating arteries supplying the central core of the brain stem. Patients are usually elderly and often have a history of hypertension or transient ischemic attacks or evidence of other atherosclerotic vascular disease. Basilar artery transient ischemic attacks are characterized by (in order of frequency of occurrence) dizziness (rarely the only symptom), diplopia, weakness and ataxia, slurred speech, and visceral sensations (nausea and vomiting).

Basilar artery occlusion causes coma in half of affected patients, and almost all present with some alteration of consciousness. Focal subtentorial signs are present from the onset, and the respiratory pattern is irregular. Pupillary abnormalities vary with the site of the lesion and include poorly reactive pupils of normal size (3 mm), pupils fixed in mid position (5 mm), or pinpoint pupils. Skew deviation of the eyes is common. Horizontal eye movements are absent or asymmetric during the doll's eye maneuver or caloric testing. Conjugate eye deviation, if present, is directed away from the side of the lesion and toward the hemiparesis. Vertical eye movements in response to the doll's eye maneuver may be intact. Symmetric or asymmetric motor signs (hemiparesis, hyperreflexia, and Babinski's sign) may be present. The cerebrospinal fluid is free of blood.

Treatment

Current opinion supports anticoagulation for progressive subtotal lesions, although evidence for the efficacy of this treatment is inconclusive.

Disposition

Hospitalize the patient for treatment and supportive care. The prognosis varies directly with the degree of brain stem injury.

2. PONTINE HEMORRHAGE

Diagnosis

Coma of apoplectic onset is the hallmark of pontine hemorrhage. Physical examination reveals many of the findings noted in basilar artery infarction, but there is no history of transient ischemic episodes preceding pontine hemorrhage. Additional features especially suggestive of pontine involvement include ocular bobbing (spontaneous brisk, periodic, mainly conjugate, downward movements of the eyes with return to mid position), pinpoint pupils, and loss of lateral eye movements. Fever as high as 39.5 °C (103 °F) or more occurs in most patients surviving for more than several hours. The cerebrospinal fluid is grossly bloody and under increased pressure. CT scan of the brain is almost always diagnostic, demonstrating high density (blood) in the brain stem.

Treatment

There is no effective treatment, and the mortality rate is high.

Disposition

Hospitalize the patient for confirmation of the diagnosis and supportive care.

3. INTRACEREBELLAR HEMORRHAGE OR INFARCTION

Diagnosis

Hypertension is the cause of intracerebellar hemorrhage in approximately three-fourths of patients. The remaining cases result from ruptured intracerebellar arteriovenous malformations. Most affected patients are over 50 years old. The clinical picture ranges from sudden brain stem compression progressing rapidly to death (a picture virtually indistinguishable from primary pontine hemorrhage) to a progressive syndrome developing over hours or even several days (as commonly seen with cerebellar infarction). The onset is sudden and characterized by headache and nausea and vomiting, with marked ataxia of gait that may progress to complete inability to walk or stand. *Caution:* Early stages of cerebellar hemorrhage are sometimes misdiagnosed as intoxication caused by use of drugs or alcohol.

Other features include small reactive pupils with conjugate gaze deviation away from the side of the lesion, preserved vertical eye movements, and an ipsilateral peripheral facial palsy in some cases. Nuchal rigidity is present in half of patients. Hemiparesis is rare and, if present, mild in degree. The incidence of ipsilateral cerebellar limb ataxia varies, but when this sign is present, it is of obvious value in locating the lesion. Cerebrospinal fluid becomes grossly bloody within several hours after intracerebellar hemorrhage.

Prompt diagnosis—preferably with CT scan of the brain (in which increased density seen on the scan represents blood in the cerebellar hemisphere)—is crucial, since surgical decompression may be lifesaving.

Treatment

The only treatment for symptomatic cerebellar hemorrhage is surgical decompression, which may dramatically reduce symptoms. Pharmacologic reduction of cerebral edema (Table 10–2) may briefly delay progression of symptoms until surgery can be performed.

If appropriately treated, lethargic or even stuporous patients may survive with minimal or no residual damage and with intact intellect. If the patient is in a deep coma, the chances for meaningful survival are small.

Disposition

Hospitalize the patient immediately for emergency surgical decompression.

4. SUBDURAL & EPIDURAL HEMATOMA (SUBTENTORIAL)

Subtentorial subdural and epidural hematomas are rare lesions with similar clinical pictures. Prompt and accurate diagnosis is important, because these potentially fatal disorders may be treated effectively.

Diagnosis

Occipital trauma frequently precedes the onset of brain stem involvement by hours to weeks.

Physical findings are those of extrinsic compression of the brain stem: vomiting, cerebellar signs with ataxia, and progressive obtundation. Nuchal rigidity may be present. Papilledema may occur in chronic cases.

In most patients, skull x-rays reveal a fracture line crossing the occipital venous sinuses. CT scan or angiography confirms the diagnosis in more than 95% of cases. Cerebrospinal fluid examination is not helpful.

Treatment & Disposition

Hospitalize the patient immediately for urgent surgical decompression.

5. "LOCKED-IN" SYNDROME

The portion of the reticular formation responsible for consciousness lies above the level of the mid pons. Therefore, "transection" of the low brain stem by basilar artery stroke, encephalitis, demyelinating disease, or an infiltrative tumor can produce an akinetic and mute state with preserved consciousness (hence "locked-in").

Diagnosis

Patients with "locked-in" syndrome are in fact awake and alert but appear comatose because they are quadriplegic and unable to speak. Decerebrate posturing or flexor spasms may be noted as well. However, one or more voluntary movements such as eye opening, vertical eye movement, or convergence are preserved. Therefore, always instruct an apparently comatose patient to "open your eyes" or "look up at my finger" at least once during the examination. *Voluntary movement of any kind is inconsistent with true coma.*

Treatment & Disposition

Hospitalize the patient for treatment and rehabilitation. Some patients will recover significant function after a month or more.

POSTICTAL STATE

Diagnosis

Coma resulting from seizure disorders is usually not a difficult diagnostic problem, since recovery of consciousness is rapid following the end of the seizure. Prolonged postictal coma (several hours) followed by several days of confusion may occur after status epilepticus, in patients with brain damage (eg, multiple cerebral infarctions, head trauma, encephalitis, mental retardation), and in patients with metabolic encephalopathy that alters consciousness and induces seizures (eg, hyponatremia, hyperglycemia).

Patients may initially be unresponsive to deep pain and exhibit sonorous respirations. The neurologic examination is usually nonfocal, although Babinski's sign may be transiently present. Uncommonly, there may be focal abnormalities (Todd's paralysis) referable anatomically to the focus of seizure activity in the brain.

Other evidence of a recent seizure may also be present, such as trauma to the tongue from biting, incontinence, or a rapidly clearing anion gap (lactic) acidosis.

The rapid resolution of coma in a patient with a witnessed seizure or known seizure disorder should suggest the diagnosis of the postictal state as the cause of coma. Coma which is at first thought to be postictal but which fails to improve should prompt an investigation for underlying processes contributing to mental status depression, including metabolic encephalopathy, underlying diffuse brain damage, encephalitis, and structural lesion. Appropriate investigations should include measurements of serum electrolytes, calcium, and magnesium; CT scan; and lumbar puncture.

Treatment

Treatment depends on the underlying cause of the seizure. The physician should be alert for metabolic causes and treat them appropriately. (See Chapter 11 for details of management.)

Disposition

Immediate hospitalization is required for all cases of status epilepticus and prolonged postictal coma and for seizures due to metabolic causes that are not quickly correctable.

Outpatient management may be possible for stable patients.

METABOLIC ENCEPHALOPATHIES

Diagnosis

Metabolic encephalopathies are characterized by a period of progressive somnolence, intoxication, toxic delirium, or agitation, after which the patient gradually sinks into a stuporous and finally comatose state. Subarachnoid hemorrhage is an exception: loss of consciousness is rapid. Headache is not an initial symptom of metabolic encephalopathy except in the case of meningitis, subarachnoid hemorrhage, or poisoning due to organophosphate compounds or carbon monoxide.

In contrast to patients with mass lesions, neurologic examination fails to reveal focal hemispheric lesions (hemiparesis, hemisensory loss, aphasia) before loss of consciousness. Neurologic findings are symmetric except in some patients with hepatic encephalopathy and hypoglycemic coma, which may be accompanied by focal signs (especially hemiparesis) that may alternate sides. Myoclonus and, during consciousness, asterixis may be present as well.

The hallmark of metabolic encephalopathy is reactive pupils (a midbrain function) in the presence of impaired function of the lower brain stem (eg, hypoventilation, loss of extraocular movements), an anatomically inconsistent set of abnormalities. Respiratory patterns in metabolic coma vary widely and may provide a further basis for establishing an etiologic diagnosis (Table 10–1).

Treatment & Disposition

Treatment depends entirely on the cause of coma. All patients require hospitalization for supportive care and specific therapy.

1. HYPOGLYCEMIA
(See also Chapter 35.)

Diagnosis

Unlike other organs, the brain relies mainly on glucose to supply its energy requirements. Abrupt hypoglycemia rapidly interferes with brain metabolism and quickly produces symptoms. Insulin and oral hypoglycemic drug overdose are the most common causes of hypoglycemia.

Signs of sympathetic nervous system activity (tachycardia, sweating, and anxiety) may warn patients of impending hypoglycemia, although these signs may be masked by propranolol and other beta-blockers and are absent in patients with diabetic autonomic neuropathy. Common neurologic abnormalities are delirium, seizures, focal signs that often alternate sides, stupor, and coma. Table 10–5 summarizes the symptoms and signs in patients undergoing insulin-induced hypoglycemic shock.

Hypoglycemic coma may be tolerated for 60–90 minutes, but once the stage of flaccidity with hyporeflexia has been reached, glucose administration within 15 minutes is mandatory to avoid irreversible damage.

Treatment & Disposition

Give glucose, 50 mL of 50% solution intravenously (adult dose). Once the diagnosis of hypoglycemia is confirmed by analysis of blood drawn before treatment, give an additional 50 mL as needed or begin an infusion of dextrose 5% in water. Patients should be observed for 1–2 hours after glucose supplementation has been discontinued to ensure that hypoglycemia does not recur before they are discharged from the hospital. In some cases, hospitalization may be necessary, especially in cases of hypoglycemia that recurs despite treatment and long-acting insulin or hypoglycemic agent overdose.

2. HYPOXEMIA

Diagnosis

Hypoxemia produces brain damage only as a result of concomitant cerebral ischemia. Cerebral blood

Table 10–5. Signs and symptoms of hypoglycemia after insulin administration.[1]

Time After Insulin Administration	Symptoms
30 minutes	Perspiration Salivation Somnolence Excitement and restlessness Tachycardia if stimulated (bradycardia if somnolent)
2–3 hours	Loss of contact with environment Myoclonus Primitive reflexes (grasping, sucking) Reactive, dilated pupils
4–5 hours	Comatose Depressed responses to pain Roving eye movements Tonic and torsional muscular spasms Extensor plantar response
5–6 hours	Decerebrate rigidity
6–7 hours	Small pupils Bradycardia Flaccid tone Depressed reflexes

[1] Modified and reproduced, with permission, from Himwich HE: *Brain Metabolism and Cerebral Disorders.* Williams & Wilkins, 1951.

flow diminishes and brain ischemia occurs when the arterial PO_2 falls to 20–45 mm Hg. In cerebral anoxia due to cardiac arrest, where the duration can be timed precisely, 4–6 minutes of asystole begins to result in permanent damage to the central nervous system. Following asystole, the pupils dilate rapidly and become fixed, and tonic posturing is observed. A few seizurelike tonic-clonic movements are common.

Treatment & Disposition

Treatment of hypoxemia depends on the cause. Support cardiac output, and maintain arterial PO_2 above 60 mm Hg by supplemental oxygen or mechanical ventilation.

Hospitalize all patients for diagnosis and treatment.

3. SEDATIVE-HYPNOTIC DRUG OVERDOSE

Sedative-hypnotic drug overdose is the most common cause of coma in patients brought to the emergency department. Barbiturates are most commonly implicated, but a similar syndrome occurs with overdose of any sedative-hypnotic drug, eg, meprobamate (Equanil, Miltown, many others), chlordiazepoxide (Librium, many others), diazepam (Valium, Valrelease, others), glutethimide (Doriden, others), ethchlorvynol (Placidyl), and methaqualone (Quaalude; although withdrawn from the market, illicit drug use is still common).

Diagnosis

In drug overdoses, intoxication precedes coma and is marked by prominent nystagmus in all directions of gaze, dysarthria, ataxia, and, with some drugs, hypotension. After the gradual onset of coma, the neurologic examination may briefly suggest an upper motor neuron lesion because of hyperreflexia, ankle clonus, or extensor plantar responses. On rare occasions, decerebrate posturing may appear briefly.

The pupillary light reflex is preserved even when respiratory depression requiring ventilatory support has occurred. Glutethimide overdose is an exception to this rule of pupillary sparing, since it regularly produces pupils fixed in mid position and unreactive to light.

Extraocular movements in response to the doll's eye maneuver are completely absent. Caloric testing may produce a delayed forced downward deviation of one or both eyes, however.

Causative drugs may be detected in samples of blood, urine, or gastric contents.

Treatment & Disposition

Almost all patients should be hospitalized. Provide supportive care, including intubation, with special attention to adequate airway protection and ventilation. See Chapter 39 for details.

4. ALCOHOL INTOXICATION

Alcohol intoxication produces a metabolic encephalopathy similar to that produced by sedative-hypnotic drugs, although nystagmus during wakefulness and early impairment of lateral eye movements are not as common. Peripheral vasodilatation is a prominent manifestation and produces tachycardia, hypotension, and hypothermia.

In individuals who are not chronic alcoholics, stupor occurs when blood alcohol levels reach 250–300 mg/dL and coma when levels reach 300–400 mg/dL. Because alcohol has significant osmotic pressure (100 mg/dL ≈ 22.4 mosm), alcohol intoxication is one cause of hyperosmolality.

Treatment & Disposition

Management is discussed in Chapter 39. Patients should be observed until improvement has occurred (normal orientation and judgment; satisfactory coordination). Hospitalize those patients with abnormalities that would normally require hospitalization (eg, metabolic abnormalities, Wernicke's encephalopathy).

5. NARCOTIC OVERDOSE

Diagnosis

In narcotic overdose, hypoventilation is almost always present, along with pinpoint pupillary constriction and absent extraocular movements in response to the doll's eye maneuver. "Pinpoint" pupils are also associated with other disorders that must be ruled out: use of miotic eye drops, pontine hemorrhage, Argyll Robertson pupils from syphilis, and organophosphate insecticide poisoning.

Narcotic intoxication is confirmed by rapid pupillary dilation and awakening after administration of a narcotic antagonist such as naloxone, 2 mg by rapid intravenous injection. *Note:* Certain overdoses, eg, propoxyphene (Darvon, many others), may not respond to 2 mg and may require up to 4 mg or more. Patients intoxicated with alcohol may awaken briefly after administration of naloxone.

The duration of action of naloxone varies with the dose and route of administration. Repeat doses are frequently necessary, especially following intoxication with long-acting narcotics (eg, methadone).

Treatment & Disposition

Treatment of drug overdose and poisoning is outlined above and discussed more fully in Chapter 39.

Hospitalization should be considered for patients

who do not recover completely in the emergency department or who have taken long-acting narcotics.

6. HEPATIC ENCEPHALOPATHY

Hepatic encephalopathy can occur in patients with severe acute or chronic liver disease. Jaundice need not be present. In the patient with preexisting liver disease, encephalopathy may develop rapidly following an acute insult such as gastrointestinal hemorrhage. Patients with surgical portacaval shunts are especially predisposed to encephalopathy.

Mental status is altered and ranges from somnolence to delirium or coma. There is increased muscle tone; hyperreflexia is common. Prominent asterixis occurs in the somnolent patient. Seizures—generalized or focal—occur infrequently. Hyperventilation with respiratory alkalosis is nearly universal and may be demonstrated by measuring arterial blood pH. Cerebrospinal fluid is normal but may appear xanthochromic in patients with serum bilirubin levels higher than 4–6 mg/dL.

Treatment & Disposition

The emergency department should provide initial supportive measures only. Hospitalization for definitive treatment is indicated for all patients.

7. DISORDERS OF ELECTROLYTES & OSMOLALITY

Diagnosis

A. Hyperosmolality and Hypo-osmolality: Coma with focal seizures is a common presentation of hyperosmolality. Consciousness is altered if serum osmolality is less than 260 mosm/kg water or greater than 330–350 mosm/kg water.

B. Hyponatremia: Delirium and seizures are common presenting features of hyponatremia. Hyponatremia may cause neurologic symptoms when serum sodium levels are below 120 meq/L, and symptoms are frequent with levels below 110 meq/L. When the serum sodium level falls rapidly, symptoms occur at higher serum sodium levels.

Treatment & Disposition

The diagnosis and treatment of these entities are discussed in Chapter 36. Hospitalization is mandatory.

8. HYPERTHERMIA & HYPOTHERMIA

Diagnosis

Hyperthermia and hypothermia are associated with symmetric neurologic dysfunction that may progress to coma. *All comatose patients must have tympanic temperature measurement or rectal temperature taken with an extended-range thermometer if the standard thermometer fails to register.*

A. Hypothermia: Internal body temperatures below 26 °C (78.8 °F) uniformly cause coma; hypothermia with core temperatures above 32 °C (89.6 °F) does not cause coma. Body temperatures between 26 and 32 °C (78.8–89.6 °F) are associated with varying degrees of obtundation. Pupillary reactivity will be sluggish below 32 °C (89.6 °F) and lost below 26.5 °C (80 °F).

B. Hyperthermia: Internal body temperatures above 41–42 °C (105.8–107.6 °F) are associated with coma and may also rapidly cause permanent brain damage. Seizures are common, especially in children.

Treatment & Disposition

If hyperthermia is present, begin to lower body temperature immediately by undressing the patient, sponging with cool water, and directing the breeze from a fan onto the patient. Further diagnostic and treatment measures are discussed in Chapter 38. Hospitalization is mandatory.

9. MENINGOENCEPHALITIS

Diagnosis

A. Prodromal Symptoms: Prodromal symptoms such as fever, headache, malaise, or upper respiratory tract symptoms are present for hours to days; 20% of patients are in a coma when first seen by a physician.

B. Headache: Headache is a common and characteristic symptom, and stuporous patients should be aroused and asked if they have a headache.

C. Meningeal Signs: The physician should look carefully for meningeal signs so that lumbar puncture can be performed if necessary and a diagnosis made as soon as possible. Can the neck be fully flexed so that the chin touches the chest (with the mouth closed), or is movement limited? Is there knee flexion, even slight, during passive neck flexion? Does the neck or contralateral knee flex during unilateral raising of the straight leg? These signs of meningeal irritation may be absent in deep coma or at the extremes of age.

D. Cerebrospinal Fluid: The cerebrospinal fluid pressure may be as high as 600 mm water. White cell counts can range from as few as 10 monocytes/mL in patients with viral meningoencephalitis to over 10,000 cells/mL, mainly PMNs, in patients with purulent bacterial meningitis. Rare patients with viral encephalitis and some patients with overwhelming bacterial meningitis show acellular cerebrospinal fluid on the first lumbar puncture, but in overwhelming bacterial meningitis, organisms may be seen on Gram-stained slides. In patients with bacterial meningitis, cerebrospinal fluid glucose is commonly below 40 mg/dL (often in the range of 5–10 mg/dL) when blood glucose is normal; in viral encephalitis, cerebrospinal fluid glucose is almost always normal.

Treatment & Disposition

Start antibiotic therapy immediately based on clinical findings and microscopic examination of cerebrospinal fluid (see Table 34–3).

Hospitalization is indicated in all patients with meningitis who present in coma.

10. SUBARACHNOID HEMORRHAGE

Blood may be found in the cerebrospinal fluid of a patient with intracerebral hemorrhage or head trauma; however, the term subarachnoid hemorrhage normally implies bleeding from a ruptured cerebral aneurysm or, less commonly, hemorrhage from a cerebral arteriovenous malformation. Aneurysmal bleeding is uncommon before age 30, whereas arteriovenous malformations may bleed much earlier, even in childhood. Ruptured mycotic aneurysm from subacute infective endocarditis is rare but may be seen at any age. About one-half of patients die within the first month following bleeding. Coma from subarachnoid hemorrhage is the result of many factors, including the contusive force of the bleeding, communicating hydrocephalus, cerebral vasospasm, altered cortical metabolic activity, and transtentorial herniation.

Diagnosis

The onset of symptoms is abrupt and accompanied by headache that is unique in the patient's experience and not necessarily severe. Consciousness is often lost at the onset. The markedly elevated blood pressure (seen in 50% of patients) is a common result of the hemorrhage and is not an indication of preceding hypertension. Decerebrate posturing or, rarely, seizures may also occur early, and moderate to marked confusion is frequent if the patient is conscious. Prominent focal signs are uncommon; bilateral extensor plantar responses occur. Meningeal irritation (as shown by nuchal rigidity) may take several hours to develop and may disappear when the patient is in deep coma. Optic fundi may show acute hemorrhages secondary to suddenly increased intracranial pressure or the more classic superficial subhyaloid (preretinal) hemorrhages.

Lumbar puncture should be performed to confirm the diagnosis of subarachnoid hemorrhage unless classic findings are seen on CT scan. Cerebrospinal fluid pressure is usually markedly elevated, often higher than 600 mm water, and the cerebrospinal fluid is grossly bloody and contains from 100,000 to more than 1 million red blood cells per microliter. In rare cases, fewer than 100,000 red cells are seen. The white blood cell to erythrocyte ratio in cerebrospinal fluid is initially the same as in the peripheral blood.

The noninfectious meningitis that results from blood in the subarachnoid space may produce a pleocytosis of several thousand white blood cells during the first 48 hours. A reduction in cerebrospinal fluid glucose resulting from this "chemical" meningitis may occur between the fourth and eighth days after hemorrhage.

Useful radiologic aids include a CT scan (which shows blood in the subarachnoid space in more than 85% of patients) and cerebral angiography (which demonstrates the site of bleeding).

Treatment

Protect the airway. Establish the diagnosis by CT scan or, if CT scan is not diagnostic, by lumbar puncture. Sedate the patient with diazepam, 5–10 mg intravenously or orally, if needed. Avoid hypotension by correcting fluid imbalance with infusion of crystalloid solutions. Obtain emergency neurosurgical consultation.

Disposition

All patients require hospitalization.

HYSTERICAL COMA

Diagnosis

Hysterical coma is a diagnosis of exclusion that should be made only after careful documentation. The general physical examination should elicit no abnormalities; neurologic examination generally reveals flaccid, symmetrically decreased muscle tone, normal and symmetric reflexes, and the normal downward response to Babinski plantar stimulation. The pupils are normal in size (2–3 mm) or occasionally larger and respond briskly to light. Lateral eye movements elicited with the doll's eye maneuver may or may not be present, since visual fixation can suppress this reflex.

Differentiating Hysterical Coma From Organic Coma

A. Eye Movements: The slow, conjugate roving eye movements of patients in metabolic coma cannot be imitated and, if present, are incompatible with a diagnosis of hysterical unconsciousness.

B. Eyelid Tone: The slow, often asymmetric and incomplete eyelid closure commonly seen in organic forms of coma following passive opening of the lids cannot be mimicked. In addition, the hysteric usually shows some voluntary muscle tone of the eyelids during passive opening by the examiner.

C. Ice-Water Caloric Response: A helpful objective test in diagnosing hysterical unconsciousness is the caloric test: there is no response at all or tonic deviation to the side of the irrigation in organic coma, but nystagmus occurs in hysterical coma. Since the quick (return) phase of nystagmus requires an intact cortex, its presence is incompatible with a diagnosis of true coma.

D. EEG: The EEG in hysterical coma is that of a normal, awake person. In coma due to other causes, it is invariably abnormal.

Treatment & Disposition

Obtain psychiatric consultation. Hospitalization may be required. See Chapter 41 for details.

CRITERIA FOR BRAIN DEATH

The most recent standards for the determination of brain death are those of the President's Commission for the Study of Ethical Problems in Medicine and Biomedical and Behavioral Research, summarized below. Both cessation and irreversibility of brain function are required for a diagnosis of brain death.

Cessation of Brain Function

A. Unreceptivity and Unresponsivity: The patient must be unresponsive to sensory input (pain and voice).

B. Absent Brain Stem Reflexes: Pupillary, corneal, and oropharyngeal responses are absent, and attempts to elicit eye movements with the doll's eye maneuver or caloric testing are unsuccessful. Respiratory responses are likewise absent, as shown by the apnea test, ie, absence of ventilatory effort after the patient's PCO_2 is permitted to rise to 60 mm Hg. PCO_2 rises at a rate of 4 mm Hg/min in the absence of ventilation. Maintain oxygenation by giving 100% oxygen by a cannula inserted into the endotracheal tube.

Irreversibility of Brain Function

A. Coma: The cause of coma must be known and adequate to explain the clinical picture.

B. Absence of Other Causes of Coma: Sedative drug intoxication, hypothermia (< 32.2 °C [90 °F]), neuromuscular blockade, and shock must be ruled out as causes of coma.

Persistence of Criteria

The criteria for brain death described above must persist for an appropriate length of time, as follows:

A. Six hours with a confirmatory isoelectric (flat) EEG.

B. Twelve hours without a confirmatory isoelectric EEG.

C. Twenty-four hours for anoxic brain injury without a confirmatory isoelectric EEG.

Note: The diagnosis of brain death in children under 5 years of age must be made with caution.

REFERENCES

Chun CH et al: Brain abscess: A study of 45 consecutive cases. Medicine 1986;65:415.

Dunne JW, Chakera T, Kermode S: Cerebellar haemorrhage—Diagnosis and treatment: A study of 75 consecutive cases. Q J Med 1987;64:739.

Edwards RH, Simon RP: Coma. Chapter 19 in: *Clinical Neurology,* 14th ed. Baker AB, Joynt RJ (editors). Harper & Row, 1986.

Executive Board, American Academy of Neurology: Position of the American Academy of Neurology on certain aspects of the care and management of the persistent vegetative state patient. Neurology 1989;39:125.

Ferbert A, Bruckmann H, Drummen R: Clinical features of proven basilar artery occlusion. Stroke 1990;21:1135.

Fischbeck KH, Simon RP: Neurological manifestations of accidental hypothermia. Ann Neurol 1981;10:384.

Fisher CM: The neurological examination of the comatose patient. Acta Neurol Scand [Suppl] 1969;36:4.

Guidelines for the Determination of Death: Report of the Medical Consultants on the Diagnosis of Death to the President's Commission for the Study of Ethical Problems in Medicine and Biomedical and Behavioral Research. Neurology 1982;32:395 and JAMA 1981;246:2184.

Helliwell M et al: Value of emergency toxicological investigations in differential diagnosis of coma. Br Med J 1979;2:819.

Higashi K et al: Five-year follow-up study of patients with persistent vegetative state. J Neurol Neurosurg Psychiatry 1981;44:552.

Kase CS et al: Lobar intracerebral hematomas: Clinical and CT analysis of 22 cases. Neurology 1982;32:1146.

Kushner MJ, Bressman SB: The clinical manifestations of pontine hemorrhage. Neurology 1985;35:637.

Levy DE et al: Predicting outcome from hypoxic-ischemic coma. JAMA 1985;253:1420.

Macdonnell RAL, Kalnins RM, Donnan GA: Cerebellar infarction: Natural history, prognosis, and pathology. Stroke 1987;18:849.

Malouf R, Brust JC: Hypoglycemia: Causes, neurological manifestations, and outcome. Ann Neurol 1985;17:421.

McCusker EA et al: Recovery from the "locked-in" syndrome. Arch Neurol 1982;39:145.

Patterson JR, Grabois M: Locked-in syndrome: A review of 139 cases. Stroke 1986;17:758.

Plum F, Posner JB: *The Diagnosis of Stupor and Coma,* 3rd ed. Davis, 1980.

Seelig JM et al: Traumatic acute subdural hematoma: Major mortality reduction in comatose patients treated within 4 hours. N Engl J Med 1981;304:1511.

Wintzen AR: The clinical course of subdural hematoma: A retrospective study of etiological, chronological and pathological features in 212 patients and a proposed classification. Brain 1980;103:855.

Syncope, Seizures, & Other Causes of Episodic Loss of Consciousness

11

Roger P. Simon, MD

I. IMMEDIATE MANAGEMENT OF LIFE-THREATENING PROBLEMS (See algorithm.)

STATUS EPILEPTICUS

Diagnosis

A prolonged seizure (lasting more than 10–15 minutes), continuous seizures, or multiple seizure episodes without intervening periods of consciousness constitute status epilepticus.

Search carefully for seizure activity in the comatose patient. Manifestations may be subtle, eg, deviation of head or eyes, repetitive jerking of fingers, hands, or one side of the face.

Immediate Measures for Patient With Active Seizures

Perform the following in the order given here.

A. Protect the Airway: Roll the patient onto one side if possible. Endotracheal intubation may be necessary. Do not waste time trying to insert a tongue blade through clenched teeth, since it does not protect the airway and may cause broken teeth.

B. Insert an Intravenous Catheter: To start diagnostic evaluation (Table 11–1), obtain blood specimens for glucose, electrolytes, magnesium, and calcium determinations; hepatic and renal function tests; and CBC; as well as 3–4 tubes of blood for possible toxicology screen or drug levels (including anticonvulsants if patient is known or suspected to be taking them).

C. Rule Out Hypoglycemia: Give glucose, 50 mL of 50% solution intravenously over 5 minutes. *Note:* If malnutrition is suspected, give thiamine, 100 mg intravenously slowly prior to, or at the same time as, glucose.

D. Give Diazepam: Give diazepam (Valium, others) once only, 5–10 mg (or lorazepam, 2–4 mg) intravenously into a peripheral vein over 1–2 minutes (adult dose). This treatment is effective in 80–90% of cases of status epilepticus, although apnea, bradycardia, or hypotension may rarely result. *Caution:* Give diazepam or lorazepam only if the patient has active seizures.

E. Administer a Loading Dose of Phenytoin: Regardless of the effect of diazepam, a maintenance drug is required. Give phenytoin (Dilantin) in normal

---

Table 11–1. Emergency evaluation of the patient with seizures.

Vital signs
  Pulse: Rule out dangerous cardiac dysrhythmia, including cardiac arrest.
  Blood pressure: Rule out postural hypotension and shock.
  Body temperature: Rule out hyperthermia (> 41–42 °C [105.8–107.6 °F]).
History
  Trauma
  Previous seizures
  Drug/alcohol use
  Medications
Physical examination
  Papilledema
  Focal neurologic signs
  Evidence of systemic disease
  Heart murmur
Laboratory and special examinations
  Serum glucose: Hypoglycemia or hyperglycemia
  Arterial blood gases: Hypoxemia, hypercapnia, acidosis
  ECG: Cardiac arrhythmia
  Serum electrolytes: Hyponatremia or hypernatremia
  Approximate serum osmolality calculation (normal range: 270–290 mosm/L):

$$\text{Osmolality} = 2(\text{Na}^+ \text{ meq/L}) + \frac{\text{Glucose mg/dL}}{18}$$

  CBC with differential
  Serum calcium and magnesium measurements
  Hepatic and renal function studies
  Lumbar puncture (if signs of increased intracranial pressure are absent)
  Blood and urine samples for toxicologic studies (if indicated)
  CT scan (if focal signs are present)

---

saline, 15–18 mg/kg by intravenous infusion at a rate of 50 mg/min or slower. Infusion of phenytoin at more rapid rates (especially if given into centrally placed intravenous lines) can precipitate cardiac arrhythmias or hypotension.

F. Measure Arterial Blood Gases and pH: Arterial blood PCO_2 is a sensitive indicator of the adequacy of ventilation (hypercapnia is present in proportion to the degree of hypoventilation). Metabolic acidosis due to lactic acidosis resulting from status epilepticus is commonly present for as long as 1 hour after a seizure, depending on the duration and vigor of muscular activity. This acidosis requires no treatment. Acidosis lasting longer than 1 hour should prompt a search for other causes of acidosis (Chapter 36).

G. Maintain Ventilation: Patients in status epilepticus or those given anticonvulsant medications that are strong respiratory depressants (eg, phenobarbital) may require endotracheal intubation to protect the airway and maintain adequate ventilation. Monitor arterial blood gas measurements to assess adequacy of ventilation ($PO_2 \geq 80$ mm Hg and PCO_2 at an appropriate level).

H. Rule Out Meningitis: Perform lumbar puncture immediately to rule out meningitis if fever (body temperature > 38.5 °C [> 101.2 °F]) or nuchal rigidity is present. However, the muscle activity of status epilepticus alone produces transient fever higher than 38.5 °C (> 101.2 °F) in 25% of patients. Status epilepticus may also produce a mild transient cerebrospinal fluid pleocytosis (< 100 cells/μL).

I. Use Alternative Drugs If Necessary: If diazepam and phenytoin fail to stop the convulsions, use alternative drugs (Table 11–2).

J. Search for the Underlying Cause of Seizure: Emergency evaluation of the patient should proceed as outlined in Table 11–1. Common causes of seizures of acute onset are listed in Table 11–3.

Prevention of Injury

Prevent injury to the patient during the seizure by padding the environment. Do not use rigid restraint (fractures may result) or insert objects into the patient's mouth during the seizure.

Treatment During Postictal State

Do not give diazepam if the patient has postictal stupor or coma rather than active seizures. Further evaluation of the patient in stupor or coma should proceed as described in Chapter 10.

Phenytoin, 15–18 mg/kg loading dose orally or intravenously (Table 11–4), should be given to all patients except those who have a short-term metabolic condition known to cause seizures, such as alcohol withdrawal or hypoglycemia, which does not require or respond to phenytoin.

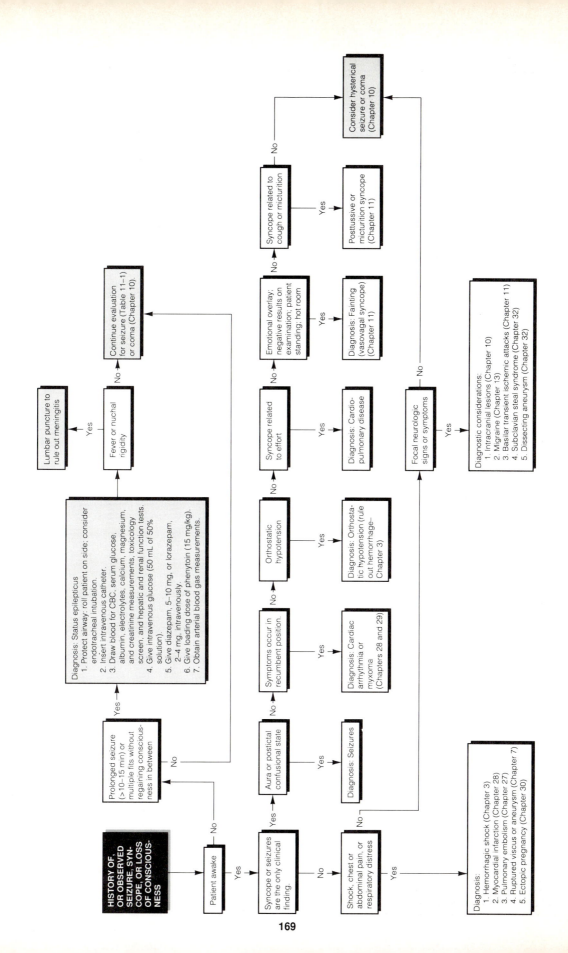

HISTORY OF OR OBSERVED SEIZURE, SYNCOPE, OR LOSS OF CONSCIOUSNESS

Patient awake

No →

Prolonged seizure (>10–15 min) or multiple fits without regaining consciousness in between

Yes →

Diagnosis: Status epilepticus
1. Protect airway; roll patient on side; consider endotracheal intubation.
2. Insert intravenous catheter.
3. Draw blood for CBC, serum glucose, albumin, electrolytes, calcium, magnesium, and creatinine measurements, toxicology screen, and hepatic and renal function tests.
4. Give intravenous glucose (50 mL of 50% solution).
5. Give diazepam, 5–10 mg, or lorazepam, 2–4 mg, intravenously.
6. Give loading dose of phenytoin (15 mg/kg).
7. Obtain arterial blood gas measurements.

↓

Fever or nuchal rigidity

Yes → Lumbar puncture to rule out meningitis

No →

Continue evaluation for seizure (Table 11–1) or coma (Chapter 10).

No (from Prolonged seizure) →

Yes →

Aura or postictal confusional state

Yes → Diagnosis: Seizures

No →

Symptoms occur in recumbent position.

Yes → Diagnosis: Cardiac arrhythmia or myxoma (Chapters 28 and 29)

No →

Orthostatic hypotension

Yes → Diagnosis: Orthostatic hypotension (rule out hemorrhage–Chapter 3)

No →

Syncope related to effort

Yes → Diagnosis: Cardiopulmonary disease

No →

Emotional overlay; negative results on examination; patient standing; hot room

Yes → Diagnosis: Fainting (vasovagal syncope) (Chapter 11)

No →

Syncope related to cough or micturition

Yes → Posttussive or micturition syncope (Chapter 11)

No → Consider hysterical seizure or coma (Chapter 10)

Syncope or seizures are the only clinical finding.

Yes (up to Aura or postictal)

No →

Shock, chest or abdominal pain, or respiratory distress

No →

Focal neurologic signs or symptoms

Yes → Diagnostic considerations:
1. Intracranial lesions (Chapter 10)
2. Migraine (Chapter 13)
3. Basilar transient ischemic attacks (Chapter 11)
4. Subclavian steal syndrome (Chapter 32)
5. Dissecting aneurysm (Chapter 32)

No → Consider hysterical seizure or coma (Chapter 10)

Yes →

Diagnosis:
1. Hemorrhagic shock (Chapter 3)
2. Myocardial infarction (Chapter 28)
3. Pulmonary embolism (Chapter 27)
4. Ruptured viscus or aneurysm (Chapter 7)
5. Ectopic pregnancy (Chapter 30)

Table 11–2. Drug treatment of status epilepticus.

Drug	Dose and Route	Advantages, Disadvantages, and Complications
First-line drug: Diazepam (Valium, others) *or* Lorazepam (Ativan, others)	10 mg intravenously (adult dose). *Do not* administer intramuscularly, because absorption is erratic. 2–4 mg intravenously.	Fast acting (lipid-soluble), short half-life intravenously (½–4 hours for diazepam; up to 16 hours for lorazepam). Respiratory depression occurs, especially if barbiturates must be added. Other complications are bradycardia and hypotension. ***Note:*** Regardless of effectiveness of diazepam, maintenance drug (phenytoin or phenobarbital) must be added to prevent recurrence of seizures.
Proceed immediately to phenytoin. Phenytoin (Dilantin, others)	1000–1500 mg (15–18 mg/kg) slowly intravenously at a rate not greater than 50 mg/min, given directly into the vein (cannot be given through dextrose-containing solutions; use saline only).	No respiratory depression. Therapeutic drug levels in the brain are achieved by the time the infusion has been completed. Effective as maintenance drug. Hypotension and cardiac arrhythmias may occur, especially in elderly patients. Infusion rate of 100 mg/min is safe during active seizures.
If seizures persist following total dose of phenytoin, immediately proceed to phenobarbital. Phenobarbital (Luminal, many others)	700 mg (10 mg/kg) intravenously at a rate of 50–100 mg/min.	Respiratory depression and hypotension common with increasing doses (intubation and ventilatory support should be immediately available). Effective as maintenance drug.
If the above is ineffective, the following third-line drugs may be tried, or one can proceed immediately to general anesthesia. Paraldehyde	Rectally: 5–10 mL diluted in 2 volumes of mineral oil *or* Intramuscularly: 5–10 mL (maximum 5 mL/site) *or* Intravenously: 0.1–0.15 mL/kg (4% solution: 200 mL paraldehyde in 500 mL normal saline).	Decomposes with storage; can cause metabolic acidosis, pulmonary hemorrhage, cardiovascular depression, and proctitis (if given rectally). Use glass syringe (paraldehyde causes plastic to break down); safely administered intravenously in 4% solution. Absorption is rapid following intramuscular administration but slow with the rectal route.
Lidocaine (Xylocaine, many others)	50 mg intravenously. If effective, then 50–100 mg diluted in 250 mL of 5% dextrose and infused at a rate of 1–2 mg/min.	Higher doses may cause seizures. Minimal adverse effects on cardiac output and evaluation. Reduce dose in congestive heart failure or liver disease.
If the above is ineffective, proceed immediately to general anesthesia. Pentobarbital (Nembutal, others)	15 mg/kg slowly intravenously; then 0.5–1 mg/kg/h.	Hypotension is limiting factor; respiratory depression is routine.
Thiopental (Pentothal)	15 mg/kg slowly intravenously, followed by 5 mg/kg/h drip.	Brain half-life less than 30 minutes; hypotension is limiting factor; respiratory depression is routine.
Amobarbital (Amytal, others)	200–1000 mg slowly intravenously.	Hypotension is limiting factor; respiratory depression is routine.

II. EVALUATION OF THE CONSCIOUS PATIENT WITH A HISTORY OF SYNCOPE

Rule Out Blood Loss

In the *awake* patient with a history of one or more episodes of loss of consciousness, first rule out acute blood loss due to various causes.

A. Measure blood pressure and pulse. **Supine hypotension** (systolic blood pressure < 90 mm Hg) or severe peripheral vasoconstriction should be considered evidence of hemorrhagic shock until proved otherwise (Chapter 3).

Orthostatic hypotension—shown by a significant fall in blood pressure or rise in pulse rate as the patient moves from lying to sitting ($\geq$ 10 mm Hg or $\geq$ 20 beats/min) or standing ($\geq$ 15 mm Hg or $\geq$ 30 beats/min) (test in both positions if possible)—is also strong evidence of hypovolemia, although the urgency of evaluation is less, since there are many conditions that can produce postural hypotension in the absence of hypovolemia (Table 11–7).

B. Gain venous access with an intravenous catheter ($\geq$ 18-gauge), and give a crystalloid solution (eg, normal saline) as needed. Obtain blood for CBC, electrolyte and glucose determinations, renal and hepatic function tests and a tube of clotted blood to be sent, if needed, for typing and cross-matching. If blood loss is suspected and the hematocrit or hemo-

Table 11–3. Common causes of seizures of acute onset.

Disorder	Comment
Primary central nervous system disorders	
Idiopathic epilepsy	Onset uncommon after age 25.
Head trauma	Especially acute trauma or when associated with depressed skull fracture or subdural hematoma.
Stroke	Especially in hemorrhagic stroke.
Central nervous system mass lesion	Primary or metastatic tumor; brain abscess; arteriovenous malformation.
Metabolic or systemic disorders	
Cerebral hypoperfusion (hypoxia)	Cardiopulmonary arrest; cardiac dysrhythmia; severe hypotension, etc (Chapters 1, 3, 28).
Meningitis, encephalitis	Acute or chronic; bacterial, viral, fungal, parasitic, etc. (Chapter 34).
Hyponatremia	Serum sodium usually less than 120 and often less than 110 meq/L (Chapter 36).
Hypoglycemia	Serum glucose usually less than 40 mg/dL (Chapter 35).
Hyperosmolality	Serum osmolalty usually greater than 300 mosm/L (Chapter 36).
Hypertensive encephalopathy	Blood pressure usually greater than 250/150 mm Hg; seizures may occur at lower pressures (usually > 160/100 mm Hg) when hypertension occurs suddenly (eg, in children with acute renal failure) (Chapter 28).
Uremic encephalopathy	
Hepatic encephalopathy	Respiratory alkalosis nearly always present.
Eclamptogenic toxemia	
Acute drug overdosage	Especially with tricyclic antidepressants, theophylline (aminophylline), phencyclidine (PCP), lidocaine, phenothiazines, isoniazid (Chapter 39).
Acute drug withdrawal	Anticonvulsants, ethanol, or sedative-hypnotic drugs (with habituation to daily doses of 600–800 mg secobarbital or its equivalent).
Benign febrile convulsions of childhood	Do not occur after age 5; always consider other causes.
Hyperthermia	Internal body temperature usually above 41–42 °C (105.8–107.6 °F); *immediate* reduction of body temperature to 39 °C (102.2 °F) is mandatory (Chapter 38).

globin is normal, a repeat determination after volume repletion may confirm blood loss. Serial CBCs may be helpful in detecting active bleeding.

C. Check stool specimens for blood (gross and microscopic).

D. Nasogastric intubation may be indicated in suspected gastrointestinal tract bleeding or in syncope with unexplained postural hypotension. *Caution:* Upper gastrointestinal tract bleeding cannot be ruled out unless the nasogastric tube aspirate contains bile. Otherwise, brisk bleeding distal to the pyloric sphincter (eg, duodenal ulcer) may be missed if the sphincter is closed (Chapter 8).

E. Consider pelvic bleeding (eg, ruptured ectopic pregnancy) or trauma, especially that which is not visually obvious, such as splenic, hepatic, retroperitoneal, or pelvic injury.

Determine Presence or Absence of Related Symptoms

A. Syncope Associated With Prominent Abdominal or Pelvic Pain: Patients with abdominal or pelvic pain may have hypovolemic syncope secondary to gastrointestinal hemorrhage, leaking aortic aneurysm, or ruptured ectopic pregnancy. Aortic dissection and rupture of a viscus into the peritoneal

cavity may also produce syncope initially by vagal stimulation or later as a result of blood loss. See Chapter 7 for further evaluation.

B. Syncope Associated With Chest Pain or Dyspnea: Consider myocardial infarction, pulmonary embolism, tension pneumothorax, or dissecting aortic aneurysm (Chapter 6).

C. Syncope Associated With Neurologic Symptoms (eg, Headache, Vertigo, Diplopia): Obtain neurologic consultation for possible basilar artery insufficiency, migraine, and subclavian steal syndrome. *Loss of consciousness as an isolated symptom is rarely if ever caused by basilar artery ischemia.*

Further Evaluation of Syncope

A detailed, accurate history from the patient, family, observers, or ambulance attendants is the most important factor in making the diagnosis. The most helpful features are the following:

A. Epileptic Aura: History of an epileptic aura preceding the syncopal attack or a period of confusion (postictal state) upon regaining consciousness strongly suggests seizures as the diagnosis. This aura must be differentiated from symptoms of decreased cerebral blood flow, eg, those occurring before a syn-

Table 11–4. Summary of anticonvulsant drug therapy.

Drug	Doses			Serum Half-Life (Normal Renal and Hepatic Function)	Serum Levels (μg/mL)		Symptoms of Toxicity	Indications
	Intravenous Loading	Oral Loading	Maintenance		Therapeutic	Toxic		
Phenytoin (Dilantin, others)	1000–1500 mg (15–18 mg/kg) directly into a large vein, not exceeding 50 mg/min. Continuous electrocardiographic monitoring is mandatory. Cannot be infused in dextrose solutions (eg, 5% dextrose in water).	1000 mg in 24 divided doses over 12–24 hours.	300–400 mg/d in a single dose or 23 divided doses.	Oral: 22 hours. Intravenous: 12 hours. (Kinetics are dose-dependent and may vary widely.)	10–20.	Above 30.	Ataxia, nystagmus, somnolence. (Nystagmus on extreme lateral gaze suggests therapeutic drug level.)	Grand mal, focal motor, and complex partial (temporal lobe) seizures.
Phenobarbital (Luminal, many others)	700 mg (10 mg/kg) over 10–20 minutes. Ventilatory support equipment must be available at bedside.	180 mg twice a day for 3 days.	90–180 mg in a single daily dose.	4 days.	10–30.	Above 40.	Ataxia, somnolence.	Grand mal, focal motor, and complex partial (temporal lobe) seizures.
Carbamazepine (Tegretol, others)	No intravenous preparation.	200 mg twice a day; increase by 200 mg daily to maintenance dose.	400 mg 2–3 times a day.	15 hours.	4–8.	Above 8.	Nausea, ataxia, diplopia.	Complex partial (temporal lobe) and grand mal seizures.
Valproic acid (Depakene, Depakote, others)	No intravenous preparation.	None.	750–2000 mg/d twice daily.	6–13 hours.	50–150.	Above 150 mg/dL.	Drowsiness and nausea at onset.	Myoclonic, photic-induced absence (petit mal) and refractory seizures.

copal episode or as a result of orthostatic hypotension or cardiac arrhythmia.

B. Position of the Patient at Time of Loss of Consciousness: Episodes beginning when the patient is lying down suggest seizure or cardiac arrhythmia, whereas orthostatic hypotension and vasovagal syncope occur when the patient is standing or sitting up.

C. Syncope Related to Active Physical Exertion: Syncope following active physical exertion is frequently noted in cardiac outflow obstruction (eg, aortic stenosis, hypertrophic obstructive cardiomyopathy [idiopathic hypertrophic subaortic stenosis], myxoma) and is elicited occasionally in patients with cardiac arrhythmias or pulmonary vascular disease (rare).

D. Other Causes of Syncope: Micturition and coughing are associated with distinctive syncopal syndromes. Simple fainting may occur during the first trimester of pregnancy and must be differentiated from syncope due to blood loss from ectopic pregnancy. Rare causes of syncope include Meniere's disease (look for associated deafness and vertigo), glossopharyngeal neuralgia (throat or neck pain), hyperventilation, and hysteria.

III. EMERGENCY TREATMENT OF SPECIFIC DISORDERS CAUSING EPISODIC LOSS OF CONSCIOUSNESS

SEIZURES (Epilepsy)

Seizures can result from a primary central nervous system disorder or may be a manifestation of a serious underlying metabolic or systemic disorder. The distinction is critical, since therapy must be directed at the underlying disorder as well as at control of the seizure. A list of common central nervous system, metabolic, and systemic disorders that may cause seizures is given in Table 11–3.

Diagnosis

Clinically, seizures are diagnosed by episodes of loss of consciousness (or depressed consciousness) associated with an **aura** preceding the seizure (50% of patients) and a period of confusion (**postictal state**) following it. The commonest type of seizure is grand mal epilepsy (generalized major motor convulsions). Firm diagnosis of subtler types of seizure (partial seizures, eg, complex partial or "temporal lobe" attacks) may require an EEG. For alcohol and drug withdrawal seizures, see Chapter 14.

Seizures, especially those of status epilepticus, are accompanied by the following clinical abnormalities:

A. Fever: Internal body temperatures as high as 42 °C (107.6 °F) may develop because of intense muscular activity. Temperatures higher than 40 °C (104 °F) should be corrected (Chapter 38).

B. Leukocytosis: The peripheral leukocyte count may reach 60,000/μL, perhaps as a result of demargination of leukocytes secondary to catecholamine release; band cells, however, are rare.

C. Acidosis: Lactic acidosis is universal after a single major motor seizure, owing to maximal muscle exertion; arterial blood pH may reach 6.8–7.1. Lactic acidosis due to seizures is transient (< 1 hour) and benign and need not be corrected. It is not associated with shifts in potassium or hyperkalemia. Acidosis does not follow hysterical seizures.

D. Trauma: Trauma occurs commonly during seizures, especially tongue and cheek bites. Fractures and joint dislocations may occur.

E. Cerebrospinal Fluid Abnormalities: Elevation of the cerebrospinal fluid leukocyte count (usually less than 50/μL and predominantly PMNs) may follow severe seizures. Infection must be ruled out by cultures.

Treatment

For treatment of status epilepticus, see p 167 and Table 11–2. Pharmacologic characteristics of the most commonly used anticonvulsant drugs are listed in Table 11–4.

Disposition

It is preferable to hospitalize all patients having seizures for the first time, or patients with focal signs, so that diagnostic studies can be performed and the patient observed. Patients with established seizure disorders may be sent home several hours after the seizures have ceased if no acute abnormalities are found. They should be referred to their regular source of medical care within a few days. Patients with **alcohol withdrawal** may have seizures for 6–12 hours following the first occurrence; 95% of any additional seizures occur during this period. No antiepileptic drugs have been shown to be effective in this syndrome. Phenytoin is clearly ineffective; phenobarbital and lorazepam, while useful in theory, have not demonstrated efficacy in controlled studies. Chronic anticonvulsant administration is not necessary for alcohol withdrawal seizures alone. (See also Chapter 14.) Hospitalization for alcohol withdrawal seizures is usually not needed if the patient can be reliably observed (eg, at a detoxification center or by family or friends) and treated with benzodiazepines.

SIMPLE FAINTS (Vasovagal Syncope)

Vasovagal disorders are exceedingly common, occur in all age groups (mean age is 40 years), and affect men and women equally. Common precipitating factors are shown in Table 11–5.

Physiologic decreases in both arterial pressure and heart rate mediated by the vagus nerve combine to produce central nervous system hypoperfusion and subsequent syncope. Prolonged cerebral hypoxia with resultant tonic-clonic movements is more likely to occur if the patient remains upright.

Diagnosis

Vasovagal episodes begin in a standing or sitting position and only rarely in a horizontal position.

A. Prodrome: The prodrome lasts from 10 seconds to a few minutes and includes weakness, lightheadedness, nausea, pallor, sweating, salivation, blurred vision, and tachycardia.

B. Syncope: Brain hypoperfusion causes dimming of vision; the patient then loses consciousness and sinks to the ground. Examination reveals an unconscious individual who is pale and sweating and who has dilated pupils and a slow, weak pulse. With loss of consciousness, bradycardia replaces tachycardia.

C. Associated Symptoms: Abnormal movements may be noted during the period of unconsciousness. These are mainly tonic or opisthotonic, but tonic-clonic activity is occasionally manifested. Urinary incontinence may occur, but tongue biting is rare.

D. Postsyncopal Findings: The patient is lucid and awake seconds to less than a minute after sinking to a recumbent position; a postictal confusional state is absent unless a convulsion has occurred. However, nervousness, dizziness, headache, nausea and vomiting, pallor, perspiration, and an urge to defecate may persist for hours.

E. Recurrence: Syncope may recur, especially if the patient stands up within 30 minutes after the attack. Syncope due to a specific precipitating factor (eg, cough) can be reproduced in the emergency department.

Treatment

Reassurance and a recommendation to avoid precipitating factors are usually all that is necessary. Cough suppression and sitting down to urinate are helpful in posttussive and micturitional syncope. Adequate nutrition and hydration should be encouraged.

Table 11–5. Common factors precipitating vasovagal syncope (fainting).

Emotional upset
Sight of blood
Sudden exposure to cold
Prolonged motionless standing
Medical or surgical procedures
Injury
Pain
Blood loss
Cough
Micturition
Migraine
Early pregnancy

Disposition

Refer the patient to an outpatient clinic or primary-care physician after a period of observation and confirmation of the diagnosis in the emergency department.

CARDIOPULMONARY SYNCOPE

A cardiovascular origin for syncope is suggested when it occurs during recumbency, during or following physical exertion, or in a patient with known heart disease. Loss of consciousness in cardiac disease is most often due to an abrupt decrease in cardiac output, with subsequent cerebral hypoperfusion producing symptoms identical to those of fainting. Such cardiac dysfunction may result from rhythm disturbances (bradyarrhythmias or tachyarrhythmias), cardiac inflow or outflow obstruction, acute myocardial infarction, intracardiac right-to-left shunts, leaking or dissecting aortic aneurysms, or acute pulmonary embolus. Table 11–6 lists some of the more common cardiopulmonary causes of syncope.

CARDIAC ARREST
(See also Chapter 1.)

Diagnosis

Loss of consciousness due to cardiac arrest (ventricular fibrillation or asystole) from any cause occurs in 3–5 seconds if the patient is standing or within 15 seconds if the patient is recumbent. The patient usually rapidly regains consciousness if adequate cardiac output is restored promptly; most patients who regain consciousness within 12 hours will recover without neurologic sequelae.

Seizures are uncommon but are more likely to occur the longer the cerebral hypoperfusion lasts. A postictal confusional state occurs in patients who have convulsed.

Treatment & Disposition

Initiate CPR; see Chapter 1 for further details. Immediate hospitalization in an intensive care unit for evaluation and treatment is required.

ACUTE MYOCARDIAL INFARCTION
(See also Chapter 28.)

Rarely, myocardial infarction is manifested by syncope without chest pain. This condition is discussed in detail in Chapter 28. Hospitalization is required in every case.

Table 11–6. Common causes of syncope due to cardiopulmonary and cerebrovascular disease.

Cardiac arrest due to any cause
Acute myocardial infarction
Cardiac dysrhythmias
  Tachyarrhythmias
    Supraventricular
      Paroxysmal atrial tachycardia
      Atrial flutter
      Atrial fibrillation
      Accelerated junctional tachycardia
    Ventricular
      Ventricular tachycardia
      Ventricular fibrillation
  Bradyarrhythmias
    Sinus bradycardia
    Sinus arrest
    Second-degree or complete (third-degree) heart block
    Implanted pacemaker failure or malfunction
  Mitral valve prolapse (click-murmur syndrome)
  Prolonged QT interval syndromes
  Sick sinus syndromes (tachycardia-bradycardia syndrome)
  Drug toxicity (especially digitalis, quinidine or procainamide, propranolol, phenothiazines, tricyclic antidepressants, potassium)
Cardiac inflow obstruction
  Left atrial myxoma or thrombus
  Constrictive pericarditis or cardiac tamponade
  Tension pneumothorax
Cardiac outflow obstruction
  Aortic stenosis
  Pulmonary stenosis
  Hypertrophic obstructive cardiomyopathy (idiopathic hypertrophic subaortic stenosis)
Severe pulmonary hypertension due to any cause
  Pulmonary hypertension
  Acute pulmonary embolus
Cerebrovascular syncope
  Basilar artery insufficiency
  Subclavian steal syndrome
  Migraine
  Takayasu's disease
  Carotid sinus syncope
Orthostatic hypotension

CARDIAC ARRHYTHMIAS
(See also Chapter 29.)

Diagnosis

See Table 11–6 for arrhythmias associated with syncope.

Palpitations, fatigue, dyspnea, or chest pain may precede loss of consciousness. Atypical chest pain (mainly nonexertional, left precordial, sharp, and of variable duration) suggests mitral valve prolapse.

Rapid ($\geq$ 160 beats/min), slow ($\leq$ 50 beats/min), or irregular pulse must be carefully investigated. Tachycardia of 180–200 beats/min will produce syncope in half of normal persons. In patients with underlying heart disease or atherosclerosis, tachycardia as slow as 135 beats/min or bradycardia as fast as 60 beats/min may result in loss of consciousness.

Chest auscultation with the patient in various positions (eg, sitting, left lateral decubitus, squatting) may disclose abnormal murmurs and clicks in the case of mitral valve prolapse.

The ECG may confirm the diagnosis of arrhythmia, heart block, sick sinus, or prolonged QT interval. However, a single ECG, obtained when the patient is asymptomatic, is frequently normal or nondiagnostic of a rhythm abnormality responsible for the syncope. A diagnosis can be firmly established only by demonstrating arrhythmias during symptomatic periods.

Treatment & Disposition

Patients with syncopal attacks thought to be due to cardiac disease should be hospitalized for a period of continuous electrocardiographic monitoring.

CARDIAC INFLOW OBSTRUCTION
(See also Chapter 28.)

Diagnosis

Patients with atrial or ventricular myxomas and atrial thrombi usually present with embolization but may also have sudden loss of cardiac output and syncope; syncope occurring with change in position is classic but uncommon. Left atrial myxoma often mimics mitral stenosis but is occasionally manifested by mitral regurgitation murmur. Mitral valve prolapse may also cause syncope.

Constrictive pericarditis or cardiac tamponade causes reduced cardiac output and may result in syncope. Any maneuver or drug that decreases heart rate or venous return will further impair cardiac output. The diagnosis is suggested by the presence of engorged neck veins, clear lung fields on chest x-ray, weak pulse, and hypotension (Chapter 28).

Tension pneumothorax reduces cardiac output by decreasing venous return and may produce syncope. There is usually a history of chest trauma or chronic pulmonary disease with bullae. Chest x-ray and physical examination confirm the diagnosis. (See Chapter 18 for details.)

Treatment & Disposition

Patients with syncope thought to be due to cardiac inflow obstruction require immediate treatment and hospitalization.

CARDIAC OUTFLOW OBSTRUCTION

1. AORTIC STENOSIS

Loss of consciousness secondary to congenital or acquired severe stenosis may occur in all age groups. Exertional syncope occurs as a result of cerebral hypoperfusion due to exercise-induced vasodilation in the presence of a fixed cardiac output. Two other pathophysiologic events are recognized: **(1)** acute transient left ventricular failure with normal sinus rhythm and (2) transient arrhythmia or cardiac standstill, causing an acute drop in cardiac output. Sudden death may result. Autonomic insufficiency also has been reported in these patients. Reflex peripheral vascular vasodilation (presumably due to left ventricular baroreceptor activity) has been demonstrated in the absence of cardiac arrhythmia.

Diagnosis

Syncope usually follows exercise and is often associated with dyspnea, anginal chest pain, and sweating. Physical findings that occur with hemodynamically severe aortic stenosis include the following:

(1) Characteristic midsystolic ejection murmur (often associated with a palpable thrill).

(2) Sustained and prolonged left ventricular lift.

(3) Paradoxically split second sound.

(4) Delayed upstroke and reduced amplitude (pulsus parvus et tardus) on the carotid pulse.

Treatment & Disposition

Promptly hospitalize all patients with symptomatic aortic stenosis (angina, congestive heart failure, or syncope) to evaluate them for possible valve replacement. Median survival time following the initial episode of syncope due to aortic stenosis in the patient who does not receive a prosthesis is 1.5–3 years.

2. PULMONARY STENOSIS

Diagnosis

Severe pulmonary stenosis may produce syncope, especially following exertion. A hemodynamic process similar to that of aortic stenosis is responsible. Physical findings include right parasternal lift, systolic ejection murmur at the upper left sternal border, a prominent fourth heart sound, and a conspicuous a wave in the jugular venous pulse.

Treatment & Disposition

Immediate hospitalization is required, since the pathophysiology and prognosis of this condition are similar to those of aortic stenosis.

3. HYPERTROPHIC OBSTRUCTIVE CARDIOMYOPATHY

Hypertrophic obstructive cardiomyopathy is also known as asymmetric septal hypertrophy or idiopathic hypertrophic subaortic stenosis (IHSS).

Diagnosis

Symptoms include syncope with exercise, dyspnea on exertion, and chest pain. Physical findings include a prominent fourth heart sound, left ventricular lift, transient arrhythmias, and systolic ejection murmur

and perhaps a thrill, both of which increase with exercise and increase with decreased left ventricular chamber size (eg, as produced during the Valsalva maneuver).

Echocardiography confirms the diagnosis.

Treatment & Disposition

Hospitalize the patient for further evaluation and treatment.

PULMONARY VASCULAR DISEASE (See also Chapter 27.)

Diagnosis

A. Pulmonary Hypertension: Syncope, often exertional, can be the presenting symptom of pulmonary hypertension. A history of dyspnea is invariably obtained as well. Signs of right ventricular failure (parasternal lift, increased pulmonary second sound [P_2], right-sided S_4, and murmurs of pulmonary and tricuspid valvular insufficiency), electrocardiographic evidence of right ventricular hypertrophy, and tachypnea are often found.

B. Massive Pulmonary Embolism: Syncope is the presenting symptom in approximately 20% of patients experiencing massive pulmonary embolism. When the patient regains consciousness after syncope, pleuritic chest pain, dyspnea, and apprehension are present. Hypotension, tachycardia, tachypnea, and significant hypoxemia frequently accompany large embolism, and death may occur.

Treatment & Disposition

Provide supplemental oxygen (10 L/min) and assisted ventilation where necessary. See Chapter 27 for further evaluation and treatment. Hospitalization is usually required.

CEREBROVASCULAR SYNCOPE

Although syncope resulting from cerebrovascular disease is often diagnosed, such an association is in fact uncommon, since consciousness is lost only when the function of both cerebral hemispheres or the brain stem reticular formation is compromised (see Table 11–6 and Chapter 10).

BASILAR ARTERY INSUFFICIENCY (See also Chapter 12.)

Diagnosis

Basilar artery transient ischemic attacks (TIAs)

usually occur after age 65 years. Loss of consciousness is a rare manifestation.

Diplopia, vertigo, dysphagia, dysarthria, lateralized sensory or motor symptoms, and sudden bilateral leg weakness suggest brain stem ischemia. Syncope is rarely if ever the initial or isolated symptom.

Transient ischemic attacks typically are of sudden onset and brief duration (seconds to minutes), but when loss of consciousness has occurred, recovery is frequently prolonged (30–60 minutes or longer).

Treatment & Disposition

Accurate diagnosis of basilar artery insufficiency is often difficult, and neurologic referral is recommended. Hospitalization is indicated, especially when syncope has occurred. Treatment with aspirin should be started; the specific effective dose has not yet been clarified.

SUBCLAVIAN STEAL SYNDROME

Diagnosis

Patients with subclavian steal syndrome present with symptoms of vertebrobasilar artery insufficiency combined with symptoms of ipsilateral upper extremity ischemia.

The diagnosis is confirmed by the episodic signs and symptoms of basilar artery ischemia: syncope, vertigo, diplopia, limb paresis, paresthesias, and ataxia. Brain stem infarction (stroke) has not been reported to result from subclavian steal syndrome alone.

Blood pressures measured in the upper extremities are nearly always unequal. The average difference is a 45-mm Hg decrease in systolic pressure in the arm supplied by the stenotic vessel.

Treatment & Disposition

If subclavian steal syndrome is suspected, elective hospitalization for arteriography and perhaps surgical correction is indicated.

MIGRAINE
(See also Chapter 13.)

Syncope occurs in 10% of patients with migraine when they stand up suddenly. The timing of attacks suggests that loss of consciousness is due to orthostatic hypotension. For details of diagnosis and treatment, see Chapter 13.

CAROTID SINUS SYNCOPE

Diagnosis

Carotid sinus syncope classically results from pressure on an abnormally sensitive carotid sinus by a tight collar, neck mass, enlarged cervical nodes, or tumor. This pressure causes vagal stimulation that slows the sinoatrial and atrioventricular nodes and inhibits sympathetic vascular tone. The resulting bradycardia and systemic hypotension may then produce syncope. Bradycardia or hypotension may also occur without syncope. The syndrome may be reproduced in the emergency department by pressure on the carotid sinus while the patient is recumbent; an ECG documents the induced bradyarrhythmia. Such pressure may also produce syncope resulting from cerebral ischemia if the examiner compresses the artery contralateral to an occluded carotid artery. Syncope is then due to cerebral hypoperfusion secondary to cerebrovascular disease and not to hypersensitivity of the carotid sinus.

Treatment

The patient with syncope should be placed supine and pressure on the carotid sinus relieved (eg, by loosening a tight collar). Further therapy is seldom required. Unusually severe or persistent bradycardia can be abolished in some cases by administration of atropine, 0.5 mg intravenously.

Disposition

Refer the patient to an outpatient clinic or primary care physician for evaluation. The patient should be told to avoid possible causes of the attacks, eg, tight collars.

ORTHOSTATIC HYPOTENSION

Orthostatic hypotension occurs more often in men than in women and is most common in the sixth and seventh decades, although it may occur even in teenagers. Orthostatic hypotension may result from multiple disorders; the more common causes are listed in Table 11–7.

Diagnosis

Syncope often occurs following rapid change to the upright position, ie, from lying to sitting or from sitting to standing. Prolonged motionless standing, especially after exercise, or standing after prolonged bed rest may also cause syncope. Patients usually describe light-headedness, dimming of vision, weakness, and a fainting sensation. True vertigo does not occur.

Blood pressure that is significantly lower (> 10 mm Hg systolic difference) when standing than when supine is diagnostic. Orthostatic tachycardia may be present as well.

A stool sample should be evaluated for the presence of blood. CBC may reveal anemia or hemoconcentration due to blood loss or dehydration, respectively.

Table 11-7. Causes of orthostatic hypotension.

Drug-induced
  Phenothiazines (chlorpromazine, etc)
  Tricyclic antidepressants (amitriptyline, etc)
  Antihypertensives
  Diuretics
  Nitrates (nitroglycerine, etc)
  Levodopa
  Monoamine oxidase inhibitors
Peripheral neuropathies (see Chapter 10)
  Diabetic
  Amyloid
Hypovolemia or hemorrhage
Addison's disease
Acute or chronic spinal cord injury
Degenerative diseases of the central nervous system
  Parkinsonism
  Shy-Drager syndrome (anhidrosis, sphincter dysfunction, impotence)
Posterior fossa tumors
Sequelae of surgical sympathectomy

Electrolyte determinations should be made to detect abnormalities produced by dehydration or drugs. Serum drug levels should be obtained as indicated.

Treatment

A. Discontinue any offending medication.

B. Encourage oral fluid intake, or administer intravenous fluids to maintain hydration.

C. Replace blood if acute blood loss is significant, and locate the source of bleeding.

D. Instruct patients to stand up gradually, elevate the head of the bed on blocks, and use elasticized support stockings.

Disposition

Hospitalize the patient (**1**) if postural hypotension is currently producing symptoms and cannot be corrected easily in the emergency department, or (**2**) if an acute underlying cause of hypotension persists (eg, vomiting, diarrhea) or warrants hospitalization in any case (eg, gastrointestinal bleeding). Otherwise, refer the patient to an outpatient clinic or primary-care physician.

MISCELLANEOUS RARE CAUSES OF STATES OF ALTERED CONSCIOUSNESS

HYPERVENTILATION

Psychogenic hyperventilation is a frequent cause of altered consciousness (faintness, light-headedness, etc) but rarely culminates in syncope. Acute anxiety is the usual cause. The disorder is usually benign, but serious cardiopulmonary causes of hyperventilation or subjective dyspnea must be ruled out (Chapter 5).

Diagnosis

A. Common symptoms include light-headedness, shortness of breath, numbness and tingling (especially circumoral or acral), muscular twitching, and in severe cases, carpal pedal spasm.

B. Positive Chvostek and Trousseau tests are noted during the acute stage.

C. Respiratory alkalosis without other abnormalities (eg, metabolic acidosis) is noted on arterial blood gas analysis.

D. Symptoms are reproduced by hyperventilating in a controlled setting (eg, emergency department).

Treatment & Disposition

Reassure the patient, and alleviate underlying anxiety. If the patient is acutely hyperventilating, ask the patient to count to 3 slowly between breaths. Patients suffering from a panic attack may benefit from alprazolam (Xanax), 0.25–0.5 mg orally. Rebreathing from a paper bag is no longer recommended because of the potential risk of hypoxia.

GLOSSOPHARYNGEAL NEURALGIA

Diagnosis

Symptoms include intermittent, agonizing unilateral paroxysmal pain localized either in the tonsillar pillars or in the external auditory meatus. Pain is triggered by pressure on the tonsillar pillars, especially during swallowing or talking.

Pain activates the glossopharyngeal-vagal reflex arc and causes transient bradyarrhythmia. The resulting cerebral hypoperfusion causes syncope.

Treatment & Disposition

See Chapter 13 for details of management.

HYSTERIA
(See also Chapter 10.)

Diagnosis

Features that suggest hysteria as the cause of episodic apparent unconsciousness are lack of any prodrome, presence of bizarre postures or movements, lack of pallor, and prolonged unconsciousness. Most patients are young and have a well-documented history of hysterical responses to stress; without such a history, a diagnosis of hysteria in a patient over 30 years of age can be made only after thorough evaluation has excluded other causes of syncope. Secondary gain may also be a factor: patients may use these episodes of unconsciousness to manipulate other people.

While the patient is unconscious, caloric testing

may be used to distinguish coma due to hysteria from coma due to structural lesions or metabolic causes. In coma of organic cause, when ice water is directed against the tympanic membrane, the eyes will remain in mid position or will tonically deviate to the side of the irrigation. In coma due to hysteria, the caloric test induces brisk nystagmus, or the patient awakens because of discomfort (Chapter 10).

Treatment & Disposition

Refer the patient to an outpatient clinic or primary-care physician for follow-up.

MENIERE'S DISEASE
(See also Chapter 26.)

Diagnosis

Recurrent attacks of severe vertigo persisting for several hours associated with tinnitus and progressive hearing loss are diagnostic of Meniere's disease. A few patients experience loss of consciousness for a few seconds at the onset of an attack.

Treatment & Disposition

Meclizine (Antivert, many others), 50 mg orally once or twice daily, is often helpful. Refer the patient to an otolaryngologist. (See Chapter 26 for details.)

REFERENCES

Seizures

Alldredge BK, Lowenstein DH, Simon RP: Placebo-controlled trial of intravenous diphenylhydantoin for short-term treatment of alcohol withdrawal seizures. Am J Med 1989;87:645.

Alldredge BK, Lowenstein DH, Simon RP: Seizures associated with recreational drug abuse. Neurology 1989; 39:1037.

Aminoff MJ, Simon RP: Status epilepticus: Causes, clinical features, and consequences in 98 patients. Am J Med 1980;69:657.

Charness ME, Simon RP, Greenberg DA: Ethanol and the nervous system. N Engl J Med 1989;321:442.

Hansotia P, Broste SK: The effect of epilepsy or diabetes mellitus on the risk of automobile accidents. N Engl J Med 1991;324:22.

Holtzman DM, Kaku DA, So YT: New-onset seizures associated with human immunodeficiency virus infection: Causation and clinical features in 100 cases. Am J Med 1989;87:173.

Kilpatrick CJ et al: Epileptic seizures in acute stroke. Arch Neurol 1990;47:157.

King DW et al: Pseudoseizures: Diagnostic evaluation. Neurology 1982;32:18.

Leppik IE (editor): Status epilepticus in perspective. Neurology 1990;40(Suppl 2):1.

Mattson RH et al: Comparison of carbamazepine, phenytoin, and primidone in partial and secondarily generalized tonic-clonic seizures. N Engl J Med 1985; 313:145.

Messing RO, Simon RP: Seizures as a manifestation of systemic disease. Neurol Clin 1986;4:563.

Messing RO, Closson RG, Simon RP: Drug-induced seizures: A 10-year experience. Neurology 1984;34: 1582.

Olsen T, Hogerhaven H, Thage O: Epilepsy after stroke. Neurology 1987;37:1209.

Pomeroy SL et al: Seizures and other neurologic sequelae of bacterial meningitis in children. N Engl J Med 1990;323:1651.

Scheuer ML, Pedley TA: The evaluation and treatment of seizures. N Engl J Med 1990;323:1468.

Temkin NR et al: A randomized, double-blind study of phenytoin for the prevention of post-traumatic seizures. N Engl J Med 1990;323:497.

Syncope

Aminoff MJ et al: Electrocerebral accompaniments of syncope associated with malignant ventricular arrhythmias. Ann Intern Med 1988;108:791.

Fujimura O et al: The diagnostic sensitivity of electrophysiologic testing in patients with syncope caused by transient bradycardia. N Engl J Med 1989;321:1703.

Hennerici M, Klemm C, Rautenberg W: The subclavian steal phenomenon: A common vascular disorder with rare neurologic deficits. Neurology 1988;38:669.

Kapoor WN: Evaluation and outcome of patients with syncope. Medicine 1990;69:160.

Kapoor WN et al: Prolonged electrocardiographic monitoring in patients with syncope. Am J Med 1987;82:20.

Kapoor WN et al: Syncope in the elderly. Am J Med 1986;80:419.

Lin JT et al: Convulsive syncope in blood donors. Ann Neurol 1982;11:525.

Lipsitz LA: Orthostatic hypotension in the elderly. N Engl J Med 1989;321:952.

Manolis AS et al: Syncope: Current diagnostic evaluation and management. Ann Intern Med 1990;112:850.

Markel ML, Waller BF, Armstrong WF: Cardiac myxoma: A review. Medicine 1987;66:114.

Perkin GD, Joseph R: Neurologic manifestations of the hyperventilation syndrome. J R Soc Med 1986;79:448.

Richards AM et al: Syncope in aortic valvular stenosis. Lancet 1984;2:1113.

Savage DD et al: Epidemiologic features of isolated syncope: The Framingham study. Stroke 1985;16:626.

Simpson RJ Jr et al: Vagal syncope during recurrent pulmonary embolism. JAMA 1983;249:390.

Sugrue DD, Wood DL, McGoon MD: Carotid sinus hypersensitivity and syncope. Mayo Clin Proc 1984;59: 637.

Zee-Cheng CS, Gibbs HR: Pure vasopressor carotid sinus hypersensitivity: Unusual cause of recurrent syncope. Am J Med 1986;81:1095.

12

Weakness & Stroke

Roger P. Simon, MD, & Mary T. Ho, MD, MPH

Disorders characterized by rapid onset of loss of motor function are discussed in this chapter. With the exception of some stroke syndromes, consciousness is not impaired by the primary disease process, although secondary respiratory insufficiency may cause hypercapnia leading to obtundation.

Caution: The major error to be avoided in dealing with patients presenting with acute weakness is misinterpreting the symptoms as psychogenic or hysterical. These patients usually are awake and alert and may not appear critically ill. They may be able to walk. *Complaints of weakness of recent onset require careful evaluation before judgments are made about the cause of symptoms.*

I. IMMEDIATE MANAGEMENT OF LIFE-THREATENING PROBLEMS ASSOCIATED WITH WEAKNESS (See algorithm.)

Stabilize Ventilation

Treat dyspnea or objective respiratory distress in a patient with weakness as a potential life-threatening emergency. Remember that respiratory muscles may be affected even though strength in the extremities is relatively unimpaired.

A. Oxygen: Give oxygen, 5 L/min, by mask or nasal prongs if breathing is labored, if there is obvious hypoventilation (patient is barely able to speak), or if there is evidence of hypoxemia (eg, cyanosis of digits). Distal extremity paresthesias and increased respiratory effort associated with the basic disease process (eg, Guillain-Barré syndrome) may support the impression of hysterical hyperventilation.

B. Laboratory Tests: Arterial blood gases, vital capacity, and maximum inspiratory force should be measured immediately. Measurements of vital capacity and maximum inspiratory force will be abnormal even before alterations in arterial blood gases occur.

C. Supported Ventilation: Frank hypoventilation ($PCO_2 > 50$ mm Hg) is an indication for emergency supported ventilation (eg, bag-mask or even

mouth-to-mouth), followed as quickly as possible by endotracheal intubation and mechanical ventilation.

Even if arterial blood gas measurements are normal or nearly normal, a markedly diminished vital capacity (< 10 mL/kg) and in particular a diminished maximum inspiratory force (< 15 cm water) in a patient with progressive weakness are indications for intubation and supported ventilation. In these cases, a delay of 1–2 hours is permissible to allow intubation under optimal conditions, as long as the patient is under close observation.

D. Hospitalization: Hospitalize every patient with complaints of dyspnea and weakness unless the vital capacity, maximum inspiratory force, and arterial blood gases remain normal during the period of observation.

Rule Out Spinal Cord Compression

Quickly assess the possibility of a mass compressing the spinal cord, since emergency operation or radiation therapy may be needed to prevent permanent paraplegia or quadriplegia.

A. Locate Level of Lesion: Acute spinal cord compression is associated with weakness and sensory loss caudad to the level of involvement. Cord-mediated functions cephalad to this level and cranial nerve examination will be normal.

1. Cervical level–Both upper and lower extremity weakness are present, but cranial nerve function is normal. Respiratory insufficiency is especially likely with high cervical cord lesions.

2. Thoracic level–Lower extremity weakness is present, but the upper extremities and cranial nerves are spared. Since spinal cord compression involves sensory as well as motor pathways, a sensory level should be carefully sought by eliciting reactions to pinprick or a cold object placed against the skin.

3. Lower spinal cord, or cauda equina, involvement–Signs and symptoms include bladder or bowel incontinence, sensory loss in sacral (saddle) distribution, and lower extremity weakness.

4. Vertebral body involvement–If spinal cord compression is due to a process that also involves the vertebral bodies (eg, metastatic tumor, epidural abscess), focal tenderness during vertebral percussion will be noted. Radiologic evidence of bony erosion or collapse of the vertebral column at the spinal cord level responsible for the abnormal neurologic findings virtually establishes the diagnosis.

B. Perform Emergency Imaging and Surgery: Patients with suspected spinal cord compression due to any cause require emergency neurosurgical consultation and imaging (preferably MRI, if available).

Caution: In case of suspected spinal cord compression, do not perform lumbar puncture in the emergency department, because it may worsen symptoms and make more difficult subsequent attempts to enter the subarachnoid space (eg, for myelography).

II. FURTHER EVALUATION OF THE PATIENT WITH WEAKNESS

After the immediate measures described above have been taken, further evaluation should proceed so as to localize the anatomic site of weakness into one of the following categories (see Table 12–1 and detailed discussions of specific disorders beginning on p 198).

SPINAL CORD DISEASE

Diagnosis

Spinal cord disease should be suspected if weakness and sensory loss are found caudad to a horizontal plane in the body. Cranial nerve examination should be normal. The most common disorders producing rapidly progressive weakness or involvement of the nervous system at the spinal cord level are essentially confined to 4 processes: (**1**) disk protrusion (Chapter 15), (**2**) spinal epidural metastases, (**3**) transverse myelitis, and (**4**) spinal epidural abscess. Other causes such as radiation myelitis and ruptured arteriovenous malformations are rare. A diagnosis of suspected spinal cord compression by abscess or tumor demands immediate confirmation by MRI or myelography and prompt surgical decompression and antibiotics for abscess and emergency radiation therapy or surgical decompression for tumor. In transverse myelitis, no such mechanical compression of the spinal cord exists, and surgery only increases the morbidity.

A. Magnetic Resonance Imaging or Myelography: MRI is the study of choice; if it is unavailable, myelography is done. Cerebrospinal fluid should be obtained only at the time of myelography, since the subarachnoid space may be difficult to enter a second time. Only a small amount of cerebrospinal fluid should be removed for study, and small volumes

of contrast media (< 2 mL) should be employed, since spinal cord herniation may follow removal or instillation of larger amounts below a complete block. If a complete block to cerebrospinal fluid flow is anticipated, the subarachnoid space should be entered above the lesion via a lateral C1-2 puncture, if possible.

B. Other Diagnostic Measures: Table 12–2 lists features helpful in differentiating the other entities causing spinal cord dysfunction. Further details about diagnosis and treatment of disk protrusion are presented in Chapter 15.

Treatment & Disposition

Hospitalize the patient, and seek immediate neurologic or neurosurgical consultation.

ANTERIOR HORN CELL INVOLVEMENT (Poliomyelitis)

Diagnosis

A. Symptoms and Signs: Poliomyelitis should be suspected if several of the following are present with weakness:

1. Asymmetric weakness with intact sensation. This asymmetry of motor involvement is virtually unique to poliomyelitis.

2. Gastrointestinal signs or symptoms.

3. Fever, headache, photophobia.

4. Meningeal signs.

B. Lumbar Puncture: Perform lumbar puncture if poliomyelitis is suspected. Spinal cord compression (abscess), transverse myelitis, and poliomyelitis are the only conditions commonly producing acute weakness associated with cerebrospinal fluid pleocytosis.

C. Differential Diagnosis: Spinal cord compression and myelitis will produce a sensory deficit. Peripheral neuropathies may spare sensory nerves; motor involvement is usually symmetric.

Treatment & Disposition

Hospitalize all patients who have a clinical diagnosis of poliomyelitis. If bulbar involvement has produced respiratory failure, support respiration with supplemental oxygen and assisted ventilation (bag-mask or endotracheal intubation).

NEUROMUSCULAR BLOCKADE

Diagnosis

A. Symptoms and Signs: Diseases affecting the neuromuscular junction are marked by early and prominent involvement of cranial nerves, causing difficulty in speaking and swallowing, facial weakness, blurred vision, diplopia, and ptosis. In-

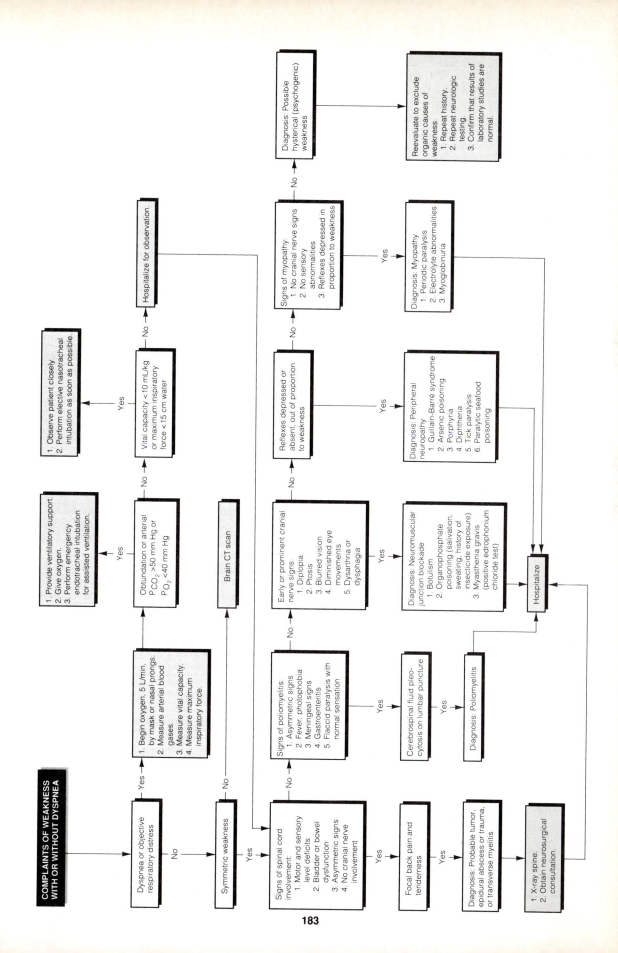

COMPLAINTS OF WEAKNESS
WITH OR WITHOUT DYSPNEA

Dyspnea or objective respiratory distress

Yes →

1. Begin oxygen, 5 L/min, by mask or nasal prongs.
2. Measure arterial blood gases.
3. Measure vital capacity.
4. Measure maximum inspiratory force.

Obtundation or arterial PCO_2 >50 mm Hg or PO_2 <40 mm Hg

Yes →

1. Provide ventilatory support.
2. Give oxygen.
3. Perform emergency endotracheal intubation for assisted ventilation.

No →

Vital capacity <10 mL/kg or maximum inspiratory force <15 cm water

Yes →

1. Observe patient closely.
2. Perform elective nasotracheal intubation as soon as possible.

No →

Hospitalize for observation.

No →

Symmetric weakness

No → Brain CT scan

Yes →

Signs of spinal cord involvement:
1. Motor and sensory level deficits
2. Bladder or bowel dysfunction
3. Asymmetric signs
4. No cranial nerve involvement

Yes →

Focal back pain and tenderness

Yes →

Diagnosis: Probable tumor, epidural abscess or trauma, or transverse myelitis

1. X-ray spine.
2. Obtain neurosurgical consultation.

No →

Signs of poliomyelitis:
1. Asymmetric signs
2. Fever, photophobia
3. Meningeal signs
4. Gastroenteritis
5. Flaccid paralysis with normal sensation

Yes →

Cerebrospinal fluid pleocytosis on lumbar puncture

Yes →

Diagnosis: Poliomyelitis

No →

Early or prominent cranial nerve signs:
1. Diplopia
2. Ptosis
3. Blurred vision
4. Diminished eye movements
5. Dysarthria or dysphagia

Yes →

Diagnosis: Neuromuscular junction blockade
1. Botulism
2. Organophosphate poisoning (salivation, sweating, history of insecticide exposure)
3. Myasthenia gravis (positive edrophonium chloride test)

No →

Reflexes depressed or absent, out of proportion to weakness

Yes →

Diagnosis: Peripheral neuropathy
1. Guillain–Barré syndrome
2. Arsenic poisoning
3. Porphyria
4. Diphtheria
5. Tick paralysis
6. Paralytic seafood poisoning

No →

Signs of myopathy:
1. No cranial nerve signs
2. No sensory abnormalities
3. Reflexes depressed in proportion to weakness

Yes →

Diagnosis: Myopathy
1. Periodic paralysis
2. Electrolyte abnormalities
3. Myoglobinuria

No →

Diagnosis: Possible hysterical (psychogenic) weakness

Reevaluate to exclude organic causes of weakness.
1. Repeat history.
2. Repeat neurologic testing.
3. Confirm that results of laboratory studies are normal.

Hospitalize

183

Table 12–1. Differential diagnosis of acute weakness by anatomic localization.

	Disease State	Location of Weakness	Cranial Nerve Involvement	Sensory Abnormalities	Meningeal Signs	Reflexes	Bladder Paralysis	Cerebrospinal Fluid
Cerebral hemispheres	Stroke.	Unilateral (ie, hemiplegia or hemiparesis).	Unilateral facial weakness.	Hemihypesthesia.	Rare.	Asymmetric; decreased acutely; then increased, with upgoing toes (Babinski's sign).	Rare.	Variable. Usually normal in thrombosis, bloody with hemorrhage.
Spinal cord	Compression by tumor or abscess; protruding disk or transverse myelitis.	Paraplegia or quadriplegia (may have a unilateral predominance).	None.	Depressed below level of lesion.	Present in one-third to one-half of patients.	Decreased acutely; then increased, with upgoing toes (Babinski's sign).	Prominent.	Highly variable: from normal to markedly increased in cells and protein. Myelographic block very common with mass lesions.
Anterior horn cell	Poliomyelitis, other enterovirus infection.	Scattered, focal, asymmetric.	10–20% of cases.	None.	Common.	Depressed in involved limbs.	Uncommon, transient.	Increased white blood cells (25–500/μL) early. Increased protein later. Glucose normal.
Peripheral nerve	Guillain-Barré syndrome, arsenical neuropathy, diphtheritic neuropathy, porphyria, tick paralysis.	Proximal or distal; usually symmetric.	Common in Guillain-Barré syndrome, especially facial muscles (seventh nerve).	Distal (stocking-glove distribution).	Rare.	Decreased or absent early and out of proportion to muscle weakness.	None.	Increased protein but may be normal acutely. Few or absent cells ("albuminocytologic dissociation").
Neuromuscular junction	Botulism, organophosphate poisoning, myasthenia gravis, aminoglycoside toxicity.	Proximal, symmetric.	Prominent and early involvement, especially eye movements. Pupils may be unreactive to light.	None.	None.	Decreased in relation to degree of muscle weakness.	None.	Normal.
Muscle	Hypokalemia, hyperkalemia, periodic paralysis, myoglobinuria, hypophosphatemia, hypermagnesemia.	Proximal, symmetric. Upper and lower extremities equally involved.	None.	None.	None.	Decreased in relation to degree of muscle weakness.	None.	Normal.

Table 12–2. Differential diagnosis of acute weakness at the spinal cord level.[1]

	Epidural Abscess	Epidural Tumor	Transverse Myelitis
Age (years)	11–77	Rare in childhood	1–65
Back pain	100%	90%	36%
Vertebral tenderness	100%	90%	58%
Fever	86%	0%	51%
White count > 10,000/µL	62%	0%	32%
Cerebrospinal fluid cells (cells/µL)	2–720	Normal	0–8800
Cerebrospinal fluid protein (mg/dL)	36–2000	82–822	18–216
Cerebrospinal fluid glucose (mg/dL)	Normal	Normal	Normal
Duration (from onset to maximum deficit)	Days to months	Hours to months	Minutes to weeks
Complete block to cerebrospinal fluid flow on myelogram	86%	81%	7%
Bony erosion or osteomyelitis (on spinal x-ray)	30–83%	85%	0%

[1]Based on 105 cases of spinal metastases, 65 cases of transverse myelopathy, and 65 cases of abscess selected from the literature.

volvement of respiratory and extremity muscles then follows. There are no sensory abnormalities, and reflexes are preserved, though responses may be depressed in proportion to the degree of weakness.

B. Etiology: Diseases causing neuromuscular blockade include botulism, myasthenia gravis, and organophosphate (insecticide or nerve gas) poisoning. Certain antibiotics (eg, aminoglycosides) may rarely cause neuromuscular blockade, but this occurs only in hospitalized patients with contributory conditions (eg, myasthenia gravis).

Differential Diagnosis

It is important to make a rapid diagnosis, since both botulism and organophosphate poisoning require immediate specific therapy.

A. Organophosphate Poisoning: Poisoning with organophosphates causes marked miosis and prominent glandular hypersecretion (sweating, salivation, lacrimation, and bronchorrhea). Most patients have been recently exposed to insecticide spraying, a fact easily elicited by questioning.

B. Botulism: Botulism affects the neuromuscular junction and causes nausea and vomiting followed by paralysis of muscles of accommodation, respiratory muscles, extraocular muscles, extremity muscles, and the lower bulbar muscles. Glandular secretion is not affected.

C. Myasthenia: Patients with myasthenia gravis usually know their diagnosis. The rare patients with undiagnosed acute myasthenia gravis should improve in response to edrophonium (Tensilon, others). Give 2 mg intravenously over 15–30 seconds; if no reaction occurs within 1 minute, give 8 mg more. Edrophonium has a rapid onset but brief duration of action, both of which permit quick assessment of cranial nerve weakness. Testing of limb muscles may require using the longer-acting cholinesterase inhibitor

neostigmine (1.5 mg intramuscularly, together with atropine, 0.5 mg intramuscularly). Edrophonium and neostigmine will not affect symptoms due to botulinus toxin or organophosphate poisoning.

Disposition

Hospitalization is mandatory for all patients with suspected neuromuscular blockade. (See Chapter 39 for treatment of organophosphate poisoning. Treatment of botulism is discussed on p 192.)

PERIPHERAL NEUROPATHY

Diagnosis

Disorders involving the peripheral nerves can produce either sensory or motor symptoms or (most often) both.

A. Symptoms and Signs: Weakness may preferentially involve either the distal or, rarely, the proximal musculature. Sensory loss is usually restricted to a distal (ie, stocking-glove) distribution. Weakness owing to cranial nerve involvement may occur but is not a common presenting feature.

Reflexes are markedly depressed or absent early; this is helpful in identifying peripheral nerve impairment even before objective weakness can be documented.

B. Laboratory Findings: Cerebrospinal fluid protein is commonly elevated, but this may not occur until days after onset. The cell count is usually normal.

Treatment

Provide supportive care (eg, respiratory support as required). None of the illnesses causing peripheral neuropathy are relieved by specific emergency therapy except for tick paralysis (p 191), which responds to the removal of the tick (usually found in the hair).

Disposition

Hospitalization is necessary for further evaluation and treatment.

MUSCLE DISEASE
(Acute Myopathy)

Diagnosis

Prompt diagnosis of primary muscle disease is important, since effective specific therapy is available for some of the conditions causing muscular weakness.

A. Symptoms and Signs: Weakness is characteristically more proximal than distal, and lower extremity weakness is often greater than that in the upper extremity. Cranial nerve and respiratory abnormalities occur in very severe cases; eye movements are spared. Objective sensory loss does not occur. Deep tendon reflexes are depressed in proportion to the muscle weakness.

B. Laboratory Findings: Collect urine for myoglobin testing (positive test for hemoglobin on dipstick in the absence of erythrocytes on microscopy; confirm by chemical assay) and blood for determination of muscle enzymes (CK, AST [SGOT]) and potassium in serum.

Treatment & Disposition

Hospitalization is generally required, although mild attacks of recurrent familial hypo- or hyperkalemic paralysis may be treated adequately in the emergency department. If hypokalemia is present, give potassium chloride, 1–2 meq/kg (equivalent to 5–10 g of potassium chloride) orally, and repeat once or twice at hourly intervals until strength is regained. Treat hyperkalemia associated with muscular weakness by infusing glucose and insulin (Chapter 36).

HYSTERIA

Hysteria as a cause of weakness can be diagnosed only after all other causes have been eliminated. A history of hysteria or psychosomatic illnesses may be helpful, but one must also search for and eliminate other causes of weakness, since organic causes of weakness are very frequently misdiagnosed initially as hysteria. Psychiatric evaluation should be obtained.

III. EMERGENCY MANAGEMENT OF SPECIFIC WEAKNESS DISORDERS

DISEASES OF THE SPINAL CORD

METASTATIC TUMOR

Diagnosis

The most common primary malignant neoplasms producing epidural metastases and spinal cord compression are breast cancer (20%), lung cancer (10%), Hodgkin's disease (10%), and prostatic cancer (7%).

A. Symptoms and Signs: Local vertebral column pain at the level of the spinal cord lesion is the presenting symptom in the vast majority of patients. This symptom usually precedes neurologic deterioration by weeks to months, but occasionally it may be present for only a few hours.

Onset of radicular radiation of the pain (involvement of the territory of a nerve root) heralds progression. Radiation of the pain may be bilateral, especially when the thoracic spine is involved. This is followed by weakness, paresthesias, and sensory impairment (especially to vibration) of the distal lower extremity. Bladder and bowel dysfunction occurs with rapid progression of symptoms over hours to days. Sensory and motor impairment soon ascends to a spinal cord level just below the site of the lesion.

B. Imaging Findings: X-rays of the spine will usually reveal bony destruction by the tumor at the involved vertebral level. Demonstrate the extent of the lesion by MRI. If a myelogram is necessary, access to the subarachnoid space above the lesion is most easily obtained via a lateral C1–2 puncture.

Treatment & Disposition

A. Patients with this diagnosis should be treated immediately with corticosteroids to reduce peritumor edema, eg, dexamethasone, 10 mg intravenously, followed by 4 mg every 6 hours intravenously or orally.

B. Obtain emergency neurosurgical and neurologic consultation.

C. Hospitalization is required for decompression by laminectomy or local radiotherapy. The latter is as effective as surgery (regardless of the tumor type) and is associated with fewer side effects.

TRANSVERSE MYELITIS

Transverse myelitis is a poorly defined entity that is usually idiopathic but may be a manifestation of a known systemic disease (eg, multiple sclerosis, systemic lupus erythematosus, vitamin B_{12} deficiency). It may also result from acute hyperextension injury of the cervical spine (central cord syndrome).

Diagnosis

A. Symptoms and Signs: The presenting symptoms are equally divided between motor weakness, sensory loss or paresthesia, and back and radicular pain. Symptoms and signs of transverse (bilateral) cord involvement may progress to a maximum level within hours. Vertebral tenderness to percussion is noted in about half of cases.

B. Imaging Findings: An MRI or myelogram is *required* to exclude a compressive lesion; myelography will almost always demonstrate free flow of contrast material.

Treatment & Disposition

Treatment is supportive only. Partial to full recovery may occur over a period of weeks to months. Hospitalization is recommended for diagnosis and supportive care. Steroid treatment is frequently used, but its benefit is uncertain.

SPINAL EPIDURAL ABSCESS

Spinal epidural abscess is one-eighth as common as transverse myelitis, but it may present with remarkably similar signs and symptoms.

Diagnosis

The most common predisposing conditions include local staphylococcal infections of the skin and surgical wounds (including intravenous sites), bacteremia, vertebral osteomyelitis, and intravenous drug abuse.

A. Symptoms and Signs: Patients are usually febrile and appear acutely ill on presentation. Focal pain and localized tenderness over the abscess are nearly constant findings. Classically, symptoms progress over a few days from local vertebral column pain to radiating radicular pain. Cord compression with weakness and sensory loss below the level of the lesion then follows.

B. Imaging Findings: Plain films of the spine reveal osteomyelitic lesions in about 85% of cases, especially in patients with symptoms of long duration (weeks). MRI or myelography will show a complete block of cerebrospinal fluid flow in over 80% of cases.

C. Laboratory Findings: Lumbar puncture (*only* at the time of myelography) should be done with great care; the operator should aspirate frequently to make certain that the needle is not advanced through the abscess, allowing pus to enter the subarachnoid space. Culture of cerebrospinal fluid is usually negative, but Gram-stained smears and cultures of pus from the abscess reveal the causative organism in almost all cases. The cerebrospinal fluid cell count, glucose, and protein content are listed in Table 12–2.

Treatment & Disposition

Hospitalization is required for emergency surgical decompression by laminectomy, abscess drainage, and intravenous antimicrobial therapy. Selected patients without significant weakness can be managed with antibiotics alone.

DISEASE OF ANTERIOR HORN CELLS

POLIOMYELITIS

Although now uncommon in the western world, poliomyelitis continues to occur in single cases or isolated epidemics in unimmunized populations. Other enteroviruses and attenuated (vaccine) strains of poliovirus may cause a similar syndrome.

Diagnosis

A. Symptoms and Signs: Poliomyelitis begins as a viral syndrome with fever, myalgias, headache, and upper respiratory or gastrointestinal symptoms. Nuchal rigidity and photophobia are common. Neurologic involvement follows this prodrome in about 1% of cases, with rapid onset of weakness that progresses over 3–5 days. Flaccid paralysis then occurs, is usually asymmetric or even unilateral, and more commonly involves the legs than the arms. Sensation is unimpaired. Cranial nerves are involved in 10–20% of cases (bulbar poliomyelitis), with the most common manifestations being facial and pharyngeal weakness; this can be unilateral. Diaphragmatic and intercostal muscle involvement may lead to respiratory failure.

B. Laboratory Findings: Lumbar puncture will show a cerebrospinal fluid cell count between 25 and 500 cells/μL, with either lymphocytes or neutrophils predominating. Cerebrospinal fluid protein and glucose are normal early. The diagnosis can be confirmed by recovery of virus (from stool, cerebrospinal fluid, or throat washings) or by demonstration of a 4-fold rise in antibody titer against the virus.

Treatment & Disposition

Hospitalization is mandatory, and public health associates should be notified promptly (by telephone, facsimile machine, or telegraph). No specific therapy is available at present.

POSTPOLIOMYELITIS SYNDROME

Diagnosis

This syndrome is characterized by the onset of new, slowly progressive weakness, fatigue, and pain in patients with a prior history of paralytic poliomyelitis years previously. Symptoms are the result of ongoing denervation of muscles involved in the prior attack that had subsequently reinnervated. Electromyography and muscle biopsy confirm active denervation.

Treatment & Disposition

Hospitalization is rarely needed, as progression of dysfunction is slow. No specific treatment is available, but physical therapy may be beneficial.

PERIPHERAL NEUROPATHIES

MONONEUROPATHIES

1. BELL'S PALSY
(Facial Weakness)
(See also Chapter 26.)

Bell's palsy is a common condition of unknown cause (although some authorities suggest a link with herpes simplex infection). Although manifestations of the disorder are dramatic, full recovery usually occurs. Recovery usually begins within 1 month, and complete resolution of symptoms occurs in 70–85% of patients. All patients with initial subtotal facial paralysis will make a cosmetically complete functional recovery.

Diagnostic features include the following:

(1) Development of symptoms over less than 24–48 hours.

(2) Unilateral involvement of the facial nerve.

(3) No signs of other nervous system involvement.

(4) Postauricular pain (not required for diagnosis).

Differential Diagnosis

The major differential diagnostic possibilities—and those of most concern to patients—are stroke and tumor. Tumors in the region of the facial nerve rarely cause sudden onset of symptoms and usually produce abnormalities of other facial nerves, resulting in decreased hearing, nystagmus, and ataxia. Facial numbness may suggest involvement of the trigeminal nerve, but patients with Bell's palsy often describe pure facial weakness in sensory terms, eg, "My face is numb."

Stroke with facial weakness is associated with weakness of the ipsilateral arm and probably the ipsilateral leg also (most easily detectable in the extensors of the arm and the flexors of the leg). Stroke produces an upper motor neuron lesion, thereby sparing the muscles of the forehead. Bell's palsy, however, involves the facial nerve itself and produces unilateral weakness of all facial muscles (those of the forehead, those responsible for eye closure, and those around the mouth). Other facial nerve functions may be involved, such as unilateral decrease of lacrimation and taste and increase in apparent intensity of sounds, eg, when talking on the telephone.

Laboratory Tests & Other Examinations

When the diagnosis is clear on clinical grounds, no further evaluation or radiographic studies (CT scans or MRI) are indicated.

Treatment & Disposition

While Bell's palsy is cosmetically disfiguring during the acute phase, the more serious concern is the risk for eye injury owing to inability to close the eyelid completely. Artificial tears should be instilled frequently during waking hours, and the lid should be taped closed (under careful instruction) when the patient is asleep to prevent corneal abrasions and ulcers. Corticosteroids have no proved effect on the ultimate recovery of motor function; however, corticosteroids such as prednisone, 40–60 mg/d orally for 10 days, decrease the postauricular pain often associated with acute Bell's palsy. All patients should be referred to a neurologist, otolaryngologist, or primary-care physician within a few days, regardless of whether or not corticosteroids have been given. Hospitalization is not required.

2. COMPRESSIVE MONONEUROPATHIES

Compressive mononeuropathies usually occur because prolonged compression of a superficial peripheral nerve interrupts blood flow, producing ischemic injury. This may result from sleep in an unusual position or from prolonged fixed position of a limb due to drug intoxication or general anesthesia.

Radial Nerve Palsy

Paralysis of the radial nerve produces complete but isolated wrist and finger drop (inability to extend the wrist or fingers) with inconsistent sensory loss over the radial portion of the dorsum of the hand. Such injuries occur from compression of the nerve against the humerus in patients sedated with alcohol or other drugs (Saturday night palsy) or during sleep with a partner (bridegroom's palsy). If the radial nerve is compressed in the axilla, as occurs in crutch palsy, the triceps muscle is affected as well, resulting in the additional finding of weakness of extension at the elbow.

Complete recovery over weeks to months is the rule.

Immediate treatment measures include splinting of the wrist or application of a sling and referral to a primary-care physician, hand specialist, or neurologist.

Ulnar Palsy

Acute injury of the ulnar nerve occurs at the elbow following fracture or dislocation. Delayed ("tardy") ulnar nerve palsies result from repeated trauma, such as resting of upper body weight on the elbows. Wasting and weakness of the hands ultimately produce a "claw" posture (hyperextension at the metacarpophalangeal joint and flexion at the interphalangeal joints that are maximal in the fourth and fifth digits). Sensory loss occurs in the ulnar border of the dorsal and palmar aspects of the hand below the wrist, extending to involve the fourth and fifth fingers. Injury to the ulnar nerve in the palm (eg, cycle-racing palsy) spares the sensory fibers.

Initial management consists of padding of the elbow and referral to a primary-care physician, hand specialist, or neurologist.

Peroneal Nerve Palsy

Nerve compression occurs at the head of the fibula as a result of acute trauma, eg, fibular fracture or sleeping with the legs crossed. The resulting footdrop produces a high-stepping gait in the involved limb, with inability to dorsiflex or evert the foot on examination. Some sensory loss may be found over the dorsum of the foot and the lateral aspects of the leg.

Lesions at the root of L5 (eg, disk disease) also produce footdrop but involve other muscles innervated by L5 as well (eg, foot invertors and knee flexors).

Immediate management in the emergency department or upon referral to the orthopedist, primary-care physician, neurologist, or physical medicine specialist consists of splinting the foot at a right angle (cock-up splint) to normalize the gait.

POLYNEUROPATHIES

1. GUILLAIN-BARRÉ SYNDROME (Infectious Polyneuritis)

Guillain-Barré syndrome is a common disease of uncertain cause involving the peripheral nerves and occurring in both sexes and all age groups, although the disease seems milder in children.

In one-half to two-thirds of cases, a mild upper respiratory infection or gastroenteritis precedes the onset of the neurologic disease by 1–3 weeks. Well-documented cases have also been recorded following surgery, other viral infections, immunization (eg, influenza vaccine), and acute glomerulonephritis or as an acute seroconversion reaction to HIV infection.

Marked hypophosphatemia can produce a nearly identical syndrome.

Diagnosis

A. Symptoms and Signs: Symmetric weakness is the major symptom. It may be either proximal or distal at onset and usually begins in the lower extremities. The weakness classically progresses in an ascending manner, involving first the lower and then the upper extremities and finally the cranial nerves within 1–3 days from onset of symptoms. The weakness does not ascend in all cases, however.

Subjective and objective sensory disturbances (numbness or paresthesias) of brief duration are common initially and may be the presenting complaint. These dysesthesias most commonly occur in a distal (stocking-glove) distribution.

Muscle pain or tenderness is also an early symptom in about half of cases.

Absence of the deep tendon reflexes (or, rarely, only distal areflexia with definite hyporeflexia of biceps and knee jerks) almost always occurs by the time of presentation to a physician. *Note:* This loss of reflexes is the most important clue to diagnosis and is found even in muscles that cannot yet be shown to be weak by objective testing.

Cranial nerve involvement is common: involvement of every nerve except nerves I and II (olfactory and optic) has been described. The nerve most commonly affected is the seventh (facial) nerve; facial weakness (usually bilateral) occurs in half of cases. Cranial nerve palsies may be the most prominent feature of the illness, as in the Guillain-Barré variant of ophthalmoplegia, ataxia, and areflexia.

Peripheral autonomic nervous system involvement also occurs and may be manifested by hypertension, tachycardia, facial flushing, postural hypotension, and electrocardiographic changes.

Respiratory musculature weakness requiring assisted ventilation occurs in 25% of cases.

B. Laboratory Findings: Increased spinal fluid pressure is seen only in severe cases. The cerebrospinal fluid cell count is normal initially in most patients, with less than 10% of patients having more than 10 leukocytes per microliter. The classic elevation in cerebrospinal fluid protein to levels as high as 100–400 mg/dL in the absence of significant pleocytosis (so-called albuminocytologic dissociation) may not be seen until several days after the onset of symptoms. These cerebrospinal fluid findings support the diagnosis of Guillain-Barré syndrome, but they are not specific and may be seen occasionally in any acute or chronic polyneuritis.

Treatment & Disposition

Endotracheal intubation and ventilatory support should be considered in the emergency department for patients in respiratory failure (see algorithm on p 183). Plasmapheresis begun within 10 days of the first symptoms in the severely affected patient may shorten the need for mechanical ventilation. Corticosteroids are ineffective and may prolong the disease in elderly patients. All patients should be hospitalized.

2. ARSENICAL NEUROPATHY

The neuropathy of arsenic poisoning is a rapidly progressive sensorimotor polyneuropathy that in many ways mimics Guillain-Barré syndrome. Common sources of arsenic include rat and ant poison and the copper acetoarsenite contained in insecticides (eg, Paris green). Fowler's solution, once used for psoriasis, also contains arsenic. Some cases, especially in patients with chronic symptoms, may represent attempted murder.

Diagnosis
A. Symptoms and Signs: Abdominal pain, nausea and vomiting, and diarrhea occur minutes to hours following ingestion. A rapidly progressive polyneuropathy ensues 7–14 days later. Symmetric ascending paresthesias, initially distal, begin in the lower extremities and progress to overt sensory loss.

Diffuse muscle aches and tenderness are common, as is a burning pain of the soles of the feet that is markedly aggravated by touching the skin. Deep tendon reflexes are depressed early and in the same distribution as the sensory loss.

Symmetric motor impairment follows as the neuropathy progresses over days to a few weeks and is typically more severe distally and in the lower extremities. The cranial nerves, rectal sphincter, and respiratory muscles are unaffected.

Cutaneous stigmas of arsenical poisoning include increased skin pigmentation and marked exfoliation (especially of the hands and feet). Mees's lines (transverse white, nonpalpable lines on the nails) are especially suggestive of arsenic poisoning but do not appear until 40–60 days after ingestion because of the slow rate of nail growth.

B. Laboratory Findings: Cerebrospinal fluid findings are similar to those seen with Guillain-Barré syndrome: Glucose and cell counts are normal, and protein is elevated, although usually less than 100 mg/dL.

The diagnosis is established by documenting elevated concentrations of arsenic in urine (upper limits of normal: 0.1 mg/24 h) or hair protected from external contamination, most commonly pubic hair (upper limits of normal: 0.1 mg/100 g of hair).

C. X-Ray Findings: If continued ingestion of arsenic is suspected, abdominal x-ray may be helpful, since arsenic is radiopaque.

Treatment
(See also Chapter 39.)
Patients with symptoms should be treated with a chelating agent to facilitate excretion of arsenic. Treatment must be started within 24 hours after ingestion to influence the course of the neuropathy.

Give dimercaprol, 3–4 mg/kg/dose intramuscularly every 4 hours for 48 hours, then 3 mg/kg every 12 hours for a total of 10 days; or penicillamine, 100 mg/kg/d orally (maximum: 1 g/d) divided into 4 doses for 5 days. The course of either may be repeated if the patient is still symptomatic. Follow urine arsenic levels, since hair and nail levels do not reflect acute changes.

Disposition
If arsenic poisoning is diagnosed or suspected, hospitalization is indicated for evaluation and treatment.

3. ACUTE INTERMITTENT PORPHYRIA

Acute intermittent porphyria is a rare inherited disorder of porphyrin metabolism producing episodic clinical symptoms, most commonly in the third to sixth decades. Women are much more frequently affected than men. Attacks are often precipitated by drugs (especially barbiturates and sulfonamides; see Table 12–3), infection, or fasting.

Diagnosis
A. Symptoms and Signs: Abdominal pain is the commonest manifestation of porphyria (85% of cases). The abdominal pain is severe, often colicky, and may be generalized or localized. Onset of pain may precede development of other signs or symptoms by several weeks. Vomiting, constipation, and abdominal distention often lead to exploratory laparotomy, even though these signs are manifestations of an autonomic peripheral neuropathy.

Table 12–3. Contraindicated and accepted drugs in treatment of acute intermittent porphyria.

Contraindicated drugs
Barbiturates (including thiopental anesthesia)
Sulfonamids
Griseofulvin
Chlordiazepoxide
Meprobamate
Phenytoin
Glutethimide
Imipramine
Ergot preparations
Methyprylon
Methsuximide
Tolbutamide
Amidopyrine-containing compounds (antipyrine)
Oral contraceptive agents
Drugs that may be safely used
Meperidine
Chlorpromazine and most other phenothiazines
Aspirin
Penicillins
Tetracyclines
Digoxin
Diazepam
Diphenhydramine

Weakness due to a predominantly motor polyneuropathy is the major neurologic manifestation. It is usually symmetric, beginning in the upper or lower extremities and most often proximally rather than distally. The neuropathy usually progresses slowly over days to weeks. Occasionally, complete flaccid quadriparesis with associated respiratory paralysis requiring mechanical ventilation occurs over a few days.

Cranial nerve involvement is common, especially the facial nerve and the nerves to the extraocular muscles. Deep tendon reflexes are depressed or absent, except for a curious preservation of the ankle jerks in some patients. Signs of sensory or autonomic neurologic involvement are usually less prominent.

Seizures, acute psychosis, hypotension, oliguria, and hyponatremia also occur. Tachycardia (> 100 beats/min) is nearly always present.

B. Laboratory Findings: Cerebrospinal fluid pressure and glucose concentration are normal; protein concentration is slightly elevated (not over 100 mg/dL), and there may be a modest pleocytosis (< 10 leukocytes per microliter). The diagnosis is established by measurement of excess urinary porphobilinogen, for which rapid qualitative determination is available with the Watson-Schwartz test.

Treatment & Disposition

Hospitalization is indicated for initiation of high-carbohydrate therapy (eg, intravenous glucose) and management of pain. Opiates, phenothiazines, and benzodiazepines (eg, diazepam) may be used safely for relief of pain and anxiety. Barbiturates are contraindicated.

4. TICK PARALYSIS

Tick paralysis is a rapidly ascending motor paralysis caused by an injected neurotoxin from the female *Dermacentor andersoni* (wood tick) and *Dermacentor variabilis* (dog tick). Symptoms begin after the ticks have been attached to the patient for 5–7 days. The disease is endemic in the southeastern and northwestern United States and in western Canada.

Diagnosis

A. Symptoms and Signs: Most cases occur in children. Neurologic symptoms begin with ataxia and lower extremity weakness, the latter progressing over 24–48 hours to involve the upper extremities and cranial nerves. Reflexes are diminished or absent early. Respiratory depression occurs and may be fatal. Distal extremity paresthesias are common, but objective sensory loss is rare.

B. Laboratory Findings: Cerebrospinal fluid and peripheral blood examinations are normal.

Treatment

The tick may be attached to any portion of the body but is most commonly hidden in long hair about the head and neck. Removal of the entire tick by application of ether, gasoline, or petroleum is followed by symptomatic improvement within hours. Complete resolution occurs within a few days to a week.

Disposition

Patients in the acute phase must be hospitalized for supportive management.

5. DIPHTHERITIC POLYNEURITIS

Diagnosis

A. Symptoms and Signs: In diphtheritic polyneuritis, the cranial and peripheral nerves are affected 2–3 weeks following infection–the cranial nerves first, especially the palate and the muscles of ocular accommodation. Although this disease is rare in the USA, it is still seen elsewhere. Involvement of the nerve supply to the pharynx, larynx, face, extraocular muscles, and extremities occurs as the illness progresses over days to weeks. Reflexes are lost early. Sensory signs are not prominent, although distal paresthesias may be noted.

Symptoms are usually maximal within 1–2 weeks. Gradual (usually complete) improvement then follows over months, although associated myocarditis may produce a significant number of deaths.

B. Laboratory Findings: Cerebrospinal fluid protein is elevated to 100–400 mg/dL. Recovery of the organisms from the pharynx or wound confirms the diagnosis, although such cultures may be negative by the time neuropathy is manifested.

Treatment & Disposition

There is no specific treatment. Administration of diphtheria antitoxin will not abort the neuropathy once symptoms have appeared. Patients must be hospitalized for supportive care.

6. PARALYTIC SEAFOOD POISONING
   (See also Chapter 38.)

Diagnosis

Saxitoxin may be present in both Atlantic and Pacific shellfish, especially between the months of May and October, and can produce a fulminating sensorimotor polyneuropathy. Numbness and tingling of the fingers, toes, and perioral region are associated with a rapidly ascending motor paralysis that can begin within minutes following ingestion. Bizarre dysesthesias (sensation that teeth are loose in their sockets; reversal of hot and cold sensation) are common and specific to saxitoxin or ciguatoxin poisoning. Ingestion of puffer fish containing tetrodotoxin may produce the same symptoms.

Treatment & Disposition

There is no available antitoxin. Supportive care (including mechanical ventilation if indicated) is followed by complete recovery. Hospitalization is indicated for infants and elderly victims and for patients with respiratory insufficiency or objective weakness.

DISEASES OF THE NEUROMUSCULAR JUNCTION

BOTULISM

Diagnosis

Clostridium botulinum toxin attacks the neuromuscular junction. Paralysis occurs mainly following the ingestion of foods contaminated with the toxin and only rarely from infected wounds. In infants, cases have resulted from colonization of the gastrointestinal tract by *C botulinum* (originating, in some cases, from ingested honey). Although commercially canned foods have caused epidemics, most cases have been due to improperly home-canned vegetables, fruits, meat, and fish. Ingestion of even a few drops of contaminated food may cause botulism. The distribution of the toxin in the contaminated vehicle may not be uniform. Fruits or vegetables contaminated with type A or B toxin will taste spoiled; other foods may not. Contaminated foods must be boiled for over 10 minutes in order for the toxin to be reliably inactivated.

A. Symptoms and Signs: Symptoms usually begin 12–48 hours following toxin ingestion and may progress over hours to days (Table 12–4). The shorter the interval between ingestion and the appearance of symptoms, the more severe the disease. The nervous system is involved in *descending* fashion, beginning with the muscles innervated by the cranial nerves. This contrasts with Guillain-Barré syndrome, in which there is usually *ascending* involvement.

Table 12–4. Symptoms and signs of botulism in approximate order of frequency.

Symptoms	Signs
Nausea and vomiting	Extraocular muscle weakness
Generalized weakness	Ptosis
Blurred vision	Bilaterally dilated and unreactive pupils
Diplopia	Dry mucous membranes
Dysphagia	Limb weakness
Dyspnea	Respiratory impairment
Dry mouth	Postural hypotension
Dizziness (especially postural)	
Constipation	
Abdominal fullness	

Nausea and vomiting are the initial symptoms in one-third of cases (prominent with type E toxin). Blurring of vision (due to paralysis of muscles of accommodation) is the most common initial neurologic symptom. Diplopia, dysphagia, and dysphonia come on in sequence as lower bulbar muscles become involved. Weakness of respiratory and extremity muscles follows as the paralysis descends. Ptosis, extraocular muscle paralysis, and pupillary dilatation and fixation follow, and then weakness of jaw and palate function. Some deep tendon reflex activity remains until muscle paralysis is complete.

Dryness of mucous membranes and orthostatic hypotension have been prominent features in some patients. Sweating, salivation, and bronchorrhea (seen in cholinesterase inhibitor poisoning) do not occur. There are no sensory abnormalities.

Infant botulism is characterized by poor feeding, poor muscle tone, episodes of aspiration, and constipation.

B. Laboratory Findings: Examination of cerebrospinal fluid and peripheral blood smears is not helpful unless a superimposed condition develops, eg, aspiration pneumonia. Specimens of blood or contaminated food should be saved for laboratory assay for botulinus toxins (available through local public health departments). Blood samples should consist of 30 mL of clotted, nonheparinized blood, which need not be centrifuged or separated but must be collected before the antitoxin is started. In infants, save a sample of stool for culture for *C botulinum* (consult the local public health department for details).

C. Electrocardiographic Findings: T wave inversions, conduction abnormalities, and ventricular arrhythmias may occur.

Treatment

A. Antitoxin: Bivalent or trivalent antitoxin should be given as soon as possible after diagnosis, even though clinical efficacy has been unequivocally demonstrated only with type E toxin. Skin testing should be performed before administration of antitoxin because of the risk of anaphylaxis. Administer one vial of antitoxin intramuscularly and one vial intravenously (dose is the same for adults and children). Repeat in 4 hours if the patient's condition worsens. Antitoxin and consultation may be obtained in the USA by telephoning the Centers for Disease Control in Atlanta: (404) 639–3311 (days) or (404) 639–2888 (nights, weekends, and holidays). The local health department should be notified immediately as well (by telegraph, facsimile machine, or telephone). Although the mortality rate has been reported to be as high as 60–70%, rapid diagnosis and adequate respiratory support should improve the outlook. Recovery of neurologic function occurs over weeks to months; complete recovery is common.

Serum sickness may develop as a result of administration of antitoxin. Neostigmine and other drugs effective in treating myasthenia gravis are not helpful in botulism.

B. Antibiotics: The treatment of wound botulism is debridement and penicillin, 300,000 units/kg/d intravenously, in addition to other measures described above. Clindamycin (30 mg/kg/d intravenously) or chloramphenicol (50 mg/kg/d intravenously) may be used in patients allergic to penicillin. Aminoglycosides may worsen neuromuscular blockade and should be avoided.

C. Additional Measures: Careful monitoring of vital capacity, maximum inspiratory force, and arterial blood gases is mandatory, since respiratory insufficiency may develop rapidly. Cathartics (eg, magnesium citrate) and enemas must be given early to remove any toxin remaining in the bowel. Emesis or gastric lavage is indicated if the contaminated food was ingested less than 6–8 hours before arrival at the emergency department. All other persons who have also eaten the suspected food should be given antitoxin, emetics, and cathartics even if they are asymptomatic.

Disposition

The patient must be hospitalized for observation and treatment.

ORGANOPHOSPHATE POISONING
(See also Chapter 39.)

Organophosphates exert their toxic effect by inhibiting acetylcholinesterase, producing stimulation and then inhibition at the myoneural junction by the uncatabolized acetylcholine. Poisoning is most commonly due to insecticides (parathion, malathion, etc) and occurs during spraying or dusting of crops. Certain poison gases used in war have a similar action.

Diagnosis

Rapidity of onset and severity of symptoms vary with the dose and route of administration; symptoms of poisoning may occur within 5 minutes to 12 hours after exposure.

A. Symptoms and Signs: (See Table 12–5.) Initial symptoms are fatigue, headache, dizziness, nausea and vomiting, and increased salivary and sweat production. Weakness of skeletal and bulbar muscles with marked fasciculations follows, and finally loss of consciousness occurs.

Examination often reveals the characteristic garlic odor of the organophosphate compound. Lacrimation is common, and pupils are pinpoint and may be unreactive to light. Muscle fasciculations and complete motor paralysis may be present.

B. Laboratory Findings: Hyperglycemia with prominent glycosuria may occur. Polymorphonuclear leukocytosis is common. Laboratory demonstration of depressed plasma and erythrocyte cholinesterase activity confirms the clinical diagnosis (Chapter 39).

Table 12–5. Manifestations of organophosphate poisoning.[1,2]

Symptoms and Signs	Severity of Poisoning		
	Severe (%)	Moderate (%)	Mild (%)
Weakness	100	100	100
Headache	100	100	95
Hyperhidrosis	100	91	91
Nausea and vomiting	100	100	77
Salivation and lacrimation	93	73	45
Miotic pupils	100	55	23
Dyspnea	100	55	14
Difficulty in walking	100	73	0
Diarrhea	64	36	36
Muscle fasciculations	100	55	0
Disturbance in speech	100	55	0
Disturbance in consciousness	100	55	0
Abdominal pain	36	36	27
Fever	64	55	0
Bronchopharyngeal secretions	71	36	0
Increase in blood pressure	71	18	0
Loss of pupillary reflex	71	0	0
Muscle cramps	64	0	0
Cyanosis	57	0	0

[1]Based on 47 cases of parathion poisoning; presented as percentage of total cases.
[2]Modified and reproduced, with permission, from Namba T et al: Poisoning due to organophosphate insecticides. *Am J Med* 1971;**50**:475.

Treatment
(See also Chapter 39.)

A. Emergency Measures: Maintain airway and respiratory function, and remove residual organophosphate by washing the skin and removing exposed clothing. Ingested organophosphates should be removed by lavage and catharsis. Induction of emesis is usually contraindicated because of the early onset of drowsiness. In this case, protect the airway, and perform gastric lavage.

B. Specific Measures:

1. Atropine, a specific antidote, is the treatment of choice; however, it does not reverse paralytic symptoms. Large doses may be required. Start with 2 mg intravenously (0.5 mg in children), followed by repeated doses of 2–4 mg every 5–10 minutes until signs of atropinization occur: flushing, mydriasis, drying of secretions, and tachycardia. The use of up to 50 mg in 24 hours is not unusual.

2. Pralidoxime (Protopam) releases organophosphates from acetylcholinesterase and should be given to all patients with significant intoxication. It should not be used for carbamate poisoning, since carbamates are not irreversibly bound to acetylcholinesterase. The dose is 20–40 mg/kg in saline intravenously over 20–30 minutes. The dose may be repeated in 6–8 hours.

Adequate renal function is a prerequisite for use of pralidoxime, since it is excreted in the urine.

Disposition

All patients except for the very mildly ill with stable or improving symptoms require hospitalization. The earlier treatment is instituted, the lower the mortality rate.

MYASTHENIA GRAVIS

Diagnosis

Musculature innervated by the cranial nerves is commonly the earliest and most severely involved in myasthenia gravis, as manifested by ptosis and by impaired eye movements, facial expressions, chewing, swallowing, and speaking. Pupillary responsiveness is preserved. There is increasing weakness on repetitive muscle use ("fatigability"). Sensory abnormalities are absent. The diagnosis in previously untreated patients is confirmed by objective and unequivocal improvement following anticholinesterase drugs, eg, edrophonium (Tensilon, others) (see p 185 for dosage); or the longer-acting neostigmine (Prostigmin) (1–1.5 mg intramuscularly; effect in 45–90 minutes). Stable myasthenic patients will be receiving one of the drug regimens listed in Table 12–6.

The acute occurrence of respiratory insufficiency or the inability to handle oropharyngeal secretions in a previously stable myasthenic patient constitutes a myasthenic crisis. Crises may be precipitated by intercurrent infection or surgery or may have no obvious cause. The subjective complaint of dyspnea in such patients demands immediate and careful evaluation.

The difference between "myasthenic" and "cholinergic" crisis is of little practical importance; the latter, however, appears to be uncommon.

Treatment

A. Immediately evaluate the need for respiratory assistance or endotracheal intubation, as described above. Temporizing with drug therapy may have disastrous consequences, as the patient may worsen within minutes.

B. Discontinue anticholinesterase therapy in the intubated patient.

C. Treat precipitating causes if present (eg, infection).

Disposition

All patients in myasthenic crisis require immediate hospitalization. Stable patients without any respiratory symptoms (not in crisis) may be treated medically (Table 12–6) and referred for outpatient care. Patients newly diagnosed as having myasthenia gravis may be hospitalized for evaluation and treatment or started on a medical regimen (Table 12–6) and referred to a clinic or private medical care.

PRIMARY ACUTE MYOPATHIES

HYPOKALEMIC PERIODIC PARALYSIS

Hypokalemic periodic paralysis is characterized by episodes of profound weakness that may occur at intervals ranging from a day to years. Episodes are often precipitated by a large carbohydrate meal or a period of strenuous exercise, especially when followed by rest or sleep.

Diagnosis

A. Symptoms and Signs: An attack of weakness usually lasts 2–24 hours. The weakness is painless and generalized, often beginning in the lower extremities and becoming more severe proximally. Paralysis of cranial and respiratory musculature is rare, and for this reason fatal episodes are uncommon. Extremity musculature is hypotonic during attacks. Reflexes are reduced in proportion to the muscle weakness. Sensory examination is normal.

B. Laboratory Findings: A markedly reduced serum potassium level (usually 2–3 meq/L) during the attack, with normal potassium levels and physical examination between episodes, confirms the diagnosis.

Treatment

A. Give potassium chloride, about 1 meq/kg orally at hourly intervals, until improvement occurs (usually within 3–4 hours). Many patients will require intravenous potassium chloride, with the rate of administration not exceeding 20 meq/h.

Table 12–6. Drug therapy of stable myasthenia gravis.

Drug	Preparation	Dose	Duration of Action
Pyridostigmine (Mestinon)	60-mg tablets.	1–4 tablets orally every 3–6 hours.	3–5 hours
Pyridostigmine (Mestinon)	180-mg sustained release capsules.	1–3 capsules orally at bedtime.	6–12 hours
Neostigmine bromide (Prostigmin)	15-mg tablets.	1–4 tablets orally every 36 hours.	2–4 hours
Neostigmine methylsulfate (Prostigmin, others)	Solution for injection, 1:1000, 1:2000, 1:4000.	1 mg (2 mL of 1:2000) intramuscularly or subcutaneously.	2–4 hours

B. The frequency and severity of attacks can be reduced with acetazolamide, 250 mg orally 2 or 3 times a day.

Disposition

Patients having acute attacks can usually be treated in the emergency department and sent home.

ACUTE ELECTROLYTE ABNORMALITIES

Profound magnesium and phosphate depletion can cause acute muscle weakness and must be particularly considered in alcohol abusers. However, the vast majority of acute clinical syndromes of muscle weakness are due to high or low serum potassium concentrations (Table 12–7). Although the onset of weakness is not well correlated with serum potassium levels, values below 3 meq/L or above 7.5 meq/L are most commonly associated with symptoms. Specific therapy is dictated by the etiologic diagnosis, but the potential for life-threatening cardiac arrhythmias from severe hypokalemia or hyperkalemia demands immediate therapy (Chapter 36).

MYOGLOBINURIA

Release of myoglobin from the body musculature may be due to many causes (Table 12–8). Weakness presumably results from loss of this contractile protein from muscle cells. Important consequences of rhabdomyolysis with myoglobinuria are acute renal failure and marked elevations of serum potassium.

Table 12–7. Disorders of serum potassium causing acute muscle weakness.

Hyperkalemia
  Potassium administration, orally or intravenously
  Renal insufficiency
  Potassium-retaining drug therapy: triamterene or spironolactone
  Acute tissue necrosis secondary to trauma or chemotherapy
  Addison's disease
  Myoglobinuria
  Rhabdomyolysis
  Hypoaldosteronism
Hypokalemia
  Gastrointestinal postassium wastage
    Chronic vomiting or nasogastric suction
    Chronic diarrhea or laxative abuse
    Villous adenoma
    Draining gastrointestinal fistulas or ureteroileostomy
  Renal potassium wastage
    Drugs (diuretics, amphotericin B)
    Hyperaldosteronism
    Cushing's disease or corticosteroid therapy
    Renal tubular acidosis
    Licorice (glycyrrhizic acid) intoxication

Table 12–8. Common causes of myoglobinuria.

Muscle compression and necrosis secondary to prolonged coma (alcoholism, drug overdose, stroke)
Vigorous exercise, especially with poor conditioning and high environmental temperature
Status epilepticus
Delirium tremens
Chronic potassium depletion
Influenza or other acute viral infections

Diagnosis

A. Symptoms and Signs: Pain and swelling of the involved muscles and weakness of the limbs occur, especially in proximal distribution. Reflexes are depressed in proportion to muscle weakness. Sensory examination is normal.

B. Laboratory Findings: The urine is red-tinged and turns dark brown on standing. Myoglobinuria may be suggested by a heme-positive (dipstick) test in erythrocyte-free urine and confirmed by specific chemical testing. Muscle enzymes (CK, AST [SGOT], LDH) are massively elevated in most cases.

Treatment

Treatment consists of hydration and administration of mannitol to ensure high urine volumes and prevent precipitation of myoglobin in renal tubules. If anuria is present, fluids should be administered cautiously. A recommended regimen is to add mannitol, 25 g (100 mL of 25% solution), and bicarbonate, 100 meq (100 mL), to 800 mL of 5% dextrose in water and administer 1 L at a rate of 200 mL/h (adult dose). Monitor urine output closely.

Disposition

Hospitalization is mandatory. Serum potassium levels should be followed closely. The prognosis of this disorder is good even with profound muscle necrosis and renal failure.

IV. IMMEDIATE MANAGEMENT OF LIFE-THREATENING PROBLEMS ASSOCIATED WITH STROKE*

Stroke is a cerebrovascular disorder resulting from impairment of cerebral blood supply by occlusion (eg, by thrombi or emboli) or hemorrhage. It is characterized by the abrupt onset of focal neurologic deficits. The clinical manifestation is dependent on the area of the brain served by the involved blood vessel.

*This section contributed by Mary T. Ho, MD, MPH

Stroke is the most common serious neurologic disorder in adults and occurs most frequently after age 60 years. The mortality rate is 40% within the first month, and 50% of patients who survive will require long-term special care.

Stabilize Ventilation

A. Establish Airway: Assess adequacy of airway and ventilation in all stroke patients, especially in the presence of depressed level of consciousness, absent gag reflex, respiratory difficulty, or difficulty managing secretions.

B. Consider Intubation: Patients with inadequate ventilation (respiratory acidosis) or difficulty managing secretions may require intubation.

Search for Head Trauma

Stroke patients may sustain head injury due to incoordination or weakness. Conversely, patients with focal neurologic findings due to head trauma may be mistakenly diagnosed as suffering from stroke. If head injury is suspected from the history or clinical findings, immobilize the spine and refer to Chapter 16 for management.

Treat Cerebral Edema

Deterioration of neurologic deficits or the presence of brainstem involvement (depressed sensorium, pupillary or extraocular movement abnormality, decorticate or decerebrate posturing) suggests significant cerebral edema and impending herniation. With the exception of temporizing measures prior to surgical decompression in cerebellar or superficial lobar hemorrhage, medical therapy for cerebral edema (see Table 10–2) associated with ischemic stroke does not alter the outcome.

Treat Seizures

See Chapter 11 for management of seizures. Consider prophylaxis for acute seizure in patients with embolic stroke or subarachnoid hemorrhage. Give intravenous phenytoin, 15–18 mg/kg at a rate not greater than 50 mg/min.

Treat Hypoglycemia

Occasionally, patients with hypoglycemia may have focal neurologic deficits that may be confused with stroke. Confirm the presence of hypoglycemia using a glucometer or reagent strips (eg, Chemstrip bG, Visidex II) before giving 50 mL of 50% dextrose solution. Stroke patients with elevated serum glucose may have a worsened outcome.

Obtain Emergency CT Scan

Emergency CT scan of the head should be obtained early. This is the most readily available method for reliably detecting the presence of hemorrhage and focal cerebral edema.

V. FURTHER EVALUATION OF THE PATIENT WITH STROKE

Accurate diagnosis and identification of the underlying etiology of the stroke are important for appropriate evaluation and treatment. Conditions that predispose to strokes should be sought and corrected. A systematic approach to the evaluation of the patient with stroke is detailed below and can be modified depending on the urgency of the patient's condition.

History

A. Determine Time Course of Deficits: Transient ischemic attacks and deficits progressive in a stepwise pattern over hours to days suggest thrombotic vascular occlusion. Abrupt onset of full neurologic deficit is characteristic of embolic stroke. Abrupt onset and rapid evolution of deficits are associated with intracerebral hemorrhage.

B. Identify Risk Factors: Hypertension, diabetes mellitus, transient ischemic attacks, hyperlipidemia, smoking, family history, and use of oral contraceptives predispose to atherosclerotic disease. Cardiac disorders (Table 12–9) such as changing cardiac rhythms (especially atrial fibrillation), dyskinetic myocardium, and valvular heart disease are associated with increased risk for embolic strokes. Bleeding dyscrasias, hypercoagulable states, blood disorders (especially sickle cell disease), and vascular disorders are also associated with a risk for stroke. Carotid artery bruits in patients with transient ischemic attacks or stroke suggest the possibility of emboli derived from atheromatous plaques. Acute stroke syndromes, especially intracerebral hemor-

Table 12–9. Sources of emboli.

Cardiac
    Changing rhythms, especially atrial fibrillation
    Valvular disease
        Rheumatic heart disease
        Valve prosthesis
        Bacterial and fungal endocarditis
        Myxomatous vegetation
        Congenital heart disease
        Mitral valve prolapse
    Atrial tumor
    Myocardial dysfunction
        Myocardial infarction
        Ventricular aneurysm
Noncardiac
    Foreign body
    Air, nitrogen, or other gases
    Fat
    Tumor
    Atheromatous material
    Thrombus

rhages, have recently been associated with cocaine and, less commonly, amphetamine use.

C. Identify Other Associated Symptoms: Severe headache and vomiting often accompany intracerebral hemorrhage. Patients with migraine headaches rarely may suffer strokes due to vascular spasm.

Physical Examination

A. General: A thorough examination may reveal the underlying cause for the stroke and direct treatment.

1. Vital signs–The body temperature should be recorded. Hypertension is a risk factor for stroke, and systolic pressure above 200 mm Hg may require treatment.

2. Head–Arteriovenous malformations may be detected by auscultation of the head for bruits. Palpate the temporal arteries for tenderness, nodularity, or absence of pulse suggestive of giant cell arteritis.

3. Eyes–Examination of the retina may reveal visible emboli in the retinal vessels. Subhyaloid hemorrhage is diagnostic for subarachnoid hemorrhage.

4. Neck–The carotid arteries should be examined for presence of bruits and reduction of pulsation. Although these findings are not specific for carotid disease, further carotid studies may be warranted to evaluate for possible carotid endarterectomy.

5. Heart–Changing cardiac rhythms and murmurs or valvular disease are associated with increased risk of embolization from the heart.

6. Skin–Ecchymosis and petechiae may suggest blood disorders or vasculitis as causative factors. Presence of recent needle tracks or subungual splinter hemorrhages suggest the possibility of septic emboli derived from infected heart valves.

B. Neurologic: A rapid neurologic examination should be performed in the emergency department and should focus on (**1**) localizing the anatomic site of deficit as an aid in determining the specific stroke syndrome (which dictates treatment) and (**2**) assessing the degree of neurologic impairment, from which improvement or worsening can be assessed.

1. Cognitive–Assess response to commands and fluency of speech. Aphasia and apraxia are associated with involvement of the cerebral cortex and anterior (carotid) circulation; lacunar infarction or disturbance of posterior (vertebrobasilar) circulation is unlikely.

2. Cranial nerves–Visual field abnormalities exclude lacunar infarction. Abnormal pupillary reflexes and ocular palsies are brainstem findings and are associated with disturbance of posterior circulation or impending brain herniation.

3. Motor–Hemiparesis can be associated with disturbance of the anterior or posterior circulation or lacunae. Generally, in anterior circulation strokes, the face, hand, and arm are more affected than the leg. In lacunar infarction and posterior circulation strokes,

this pattern is less common. Hemiparesis involving one side of the face and the other side of the body is due to disturbance of posterior circulation.

4. Sensory–Hemisensory deficits without associated motor involvement are usually due to lacunar infarcts. Astereognosis (inability to identify objects by touch) and agraphesthesia (inability to recognize figures traced on the skin) are cortical sensory deficits and are due to disturbance of anterior circulation.

5. Cerebellar–Hemiataxia suggests involvement of the cerebellum or the brainstem, or lacunar infarction deep in white matter.

Laboratory Tests

A. Blood Tests: The following blood tests should be obtained in most patients with focal neurologic deficits:

1. Complete blood count and platelet count to detect blood dyscrasias, and prothrombin time (PT) and partial thromboplastin time (PTT) for coagulation disorders.

2. Glucose level, since both hyperglycemia and hypoglycemia may cause focal neurologic findings that can mimic stroke.

3. Erythrocyte sedimentation rate to detect vasculitis or arteritis.

4. Serologic test for syphilis.

5. Toxicologic screen if drug use is suspected.

B. Electrocardiogram: An ECG may reveal new arrhythmias or reversion to a normal rhythm, both of which are associated with increased risk for emboli. Presence of myocardial infarction or persistent changes suggestive of a ventricular aneurysm also increase the risk for stroke.

C. CT or MRI Scan: These studies are essential for localizing the lesion, distinguishing hemorrhagic from occlusive stroke, and identifying other intracranial disease, such as tumor or abscess, that can be confused with strokes. A CT or MRI scan should be obtained in any stroke patient.

D. Lumbar Puncture: Occasionally, in patients suspected of having subarachnoid hemorrhage but whose CT scan is negative or equivocal, a lumbar puncture may be diagnostic (the cerebrospinal fluid is bloody or the supernatant is xanthochromic). Lumbar puncture is often useful in patients with meningoencephalitis and vasculitis.

Caution: In patients with focal neurologic findings, a CT or MRI scan should be performed prior to lumbar puncture.

E. Vascular Studies: Cerebral angiography may be indicated in patients suspected of having a surgically correctable condition such as cerebral aneurysm, arteriovenous malformation, and carotid atherosclerosis or stenosis. Noninvasive vascular studies such as ophthalmodynamometry, doppler sonography, thermography, and ultrasonic studies may be useful to identify patients with suspected carotid atherosclerotic disease who may need angiography.

VI. MANAGEMENT OF SPECIFIC STROKE SYNDROMES

HEMORRHAGIC STROKE

SUBARACHNOID HEMORRHAGE
(See also Chapter 10.)

Bleeding occurs within the subarachnoid space and is usually due to a ruptured cerebral aneurysm or, less commonly, an arteriovenous malformation. Arteriovenous malformations tend to bleed earlier than aneurysms, often becoming symptomatic in childhood or before age 30 years.

Diagnosis
Abrupt onset of severe headache often accompanied by vomiting is the classic presentation, but the headache is not invariably severe; it is, however, unique in quality in the patient's experience. As bleeding is within the subarachnoid space, focal neurologic deficits are usually absent. Depressed mentation, ranging from lethargy to coma, is common. Signs of meningeal irritation (nuchal rigidity, Kernig's sign, or Brudzinski's sign) develop within several hours after onset of bleeding. Preretinal (subhyaloid) hemorrhage may be present. Hypertension, cardiac arrhythmias, and ST segment and T wave abnormalities of the ECG may occur as a result of the hemorrhage.

A CT scan should be obtained and is diagnostic in approximately 85% of cases. When CT scan is negative or nondiagnostic and subarachnoid hemorrhage is suspected, lumbar puncture should be performed. In this setting, bloody or xanthochromic cerebrospinal fluid is diagnostic.

Treatment & Disposition
Initial treatment should include analgesia and bed rest. Blood pressure should be maintained in the physiologic range for the patient; avoid hypotension, which can worsen ischemia. Bed rest is usually adequate treatment for hypertension and is the only protection against vasospasm. Begin prophylactic anticonvulsant therapy with phenytoin, 15–18 mg/kg intravenously in a loading dose. Obtain emergency neurosurgical consultation. Early surgery is the best defense against rerupture. All patients should be hospitalized.

INTRACEREBRAL HEMORRHAGE
(See also Chapter 10.)

Bleeding occurs primarily in the brain parenchyma, although blood appears in the cerebrospinal fluid in the majority of patients. Symptoms are due to mass effect of the hematoma with displacement and compression of adjacent brain tissue. The most common cause is damage of intracerebral arterioles by long-standing systemic hypertension. Other causes include anticoagulation or thrombolytic therapy, bleeding diathesis, neoplasms, cerebral amyloid angiopathy, infections, and arteriovenous malformations.

Diagnosis
Clinical findings depend on the site of the hemorrhage but occur abruptly and progress within minutes to a few hours. Headache and vomiting are frequent symptoms. Focal neurologic deficits are prominent, since most bleeding sites abut the basal ganglia, thalamus, and internal capsule. Abrupt onset of coma and prominent brainstem findings (pinpoint pupils, absent extraocular movements) is characteristic of pontine hemorrhage. A CT scan is diagnostic.

Ataxia and cerebellar abnormalities, with absent or mild hemiparesis, are characteristic of cerebellar hemorrhage. It is particularly important to diagnose hypertensive intracerebellar hemorrhage rapidly, since fatal brainstem compression may occur rapidly; emergency surgical decompression can be lifesaving. Because the clinical differentiation from acute vestibular dysfunction may be difficult, patients with sudden onset of disequilibrium and vomiting may need a CT scan of the brain to exclude cerebellar hemorrhage.

Treatment & Disposition
Treatment is mainly supportive, consisting of airway management. Reduction of cerebral edema with fluid restriction, hyperventilation, and osmotic diuresis is rarely effective except as a temporizing measure prior to surgery. *Emergency neurosurgical consultation should be obtained for evacuation of clot in intracerebral or superficial cortical hemorrhages with mass effect.*

OCCLUSIVE STROKE

Occlusive strokes, comprised of thrombotic, embolic, and lacunar occlusions, account for over 75% of all strokes and result in cerebral ischemia or infarction. A variety of disorders of blood, blood vessels, and heart can cause occlusive strokes, but the most common by far are atherosclerotic disease (especially of the carotid and vertebrobasilar arteries) and cardiac abnormalities. Risk factors for atherosclerosis are often present and include smoking, hypertension, coronary artery disease, hyperlipidemia, diabetes mellitus, family history of stroke, and oral contraceptive use.

THROMBOTIC STROKE

Diagnosis
Occurrence of transient ischemic attacks preceding the stroke is the hallmark of thrombotic stroke. The neurologic deficits may evolve over minutes to hours or days and are typical for a specific vascular distribution. Motor and sensory pathways are impaired. Headache and vomiting are rare. The diagnosis is made on the basis of the clinical findings and exclusion of hemorrhage by CT scan or lumbar puncture. MRI and repeat CT scan at 48–72 hours will often confirm the diagnosis when the initial study is normal.

Treatment & Disposition
For completed strokes with major deficits, the treatment is largely supportive. Specific treatment depends on the temporal evolution of the stroke (see Transient Ischemic Attacks, Progressive Stroke, and Completed Stroke, below). All patients should be hospitalized. For patients with transient ischemic attacks or mild fixed deficits who have high-grade (> 70%) carotid artery stenosis, endarterectomy is the treatment of choice. In most cases, elevated blood pressure should not be treated acutely, since this may result in decreased perfusion to the ischemic brain region where autoregulation of cerebral blood flow is impaired.

EMBOLIC STROKE

Diagnosis
The stroke syndrome that can be clinically recognized as embolic is that of cardiac origin. Stroke due to emboli from other arteries (eg, the carotid artery) cannot easily be distinguished clinically from strokes due to other causes. Symptoms of embolic stroke are apoplectic in onset. Prior episodes of transient ischemic attacks are notably absent. Neurologic deficits may be similar to those produced by thrombotic stroke. However, involvement of the area supplied by an end artery (posterior cerebral, anterior cerebral, or inferior division of the middle cerebral arteries) suggest an embolic cause. Occasionally, multiple emboli occur and deficits reflecting involvement of more than one vascular distribution will be found. Such findings are highly suggestive of emboli from a cardiac source, especially when both cerebral hemispheres are affected. The diagnosis can be made with certainty when neurologic symptoms occur abruptly without preceding episodes of transient ischemic attacks, a source of emboli can be identified (eg, acute myocardial infarction, atrial fibrillation), and primary

intracortical hemorrhage is excluded by CT scan or lumbar puncture. Common sources of emboli from cardiac and noncardiac sources are listed in Table 12–9.

Treatment & Disposition
Patients with embolic stroke from cardiac causes should receive anticoagulation therapy, if not contraindicated, to prevent further emboli. The risk of recurrent emboli is highest within the first hour of the initial event and remains elevated for up to 2 weeks. Administer intravenous heparin in a 5000–10,000 unit bolus, followed by continuous infusion of 1000 units per hour adjusted to maintain activated PTT at twice normal. The underlying cause of emboli should be corrected, if possible. Caution should be used in patients with large areas of infarcted brain, as the risk of hemorrhage into the region of infarction is significant.

All patients should be hospitalized.

LACUNAR STROKE

Diagnosis
Lacunar stroke results from occlusion of the small penetrating arteries of the brain by lipohyalinotic deposits, which are a product of long-standing hypertension. The areas of infarction are generally small, and multiple old infarct sites may also be identified on CT scan. The clinical findings are distinct and may range from pure motor or pure sensory deficits to incoordination and clumsiness of the hand or ataxia of the arm or leg. Computed tomographic scan is often normal or may show small lucencies in the affected areas, usually in the internal capsule, pons, cerebellum, or subcortical white matter.

Treatment & Disposition
Treatment is supportive and consists mainly of blood pressure control. The prognosis is generally good. Patients should usually be hospitalized for observation.

ARTERIAL DISSECTION

Diagnosis
An acute progressive syndrome of carotid or vertebral artery ischemia almost invariably associated with anterior or posterior neck pain should suggest carotid or vertebral artery dissection, respectively. A history of recent neck trauma is frequent and may be relatively trivial, such as chiropractic manipulation. Angiography is diagnostic and shows the markedly reduced intravascular lumen caused by dissection of the intimal layer, producing the characteristic "string sign."

Treatment & Disposition

Surgical intervention is not indicated. Vessels recanalize spontaneously over months. Current opinion favors anticoagulation acutely and for several months thereafter to reduce the potential for distal embolization of platelet aggregates formed on the damaged vessel wall.

TRANSIENT ISCHEMIC ATTACKS (TIA)

Diagnosis

Neurologic deficits occur suddenly and persist from minutes to hours but completely resolve within 24 hours. These episodes are caused by small platelet, fibrin, or atheromatous emboli originating in extracranial vessels or the heart. Clinical findings depend on the area of the brain affected. Transient monocular blindness due to embolus in the retinal artery (amaurosis fugax) usually signifies ipsilateral carotid artery disease, but unlike hemispheric transient ischemic attack, amaurosis fugax is associated with less risk for subsequent carotid stroke.

Treatment

Transient ischemic attacks may be harbingers of impending stroke, with one-third of patients suffering a stroke within 5 years; 20% of these occur within 1 month and 50% within 1 year. Treatment is directed at identifying and correcting the underlying cause (eg, treat hypertension, evaluate for carotid endarterectomy). Specific treatments include the following.

A. Aspirin: Aspirin, 325 mg orally once daily, appears to reduce the risk of stroke in patients with prior strokes or transient ischemic attacks. In all other cases, the effect of treatment with aspirin is unclear. Other antiplatelet agents (sulfinpyrazone, dipyridamole) are not as effective and do not appear to enhance the effect of aspirin.

B. Anticoagulants: Effectiveness of heparin or warfarin for noncardiac causes of transient ischemic attacks remains unclear. The risk of hemorrhage in general—and intracerebral hemorrhage in particular—must be weighed against any possible advantage. Anticoagulants should be used only in patients who do not tolerate or fail to respond to aspirin therapy. Treatment should be continued only for 2–3 months; longer periods of treatment do not have any additional benefit.

C. Carotid Endarterectomy: Patients with symptomatic (eg, transient ischemic attacks in the carotid artery territory), atherosclerotic, high-grade stenosis in the extracranial internal carotid artery benefit from carotid endarterectomy. Noninvasive vascular studies should be performed in patients with hemispheric carotid transient ischemic attacks who are surgical candidates. Patients with > 70% stenosis

should undergo carotid angiography to determine eligibility for carotid endarterectomy.

D. Antihypertensive Medication: Hypertension is the major risk factor for future stroke and should be promptly corrected.

Disposition

Most patients with transient ischemic attacks should be hospitalized. Patients who have had recent prior thorough evaluation for transient ischemic attacks or who are not candidates for therapy should be referred to their primary physician for outpatient follow-up.

REVERSIBLE ISCHEMIC NEUROLOGIC DEFICIT (RIND)

Neurologic deficits persist for over 24 hours but resolve completely within 4 weeks, usually within 2–3 days. This syndrome cannot be differentiated from a completed stroke in the emergency department. Treatment should be identical to that for a transient ischemic attack.

PROGRESSIVE STROKE (Stroke in Evolution)

Diagnosis

Neurologic deficits continue to progress over time.

Treatment & Disposition

Emergency CT scan must be obtained to detect hemorrhage, cerebral edema, and nonvascular causes of focal neurologic deficits. Anticoagulation therapy with intravenous heparin is currently the standard mode of therapy. However, except in the case of vertebrobasilar ischemia, recent studies have cast doubt on the effectiveness of anticoagulants in the treatment of progressive ischemic strokes.

All patients should be hospitalized.

COMPLETED STROKE

Diagnosis

Neurologic deficits are stable. Improvement may occur over the subsequent weeks as edema associated with the infarct resolves, but residual motor deficits and language abnormalities that remain unchanged after 3 weeks and 3 months, respectively, will persist.

Treatment & Disposition

Treatment is primarily supportive. There is some evidence that the incidence of subsequent strokes may decrease when aspirin is administered chronically. Anticoagulation therapy is not recommended. However, if a persistent source of cardiac emboli is present (eg, prosthetic heart valve, rheumatic valvular disease, atrial or ventricular thrombus) anticoagulation therapy, if not contraindicated, should be initiated immediately to prevent subsequent embolic strokes. While hemorrhage into the infarct may occur, the outcome is not adversely affected except in large infarctions. Systolic hypertension below 200 mm Hg should not be treated if asymptomatic. Reduction in systemic blood pressure can worsen cerebral ischemia and extend the area of cerebral infarct.

All patients should be hospitalized.

REFERENCES

Weakness

Asbury AK, Cornblath DR: Assessment of current diagnostic criteria for Guillain-Barré syndrome. Ann Neurol 1990;27(Suppl):S21.

Baker AS et al: Spinal epidural abscess. N Engl J Med 1975;293:463.

Cashman NR et al: Late denervation in patients with antecedent paralytic poliomyelitis. N Engl J Med 1987; 317:7.

Center for Disease Control News: Diagnosis and treatment of botulism. J Infect Dis 1971;124:108.

Engel AG: Myasthenia gravis and myasthenic syndromes. Ann Neurol 1984;16:519.

Griggs RC, Engel WK, Resnick JS: Acetazolamide treatment of hypokalemic periodic paralysis. Ann Intern Med 1970;73:39.

Hughes JM et al: Clinical features of type A and type B food-borne botulism. Ann Intern Med 1981;95:442.

Johnson R, Jong EC: Ciguatera: Caribbean and Indo-Pacific fish poisoning. West J Med 1983;138:872.

Koffler A, Friedler RM, Massry SG: Acute renal failure due to nontraumatic rhabdomyolysis. Ann Intern Med 1976; 85:23.

Layzer RB: Neuromuscular manifestations of systemic disease. In: *Contemporary Neurology.* Vol. 25. Davis, 1985.

Leys D et al: Decreased morbidity from acute bacterial spinal epidural abscesses using computed tomography and nonsurgical treatment in selected patients. Ann Neurol 1985;17:350.

Lotti M, Becker CE, Aminoff MJ: Organophosphate polyneuropathy: Pathogenesis and prevention. Neurology 1984;34:658.

McKhann GM: Guillain-Barré syndrome: Clinical and therapeutic observations. Ann Neurol 1990;27 (Suppl):S13.

McQuillen MP, Cantor HE, O'Rourke JR: Myasthenic syndrome associated with antibiotics. Arch Neurol 1968;18: 402.

Ropper AH, Poskanzer DC: The prognosis of acute and subacute transverse myelopathy based on early signs and symptoms. Ann Neurol 1978;4:51.

Schmitt N, Bowmer EJ, Gregson JD: Tick paralysis in British Columbia. Can Med Assoc J 1969;100:417.

Wadia RS et al: Neurological manifestations of organophosphorus insecticide poisoning. J Neurol Neurosurg Psychiatry 1974;37:841.

Stroke

Boston Area Anticoagulation Trial for Atrial Fibrillation Investigators: The effect of low-dose warfarin on the risk of stroke in patients with nonrheumatic atrial fibrillation. N Engl J Med 1990;323:1505.

Bougousslavsky J et al: Migraine stroke. Neurology 1988; 38:223.

Bousser MG et al: Cerebral venous thrombosis: A review of 38 cases. Stroke 1985;16:199.

Caplan L: Intracerebral hemorrhage revisited. Neurology 1988;38:624.

Cerebral Embolism Task Force: Cardiogenic brain embolism: The second report of the Cerebral Embolism Task Force. Arch Neurol 1989;46:727.

Grotta JC: Current medical and surgical therapy for cerebrovascular disease. N Engl J Med 1987;317:1505.

Hart RG, Easton JD: Dissections of cervical and cerebral arteries. Neurol Clin 1983;1:155.

Kaku DA, Lowenstein DH: Emergence of recreational drug abuse as a major risk factor for stroke in young adults. Ann Intern Med 1990;113:821.

Kittner SJ et al: Infarcts with a cardiac source of embolism in the NINCDS stroke data bank: Historical features. Neurology 1990;40:281.

Levine SR et al: Cerebrovascular complications of the use of the "crack" form of alkaloidal cocaine. N Engl J Med 1990;323:699.

Levy DE: How transient are transient ischemic attacks? Neurology 1988;38:674.

Levy DE et al: Predicting outcome from hypoxic-ischemic coma. JAMA 1985;253:1420.

Markel ML, Waller BF, Armstrong WF: Cardiac myxoma: A review. Medicine 1987;66:114.

Peterson P et al: Placebo-controlled, randomised trial of warfarin and aspirin for prevention of thromboembolic complications in chronic atrial fibrillation: The Copenhagen AFASAK study. Lancet 1989;1:175.

Rolak LA, Gilmer W, Strittmatter WJ: Low yield in the diagnostic evaluation of transient ischemic attacks. Neurology 1990;40:747.

Stroke Prevention in Atrial Fibrillation Study Group Investigators: Preliminary report of the stroke prevention in atrial fibrillation study. N Engl J Med 1990;322:863.

Werdelin L, Juhler M: The course of transient ischemic attacks. Neurology 1988;38:677.

Wipf JE, Lipsky BA: Atrial fibrillation: Thromboembolic risk and indications for anticoagulation. Arch Intern Med 1990;150:1598.

13

Headache

Roger P. Simon, MD

IMMEDIATE EVALUATION & MANAGEMENT OF HEADACHE CAUSED BY LIFE-THREATENING CONDITIONS
(See algorithm.)

Has Head Trauma Occurred?

If recent head trauma has occurred, evaluation of this problem takes precedence (Chapter 16).

Have Seizures Occurred?

Patients may have headache following one or more grand mal seizures. However, because the seizures may themselves be due to serious underlying disease (eg, subdural hematoma), evaluation of this problem takes precedence (Chapter 11).

Are There Focal Neurologic Abnormalities?

The presence of new focal neurologic abnormalities with headache, especially if papilledema is present as well, is strongly suggestive of a mass lesion (tumor, hematoma, abscess). CT scan, MRI, or angiogram should be done as soon as practical to make the diagnosis. Further evaluation is discussed in Chapter 12.

Is Headache New or of Recent Origin?

The single most important item of information to obtain from a patient with headache is whether the headache is new. A new headache is one occurring in a patient without a history of headaches, or a novel pattern or quality of pain in a patient with a history of headaches. New headaches demand immediate careful evaluation.

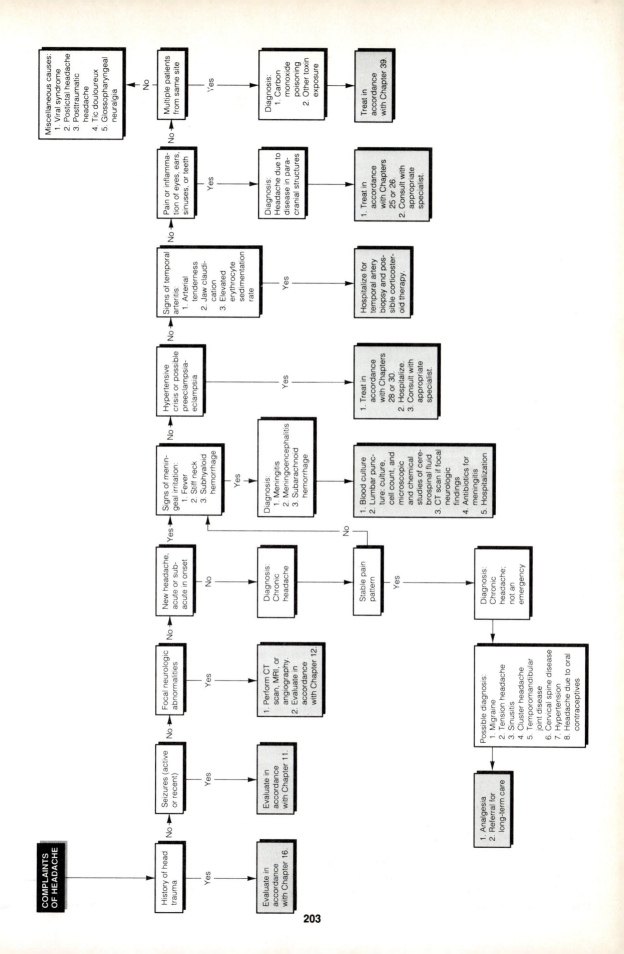

COMPLAINTS
OF HEADACHE

History of head
trauma

Yes → Evaluate in
accordance
with Chapter 16.

No ↓

Seizures (active
or recent)

Yes → Evaluate in
accordance
with Chapter 11.

No ↓

Focal neurologic
abnormalities

Yes → 1. Perform CT
scan, MRI, or
angiography.
2. Evaluate in
accordance
with Chapter 12.

No ↓

New headache,
acute or sub-
acute in onset

No → Diagnosis:
Chronic
headache → Stable pain
pattern

Yes → Diagnosis:
Chronic
headache;
not an
emergency

↓

Possible diagnosis:
1. Migraine
2. Tension headache
3. Sinusitis
4. Cluster headache
5. Temporomandibular
joint disease
6. Cervical spine disease
7. Hypertension
8. Headache due to oral
contraceptives

↓

1. Analgesia
2. Referral for
long-term care

No (from Stable pain pattern) ↑

Yes ↓ (New headache)

Signs of menin-
geal irritation:
1. Fever
2. Stiff neck
3. Subhyaloid
hemorrhage

Yes → Diagnosis:
1. Meningitis
2. Meningoencephalitis
3. Subarachnoid
hemorrhage

→ 1. Blood culture
2. Lumbar punc-
ture: culture,
cell count, and
microscopic
and chemical
studies of cere-
brospinal fluid
3. CT scan if focal
neurologic
findings
4. Antibiotics for
meningitis
5. Hospitalization

No ↓

Hypertensive
crisis or possible
preeclampsia-
eclampsia

Yes → 1. Treat in
accordance
with Chapters
28 or 30.
2. Hospitalize.
3. Consult with
appropriate
specialist.

No ↓

Signs of temporal
arteritis:
1. Arterial
tenderness
2. Jaw claudi-
cation
3. Elevated
erythrocyte
sedimentation
rate

Yes → Hospitalize for
temporal artery
biopsy and pos-
sible corticoster-
oid therapy.

No ↓

Pain or inflamma-
tion of eyes, ears,
sinuses, or teeth

Yes → Diagnosis:
Headache due to
disease in para-
cranial structures

→ 1. Treat in
accordance
with Chapters
25 or 26.
2. Consult with
appropriate
specialist.

No ↓

Multiple patients
from same site

Yes → Diagnosis:
1. Carbon
monoxide
poisoning
2. Other toxin
exposure

→ Treat in
accordance
with Chapter 39.

No ↓

Miscellaneous causes:
1. Viral syndrome
2. Postictal headache
3. Posttraumatic
headache
4. Tic douloureux
5. Glossopharyngeal
neuralgia

Is the Complaint Consistent With Meningitis or Meningeal Irritation?

If the headache is acute (sudden) or subacute (hours to days) in onset, subarachnoid hemorrhage (with resultant irritative [chemical] meningitis) or meningitis must be suspected. The usual manifestations are signs of meningeal irritation (stiff neck; positive Kernig and Brudzinski signs) (see below) and fever (usually absent in subarachnoid hemorrhage). These findings may be minimal or even absent in very young or very old patients. Seizures, confusion, or coma may be present as well. Subarachnoid hemorrhage should be strongly suspected in a patient with abrupt onset of headache that is unique to the patient's experience, especially if meningeal irritation or focal neurologic findings are present. Subhyaloid (preretinal) hemorrhages may be present after subarachnoid hemorrhage and are fairly specific to that condition (see Chapters 10 and 12). An emergency CT scan is required; if the diagnosis is still unclear, lumbar puncture should be performed. If meningitis is also a possibility, antibiotic therapy should be started as soon as possible (based on microorganisms most common for each age group) and before the CT scan is obtained (see Chapter 34).

Meningitis should be strongly suspected in a patient who presents with headache accompanied by fever, especially if signs of meningeal irritation are present. A lumbar puncture should be performed immediately and antibiotics begun as soon as possible (ie, within 30 minutes of arrival in the emergency department) (see Chapter 34).

If there are signs of altered mental status or if there are focal neurologic findings in a patient with fever, a brain abscess should be suspected. Lumbar puncture should be delayed until a CT scan is performed.

Is Headache Due to Hypertensive Encephalopathy or Preeclampsia-Eclampsia?

Moderate elevations of blood pressure alone seldom cause headache; however, severe hypertension as seen in hypertensive crises and eclampsia is associated with headache. If hypertension is present and the patient is pregnant or has signs of cerebral dysfunction (confusion, obtundation, or coma) or other end-organ damage (retinitis; nephritis with proteinuria), a life-threatening emergency exists. *Note:* In pregnancy, a slight increase in blood pressure may be more significant than in the nonpregnant patient. See Chapter 28 (hypertensive crisis) or Chapter 30 (eclampsia).

Is This Temporal Arteritis?

Temporal arteritis, a rare but treatable disease with serious sequelae, must be considered in every elderly patient with new headache. The principal manifestations are headache with temporal artery tenderness (not found in every case) and a markedly accelerated erythrocyte sedimentation rate. Sudden monocular blindness may occur. If this condition is suspected, hospitalization is warranted to confirm the diagnosis by means of temporal artery biopsy and to begin therapy. For details of diagnosis and management, see p 209.

Is Headache Due to Disease in Paracranial Structures?

New or acute headaches are often caused by disease in the eyes, ears, sinuses, or teeth. Look carefully for iritis or acute glaucoma (Chapter 25), sinusitis, otitis media, or dental caries or abscess (Chapter 26). Treatment should be focused on the primary condition.

Are There Multiple Patients From the Same Vicinity?

Multiple patients from the same vicinity with complaint of headache suggest carbon monoxide poisoning or other toxin exposure. Patients should be questioned specifically about heating sources (eg, gas heat or oven), burning materials (eg, charcoal) in poorly ventilated areas, use of household cleaners, or other chemical exposure. Specific treatment of carbon monoxide poisoning and other toxin exposure is discussed in Chapter 39.

Disposition

Even after careful initial history and physical examination, the diagnosis may not be apparent in the patient with new headache. Patients with recent onset of new headache should be hospitalized if there is any suspicion of a life-threatening process. Increasing severity of subacute headache over days or weeks, even without focal signs, suggests serious intracranial disease, and the patient should be referred immediately for diagnostic procedures. Subacute headaches without progressive symptoms and chronic headaches may be evaluated on a nonemergency basis.

APPROACH TO THE DIAGNOSIS OF HEADACHE

Pain-Sensitive Structures & Their Projections

Headache is caused by traction, displacement, inflammation, or distention of pain-sensitive structures in the head or neck. Disorders of the scalp, teeth, eyes, and ears and of the mucous membranes of the nose, sinuses, and oropharynx can produce pain. Pain-sensitive structures about the calvarium include the scalp and its blood vessels, the neck muscles, and the upper cervical nerves. The skull, brain, and most of the dura are not pain-sensitive. In general, discrete intracranial lesions above the cerebellar tentorium produce pain in trigeminal distribution (anterior to ears), whereas lesions in the posterior fossa project pain to the second and third cervical dermatomes (posterior to ears).

History

A. Time of Onset: Chronic headache (duration of months or more) is usually not due to a serious disorder, but headache of acute onset or of a changing pain pattern demands prompt evaluation in the emergency department. If the patient has a chronic headache disorder, determine if the present headache differs from or is identical to the patient's chronic problem.

Although the sudden onset of pain or "the worst headache I ever had in my life" typifies subarachnoid hemorrhage, the associated headache will be unique but *need not be severe.*

B. Precipitating Factors:

1. Tension headache–Tension, emotional stress, fatigue.

2. Migraine–Hunger, nitrite-containing foods (hot dogs, salami, sausage), chocolate, cheddar cheese, bright lights, menses.

3. Cluster variant of migraine–Alcohol.

4. Glossopharyngeal neuralgia, tic douloureux, and the jaw claudication of temporal arteritis–Chewing and eating.

C. Location of Pain:

1. Migraine or the cluster variant–Hemicranial or retro-ocular pain.

2. Tension headaches–Commonly diffuse, occipital, or bandlike pain.

3. Mass lesion headaches– Often focal ("right here").

4. Tic douloureux–Lancinating pain localized to the second or third division of the trigeminal nerve.

5. Postherpetic neuralgia– Burning pain confined to the distribution of one or more divisions of the trigeminal nerve.

6. Glossopharyngeal neuralgia– Pharynx and external auditory meatus are frequent locations.

D. Quality of Pain:

1. Migraine headaches are commonly described as throbbing and are often preceded by prodromal symptoms or auras, eg, scintillating scotomas or other visual changes.

2. Tension headaches and the pain produced by mass lesions are usually steady.

3. Trigeminal neuralgia and glossopharyngeal neuralgia have a shooting or lancinating character.

E. Timing:

1. Mass lesion headaches are commonly maximal on awakening.

2. Cluster headaches frequently awaken patients from sleep and often recur at the same time of day or night.

3. Tension headaches may develop at regular intervals, especially with recurrent stressful situations.

F. Factors Influencing Severity:

1. Migraine headaches are frequently relieved by pressure on the ipsilateral temporal or carotid artery; by darkness, sleep, or vomiting; or during pregnancy.

2. Intracranial mass lesion headaches are often exacerbated by events such as coughing and sneezing that transiently raise intracranial pressure.

G. Associated Symptoms:

1. Nausea or vomiting is common with migraine and posttraumatic headache syndromes and may be seen late in the course of mass lesions.

2. Photophobia is prominent with migraine headache but occurs also with meningitis, especially viral (aseptic) meningitis.

3. Myalgias of paracranial muscles (eg, posterior neck muscles) often accompany tension headaches and viral syndromes.

4. Rhinorrhea and lacrimation during headache typify the cluster variant of migraine and are ipsilateral to the pain.

5. Loss of consciousness may occur with migraine (vasovagal syncope) and glossopharyngeal neuralgia (bradyarrhythmia).

Physical Examination

A. Vital Signs:

1. Fever–The presence of fever supports a diagnosis of meningitis, encephalitis, or headache associated with viral infection. A low-grade fever may also occur in temporal arteritis.

2. Blood pressure–Hypertension per se rarely causes headache, but chronic hypertension is the major risk factor for stroke, especially intracerebral hemorrhage, and stroke may be associated with acute headache. Blood pressure may be markedly elevated during hypertensive encephalopathy or as a result of preeclampsia-eclampsia, subarachnoid hemorrhage, or brain stem stroke.

B. Skin:

1. Neurofibromas or café au lait spots of Recklinghausen's disease may be associated with benign or malignant intracranial tumors.

2. Cutaneous angiomas sometimes accompany arteriovenous vascular malformations of the central nervous system; rupture results in subarachnoid hemorrhage and acute headache.

C. Scalp and Head:

1. Temporal arteries–Note nodularity or tenderness compatible with temporal arteritis.

2. Sinuses– Note tenderness, erythema of overlying skin, or nasal discharge.

3. Temporomandibular joints–Look for tenderness or limitation of motion.

4. Orbits–A bruit heard when the stethoscope is

placed on the eyeball over closed eyelids may suggest intracranial arteriovenous malformation.

D. Neck and Back:

1. Muscle spasm– Cervical muscle spasm may be a sign of tension or may occur with migraine.

2. Meningeal signs–Can the patient touch chin to sternum? If not, is the limitation of motion mainly in the anteroposterior direction, suggesting meningeal irritation, or in all directions, as is common with cervical spine disorders? Is there any discomfort, neck flexion, or contralateral knee flexion during straight leg raising (Kernig's sign)? Most importantly, is there even slight flexion of the knee (Brudzinski's sign) during passive neck flexion?

a. Lumbar puncture– *Any evidence of meningeal irritation in a patient with acute headache demands lumbar puncture to rule out meningitis and subarachnoid hemorrhage.* The only exception to this rule is the presence of obvious lateralizing findings suggesting a mass lesion (brain abscess, tumor), in which case confirmatory studies (CT scan, MRI, or angiogram) should be done first. If there will be a delay (> 1 hour) in obtaining the CT scan, begin antimicrobials (see Table 34–3).

b. Absence of meningeal signs–It is important to realize that meningeal signs may be absent or difficult to demonstrate in the early stages of subacute meningitis (eg, tuberculous meningitis), that several hours may elapse before evidence of meningeal irritation develops after subarachnoid hemorrhage, and that these signs disappear if the patient lapses into deep coma. Meningeal signs may also be minimal in the very young or very old.

E. Neurologic Examination: Unilateral cranial nerve, cerebellar, motor, or reflex abnormalities suggest a diagnosis of intracranial mass lesion.

F. Miscellaneous Physical Findings:

1. Papilledema, the hallmark of increased intracranial pressure, should always be sought.

2. Superficial preretinal (subhyaloid) hemorrhages are characteristic of subarachnoid hemorrhage in adults but may be seen with subdural hematoma in children.

3. Acute confusion or altered consciousness is common after subarachnoid hemorrhage and with purulent meningitis.

G. Special Signs: It is helpful to observe the patient for diagnostic signs during a headache.

1. Ipsilateral conjunctival injection, lacrimation, and rhinorrhea support a diagnosis of cluster headache.

2. Scalp tenderness is characteristic of migraine headache, subdural hematoma, and temporal arteritis. A diagnostically helpful feature of migraine is reduction of headache pain by compression of the carotid or superficial temporal artery ipsilateral to the pain.

MANAGEMENT OF SPECIFIC DISORDERS CAUSING ACUTE HEADACHE

SUBARACHNOID HEMORRHAGE

Subarachnoid hemorrhage is a serious emergency and is discussed in Chapter 10. Hospitalization is required.

CEREBROVASCULAR ACCIDENT (Stroke) (See also Chapter 12.)

Diagnosis

Thrombotic or embolic strokes may be associated with mild to moderate nonthrobbing headaches that are mainly contralateral to the paralysis. The headache may precede or accompany the stroke.

Treatment & Disposition

Treat stroke as described in Chapter 12. Hospitalize the patient for evaluation and treatment.

MENINGITIS & MENINGOENCEPHALITIS (See also Chapter 34.)

Diagnosis

Headache, confusion, and nuchal rigidity developing over hours to days are classic features of meningitis (infectious, carcinomatous, or irritative [chemical]). However, in rapidly progressive pyogenic meningitis, fever and altered consciousness are the most prominent presenting signs. In patients with subacute meningitis (eg, cryptococcosis, tuberculosis), headache is an early symptom that may precede nuchal rigidity and other meningeal signs. The headache of meningitis is continuous and throbbing and, although generalized, usually most prominent over the occiput. The pain is increased by head shaking, jugular vein compression, or any other maneuver that increases intracranial pressure (eg, coughing, sneezing, straining at stool). Pain is not relieved by changes in posture. Neck stiffness and other signs of meningeal irritation must be sought with care, since they may not be obvious early.

If meningitis or meningoencephalitis is suspected, perform **lumbar puncture** (Chapter 46), and obtain blood for culture. Relative contraindications to lumbar puncture are **(1)** papilledema and **(2)** prominent focal neurologic findings, suggesting mass lesion.

Treatment

A. Antimicrobials: Begin antibiotics immediately after taking samples of blood and cerebrospinal fluid for culture if bacterial meningitis is suspected. If lumbar puncture must be delayed for anatomic studies (CT scan), obtain 2 blood culture samples, and begin antimicrobials; perform lumbar puncture, and culture cerebrospinal fluid as soon as possible. The choice of drug depends on the clinical circumstances and the results of Gram's stain and culture of cerebrospinal fluid (see Table 34–3).

B. Supportive Care: General supportive care should be initiated in the emergency department as well. Protect the patient's airway, and provide padded bed rails or restraints for agitated or delirious patients. If seizures have occurred, anticonvulsant therapy should be started (Chapter 11). Avoid overhydration, which may worsen cerebral edema. Avoid osmotic diuretic agents (eg, mannitol), which have not been established as beneficial (and may be harmful) in pyogenic meningitis. Concomitant corticosteroid treatment in purulent meningitis has been shown in children to decrease the incidence of residual hearing impairment.

Disposition

Immediate hospitalization is warranted except perhaps in the case of a patient with aseptic (viral) meningitis who appears well and can be observed at home by a third party.

POSTICTAL HEADACHE

Diagnosis

Headache may occur after grand mal seizures. Care must be taken to exclude conditions causing both seizures and headache (eg, meningitis, mass lesions).

Treatment & Disposition

Analgesia is rarely needed. Hospitalization is not required. Provide follow-up if necessary for management of seizures.

POSTURAL (POST-LUMBAR PUNCTURE) HEADACHE

Diagnosis

Postural headache may follow lumbar puncture, especially if a large needle is used. This type of headache is worse in the upright position and nearly absent in recumbency. An identical idiopathic headache syndrome also occurs.

Treatment & Disposition

Recumbency for 18–24 hours, good hydration, and analgesics are usually sufficient management. Brief hospitalization may be required to ensure recumbency.

For more persistent cases, refer the patient to an anesthesiologist for an epidural blood patch at the site of the puncture (epidural injection of autologous blood at the site of the puncture will clot to seal the dural opening and prevent further leakage of cerebrospinal fluid).

MANAGEMENT OF SPECIFIC DISORDERS CAUSING SUBACUTE HEADACHE

POSTTRAUMATIC HEADACHE

Diagnosis

Headache caused by head injury may begin immediately or many days after the traumatic event, and symptoms are not necessarily proportionate to the severity of the inciting event. Persistent worsening of headache, particularly after trauma, suggests subdural hematoma (Chapter 16). Associated dizziness, vertigo, insomnia, depression, and personality change may occur. This constellation of symptoms is referred to as posttraumatic syndrome. Posttraumatic headache usually presents no special diagnostic or distinguishing features, although it may be suggestive of tension headache or migraine. Pain usually remits after days to weeks but occasionally persists for years.

Treatment & Disposition

Treatment for tension or migraine headache should be tried as dictated by the character of the headache. Refer the patient to a neurologist if headache persists. Hospitalization is not indicated unless rapid worsening of symptoms suggests an intracranial mass lesion (eg, subdural hematoma).

TIC DOULOUREUX (Trigeminal Neuralgia)

Diagnosis

In this syndrome, lightninglike stabs of excruciating pain characteristically recur over seconds to minutes and spontaneously abate. Occurrence during sleep is rare. Sensory stimulation (touch, cold, wind, talking, chewing, etc) of "trigger zones" about the cheek, nose, or mouth precipitates paroxysms of pain. Pain-free intervals may last minutes to weeks, but permanent spontaneous remission is rare. Pain is confined mainly to areas supplied by the second or third divisions of the trigeminal nerve (maxillary and mandibular areas of the face). Physical examination must show no abnormalities of trigeminal nerve function (facial sensation, muscles of mastication, corneal reflex) that would support a diagnosis of posterior fossa lesions. Involvement of the first division of the trigeminal nerve (the forehead) or bilateral disease occurs in less than 5% of cases.

Tic douloureux usually develops after the fourth decade.

Treatment

Phenytoin, 250 mg intravenously over 5–10 minutes, will abort an acute attack. Remission of symptoms with carbamazepine (Tegretol, others), 400–1200 mg/d orally in 2–3 divided doses, occurs in so many patients that it has been used as a diagnostic test. Begin with 200 mg orally twice daily, and increase by 200 mg every other day until the patient is pain-free or side effects develop.

Baclofen (Lioresal, others) is also beneficial and has synergistic effects when used with carbamazepine or phenytoin. Begin with 5–10 mg orally 3 times daily, and increase by 10 mg every other day until the patient is pain-free or side effects (eg, dizziness, gastrointestinal upset) occur. The usual maintenance dosage is 50–60 mg/d in 4–8 divided doses. Abrupt cessation of baclofen can cause seizures or hallucinations; the dosage should be decreased gradually.

Disposition

Neurologic referral for evaluation and treatment is appropriate.

INTRACRANIAL MASS
(Brain Tumor)

Diagnosis

Headache due to primary or metastatic intracranial tumor is usually mild to moderate in severity and described as deep, aching, and initially intermittent. Pain is maximal on awakening and during episodes of increased intracranial pressure (eg, coughing, sneezing, or straining at stool). Headaches increase in frequency and duration over weeks to months and become associated with focal neurologic signs. One-third to one-half of patients with brain tumor present with this classic history.

A CT or MRI scan will confirm the diagnosis.

Treatment & Disposition

If an intracranial mass lesion is suspected as the cause of headache, urgent neurologic or neurosurgical consultation is indicated. Hospitalization may be required for initiation of treatment. The distinction between primary and metastatic tumor is essential, since treatment differs.

PSEUDOTUMOR CEREBRI
(Benign Intracranial Hypertension)

Diagnosis

A diffuse increase in intracranial pressure due to decreased cerebrospinal fluid absorption, producing headache and papilledema without focal neurologic signs, may be a result of many nonneoplastic disease states and is thus termed pseudotumor cerebri. Women are much more commonly affected than men; the peak incidence occurs in the third decade. Diffuse headache is almost invariably a presenting symptom. Complaints of diplopia and blurred vision or transient visual obscuration occur in 60% of cases. Moderate to severe papilledema is seen in over 40% of affected persons. The course in idiopathic cases is generally self-limited over several months, but visual loss may occur. Disorders associated with pseudotumor cerebri are listed in Table 13–1. Differentiation from space-occupying intracerebral mass lesions is critical.

Treatment & Disposition

Hospitalization is necessary for evaluation and treatment.

HEADACHE ASSOCIATED WITH
ORAL CONTRACEPTIVES

Diagnosis

New headaches or exacerbation or diminution of preexisting headaches of diverse cause often occurs in patients taking oral contraceptives. The pain is commonly migrainous in type, but tension headaches may also be induced. Headache associated with use of contraceptive pills may begin weeks to years after starting the medication. Of great concern is the small but significant increased risk of stroke in these patients.

Table 13–1. Some causes of pseudotumor cerebri syndrome.

Intracranial venous obstruction
Venous sinus thrombosis
Polycythemia vera
Endocrine dysfunction
Obesity
Pregnancy
Menarche
Oral contraceptives
Corticosteroids (excess, deficiency, or withdrawal)
Hypoparathyroidism
Drug therapy (primarily children)
Hypervitaminosis A
Antibiotics (tetracycline, chloramphenicol)
Miscellaneous
Chronic hypercapnia
Meningeal inflammation
Intrathoracic venous obstruction
Idiopathic

Specific contraceptive hormone combinations vary significantly in their propensity to produce headache; there is no agreement regarding the causative components. A combination of a weak estrogen with a weak progesterone may be associated with less frequent headaches.

Treatment & Disposition

Discontinue oral contraceptives if headache is not alleviated early with aspirin or nonnarcotic analgesics. Hospitalization is not warranted, but referral for neurologic consultation may be indicated.

TEMPORAL ARTERITIS
(Giant Cell Arteritis)

Diagnosis

Temporal arteritis affects women twice as frequently as men and is uncommon before age 50. Nonspecific signs and symptoms are typical: malaise, myalgia, weight loss, arthralgia, and fever. The headache is classically of rapid onset, unremitting, and located over the temporal arteries. It is often unilateral as well. Associated scalp tenderness may be a prominent complaint, especially when the patient lies with her head on a pillow or brushes her hair. Pain during chewing (jaw claudication) is strongly suggestive of temporal arteritis. Permanent unilateral blindness, usually sudden in onset, occurs in about half of patients if treatment is delayed; half of patients so affected go on to develop bilateral blindness.

The temporal arteries may be normal on examination, although focal tenderness, thickening, nodularity, or decreased pulsation may be found. The diagnosis should be suspected if the erythrocyte sedimentation rate is markedly accelerated (100 mm/h or more).

The diagnosis can be established by demonstration of vasculitis in biopsy specimens of an affected artery. The biopsy specimens must be carefully examined (multiple sections) because involvement is segmental.

Treatment

Temporal arteritis responds dramatically to corticosteroid treatment. Begin prednisone, 40–60 mg/d orally, as soon as the diagnosis is suspected. Biopsy should be obtained within 2–3 days after beginning corticosteroids. Nonsteroidal anti-inflammatory agents may alleviate symptoms but have no effect on the arteritis and do not prevent blindness.

Disposition

Hospital admission is urgently indicated for evaluation and treatment, since patients may develop sudden blindness at any time.

GLOSSOPHARYNGEAL NEURALGIA

Diagnosis

Glossopharyngeal neuralgia is characterized by attacks of paroxysmal pain similar to tic douloureux but localized to the oropharynx, tonsillar pillars, base of the tongue, or auditory meatus. Men are more commonly affected than women, and symptoms occur at a somewhat younger age than is the case with tic douloureux. Trigger areas are usually found around the tonsillar pillars. Symptoms are initiated by swallowing (especially hot or cold liquids) or by talking and may be accompanied by loss of consciousness as a result of transient bradyarrhythmia (Chapter 11). The diagnosis is established by the classic history and by stimulation of the trigger zone to produce the pain. Topical anesthesia to the trigger area blocks the pain response.

Treatment & Disposition

Carbamazepine (Tegretol, others), 400–1000 mg/d orally in 2–3 divided doses, often dramatically relieves pain and prevents syncopal attacks. Neurologic referral is indicated. Hospitalization is not required unless life-threatening syncopal attacks are occurring.

MANAGEMENT OF SPECIFIC DISORDERS CAUSING CHRONIC HEADACHE

TENSION HEADACHE

Diagnosis

In tension headache, women are affected 3 times as commonly as men, and the age at onset is usually between the third and fifth decades. Headaches are often associated with emotional stress and have no prodrome. The pain typically comes on gradually; is bilateral, occipital, or frontal in location; and is described as a tight band or pressure about the head. The pain is constant and nonthrobbing and persists for hours or for the entire day. Nausea and photophobia are frequent accompanying symptoms but are milder than with migraine. Muscle spasm, especially nuchal-occipital, is usually present. About half of patients have headaches 10–30 times a month, and about one-fifth are never completely free of headache. Results on neurologic examination are normal.

Treatment

Simple analgesics (aspirin, acetaminophen, or other nonsteroidal anti-inflammatory drugs) should be tried first. Psychologic support to decrease precipitating factors and physical therapy (eg, local heat and massage) are often helpful for muscle spasm. Success has been reported with diazepam (Valium, others), 5 mg orally no more than 3 times a day; or amitriptyline (Elavil, many others), 25 mg orally 3 times daily or 75 mg at bedtime; or combination therapy with both drugs if necessary.

Disposition

If simple measures are not successful, neurologic referral may be necessary.

MIGRAINE

Migraine headache is a disorder of neurohumoral function associated with (but not caused by) spasm followed by dilatation of branches of the external carotid artery. Most cases occur in women, there is an inherited predisposition, and onset may be as early as the first decade. Recurrent vomiting during childhood may be the earliest manifestation of migraine. A family history of migraine is commonly present.

Diagnosis

Migraine may be called "classic" or "common" migraine.

Classic migraine headache is preceded by transient neurologic symptoms (the aura). The most common auras are visual disturbances: hemianopic field defects, scotomas, and scintillations that enlarge and spread peripherally. As the aura fades, vasodilatation occurs, producing the headache; however, aura can occur without headache. Migraine is said to be hemicranial, but half of migraine headaches are bilateral, and some are occipital. **Common** migraine headache lacks the classic aura and is bilateral in over half of cases.

The pain is throbbing in most cases. Associated symptoms in both classic and common migraine include nausea and vomiting, photophobia, and, less often, fluid retention, diarrhea, light-headedness, and fainting. Continuing pain may cause cervical muscle contraction, leading to an erroneous diagnosis of tension headache. Scalp tenderness may occur. A useful diagnostic test during the headache is easing of the pain by compression of the ipsilateral carotid or superficial temporal artery.

Attacks may be precipitated by certain foods such as tyramine-containing cheeses, wine, meat with nitrite preservatives, chocolate containing phenylethylamine, and monosodium glutamate (a flavor enhancer). Fasting, emotion, menses, drugs (especially oral contraceptive agents and vasodilators such as nitroglycerin), and bright lights may also trigger attacks. Over half of patients experience no more than one attack a week lasting less than a day. Remissions are common during pregnancy and after menopause.

Treatment

A. Ergot preparations (Table 13–2) must be given at the *first sign of onset* to be maximally effective. Rapid absorbable forms (eg, sublingual, aerosol) are therefore more effective than oral preparations. In the emergency department, with the headache well-established, parenteral preparations such as D.H.E. 45 should be used. This nonopioid is especially useful if drug-seeking behavior is an issue. Nausea is a common side effect of these drugs, and pretreatment with an antiemetic is necessary. Ergot preparations are contraindicated in the presence of pregnancy, hypertension or atherosclerosis, especially coronary atherosclerosis.

B. Phenothiazines are often effective in alleviating well-established headaches and are becoming the initial drug of choice in the treatment of migraine in the hospital or clinic setting. They are especially useful if drug-seeking behavior is suspected. They should be used for their antiemetic effect before treatment with parenteral dihydroergotamine, since the headache may abate with phenothiazines alone. Sedation and occasionally hypotension or extrapyramidal side effects (eg, torticollis) may occur. Give prochlorperazine (Compazine), 5–10 mg, or chlorpromazine, 12.5 mg intravenously; repeat in 20–30 minutes as needed.

C. Well-established vascular headaches often respond only to narcotic analgesics (eg, meperidine, 75–100 mg intramuscularly), and these are the only clearly safe drugs during pregnancy (meperidine, 50-mg tablets, 1–2 orally as needed).

D. Place the patient at bed rest in a quiet, dark room.

E. Prophylactic drugs (eg, methysergide) should not be initiated in the emergency department.

Table 13–2. Ergot preparations effective in the early treatment of vascular headache syndromes (migraine, cluster headache).

Parenteral
Dihydroergotamine mesylate (D.H.E. 45), 0.5–1 mg intramuscularly or intravenously (with prochlorperazine, 5 mg intravenously or 10 mg intramuscularly 10 minutes beforehand). Repeat in 1 hour if necessary.

Nonparenteral
Ergotamine tartrate aerosol (Medihaler), 1–2 puffs.

Ergotamine tartrate sublingual (Ergomar, Ergostat, Wigrettes), 2-mg tablets; 1–3 tablets sublingually.
Ergonovine maleate (ergotrate maleate), 0.2-mg tablets; 2–6 tablets at onset and 2 per hour thereafter.

Ergotamine (1 mg) with caffeine (100 mg) (Cafergot, others), 1–4 tablets orally at onset. Repeat in 20 minutes if no relief.

Cafergot suppositories, ½–1 per rectum.

Contraindications to ergot preparations
Atherosclerotic vascular disease (peripheral or cardiac).

Pregnancy.

Coexisting serious systemic infection.

Disposition

Referral to a neurologist or primary-care physician is indicated. Hospitalization (other than a brief stay in the emergency department for parenteral medication) is rarely needed.

CLUSTER HEADACHE

Diagnosis

Cluster headache is a distinct migraine variant that is more common in men than in women. Cluster headaches begin later in life than migraine headaches, 70% beginning between ages 11 and 30. There is no family history of similar headache. The headaches present as episodes of severe, unilateral (usually periocular), constant, nonthrobbing headaches that last from 10 minutes to a few hours. The headache may begin as a burning sensation over the side of the nose or as a feeling of pressure behind the eye. Ipsilateral conjunctival injection, lacrimation, nasal stuffiness, or Horner's syndrome may accompany the attack. Headaches commonly occur at night, awakening the patient from sleep and recurring 1–3 times daily, often at nearly the same time for a period of weeks to 2–3 months. Episodes may be precipitated by alcohol or vasodilator drugs. A nitroglycerin challenge can be diagnostic, producing a typical headache in 30–60 minutes.

Treatment

Treatment is difficult, because the symptoms progress rapidly and are well established by the time the patient has awakened from nocturnal attacks.

A. Narcotic analgesics are required for pain relief (eg, meperidine, 50–100 mg intramuscularly) in the emergency department.

B. Rapidly acting forms of ergot preparations (sublingual or aerosol) also are effective early in treatment (Table 13–2).

C. Prednisone, 40 mg/d orally and tapered over 21 days, is usually effective in preventing or ameliorating further attacks.

Disposition

Neurologic referral is indicated.

HEADACHE DUE TO HYPERTENSION

Headache is not a prominent feature of chronic hypertension. True hypertensive headaches are mild, bilateral, primarily occipital, and maximal on awakening. The pain decreases over the course of the day with or without analgesics. The acute onset of headache and severe blood pressure elevation are components of hypertensive crisis (Chapter 28) and also are commonly present following subarachnoid hemorrhage.

POSTHERPETIC NEURALGIA

Diagnosis

A severe, constant, burning, dysesthetic pain occurring in a dermatome previously affected by zoster may present as headache when a cephalic dermatome is involved. Examination discloses decreased cutaneous sensitivity in the involved skin.

Treatment

Acute herpetic pain (occurring coincidentally with rash) is best treated with analgesics or nerve blocks. In elderly patients, corticosteroids (eg, prednisone, 60 mg/d orally and tapered over 2–3 weeks) may decrease the incidence of postherpetic neuralgia. Established postherpetic neuralgia responds best to tricyclic antidepressants in combination with a substituted phenothiazine (eg, Triavil, one tablet at bedtime). Nonnarcotic analgesics can be used as well.

Capsaicin cream (0.025%), applied to painful skin 3–4 times daily, has been used to deplete the pain neurotransmitter, substance P. Transient burning may occur.

Disposition

Patients with chronic postherpetic neuralgia requiring more than nonnarcotic analgesics should be referred to a neurologist.

REFERENCES

Bell R et al: A comparative trial of three agents in the treatment of acute migraine headache. Ann Emerg Med 1990;19:1079.

Callahan M, Raskin NH: A controlled study of dihydroergotamine in the treatment of acute migraine headache. Headache 1986;26:168.

Caviness VS Jr, O'Brien P: Current concepts: Headache. N Engl J Med 1980;302:446.

Diamond S, Dalessio DJ: *The Practicing Physician's Approach to Headache,* 3rd ed. Williams & Wilkins, 1982.

Diamond S (editor): Headache. Med Clin North Am 1991; 75:521.

Gallagher RM: Emergency treatment of intractable migraine. Headache 1986;26:74.

Jamieson M: Clinical algorithms: Headache. Br Med J 1984;288:1281.

Katusic S et al: Incidence and clinical features of trigeminal neuralgia, Rochester, Minnesota, 1945–1984. Ann Neurol 1990;27:89.

Lance JW: Headache. Ann Neurol 1981;10:1.

Olesen J et al: Timing and topography of cerebral blood flow, aura, and headache during migraine attacks. Ann Neurol 1990;28:791.

Portenoy RK, Duma C, Foley KM: Acute herpetic and postherpetic neuralgia: Clinical review and current management. Ann Neurol 1986;20:651.

Raskin NH: Chemical headaches. Annu Rev Med 1981;32:63.

Raskin NH: *Headache,* 2nd ed. Churchill Livingstone, 1988.

Raskin NH: Headaches associated with organic diseases of the nervous system. Med Clin North Am 1978;62:459.

Raskin NH, Appenzeller O: Headache. Mod Probl Intern Med 1980;19:1. [Entire issue.]

Raymond JR, Raymond PA: Post–lumbar puncture headache: Etiology and management. West J Med 1988;148:551.

Shinnar S, D'Souza BJ: The diagnosis and management of headache in childhood. Pediatr Clin North Am 1982; 29:79.

Symposium on headache and related pain syndromes. Med Clin North Am 1978;63:427.

Delirium & Acute Confusional States

14

Roger P. Simon, MD

IMMEDIATE MANAGEMENT OF LIFE-THREATENING PROBLEMS
(See algorithm.)

Delirium and acute confusional states are among the most difficult problems confronting the emergency physician. Confused patients are often uncooperative or combative, making evaluation difficult. Symptoms and signs may be manifestations of a life-threatening underlying condition demanding prompt diagnosis and treatment to prevent irreversible brain damage (Table 14–1). Although evaluation may be difficult, every patient with an acutely altered state of consciousness must be examined and a history taken so that the cause can be established, if possible, in the emergency department. If the diagnosis cannot be established with certainty, the patient should be hospitalized.

Immediate Measures
  A. Maintain airway; clear secretions as needed. Begin oxygen, if necessary, 5–10 L/min, by mask or nasal prongs.
  B. Restrain the patient only if necessary.
  C. Insert a large-bore (≥ 18-gauge) intravenous catheter.
  D. Draw blood for CBC; serum glucose, electrolyte, calcium, and magnesium determinations; and hepatic and renal function tests. Reserve one tube of clotted blood for toxicology screen.
  E. Administer the following intravenously: (**1**) thiamine, 100 mg by slow bolus injection; (**2**) 50% dextrose in water, 50 mL over 3–5 minutes; and (**3**)

Table 14–1. Conditions associated with acute confusion or delirium that may cause rapid cerebral damage.

Hypoglycemia
Wernicke's encephalopathy
Hypotension and shock
Respiratory failure (hypercapnia or hypoxemia)
Hyperthermia or hypothermia
Meningitis or encephalitis
Stroke
Mass lesions (including intracranial bleeding)
Poisoning (methanol, ethylene glycol, carbon monoxide)

naloxone (Narcan, others), 2 mg by bolus injection. *Caution:* Administration of glucose may worsen brain injury by increasing lactate in ischemic areas. *Do not* give glucose to patients during the acute phases of stroke or after cardiac arrest if serum glucose is normal.

F. Treat Shock: Hypotension and shock with associated peripheral hypoperfusion may be associated with delirium or confusion. Treat shock with immediate intravenous administration of crystalloid solutions unless the patient is in cardiogenic shock, and follow with more specific measures (Chapter 3).

G. Correct Respiratory Failure: Either hypoxemia or hypercapnia that develops abruptly may be associated with delirium. Assess ventilatory status by means of arterial blood gases, and correct hypoxemia or hypercapnia by administration of oxygen, assisted ventilation, or both, as needed (Chapter 5).

H. Treat Hyperthermia or Hypothermia: Markedly elevated body temperatures (40.6 °C [105 °F]) may be associated with delirium or acute confusional states. Hypothermia is likely to produce confusion at body temperatures below 32.2 °C (90 °F) and unconsciousness at temperatures below 26.6 °C (80 °F). Treat by lowering or raising core temperature (Chapter 38).

I. Treat Severe Hypertension: Severe hypertension (when associated with papilledema and encephalopathy) is a medical emergency requiring rapid reduction of diastolic pressure toward 100 mm Hg (Chapter 28). The diagnosis of hypertensive encephalopathy must be firmly established before antihypertensive therapy is started, however, since reduction of blood pressure in states of cerebral ischemia can severely exacerbate ischemic brain injury.

Initial Evaluation

A. Obtain complete vital signs, including temperature.

B. Assess for shock (peripheral hypoperfusion).

C. Obtain results of arterial blood gas and pH determinations.

D. Does the delirium lighten after administration of intravenous glucose, thiamine, and naloxone? If so, consider the following possibilities:

1. Hypoglycemia (diagnosis is confirmed by finding of low serum glucose).

2. Wernicke's encephalopathy (look for associated alcoholism, malnutrition, ataxia, ophthalmoplegia, and peripheral neuropathy).

3. Opiate overdose (diagnosis is confirmed by positive response to naloxone and toxicology screen).

Further Evaluation
(See Table 14–2.)

A. Examination and Diagnostic Tests:

1. Obtain a brief history from the patient, family, friends, neighbors, ambulance attendants, or bystanders. Ask in particular about prior episodes of confusion or delirium, duration and other features of the present episode, drug usage, and previous illness.

2. Perform a general physical examination, and look especially for signs of trauma, meningeal irritation, and cardiac disease. Complete a basic neurologic examination, including tests of orientation and memory.

3. Send blood to the laboratory for CBC; serum electrolyte, glucose, calcium, and magnesium determinations; renal and liver function tests; carboxyhemoglobin level; and toxicology studies.

4. Obtain urine for urinalysis and toxicology studies.

5. Obtain an ECG in order to seek any abnormalities that might suggest a cardiac cause of the confusional state (eg, myocardial infarction, cardiac arrhythmias, prolonged intervals, etc). T-wave changes, however, are nonspecific and may be seen with acute intracranial events.

6. Special studies may be indicated based on the results of history and physical examination (eg, lumbar puncture for cerebrospinal fluid in the patient with confusion and fever or signs of meningeal irritation).

7. Administer an activated charcoal slurry (50–100 mg of activated charcoal admixed with water or sorbitol), and consider gastric lavage if ingestion or overdose of a toxin is a diagnostic possibility or if no other cause of the confusional state is found (Chapters 39 and 46).

B. Trauma: If there is evidence of trauma—even if the head itself appears uninjured—the possibility of traumatic brain damage (eg, subdural or epidural hematomas) should be considered. CT scan may be indicated (Chapter 16). Hospitalization is required even if no specific abnormality is found.

C. Meningeal Irritation: Look first for signs of meningitis due to infection or subarachnoid hemorrhage. Headache is common and may not be severe. Fever is common in infectious meningitis but is absent in the initial stage of subarachnoid hemorrhage. Signs of meningeal irritation (meningismus: stiff neck, positive Kernig's and Brudzinski's signs) are almost invariably present in meningitis or subarach-

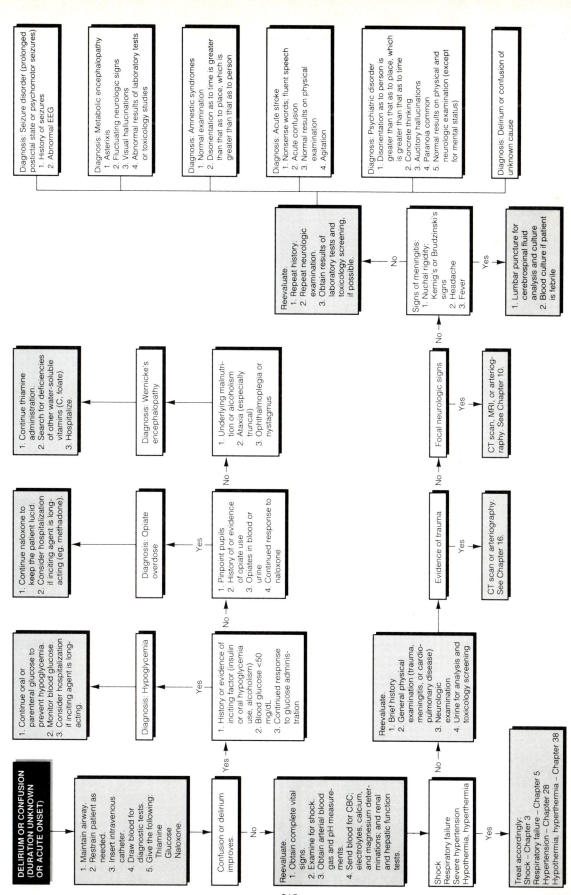

Table 14–2. Differential diagnosis of conditions causing delirium or confusion.

Etiologic Category	Clinical Findings
Central nervous system mass lesion (subdural hematoma, cerebral infarction, brain tumor)	Somnolence; neurologic examination shows focal or asymmetric abnormality. Posterior nondominant parietal lobe strokes present with an agitated delirium, without hemiparesis.
Meningitis or meningoencephalitis Infectious, carcinomatous, or chemical meningitis secondary to subarachnoid hemorrhage	Headache, fever, meningeal signs, cerebrospinal fluid pleocytosis.
Seizure disorders Confusional states following seizures (postictal states) Psychomotor status epilepticus	History or evidence of seizures, especially seen in seizure patients with superimposed metabolic abnormality, encephalitis, or diffuse cerebral damage, in whom postictal state may be prolonged.
Amnestic states	Findings confined to recent memory loss.
Fluent aphasias	Sudden onset; patient alert; mild right hemiparesis (may be absent). Excessive speech with frequent word substitutions and nonsense phrases.
Psychiatric disease (thought disorders and hysteria)	Paranoia prominent; auditory hallucinations common; disorientation as to person which is greater than that as to place, which in turn is greater than that as to time. Recent memory preserved.
Head trauma (acute posttraumatic delirium, postconcussion syndrome)	Recent history or evidence of head trauma.
Metabolic encephalopathy; drug intoxication or withdrawal	Fluctuations in mental status (lucid intervals); asterixis; myoclonus; tremor; visual hallucinations; disorientation as to time which is greater than that as to palce, which in turn is greater than that as to person; nystagmus.

noid hemorrhage except in very young or very old patients. The most helpful diagnostic maneuver is passive flexion of the patient's neck, which elicits reflex knee flexion (usually unilateral) if meningeal irritation is present (positive Brudzinski's sign). Perform lumbar puncture immediately in patients with meningismus in the absence of signs of increased intracranial pressure (papilledema, focal neurologic findings) for evaluation of cerebrospinal fluid (Chapter 13). Bacterial meningitis requires urgent treatment (Chapter 34).

D. Focal Neurologic Findings: (See Table 14–2.) Although focal signs may be found in metabolic brain disease (notably the fluctuating hemiparesis that may occur with hypoglycemia and hepatic encephalopathy), such asymmetric findings should be assumed to reflect a structural brain lesion until proved otherwise; appropriate neurologic or neurosurgical consultation should be obtained (Chapter 10).

The principal differential diagnostic considerations are **cerebrovascular accidents** (thrombotic or embolic) and **mass lesions**. Lumbar puncture is contraindicated, and the patient should be evaluated with CT scan (preferable) or angiography (less desirable). See Chapter 10 for further details.

In patients with fever and focal neurologic findings, a brain abscess must be considered along with meningitis and encephalitis. A lumbar puncture is contraindicated until a CT scan has eliminated the possibility of a mass lesion. To avoid delay of needed

treatment for possible meningitis while awaiting the results of the CT scan, obtain blood cultures, and begin antibiotics immediately (Chapter 34).

E. Other Causes of Delirium or Confusion: Once life-threatening conditions have been ruled out, a more specific diagnosis can be attempted. Main causes are shown in Table 14–2 and described below. Delirium or confusion occurring in patients with AIDS is discussed in Chapter 34.

EMERGENCY MANAGEMENT OF SPECIFIC DISORDERS

SEIZURE DISORDERS
(See Chapter 11.)

1. PROLONGED POSTICTAL STATES

Diagnosis

The diagnosis of delirium arising from seizure disorders is based on the following: (1) a seizure that has been witnessed, (2) past history of seizure disorder, (3) gradually clearing mental status (ie, postictal confusion), and (4) an anion-gap metabolic acidosis that resolves within 1 hour. Prolonged postictal confusion may occur in patients who have superimposed metabolic encephalopathy (eg, hyponatremia, hyperosmolality), underlying diffuse brain damage (eg, following multiple cerebrovascular accidents or head trauma), or encephalitis. Patients with a mental status that fails to improve should be examined for underlying processes that may be contributing to mental status depression; a CT scan should be done to search for possible structural causes.

Treatment & Disposition

Hospitalize for observation until recovery has occurred, and give anticonvulsants to prevent further seizures (Chapter 11).

2. PSYCHOMOTOR STATUS EPILEPTICUS

Diagnosis

Psychomotor (temporal lobe) status epilepticus may also present as a prolonged state of acute confusion. Delusions, hallucinations, automatisms, and other bizarre behavior may also be prominent and may mimic acute schizophrenia.

The diagnosis of status epilepticus is confirmed by an EEG showing seizure activity.

Treatment & Disposition

Administer parenteral anticonvulsants, and hospitalize for observation (Chapter 11).

METABOLIC ENCEPHALOPATHIES

1. SYSTEMIC METABOLIC DISORDERS

Systemic metabolic disease, acute drug intoxication, or sedative-hypnotic drug withdrawal can produce an altered mental status ranging from florid, agitated delirium to lethargy or coma. Marked fluctuation in the patient's mental state with intermittent periods of lucidity, without focal abnormalities, is characteristic of metabolic encephalopathy. A history of systemic illness (Table 14–3) or drug ingestion should be sought in every patient with a confusional state. Helpful clinical findings include the following:

(1) Symmetric nystagmus is found in sedative-hypnotic drug and phencyclidine ingestion.

(2} Asterixis is most commonly associated with hepatic or renal insufficiency.

(3) Hallucinations occur in metabolic disorders and are typically visual, as exemplified by delirium tremens.

(4) Orientation as to time is lost early in metabolic encephalopathy and is followed later by loss of orientation as to place, but orientation as to person is

Table 14–3. Systemic illnesses associated with confusion due to metabolic encephalopathy.

Renal	Respiratory
Renal failure with azotemia	Hypercapnia
Electrolyte	Hypoxemia
Hypernatremia	**Cardiac**
Hyponatremia	Heart failure
Dehydration	Endocarditis
Hypercalcemia	**Other**
Hypocalcemia	Sepsis
Hyperglycemia	Shock
Hypoglycemia	Drug ingestion
Hypermagnesemia	Thiamine deficiency
Hypomagnesemia	(eg, Wernicke-Korsakoff's syn-
Hepatic	drome)
Hepatic failure	Hyperthyroidism
Lactic acidosis	Hypothyroidism

almost invariably preserved. This characteristic pattern of metabolic brain disease contrasts with that of psychiatric disorders, in which patients may know the correct day and date but are uncertain who or where they are.

(5) Arterial blood gas and pH measurements may suggest a metabolic cause for acute confusional states and are useful in distinguishing the metabolic causes of coma. See Table 10–1 for some characteristic arterial blood gas and pH abnormalities associated with the more common metabolic encephalopathies.

Seek and correct the cause of the metabolic disorder. Hospitalize the patient for treatment and diagnosis as indicated.

2. DRUG WITHDRAWAL SYNDROMES (Ethanol & Other Sedative-Hypnotic Drugs)

Several well-recognized syndromes are associated with acute withdrawal from alcohol, barbiturates, or other sedative-hypnotic drugs (Table 14–4). In one series of 266 patients seen at Boston City Hospital with manifestations of acute alcohol withdrawal, diagnoses were as follows:

Acute alcoholic tremulousness, 35%

Acute intoxication (inebriation, stupor, or combative states), 21%

Alcohol withdrawal seizures, 12%

Tremor and transitory hallucinations, 11%

Typical delirium tremens, 5%

Atypical delirious-hallucinatory states, 4%

Acute auditory hallucinations, 2%

Other miscellaneous manifestations, including Wernicke-Korsakoff's syndrome, 21%

Acute tremulous and hallucinatory states that are distinct from delirium tremens are more common and less serious than delirium tremens and are seen within the first 6–36 hours following relative or absolute abstinence from alcohol, whereas classic delirium tre-

Table 14–4. Sedative drugs reportedly followed by clinical abstinence syndromes after withdrawal from excessive dosage.

Barbiturates (phenobarbital, many others)
Alcohol
Meprobamate (Equanil, Miltown, others)
Glutethimide (Doriden, others)
Methyprylon (Noludar)
Ethinamate (Valmid)
Ethchlorvynol (Placidyl)
Benzodiazepines (eg, chlordiazepoxide [Librium, many others], diazepam [Valium, many others])

mens syndrome typically appears after 3–4 days of abstinence (range: 24 hours to 5 days or more).

Diagnosis

A. Delirium Tremens: *Note:* Delirium tremens is an uncommon but life-threatening illness that requires prompt recognition and treatment for the best outcome. Symptoms and signs include the following:

1. Profoundly delirious state associated with tremulousness and agitation.

2. Excessive motor activity (most notable as a tremor affecting the face, tongue, and extremities but that may also involve speech) and purposeless activity such as picking at the bedclothes.

3. Hallucinations, classically visual rather than auditory, are a prominent feature, especially if patients are specifically asked, "What do you see? What's over there? Is there anything frightening you?" These patients may be quite suggestible and may be persuaded to light an imaginary cigarette or identify the color of a nonexistent piece of string.

4. Autonomic nervous system hyperactivity: tachycardia, dilated pupils, fever, and hyperhidrosis.

5. Loss of orientation as to time and place. Such patients are often oblivious to the most obvious features of the surrounding environment (eg, they do not know whether they are in bed or on a chair or wearing a suit or pajamas).

6. Duration of delirium tremens is less than 24 hours in 15% of cases and less than 3 days in over 80%.

B. Withdrawal Seizures: Withdrawal seizures, a syndrome distinct from delirium tremens, may result from abrupt decrease or cessation of alcohol consumption. About 90% of such convulsions occur between 6 and 48 hours after abstinence, and 30% of patients having withdrawal seizures subsequently develop delirium tremens.

Since delirium tremens requires a longer period of abstinence than withdrawal seizures, pure withdrawal seizures (ie, those occurring only during periods of alcohol withdrawal) always occur before delirium tremens. Therefore, any seizures occurring after delirium tremens must be assumed to be due to some cause other than alcohol withdrawal, and further evaluation is required (Chapter 11).

C. Sedative-Hypnotic Drug Withdrawal: A syndrome nearly identical to delirium tremens but somewhat more protracted may follow withdrawal from short-acting barbiturates or other sedative-hypnotic drugs (Table 14–4) in habituated patients. These drug-induced withdrawal reactions occur only when the patient has become habituated to large doses of the drug, eg, secobarbital, in the range of 1 g daily taken over a period of 1 month or more.

Treatment

A. Delirium Tremens:

1. Note temperature, pulse, and blood pressure, and record results twice hourly to monitor for hyperpyrexia and hypotension. Consider lumbar puncture to rule out meningitis if fever or meningismus is present.

2. Fluid requirements on the first day of treatment may be as high as 4–10 L because of profound dehydration. Intravenous fluid should contain glucose to prevent hypoglycemia.

3. Thiamine, 100 mg/d, prevents Wernicke's encephalopathy. Other water-soluble vitamins (B complex and C) should also be given.

4. Judicious use of sedative drugs does not eliminate established delirium but does protect the patient against self-induced trauma and permit continued treatment. Sedatives (eg, a benzodiazepine) may also prevent patients with impending delirium tremens from developing a full-blown case. Diazepam is the drug of choice.

a. Initial dose–A suggested regimen is diazepam (Valium, others), 10 mg intravenously given over at least 2 minutes, followed by 5 mg intravenously every 5 minutes until the patient is calm. The total dose required to calm a patient may be as high as 200 mg (rarely, even 700 mg or more). Drug-induced hypotension and respiratory depression during administration of diazepam for delirium tremens are uncommon if adequate hydration is maintained and overzealous treatment avoided. After delirium tremens has been controlled, the patient may sleep uninterruptedly for up to 36 hours but can nonetheless be easily aroused.

b. Maintenance doses–Administer diazepam, 5–10 mg intravenously or orally as needed. Avoid intramuscular administration, because absorption by this route is erratic. Sedation is achieved within a few minutes following intravenous injection but may be delayed for 3 hours or longer following intramuscular injection if there is associated obesity, hyperpyrexia, or complicating illness (eg, pneumonia).

5. Do not administer ACTH or corticosteroids for delirium tremens; they are ineffective and potentially harmful.

6. Phenothiazines have been used and may promptly control hallucinatory symptoms; however, these drugs are not recommended, because they may cause hypotension or precipitate seizures.

7. The concomitant administration of beta-blocking drugs decreases the associated autonomic hyperactivity.

B. Withdrawal Seizures: Pure withdrawal seizures are self-limited and usually do not require anticonvulsant therapy. Observation is necessary, since about 60% of patients will have more than one seizure, 95% of which will occur within 12 hours after the initial seizure and 80% within 6 hours. Repetitive alcohol withdrawal seizures can be pharmacologically controlled with a single loading dose of phenobarbital (750 mg, intravenously slowly); phenytoin is ineffective. Patients with withdrawal seizures, unless previously investigated, should receive outpatient follow-up. Most should be investigated at least once for structural causes. Hospitalization is rarely required.

C. Sedative-Hypnotic Drug Withdrawal: Give short-acting barbiturates (eg, pentobarbital) and then switch to the equivalent dose of a long-acting barbiturate (eg, phenobarbital), from which withdrawal can be accomplished gradually and safely.

1. Initial dose—For withdrawal symptoms, give pentobarbital, 300 mg orally, repeated every 2 hours; or 200 mg intramuscularly, repeated every 15–30 minutes; or 0.03–0.04 mg/kg/min by intravenous infusion, until the patient becomes sleepy.

2. Maintenance dose—Once the patient is sleepy but can still be aroused, give phenobarbital, 30 mg orally for every 100 mg of pentobarbital required for sedation (500 mg maximum). Then taper the dose of phenobarbital at a rate of 30 mg/d over a maximum period of 10 days.

Disposition

Hospitalization is indicated for all patients with sedative-hypnotic drug withdrawal who have active delirium tremens or possible impending delirium tremens (tremor, tachycardia, and agitation). Patients with more benign withdrawal states (tremulousness alone, hallucinatory states other than delirium tremens, withdrawal seizures) may be sent home after 6–12 hours of observation and treatment in the emergency department.

3. WERNICKE'S ENCEPHALOPATHY (Acute Thiamine Deficiency)

Diagnosis

Wernicke's encephalopathy is a medical emergency characterized by ophthalmoplegia, ataxia, and confusion. Most cases are associated with alcoholism, malnutrition, or both. Failure to initiate prompt thiamine therapy in a patient with any of these features may result either in death or in permanent neuropathy or loss of cognitive function.

A. Ocular Abnormalities:

1. Nystagmus (horizontal alone or horizontal and vertical; isolated vertical nystagmus is rare).

2. Bilateral lateral rectus muscle (sixth cranial nerve) palsies and conjugate gaze palsies. Other types of ophthalmoplegia may occur.

3. The response to irrigation of the external ear canal with ice water (caloric test) is invariably abnormal and reveals unilateral or bilateral absence of ocular movement.

B. Ataxia:

1. Ataxia is similar to that associated with alcoholic cerebellar degeneration. Truncal ataxia is most common, with a wide-based, unsteady gait as the major finding.

2. Limb ataxia is less common than ataxia of gait and affects the lower extremities much more than the upper extremities.

C. Confusion:

1. Frank delirium occurs in about 20% of cases.

2. Blatant apathy, manifested as inattention, drowsiness, and decreased spontaneous speech, is present in most cases.

3. In the recovery phase, Korsakoff's psychosis may become more prominent, with marked impairment of recent memory and inability to retain new information. Confabulation is common.

D. Cardiovascular Abnormalities: Tachycardia, exertional dyspnea, minor electrocardiographic abnormalities, and orthostatic hypotension are common. Overt beriberi heart disease with heart failure is rare.

E. Neuropathy: Peripheral neuropathy is associated with Wernicke's encephalopathy in approximately 80% of cases.

Treatment

A. Vitamins: Give thiamine, 100 mg intravenously, immediately upon diagnosis of Wernicke's encephalopathy. Patients should be hospitalized and thiamine continued in doses of 50 mg/d intravenously until adequate diet and bowel function are reestablished. Other water-soluble vitamins (B complex and C) should also be given, since multiple deficiencies are common in these patients. The need for folate or vitamin B_{12} should be assessed based on the CBC (presence of hypersegmented PMNs and macrocytosis). Deficiencies of fat-soluble vitamins (A, D, and E) are rare.

Magnesium deficiency is common in alcohol withdrawal states, and magnesium should be replaced based on blood levels (Chapter 36).

B. Bed Rest: Bed rest is necessary because of the patient's fragile cardiovascular status (deaths have been reported following trivial physical exertion).

C. Outcome: With thiamine therapy, oculomotor abnormalities may begin to improve within minutes to hours, and complete recovery will occur within 1–4 weeks, except for persistent lateral gaze nystagmus. Global confusional state, ataxia, peripheral neuropathies, and Korsakoff's psychosis in particular clear much less quickly, and permanent disability is common.

Disposition

All patients with thiamine deficiency syndromes should be hospitalized for supportive care and continued administration of thiamine.

4. DRUG INTOXICATION

Centrally Acting Anticholinergic Drugs

Intoxication with a wide variety of anticholinergic medications that penetrate the central nervous system may produce agitated and confusional states. Representative medications (prescription and over-the-counter) are listed in Table 14–5.

Delirium, psychosis, anxiety, hallucinations, breathlessness, hyperactivity, disorientation, seizures, and coma are typically associated with signs of peripheral cholinergic blockade: tachycardia, mydriasis, hyperpyrexia, urinary retention, decreased bowel motility, decreased sweating, and decreased bronchial, pharyngeal, and salivary secretions. The patient is hot, dry, red, and "mad as a hatter."

Treatment is discussed in Chapter 39. Hospitalization is required for supportive care.

Stimulants & Hallucinogenic Drugs

Some commonly abused drugs can cause an agitated confusional state, eg, cocaine, amphetamine, LSD (lysergic acid ethylamide), jimsonweed, and PCP (phencyclidine). Cocaine is currently the most frequent culprit and can produce agitation, anxiety, depression, psychosis, paranoia, suicidal ideation, or any combination of these conditions. Symptoms are independent of the route of drug administration. Treatment is discussed in Chapter 39. Short-term psychiatric admission often is required.

REYE'S SYNDROME

Reye's syndrome, an encephalopathy associated with fatty degeneration of the liver, is a major cause of delirium progressing to coma in infants and children. The degree of central nervous system impairment does not correlate well with the degree of hepatic dysfunction. The disease is extremely rare in individuals over the age of 20 years. Seasonal occurrence from November to April with a peak incidence in February has been noted. There may be a history of a preceding viral illness. Epidemiologic evidence has firmly linked Reye's syndrome with chickenpox and influenza virus infections. An association between

Table 14–5. Drugs that may cause a central anticholinergic syndrome. Only selected representatives from each group are listed.

Anticholinergics
Atropine (eg, belladonna, Donnatal)
Scopolamine (also found in jimsonweed [*Datura* sp])

Tricyclic antidepressants
Amitriptyline (Elavil, many others)
Doxepin (Adapin, Sinequan, others)
Imipramine (Tofranil, many others)

Phenothiazines
Chlorpromazine (Thorazine, many others)
Trifluoperazine (Stelazine, many others)
Thioridazine (Mellaril, many others)

Antihistamines
Chlorpheniramine (Ornade, Teldrin, many others)
Diphenhydramine (Benadryl, many others)
Promethazine (Phenergan, many others)

Ophthalmic preparations
Atropine, 1% ophthalmic solution
Cyclopentolate (AK-Pentolate, Cyclogyl, others)
Tropicamide (Mydriacyl, others)

Antispasmodics
Methantheline (Banthine)
Propantheline (Pro-Banthine, others)

Antiparkinsonism agents
Benztropine (Cogentin, many others)
Biperiden (Akineton)
Trihexyphenidyl (Artane, others)

Over-the-counter drugs (hypnotics, analgesics)
Sominex (diphenhydramine)
Sleep-Eze (diphenhydramine)
Contac (chlorpheniramine)
Dristan (chlorpheniramine)

Reye's syndrome and the use of salicylates during an antecedent illness has been demonstrated.

Diagnosis

Illness begins with protracted vomiting and delirium that progresses to coma within 2 days. Seizures are common but are usually self-limited. Decerebrate posturing is common, but focal neurologic signs are rare once coma is established. Sustained hyperventilation and hepatomegaly are usually noted. Cerebrospinal fluid examination reveals normal protein and cell count. Blood glucose is frequently reduced because of hepatic failure and may be reflected in low levels of cerebrospinal fluid glucose. Serum transaminase and blood ammonia levels are characteristically elevated. Prothrombin time is prolonged. Serum bilirubin is normal, so that icterus makes the diagnosis of Reye's syndrome doubtful.

Treatment & Disposition

Hospitalization is invariably required for control of intracranial pressure and supportive care. Early placement of an intracranial pressure monitor and measures to lower intracranial pressure may be helpful (Chapter 6). There is no specific treatment.

AMNESTIC SYNDROMES

1. AMNESTIC EPISODES

Diagnosis

The neurologic abnormality of memory loss is easily missed unless recall is specifically tested. Confused patients may present with only memory loss and no alteration of consciousness; the general physical examination may be entirely normal. Such patients have markedly abnormal recent memory (eg, they cannot remember 3 objects after 60 seconds or even 30 seconds). Other cognitive functions and past memory are relatively intact. Such patients are confused about where they are and what they are doing.

The causes and differential diagnosis of the amnestic syndromes are presented in Table 14–6. The history, cerebrospinal fluid examination, CT scan or MRI, clinical course, or associated findings establish the cause in most cases.

Treatment & Disposition

Administer thiamine, 100 mg intravenously, since Wernicke's syndrome is a diagnostic possibility. All patients with new onset of memory loss should be hospitalized for evaluation.

2. TRANSIENT GLOBAL AMNESIA

Diagnosis

Transient global amnesia occurs suddenly in previously normal middle-aged or elderly patients. Men are affected more frequently than women. Episodes of amnesia occur without warning and without associated headache or findings suggesting epilepsy. Cerebrovascular disease affecting thalamic or temporal

Table 14–6. Causes of amnestic syndromes.[1]

Amnesia of sudden onset with gradual but incomplete recovery
Bilateral hippocampal or thalamic infarction
Diencephalic or bilateral temporal lobe injury following subarachnoid hemorrhage
Brain injury due to hypoxemia
Slowly progressive amnestic states
Third ventricular tumors
Alzheimer's disease and other degenerative disorders
Amnesia of sudden onset and transient duration
Temporal lobe seizures
Postconcussive states
Transient global amnesia
Hysteria
Amnesia of subacute onset with variable recovery
Wernicke-Korsakoff's syndrome
Herpes simplex encephalitis
Granulomatous meningitis (tuberculosis, sarcoidosis, etc)

[1]Modified and reproduced, with permission, from Victor M: The amnesic syndrome and its anatomical basis. *Can Med Assoc J* 1969; **100**:1115.

lobe structures is the most likely cause. The results of laboratory studies are completely normal.

During an attack, agitation is not a feature. Patients' responses to the illness are variable: some may be unaware of their deficit, but most realize that "something is wrong"; a few may recognize that their memory is impaired. During these episodes, patients may repeatedly ask the same questions regarding their current condition.

The period of retrograde amnesia varies from a day to a few months or even years. Recovery usually occurs within hours, but amnesia for the entire episode is total and permanent.

Treatment & Disposition

No specific treatment is available. Hospitalization is indicated, in part to prevent injury.

ACUTE STROKES
(Cerebrovascular Accidents)

1. FLUENT APHASIA

Lesions of the dominant posterior frontal lobe may produce a nonfluent (expressive) aphasia and prominent right hemiparesis. Lesions in a more posterior location may partially or completely spare motor function but produce a fluent (receptive) aphasia easily mistaken for confusion or delirium. Such lesions occur suddenly and are usually caused by embolic strokes in patients at risk of stroke (eg, the elderly or those with valvular or ischemic heart disease predisposing to embolization).

Diagnosis

Patients talk volubly. Their speech is well-articulated and grammatically correct but has little content. Sentences are characterized by word substitutions (eg, "glass" instead of "clock"); replacement of real words by nonsense words (eg, "dreislen" for "finger"); and substitution of explanatory phrases for words that cannot be recalled (eg, "the thing you write with" for "pen").

Deficits of comprehension are evident. Patients are unable, for example, to carry out the command, "Put your left hand on your right ear," or to repeat the simple phrase, "No *ands, ifs,* or *buts.*"

The isolated inability to name objects (anomia) without deficits of comprehension and repetition may represent a form of fluent aphasia due to a structural lesion but most commonly occurs with metabolic encephalopathies of any cause.

Treatment & Disposition

Hospitalization is indicated for new cases to provide supportive care and determine the cause of the aphasia. A CT scan should be obtained. Emboli with an origin in the heart are a common cause and require short-term treatment with anticoagulants. Chronic cases do not require hospitalization.

2. AGITATED CONFUSION

Diagnosis

The acute onset of an agitated confusional state may occur with infarctions of the inferior division of the right middle cerebral artery. Such strokes spare motor cortex, so that localizing signs, eg, hemiparesis, are mild or absent. A homonymous hemianopia may be present on examination. The diagnosis is suggested by the abrupt onset of agitated confusion and is confirmed by CT scan or MRI. Embolus with an origin in the heart is common.

Treatment & Disposition

Hospitalize the patient for treatment and observation. Evaluation for the source of the embolus and treatment with anticoagulants may be indicated.

CONFUSION ASSOCIATED WITH PSYCHIATRIC DISEASE

Differentiation between organic and psychiatric causes of confusion (psychosis or hysteria) may be difficult. If careful evaluation (described below) is performed, few patients with metabolic diseases will be improperly diagnosed as having psychiatric illness. Additional useful differential features are outlined in Table 14–7.

1. PSYCHOTIC CONFUSIONAL STATES

Diagnosis

Patients with bona fide psychotic disorders (eg, schizophrenia) usually demonstrate the following characteristic patterns of confusion:

(1) They may be fully oriented or, if disoriented, exhibit a disorientation as to person that is at least as great as or greater than their disorientation as to time and place. In organic brain disease, on the other hand, disorientation as to time and place is invariably greater than that as to person.

(2) Psychotic patients usually retain recent memory and are able to perform simple calculations and other cognitive tasks adequately. In contrast, these functions are rarely preserved in organic confusional states.

(3) Hallucinations tend to be auditory in psychotic states rather than visual (the latter being found in organic brain disease). However, hallucinations may not be mentioned unless the patient is specifically asked about them, eg, "Do voices ask you to do strange things? Does God talk to you?" Psychotic patients may report hearing their own thoughts as "broadcasts," have feelings of thought insertion, and experience somatic unreality.

Treatment & Disposition

Psychiatric consultation should be obtained. Hospitalization in a secure ward is required for patients with acute psychosis or abrupt worsening of chronic psychosis. Parenteral antipsychotics, eg, haloperidol (Haldol, others), 5–10 mg intramuscularly every 30 minutes to 1 hour, should be given until the patient shows improvement. Chlorpromazine (Thorazine,

Table 14–7. Differentiating features of organic and psychiatric disorders of mentation.

Features	Organic	Psychiatric (Hysteria or Psychosis)
Age	Any; older more susceptible.	Younger; puberty to mid 30s.
Premorbid personality	Any.	Previous functional illness common.
Onset	Often acute.	Usually gradual and insidious.
Weakness, fatigue	Rare.	Common.
Level of awareness	Fluctuates between confusion and lucidity.	Usually consistent.
Hallucinations	Common; predominantly visual, tactile, and olfactory.	Common; predominantly auditory.
Orientation	Impaired: disorientation as to time is greater than that as to place, which in turn is greater than that as to person.	Impaired: disorientation to person is greater than that as to place, which is greater than that as to time; may be unimpaired, however.
Memory	Usually affected; recent memory more affected than remote memory.	Total amnesia, including self-identity; or memory may be completely unimpaired.
Other evidence of organic central nervous system disease	Present.	Usually absent.
EEG	Frequently abnormal, usually slow.	Usually normal.
Asterixis and multifocal myoclonus	Diagnostic if present.	Never seen.

many others), 25–50 mg intramuscularly, is equally effective but is less commonly used because of side effects of sedation and postural hypotension. See Chapter 41 for details of treatment.

2. HYSTERIA

Diagnosis

Hysteria is a diagnosis of exclusion and should be made only after all other possibilities have been ruled out. The differential features listed in Table 14–7 are helpful, but few guidelines are absolute. It is useful to remember that amnesia is probably the most common hysterical disturbance of mental function. Hysterical amnesia usually includes the inability both to form new memories and especially to recall any past experience with certainty. For example, such patients often deny knowledge of their own name, a finding which in an awake and alert person is essentially restricted to the hysterical personality. The disparity between alleged mental incapacity and the ability to function in the immediate surroundings is often quite striking.

The most helpful differentiating features on physical examination are asterixis and myoclonus, which, when present, point to a metabolic cause of the symptoms. Asterixis and myoclonus do not occur as features of psychiatric or hysterical illness.

An EEG is often helpful in diagnosis, since it is nearly always normal in psychiatric disease and is frequently abnormal (usually slowed) in organic or metabolic disease. The presence of very fast beta wave activity on the tracing may be seen with sedative-hypnotic drug intoxication and provides a helpful clue to proper diagnosis.

Treatment & Disposition

Refer the patient for psychiatric consultation. Anxiolytics, eg, diazepam (Valium, others), 5–10 mg orally, may be helpful. Hospitalization may be required if a protected home environment is not available.

CONFUSIONAL STATES OF UNCERTAIN CAUSE

Even after all the above diagnoses have been considered, there are still many patients in confusional states for whom no clear diagnosis can be established in the emergency department. These patients, especially the elderly, are often found to be suffering from subclinical mild metabolic or drug-induced abnormalities or infection, and correction of the underlying disorder may restore patients to their customary normal state. Hyperthyroidism or hypothyroidism must be considered, especially in elderly patients.

Hospitalization is indicated for further evaluation of all patients with confusional states of uncertain cause.

REFERENCES

Charness ME, Simon RP, Greenberg DA: Ethanol and the nervous system. N Engl J Med 1989;321:442.

Geschwind N: Aphasia. N Engl J Med 1971;284:654.

Khantzian EJ, McKenna GJ: Acute toxic and withdrawal reactions associated with drug use and abuse. Ann Intern Med 1979;90:361.

Larson EB et al: Adverse drug reactions associated with global cognitive impairment in elderly persons. Ann Intern Med 1987;107:169.

Logan WJ: *Neurological Aspects of Hallucinogenic Drugs.* Vol 13 of: *Advances in Neurology.* Friedlander WJ (editor). Raven Press, 1975.

Lowenstein DH et al: Acute neurologic and psychiatric complications associated with cocaine abuse. Am J Med 1987;83:841.

McArthur JC: Neurologic manifestations of AIDS. Medicine 1987;66:407.

Miller JW et al: Transient global amnesia: Clinical characteristics and prognosis. Neurology 1987;37:733.

Pearlson GD: Psychiatric and medical syndromes associated with phencyclidine (PCP) abuse. Johns Hopkins Med J 1981;148:25.

Plum F, Posner JB: *The Diagnosis of Stupor and Coma,* 3rd ed. Davis, 1980.

Pruitt AA et al: Neurologic complications of bacterial endocarditis. Medicine 1978;57:329.

Reich P, Gottfried LA: Factitious disorders in a teaching hospital. Ann Intern Med 1983;99:240.

Reuler JB et al: Wernicke's encephalopathy. N Engl J Med 1985;312:1035.

Roy-Byrne PP, Hommer D: Benzodiazepine withdrawal: Overview and implications for the treatment of anxiety. Am J Med 1988;84:1041.

Thompson W, Johnson AD, Maddrey L: Diazepam and paraldehyde for treatment of severe delirium tremens: A controlled trial. Ann Intern Med 1975;82:175.

Tunkel AR, Wispelwey B, Scheld WM: Bacterial meningitis: Recent advances in pathophysiology and treatment. Ann Intern Med 1990;112:610.

Victor M: The amnesic syndrome and its anatomical basis. Can Med Assoc J 1969;100:1115.

Whitley RJ: Viral encephalitis. N Engl J Med 1990;323:242.

15

Arthritis & Back Pain

Peter G. Trafton, MD

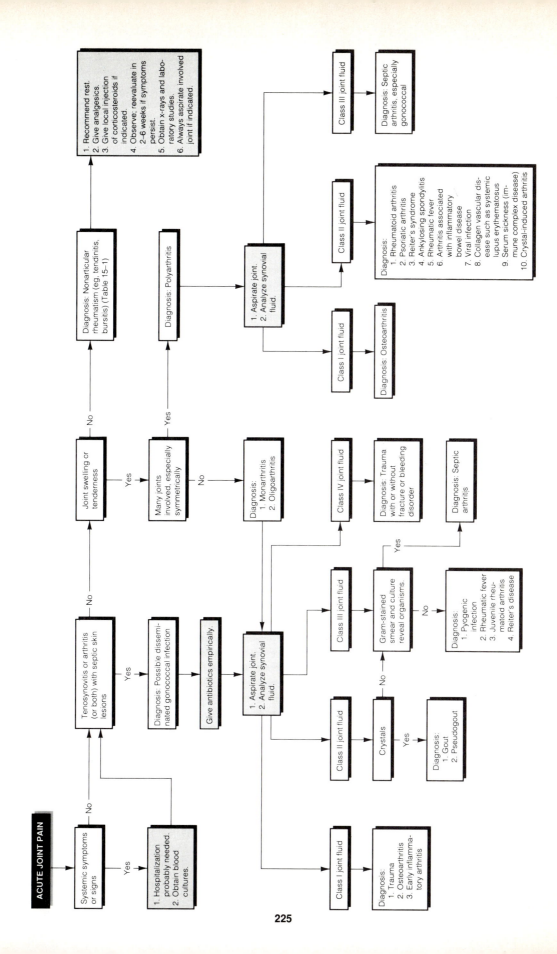

ACUTE JOINT PAIN

Systemic symptoms or signs

No →

Yes ↓

1. Hospitalization probably needed.
2. Obtain blood cultures.

Tenosynovitis or arthritis (or both) with septic skin lesions

No

Yes ↓

Diagnosis: Possible disseminated gonococcal infection

Give antibiotics empirically.

Joint swelling or tenderness

No → Diagnosis: Nonarticular rheumatism (eg, tendinitis, bursitis) (Table 15–1)

Yes ↓

1. Recommend rest.
2. Give analgesics.
3. Give local injection of corticosteroids if indicated.
4. Observe: reevaluate in 2–6 weeks if symptoms persist.
5. Obtain x-rays and laboratory studies.
6. Always aspirate involved joint if indicated.

Many joints involved, especially symmetrically

Yes → Diagnosis: Polyarthritis

No ↓

Diagnosis:
1. Monarthritis
2. Oligoarthritis

1. Aspirate joint.
2. Analyze synovial fluid.

Class I joint fluid → Diagnosis:
1. Trauma
2. Osteoarthritis
3. Early inflammatory arthritis

Class II joint fluid → Crystals

Yes → Diagnosis:
1. Gout
2. Pseudogout

No

Class III joint fluid → Gram-stained smear and culture reveal organisms.

Yes → Diagnosis: Septic arthritis

No → Diagnosis:
1. Pyogenic infection
2. Rheumatic fever
3. Juvenile rheumatoid arthritis
4. Reiter's disease

Class IV joint fluid → Diagnosis: Trauma with or without fracture or bleeding disorder

1. Aspirate joint.
2. Analyze synovial fluid.

Class I joint fluid → Diagnosis: Osteoarthritis

Class II joint fluid → Diagnosis:
1. Rheumatoid arthritis
2. Psoriatic arthritis
3. Reiter's syndrome
4. Ankylosing spondylitis
5. Rheumatic fever
6. Arthritis associated with inflammatory bowel disease
7. Viral infection
8. Collagen vascular disease such as systemic lupus erythematosus
9. Serum sickness (immune complex disease)
10. Crystal-induced arthritis

Class III joint fluid → Diagnosis: Septic arthritis, especially gonococcal

225

I. EVALUATION OF THE PATIENT WITH ACUTE ARTHRITIS (See algorithm.)

Is the Patient Systemically Ill?

Whenever a patient with acute joint pain also presents with fever, rigors, systemic symptoms, or signs of involvement of additional organ systems, careful evaluation is necessary to rule out potentially life-threatening processes such as infection or diffuse vasculitis.

Hospitalization and consultation for evaluation of rheumatic or infectious disease are usually required for patients with arthritis and systemic symptoms. Obtain blood cultures, and perform the evaluation outlined below.

Is This Disseminated Gonococcal Infection?

In young adults, hematogenous gonococcal infection is one of the commonest causes of acute arthritis. Arthritis may be the sole manifestation of disseminated gonococcal infection, or skin lesions and acute tenosynovitis may accompany the arthritis. Skin lesions are few and are found on the extremities, frequently around a joint, and are pustular or hemorrhagic, rarely bullous. Gram-stained smears of material contained in the pustules may reveal gram-negative diplococci within PMNs. Tenosynovitis classically involves tendons of the hand or foot. The primary (mucosal) site of gonococcal infection is often asymptomatic. If disseminated gonococcal infection is suspected, culture of blood and secretions from the pharynx, rectum, and urethra or cervix should be obtained.

Is There Arthritis on Joint Examination?

Ascertain by careful examination whether acute joint pain is due to an intra-articular process. Is there redness, heat, effusion, synovial thickening, bony enlargement, or painful limitation of active and passive motion? If the joint itself is not involved—although acute pain is localized to the region of the joint—cellulitis, tenosynovitis, bursitis, or other periarticular lesions should be considered.

If It Is Not Arthritis, What Is It?

The shoulders and upper extremities are the site of acute painful non–intra-articular processes more often than are other parts of the body. Table 15–1 lists the common syndromes of nonarticular rheumatism.

These disorders are described more fully later in this chapter.

Is the Process Oligoarticular or Polyarticular?

Involvement of 1–3 joints in an asymmetric pattern is generally considered characteristic of oligoarthritis, although this asymmetric involvement may occur early in some polyarticular conditions such as juvenile rheumatoid arthritis. Common causes of oligoarthritis include infection, crystal deposition (eg, gout), and trauma. The polyarthritis syndromes involve many joints, usually in a symmetric fashion.

Perform Arthrocentesis

If one of the affected joints is acrally located (eg, wrist, elbow, knee, ankle), arthrocentesis should be attempted in the emergency department, using local anesthesia (Chapter 46). Arthrocentesis of shoulders and hips is best done by a specialist. Occasionally, fluoroscopic control with dye injection is necessary to ensure that the joint space (rather than a bursa) has been entered. The joint fluid should be analyzed and the results used to classify the arthritis according to the scheme in Table 15–2.

Classification of Arthritis (See Table 15–2.)

A. Noninflammatory (Class I): Acute arthritis in the presence of normal joint fluid usually indicates trauma, osteoarthritis, or osteochondritis dissecans. Rarely, early joint aspiration in inflammatory arthritis produces a similar result.

B. Inflammatory (Class II): Inflammatory arthritis may be present in acute gout or pseudogout or in a variety of "collagen vascular" or "allergic" arthritides such as Reiter's syndrome, rheumatoid arthritis, and rheumatic fever. Gram's stain and culture of synovial fluid should be done to rule out early infectious arthritis.

C. Septic (Class III): Purulent joint fluid (class III) is seen almost exclusively in bacterial and fungal infections. Gram's stain of joint fluid may help to identify the causative organism before cultures become positive.

D. Hemorrhagic (Class IV): Hemorrhagic joint fluid is seen in trauma with or without fracture; the presence of fat globules suggests fracture. A tear in the anterior cruciate ligament is the commonest cause of hemarthrosis in the knee when no fracture is present. Also frequent are peripheral meniscus tears and patellar dislocations (with medial retinaculum tears). Hemorrhagic effusion is more likely to be associated with acute pain than is the noninflammatory effusion that can occur with minor joint trauma. Hemorrhagic fluid is also seen in the hemorrhagic diatheses, including hemophilia, in pigmented villonodular synovitis, and in association with hemangioma and other synovial neoplasms. Any of these disease processes

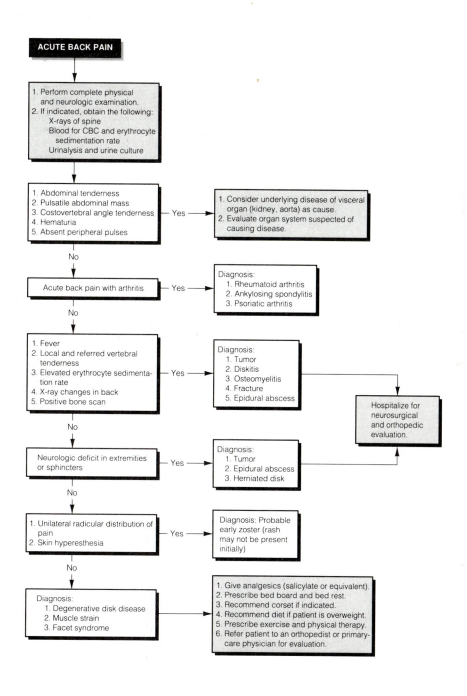

ACUTE BACK PAIN

1. Perform complete physical
   and neurologic examination.
2. If indicated, obtain the following:
     X-rays of spine
     Blood for CBC and erythrocyte
       sedimentation rate
     Urinalysis and urine culture

1. Abdominal tenderness
2. Pulsatile abdominal mass
3. Costovertebral angle tenderness
4. Hematuria
5. Absent peripheral pulses

— Yes →

1. Consider underlying disease of visceral
   organ (kidney, aorta) as cause.
2. Evaluate organ system suspected of
   causing disease.

No

Acute back pain with arthritis

— Yes →

Diagnosis:
  1. Rheumatoid arthritis
  2. Ankylosing spondylitis
  3. Psoriatic arthritis

No

1. Fever
2. Local and referred vertebral
   tenderness
3. Elevated erythrocyte sedimentation rate
4. X-ray changes in back
5. Positive bone scan

— Yes →

Diagnosis:
  1. Tumor
  2. Diskitis
  3. Osteomyelitis
  4. Fracture
  5. Epidural abscess

Hospitalize for
neurosurgical
and orthopedic
evaluation.

No

Neurologic deficit in extremities
or sphincters

— Yes →

Diagnosis:
  1. Tumor
  2. Epidural abscess
  3. Herniated disk

No

1. Unilateral radicular distribution of
   pain
2. Skin hyperesthesia

— Yes →

Diagnosis: Probable
early zoster (rash
may not be present
initially)

No

Diagnosis:
  1. Degenerative disk disease
  2. Muscle strain
  3. Facet syndrome

1. Give analgesics (salicylate or equivalent).
2. Prescribe bed board and bed rest.
3. Recommend corset if indicated.
4. Recommend diet if patient is overweight.
5. Prescribe exercise and physical therapy.
6. Refer patient to an orthopedist or primary-
   care physician for evaluation.

Table 15–1. Some common syndromes of nonarticular rheumatism.

	History	Findings	X-Rays	Diagnosis	Treatment[1]
Shoulder	Severe pain, subacromial with or without midarm pain, worse with abduction.	Point tenderness in rotator cuff. Painful abduction.	Negative, or calcific deposit overlying greater tuberosity.	Rotator cuff tendinitis (subacromial bursitis).	Local infiltration of corticosteroid. Physical thereapy to preserve motion.
	Overuse. Pain and decreased motion of shoulder.	Resistance to elbow flexion and extension reproduces pain. Point tenderness over bicipital groove.	Negative, or calcium in bicipital tendon.	Bicipital tendinitis.	Anti-inflammatory drugs. Rest. Local infiltration of corticosteroid.
Elbow	Sharp lateral pain radiating posteriorly to wrist with lifting and twisting.	Point tenderness over lateral epicondyle or radial head.	Negative; rarely shows calcium.	Tennis elbow (lateral epicondylitis).	As above. Eliminate or modify activity causing pain.
	Overuse. Trauma, often seemingly trivial. Swelling and pain over olecranon. Male.	Swollen, hot, tender olecranon bursa. Aspirate reveals purulent material.	Negative.	Olecranon bursitis (infection, trauma, gout).	Needle drainage. Hospitalization. Specific therapy (for staphylococcal infection, gout).
Wrist	Moderate pain with use of thumb and grip on radial side of wrist.	Positive Finkelstein test. Tender swelling over extensor digitorum brevis and abductor pollicis longus tendon sheath.	Negative.	De Quervain's stenosing tenosynovitis.	Usually responds to local corticosteroid injection. Splint early; then mobilize.
Hip	Pain over hip and thigh.	Swelling and tenderness over greater trochanter.	Negative.	Trochanteric bursitis.	Rest. Local corticosteroid infiltration.
Knee	Swollen knee; pain occasionally.	Swelling and slight tenderness over prepatellar bursa.	Negative.	Prepatellar or infrapatellar bursitis (housemaid's knee).	Rest. Local injection of corticosteroids for resistant cases.
	Tender patella; swelling variable.	Tenderness of patella.	Negative.	Patellofemoral chondromalacia.	Rest, anti-inflammatory drugs. Eliminate activity causing pain.

[1]Nonsteroidal anti-inflammatory agents such as ibuprofen or naproxen may be useful in any of these conditions.

Table 15–2. Classification of abnormal synovial fluid.

Type of Joint Fluid	Viscosity	Clarity	Color	Leukocyte Count (per μL)	Gram's Stain and Culture	Other Findings
Normal	High	Clear	Light yellow	< 200	Negative	. . .
Noninflammatory (class I)	High	Clear	Light yellow	200–2000	Negative	. . .
Inflammatory (class II)	Low	Cloudy	Dark yellow	> 2000	Negative	Crystals are diagnostic of gout or pseudogout (differentiate with polarizing microscopt); usually seen with class II joint fluid.
Septic (class III)	Low	Cloudy	Dark yellow	Usually > 40,000	Usually positive[1]	Bacteria on culture or Gram-stained smear. Usually seen with class III joint fluid but may be seen with class II; rarely, class I.
Hemorrhagic (class IV)	Variable	Cloudy	Pink-red	Usually >2000[2]	Negative	Fat globules strongly suggest intra-articular fracture and are usually seen with class IV joint fluid.

[1]Commonest exception is gonococcal infection (only about 25% of cases have positive culture or Gram's stain).
[2]Many red cells also found.

may be associated with acute joint pain, because blood within the joint space generally causes an inflammatory reaction.

II. EMERGENCY TREATMENT OF SPECIFIC CONDITIONS CAUSING ACUTE ARTHRITIS

MONARTHRITIS OR OLIGOARTHRITIS

TRAUMATIC ARTHRITIS

Diagnosis

Severe joint pain associated with trauma is usually related temporally to an obvious injury. Mild pain may occur some time after the injury, particularly if the injury is minor and goes unnoticed. Fever and other systemic signs are not present unless there have been multiple traumatic injuries. The presence of noninflammatory or hemorrhagic synovial fluid confirms the diagnosis. Because patients with septic arthritis may also give a history of recent trauma, Gram's stain and culture of fluid should be performed.

The presence of many small fat globules in hemorrhagic joint fluid strongly suggests intra-articular fracture; x-rays, including special views as indicated, should be carefully scrutinized to locate occult fractures. Well-localized tenderness over a bone, as opposed to a joint capsule or a ligament, is an important sign of fracture (Chapter 22). Scaphoid (carpal navicular) fractures are particularly difficult to locate and require special views and careful correlation with clinical findings (eg, localized tenderness in the anatomic snuffbox). X-rays that show only joint effusion or periarticular soft tissue swelling are consistent with occult fractures or other joint injuries such as spontaneously reduced dislocations, ligamentous injuries, meniscus tears, avulsion fractures, and osteochondral fractures. Careful examination is therefore required.

Joint effusions that accumulate immediately following trauma are uniformly hemorrhagic and usually do not require arthrocentesis for diagnostic purposes. Because occult fracture is a common cause of the effusion, contamination of the joint space during arthrocentesis would result in a compound fracture with an increased risk of complications. Therefore, acute traumatic effusions should be aspirated only if they are markedly painful and tense to reduce discomfort, and then only with the strictest aseptic technique.

Treatment & Disposition

Splinting, protection from weight bearing, and follow-up care are essential. Analgesia may be needed. See Chapter 22 for more specific details and guidelines for treatment and disposition.

ACUTE GOUTY ARTHRITIS

Diagnosis

Patients with acute gouty arthritis have oligoarthritis with class II or class III joint fluid and urate crystals in the synovial fluid.

A. Symptoms and Signs: There is sudden onset of warmth, hyperemia, induration, and extreme pain in a joint, most commonly the metatarsophalangeal joint of the great toe (podagra); the next most commonly involved is the knee (gonagra). Although most patients present with only one painful joint, up to 5% may present with 2, 3, or more involved joints.

B. Laboratory Findings: Elevated serum uric acid concentration is supporting evidence of gouty arthritis, although during an acute attack, the serum urate level may be normal. Definitive diagnosis requires use of a polarizing microscope to demonstrate characteristic negative birefringence of urate crystals in the synovial fluid. The presence of tophi from which urate can be aspirated also strongly supports the diagnosis, as does a history of uric acid nephrolithiasis.

Treatment

A. Nonsteroidal Anti-Inflammatory Drugs: Indomethacin or other nonsteroidal anti-inflammatory agents may be indicated if a diagnosis of arthritis is well established. Aspirin is contraindicated, because small doses may cause hyperuricemia.

1. Indomethacin–Give 50 mg orally every 6 hours for 3–4 doses; then reduce to 25 mg 3–4 times daily for 4–5 days. Peptic ulcer disease is a contraindication to indomethacin.

2. Other drugs–Ibuprofen, 600 mg orally every 6 hours; naproxen, 750 mg orally followed by 250 mg every 8 hours; fenoprofen, 600 mg orally every 6 hours; and sulindac, 200 mg orally twice daily are also effective in acute gout.

3. Phenylbutazone–Give 100 mg orally 3–4 times daily for 1–2 days; then reduce the dose. Phenylbutazone is contraindicated in patients with peptic ulcer disease. *Caution:* Because of the risk of agranulocytosis, and aplastic anemia, phenylbutazone is not recommended as initial therapy for any indication. It should be reserved for use only when all safer forms of therapy have failed and the potential benefit outweighs potential risks.

B. Colchicine: Oral or intravenous colchicine administered *early* in the course of acute arthritis provides dramatic relief in 85–90% of patients; an additional 5% show partial response. Response to colchicine also strongly supports a diagnosis of gout.

1. Oral treatment–Give colchicine, 0.5 mg every hour (or 1 mg every 2 hours) until pain has resolved or until nausea or diarrhea supervenes. The usual dose is 4–8 mg.

2. Intravenous treatment–Gastrointestinal toxicity can be reduced by giving colchicine, 1–2 mg intravenously in 50 mL of normal saline over 20 minutes; repeat this dose every 6 hours until the patient is asymptomatic or to a total dose of 4 mg.

Disposition

Hospitalization is rarely necessary. The patient should receive follow-up evaluation in a few days.

ACUTE PSEUDOGOUT

Diagnosis

Patients with acute pseudogout have acute oligoarthritis with class II joint fluid and calcium pyrophosphate crystals in the synovial fluid. Pseudogout simulates gout in middle-aged or elderly patients. It differs from gout in that the knee is the most commonly involved joint.

Serum uric acid levels are usually normal.

Chondrocalcinosis may be present, although not necessarily in the acutely involved joint. Radiopaque deposits are seen most commonly in the cartilage of the acromioclavicular joint, the intervertebral disks, and the symphysis pubica. Deposits may also be seen in the knee joint but not as a manifestation of the acute arthritis. Chondrocalcinosis also frequently occurs in severe osteoarthritis, hyperparathyroidism, alkaptonuria, hemochromatosis, Wilson's disease, acromegaly, and possibly gout. The presence of chondrocalcinosis, however, whether located in the inflamed joint or not, is not diagnostic. Definitive diagnosis depends on the presence of calcium dihydrate (pyrophosphate) crystals in synovial fluid.

Treatment

Aspiration of the joint is often adequate for relief of symptoms. The use of intra-articular corticosteroids or oral indomethacin or other nonsteroidal antiinflammatory agents may be helpful (see Acute Gouty Arthritis, above). Unlike patients with gouty arthritis, patients with acute pseudogout rarely respond to colchicine.

Disposition

Hospitalization is rarely necessary. Refer the patient to a primary-care physician.

SEPTIC ARTHRITIS

Septic arthritis is one of the more common causes of oligoarthritis, but often only one joint is affected. The most frequent pathogen is the gonococcus, which, although difficult to demonstrate in joint fluid, often produces typical pustular skin lesions or tenosynovitis. Other common pathogens are the pyogenic cocci (*Staphylococcus aureus,* streptococci) and aerobic gram-negative bacteria (eg, meningococci; *Haemophilus influenzae*). Less common forms of septic arthritis include those caused by *Mycobacterium tuberculosis,* fungi *(Coccidioides immitis, Blastomyces dermatitidis, Cryptococcus neoformans),* and spirochetes (eg, Lyme disease spirochete, *Treponema pallidum*).

Diagnosis

Patients with septic arthritis show evidence of infection in the joint (bacteria on Gram-stained smear or culture, or rapid response to antimicrobial therapy). Class III joint fluid is usually present.

A. Symptoms and Signs: Septic arthritis usually presents as a severe monarticular process characterized by marked pain, erythema, and tenderness. Its onset is usually less precipitous than that of gout. A few patients with staphylococcal or gonococcal arthritis may present with 2 or more involved joints. Acute migratory oligoarthritis followed in 1–2 days by acute arthritis localized to 1 or 2 joints is especially suggestive of gonococcal arthritis. If multiple joints are involved in septic arthritis, the distribution is usually asymmetric. Systemic symptoms and signs of infection (eg, fever, chills, leukocytosis) are common but not invariable.

B. Laboratory Findings: A definitive diagnosis is established by demonstrating the infecting organism in synovial tissue or joint fluid.

Joint fluid shows high leukocyte counts, usually over 40,000/µL. The higher the white blood cell count in joint fluid, the greater the likelihood of bacterial or fungal arthritis. The glucose content of synovial fluid is usually reduced but may occasionally be normal. If no antimicrobial therapy has been given, smears and cultures of joint fluid usually reveal organisms.

In gonococcal arthritis, however, Gram-stained smears and even cultures of joint fluid are frequently negative, though in most cases, cultures of exudate from the cervix, urethra, pharynx, or rectum demonstrate gonococci. In gonococcal arthritis, the diagnosis may also be confirmed by prompt response to antimicrobial therapy (Chapter 34).

Treatment

A. Aspiration of the joint is essential. Obtain cultures of blood and joint fluid. If gonococcal arthritis is suspected, cervical, urethral, and possibly pharyngeal and rectal cultures should be obtained. If sepsis is considered likely, as much fluid as possible should be removed from the joint.

B. Begin an antibiotic deemed appropriate based on clinical findings and Gram-stained smears. If the causative organism cannot be determined with reasonable certainty from a Gram-stained smear and the clinical setting, begin treatment with an antibiotic effective against staphylococci, pneumococci, gonococci, and gram-negative organisms. Particularly in older patients with underlying disease, give nafcillin, 150 mg/kg/d intravenously in 4–6 divided doses; and gentamicin, 3–5 mg/kg/d intravenously or intramuscularly in divided doses every 8 hours, until the results of culture and sensitivity studies are available to dictate any changes required in antimicrobial therapy. Alternatively, a first- or second-generation cephalosporin may be used (eg, ceftriaxone, 2 g intravenously once daily or in 2 divided doses every 24 hours). The treatment of gonococcal arthritis is discussed in more detail in Chapter 34.

Disposition

All patients with suspected or documented septic arthritis should be hospitalized. A patient with mild gonococcal arthritis can often be discharged early and given antibiotics to be taken orally, provided that the patient is reliable and careful follow-up can be ensured.

OLIGOARTHRITIS OR POLYARTHRITIS

OSTEOARTHRITIS
(Degenerative Joint Disease)

Diagnosis

Osteoarthritis generally presents as polyarthritis of insidious onset, although oligoarthritis and monarthritis may occur and symptoms may worsen acutely. The pain is improved by rest and worsened by activity. Examination shows minimal evidence of systemic manifestations or joint inflammation, but joint crepitus is often present. Clinical and laboratory signs of inflammation are absent. The x-ray findings are characteristic and include narrowed joint spaces, osteophytes, and bony cysts.

Treatment & Disposition

For routine cases, reassurance, nonsteroidal anti-inflammatory agents (eg, aspirin, 650–975 mg every 4–6 hours), rest, and referral (if necessary) to a source of long-term care are all that is required. Crutches may be necessary if a weight-bearing joint is severely involved.

Hospitalization may be warranted for the patient with disabling active osteoarthritis or for the occasional patient with osteoarthritis who presents with acute oligoarthritis. In the latter case, hospitalization to rule out infectious arthritis is advisable.

RHEUMATIC FEVER & POSTSTREPTOCOCCAL ARTHRITIS

Rheumatic fever or poststreptococcal arthritis may occasionally present as acute monarticular joint pain, particularly before the disease spreads to involve other joints. Patients with rheumatic fever often have other features such as carditis, erythema marginatum rheumaticum, or characteristic subcutaneous nodules. These signs are not seen in poststreptococcal arthritis. The erythrocyte sedimentation rate is elevated, and evidence of recent group A streptococcal infection (positive culture or elevated antistreptococcal antibodies [ASO, etc]) is found in both conditions. The patient should be hospitalized if rheumatic fever is suspected. The diagnosis is established on the basis of combined clinical and laboratory features as outlined in Table 15–3 (Jones criteria).

RHEUMATOID ARTHRITIS

Diagnosis

Although rheumatoid arthritis usually begins insidiously and involves several joints, it may present as acute monarthritis. Juvenile rheumatoid arthritis, whether of adult or childhood onset, is more likely to present as a single painful joint than is classic rheumatoid arthritis. Early x-ray studies and laboratory tests are not helpful, especially in the juvenile variant. An elevated erythrocyte sedimentation rate may be the only abnormality. At this stage, a careful history is the most important diagnostic tool. Continued observation for several weeks may be necessary to establish the diagnosis.

Treatment & Disposition

See Rheumatoid Arthritis, below.

Table 15–3. Jones criteria for diagnosis of rheumatic fever.[1]

Major criteria
  Pericarditis, myocarditis, or endocarditis
  Chorea
  Subcutaneous nodules
  Erythema marginatum
  Polyarthritis
Minor criteria
  Fever
  Malaise
  Arthralgias
  Laboratory findings: leukocytosis, elevated sedimentation rate, evidence of preceding streptococcal infection (increased titer of antistreptolysn O)
  History of rheumatic fever or rheumatic heart disease

[1]The presence of 2 major or one major and 2 minor criteria with supporting evidence of recent infection with group A streptococcus indicates a high probability of rheumatic fever.

POLYARTHRITIS

RHEUMATOID ARTHRITIS

Diagnosis

Rheumatoid arthritis generally presents as a symmetric, chronic polyarthritis with prominent involvement of proximal interphalangeal and metacarpophalangeal joints, often with deformity.

A. Symptoms and Signs: Rheumatoid arthritis is probably the most common cause of subacute joint pain involving multiple joints in the adult. Symmetric involvement is characteristic; however, the disease may begin with asymmetric involvement and remain asymmetric for some time. Early in the disease, joint swelling is chiefly intra-articular secondary to effusion. Periarticular soft tissue swelling is a later phenomenon. Involvement of the proximal interphalangeal and metacarpophalangeal joints suggests the diagnosis, as does the presence of subcutaneous nodules (if they are definitely not tophi).

B. Laboratory Findings: Rheumatoid factor may be present at onset, but a negative test does not rule out rheumatoid arthritis. Hypergammaglobulinemia and an elevated erythrocyte sedimentation rate are also common.

C. X-Ray Findings: In subacute presentation, early x-ray examination generally reveals only soft tissue swelling. Juxta-articular osteoporosis and erosions are seen later.

Treatment

Nonsteroidal anti-inflammatory agents are the mainstay of treatment.

A. Aspirin: Aspirin is the drug of choice unless the patient is intolerant or allergic. The usual dose for adults is 975 mg (3 tablets) 4 times a day. The dose is adjusted upward or downward based on patient response and tolerance. A serum aspirin concentration over 20 mg/dL or a dose just under that which causes tinnitus is the goal.

B. Other Drugs: If the patient cannot take aspirin or shows inadequate response to the maximum tolerated dose, one of the following agents should be tried: naproxen, 250–500 mg 2 times a day; indomethacin, 25–50 mg 3–4 times a day; or similar drugs in comparable doses (ibuprofen, tolmetin, fenoprofen, sulindac, piroxicam).

Disposition

The patient should be referred early to a rheumatologist or an internist with an interest in rheumatic disease. Severe systemic involvement (eg, disabling polyarthritis, fever, or weight loss) or vasculitis may warrant hospitalization.

PSORIATIC ARTHRITIS

Diagnosis

Most patients with psoriatic arthritis have characteristic skin and nail lesions (pitting) at the time they present with acute joint pain. In rare instances, arthritis may precede all other manifestations of psoriasis (although even then nail pitting may be present on careful examination). Involvement of the distal interphalangeal joints— if Heberden's nodes can be ruled out—supports the diagnosis. Psoriatic arthritis is usually asymmetric and often involves weight-bearing joints.

Treatment & Disposition

Treatment for mild to moderately severe disease consists of aspirin or other nonsteroidal anti-inflammatory agents (see Rheumatoid Arthritis, above). Severe skin and joint involvement requires hospitalization.

REITER'S SYNDROME

Diagnosis

Acute arthritis due to Reiter's syndrome is usually accompanied by several other manifestations, including urethritis, conjunctivitis, circinate balanitis, other mucous membrane lesions, and keratoderma blennorrhagicum. Heel tenderness may be prominent. When several of these symptoms occur simultaneously with the arthritis, the diagnosis of Reiter's syndrome can be made with confidence. Reiter's syndrome generally occurs in young men and presents with asymmetric involvement of weight-bearing joints; arthrocentesis demonstrates class II (inflammatory) joint fluid. X-ray may show periosteal new bone formation at the insertion of the Achilles tendon and elsewhere.

There are no specific abnormalities on laboratory tests, although the diagnosis is supported if HLA-B27 antigen is found on histocompatibility typing.

The simultaneous occurrence of Reiter's syndrome and gonococcal infection is common; therefore, the presence of gonococci on a urethral smear does not rule out Reiter's syndrome, particularly if the arthritis fails to respond quickly to antibiotic therapy.

Treatment & Disposition

There is no specific therapy, but nonsteroidal anti-inflammatory agents, including aspirin and indomethacin, should be employed for symptomatic relief. Referral for long-term follow-up should be made, with hospitalization reserved for those who are acutely ill with systemic symptoms and severe or multiple joint involvement.

ANKYLOSING SPONDYLITIS

Diagnosis

In patients with ankylosing spondylitis, acute joint

pain can occur before any overt evidence of back involvement. Most patients, however, demonstrate radiographic changes in the lumbar spine or sacroiliac joints at the time they present with peripheral arthritis. Restricted chest expansion may be an early clinical finding; limitation of back motion also occurs. The hips, shoulders, and knees are the most common sites of involvement. Ankylosing spondylitis should be considered in males between 15 and 30 years of age with acute joint pain who give a history of unremitting chronic low back discomfort over 3 months or longer that is worse in the morning and improves with activity. The following test can be performed during the physical examination; if the test is positive, it is supportive of the diagnosis. With the patient standing erect, draw a vertical line 10 cm long along the spine from the T12 vertebra to the L3 vertebra (approximately). Ask the patient to bend as far forward as possible, and measure the line again. If the line does not lengthen to more than 13 cm, the test is positive. Such patients have inflammatory (class II) joint fluid on arthrocentesis. An elevated erythrocyte sedimentation rate is common. A positive family history is common, and there is a strong correlation with the presence of HLA-B27 antigen.

Treatment & Disposition

Appropriate treatment includes anti-inflammatory therapy, bed rest, and referral to a rheumatologist for follow-up and appropriate long-term care.

VIRAL ARTHRITIS

Acute symmetric polyarthritis occurs in rubella, early viral hepatitis, Chikungunya, O'nyong-nyong fever, mumps, and, rarely, in other viral infections. It can also occur after immunization for rubella.

Diagnosis

Joint pain is usually not severe, but it may be of acute onset, and the presentation often mimics that of rheumatoid arthritis. Careful history taking helps in the diagnosis; the patient should be asked about recent immunization or exposure to persons with viral infections. Arthritis may precede the overt systemic disease, occur concurrently, or persist following acute infection.

If arthritis associated with hepatitis is the working diagnosis, tests for HBsAg and complement levels may be useful, since patients with hepatitis B often are HBsAg-positive and hypocomplementemic during the arthritic stage. Results of liver function tests are also frequently abnormal.

Treatment & Disposition

Appropriate treatment of the articular manifestations of viral arthritis is symptomatic and includes rest and anti-inflammatory agents. Refer patients to their usual source of medical care for follow-up.

SERUM SICKNESS (Immune Complex Disease)

Diagnosis

Arthritis is a common symptom of serum sickness. A history of penicillin administration 7–15 days before the onset of arthritis is common in patients with serum sickness, although administration of other drugs or heterologous serum may also produce the disease. The arthritis is often accompanied by urticaria and other skin rashes. Glomerulonephritis may occur. Diagnosis may be difficult when the rash does not appear. Diagnosis may also be obscured if the patient has recently received an inadequate course of penicillin for either group A streptococcal pharyngitis or gonococcal disease; either rheumatic fever or gonococcal arthritis may mimic serum sickness on presentation.

Treatment & Disposition

Appropriate treatment includes stopping administration of the offending antigen and starting treatment with anti-inflammatory drugs and bed rest. Oral corticosteroids may be beneficial. Hospitalization may be advisable.

SYSTEMIC LUPUS ERYTHEMATOSUS

Diagnosis

Acute onset of joint pain is not common in systemic lupus erythematosus, but it may occur. Patients usually also have fever, rash, polyserositis, or other features of the disease. When patients present with several obvious symptoms of systemic lupus erythematosus, diagnosis is not difficult. Diagnosis in patients who present only with arthritis requires demonstration of a positive antinuclear antibody test or anti–double-stranded DNA.

Treatment & Disposition

The acute arthritis of systemic lupus erythematosus is treated with nonsteroidal anti-inflammatory agents. Patients should be referred to a rheumatologist for diagnostic evaluation and appropriate care.

INTESTINAL ARTHRITIS

Arthritis associated with ulcerative colitis or regional enteritis has clinical findings similar to those of psoriatic arthritis. Treatment and disposition are similar also.

NONARTICULAR RHEUMATISM

Joint pain and periarticular swelling and tenderness mimicking arthritis may often be due to inflammation of periarticular structures (bursae and tendons). The clinical features of the common tendinitis and bursitis syndromes are set forth in Table 15–1.

TENDINITIS

Diagnosis
In tendinitis, the tendon and tendon sheath are inflamed. There is pain and tenderness over the course of the involved tendon, and active or passive movement of the tendon within its sheath also causes pain. Tendinitis may be idiopathic, traumatic, or infectious in origin. Infectious (septic) tenosynovitis is a true surgical emergency that involves flexor tendons in the hand. A small penetrating wound of a digital flexion crease is typically present. Organisms most commonly involved are *Staphylococcus aureus* and *Streptococcus.* There is marked pain and tenderness along the course of the tendon sheath, with exquisite pain on passive stretching of the tendon. Swelling, erythema, and in some cases, fever may be associated. (See Infections in Chapter 23.) Acute peritendinous inflammation in the ankle or wrist may be associated with gonococcemia.

Treatment
A. Adjunctive Measures: Rest, effective splinting, and ice as needed are the mainstays of treatment. Oral anti-inflammatory agents, local ultrasound treatments, and an exercise program to maintain joint motion and build muscle strength are helpful.

B. Local Injection: Local injection of anesthetic and depot glucocorticoid preparations may be appropriate for some patients (see Bursitis, below). This should not be attempted, however, by an individual unskilled in the procedure, as complications can result (eg, local atrophy and rupture of the tendon) if corticosteroids are errantly injected into a weight-bearing tendon.

C. Antimicrobials: The occasional pyogenic tendinitis (usually due to the gonococcus) must be treated with antimicrobials. A cephalosporin (eg, cefazolin, 60 mg/kg/d intramuscularly or intravenously in 3 divided doses) is satisfactory empiric therapy while the results of cultures are pending. Septic tenosynovitis usually requires hospitalization. If a tendon of the hand is involved, consultation with a hand surgeon should be obtained because decompression and debridement of the tendon sheath may be necessary.

Disposition
Most patients with tendinitis can be treated on an outpatient basis, with referral to a rheumatologist or orthopedist as necessary. Patients with pyogenic tendinitis usually require hospitalization and surgical drainage.

BURSITIS

Diagnosis
Bursitis is inflammation of the synovial cavities that surround joints and allow free movement of soft tissue juxta-articular structures. Like tendinitis, bursitis may be due to trauma ("housemaid's knee," or prepatellar bursitis) or infection (most commonly found in the olecranon bursa) or may be idiopathic. Clinical findings are pain, tenderness, and swelling of the involved bursa.

Treatment
A. Aspiration: The bursa should be aspirated for diagnosis and treatment.

B. Antibiotics: Septic bursitis (most commonly of the olecranon bursa) is usually due to *S aureus* and pending results of culture and susceptibility testing, should be treated with a penicillinase-resistant, beta-lactamase–resistant antimicrobial (eg, nafcillin, 150 mg/kg/d intravenously in 4–6 divided doses; or cefazolin, 60 mg/kg/d intramuscularly or intravenously in 3 divided doses).

C. Anti-inflammatory Agents: If an aseptic but inflammatory process is present, rest the affected area, give anti-inflammatory agents (indomethacin, 25–50 mg orally 3 times a day; ibuprofen, 400–600 mg orally 4 times a day; or naproxen, 375–500 mg twice daily), and maintain range of motion.

D. Corticosteroid Injection: Locally injected corticosteroids are useful in treatment of *aseptic* bursitis. It is desirable to obtain a negative culture or Gram's-stain smear prior to injection. The procedure is to infiltrate the area with 1% lidocaine (typically 0.5–2 mL) and follow with injection of methylprednisolone acetate (or equivalent) into the bursa: 5–10 mg of methylprednisolone for small bursae, 10–40 mg for medium bursae, and 20–80 mg for large bursae.

E. Surgery: Pyogenic bursitis may require incision and drainage. This should be considered whenever an abscesslike collection of pus is present.

Disposition
Patients with septic bursitis require hospitalization. Patients with aseptic bursitis may be discharged but should be seen by a primary-care physician for follow-up within 3–4 days.

III. EVALUATION OF THE PATIENT WITH ACUTE BACK PAIN (See algorithm.)

Perform Baseline Evaluation

An established routine for evaluating patients with acute back pain will ensure that the emergency physician does not miss life-threatening disease. Patients who do not fit into the categories mentioned below have acute back pain due to degenerative disk disease, facet syndrome, strains, and sprains, etc, without underlying disease.

A. History:

1. Is there trauma or a precipitating event?–Often the patient reports trauma or a precipitating event causing acute back pain. In patients with chronic or recurrent back problems, even minor trauma such as a cough or a sneeze can cause acute back pain.

2. Is there visceral disease?–The emergency physician's first goal should be to exclude nonorthopedic causes of back pain (Table 15–4). Evaluation and treatment should focus on the organ thought to be involved.

3. Is there associated arthritis?–When back pain is associated with arthritis (oligo- or polyarthritis), both disorders are usually due to the same cause; eg, ankylosing spondylitis commonly causes peripheral and vertebral arthritis concurrently. Evaluate and treat these patients as if they had acute arthritis.

4. Are systemic symptoms present?–Fever, weight loss, night sweats, or symptoms of other organ involvement (eg, jaundice, pleural effusions) may indicate infection (osteomyelitis, diskitis) or metastatic tumor. In these cases, radiologic abnormalities (vertebral radiolucencies or compression fractures) are common but not always present. A history consistent with potentially metastatic malignancy requires a thorough, well-documented neurologic examination to exclude spinal cord involvement.

5. Is there a neurologic deficit?–A new neurologic deficit of the lower extremities or (rarely) the upper extremities in association with back pain may indicate cord compression due to infection, tumor, or disk disease and calls for vigorous management. Seek consultation with a neurosurgeon or neurologist immediately, and consider myelography. Such patients may require hospitalization for diagnosis and treatment.

6. Is there radicular distribution of pain?–Unilateral radicular pain suggests preeruptive zoster. If tests besides those for zoster are negative, refer the patient for follow-up care after providing appropriate analgesics.

B. Examination: Examine the back for deformity, tenderness, and range of motion; test for limitation of straight-leg raising and evaluate gait. Also examine the heart, peripheral pulses, lungs, and abdomen. Perform a neurologic evaluation that includes reflexes, muscle strength, sensory examination of the legs and perineum, and assessment of rectal sphincter strength.

C. X-Ray and Laboratory Studies: If indicated by abnormal results on history or physical examination, obtain x-rays of the back, CBC with differential, erythrocyte sedimentation rate, and urinalysis with culture. A bone scan is more sensitive than radiographs for locating occult focal lesions (tumor or infection). Uncomplicated low back pain that is of musculoskeletal origin, of less than 1 month's duration, and not associated with signs of infection, metastatic disease, or trauma usually does not require x-rays or blood tests.

D. Disposition: See below under specific conditions.

Table 15–4. Nonorthopedic (visceral) causes of acute back pain.

Diagnosis	Common Clinical Findings
Pyelonephritis	Flank pain, fever, pyuria, dysuria.
Nephrolithiasis	Flank pain, hematuria.
Abdominal aortic aneurysm	Hypotension, pulsatile mass, abnormal plain film or abdominal x-ray.
Aortic dissection	Absent pulses, hematuria, abnormal chest x-ray.
Pancreatitis	Elevated serum and urine amylase; tender abdomen, pancreatic calcification.
Ruptured abdominal viscus	Tender abdomen, air under diaphragm.

IV. EMERGENCY TREATMENT OF SPECIFIC CONDITIONS CAUSING BACK PAIN

TRAUMATIC BACK PAIN

Back pain associated with recent trauma may imply a fracture or dislocation of the thoracic or lumbar spine. The patient should be kept immobilized on a long spine board or equivalent stretcher and carefully examined for other associated injuries. Neurologic function (including anal sphincter contraction) should be documented and thoracic and lumbar spine x-rays obtained. Other evaluation and treatment should proceed as indicated depending on the injuries present (Chapters 4 and 21).

CHRONIC DEGENERATIVE DISK DISEASE

Diagnosis

A. Symptoms: Most patients are 35–55 years of age. The pain of chronic degenerative disk disease is typically a deep steady pain in the mid or low back that may be episodic. It is commonly unilateral and may radiate into the buttocks and posterior thigh. Pain is relieved by bed rest and aggravated by bending and lifting but is usually not worsened by sneezing or coughing. Night pain is unusual. Neurologic symptoms are absent.

B. Physical Examination: The physical examination may show normal results or may disclose one or more of the following: increased lumbar lordosis, protuberant abdomen, scoliosis, limited back motion, asymmetric lateral bending, local deep tenderness, or tight hamstring muscles. Tenderness to deep percussion, neurologic deficit, and positive sciatic stretch tests are not present.

C. Laboratory Findings: CBC, urinalysis, and erythrocyte sedimentation rate, if obtained, are all normal.

D. X-Ray Findings: X-rays, if obtained, may be normal or may have one or more of the following signs of degenerative disk disease: disk space narrowing, horizontal anterior osteophytes, spondylolisthesis, posterior facet subluxation, sclerosis, spurs.

Treatment

A. Analgesics: Give aspirin or equivalent (eg, nonsteroidal anti-inflammatory agents); if narcotics are required, consider hospitalization.

B. Bed Rest: Institute bed rest in the semi-Fowler position (a pillow under the knees when the patient is supine) or fetal position on one side on a firm mattress over a bed board.

C. Muscle Relaxants: If spasm of the lumbar musculature is present, striated muscle relaxants (eg, methocarbamol, others) for the first several days may be helpful. These agents may cause sedation.

D. Corset: Use a corset in ambulatory patients as a temporary substitute for poor abdominal musculature. A corset is also useful in elderly or pregnant women.

E. Diet: Weight loss is important if obesity is a causative factor in low back strain (common).

F. Exercise: Send the patient for physical therapy instruction in graded exercise and amelioration of pain through heat or ice and massage, etc.

Disposition

Hospitalization is rarely required. Refer the patient to a primary-care physician or orthopedist.

ACUTE INTERVERTEBRAL DISK HERNIATION, RUPTURE, OR EXTRUSION (Without Neurologic Involvement)

Acute lumbar disk herniation, rupture, or extrusion represents an acute episode in a chronic degenerative process. Patients may have a history of chronic episodic low back pain.

Diagnosis

Pain usually begins abruptly, often with trivial trauma such as sneezing. The pain is often described as stabbing or shooting, worse with sneezing or coughing, and often incapacitatingly severe. Radiation in the distribution of the sciatic nerve is common. The physical findings are similar to those of degenerative disk disease, with the addition of severe paravertebral muscle spasm. Sciatic stretch tests may be positive. Neurologic function, including sensation and deep tendon reflexes, is intact. X-rays and the results of laboratory studies are usually normal.

Treatment & Disposition

Acute lumbar disk herniation usually requires complete bed rest and narcotic analgesics (for the first day or so). Additional measures are as described for chronic degenerative disk disease, above (ie, aspirin, nonsteroidal anti-inflammatory agents, muscle relaxants). Unless *ideal* support is available at home, the patient requires hospitalization. Bed rest is frequently required for 3–4 weeks, although most patients are significantly improved within 2 weeks.

ACUTE INTERVERTEBRAL DISK HERNIATION, RUPTURE, OR EXTRUSION (With Neurologic Involvement)

Diagnosis

The clinical picture is identical to that of acute lumbar disk herniation with the addition of neurologic deficits (Table 15–5). The levels most frequently involved are the L5–S1 and L4–5 disks. A single disk rupture may involve 2 roots; or, if it is central and affects several roots, it may produce an acute cauda equina syndrome with impaired bladder and rectal sphincter function.

Treatment & Disposition

Mild cases may be managed on an outpatient basis with strict bed rest and other measures as outlined for disk herniation without neurologic involvement, above. Neurosurgical or orthopedic consultation should be obtained, and follow-up should be arranged in 7–10 days.

Table 15–5. Neurologic findings in herniated lumbosacral disk.

Disk	Root	Motor Findings	Sensory Findings	Reflexes	Sciatic Stretch Tests
L5–S1	S1	Weak foot evertors and plantar flexors.	Decreased response on lateral side of foot and leg.	Achilles jerk depressed or absent.	Strongly positive.
L4–5	L5	Weak extensor hallucis longus.	Decreased response on mid dorsum of foot.	No changes.	Moderately positive.
L3–4	L4	Weak knee extension.	Decreased response on medial foot and anteromeidal leg.	Knee jerk depressed or absent.	May be negative.

Moderate to severe cases require hospitalization for bed rest, traction, pain control, and neurosurgical or orthopedic consultation.

CT scan and MRI are useful diagnostic tools in the evaluation of sciatica and radiculopathy but are generally indicated only if surgery is being considered.

STRAINS & SPRAINS

Although some episodes of back pain during or after heavy lifting may represent true muscle pull or ligamentous strain, the clinical picture is the same as that in patients with degenerative disk disease. Most patients with strains or sprains have some element of degenerative disk disease.

FACET SYNDROME

Excessive overriding of lumbar or thoracic facets usually occurs as a consequence of disk space narrowing associated with degenerative disk disease. Facet syndrome is unusual and episodic and is characterized by the onset of acute scoliosis after asymmetric lifting. The diagnosis is usually made by exclusion. Patients should be instructed in the fundamentals of proper back care; they may respond to spinal manipulation.

DISKITIS, OSTEOMYELITIS, & EPIDURAL & PARASPINOUS ABSCESS
(See also Chapter 34.)

Disk space infections today are most commonly seen in intravenous drug abusers but occur sporadically in other patients. The organism most commonly implicated is *S aureus*.

Diagnosis

Patients with disk space infections characteristically have night pain, cough pain, tenderness on percussion, fever, and an elevated erythrocyte sedimentation rate. The physician should be alert for the rare low-grade presentations of tuberculous and fungal diskitis. Systemic evidence of infection is usually (not always) present.

The typical x-ray changes of disk space narrowing with adjacent vertebral end-plate destruction do not appear until 10–14 days after onset of symptoms. Bone scans are usually positive early in the illness before x-ray changes appear. Epidural or paraspinous abscess may appear as an ill-defined mass on x-ray. CT scan or MRI is useful in helping to establish the diagnosis.

Treatment & Disposition

Treatment of vertebral osteomyelitis requires hospitalization for orthopedic consultation, needle aspiration for bacteriologic diagnosis, bed rest, and appropriate antibiotics. Occasionally surgical drainage is required.

A neurologic deficit in association with signs of vertebral diskitis or osteomyelitis often means that an epidural or paraspinous abscess is present. Epidural or paraspinous abscess is a *major emergency* demanding immediate neurosurgical and orthopedic consultation and hospitalization for CT scan or myelogram and possible surgery.

ANKYLOSING SPONDYLITIS

See above for details of diagnosis, treatment, and disposition.

NEOPLASM

Metastatic tumor is the most common neoplastic process causing back pain. Bone marrow tumors such as multiple myeloma are second in frequency. Primary tumors of the spinal column or spinal cord are rare.

Fifty percent of bone must be lost before a lesion is evident on plain x-ray films. Multiple lesions are common. Bone scan is more sensitive for early diagnosis.

Clues to diagnosis are night pain in the absence of day pain, a history of insidious and progressive pain that has not responded to conservative measures, an elevated erythrocyte sedimentation rate, significant anemia, proteinemia, and findings in other organ systems that suggest neoplasm.

ZOSTER

Preeruptive zoster may mimic degenerative disk disease. The pain of zoster is burning and dysesthetic, however, with striking unilateral radicular distribution that does not cross the midline. Skin hyperesthesia over the painful area is the earliest physical finding. See Chapter 40 for details.

REFERENCES

Bluestone R: Diagnosis of rheumatic disease. Postgrad Med (March) 1979;65:64.

Boss GR, Seegmiller JE: Hyperuricemia and gout: Classification, complications and management. N Engl J Med 1979;300:1459.

Condemi JJ: The autoimmune diseases. JAMA 1987;258:2920.

Deyo RA: Conservative therapy for low back pain: Distinguishing useful from useless therapy. JAMA 1983;250:1057.

Eismont FJ et al: Pyogenic and fungal vertebral osteomyelitis with paralysis. J Bone Joint Surg [Am] 1983;65A:19.

Goldenberg DL, Reed JI: Bacterial arthritis. N Engl J Med 1985;312:764.

Ho G Jr, Tice AD, Kaplan SR: Septic bursitis in the prepatellar and olecranon bursae: An analysis of 25 cases. Ann Intern Med 1978;89:21.

Lo B: Hyperuricemia and gout. West J Med 1985;142:104.

Shearn MA, Hellmann DB: Arthritis and musculoskeletal disorders. Chapter 15 in: *Current Medical Diagnosis & Treatment 1991*. Schroeder SA et al (editors). Appleton & Lange, 1991.

Sternbach GL: Evaluation of the knee. J Emerg Med 1986;4:133.

Section II.
Trauma Emergencies

Head Trauma

16

Henry M. Bartkowski, MD, PhD

IMMEDIATE MANAGEMENT OF LIFE-THREATENING PROBLEMS IN THE PATIENT WITH HEAD INJURY

Immobilize Cervical Spine

About 2–5% of patients with blunt head trauma have associated neck injury, but penetrating wounds of the head very rarely are accompanied by neck injury. Therefore, if head injury is the result of blunt trauma, the cervical spine should be immobilized until cervical spine x-rays can be obtained unless the patient is fully alert and has no neck pain or tenderness or other major injury.

The patient should be supine on a rigid long spine board (fireman's board) with the neck in a neutral position (not bent). Adequate immobilization requires combined use of a rigid cervical collar and lateral sandbags or neck rolls connected by tape across the forehead. Studies have shown that there may be significant movement of the cervical spine if a collar alone is used. If the patient needs to be turned, have someone hold the head, and logroll the patient, maintaining axial orientation. Axial traction using a halter with 3-kg (7-lb) traction provides excellent immobilization (see Fig 21–1) but may not be available in most emergency departments.

Establish Airway & Ventilation

Hypercapnia ($PCO_2 > 40$ mm Hg) and hypoxemia

(PO_2 < 70 mm Hg) increase both cerebral blood flow and intracranial pressure, aside from their other deleterious effects. Arterial blood gas measurements provide the best overall indication of the adequacy of the airway and ventilation and should be repeated as needed.

A. Identify Airway Problems: Problems in the airway may be manifested by gurgling or stertorous respirations, apnea, or cyanosis. Even with an adequate airway, brain injury itself may depress ventilation to the point of cyanosis or apnea. More subtle degrees of respiratory distress may be demonstrated only by arterial blood gas measurements, which should be obtained frequently. A reasonable goal is good oxygenation (PO_2 ≥ 80 mm Hg) with slight hypocapnia (PCO_2 ≤ 25 mm Hg).

B. Remove Obstruction, and Give Oxygen:

1. Using a tonsil sucker, clear the mouth and upper airway of obvious foreign material.

2. Position the head gently, and avoid moving the cervical spine.

3. Insert a nasal airway, and support respiration with a bag-mask combination and supplemental oxygen.

4. Endotracheal intubation should be performed if adequate ventilation or oxygenation cannot be provided by other means. It should be used to protect the airway in a patient with a depressed or absent gag reflex or to provide hyperventilation in a patient with increased intracranial pressure. Nasotracheal intubation is usually safer than orotracheal intubation in cases of suspected cervical spine injury but is technically more difficult and time-consuming and should be avoided in patients with midface fractures. If nasotracheal intubation is not possible, orotracheal intubation should be performed with careful axial cervical traction applied manually and care taken not to hyperextend the neck.

5. Rarely, it will be impossible to develop or maintain an orotracheal or nasotracheal airway in patients with severe facial trauma and distortion of normal anatomic relationships or in the presence of a laryngeal fracture. In these cases, direct intubation of the trachea through cricothyrotomy or tracheostomy is indicated (Chapter 46).

Establish Satisfactory Circulation

A. Cardiac Arrest: Perform CPR if no pulse is detected (Chapter 1).

B. Shock or Hypotension:

1. Examine the patient for hypotension or shock (cool, clammy skin). Head injury alone is rarely a cause of hypotension or shock unless there has been extensive blood loss from scalp lacerations or associated spinal cord injury. However, shock can cause abnormal mentation, which in the presence of head trauma can complicate diagnosis and management.

2. Treat shock or hypotension by inserting one or more large-bore (≥ 16-gauge) intravenous cannulas

and beginning rapid intravenous infusion of crystalloid solution (normal saline or lactated or acetated Ringer's injection). Up to 3 L of crystalloid solution may be given (adult dose) before red cell transfusions are required. If hypotension or shock does not respond to the administration of fluid, provide further treatment as outlined in Chapter 3. Stop external hemorrhage by compression (Raney clips may be used on the edges of a lacerated scalp, and hemostats may be used on the edges of the galea of the scalp). Use of a pneumatic antishock garment (eg, MAST) to control hypotension does not adversely affect central nervous system function.

If blood pressure is normal and no other injuries require infusion of crystalloid solution, avoid giving excess fluids (especially free water, eg, 5% dextrose in water) that might increase cerebral edema.

MANAGEMENT OF OTHER SYMPTOMS

Temperature

A. Fever: Elevated body temperature causes increased cerebral blood flow and intracranial pressure. Antipyretics and, if necessary, mechanical cooling (eg, cooling blankets, ice-water sponge baths) should be instituted to control body temperature quickly; the cause of fever should be found and treated specifically, if possible.

B. Hypothermia: Subnormal body temperature may protect against cerebral edema and need not be rapidly corrected (Chapter 38).

Systemic Hypertension

Treat systemic hypertension by reducing intracranial pressure, not by giving antihypertensive medications. The hypertension is a reflex response that attempts to maintain cerebral perfusion in the presence of raised intracranial pressure.

Cerebral Edema

A. Hyperventilation: Hyperventilation by means of an endotracheal airway (PCO_2 ≤ 25 mm Hg) produces cerebral vasoconstriction and helps control cerebral swelling. It is one of the most effective means of rapidly lowering increased intracranial pressure.

B. Diuretics: Osmotic diuretics such as mannitol, 500 mL of 20% solution given intravenously over 15–30 minutes, reduce brain bulk for several hours. Mannitol should be given *only* if a more definitive diagnostic step (eg, CT scan, MRI, or angiography) or therapeutic procedure (eg, operation) follows closely. Other diuretics (eg, furosemide, urea, glycerol) offer no advantages over mannitol.

C. Emergency Bur Holes: Occasionally, abrupt clinical deterioration in the patient with head trauma requires emergency surgery as a lifesaving measure before specific diagnosis can be reached. For example, abrupt change (over minutes) from wakefulness to clinical findings characteristic of transtentorial herniation (dilated, fixed pupil; extensor rigidity of extremities; coma) despite maximal measures to combat cerebral edema justifies having a surgeon drill exploratory bur holes immediately even though a specific diagnosis has not yet been made. Drilling of bur holes should be done in an operating room.

D. Corticosteroids: Although corticosteroids control cerebral swelling in some situations (eg, brain tumor), they have been shown to be *ineffective* for posttraumatic cerebral edema, and the author feels they should not be used.

Seizures
(See also Chapter 11.)

If the patient has seizures, they must be controlled without delay. An intravenous bolus injection of diazepam, 5–10 mg (for adults) over 1–2 minutes, usually controls persistent seizures. *The dose should not be repeated.* Respiratory depression is uncommon even with larger doses of diazepam, but mentation is impaired temporarily, which limits the value of subsequent neurologic examinations. Follow diazepam with a loading dose of phenytoin (see below and Chapter 11).

Patients with evidence of intracranial blood (subarachnoid, intraparenchymal, or subdural hemorrhage) on CT scan or MRI should receive phenytoin. Some authorities recommend giving prophylactic phenytoin if injury is severe (eg, if coma is present), even if there is no evidence of seizures or intracranial blood. Give phenytoin, 15–18 mg/kg intravenously, at a rate no faster than 50 mg/min.

Tetanus Prophylaxis

All patients with open wounds should receive tetanus toxoid, 0.5 mL intramuscularly, if a reliable history of tetanus immunization within the past 5–10 years cannot be obtained. Patients without prior tetanus immunization should also receive tetanus immune globulin (eg, Hyper-Tet). (See Chapter 24.)

Prophylactic Antibiotics

A. Open Wounds of the Cranium: Patients with open cranial wounds, (eg, gunshot wounds, open depressed skull fractures) should be given prophylactic antibiotics as soon as possible. Give nafcillin, 200 mg/kg/d intravenously in 4–6 divided doses.

B. Basilar Skull Fractures: Basilar skull fractures, even those with cerebrospinal fluid otorrhea or rhinorrhea, do not require prophylactic antibiotics, since no good evidence exists to support their use. If the patient develops fever, meningismus, or deteriorating mental status, then cerebrospinal fluid should be obtained for culture (by lumbar puncture if a mass lesion has been ruled out), and the patient should be started on penicillin G, 20–24 million units intrave-

nously in 6 divided doses. Antibiotic treatment should be altered appropriately based upon results of culture and susceptibility testing. An alternative regimen is cefuroxime, 1.5 g intravenously every 8 hours (children, 100–150 mg/kg/d in 3 divided doses).

Analgesics

Most patients with head injuries do not require and should not be given analgesics, because these drugs may interfere with serial neurologic evaluations. If associated injuries cause significant pain, the emergency physician should not hesitate to administer analgesics. Narcotics are preferred, since their effects may be quickly reversed if there is doubt about results of neurologic examination.

HOSPITALIZATION

General indications for hospitalization after head injury include the following:

(1) Seizures.

(2) Skull fractures.

(3) Abnormal mental or neurologic status, especially if the condition is either new or worsening.

(4) Associated medical or surgical disease, even if the underlying condition might not necessarily require hospitalization.

(5) Living situation that prevents effective home management of injury (eg, patient lives alone).

(6) A patient who has experienced a brief period of unconsciousness and has normal findings on CT scan or MRI may be discharged if adequate home management can be ensured. Patients experiencing prolonged loss of consciousness (> 5 minutes) usually require admission to the hospital.

FURTHER EVALUATION OF THE PATIENT WITH HEAD INJURY

Brief History

A brief history should be obtained from the patient, friends, bystanders, police, or ambulance attendants. The circumstances of the injury—loss of consciousness, drug intoxication, chest pain, seizures, etc, prior to or shortly after injury—are important and may influence management. As with any other injury, inquire about previous illnesses, previous head trauma or chronic seizure disorders, allergies, and current medications.

Physical Examination

Brief general physical examination should precede specific assessment of neurologic function.

A. Obtain complete vital signs, including core temperature.

B. Inspect the head, and palpate carefully for scalp lacerations, subgaleal hematomas, ecchymoses, and deformity. *Do not rely on skull x-rays as a substitute for careful examination of the skull.* Unless hair is combed out, it may obscure these lesions (rarely, hair may be so matted that it must be shaved off to inspect the scalp).

C. Inspect neck, chest, abdomen, back, and extremities—tenderness, pain, and deformity are often signs of associated injuries that require specific early treatment.

Neurologic Examination

The emergency department neurologic examination should be brief and consistent in format and should be repeated at regular intervals. The neurologic examination is designed to assess the following functions:

A. Mentation: The spectrum of mentation includes all levels of consciousness from alert to comatose.

1. An **alert** patient responds appropriately to a variety of external stimuli.

2. A patient in **coma** fails to respond normally to any external stimuli, including deep pain.

3. Gradation between these extremes is best described by specific responses to specific questions or sensory stimuli, eg, "Patient is sleepy but arouses to loud voice. Knows name and location, but not time or reason for being here." Avoid vague terms to describe states of consciousness (eg, obtunded, semicoma, semistupor, lethargy), since these terms may be used differently by different examiners.

B. Movement: Movement of extremities should be graded as follows:

1. Normal movement means that the patient moves all extremities spontaneously, purposefully (ie, in response to commands), and with full strength.

2. Paralysis denotes inability of a conscious patient to move the extremity either spontaneously or in response to commands or painful stimuli (stimuli should be applied both directly to the extremity and to the trunk, since failure to move may be secondary to hypesthesia of the extremity). Failure to move at all, either spontaneously or in response to an unpleasant stimulus, may indicate paralysis due to a structural lesion or metabolic cause (eg, drug overdose). Often failure to respond is simply due to an inadequately painful stimulus.

3. Gradation between these extremes should be described precisely, eg, "Patient extends right arm and leg, flexes left arm, and extends left leg in response to supraorbital pressure." Avoid broad descriptive terms such as "paraparesis" or "decerebrate posturing."

C. Sensation: Sensory examination for head trauma in the emergency department is usually restricted to observing the response to pain (ie, whether movement occurs or pain is felt). If mentation is impaired, more sophisticated sensory testing is fruitless.

D. Tendon Reflexes: Testing of peripheral reflexes is useful, since it assesses both sensory input and motor output and is readily reproducible. Tendon reflexes are abnormal only if they are asymmetric or absent. Plantar responses have diagnostic value only if they are asymmetric.

E. Brain Stem Reflexes and Eye Examination:

1. Pupils–Pupillary constriction in response to light occurs if the optic nerve (cranial nerve II), oculomotor nerve (cranial nerve III), and intermediary midbrain nuclei are intact and functioning normally. The pupils are under control of the autonomic nervous system as well, since they constrict in response to parasympathetic (vagal) discharge and dilate in response to sympathetic nervous activity.

a. Lack of response–Failure to constrict to light may indicate interruption of this important reflex arc anywhere along its course, eg, from third nerve compression during transtentorial herniation. Other common causes of an apparently nonreactive pupil include prior eye surgery, presence of a glass eye, blindness from intraocular disease, and drugs (eg, pilocarpine, heroin, amphetamines).

b. Dilated or constricted pupils–Pupillary dilatation may occur when transtentorial compression occurs and parasympathetic tone of the pupil is totally lost. Conversely, pinpoint pupils after head injury may indicate loss of sympathetic tone resulting from a lesion in the brain stem caudal to the oculomotor nuclei (eg, pontine hemorrhage).

2. Eye movements–The range of extraocular movement is the best single test of brain stem function. If eye movements are full and spontaneous, then the third, fourth, and sixth cranial nerves and their nuclei within the brain stem are intact.

Specific palsies can be readily identified in the awake patient: diplopia is a good clue, because it is obvious to the patient. If eye movements are not spontaneous, stimulation of the vestibular apparatus (cranial nerve VIII) by ice-water lavage of the ear canals produces full eye movements to the side of the stimulus if cranial nerves III, IV, VI, and VIII and their connecting brain stem tracts (medial longitudinal fasciculi) are intact.

In patients with suspected injuries to the neck, avoid the doll's eye maneuver because of possible injury to the spinal cord. Caloric testing is safer and more reliable in this situation.

3. Fundi–The ocular fundi may show papilledema, subhyaloid hemorrhages, or other signs of head trauma (eg, retinal detachment). Papilledema noted soon after head injury is uncommon, because several hours must usually elapse before it becomes clinically obvious. Subhyaloid hemorrhages, on the other hand, are a reliable sign of subarachnoid hemorrhage and intracranial bleeding.

4. Corneal sensation and facial mobility–Corneal sensation and facial mobility (governed by cranial nerves V and VII, respectively) are readily tested by touching the cornea and observing the resulting eye blink. A normal corneal reflex requires that the trigeminal and facial nerves, their brain stem nuclei, and the connecting pontine fibers between them be intact.

5. Ciliospinal reflex–The ciliospinal reflex is positive when the pupils dilate in response to a painful stimulus, usually a pinch on the back of the neck. The positive reflex indicates that the spinothalamic tracts and their connections to sympathetic fibers in the brain stem are intact.

6. Brain stem reflexes–The ability to cough or gag when the trachea or posterior pharynx is stimulated is evidence of intact caudal brain stem nerves and reflex arcs (cranial nerves IX and X).

F. Olfaction and Visual Acuity: Smell is commonly disturbed after head trauma, usually as a result of injury to the olfactory nerves, but testing the sense of smell in the emergency department is of limited usefulness, since function of these sensory nerves can only be tested easily in awake, cooperative patients. Visual field and acuity testing similarly requires an awake, cooperative patient.

Rectal Examination

Rectal examination is an essential part of the emergency assessment of head injury. Rectal sphincter tone is present if the injury is intracranial only; if there is coexisting spinal cord injury, the anal sphincter has little or no muscle tone. Coexisting head and spinal cord injuries should always be suspected until proved otherwise.

Repeat Neurologic Examinations

Neurologic examination is helpful only if it is repeated often enough to establish a diagnosis, suggest further diagnostic steps, or clearly indicate a trend in neurologic function. The results of each examination may be seen as a point on a curve showing neurologic function with time. If successive examinations indicate improvement, further specialized testing may not be necessary. Failure to improve—verified by repeated examinations—indicates that additional studies are necessary, as does progressive deterioration from a baseline established by examination done on arrival in the emergency department. The Glasgow Coma Scale (see Fig 4–1A) is a frequently used scoring device that correlates well with outcome from head injury. The maximum score of 15 indicates that the patient is alert and awake, and the lowest score of 3 indicates that the patient is flaccid, mute, and unconscious.

Laboratory Tests

If hospital admission is necessary, routine studies should include CBC, urinalysis, serum electrolyte de-terminations, serum osmolality, blood glucose measurements, and tests of renal function; arterial blood gas measurements are essential if respiration or circulation is abnormal.

Radiologic Examination

A. Cervical Spine: X-rays, particularly a portable lateral view, are useful to rule out bony neck injury, thus simplifying subsequent management. Films should show all of the cervical vertebrae (Chapter 21).

B. Chest: A plain chest film should be obtained in all patients with head trauma who require hospitalization.

C. CT Scan:

1. A CT scan is the study of choice for a patient with suspected neurologic injury. Intracranial hematomas, skull fractures, and parenchymal abnormalities are visualized quickly and easily. Indications for CT scan include seizures, abnormal mental status, abnormal neurologic examination, or signs of skull fracture. Brief loss of consciousness alone or mild amnesia in an awake, alert patient is a low-yield indication and does not require CT scan if adequate observation can be provided. As an alternative, an MRI may be obtained, although bone is visualized more clearly on a CT scan. Cerebral angiography is rarely used in the diagnostic evaluation of head trauma unless specific vascular injury is suspected or facilities for CT scan or MRI are unavailable.

2. Indications for skull x-rays are few with the increasing availability of CT scanning. A skull x-ray is indicated if physical examination suggests bony depression, if there is evidence (by history or physical examination) of penetrating trauma, or if subgaleal hematoma is present.

Special Studies

A. Lumbar Puncture: *Lumbar puncture should not be done when head injury is an obvious or likely diagnosis.* Abnormal results on lumbar puncture, with either bloody or xanthochromic fluid or elevated cerebrospinal fluid pressures, do not localize or define an intracranial abnormality. Conversely, normal results on lumbar puncture do not exclude the possibility of intracranial hematoma.

B. Other Studies: Studies of limited value in early management of head injury include echoencephalography, electroencephalography, radionuclide brain scan, air contrast studies, and conventional tomography.

EMERGENCY TREATMENT OF SPECIFIC HEAD INJURIES

SCALP INJURIES

1. LACERATIONS
(See also Chapter 24.)

Diagnosis & Treatment

A. Position the patient so that the laceration is easily accessible and can be seen in good light.

B. Clip or shave around the laceration to facilitate inspection and reduce the rate of infection after closure.

C. Irrigate the wound copiously with normal saline; do not use antiseptics or soap.

D. Control bleeding with direct pressure or the use of clips (eg, Raney clips) on scalp margins or hemostats on galeal edges, and palpate the base of the wound for an underlying skull fracture. Inspect for foreign bodies and devitalized tissue that must be removed.

E. Obtain skull x-rays, if indicated, *before* closing the wound.

F. If the wound is less than 12 hours old and not grossly contaminated, closure may be performed in layers using absorbable and nonabsorbable synthetic sutures.

G. Do *not* close lacerations over skull fractures: these are open skull fractures and require neurosurgical consultation and may necessitate repair in an operating room.

Disposition

Patients with scalp lacerations without complicating skull fracture or intracranial injury may be discharged from the emergency department and referred for follow-up within 3–5 days.

2. HEMATOMA
(Subgaleal Hematoma)

Diagnosis

Scalp hematoma suggests underlying fracture and requires careful palpation and tangential x-ray (ie, x-ray beam parallel to area of skull surrounding the fracture) to rule out bony abnormalities.

Treatment

Infants and young children may lose significant amounts of blood beneath the scalp and may require transfusion to restore adequate blood volume. Needle aspiration of large collections of blood is not war-

ranted. Subgaleal hematomas in adults or older children rarely require specific treatment.

Disposition

The rare patient with subgaleal hematoma without underlying skull fracture may be discharged and referred for follow-up within 5–7 days. Other patients must be hospitalized.

SKULL FRACTURE

Skull fracture does not necessarily mean severe brain injury; however, it is better to assume that injury is substantial and hospitalize the patient for observation overnight.

1. CLOSED FRACTURES

Diagnosis

Closed fractures are most frequently detected on x-ray (Fig 16–1) or a CT scan, although some may be evident through direct or indirect physical findings (crepitation on palpation of an injury, Battle's sign, etc).

A closed skull fracture has little potential for infection, but there is a significant chance of associated intracranial hematoma. Diploetic, meningeal, and pericranial vessels are disrupted by any skull fracture, with resulting epidural and subperiosteal bleeding.

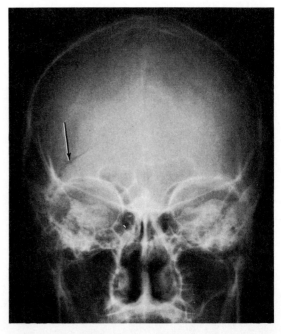

Figure 16–1. Closed linear skull fracture (arrow) with suture diastasis secondary to blunt trauma.

Nearly all epidural hematomas of clinical consequence are accompanied by a skull fracture on the same side. About 60% of patients with subdural hematoma have skull fractures, but not consistently on the same side as the clot.

Treatment & Disposition

Treat intracranial injury as discussed below under Brain Injury. Hospitalization of patients with acute injuries for observation for a minimum of 24 hours is indicated. If the fracture is definitely more than a week old and there are no abnormal symptoms or signs, referral to a neurologist or neurosurgeon is satisfactory.

2. OPEN FRACTURES

Diagnosis

Open fractures underlie open scalp wounds and differ from closed fractures only in that they may be diagnosed by direct palpation and have potential for serious infection. All penetrating trauma of the skull must be classed as open fracture.

Treatment & Disposition

Hospitalize the patient for debridement and closure in an operating room. Antimicrobial prophylaxis should be started in the emergency department, eg, nafcillin, 200 mg/kg/d intravenously in 4–6 divided doses.

3. DEPRESSED FRACTURES

Diagnosis

Depressed fractures are best detected by gentle palpation of the depressed bony fragments through intact or lacerated scalp, or by tangential x-ray of the skull (Fig 16–2). The degree of injury to the underlying dura or brain varies. CT scan will show depressed bone fragments as well as brain underlying the fracture.

Treatment & Disposition

A. Do not attempt to treat the wound in the emergency department.

B. Begin antimicrobials as for open skull fractures, above.

C. Hospitalize for operative inspection and repair.

4. BASILAR SKULL FRACTURES

Diagnosis

Basilar skull fractures are frequently not seen directly on x-ray unless detailed tomographic films or CT scans are obtained. Clinical signs include (**1**) hemotympanum (early); (**2**) mastoid ecchymosis (Battle's sign; appears hours to days after injury); (**3**) bilateral or unilateral periorbital ecchymoses ("raccoon eyes"; delayed); (**4**) impaired hearing; (**5**) facial palsy on same side as fracture; and (**6**) blood or cerebrospinal fluid in the nasal sinuses or ear canal (indirect signs of basilar skull fracture).

Treatment & Disposition

Hospitalize the patient for observation. Cerebrospinal fluid otorrhea or rhinorrhea may develop.

CEREBROSPINAL FLUID LEAK

Diagnosis

Cerebrospinal fluid rhinorrhea or otorrhea occurs when injury has penetrated the arachnoid, dura, bone, periosteum, and sinus mucosa.

A. Cerebrospinal fluid emerging from the nose or ear implies basilar skull fracture and an open wound. Clear or blood-tinged fluid emerging from the ear or nose should be assumed to be cerebrospinal fluid; *there is no reliable method available in the emergency department for distinguishing cerebrospinal fluid from nasal mucus.* The use of glucose indicator sticks is associated with a high incidence of false-positive results.

B. Radiographic signs include a fracture line, displaced bone, pneumocephalus, and fluid in the sinuses.

Treatment & Disposition

Hospitalize for observation, fluid restriction, and elevation of the head (15–20 degrees). Give acetazolamide, 15 mg/kg/d orally in 4 divided doses. Persistent leaks, especially if associated with infection, many require surgical closure.

BRAIN INJURY

The essence of early management of significant head injury is recognizing the presence of an intracranial mass through the use of repeated neurologic evaluations. Some helpful differentiating features are given in Table 16–1. Definitive diagnosis, which formerly required invasive procedures such as cerebral angiography, can now be accomplished noninvasively and quickly with CT scan or MRI.

1. MASS LESIONS

Diagnosis

A. Epidural Hematoma: Nearly all patients with significant epidural hematomas have progressively deteriorating neurologic function and skull fracture. A brief lucid interval after initial uncon-

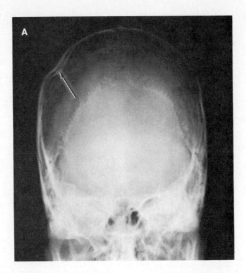

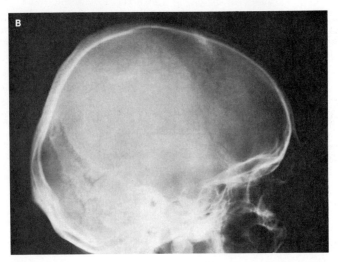

Figure 16–2. Depressed skull fracture (arrow) much better seen on anteroposterior view *(A)* than on lateral view *(B)*.

sciousness is a typical clinical feature. Epidural hematomas usually appear in the temporoparietal region but may occur in the frontal and occipital areas and in the posterior fossa (Fig 16–3).

B. Subdural Hematoma: Progressive loss of neurologic function after trauma, with or without associated skull fracture, is typical of acute subdural hematomas. The clinical course may be precipitous or insidious. Underlying brain is often contused and hemorrhagic. Expansion of the hematoma, combined with development of edema in the brain parenchyma, accounts for progressive deterioration in many patients (Fig 16–4).

C. Parenchymal Hematoma: Although intraparenchymal hematoma is not as common as subdural hematoma, it has the same clinical effect as subdural hematoma: progressive neurologic deterioration caused by the mass itself and by the brain

edema surrounding the lesion. Lateralizing neurologic signs (eg, hemiparesis, visual field deficit) with or without impaired mentation are characteristic early findings (Fig 16–5).

Treatment

Obtain immediate neurosurgical consultation for patients with identifiable posttraumatic mass lesions, since operation probably will be required. Surgery is mandatory if neurologic signs worsen. Some patients with small hematomas and stable or improving neurologic signs may be closely monitored with neurologic examinations. A neurosurgeon should be familiar with the patient's condition so that surgery can be performed promptly if symptoms worsen.

Disposition

All patients with brain injury following trauma re-

Table 16–1. Differentiating features of posttraumatic head injury syndromes.

Diagnostic Method	Common Clincal Findings	
	Mass Lesion (Subdural Hematoma, etc)	Diffuse Lesions (Cerebral Contusions, etc)
History	Focal symptoms.	Nonfocal symptoms.
Examination	Early focal signs: pupillary asymmetry or focal motor or sensory deficits.	Symmetric neurologic defects.
	Deteriorating condition as indicated by results on neurologic examination.	Stable or improving condition as shown by results on neurologic examination.
CT scan or angiogram	Focal defects.	Brain edema.

quire hospitalization according to the general guidelines given earlier in this chapter.

2. DIFFUSE LESIONS

Diagnosis

A. Concussion: The term concussion denotes brain injury that does not result in identifiable neuropathologic changes. Concussion affects only mentation, with return of consciousness moments or

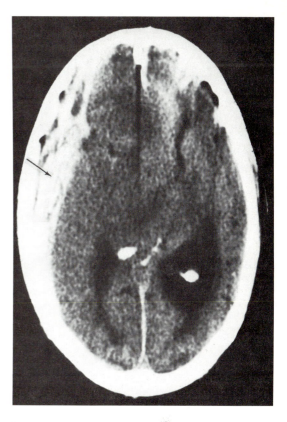

Figure 16–4. CT scan of acute subdural hematoma (arrow). The subdural hematoma is concave to the surface of the cerebral hemisphere. Significant midline shift is present.

minutes after impact. Motor function and brain stem reflexes are not impaired. CT scan is normal.

B. Contusions, Ischemia, and Hypoxemia: Contusions, ischemia, and hypoxemia have the same effect on brain tissue, ie, swelling and diffuse loss of neurologic function. However, focal abnormalities may develop if brain swelling is sufficient to cause tentorial herniation. If contusion is localized (eg, beneath a depressed fracture), mentation is often normal, although motor and sensory function may be impaired. If contusion is widespread, mentation is impaired as well. Ischemia may be similarly localized or diffuse. Hypoxemia primarily affects mentation and may be superimposed upon traumatic brain injury, particularly if the airway has been compromised as a result of injury.

Treatment

Conservative, nonoperative supportive care is best for most patients with diffuse lesions. Intracranial pressure monitoring should be utilized in unconscious patients.

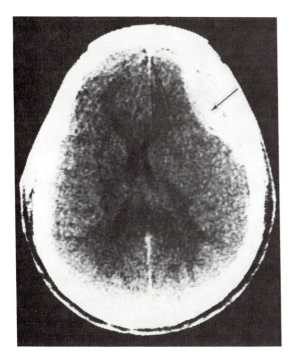

Figure 16–3. CT scan of acute epidural hematoma (arrow) with typical lenticular shape. Considerable midline shift is evident.

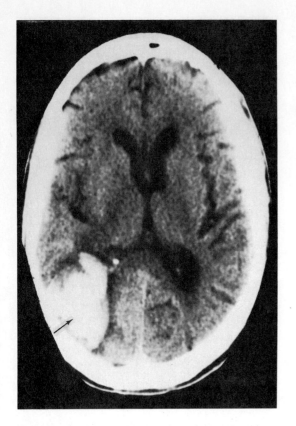

Figure 16–5. CT scan of acute intracerebral hematoma (arrow). Significant shift of the choroid plexus is present.

Disposition

See Mass Lesions, above.

3. BRAIN LACERATIONS

Diagnosis

Lacerations of the brain may result either from severe blunt trauma—in which case they are often multiple or else confined to a single area under a depressed skull fracture—or from penetrating trauma. Multiple small lacerations give a clinical picture of diffuse brain injury. Single lesions may produce focal findings, although usually not with neurologic deterioration, as occurs with mass lesions.

Treatment

Open lacerations require operative debridement; closed lacerations, as evidenced on CT scan or MRI, may be managed with supportive care and management of associated problems—subdural hematoma, cerebral edema, etc.

Disposition

See Mass Lesions, above.

MINOR HEAD INJURIES

Most head injuries seen in the emergency department are mild. They are characterized by a minor mechanism of injury in an alert, awake patient who has normal findings on neurologic examination. If loss of consciousness has occurred, it has been for a brief period and there is no associated amnesia. On physical examination, there are no signs of skull fracture. Such patients have a low incidence of complications and do not require CT scan, MRI, or skull x-rays, They may be discharged provided written after-care instructions are given (see box) directly to a responsible adult who understands the instructions and will observe the patient in an appropriate setting (ie, with quick access to emergency medical services).

No patient should be discharged if he or she is intoxicated. If doubt exists, it is always better to observe the patient in the emergency department for 4–6 hours or in the hospital, as home observation is notoriously unreliable in these cases.

Head Injury After-Care Instructions

Although no evidence of serious head injury appears to be present at this time, delayed signs may appear many hours after the injury has occurred. Therefore, a responsible person should remain with and observe the patient for the first 24 hours.

1. The patient should be awakened every 2 hours to ensure that he or she is arousable to a normal state of alertness.
2. The patient should engage in a decreased level of activity for the first 24 hours after injury.
3. No alcohol, sedatives, or pain relievers other than acetaminophen (Tylenol, others) should be given for 48 hours.

Bring the patient to the emergency department or call an ambulance (or call 9–1–1, if available) immediately if any of the following occur:

1. Unusual drowsiness or confusion.
2. Difficulty in waking the patient (awaken every 2 hours the first night).
3. Continuous vomiting.
4. Blurred vision.
5. Continued severe headache, not relieved by acetaminophen.
6. Stiffness of neck.
7. Bleeding or clear fluid dripping from ears or nose.
8. Noticeable new weakness of either arm or leg.
9. Seizures.
10. Unequal pupils (one large, one small).

POSTCONCUSSIVE HEADACHE

See Chapter 13.

ASSOCIATED INJURIES

Neck
(See also Chapter 21.)

About 5–10% of patients with serious head injuries have associated neck injuries; only careful evaluation confirms their coexistence. Neck injury must be assumed to be present until proved otherwise, both by physical examination and lateral cervical spine x-rays or other diagnostic methods (eg, CT scan). These studies should be performed as early as possible.

Craniofacial & Eye Injuries
(See also Chapters 17, 25, and 26.)

Injuries of the face, eyes, and ears are commonly associated with head trauma as well. See specific chapters for details.

Multiple Injuries
(See also Chapter 4.)

Many patients with head injury have other injuries also. Priorities of diagnosis and treatment must follow a simple rule: *the most serious first* and in accordance with the mnemonic for life-support priorities: *A:* airway, *B:* breathing and ventilation, and *C:* circulation. Meticulous care of head injury is worthless if life-threatening injuries elsewhere compromise ventilation and perfusion.

REFERENCES

Bakay L, Glasauer FE: *Head Injury.* Little, Brown, 1980.

Bartkowski HM, Pitts LH: Neurologic injury. In: *Current Therapy of Trauma 1983–1984.* Trunkey DD, Lewis FR (editors). Mosby, 1984.

Bayless P, Ray VG: Incidence of cervical spine injuries in association with blunt head trauma. Am J Emerg Med 1989;7:139.

Becker DP et al: Outcome from severe head injury with early diagnosis and intensive management. J Neurosurg 1977; 47:491.

Freed HA: Posttraumatic skull films: Who needs them? Ann Emerg Med 1986;15:233.

Hesselink JR et al: MR imaging of brain contusions: A comparative study with CT. AJR 1988;150:1133.

Hoyt DB, Hollingsworth-Fridlund P (editors): Head injuries. (Symposium.) Trauma Q 1985;2:1. [Entire issue.]

Israel RS et al: Hemodynamic effects of mannitol in a canine model of concomitant increased intracranial pressure and hemorrhagic shock. Ann Emerg Med 1988;17:560.

Jamieson KG: *A First Notebook of Head Injury,* 2nd ed. Butterworth, 1971.

Jennett B, Teasdale G: *Management of Head Injuries.* Davis, 1981.

Langfitt TW: Measuring the outcome from head injuries. J Neurosurg 1978;48:673.

Masters SJ et al: Skull x-ray examinations after head trauma: Recommendations by a multidisciplinary panel and validation study. N Engl J Med 1987;316:84.

Mayer TA, Walker ML: Pediatric head injury: The critical role of the emergency physician. Ann Emerg Med 1985;14:1178.

O'Malley KF, Ross SE: The incidence of injury to the cervical spine in patients with craniocerebral injury. J Trauma 1988;28:1476.

Peyster RG, Hoover ED: CT in head trauma. J Trauma 1982;22:25.

Plum F, Posner JB (editors): *Diagnosis of Stupor and Coma,* 3rd ed. Davis, 1980.

Ringenberg BJ et al: Rational ordering of cervical spine radiographs following trauma. Ann Emerg Med 1988; 17:792.

Roberge RJ et al: Selective application of cervical spine radiology in alert victims of blunt trauma: A prospective study. J Trauma 1988;28:784.

Saunders CE, Cota R, Barton CA: Reliability of home observation for victims of mild closed-head injury. Ann Emerg Med 1986;15:160.

Simpson DA et al: Extradural hematoma: Strategies for management in remote places. Injury 1988;19:307.

Tyson GW: The concussed patient. Compr Ther 1985; 11:62.

17   Maxillofacial & Neck Trauma

Roger L. Crumley, MD

I. IMMEDIATE MANAGEMENT OF LIFE-THREATENING PROBLEMS

Emergency management of life-threatening associated conditions is described in Chapter 4.

ENSURE AIRWAY

Evaluate the pharyngeal, laryngeal, and tracheal components of the airway in patients with head and neck trauma. The head and neck should be stabilized with sandbags and not moved until the condition of the cervical spine can be assessed.

Caution: Patients with suspected neck injuries must be under constant observation and must never be sent to the x-ray department or any area where constant medical attention is not available. Edema and hematoma may worsen within a few minutes, causing total airway obstruction. Whenever possible, the emergency physician should accompany the patient to the next department or hospital area. Any patient with subcutaneous emphysema, hoarseness, or persistent pain in the laryngeal area (signs and symptoms of laryngeal fracture) must automatically be included in this high-risk group, and such patients should have a tracheotomy set with them at all times.

Pharyngeal Airway Injury

Massive injuries of the tongue or mandible may compromise or obliterate the pharyngeal airway.

If there is no air exchange, immediately clear the oral cavity and pharynx of blood and loose teeth while preparing a laryngoscope for emergency intubation (Chapter 46). Cricothyrotomy (Chapter 46) or tracheotomy should be considered if cervical spinal injury is suspected, because laryngoscopy may cause spinal cord injury in such cases.

Laryngeal Airway Injury

If there is evidence of injury below the level of the hyoid bone with compromise of the airway, assume that laryngeal fracture or laryngotracheal crush injury is present.

Cricothyrotomy (Chapter 46) is the most rapid method of creating an emergency airway in patients with pharyngeal or laryngeal airway obstruction when laryngoscopy is difficult, delayed, or contraindicated. After a small-bore endotracheal tube is inserted through the cricothyrotomy, a standard tracheotomy should be performed. Failure to convert the cricothyrotomy to a tracheotomy increases the risk of injury to the cricoid cartilage with subsequent subglottic stenosis.

Tracheal Airway Injury

If there is injury below the cricothyroid membrane, a standard tracheotomy will be necessary to bypass the obstructive lesion.

In patients with no air exchange, it is permissible to attempt orotracheal intubation for 60 seconds, but it must be emphasized that preparations must be going forward simultaneously for cricothyrotomy or the actual tracheotomy procedure itself.

Intubation of the Trachea Through a Traumatic Opening

Occasionally, patients will come to the emergency department with impending asphyxia and with a gaping wound of the lower anterior neck. In some of these patients, removal of dressings and clots in the wound exposes a traumatic defect of the trachea that can be intubated easily. Patients with dashboard injuries or "clothesline-fence" snowmobile or motorcycle injuries often present with laryngotracheal separation immediately above or below the cricoid cartilage. If the wound is closed (no laceration), immediate tracheotomy is the preferred method of airway management, since peroral intubation may precipitate airway obstruction and cause death. If the wound is open, direct intubation through the wound is also possible in these cases.

Nasogastric Intubation

In patients with depressed mental status, once the airway is established and secured, a nasogastric tube may have to be inserted to empty the stomach of food and blood.

STOP BLEEDING

Control Hemorrhage

Patients with neck trauma (penetrating or blunt) may have rapidly expanding cervical hematomas from arterial or venous bleeding. Hematomas may cause airway obstruction and death if not recognized and treated. Facial and neck wounds may also be associated with external arterial or venous bleeding. Do not remove penetrating weapons left in the wound, since they may be preventing further hemorrhage.

A. Pressure: If venous oozing occurs, apply a pressure dressing in the emergency department. Do not encircle the neck with a "wraparound dressing," since it may act as a noose if edema worsens or a cervical hematoma expands.

B. Pressure and Clamping: If major arterial bleeding occurs in an open wound, try applying pressure first. If that fails—and only then—hemostats may be applied carefully under direct vision. Clamping of large amounts of soft tissue without good visualization is contraindicated, since the vagus nerve or phrenic nerve may be included in the clamp (Fig

17–1). A firm pressure dressing is the safest hemostatic agent.

C. Tracheotomy: Exsanguinating oral hemorrhage after penetrating trauma may be controlled by endotracheal intubation through a cricothyrotomy or tracheotomy (with immediate inflation of the cuff to prevent aspiration), followed by pharyngeal packing.

Treat Shock

If hypovolemic shock is present as a result of bleeding from face or neck injuries, it is managed with infusion of intravenous crystalloid solution or blood as described in Chapter 3. Briefly—

A. Insert 2 or more large-bore ($\geq$ 16-gauge) intravenous catheters.

B. Draw blood for CBC, blood glucose and serum electrolyte determinations, and renal function tests, and submit a tube of clotted blood for typing and cross-matching.

C. Infuse crystalloid solution (up to 2–3 L in 30–60 minutes) to support blood pressure and urine output.

D. Insert a urinary catheter to monitor urine output.

STABILIZE CERVICAL SPINE

While the airway and bleeding are being managed, it is important that the emergency physician be thinking about the cervical spine. Unless the physician is certain that the cervical spine is intact, the patient's head should not be moved. The standard head position during laryngoscopy includes flexion in the area of the sixth and seventh cervical vertebrae and extension at the atlanto-occipital joint. Fractures in either of these regions may produce spinal cord injury if positioning for laryngoscopy is carried out. Consequently, in patients with tenderness of the cervical spine who require emergency restoration of the airway, nasotracheal intubation with fiberoptic visualization of the larynx is preferred. If nasotracheal intubation cannot be performed, a cricothyrotomy should be strongly considered.

Stabilization of the head with tape and lateral neck rolls (on a rigid spine board) should be standard emergency department technique before cervical spine x-rays are taken (a portable film is adequate). Lateral and anteroposterior cervical spine x-rays or CT scans should be taken in all patients with head or neck trauma as soon as the airway is established and bleeding or shock is controlled. See Chapter 21 for further evaluation and management.

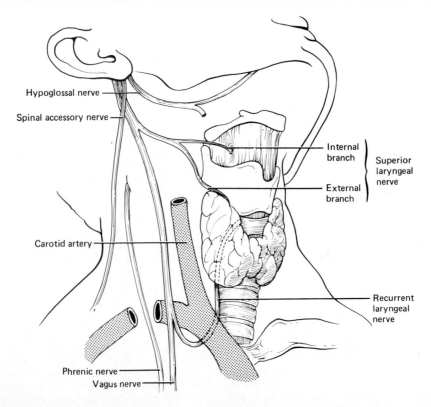

Figure 17–1. Location of nerves passing through the anterior neck that are susceptible to injury from penetrating trauma.

II. FURTHER DIAGNOSIS & EVALUATION

NECK TRAUMA

Type of Trauma

A. Penetrating Injury:

1. Knife wounds–If the penetrating instrument is still in situ, *leave it there,* and obtain posteroanterior and lateral neck films or CT scan to determine its exact location (Fig 17–2). Even if the assailant has withdrawn the knife blade, it is useful to know its length and shape as well as the direction from which the blade entered. Knowing the direction and depth of the injury provides information about what structures have been injured and may eliminate the need for surgical exploration.

2. Bullet wounds–Trauma from high-velocity missiles cannot be accurately assessed externally. Bullets frequently do not travel in a straight line, since they may be deflected or fragmented by bone. Bullets with high kinetic energy cause cavitation, with tissue injury remote from the missile track. Thus, all high-velocity missile injuries require surgical exploration, often with other diagnostic tests such as angiography or esophagoscopy.

B. Blunt Trauma: Blunt trauma to the neck is associated primarily with injury to the cervical spine and airway. Vascular and esophageal injuries are rare. Thus, careful assessment in the emergency de-partment can identify the need for surgical exploration.

Anatomic Location

The neck may be divided into 3 zones: zone I is the area of the neck from the angle of the mandible upward, zone II is the area between the angle of the mandible and the lower border of the cricoid cartilage, and zone III is the area below the lower border of the cricoid cartilage.

Wounds that penetrate the platysma should not be probed in the emergency department; they should be explored in the operating room.

Airway Injury

Airway injury may be manifested by an air leak, subcutaneous or mediastinal emphysema, or pneumothorax, indicating frank airway laceration. Stridor, hoarseness, painful phonation, and hemoptysis and hemothorax may also indicate airway injury (pharynx, larynx, or trachea). Posteroanterior and lateral neck and chest x-rays or CT scans are therefore essential to the evaluation of neck injury. Direct or indirect laryngoscopy must be performed before surgery to determine the exact nature of the airway injury.

Esophageal Injury

Injuries to the upper esophagus are associated with soft tissue crepitus, dysphagia, odynophagia, and drooling. Evaluate with an esophagogram, using water-soluble contrast medium (eg, Gastrografin), and look for dye extravasation as evidence of esopha-

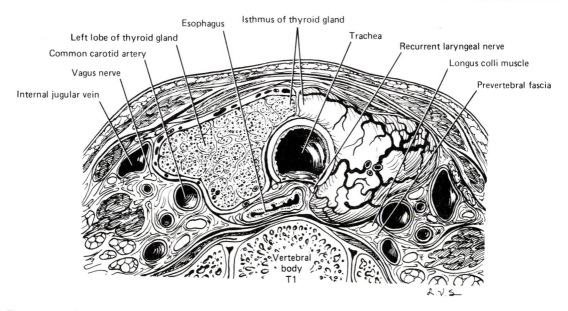

Figure 17–2. Cross section of the anterior neck at the level of C6, looking down from above, showing structures that may be injured.

geal injury. Esophagoscopy is virtually always necessary.

Vascular Injury
(See also Chapter 32.)

Vascular injury may be immediately apparent if there is external bleeding or a cervical hematoma, or it may be hidden if bleeding occurs into the pleural space. Neurologic deficit may indicate intracranial vascular insufficiency.

Suspected vascular injuries require either neck exploration in the operating room or angiography for evaluation (Chapter 32). Injuries occurring in zone I or zone III usually require angiography. Zone III injuries may require thoracotomy to control hemorrhage.

Nerve Injury
(See Fig 17–1.)

Assess the nerves in the neck susceptible to injury.

A. Vagus, Recurrent Laryngeal: Record the character of the patient's voice, and examine the vocal cords via indirect (mirror) or fiberoptic laryngoscopy.

B. Spinal Accessory: Test for function of the sternocleidomastoid and trapezius muscles.

C. Hypoglossal: Test for deviation of the protruded tongue to the side of the injury.

D. Phrenic: Assess movement of the diaphragm on chest examination or by x-ray.

Disposition

Patients with **penetrating trauma** of the neck should be hospitalized unless local exploration of the wound shows it to be superficial to the platysma. Patients with **blunt trauma** with no evidence of significant injury (by physical examination and x-rays of the neck and chest) may be safely discharged to home care.

FACIAL TRAUMA

Type of Injury

Most facial injuries consist of blunt trauma or cutting injury of the superficial soft tissue (lacerations, etc). High-velocity missile injuries of the face usually involve the central nervous system, and such injuries take priority for management (Chapter 16).

Airway Injury

Severe trauma to the lower face may compromise the airway. If obvious measures such as suction or pulling the tongue forward do not correct the problem, diverting the airway around the injury by performing endotracheal intubation, cricothyrotomy, or tracheotomy is preferred.

Vascular Injury

Bleeding from facial injuries typically is profuse but rarely causes hypovolemia or shock. *Control*

bleeding by direct pressure only; hemostatic clamping may injure important nonvascular structures.

Nerve Injury

Blunt or penetrating trauma may injure branches of the trigeminal, facial, auditory, lingual, or hypoglossal nerves. The best chance to diagnose such injuries is often in the emergency department before edema and pain worsen. A careful assessment of both motor and sensory function of these nerves, especially the facial nerve, is imperative.

A. Facial Nerve: Branches of the facial nerve can be tested by these maneuvers:

1. Temporal branch (to the frontalis muscle)–Ask patient to wrinkle forehead.

2. Zygomatic branch (to the orbicularis oculi muscle)–Ask patient to squeeze eyes shut tightly.

3. Buccal branch (to the smile muscles)–Ask patient to wrinkle nose, elevate upper lip, smile, and "show your teeth."

4. Marginal mandibular branch (to the lower lip depressors)–Ask patient to pucker or whistle.

5. Cervical branch– Ask patient to wrinkle the neck.

B. Trigeminal Nerve: Test for sensation over the entire face and upper neck.

C. Auditory Nerve: Test hearing in both ears.

D. Lingual Nerve: Test for sensation on both sides of the anterior tongue.

E. Hypoglossal Nerve: Test for ability to protrude tongue in midline and to both sides.

Parotid Gland Injury

An irregular quadrilateral area connecting the tragus, the angle of the mandible, the lateral commissure of the mouth, and the lateral canthus of the eye bounds an area where lacerations are most apt to injure Stensen's duct or branches of the facial nerve (Fig 17–3). Stensen's (parotid) duct courses anteriorly from the parotid gland in the preauricular area through the cheek to enter the buccal mucosa near the maxillary (upper) molar teeth. The initial evaluation of Stensen's duct requires only gentle probing with lacrimal probes, entering through the buccal surface. If the end of the probe appears in the cheek laceration, Stensen's duct has been disrupted and requires surgical repair. If lacerated and unrepaired, the duct will spill saliva into the cheek or externally, creating a troublesome salivary fistula. This complication is easy to prevent but difficult to treat.

Mouth Injuries

Test for pain on jaw movement or biting, feel for crepitus on movement of upper or lower teeth, and look for obvious malocclusion indicating fracture of the mandible or maxilla. Look for loose or fractured teeth. Inspect the buccal mucosa, tongue, floor of mouth, teeth, palate, and pharynx for evidence of injury. Grasp the upper alveolar bone, and check for

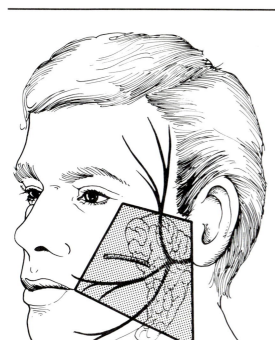

Figure 17–3. Area of the face where facial lacerations may injure the parotid gland, Stensen's duct, or facial nerve branches.

Table 17–1. Radiologic evaluation of facial injuries.[1]

Site of Suspected Injury	X-Ray Views
Mandible	Panorex or pantomogram (use lateral oblique, posteroanterior, and reverse Towne view if Panorex is unavailable, axial CT scan
Maxilla (Le Fort)	Waters (stereo technique), axial CT scan
Zygoma (tripod)	Waters, CT scan
Zygomatic arch	Submentovertex (base) axial CT scan
Orbital floor (blowout)	Waters, orbital floor tomogram or poly-tomogram, coronal CT scan
Nose	None
Frontal sinus	Caldwell, lateral, Waters, or coronal and axial CT scan
Temporal bone (basilar skull fracture)	Mastoid series (Stenver, Law, Mayer) anteroposterior and lateral poly-tomograms, CT scan

[1]Routine sinus (facial) x-ray series includes Waters, Caldwell, lateral, and submentovertex (base) views.

movement that suggests a maxillary or fracture. Palpate the remainder of the face to determine if other areas are potentially fractured. Obtain x-rays as indicated (Table 17–1).

Eye Injury
(See also Chapter 25.)

Look for obvious injury to the globe. Either enophthalmos or complaints of diplopia should arouse suspicion of orbital bone fracture.

Bilateral periorbital hematomas ("raccoon eyes") are a sign of anterior basilar skull or ethmoid bone fracture, and a search for cerebrospinal fluid rhinorrhea should be made. Cerebrospinal fluid rhinorrhea may accompany closed head or maxillofacial injury. It should be suspected whenever clear fluid or watery bloodstained fluid drains from the nose. If cerebrospinal fluid rhinorrhea is suspected, a CT scan followed by ENT and neurosurgical consultation are indicated. There is no reliable method available in the emergency department for distinguishing cerebrospinal fluid from nasal mucus. The use of glucose indicator sticks is associated with a high incidence of false-positive results.

Nasal Injury

Inspect the nose for obvious deformity or septal hematoma. Palpate for the presence of nondisplaced fracture. If active epistaxis is present (infrequent), use packing or cautery to control the bleeding. Look for cerebrospinal fluid rhinorrhea (see above), which, if present, is an automatic indication for hospitalization.

Ear Injury

Inspect the external ear, ear canal, and tympanic membrane. Test hearing if possible. A direct blow to the external ear may produce otohematoma, auricular laceration, ossicular disruption, or perforated tympanic membrane (conductive hearing loss). Blunt head trauma may fracture the temporal bone (basilar skull fracture; see Chapter 16), which is associated with hemotympanum or blood in the external canal, postauricular hematoma (Battle's sign), cerebrospinal fluid otorrhea, facial nerve palsies, or sensorineural hearing loss.

Disposition

Most patients with extensive or open fractures or with serious injuries of the eye, ear, or salivary gland should be hospitalized. Uncomplicated fractures of the mandible, maxilla, and nasal bone—as well as contusions or lacerations of skin—may be managed without hospitalization. (See specific injuries for details.)

III. EMERGENCY MANAGEMENT OF SPECIFIC INJURIES

FACIAL FRACTURES

MANDIBULAR FRACTURES

With the exception of the nasal bones, the mandible is by far the most frequently fractured facial bone. Initial evaluation of the patient with mandibular fracture must include those points mentioned below. The oral cavity must be cleaned and suctioned of foreign bodies and debris, and a patent airway ensured. Laryngeal, cervical spine, and intracranial injuries must be sought first and treated. Failure to recognize a mandibular fracture may result in serious sequelae such as osteomyelitis, permanent malocclusion, or nonunion.

Diagnosis

A. Mandibular fractures may be detected simply by the presence of gross facial asymmetry on inspection or by malocclusion.

B. Pain is always present following mandibular fracture and may be so severe that the patient will refuse to open or close the jaw. The patient will usually point to the fracture site when asked to localize pain associated with mandibular movement. Having the patient bite down on 2 tongue blades will usually cause pain at the fracture line.

C. Tenderness is best ascertained by bidigital examination with the examiner's thumbs in the mouth on the teeth or dental alveoli (in edentulous patients). The fingers then palpate externally along the lower border of the mandible. By "rocking" the mandible from side to side, the physician can sense mobility in the midline area.

D. X-ray evaluation for mandibular fracture should include a Panorex examination, which gives a panoramic view of the entire mandible on one film and will usually show all fractures present. If Panorex technology is unavailable (or if patients with multiple injuries cannot be positioned properly), lateral oblique, posteroanterior, and reverse Towne views or an axial CT scan are often sufficient (Table 17–1). Types of fractures by location are shown in Fig 17–4.

Treatment

Once the diagnosis of mandibular fracture has been established, the following measures should be carried out:

A. Tetanus Prophylaxis: Give tetanus toxoid or tetanus-diphtheria toxoid as needed (Chapter 24).

B. Antibiotics: Give aqueous procaine penicillin, 2–4 million units intramuscularly initially; then penicillin V, 500 mg orally every 6 hours. Alternatively, give aqueous penicillin G, 10–12 million units/d intravenously in 4–6 divided doses. Clindamycin (450 mg orally or intravenously 3 times a day) or erythromycin (500 mg orally or intravenously 4 times a day) may be substituted in patients allergic to penicillin.

C. Barton Bandage: To provide comfort and initial stabilization of the fracture, a Barton bandage should be applied. This is simply a wraparound gauze or Kerlix dressing that passes under the mandible and

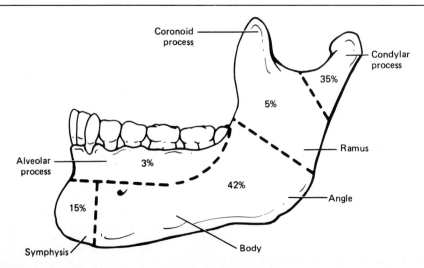

Figure 17–4. Regions of the mandible, showing fracture sites by frequency of involvement. (Redrawn and reproduced, with permission, from Dingman RO, Natvig P: *Surgery of Facial Fractures.* Saunders, 1964.)

over the top of the head so as to close the mandible. Care must be taken, however, to maintain airway patency.

Disposition

Ideally, patients with mandibular fractures should be treated definitively in the emergency department before discharge. If necessary, however, patients with simple mandibular fractures may be discharged and referred to an otolaryngologist, plastic surgeon, or oral surgeon within a few days for definitive treatment. Provide adequate analgesics, and instruct the patient to drink plenty of liquids with a straw.

Patients with open or severely displaced mandibular fractures should be seen by the maxillofacial consultant and hospitalized for treatment.

MAXILLARY (LE FORT) FRACTURES

Le Fort fractures are fractures of the maxilla and associated structures in the middle third of the face. Most result from blunt trauma (primarily fistfights and motor vehicle accidents). Le Fort fractures are usually bilateral and are frequently associated with other facial and intracranial injuries.

Clinical Findings

The most helpful clinical findings are malocclusion, local tenderness, and maxillary mobility. The latter finding is elicited by grasping and rocking the anterior portion of the maxilla intraorally with one hand while stabilizing the head with the other hand. Motion is elicited in bilateral maxillary fractures if they are not seriously impacted. Diagnosis is confirmed by a Waters view x-ray using stereo technique or by CT scan (Table 17–1). Le Fort fractures can be classified into 3 types (Fig 17–5). Management and complications are different for each type.

1. LE FORT I FRACTURE

Diagnosis

Le Fort I fracture is essentially a maxillary alveolar fracture in which the fracture line extends from the posterior portion of the maxilla behind the molars horizontally across the lateral wall of the maxillary sinus anterior to the piriform aperture (Fig 17–5A). When bilateral, this fracture essentially separates the maxillary teeth and alveolar bone from the rest of the maxilla and face. There are usually no airway complications with such a fracture.

Treatment

No specific emergency treatment is indicated; patients with Le Fort I fractures should be seen by the maxillofacial consultant (otolaryngologist, plastic

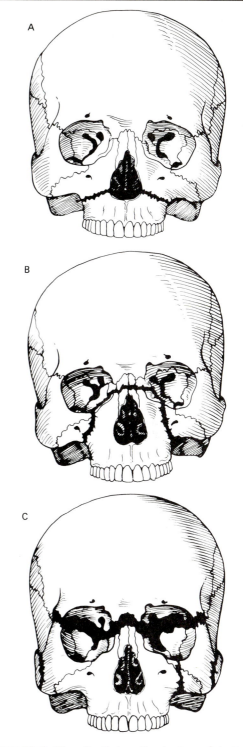

Figure 17–5. Sites of Le Fort maxillary fractures. **A:** Le Fort I fracture. **B:** Le Fort II fracture. **C:** Le Fort III fracture. The left side shows a common variant of Le Fort III fracture, in which the zygomatic bone is dislodged as a free fragment. (Redrawn and reproduced, with permission, from Song IC, Bromberg BE: Maxillofacial fractures. Chapter 26 in: *Quick Guide to Surgical Emergencies.* Shaftan GW, Gardner B [editors]. Lippincott, 1974.)

surgeon, or oral surgeon) in the emergency department for definitive repair. Give adequate analgesics.

Disposition

Patients with uncomplicated Le Fort I fractures may be discharged and referred for definitive treatment within a few days if specialist care in the emergency department is not feasible. Patients with complex or open fractures should be hospitalized.

2. LE FORT II FRACTURE

Diagnosis

Le Fort II fracture lines are similar to those of Le Fort I except that the bony nasal skeleton and the middle one-third of the face are included. For this reason, the fracture is sometimes called a "pyramidal fracture" (Figs 17–5B and 17–6). Once again, occlusion is altered by displacement of the maxillary teeth. Examination usually reveals ecchymosis of the nasal dorsum, the lower eyelids, and the maxillary gingival buccal sulcus. Since these fracture lines may traverse the bony infraorbital nerve canal, there may be hypesthesia below the lower eyelid. The face may appear elongated, and the anterior portion of the mid face will be mobile relative to the forehead. Facial x-rays will reveal fluid levels in the maxillary sinus.

The best routine x-ray view for visualizing these fractures is the Waters view (Fig 17–6). However, CT scans are preferred and in most centers have become the procedure of choice.

Treatment

No specific immediate treatment is necessary. Provide adequate analgesics.

Disposition

Patients with Le Fort II fractures should be hospitalized, if possible, for definitive repair. Repair may be delayed for several days without affecting the final outcome, but this determination should be made by the maxillofacial consultant.

3. LE FORT III FRACTURE (Craniofacial Disjunction)

Diagnosis

In Le Fort III fracture, the entire facial skeleton (including the zygoma, infraorbital rim, nasal skeleton, maxillary alveoli, and teeth) is dislocated from the base of the skull. The fracture lines usually traverse the lateral orbital rim and orbital wall, passing posteriorly to the inferior orbital fissure. The lines then pass medially across the glabellar region (bridge of nose). In addition, the zygomatic arches are also fractured. In some patients, the zygoma may become completely separated by fracture lines (Fig 17–5C, left side). Patients with Le Fort III fracture tend to have massive facial edema and ecchymosis and occasionally airway obstruction secondary to dissection of hematoma into the palate, pharyngeal walls, or tonsillar pillars. Patients frequently have associated mandibular fractures with posterior prolapse of the tongue and hematoma formation.

Treatment

A. Secure airway. Perform orotracheal intubation or cricothyrotomy if the airway has been compromised by edema or hematoma.

B. Provide adequate analgesics.

Disposition

In virtually all cases, a maxillofacial consultant should examine the patient in the emergency department to determine the need for hospitalization.

ZYGOMATIC ("TRIPOD") FRACTURES

Malar complex (zygomaticomaxillary) fracture most commonly results from lateral-to-medial force applied to the face, frequently by the fist of an intoxicated combatant. There are 3 fracture lines—hence the name tripod fracture (Figs 17–7 and 17–8). The lateral orbital rim is fractured at the frontozygomatic suture. The orbital floor is disrupted, with the anterior end of the fracture line passing across through the zygomaticomaxillary suture line or the infraorbital foramen. The third fracture is through the zygomatic arch. When associated with tripod fracture, the orbital floor fracture line is not a blowout fracture and should not be confused with one.

Diagnosis

Epistaxis occurs, since the bony floor of the orbit is also the roof of the maxillary sinus. Periorbital edema

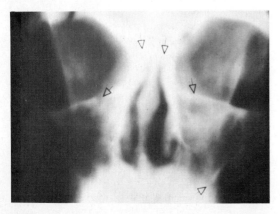

Figure 17–6. Le Fort II (pyramidal) fracture shown by tomography in a Waters projection. Arrows show fracture lines.

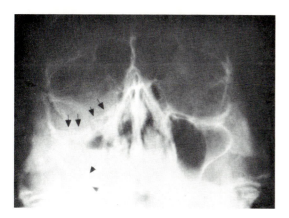

Figure 17–7. Zygomatic (tripod) fracture shown in a Waters view x-ray. Arrows show fracture lines.

and ecchymosis are present. Examination and palpation show flattening of the normal malar prominence and depression or separation of the lateral or inferior orbital rim.

Facial paresthesias or hypesthesias of the upper lip and cheek occur if the infraorbital nerve is damaged at the infraorbital foramen or more posteriorly in the orbital floor, where the infraorbital canal constitutes an area of weakness. Diplopia may be present as a result of orbital hematoma or slight displacement of the eyeball. Herniation of orbital contents into the antrum (maxillary sinus) is less common in tripod frac-

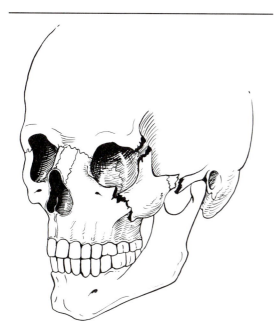

Figure 17–8. Diagram of a tripod fracture. Note disruption of both the lateral orbital rim and the orbital floor, as well as the zygomatic arch.

ture than in orbital blowout fracture. Subcutaneous emphysema of the face indicates that the fracture has extended into the paranasal sinuses.

X-ray confirmation is readily obtained with a routine facial x-ray (Waters, Caldwell, lateral, base, or submentovertex views; Table 17–1 and Fig 17–7) or CT scan.

Treatment

A. Control epistaxis with nasal packing or cautery, and provide adequate analgesics.

B. Administer antimicrobials if fracture extends into the sinuses. Penicillin, 150,000–200,000 units/kg/d intravenously in 4–6 divided doses, is the drug of choice. Doxycycline, 100 mg intravenously every 12 hours, may be used for adults with penicillin allergy.

Disposition

Before being discharged from the emergency department, the patient should be examined by a maxillofacial consultant to determine the need for hospitalization. Ophthalmologic consultation is also advisable.

In general, simple closed fractures of the zygomatic arch alone do not require further specific treatment or hospitalization. True tripod fractures—especially those that are open or displaced, or with displacement of orbital contents—require open reduction under general anesthesia. Although these patients may be discharged from the emergency department for definitive repair within 10 days, it is preferable to hospitalize them at the time of initial evaluation.

ORBITAL FLOOR ("BLOWOUT") FRACTURES

Pure blowout fracture results from blunt anteroposterior force directed against the eyeball. Intraocular pressure rises markedly and is exerted in all directions. The orbital floor gives way because it is the weakest component of the orbital skeleton. Orbital fat, bone from the orbital floor, and occasionally extraocular muscles may be forced into the maxillary antrum. For this reason, ocular injuries and complications are more extensive with this fracture than with any other fracture. Because the infraorbital rim is not involved by the fracture, tenderness may not be palpable on the face, and the diagnosis may be missed if the physician is not aware of the fracture and its mechanism. Unrepaired blowout fractures may result in permanent diplopia or disfiguring enophthalmos.

Impure blowout fracture results from anteroposterior blunt force similar to that causing pure blowout fracture, but in this instance the force is also exerted against the infraorbital rim, producing a fracture. Impure blowout fracture is more common than pure blowout fracture. Because the force is dissipated by the rim fracture, the globe usually sustains less trauma, with the result that ocular complications (hyphema, retinal detachment, commotio retinae, lens dislocation, etc) are less common than in pure blowout fractures.

Diagnosis

Suspect blowout fracture in any patient who has sustained blunt ocular or periorbital trauma. Diplopia and restricted upward gaze may confirm ocular muscle entrapment as a result of the fracture. Infraorbital nerve injury with infraorbital hypesthesia is common in both pure and impure blowout fracture. Epistaxis may be present from laceration of the mucosa of the roof of the maxillary sinus.

Ocular injuries are usually associated with pure blowout fractures. Palpable fracture of the infraorbital rim occurs with impure blowout fractures and is absent in pure blowout fractures.

Facial x-rays usually reveal fracture fragments and soft tissue prolapsed into the superior portion of the maxillary sinus. Occasionally, opacification or an air-fluid level in a maxillary sinus (Waters view) may be the only sign. Coronal CT scans of the orbital floor are often helpful in delineating the exact extent of the fracture (Fig 17–9).

Treatment & Disposition

Obtain consultation with an otolaryngologist and

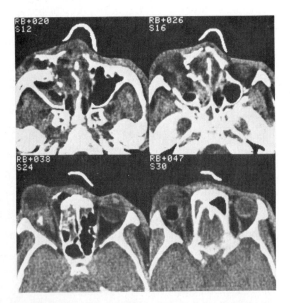

Figure 17–9. Orbital blowout fracture (impure type) on CT scan. Sequential horizontal cuts through the mid skull show blowout fracture of the right orbit, with rupture of the orbital contents into the maxillary sinus (upper left frame). Edema of the orbital contents is causing protrusion of the right eyeball (lower left frame).

ophthalmologist before discharging the patient from the emergency department.

Patients with blowout fractures and orbital entrapment (ie, diplopia or limitation of ocular mobility) should be hospitalized for exploration of the orbital floor under general anesthesia. Reduction and internal fixation of associated facial fractures may have to be performed simultaneously.

Patients with orbital floor or rim fractures with no limitation of ocular mobility and without associated injury of the globe (Chapter 25) may be discharged from the emergency department and referred to an otolaryngologist to be seen within a few days.

NASAL FRACTURES

The nasal bones are sometimes fractured laterally in one fragment, but more commonly there is impaction of the nasal skeleton into the piriform aperture (bony nasal vault), requiring that the septum and nasal bones be disimpacted anteriorly before they can be reduced laterally. Open nasal fractures are rare.

Diagnosis

There is a history of a blow to the nose, often associated with epistaxis. Tenderness, crepitation, or movement of nasal bones on palpation is present. Septal hematoma may be found on examination.

X-rays of the nasal bones seldom provide additional information and are not recommended for routine use.

Treatment

Patients with nasal fractures without deformity or septal hematoma may be treated with analgesia alone; give acetaminophen (Tylenol) with codeine or its equivalent. If airflow obstruction develops in nasal passages or if obvious deformity is revealed when the swelling subsides, the patient should be referred to an otolaryngologist within 3–5 days. Ideally, nasal fractures with deformity but no associated soft tissue swelling should be reduced immediately before swelling develops. If swelling develops, reduction should be delayed until the swelling subsides, usually in 3–5 days. Reduction should not be delayed beyond 10–14 days.

A. Provide Anesthesia: Most fractures can be reduced following topical intranasal anesthesia with cocaine. Roll cotton pledgets into a cylindric shape, and soak in 4% cocaine solution. Insert with nasal forceps into the upper and lower nasal cavities, and leave in place for about 15 minutes. Occasionally, topical anesthesia must be supplemented by injected local anesthetic. General anesthesia is preferred in children.

B. Reduce Fracture: Simple, laterally displaced fractures may be reduced by exerting thumb pressure on the nose in the direction opposite to the initial fracture force.

Comminuted fractures must be manipulated anteriorly and laterally. This is most easily done with a Kelly clamp or Asche septal forceps inserted in the nose up the fracture site (Fig 17–10). If the nose then has normal external configuration, reduction is successful and should be maintained by applying tape over the nose, perhaps supplemented by an anterior nasal pack of petrolatum-impregnated gauze.

If the fracture has been reduced or if it was nondisplaced, arrange for otolaryngologic consultation within 3 days. If the emergency physician cannot achieve adequate reduction of a nasal fracture, an otolaryngologist should be consulted immediately. Simple lacerations without associated septal dislocation should be copiously irrigated and closed primarily. Antimicrobial prophylaxis (see below) should be given. Deep or complex lacerations or those associated with septal deviation or nasal deformity should not be repaired until the otolaryngologist or plastic surgeon has examined the patient. Dislocated cartilage can often be repaired and reduced through such lacerations.

C. Drain Hematomas: Septal hematomas should be drained by incision through the anterior nasal mucosa at the time of fracture reduction. If septal hematoma is allowed to persist and results in abscess formation, the entire septal cartilage may be lost, resulting in a disfiguring "saddle" deformity of the nose. Give antimicrobial prophylaxis, eg, ampicillin or erythromycin, 500 mg orally 3 or 4 times a day.

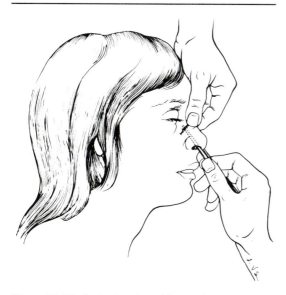

Figure 17–10. Reduction of nasal fracture by anterior traction with forceps. (Redrawn and reproduced, with permission, from Wang MK, Macomber WB: Maxillofacial injuries. Chapter 14 in: *Emergency Room Care,* 4th ed. Echert C [editor]. Little, Brown, 1981.)

Disposition

Hospitalization is rarely required for nasal fractures. Patients should be told that the nasal air passages may become narrowed on one side or the other, thereby requiring septorhinoplasty at a later date.

FRONTAL SINUS FRACTURES

Frontal sinus fractures most commonly result from motor vehicle trauma in which the patient's head strikes the dashboard. Patients with frontal sinus fractures require thorough head, neck, and neurologic examination, including ophthalmologic consultation. If there are variations in the level of consciousness, neurosurgical consultation should be obtained immediately. Fractures of the posterior wall of the frontal sinus may cause dural tears or brain injury, while fractures of the floor of the sinus often injure the nasofrontal duct.

Diagnosis

There will usually be a history as well as evidence of trauma to the forehead. Cerebrospinal fluid rhinorrhea is common following fractures of the posterior wall of the frontal sinus, and a specific note about its presence or absence should be entered in the emergency department record. Epistaxis may represent associated direct nasal trauma or frontal sinus hemorrhage.

Standard sinus x-rays should be taken as soon as possible. Caldwell, Waters, and lateral views usually reveal fractures of the frontal sinus. Fractures of the posterior wall of the frontal sinus are usually best seen on the lateral view. Axial CT scan is often the best way of demonstrating sinus fractures.

Associated injuries frequently include other facial fractures, depressed skull fractures, and orbital fractures.

Treatment

A. When brisk hemorrhage from the nasal cavity accompanies these fractures, it is acceptable to pack the anterior nasal vault tightly with 1.25-cm (½-in) iodoform gauze. Elevation of the head will reduce venous pressure and bleeding while the patient's condition stabilizes or arrangements are made for surgery.

B. Obtain urgent otolaryngologic and neurosurgical consultation.

C. If the fracture is open, the wound should be covered with saline-soaked gauze. Avoid manipulation of bony fragments in the emergency department, since this may produce further dural injury.

D. Give penicillin, 2 million units intravenously every 4 hours; or doxycycline, 100 mg intravenously every 12 hours (for an adult allergic to penicillin). Antibiotics are needed because the fracture lines cross the contaminated mucosal surfaces of the nose and sinus.

E. Surgery is indicated for cerebrospinal fluid rhinorrhea, open fractures, markedly displaced fractures, and fractures involving the posterior wall or floor of the sinus.

Disposition

All patients with frontal sinus fractures should be hospitalized.

TEMPORAL BONE FRACTURES
("Basilar Skull Fracture")

Most "basilar skull fractures" include temporal bone fractures. The temporal bone is shaped like a pyramid with its base directed laterally and its apex medially. Because it houses the cochlea, vestibule, facial nerve canal, jugular vein, and internal carotid artery, fractures through the temporal bone may have serious sequelae.

Diagnosis is based on the history of trauma and the presence of bleeding; ecchymosis of the external ear, mastoid tip (Battle's sign), or ear canal; bilateral, periorbital ecchymoses ("raccoon eyes"); hemotympanum; hearing loss (conductive or sensorineural); or anosmia. *Note: Routine x-rays often fail to demonstrate a fracture.* A CT scan is most useful in identifying associated intracranial abnormalities.

Clinical features depend on the type of fracture. Because basilar skull fractures may be associated with intracranial bleeding, brain injury, or subsequent meningitis, neurosurgical consultation, in addition to otolaryngologic consultation, should be obtained for all patients with suspected temporal bone fracture.

1. TYMPANIC BONE FRACTURES

The anterior face of the tympanic bone is the glenoid fossa of the temporomandibular joint. Hence, the mandibular condyle may be driven posteriorly into the middle ear or to the external auditory canal. Patients with facial trauma who have ecchymosis, bleeding, or lacerations of the anterior external auditory canal often have such a fracture. A CT scan or mastoid x-rays confirm the diagnosis.

Treatment

The ear canal is anesthetized by injection of local anesthetic, and tympanic bone displacement is reduced by means of a metal speculum in the ear canal. This procedure is usually performed by an otolaryngologist.

Disposition

Hospitalization is not usually necessary unless there are associated injuries.

2. LONGITUDINAL FRACTURES

Longitudinal fractures are so named because the fracture line parallels the long axis of the temporal bone (petrous pyramid). These fractures account for 80% of all fractures of the temporal bone. The tympanic membrane is frequently torn, and a step-off may be seen in the roof of the external auditory canal. Ossicular chain dislocation with conductive hearing loss is frequent. The hearing loss in longitudinal fractures is usually conductive rather than sensorineural, since the fracture line does not traverse the cochlea. When there is facial nerve paralysis, it is usually delayed. Delayed facial paralysis implies a better prognosis than does immediate paralysis, which indicates lacerations or other disruption of the nerve trunk and thus requires surgical exploration of the bony nerve canal as soon as the patient's condition permits.

Treatment & Disposition

Obtain urgent otolaryngologic consultation. All patients with this injury require hospitalization.

3. TRANSVERSE FRACTURES

Although less frequent than longitudinal fractures, the transverse fracture causes more severe injuries to the contents of the temporal bone. It usually starts near the internal auditory canal and runs a course perpendicular to the longitudinal axis of the temporal bone. Consequently, these fractures frequently traverse the cochlea, resulting in complete sensorineural hearing loss. Facial nerve injuries occur in over half of patients, and paralysis is commonly immediate, requiring exploration of the facial nerve canal.

Treatment & Disposition

Patients with suspected transverse temporal bone fractures require hospitalization for evaluation and surgery. Immediate otolaryngologic consultation should be obtained.

TOOTH INJURIES

AVULSION OF TEETH

Stop gingival bleeding with pressure. Wash the tooth with saline, and replace it immediately in the tooth socket. Obtain emergency oral surgical consultation, since avulsed teeth can be successfully reimplanted in some cases. For this reason, an attempt should be made to retrieve avulsed teeth from the scene of the accident.

SUBLUXATION OF TEETH

Gently manipulate the tooth back into its proper position. Obtain oral surgical consultation, since the loose tooth will have to be immobilized until it has reattached to periodontal and gingival tissues.

TOOTH FRACTURES

Exposure of the pulp or dentin is exquisitely painful, and a dentist should cover the tooth with a temporary plastic crown affixed with zinc oxide–eugenol paste. Follow-up care should be provided by the patient's regular dentist within a few days.

EXTERNAL EAR TRAUMA

OTOHEMATOMA

Diagnosis
Bleeding between the auricular cartilage and the perichondrium frequently follows contusions or other injuries to the auricle. Such injuries are frequent in boxers and wrestlers. If untreated, they will result in cauliflower ear deformity, since blood under the perichondrium results in proliferative scarring and new cartilage formation.

Treatment
Treatment consists of aspiration or incision and drainage of hematomas, followed by application of saline-soaked cotton balls that conform to the auricular formation. Antibiotic (eg, gentamicin) ointment applied to the ear may be helpful. A firm compression dressing should be wrapped around the head to prevent further hematoma formation.

Disposition
The patient should be seen by an otolaryngologist within 1–2 days. No specific instructions need be given. Hospitalization is not required.

LACERATIONS OF THE AURICLE

Diagnosis & Treatment
Lacerations of the auricle result in deformity if not meticulously repaired. Debridement of devitalized tissue is important. Approximation of lacerated cartilage and perichondrium should be performed with a single layer of 5–0 chromic catgut or synthetic absorbable sutures (eg, polyglycolic acid) on a small (Ethicon P-1 or similar) needle. This layer is fol-

lowed by 6–0 nylon skin sutures or skin tapes. Apply a petrolatum gauze dressing under slight pressure.

Disposition
Patients with extensive lacerations of the auricle should be hospitalized for repair in the operating room. Smaller lacerations repaired in the emergency department should be inspected by an otolaryngologist or plastic surgeon in 1–2 days.

MIDDLE & INNER EAR DISORDERS FOLLOWING HEAD TRAUMA

CEREBROSPINAL FLUID OTORRHEA

Diagnosis
Cerebrospinal fluid otorrhea often results from minimal head injuries. Small cracks in the tegmen tympani (roof of the middle ear) provide a route for leakage of cerebrospinal fluid into the middle ear cavity. If the eardrum has a chronic perforation or has been torn at the time of injury, such leaks will result in cerebrospinal fluid *otorrhea*. This flow is best demonstrated in the head-down position. If the eardrum is intact, however, the fluid may pass through the auditory tube and produce cerebrospinal fluid *rhinorrhea*. In either case, meninigitis (usually due to pneumococci) is a potential complication. A CT scan will help diagnose the injury and eliminate the possibility of associated intracranial bleeding or brain injury.

Treatment & Disposition
Hospitalization and neurosurgical consultation are indicated for all patients with suspected leakage of cerebrospinal fluid. Prophylactic antibiotics have not been shown to be of benefit and are not recommended.

FACIAL NERVE PARALYSIS

Diagnosis
Facial nerve paralysis may result from a small temporal bone fracture. The facial nerve passes through the middle ear cavity, where it is exposed to risk of injury from foreign bodies introduced through the ear canal as well as fractures. Schirmer's test (comparison of rate of tear flow in the 2 eyes) determines the location of injury to the nerve: if lacrimation is decreased on the side of the facial paralysis, the injury to the facial nerve is proximal to the middle ear por-

tion of the nerve. This test should be performed by an otolaryngologist.

Treatment & Disposition

Patients with temporal bone fractures and immediate facial paralysis should be hospitalized and otolaryngologic consultation obtained immediately. Delayed paralysis should be followed daily by the otolaryngologist to determine whether operation is required.

CONDUCTIVE HEARING LOSS

Diagnosis

Disarticulation of the ossicular chain may result from head injuries with or without temporal bone fracture. One or more of the tiny ossicles may be jarred free from attachments and prevent normal function of the middle ear conduction mechanism. Such patients complain of acute loss of hearing. There may or may not be evidence of temporal bone fracture. If a step-off is seen at 12 o'clock at the medial end of the ear canal, it is further evidence of such an injury. Bone conduction is greater than air conduction in tuning fork tests. Audiometric examination reveals whether a coexisting sensorineural hearing loss is also present.

Treatment & Disposition

Such patients should be referred to an otolaryngologist within a few days for surgical reconstruction of the ossicular chain in the middle ear. Immediate hospitalization is not required.

SENSORINEURAL HEARING LOSS

Diagnosis

More severe temporal bone fractures may produce sensorineural hearing loss due to fractures that traverse the cochlea. Such hearing losses are often total, and patients have severe vertigo during the first few days following injury.

Treatment & Disposition

Intravenous diazepam (2–5 mg over 5–10 minutes) is an effective labyrinthine suppressant for control of vertigo in such patients. The patient should be hospitalized for evaluation and urgent otolaryngologic consultation.

VERTIGO

Diagnosis

Some patients with head injuries complain of vertigo even though x-rays show the temporal bone to be intact. These symptoms are thought to result from jar-

ring of the delicate membranous inner ear structures within the bony labyrinth. In most instances, the vertigo is described as difficulty in walking or as a "floating" sensation. Occasionally, vertigo is so severe as to be associated with nystagmus.

Treatment & Disposition

Symptoms diminish as time passes. Reassurance and sedation with diazepam, 2–5 mg orally 2–4 times daily, or meclizine, 25 mg orally 3–4 times daily, are usually all that is required. Hospitalization is rarely necessary. The patient may be referred to an otolaryngologist for follow-up in 5–7 days.

CARE OF FACIAL LACERATIONS
(See also Chapter 24.)

Closure of Lacerations

Careful, painstaking closure of facial lacerations with fine suture material will give gratifying results. If the emergency physician has insufficient time for meticulous care of these wounds, help should be requested from a consultant surgeon with available suture material and access to an operating room if necessary.

Some parts of the face require more precise tissue approximation than others. Lacerations involving the hairline, eyebrows, eyelids, nasal dorsum, nasolabial folds, nostril rims, columella, and philtrum should be closed with exact approximation of anatomic lines and structures.

Injuries to the upper and lower lip are extremely common and likewise require precise repair. A soaking wet gauze sponge should be used to clean the lip of all blood and foreign debris. The vermilion border can be seen most easily if left wet. Closure of lacerations of this area should begin with placement of a small "sentinel" suture to align this border. The repair then progresses in either direction from it.

Replacement of Avulsed Tissue

Debridement of "devitalized" pieces of tissue should be done with caution and conservatism. Likewise, small avulsed pieces of external ear, nose, or facial soft tissue with skin may be cleaned, debrided, and replaced with a reasonable chance for survival. Larger pieces, as in total or subtotal avulsion of the external ear or scalp, are best reattached by microvascular techniques in the operating room. The physician should ask the patient with an avulsion injury if a friend or relative can return to the scene of the accident to retrieve lost fragments of tissue.

Delay in Closing Lacerations

In general, lacerations of the eyelids, lateral orbital region, nasal dorsum, and mandibular region should not be closed until x-rays of the facial bones have been taken. The otolaryngologist or maxillofacial consultant may prefer reduction and fixation of the fracture fragments through these lacerations.

Because of the rich blood supply of the area, it is acceptable to close facial lacerations as much as 12 hours after injury when necessary. When delayed closure is necessary, the wound should be packed open with saline sponges and the use of antibiotics considered (eg, dicloxacillin, 500 mg orally 4 times a day). Pressure dressings can be used to control hemorrhage, or hemostats may be applied if bleeding vessels can be identified.

Repair Technique

Repair of facial lacerations should always be done in layers. There is no "rule" for numbers of layers or type of suture technique. In general, however, in most severe facial lacerations, careful approximation of muscle with fine absorbable suture (4–0 or 5–0 chromic catgut, Dexon, or Vicryl) will stabilize the wound and make skin closure more accurate and cosmetically satisfactory. Small bites of the needle are appropriate, and nerves and vessels must be carefully avoided.

The subcutaneous tissue should always be sutured, care being taken to "bury" the knot (see Fig 24–9). The superficial passage of the needle should be very close to the skin edge, so that after this layer is complete, the skin is already approximated and the skin sutures serve only to ensure accuracy of repair.

Facial skin should be sutured with 6–0 nylon or polypropylene on a nontraumatic reverse cutting needle. An important aspect of plastic closure of such lacerations is the angle of entry of the needle into the skin and the eversion that is produced by each suture (see Fig 24–10). Since the subcuticular layer has already approximated the skin, the skin sutures need not be tied tightly. A surgeon's knot (2 loops) should be tied and pulled down loosely so that the skin edges just touch. The next loop of suture should be tied with the opposite twist, so that a square knot results. If this second loop is not tied down tightly, a small loop results between the first (surgeon's) knot and the second loop; this is thought to reduce tissue strangulation when wound edema causes the skin edges to swell against the sutures. At least 2 additional knot loops should be tied on top of this second knot.

For linear lacerations, a running (uninterrupted) suture is acceptable. The same important principles of an everting needle angle and gentle tension will give the most cosmetic repair.

Facial skin sutures should be removed not later than the fourth day. An ophthalmic suture scissor or a No. 11 Bard-Parker blade is best for removing these fine sutures. After suture removal, both sides of the laceration should be painted with tincture of benzoin and the wound closed with adhesive dressings (eg, Steri-Strips) so that the opposing edges of the wound are pulled together. This will eliminate any tension on the closure and minimize widening and hypertrophy of the scar. The patient should be told that facial scars mature for 12 months and that facial scar revision may be done after that time.

REFERENCES

Busuito MJ, Smith DJ Jr, Robson MC: Mandibular fractures in an urban trauma center. J Trauma 1986;26:826.

Converse JM: *Surgical Treatment of Facial Injuries,* 3rd ed. Williams & Wilkins, 1974.

Dingman RO, Natvig P: *Surgery of Facial Fractures.* Saunders, 1964.

Foster CA, Maisel RH, Meyerhoff WL: Head and neck trauma: Initial evaluation, diagnosis and management. Minn Med 1981;64:85.

Gussack GS, Jurkovich GJ: Treatment dilemmas in laryngotracheal trauma. J Trauma 1988;28:1439.

Holt GR: Pages 333–343 in: *Otolaryngology--Head and Neck Surgery.* Cummings C et al (editors). Mosby, 1986.

Kellerman R, Schilli W: Plate fixation of fractures of the mid and upper face. Otolaryngol Clin North Am 1987;20:559.

Mafee MF: Radiology of maxillofacial trauma. Top Emerg Med 1983;5:28.

Mathog RH: *Maxillofacial Trauma.* Williams & Wilkins, 1983.

Meyerhoff WM et al: *Surgery of Facial Fractures.* Manual of American Academy of Otolaryngology: Head & Neck Surgery. American Academy of Otolaryngology, 1980.

Ordog GJ et al: Shotgun "birdshot" wounds to the neck. J Trauma 1988;28:491.

Schultz RC, de Camara DL: Athletic facial injuries. JAMA 1984;252:3395.

Sheely CH II, Mattox KL, Beall AC Jr: Management of acute cervical tracheal trauma. Am J Surg 1974;128:805.

Walton RL et al: Maxillofacial trauma. Surg Clin North Am 1982;62:73.

Williams CN, Cohen M, Schultz RC: Intermediate and long-term management of gunshot wounds to the lower face. Plast Reconstr Surg 1988;82:433.

Wood J, Fabian TC, Mangiante EC: Penetrating neck injuries: Recommendations for selective management. J Trauma 1989;29:602.

Yealy DM, Paris PM: Recent advances in airway management. Emerg Med Clin North Am 1989;7:83.

18

Chest Trauma

Melvin D. Cheitlin, MD, & Donald D. Trunkey, MD

EMERGENCY MANAGEMENT OF LIFE-THREATENING PROBLEMS

IMMEDIATE EVALUATION & TREATMENT
(See algorithm.)

The measures described below should be instituted simultaneously, if possible.

Ensure Adequate Airway
A. Perform Intubation: If necessary, intubate the patient (Chapter 46). Facial or neck injuries or upper airway obstruction may prevent adequate ventilation by bag-mask. In these cases, immediate endotracheal intubation or cricothyrotomy (Chapter 46) is necessary. If the patient is in respiratory distress (gasping respirations, tachypnea, cyanosis, or flail

chest), the first priority is to provide adequate ventilation.
B. Begin Oxygen: Assist ventilation with a bag-mask combination, and give supplemental oxygen at a rate of 10 mL/min.

Assess Ventilation
A. Relieve Hemothorax or Pneumothorax: Examine the chest for penetrating wounds, and listen for unilateral decreased breath sounds. Look for a deviated trachea. If hemothorax or pneumothorax is thought to be present, immediate tube thoracostomy should be performed (Chapter 46). If significant (> 1000 mL) hemothorax is present, consider autotransfusion (Chapter 46).
B. Support Flail Chest: Assist ventilation. If flail chest is contributing to respiratory distress, provide assisted ventilation until the patient's condition permits accurate assessment of respiratory function. Endotracheal intubation is usually necessary.

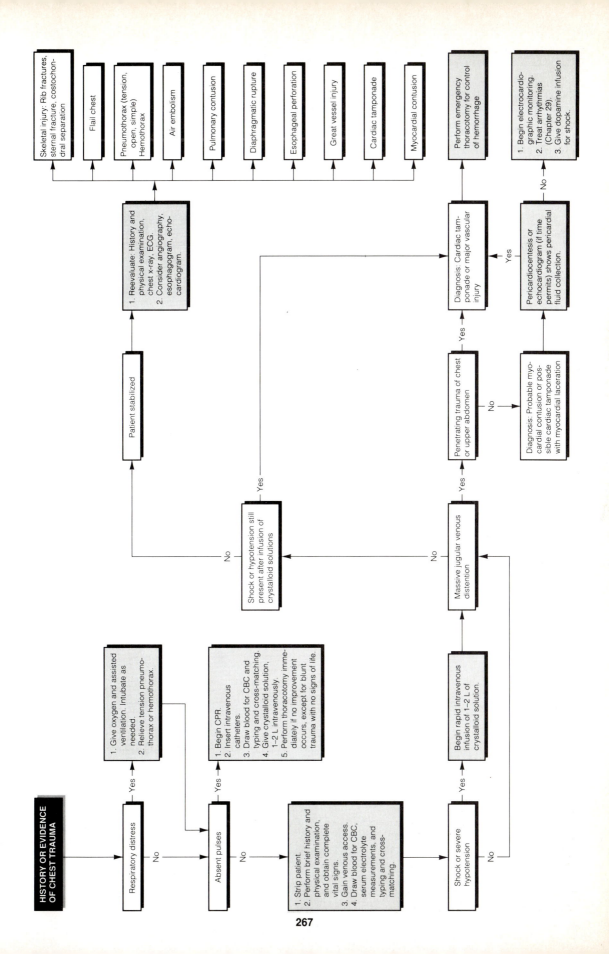

HISTORY OR EVIDENCE OF CHEST TRAUMA

Respiratory distress
— Yes → 1. Give oxygen and assisted ventilation. Intubate as needed.
2. Relieve tension pneumothorax or hemothorax.
— No →

Absent pulses
— Yes → 1. Begin CPR.
2. Insert intravenous catheters.
3. Draw blood for CBC and typing and cross-matching.
4. Give crystalloid solution, 1–2 L intravenously.
5. Perform thoracotomy immediately if no improvement occurs, except for blunt trauma with no signs of life.
— No →

1. Strip patient.
2. Perform brief history and physical examination, and obtain complete vital signs.
3. Gain venous access.
4. Draw blood for CBC, serum electrolyte measurements, and typing and cross-matching.

Shock or severe hypotension
— Yes → Begin rapid intravenous infusion of 1–2 L of crystalloid solution.
— No →

Massive jugular venous distention
— Yes → Penetrating trauma of chest or upper abdomen
— No →

Penetrating trauma of chest or upper abdomen
— Yes → Diagnosis: Cardiac tamponade or major vascular injury
— No → Diagnosis: Probable myocardial contusion or possible cardiac tamponade with myocardial laceration

Diagnosis: Probable myocardial contusion or possible cardiac tamponade with myocardial laceration → Pericardiocentesis or echocardiogram (if time permits) shows pericardial fluid collection

Pericardiocentesis or echocardiogram (if time permits) shows pericardial fluid collection
— Yes → Diagnosis: Cardiac tamponade or major vascular injury
— No → 1. Begin electrocardiographic monitoring.
2. Treat arrhythmias (Chapter 29).
3. Give dopamine infusion for shock.

Diagnosis: Cardiac tamponade or major vascular injury → Perform emergency thoracotomy for control of hemorrhage

Shock or hypotension still present after infusion of crystalloid solutions
— No →
— Yes → Patient stabilized → 1. Reevaluate: History and physical examination, chest x-ray, ECG. 2. Consider angiography, esophagogram, echocardiogram.

Skeletal injury: Rib fractures, sternal fracture, costochondral separation

Flail chest

Pneumothorax (tension, open, simple) Hemothorax

Air embolism

Pulmonary contusion

Diaphragmatic rupture

Esophageal perforation

Great vessel injury

Cardiac tamponade

Myocardial contusion

267

Assess Adequacy of Circulation

Palpate for the presence of pulses, and look for signs of shock (Chapter 3). Stop gross external hemorrhage.

A. Immediate Measures: If no pulse is palpable, begin CPR (Chapter 1). Insert 2 large-bore intravenous lines. One central line should be placed (femoral vein is preferred if CPR is in progress) and one cutdown should be performed if immediate access is not available through antecubital veins. Draw blood for CBC, serum creatinine and serum electrolyte measurements, and typing and cross-matching. Begin rapid administration of intravenous crystalloid solution (up to 2 L in 15 minutes) to restore perfusion. Stop obvious external blood loss with gentle finger or palm pressure.

B. Thoracotomy: If pulses are absent or profound shock (eg, systemic blood pressure < 60 mm Hg) persists despite vigorous resuscitation, an immediate thoracotomy should be performed for open chest cardiac compression to relieve cardiac tamponade; control bleeding from the great vessels, and cross-clamp the descending aorta. Patients who are likely to benefit from emergency thoracotomy are victims of penetrating trauma (stab wounds or small-caliber hand guns) who exhibited signs of life during transport to the hospital or in the emergency department (survival is around 5%). Victims of blunt trauma without signs of life in the emergency department are unlikely to survive, and emergency thoracotomy is unnecessary. The procedure should only be performed if adequate surgical backup is available.

Evaluate & Treat
Hypotension & Shock
(See Chapter 3.)

Blood loss is the cause of hypotension and shock in most cases and may result from thoracic injury itself or concurrent intra-abdominal injury. The physician should remember that clinically inapparent massive bleeding may occur into the retroperitoneum or deep muscles of the thigh. Other causes of hypotension include cardiac tamponade (especially with penetrating trauma), myocardial contusion (especially with blunt trauma), and central nervous system injury (rare).

A. Examine and Evaluate the Patient: Completely strip the patient, and quickly examine the entire chest (and body) for obvious injuries. Record vital signs. Repeat blood pressure and pulse measurements in the sitting position (if there is no evidence of vertebral injury) if they are normal while the patient is supine.

Watch for persistent hypotension or shock with central plethora (jugular venous distention), which suggests cardiac tamponade or myocardial contusion. *Note: Even with cardiac tamponade, central venous pressure may not be elevated if blood volume is low because of hemorrhage.* Only when blood volume is restored will jugular venous pressure rise.

B. Establish Intravenous Access: Insert 2 large-bore (≥ 16-gauge) intravenous lines, and draw blood for CBC, serum electrolyte measurements, renal function tests, and typing and cross-matching. Administer 1–2 L of crystalloid solution (eg, balanced salt solution) intravenously over 10–15 minutes. Improvement in blood pressure after these measures without development of jugular venous distention suggests hypovolemic shock.

C. Determine Type of Injury:

1. Penetrating trauma–If the patient has sustained penetrating trauma, suspect cardiac tamponade, and perform immediate pericardiocentesis (Chapter 46). If vital signs do not improve, if the wound is directly over the heart, or if the path of the blow or trajectory of the missile suggests cardiac injury, perform *immediate* left anterolateral thoracotomy and pericardiotomy to relieve tamponade and control bleeding. Remember that exit or entrance wounds remote from the heart (lateral chest, abdomen) can be associated with cardiac injury.

2. Blunt trauma–If the patient has sustained blunt chest trauma, suspect myocardial contusion, particularly with deceleration-type injuries, a sternal fracture, flail chest, etc, and confirm the diagnosis with an ECG and measurement of cardiac isoenzymes. Two-dimensional echocardiography has been useful in identifying wall motion abnormalities associated with significant myocardial contusion. Although radionuclide angiography also demonstrates wall motion abnormalities with contusion, it is rarely available in the emergency room. Remember that cardiac laceration and cardiac tamponade may occur with nonpenetrating trauma, although less commonly than with penetrating trauma.

D. Insert a nasogastric tube and urinary catheter.

E. Obtain a chest x-ray (portable upright film, if possible).

Reevaluate Status of Shock

Patients who, despite volume replacement, remain in shock because of intrathoracic blood loss or cardiac tamponade require immediate thoracotomy for definitive management. When the source of blood loss does not originate within the chest, reexamine the patient for possible abdominal injuries.

Patients who recover from shock should receive more thorough evaluation with repeated physical examinations, other x-rays, angiography, or CT scan, as indicated.

Treat Pain

Patients with chest trauma who are in severe pain should be given morphine, 1–4 mg intravenously every 10–15 minutes, until pain is relieved. Monitor arterial blood gases if the patient is not on assisted ventilation.

FURTHER MANAGEMENT OF CHEST TRAUMA

1. PENETRATING CHEST TRAUMA

Mechanisms of injury in penetrating abdominal trauma are discussed extensively in Chapter 19. In contrast to penetrating abdominal trauma, about 80% of penetrating chest injuries can be managed conservatively without operation, since most injuries to pleura and lungs can be managed by tube thoracostomy alone. Only penetrating injuries of the heart or great vessels routinely require surgery.

Diagnosis

A. Symptoms and Signs: Clinical findings depend entirely on the organ injured. Common presenting signs include the following:

1. Hypotension or shock–Hypotension or shock may be due to blood loss into the pleural space or to impaired venous return (tension pneumothorax or cardiac tamponade).

2. Respiratory distress–Respiratory distress is usually due to pneumothorax or hemopneumothorax and is occasionally due to disruption of the tracheobronchial tree, flail chest, or pulmonary contusion. The patient may be tachypneic because pain from a fractured rib may limit inspiratory excursion. Respiratory distress on occasion can be secondary to left heart failure.

3. Neurologic abnormalities–Neurologic abnormalities may result from air embolism, arterial injury, or hypoxemia.

B. History: Elicit as much information as possible about the mechanism of injury (weapon, direction and depth of penetration, interval between injury and hospitalization, etc). Also inquire about prior illnesses (especially cardiac), injuries, allergies, and drug use.

C. Physical Examination: Look for signs of pneumothorax, tension pneumothorax, hemothorax, and cardiac tamponade. Record location and size of wounds (do not attempt to judge entrance and exit wounds or probe the wound track). Auscultate the heart for possible pericardial friction rub, mediastinal "crunch" due to air in the mediastinum, and murmurs. Examine the abdomen to rule out abdominal injury.

D. X-Ray and Electrocardiographic Examination and Laboratory Tests: Obtain a chest x-ray (preferably an upright view) to examine for air in the mediastinum or under the diaphragm and identify thoracic injuries. An ECG, hematocrit, arterial blood gas measurements, and urinalysis are also necessary.

Treatment

A. Treat respiratory distress, cardiac arrest, and shock as described above. Relieve pneumothorax or hemothorax (discovered on chest x-ray) with tube thoracostomy. Use autotransfusion for patients with hemothoraces of more than 1 L (Chapter 46).

B. Treat cardiac tamponade. In patients in unstable condition, perform immediate thoracotomy for pericardiotomy, and control myocardial injury with a finger or hand. The chest wall should be disinfected before general anesthesia is administered. Patients with cardiac tamponade may develop shock when anesthesia is started. Pericardiocentesis (Chapter 46) may be substituted as a temporizing measure only.

In patients in stable condition, obtain an echocardiogram to confirm the diagnosis. Diagnostic pericardiocentesis may be used if echocardiography is not immediately available. Remember that blood accumulating rapidly in the pericardial sac may clot and give false-negative results on pericardiocentesis.

C. Search for occult injury. Perform aortography for possible vascular injury if injury to the aorta or another artery is suspected on the basis of widened mediastinum, pulse deficit, or site of injury. A swallow of water-soluble contrast medium or esophagoscopy is useful to detect possible esophageal perforation (suspicion is based on the nature and trajectory of the injury or the presence of air in the mediastinum).

All penetrating injuries of the lower third of the chest need evaluation for laceration of the diaphragm and possible intra-abdominal injury, since these injuries require immediate operative repair.

Disposition

Hospitalize all patients with penetrating chest trauma.

2. BLUNT CHEST TRAUMA

Mechanisms of injury in blunt abdominal trauma are discussed in Chapter 19. Most blunt chest trauma results from vehicular accidents, and most injuries do not require surgery.

Diagnosis

A. Symptoms and Signs: Symptoms and signs are similar to those seen with penetrating trauma. Sustained crushing injuries to the chest, such as those occurring when a victim is pinned under a car for a long time, cause traumatic asphyxia. The victim appears seriously ill, with ocular and cutaneous hemorrhages and a violaceous skin tone, but serious internal injuries are not necessarily present.

If the patient has been found behind a *bent* steering wheel and was not wearing a seat belt, the physician should suspect sternal fractures, myocardial contusion, hemothorax, or coexisting upper abdominal injury.

Deceleration injuries may cause cardiac contusion or disruption of the great veins or even of the aorta with no sign of external thoracic injury.

B. History: Elicit as much information as possible about the mechanism of injury from the patient or witnesses. A description of the patient's position in the vehicle, the presence or absence of restraints, the speed at which the vehicle was traveling, damage to the steering wheel, and details of the patient's extrication from the vehicle will help to determine the type and extent of injuries.

Also inquire about prior illnesses (especially cardiac), injuries, allergies, or drug use.

C. Physical Examination: After ensuring an adequate airway and providing oxygen and ventilation, inspect the chest wall carefully, and look for rib or sternal fractures, costochondral separations, and paradoxical motion (flail chest). Auscultate the chest to detect hemothorax or pneumothorax and the heart for the presence of murmurs, mediastinal "crunch," or pericardial friction rubs. Examine the neck veins to evaluate central venous pressure. Examine the upper abdomen to detect coexisting intra-abdominal injury. Evaluate all patients for ruptured diaphragm (see below). Obtain blood pressure readings in both arms.

D. X-Ray and Electrocardiographic Examination and Laboratory Tests: Obtain a chest x-ray, and look for widened mediastinum (possible vascular injury), pulmonary infiltrates (or other evidence of possible lung contusion), rib fractures, and hemopneumothorax. Examine the ECG for QRS and ST–T wave abnormalities and arrhythmias (including atrioventricular block and bundle branch block) suggesting myocardial contusion. Draw blood for CBC, hematocrit, and arterial blood gas determinations.

Treatment

A. Treat respiratory distress, cardiac arrest, and shock as described above.

Provide analgesia (intravenous morphine in 1- to 4-mg doses, repeated as necessary) unless associated head trauma is present. Provide assisted ventilation for flail chest injuries, and perform tube thoracostomy to relieve pneumothorax or hemothorax (Chapter 46).

B. Treat cardiac arrhythmias. Most life-threatening arrhythmias following blunt chest trauma are ventricular and should be managed initially with lidocaine (loading dose of 1 mg/kg by bolus intravenous injection, followed by 1–4 mg/min by intravenous infusion). Unifocal premature ventricular contractions, even if frequent, do not need treatment if there is no other sign of myocardial contusion, if there is no history of previous underlying heart disease, especially with reduced left ventricular function, and if the contractions are asymptomatic. Atrial fibrillation and, less often, atrial flutter can be seen after trauma. If the ventricular response is rapid with reduction in blood pressure, cardioversion is indicated. If no hemodynamic instability is present, intravenous digoxin can be administered. If the ventricular rate is below 120/min, no immediate therapy is necessary. (See

Chapter 29 for details of treatment of cardiac arrhythmias.)

C. Intubate the disrupted tracheobronchial tree by selective intubation of the right or left main stem bronchus distal to the injury (see below).

Disposition

Patients with fractures of the sternum or 3 or more ribs should be hospitalized, as should those in whom serious abnormalities are revealed on evaluation. Patients with suspected myocardial contusion should be hospitalized and monitored for arrhythmias. Although there is increasing evidence that patients with suspected myocardial contusion without hemodynamic instability, signs of heart failure, or sustained arrhythmias and without other injuries have a benign course, if a diagnosis of suspected myocardial contusion is made, the patient should be hospitalized. Without other indications for admission to an ICU and without sustained arrhythmias, patients may be admitted for observation to a step-down unit and offered a ward bed. In the absence of congestive heart failure, tamponade, pericardial friction rub, or electrocardiographic evidence of myocardial infarction, the diagnosis of suspected myocardial contusion is difficult to make with certainty in the emergency room. It frequently depends on ST–T changes or arrhythmias on the ECG or the presence of a murmur, all of which are nonspecific for myocardial contusion. Two-dimensional echocardiography along with serial CK-MB enzymes may be diagnostic but usually are not immediately available in the emergency department. Most such patients have no complications in the hospital. The course recommended is necessary at present for medicolegal reasons. Other patients should be referred to an outpatient clinic or their regular physician within 2–3 days.

EMERGENCY TREATMENT OF SPECIFIC INJURIES

RIB & STERNAL FRACTURES & COSTOCHONDRAL SEPARATIONS

Diagnosis

A. Symptoms and Signs: Rib fractures are best recognized by localized chest pain and tenderness that may worsen with movement or respiration.

Palpation over the site of fracture will reproduce the pain and will often produce an audible crunching sound as the rib ends ride over each other. Costochondral separations have symptoms and signs similar to those of rib fracture (tenderness is found over costochondral junctions).

B. X-Ray Examination: Obtain a chest x-ray to search for complications (eg, hemothorax or pneumothorax) and *not* to look specifically for rib fractures, since the chest x-ray is less sensitive than physical examination in this regard. X-rays may show no abnormalities in costochondral separations. (Calcified costochondral junctions in the elderly may show on x-ray.)

C. Associated Complications: Some chest wall fractures are commonly associated with serious visceral injury.

1. First and second ribs–The first and second ribs are rarely injured except by severe trauma; associated neurovascular injuries are common, and aortic arch arteriography should be considered.

2. Left lower ribs–Left lower rib injury is associated with splenic rupture in 20% of cases.

3. Right lower ribs–Right lower rib injury is associated with hepatic injury in 10% of patients.

4. Sternal fractures–Sternal fracture is commonly associated with myocardial contusion.

5. Multiple fractured ribs–Fractures of more than 3 ribs are associated with an increased incidence of lung contusion (although contusion may occur without rib fractures, especially in the young). Atelectasis and pneumonia may follow, because pain causes hypoventilation and inadequate coughing.

6. Open fractures–Visceral injury is common with open fractures, since significant force is required to produce an open fracture; operative debridement is required (Chapter 22).

Treatment

Caution: Do not tape the chest to reduce pain, since this predisposes to atelectasis and pneumonia. Give adequate analgesia (codeine or morphine if required). Encourage coughing and deep breathing to prevent atelectasis. An incentive spirometer may be helpful.

Disposition

A. Patients with any of the following conditions should be hospitalized: fractures of multiple ribs, fractures of the first and second ribs, suspected visceral injury (splenic or liver lacerations, etc), sternal fractures, or antecedent physiologically significant chronic pulmonary disease (increased risk of respiratory failure and pneumonia, even from seemingly minor chest injuries). If parenteral analgesics are required for adequate pain relief, the patient should be hospitalized.

B. Patients with fractures of 1–3 ribs without chronic pulmonary disease and without suspected visceral injury may be discharged. Provide analgesia and instructions to prevent atelectasis (eg, coughing, deep breathing, incentive spirometer). A follow-up appointment should be arranged within a few days in most cases.

FLAIL CHEST

Diagnosis

When many ribs are fractured, especially at multiple sites, a portion of the chest wall may become mechanically unstable. When negative intrathoracic pressure is developed during inspiration, the unstable (flail) segment moves inward and markedly reduces tidal volume. This paradoxical movement of the flail segment on respiration (inward movement with inspiration) is due to instability of all or a portion of the chest.

Surprisingly, there may be few or no associated injuries of the intrathoracic or abdominal viscera.

Clinical findings include pain and other symptoms and signs of multiple rib fractures. Dyspnea or respiratory distress is present to some degree. Frank respiratory failure may occur if the flail segment is large. With marked flail chest, the patient may initially be able to compensate for reduced tidal volume by hyperventilating; therefore, the patient's respiratory status may be satisfactory when the patient is first seen in the emergency department. When fatigue develops, however, respiratory failure may supervene.

Treatment

Provide supplemental oxygen delivered by a bag-mask combination initially. Approximately 50% of patients will require immediate endotracheal intubation. Monitor ventilatory function with arterial blood gas measurements. Provide analgesia (eg, intravenous morphine in increments of 1–4 mg). Morphine relieves anxiety as well. External chest wall supports (taping, rib tongs, etc) are not indicated and may be harmful. Many patients can be treated with continuous epidural analgesia and will not require ventilator management.

Disposition

Hospitalization in an intensive care unit is required in every case. The need for prolonged assisted ventilation should be assessed in that setting.

PNEUMOTHORAX
(Including Tension Pneumothorax)

Either blunt or penetrating chest trauma may cause pneumothorax, as may penetrating abdominal injuries that cross the diaphragm. Pneumothorax may result from chest wall injury that allows air to enter the pleural space (see Open Pneumothorax, below) or, more commonly, from lung injury. If injury allows air to enter the pleural space on inspiration but not to escape on expiration, tension pneumothorax results.

Uncomplicated unilateral pneumothorax, even with complete collapse of one lung, is not an immediate threat to life in an otherwise healthy individual, although the patient may be quite uncomfortable. Oxygen and carbon dioxide exchange remains relatively unimpaired. In a patient with severe preexisting chronic lung disease, however, unilateral simple pneumothorax may be life-threatening.

Tension pneumothorax may be rapidly fatal. Rising intrathoracic pressure impedes venous return, and hypotension and shock ensue. *Thus, death from tension pneumothorax results both from circulatory compromise as well as from lung collapse and ventilatory failure.*

Diagnosis

Pneumothorax is characterized by sudden chest pain that may be referred to the shoulder and is associated with dyspnea. Hyperresonance, decreased chest motion, and decreased breath and voice sounds are noted on the involved side. Chest x-ray shows air in the pleural space that may or may not be under increased pressure. Shift of the trachea and mediastinum away from the involved side occurs in some but not all cases of tension pneumothorax. Hypotension or shock may be present and requires evaluation for possible blood loss.

Treatment

A. Respiratory Support: Provide respiratory support with assisted ventilation and supplemental oxygen if necessary. Monitor arterial blood gases.

B. Tension Pneumothorax: Perform thoracostomy *at once* through an anterior axillary line incision in the fourth or fifth intercostal space (Chapter 46). *Note:* A high anterior thoracostomy (eg, first or second intercostal space in the midclavicular line) is not recommended. If a chest tube is not immediately available, use a large-bore (≥ 16-gauge) needle. Alternatively, if tension pneumothorax is present, make an incision in the skin and intercostal muscles with a scalpel, and decompress the pleural space by inserting a finger or a clamp. If a penetrating wound is already present, it may be held open with a finger or a clamp to relieve the pressure. Definitive tube thoracostomy should be done as soon as possible.

C. Simple Pneumothorax: Confirm the diagnosis by chest x-ray. Perform tube thoracostomy as soon as possible. Recently, simple, uncomplicated pneumothoraces have been shown to be successfully treated in many cases by catheter aspiration. The patient is then observed in the emergency department for 6 hours. If reexpansion is maintained on follow-up chest x-ray, the patient may be discharged. However, patients who require surgery for other injuries, are unstable, or require monitoring or ventilatory support should receive a tube thoracostomy.

Disposition

Hospitalize all patients with traumatic pneumothorax unless they have simple, uncomplicated pneumothoraces successfully treated by catheter aspiration.

OPEN PNEUMOTHORAX ("Sucking Chest Wound")

Diagnosis

Large penetrating injuries of the thorax result in immediate pneumothorax on the affected side. Patients are in respiratory distress and have an obvious chest wound through which air moves on respiration. With smaller wounds, a valvelike effect may allow entry of air on inspiration but not exit on expiration. The result is rapidly progressive tension pneumothorax. Hemothorax is commonly associated with traumatic open pneumothorax.

Treatment

A. Relieve possible tension pneumothorax by opening small wounds with a gloved finger or a clamp. The outward rush of air relieves the tension. Cover the wound with an occlusive dressing (eg, petrolatum gauze) taped on 3 sides to temporarily seal the wound and prevent further development of tension pneumothorax.

B. Support respiration with assisted ventilation (if required) and supplemental oxygen. Perform tube thoracostomy through the fifth or sixth intercostal space in the midaxillary line as quickly as possible (Chapter 46).

C. Evaluate for blood loss, and begin volume replacement. Hypotension persisting after relief of tension pneumothorax suggests hypovolemia. If there is coexisting hemothorax of 1 L or more, consider autotransfusion (Chapter 46).

Disposition

Hospitalization is required in all cases.

HEMOTHORAX

Diagnosis

Injury to the chest wall, great vessels, or lung from penetrating (or less commonly, blunt) trauma may result in intrapleural bleeding or hemothorax. Some degree of pneumothorax is usually present as well. In addition to the findings associated with pneumothorax, fluid is found on chest examination or on x-ray. Depending on the amount of blood lost, hypotension or shock may be present.

Treatment

A. Perform tube thoracostomy in the midaxillary line in the fourth or fifth intercostal space (Chapter 46). Removal of blood and clot in the pleural space often coapts the edges of the pleura and slows blood loss.

B. Insert 2 large-bore (≥ 16-gauge) intravenous lines, preferably including one venous cutdown. Draw blood for CBC, and send clotted blood for typing and cross-matching of 8 units of whole blood.

Begin fluid replacement with intravenous infusion of crystalloid solution to rapidly restore and maintain adequate blood pressure (Chapter 3).

C. Autotransfusion of blood removed from the pleural space (Chapter 46) should be considered if there is 1 L or more of blood in the pleural space and if ipsilateral gastrointestinal tract injury can be ruled out (contiguous gastrointestinal tract injury may contaminate pleural blood). If autotransfusion is performed, the blood should be collected in anticoagulant and re-administered through a blood filter. All emergency departments that care for patients with major trauma should have an autotransfusion device ready for use.

Disposition

Hospitalize all patients. Initial blood loss in the pleura of more than 1–1.5 L or continued blood loss (> 250 mL/h) after chest tube replacement requires surgery.

AIR EMBOLISM

Diagnosis

A. Left-sided or Systemic Air Embolism: Air embolism occurs when trauma creates communication between pulmonary veins and lung airways. When airway pressures exceed venous pressures, air is forced into the pulmonary venous system, where it is "embolized" into the systemic arterial tree. Air embolization occurs most often after penetrating trauma, but it may occur after blunt trauma and has occurred spontaneously in scuba divers breathing pressurized gas mixtures.

Accurate diagnosis is difficult, but air embolism should be suspected if any of the following is present in the patient with chest trauma:

(1) Focal neurologic abnormalities in the absence of head trauma.

(2) Air bubbles in retinal vessels on funduscopic examination.

(3) Cardiovascular collapse shortly after institution of positive pressure ventilation.

(4) Air or froth in arterial blood gases not due to technical error in laboratory handling (air embolization of this degree is usually fatal).

B. Right-Sided or Pulmonary Air Embolism: Iatrogenic air embolism to the pulmonary circulation and right side of the heart may occur during catheterization of central veins if the catheter lumen is not kept occluded. Air embolism to the right side of the heart may be minimized by performing venipuncture and catheter insertion with the patient in the reversed Trendelenburg (head-down) position and by having the patient perform a Valsalva maneuver during catheter insertion. Air embolism is most likely to occur after the sheath is inserted into the subclavian or internal jugular vein during the insertion or changing of catheters or pacemaker leads.

Treatment

Administer 100% oxygen (rebreathing mask or endotracheal tube). Support circulation with intravenous infusion of crystalloid solution. If cardiovascular collapse occurs, the patient should be placed in Trendelenburg in the left lateral decubitus position if air embolism is right-sided. If it is left-sided, immediate thoracotomy on the side of air entry with clamping on the hilum of the lung may be lifesaving.

Disposition

Hospitalize the patient at once.

RUPTURED TRACHEOBRONCHIAL TREE

Diagnosis

Rupture of the structures of the tracheobronchial tree occurs primarily as a result of severe blunt trauma and less commonly from penetrating trauma. Compressive shear forces generated in such trauma break the large airways, most commonly at the distal trachea or proximal main stem bronchi.

Clinical findings include respiratory distress, pneumomediastinum, subcutaneous emphysema, and often pneumothorax. Hemoptysis is common. Suspect rupture of structures of the tracheobronchial tree when there is a large persistent air leak after tube thoracostomy or if hypercapnia persists despite adequate ventilation. Disruption of the tracheobronchial tree is identified at bronchoscopy or surgery.

Treatment

Provide suction to keep the airway clear, and administer oxygen, 5–10 L/min, by mask or nasal prongs. Treat associated pneumothorax, if present, with tube thoracostomy, and perform bronchoscopy to identify the site of the tear. Intubate the airway *distal* to the disruption to maintain ventilation and reduce the air leak. Intubation may be attempted without prior bronchoscopy if a bronchoscopist is not immediately available.

Disposition

Hospitalize all cases for definitive surgical repair.

PULMONARY CONTUSION

Pulmonary contusion is a "bruise" of the lung underlying blunt chest trauma. It is often associated with rib fractures, although young people with flexible rib cages may not have associated fractures. It may also occur surrounding high-velocity bullet tracts.

Diagnosis

There are no specific clinical findings, although

chest pain, dyspnea, and pulmonary infiltrates on chest x-ray are common, and hypoxemia may be evident from arterial blood gas analysis. Pulmonary infiltrates may become more extensive for several days following injury but clear spontaneously without sequelae.

Treatment

Provide supplementary oxygen or ventilatory support as needed. Do not administer corticosteroids, diuretics, or salt-poor albumin, since their efficacy is unproved.

Disposition

Hospitalize the patient to provide respiratory support.

DIAPHRAGMATIC RUPTURE

Diaphragmatic rupture may occur from penetrating or blunt trauma of either the chest or the abdomen. Displacement of the abdominal viscera into the chest may occur, with serious sequelae.

Diagnosis

The diagnosis is not easily made, since about one-third of patients have a normal chest x-ray. However, misdiagnosis may have serious consequences, since diaphragmatic eventration may occur, with later displacement of viscera into the chest. Suspect diaphragmatic injury based on the location and trajectory of the injury. Borborygmi occasionally may be heard in the chest.

The x-ray commonly shows hemothorax, pneumothorax, elevated hemidiaphragm, and, at times, stomach or other bowel parts in the chest. The picture may be confused with that of pneumothorax; passage of a nasogastric tube helps confirm the diagnosis if the stomach is in the chest. Penetrating injuries to the lower chest or upper abdomen should increase the index of suspicion for possible diaphragmatic injury. A CT scan often is diagnostic.

Treatment

Treat associated injuries. Perform tube thoracostomy for hemothorax or pneumothorax (perforate the parietal pleura with a relatively blunt object, such as a finger, to avoid inserting the thoracostomy tube into displaced bowel). Insert a nasogastric tube, and connect it to suction.

Disposition

Hospitalize the patient for surgical repair of the rupture.

ESOPHAGEAL PERFORATION

The esophagus is well protected and is rarely injured by penetrating trauma and extremely rarely by blunt trauma. However, when injury does occur, clinical findings may not be apparent initially. Failure to detect esophageal perforation may result in life-threatening neck or mediastinal infection.

Diagnosis

Clinical findings depend on the location of injury. In cervical esophageal perforation, the patient will complain of difficulty in swallowing and pain on motion of the head. In thoracic esophageal perforation, there may be no symptoms initially. When findings are present, they may include pneumomediastinum, pneumothorax, pleural effusion, fever, and chest pain.

Definitive diagnosis is made by an esophagogram using water-soluble x-ray contrast medium, although about 30% of injuries will be missed with this test. Esophagoscopy should be considered if the esophagogram is negative and perforation is strongly suspected.

Treatment

A. Give morphine, 2–4 mg intravenously, for pain; the dose may be repeated.

B. Begin infusion of crystalloid solution through a large-bore ($\geq$16-gauge) intravenous cannula to support blood pressure.

C. Begin prophylactic intravenous antibiotics (penicillin, 200,000 units/kg/d; or clindamycin, 40 mg/kg/d).

D. Insert a nasogastric tube and connect to suction.

E. Perform tube thoracostomy if associated pneumothorax or pleural effusion is present.

F. Obtain urgent surgical consultation.

Disposition

Hospitalize the patient for surgical closure of the defect and antimicrobial therapy.

GREAT VESSEL INJURIES
(See also Chapter 32.)

Injury to intrathoracic large arteries or veins may occur from either penetrating or blunt trauma. Common sites of aortic injury from blunt trauma include the aortic root and the descending aorta at the origin of the ductus arteriosus and at the diaphragm. These injuries are fatal in a few minutes—only 15% of patients with thoracic aortic injuries reach the hospital alive—unless the defect is small or unless pressure by the surrounding tissue temporarily arrests bleeding. It is not uncommon for the aortic intima and media to be fractured circumferentially, with only the adventitia and surrounding mediastinal tissues serving to prevent fatal hemorrhage. In these cases, the patient may appear relatively well, yet failure to recognize and treat the vascular injury often results in exsanguination later.

Diagnosis

Note: One-third of cases have no visible external trauma to the chest.

Clinical findings include progressive hypotension and shock, hemothorax, mediastinal widening or obscuration of the shadow of the aortic arch, obliteration of the aortopulmonary window, deviation of the trachea or nasogastric tube, obscuration of the paratracheal stripe, fractures of the first or second rib or sternum, and left apical "cap" (fluid in the apical pleural space).

Aortography confirms the diagnosis in stable patients. CT scanning can fail to diagnose aortic rupture and should not be used in place of aortography.

Treatment & Disposition

A. Hospitalize the patient at once. Insert at least 2 large-bore (≥ 16-gauge) intravenous lines, of which at least one should be a venous cutdown. Draw blood for CBC, and send clotted blood for typing and cross-matching (reserve 12 units of whole blood). Begin rapid intravenous administration of crystalloid solution to restore and maintain blood pressure. Universal donor or type-specific blood may be required if initial bleeding is very brisk or if the hematocrit is low initially or drops rapidly with infusion of intravenous crystalloid solutions.

B. Drain hemothorax with tube thoracostomy, utilizing autotransfusion if there are no contraindications and the volume of blood in the chest is 1 L or more (Chapter 46).

C. Perform immediate thoracotomy for repair of vascular injury in the hemodynamically unstable patient. In the patient with stable vital signs and adequate blood pressure and perfusion, aortography must be performed before surgery to define the extent of injury.

CARDIAC TAMPONADE

Cardiac tamponade occurs when arterial, ventricular, or, rarely, atrial injury (almost always due to penetrating trauma) causes blood to leak into the pericardial sac. Because the pericardium is nondistensible, intrapericardial pressure gradually increases, resulting in increased resistance to diastolic filling of both ventricles, collapse of the right atrium, and, finally, a drop in cardiac output. Hypotension and then shock result.

Diagnosis

There is evidence of penetrating chest trauma or penetrating injury of the upper abdomen or back. Jugular venous distention occurs and is often massive. *Note: Remember that jugular venous distention will not occur in the presence of coexisting severe hypovolemia.* Progressive hypotension and shock are found. The cardiac silhouette is usually not enlarged on chest x-ray. If coronary artery laceration has occurred, an ECG may show myocardial infarction.

Treatment

A. Adequate fluid replacement with crystalloid solutions is imperative, since increasing venous pressure may temporarily sustain ventricular filling and may temporarily reverse the hemodynamic abnormalities in tamponade. Give 1–2 L of crystalloid solution intravenously over 15–30 minutes if severe hypotension or shock is present; otherwise, infuse at a rate of 200 mL/h.

B. Provide respiratory support as required, including supplemental oxygen (5–10 L/min).

C. Relieve tamponade. If the diagnosis is merely suspected or if the patient has stable blood pressure, the diagnosis may be confirmed and the pressure relieved by pericardiocentesis (Chapter 46); a small needle should *not* be used, since partially clotted blood in the pericardium may fail to pass through the needle, causing false-negative results on pericardial aspiration. Aspiration of nonclotting blood is diagnostic. With rapid, fresh bleeding, however, clotting may still occur. When time and resources permit, an echocardiogram is useful to confirm the diagnosis and guide needle placement. Cardiac tamponade may recur after needle aspiration.

In the patient with severe shock in whom tamponade is virtually assured, emergency left anterolateral thoracotomy and pericardiotomy should be performed in the emergency department to allow direct control of myocardial injury by the physician's finger. The patient can then be transferred to the operating room for surgical closure.

Disposition

Hospitalize the patient for definitive surgical repair.

MYOCARDIAL CONTUSION & LACERATION

Blunt chest trauma may cause myocardial injury varying from microscopic intramural bleeding to frank myocardial infarction. The consequences of this type of myocardial injury depend on the amount of myocardium involved and are identical to those of myocardial infarction: depressed cardiac output and arrhythmias immediately following injury, with cardiac rupture and ventricular aneurysms occurring as late complications. The stress of trauma may precipitate myocardial infarction in individuals with preexisting coronary artery disease.

Because the right ventricle is anterior and substernal, contusion of the right ventricle occurs frequently with and without left ventricular contusion. If the contusion is large, evidence of right ventricular failure can be present (elevation of jugular venous pressure, the systolic murmur of tricuspid insufficiency, and right-sided S_4 and S_3 sounds).

Although myocardial and coronary lacerations result chiefly from penetrating trauma, they may result from nonpenetrating trauma as well. Usually, when the forces of injury are severe enough to cause myocardial laceration, the tears are extensive and rapidly fatal. However, ventricular, atrial, or great vein lacerations with nonpenetrating trauma may occur and result in cardiac tamponade. Usually in these patients, cardiac tamponade is not relieved by needle aspiration or it rapidly recurs, and emergency thoracotomy is required.

Injuries to any of the cardiac valves may occur from penetrating and nonpenetrating trauma and may result in the classic murmurs of valvular insufficiency as well as in the clinical picture of acute valvular insufficiency. With nonpenetrating trauma, mitral insufficiency results from injury to or rupture of the papillary muscle. Aortic insufficiency is usually caused by tearing of an aortic cusp.

With acute aortic or mitral insufficiency, the patient usually presents with congestive heart failure or pulmonary edema. Remember that heart size in these patients may be only slightly enlarged, so that the cardiac silhouette on x-ray may seem normal despite the presence of pulmonary congestion or pulmonary edema. Marked elevation of left ventricular filling pressure as well as of left atrial and pulmonary artery pressures occurs with the sudden volume overload. The sudden elevation in pulmonary artery pressure may cause right ventricular failure. The suddenly dilated left ventricle contained within the relatively inelastic normal pericardium interferes with the filling of the right ventricle, thereby elevating right ventricular filling pressure.

In nonpenetrating injury, right-sided valvular insufficiency may occur, usually as a result of rupture of the right ventricular papillary muscle or (rarely) the tearing of the pulmonary cusps. The murmur of tricuspid insufficiency may be subtle. The murmur may be nonpansystolic, short, early, or late systolic, or may even be absent. If tricuspid insufficiency is severe, there is usually a large v wave visible in the neck veins.

With nonpenetrating injury, rupture of the ventricular septum may occur, usually resulting in a loud systolic murmur that occurs along the left sternal border or at the apex, depending on the site of rupture of the septum and the direction of the jet of blood. There is volume overload of the left ventricle, and pulmonary congestion and congestive heart failure usually occur as well.

Diagnosis

Clinical findings include chest pain (either from chest wall injury or myocardial ischemia), cardiac arrhythmias (both atrial and ventricular) as well as atrioventricular and bundle branch conduction blocks, and signs of myocardial muscle damage, eg, elevated CK-MB isoenzymes or elevated ST segments on the ECG. However, the ECG may be normal or show only nonspecific ST–T abnormalities. Heart failure or cardiogenic shock may be present but, in the absence of septal rupture or acute valvular regurgitation, is rare and indicates massive myocardial contusion. Third or fourth heart sounds or murmurs consistent with septal rupture or mitral insufficiency may be heard.

Two-dimensional echocardiography, which may be readily available, can demonstrate the presence and extent of wall motion abnormalities in the areas of myocardial contusion. Intravenous injection of agitated blood-saline mixture during 2-dimensional echocardiography introduces microbubbles that opacify the right atrium and ventricle and can detect the presence and site of intracardiac shunts. Radionuclide angiography with imaging of the right and left ventricals in multiple views can also show wall motion abnormalities but is less readily available in most emergency departments.

Treatment

Administer oxygen, 5 L/min, by mask or nasal prongs. Give analgesia (eg, morphine, 4 mg intravenously) immediately, and repeat as needed. Gain intravascular access. Treat arrhythmias, heart failure, or shock (Chapters 28 and 29), and provide continuous electrocardiographic monitoring. With severe aortic or mitral valvular regurgitation, intravenous nitroprusside can be started as a preload and afterload reducing agent at 10 µg/min and increased by 5–10 µg/min every 5 minutes until the desired effect is achieved or the blood pressure begins to fall. With acute mitral regurgitation, counterpulsation can be helpful.

Disposition

Hospitalize in a coronary care or intensive care unit with continuous cardiac monitoring.

As previously stated, the diagnosis of isolated myocardial contusion without hemodynamic instability and without electrocardiographic evidence of acute infarction, sustained arrhythmias, congestive heart failure, tamponade, or pericardial friction rub is difficult to make with certainty, and the subsequent course is benign in most cases. Hospitalization when a diagnosis of suspected myocardial contusion is made can be elsewhere than in the ICU and is required at present for medicolegal reasons.

TRAUMATIC ASPHYXIA

Diagnosis

Sustained crushing injury of the chest or abdomen causes venous hypertension of the upper body and face. Patients have a distinctive violaceous edema of the skin, often with cutaneous and subconjunctival hemorrhages and epistaxis. Other internal injuries are common, and signs should be carefully sought, especially clinical or laboratory findings suggesting cardiac injury. Chest x-ray is mandatory.

Treatment & Disposition

In the absence of other injuries, no specific therapy is required. Normal skin color gradually returns. Hospitalization for 1 or 2 days is advisable.

REFERENCES

Antunes MJ, Fernandes LE, Oliviera JM: Ventricular septal defects and arteriovenous fistulas with and without valvular lesions, resulting from penetrating injury of the heart and aorta. J Thorac Cardiovasc Surg 1988;95:902.

Baker CC, Thomas AN, Trunkey DD: The role of emergency room thoracotomy in trauma. Trauma 1980;20:848.

Baxter BT et al: Emergency department thoracotomy following injury: Critical determinants for patient survival. World J Surg 1988;12:671.

Bodai BI et al: Emergency thoracotomy in the management of trauma: A review. JAMA 1983;249:1891.

Cheitlin MD, Abbott JA: The internist's role in the recognition and management of cardiovascular trauma. Med Clin North Am 1979;63:201.

Demas C et al: The intra-aortic balloon pump as an adjunctive therapy for severe myocardial contusion. Am J Emerg Med 1987;5:499.

Demetiades D et al: Penetrating injuries of the diaphragm. Br J Surg 1988;75:824.

Dubrow TJ et al: Myocardial contusion in the stable patient: What level of care is appropriate? Surgery 1989;106:267.

Fabian TC et al: Myocardial contusion in blunt trauma: Clinical characteristics, means of diagnosis, and implications for patient management. J Trauma 1988;28:50.

Feliciano DV et al: Civilian trauma in the 1980s: A 1-year experience with 456 vascular and cardiac injuries. Ann Surg 1984;199:717.

Frazee RC et al: Objective evaluation of blunt cardiac trauma. J Trauma 1986;26:510.

Hiatt JR, Yeatman LA: The value of echocardiography in blunt chest trauma. J Trauma 1988;28:914.

Keller KD, Shatney CH: Creatine phosphokinase–MB assays in patients with suspected myocardial contusion: Diagnostic test or test of diagnosis? J Trauma 1988;28:58.

King RM et al: Cardiac contusion: A new diagnostic approach utilizing two-dimensional echocardiography. J Trauma 1983;23:610.

Kram HB et al: Diagnosis of traumatic thoracic aortic rupture: A 10-year retrospective analysis. Ann Thorac Surg 1989;47:282.

Lindenbaum GA et al: Value of creatine phosphokinase isoenzyme determinations in diagnosis of myocardial contusion. Ann Emerg Med 1988;17:885.

Marshall WG Jr, Bell JL, Kouchoukos NT: Penetrating cardiac trauma. J Trauma 1984;24:147.

Miller FB, Shumate CR, Richardson JD: Myocardial contusion: When can the diagnosis be eliminated? Arch Surg 1989;124:805.

Mirvis ST et al: Imaging diagnosis of traumatic aortic rupture: A review and experience at a major trauma center. Invest Radiol 1987;22:187.

Newman RJ, Jones IS: A prospective study of 413 consecutive car occupants with chest injuries. J Trauma 1984;24:129.

Potkin RT et al: Cardiac contusion: Evaluation of noninvasive tests of cardiac damage in suspected cardiac contusion. Circulation 1982;66:627.

Robbs JV, Baker LW: Cardiovascular trauma. Curr Probl Surg 1984;21:1.

Rosenbaum RC, Johnson GS: Posttraumatic cardiac dysfunction in assessment with radionuclide ventriculography. Radiology 1986;160:91.

Sturaitis M et al: Lack of significant long-term sequelae following myocardial contusion. Arch Intern Med 1986;146:1756.

Wojcik JB, Morgan AS: Sternal fractures: The natural history. Ann Emerg Med 1988;17:917.

Woodring JH, King JG: The potential effects of radiographic criteria to exclude aortography in patients with blunt chest trauma: Results of a study of 32 patients with proved aortic or brachiocephalic arterial injury. J Thorac Cardiovasc Surg 1989;97:456.

19

Abdominal Trauma

Donald D. Trunkey, MD

IMMEDIATE MANAGEMENT OF LIFE-THREATENING PROBLEMS (See algorithm.)

Assess Severity, & Give Immediate Necessary Care

A. Ensure Adequate Airway: Intubate if necessary (Chapter 46), and administer oxygen. The cervical spine should be immobilized if cervical spine injury is possible.

B. Assess Ventilation: Auscultate the chest for the presence of symmetric breath sounds. Look for flail segments and obvious chest wounds, and perform thoracostomy as indicated for pneumothorax (Chapter 18).

C. Assess Adequacy of Circulation: Palpate for the presence of pulses, look for signs of shock (Chapter 3), and stop gross external hemorrhage. If no pulses are present, insert 2 large-bore intravenous lines, and rapidly administer 1–2 L of crystalloid solution to restore perfusion. If rapid fluid administration fails to resuscitate the patient, perform emergency thoracotomy for open chest cardiac compression to relieve tamponade, and cross-clamp the aorta (Chapter 46).

D. Briefly Assess Neurologic Status: Check pupillary size and reactivity to light, and determine the level of responsiveness to stimuli.

E. Undress the Patient: Remove all clothing from the patient, and quickly examine the entire body for obvious injuries. Do not remove embedded penetrating objects, because they may be blocking injured blood vessels and thus serving a useful hemostatic function.

F. Begin Resuscitative Measures, and Obtain Vital Signs.

Treatment of Patients in Shock

Treat shock or impending shock (supine hypotension). (See Chapter 3 for more detailed discussion.) Briefly—

1. Place patient supine.

2. Insert 2 or more large-bore ($\geq$ 16-gauge) intravenous catheters or venous cutdowns.

3. Obtain blood for CBC, serum creatinine, electrolyte, and amylase measurements, and blood glucose determinations.

4. Type and cross-match for 6 units of whole blood.

5. Immediately begin a rapid infusion of crystalloid solution, and carefully monitor blood pressure. If more than 3 L of crystalloid solution is required to maintain adequate blood pressure in a trauma victim, cross-matched, type-specific, or universal donor

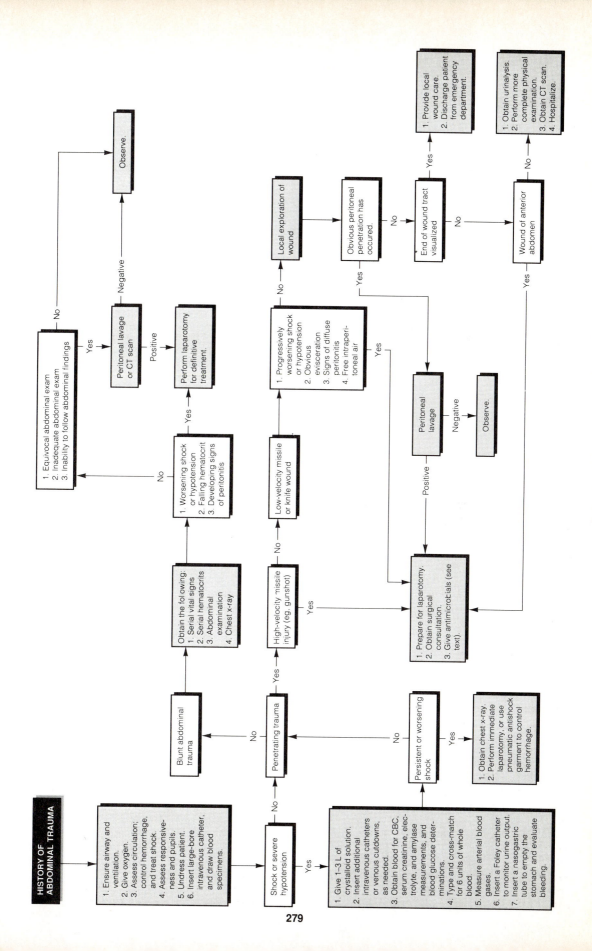

HISTORY OF
ABDOMINAL TRAUMA

1. Ensure airway and ventilation.
2. Give oxygen.
3. Assess circulation; control hemorrhage, and treat shock.
4. Assess responsiveness and pupils.
5. Undress patient.
6. Insert large-bore intravenous catheter, and draw blood specimens.

Shock or severe hypotension

Yes

1. Give 1–3 L of crystalloid solution.
2. Insert additional intravenous catheters or venous cutdowns, as needed.
3. Obtain blood for CBC, serum creatinine, electrolyte, and amylase measurements, and blood glucose determinations.
4. Type and cross-match for 6 units of whole blood.
5. Measure arterial blood gases.
6. Insert a Foley catheter to monitor urine output.
7. Insert a nasogastric tube to empty the stomach and evaluate bleeding.

Persistent or worsening shock

Yes

1. Obtain chest x-ray.
2. Perform immediate laparotomy, or use pneumatic antishock garment to control hemorrhage.

No

No

Penetrating trauma

Yes

High-velocity missile injury (eg, gunshot)

No

Low-velocity missile or knife wound

Yes

1. Progressively worsening shock or hypotension
2. Obvious evisceration
3. Signs of diffuse peritonitis
4. Free intraperitoneal air

No

Local exploration of wound

Obvious peritoneal penetration has occured.

No

End of wound tract visualized

Yes

1. Provide local wound care.
2. Discharge patient from emergency department.

No

Wound of anterior abdomen

No

1. Obtain urinalysis.
2. Perform more complete physical examination.
3. Obtain CT scan.
4. Hospitalize.

Yes

Yes

Peritoneal lavage

Positive

Negative

Observe.

1. Prepare for laparotomy.
2. Obtain surgical consultation.
3. Give antimicrobials (see text).

Yes

Blunt abdominal trauma

Obtain the following:
1. Serial vital signs
2. Serial hematocrits
3. Abdominal examination
4. Chest x-ray

No

1. Worsening shock or hypotension
2. Falling hematocrit
3. Developing signs of peritonitis

Yes

Peritoneal lavage or CT scan

Positive

Perform laparotomy for definitive treatment.

Negative

No

1. Equivocal abdominal exam
2. Inadequate abdominal exam
3. Inability to follow abdominal findings

Yes

No

Observe.

279

whole blood (in that order of preference) should be substituted and given at comparable rates of infusion.

6. Measure arterial blood gases: poor tissue perfusion will be reflected as metabolic acidosis and poor ventilation by hypoxemia and hypercapnia.

7. Insert a Foley catheter to monitor urine output if no contraindications exist (meatal bleeding, scrotal hematoma, or malpositioned prostate).

8. Insert a nasogastric tube to empty the stomach and evaluate bleeding.

Treatment of Patients Not in Shock

1. Place patient supine.

2. Insert one large-bore intravenous catheter.

3. Draw blood for CBC and amylase (obtain and hold specimens for blood typing and cross-matching, serum electrolytes, and creatinine).

4. Obtain a urine specimen (spontaneously voided).

Complete the Examination

In patients not in shock or in whom signs of shock regress with administration of intravenous fluids, a more complete evaluation is in order depending on the type of trauma.

Traumatic injury to the abdomen is often accompanied by other injuries. (See Chapter 4 for management of the patient with multiple injuries.) In most patients, a portable chest x-ray and anteroposterior view of the pelvis are indicated and should be obtained as soon as possible. If cervical spine injury is a possibility, obtain cervical spine x-rays as well. Patients who remain in shock should have an immediate exploratory laparotomy if no other source of blood loss can be promptly identified. If laparotomy cannot be performed promptly in a patient with persistent shock, a pneumatic antishock garment (eg, MAST) may preserve heart and brain perfusion for an hour or so until definitive surgery can be undertaken. Additional infusion of crystalloid solution or blood will also help sustain blood pressure.

EMERGENCY MANAGEMENT OF MAJOR TYPES OF ABDOMINAL INJURIES

PENETRATING ABDOMINAL TRAUMA

Classification & General Considerations

Penetrating abdominal wounds are classified as high-velocity or low-velocity. In civilian practice, penetrating abdominal injuries consist mostly of gunshot wounds and knife wounds. Penetrating wounds may occur also in the course of bomb attacks or in "freak" construction or industrial accidents.

A. Gunshot Wounds:

1. Rifle and handgun wounds–Bullets cause injury by a combination of penetration and local dissipation of kinetic energy. The amount of energy that the missile imparts to tissues largely determines the degree of injury. The kinetic energy of a missile equals its mass times the square of its velocity divided by twice the force of gravity. Therefore, small increments in velocity result in large increases in kinetic energy. Civilian handguns may achieve muzzle velocities of 152–609 meters per second (m/s) (500–2000 feet per second [f/s]), whereas the muzzle velocity of military and civilian rifles may exceed 914 m/s (3000 f/s). The amount of energy imparted to tissue is estimated as kinetic energy upon impact minus kinetic energy upon exit. To cause maximal injury, therefore, a bullet must dissipate all of its energy into the tissue, with no residual exit energy. For this reason, bullets may be designed to disintegrate upon impact, eg, soft-point and hollow-nose bullets. Disintegrating missiles fired at high muzzle velocity cause extensive tissue damage and may result in a temporary cavity 30 times the size of the entering bullet. Additional damage is caused by the yawing motion of the missile as it passes through tissue and by secondary missiles of bone or bullet fragments.

2. Shotgun wounds–Shotgun blasts cause devastating injuries, particularly at close range. Sherman and Parrish have classified shotgun wounds into 3 categories: type I, sustained at long range (> 6.4 meters [> 7 yards]); type II, sustained at close range (2.7–6.4 meters [3–7 yards]); and type III, sustained at very close range (< 2.7 meters [< 3 yards]). **Type I injuries** usually present as scatter types, and wounds from guns fired from a distance of more than 37 meters (40 yards) may not even penetrate visceral cavities. At 18.3 meters (20 yards), the probability of penetration is increased, but nonoperative management may still be warranted. **Type II injuries** usually involve damage to deep structures, and operation is required. **Type III wounds** are massive and associated with a high mortality rate (85–90%) despite aggressive operative management.

B. Knife Wounds, etc: Penetrating injuries caused by missiles entering at low velocity (arrows) or sharp instruments (knives, etc) cause injury by local tissue disruption in the track of the weapon. Therefore, the physician is often better able to predict the extent of internal injuries than is the case with gunshot wounds. The exceptions are penetrating injuries induced by sexual play; the patient may not give an accurate history, and entrance wounds within the vagina or rectum may be overlooked.

Note: If a penetrating missile enters the peritoneal cavity, surgery is indicated.

Diagnosis

See algorithm on p 279. The clinical findings depend on the type of weapon used, the organs injured, and the time elapsed from injury to hospitalization. No well-defined syndromes are associated with penetrating trauma of the abdomen other than hemorrhagic shock.

A. History: Obtain as much information as possible from the police, paramedics, the patient, or witnesses regarding the weapon used, the distance from which it was fired, the angle of entry, the amount of blood lost at the scene, and the time elapsed from injury to arrival at the emergency department. This information can be used to predict the type and severity of injuries.

Note: If possible, obtain information about allergies, drug use (prescription or illicit drugs, alcohol), and previous illnesses or injuries.

B. Physical Examination:

1. Verify adequacy of ventilation, and assess for shock. Check vital signs. Check for hypotension: weak and rapid pulse; cold, clammy skin; or pallor.

2. Completely examine all body surfaces, including the anus, rectal folds, and vagina, for penetrating injuries. Digital rectal examination should be performed in all patients unless there is an obvious perirectal wound. No attempt should be made to identify injuries as exit or entry wounds. The clinician is often in error, and a forensic pathologist is needed to make a more accurate determination.

3. Examine the abdomen for rigidity or involuntary guarding, which may signify serious visceral injuries.

4. Repeated examinations, accurately recorded, are helpful in evaluating patients who have minimal abdominal findings initially.

C. X-Ray and Laboratory Studies:

1. Chest x-ray–The chest x-ray is one of the most important tests in evaluating the victim of abdominal trauma. The chest x-ray will detect many associated intrathoracic injuries, and if performed with the patient in the upright position, it may show free peritoneal air below the diaphragm.

2. Blood tests–Obtain blood for CBC and typing and cross-matching. Measurements of serum electrolytes and amylase and tests of renal and hepatic function are often performed as well and may be helpful in subsequent management of seriously ill patients.

3. Arterial blood gas measurements and pH–Look for metabolic acidosis as an early clue to impending shock. Assess adequacy of ventilation.

4. Urinalysis–Hematuria indicates possible urologic injury, so that an emergency intravenous urogram, cystogram, or urethrogram may be required (Chapter 20).

Treatment

A. Supportive Care:

1. Ensure adequate ventilation, and administer supplemental oxygen.

2. Correct hypovolemia with intravenous infusion of crystalloid solution. Use whole blood (typed and cross-matched, if possible) when the hematocrit falls below 25% or if more than 3 L of crystalloid solution is required to maintain adequate blood pressure.

3. Type and cross-match for 6 units of whole blood.

4. Insert a Foley catheter to monitor urine output.

5. Insert a nasogastric tube connected to intermittent suction to drain stomach contents and to assess possible gastric injury.

6. Obvious evisceration should be temporarily managed by placing a sterile petrolatum-impregnated gauze bandage directly over the bowel and covering it with a sterile dressing. Attempts to reduce the bowel in the emergency department may cause further injury.

7. Antimicrobial prophylaxis should be started immediately if small or large bowel injury is suspected. Drugs active against both aerobic and anaerobic organisms are required. Some recommended regimens are set forth in Table 19–1; the author prefers either cefoxitin or clindamycin plus tobramycin.

B. Evaluation for Laparotomy: (See algorithm.) Almost all patients with penetrating abdominal injuries will require laparotomy. The decision to perform exploratory surgery can be based on the history and physical examination in most cases. *Caution:* Do not perform peritoneal lavage or contrast x-rays of the missile track, since these procedures are not helpful in determining the need for laparotomy.

1. Gunshot wounds–If the wound is over the abdomen, the missile is assumed to have entered the abdomen, and exploratory laparotomy is indicated. Very rarely, spent high-velocity missiles or low-velocity bullets (eg, air gun pellets) will not penetrate

Table 19–1. Antimicrobials for prevention of infection after penetrating abdominal trauma.

Drug	Dose
Cefoxitin	150 mg/kg/d intravenously in 4–6 divided doses.
Chloramphenicol	60 mg/kg/d intravenously.
Clindamycin[1] plus	40 mg/kg/d intravenously in 3 divided doses.
Tobramycin[2] or	5 mg/kg/d intravenously in 3 divided doses.
Gentamicin	5 mg/kg/d intravenously in 3 divided doses.
Penicillin (may be added to any of the above regimens for activity against enterococci)	200,000 units/kg/d intravenously in 4–6 divided doses.

[1]Metronidazole may be substituted for clindamycin. Give 15 mg/kg over 1 hour (loading dose), then 10 mg/kg every 8 hours. Penicillin (as above) must be combined with this regimen.

[2]A second- or third-generation cephalosporin (eg, cefuroxime, 75 mg/kg/d in 4 divided doses) may be substituted for the aminoglycoside.

the peritoneum. This can be confirmed by exploring the wound locally and thereby avoiding laparotomy.

2. Knife wounds–If peritoneal penetration is not obvious on inspection (eg, knife buried to the hilt in the abdomen) and the patient does not have signs of peritoneal inflammation, local exploration of the wound to determine if it is deep enough to have penetrated the peritoneum may be justified. If the posterior rectus sheath or deeper structures have been penetrated, laparotomy should be performed. Studies have found that a negative peritoneal lavage may be useful in identifying a subset of patients who may be treated nonoperatively with hospitalization and observation. Knife wounds of the back are less likely to perforate the peritoneum than are those of the anterior abdomen. Adjunctive diagnostic tests, including CT scan and arteriography, should be considered to determine the need for surgery.

Penetrating wounds to the thorax below the nipple line require an evaluation of the abdomen for diaphragmatic penetration. A peritoneal lavage with ≥ 5000 RBC/mL indicates the need for exploratory laparotomy.

Disposition

All patients with penetrating abdominal trauma must be hospitalized.

Laparotomy is indicated if peritoneal penetration is documented or strongly suspected based on an estimate of the missile tract, if hypovolemia or peritoneal signs are present initially or if they develop, or if peritoneal lavage is positive.

Patients with minor abdominal wounds, which fail to penetrate the posterior rectus sheath, may have their wounds treated and be discharged. All patients with gunshot wounds should be hospitalized.

BLUNT ABDOMINAL TRAUMA

Classification
(See Table 19–2.)

Blunt injury can be caused by direct impact, deceleration, rotary forces, or shear forces.

A. Direct Impact: Direct impact may cause significant injury. Severity of injury can be estimated by knowing the force and duration of impact, the mass of the patient, and the surface area of the point of contact. Common injuries resulting from direct impact include splenic rupture and liver fractures.

B. Deceleration: Deceleration injuries are most often associated with high-speed motor vehicle accidents and falls from heights. As the body impacts, the organs continue to move forward at decreasing velocity, tearing vessels and tissues from points of attachment. Common injuries include duodenal and aortic rupture.

C. Rotary Forces: Rotary forces also tend to

Table 19–2. Patterns of injury in blunt abdominal trauma.

Site of Primary Injury	Risk of Associated Injuries		
	High	Medium	Low
Right lower chest	Liver	Diaphragm Kidney	Gallbladder Right colon
Left lower chest	Spleen Diaphragm	Kidney Pancreas	Colon
Epigastrium	Duodenum Heart	Pancreas Liver Spleen	Colon Stomach
Pelvis	Bladder Urethra Uterus (third trimester)	Rectum Large arteries and veins Genitalia	Sigmoid colon Ureter
Abdominal wall	Small bowel Colon	Pancreas Duodenum	Stomach
Thoracic and lumbar spine	Kidney	Spleen Liver	Large arteries and veins Pancreas Duodenum

cause tearing injuries resulting from a tumbling type of action.

D. Shear Forces: Shear forces are common in degloving injuries or when the victim is run over by a heavy vehicle. In the latter instance, as the vehicle passes over the abdominal cavity, the skin and subcutaneous tissues are pushed forward, tearing nutrient blood vessels. Extensive soft tissue loss is common in such cases.

Diagnosis

Blunt abdominal trauma may produce serious injuries that are difficult to diagnose because of their insidious clinical manifestations. Three general modes of presentation of blunt abdominal trauma are described briefly below.

A. Symptoms and Signs:

1. Associated injuries syndrome–Most patients with abdominal trauma present with signs or symptoms of associated injuries: rib fractures, pelvic fractures, abdominal wall injuries, or fractures of the thoracic or lumbar spine. Symptoms of these associated injuries should arouse a suspicion that major intra-abdominal trauma has occurred (Table 19–2). For example, 20% of patients with fractures of the left lower ribs have ruptured spleens.

2. Hypotensive shock syndrome–Intra-abdominal injuries may present as unexplained hypotension or shock (Chapter 3). Hypovolemic shock may be the sole presenting sign of trauma to organs such as the spleen, liver, or kidneys. The most important rule to remember regarding blunt trauma is this: *If the patient has unexplained hypotension or shock and the chest x-ray is normal, intra-abdominal bleed-*

ing must be assumed until the contrary is proved by laparotomy, peritoneal lavage, or CT scan.

3. Peritonitis syndrome–Blunt abdominal trauma may present as peritonitis. Peritonitis implies that a hollow viscus has been disrupted or that the pancreas has been injured. Fever, tachycardia, diffuse abdominal pain and tenderness, and ileus are the commonest findings.

B. Evaluation:

1. History–Obtain as much information as possible from police, paramedical personnel, the patient, or witnesses. In evaluation of a patient who has been involved in a motor vehicle accident, a description of the patient's position in the vehicle, the presence or absence of passive or active restraints, the speed of the vehicle on impact, and details of extrication following the crash provide clues to the type and extent of injuries sustained. For example, if the patient is found behind the steering wheel and it is bent, significant blunt trauma to the upper abdomen and chest is likely to have occurred, and the physician should suspect duodenal, pancreatic, or cardiac injury (Table 19–2).

Note: If possible, inquire about allergies, drug usage (prescription or illicit drugs, alcohol), and previous injuries or illnesses.

2. Examination–

a. Measure vital signs, and—in the absence of signs of spinal injury—note whether there are orthostatic changes in blood pressure or pulse that suggest hypovolemia.

b. Examine all body surfaces for bruises or abrasions that may be due to blunt trauma.

c. Examine the abdomen for rigidity or involuntary guarding that would indicate serious visceral injury. Repeated examinations, accurately recorded, are helpful in evaluating patients with minimal abdominal findings initially. *Obtunded or intoxicated patients may have normal results on abdominal examination despite significant intra-abdominal injury.*

d. Insert a nasogastric tube to decompress the stomach and to determine if blood is present, which would indicate gastric injury.

e. Perform a rectal examination, and look for signs of anorectal injury and prostate malposition. Obtain a stool sample to test for occult blood.

f. In women, perform vaginal examination.

g. Examine the chest and pelvis for associated fractures.

h. Evaluate for genitourinary injury (Chapter 20). Briefly, if there is no apparent injury to the external genitalia, scrotal hematoma, prostate malposition, or meatal blood, attempt to pass a Foley catheter. If resistance is encountered, a urethrogram should be obtained before any further attempt is made to insert the catheter. Likewise, if obvious injury to the external genitalia has occurred, a urethrogram should be obtained first. If the catheter passes easily and hematuria is observed (either grossly or microscopically),

a biplane cystogram is then indicated in the stable patient, followed by excretory urography (Chapter 20).

C. X-Ray and Laboratory Studies:

1. Chest x-ray (preferably in the upright position) should be obtained to exclude injury to the lower chest.

2. Hematocrit (especially serial determinations) should be obtained. Send blood for typing and cross-matching.

3. Arterial blood gas measurements and pH determinations are helpful (acidosis indicates poor visceral perfusion due to shock).

4. Serum amylase is an insensitive and nonspecific test for pancreatic injury; however, a markedly elevated serum amylase level (3 times normal) may be a clue that significant intra-abdominal injury has occurred.

5. If the urine dipstick is positive for blood, a specimen should be sent for microscopic analysis. Persistent hematuria (> 50 RBC per high-power field) on urinalysis indicates genitourinary injuries and suggests the need for a cystogram and excretory urogram (Chapter 20).

6. Serum electrolyte determinations and tests of renal and hepatic function may be useful in the subsequent management of seriously ill patients.

D. Special Studies:

1. Peritoneal lavage–(See Chapter 46 for technique.) Lavage of the peritoneal cavity is used to determine if intraperitoneal bleeding or, less commonly, fecal soilage has occurred. It is reasonably sensitive and specific, although both false-positive and false-negative results do occur.

a. Indications–The following are indications for peritoneal lavage:

(1) Inability to adequately evaluate the abdomen (spinal cord trauma or altered mentation, alcohol or drug intoxication).

(2) Equivocal abdominal examination.

(3) Unexplained blood loss or hypotension.

(4) Selected cases of penetrating abdominal trauma.

(5) Low thoracic penetrating chest wounds.

(6) Patients who will be unavailable for close monitoring (eg, those undergoing special studies or those undergoing general anesthesia for other injuries).

b. Positive lavage–A lavage is considered positive if the effluent has one or more of the following characteristics:

(1) 10–15 mL gross blood on initial aspiration.

(2) Effluent hematocrit > 2%.

(3) RBC > 100,000/mL (unspun 50,000–100,000/mL is considered equivocal; 5000/mL in penetrating chest trauma).

(4) WBC > 500/mL (unspun).

(5) Bile, fecal material, or bacteria present on Gram's stain.

2. Gastrointestinal contrast studies–Esophagograms, upper gastrointestinal tract series, and enemas using a water-soluble contrast agent may be useful for patients with suspected visceral injuries (eg, stomach, duodenum, sigmoid colon).

3. CT scan—CT scan is very effective in detecting injuries to the liver, spleen, pancreas, and kidneys. The CT scan is probably the only useful noninvasive test for diagnosis of pancreatic injuries, and it is very helpful in disclosing retroperitoneal injury. However, CT scanning may miss hollow viscus injuries that would be detected by peritoneal lavage. It also requires 2–3 hours to complete compared with 30 minutes for lavage.

The CT scan should be utilized primarily in hemodynamically stable patients with equivocal symptoms or in those in whom the possibility of intra-abdominal injury is uncertain (eg, the unconscious or intoxicated patient). It should *not* be utilized for unstable patients or those with obvious intra-abdominal injury, in whom exploratory laparotomy will almost certainly be necessary; the delay associated with performing the CT scan may be fatal.

Treatment

A. Supportive Measures:

1. Ensure adequate ventilation, and administer supplemental oxygen at a rate of 5 L/min by mask or nasal prongs.

2. Correct hypovolemia with intravenous infusion of crystalloid solution. Follow with whole blood (typed and cross-matched, if possible) if the hematocrit falls below 25% or if more than 3 L of crystalloid solution is required for volume replacement.

3. Insert a Foley catheter to monitor urine output. Perform urethrography first if there are obvious injuries to the external genitalia or if resistance is met in passing the Foley catheter (Chapter 20).

4. Insert a nasogastric tube to drain the stomach contents.

5. Type and cross-match for 6 units of whole blood.

B. Evaluation for Laparotomy: Laparotomy should be performed as soon as possible if there is involuntary guarding of the abdomen due to peritonitis; if there is unexplained, persistent hypotension or falling hematocrit; or if abnormal results are obtained on special tests such as peritoneal lavage, CT scan, or upper gastrointestinal x-ray with a water-soluble contrast medium.

Laparotomy should be considered if the patient has persistent abdominal pain or involuntary guarding. Such patients should be hospitalized for observation or further diagnostic tests.

Disposition

Patients with minor blunt trauma to the abdomen with resolution of symptoms and no evidence of blood loss may be sent home with instructions to return if there are any recurrent symptoms, light-headedness, syncope, or sudden abdominal pain.

Hospitalization is mandatory for all other patients, including those with negative results of peritoneal lavage.

EMERGENCY MANAGEMENT OF SPECIFIC ABDOMINAL INJURIES

SPLENIC RUPTURE

Diagnosis

Rupture of the spleen is the commonest injury resulting from blunt abdominal trauma. It may also occur as a result of penetrating trauma to the left upper quadrant. In patients with pathologically enlarged spleens (eg, from infectious mononucleosis), splenic rupture may occur from relatively trivial injury. Delayed rupture of contained subcapsular hematoma can occur several days after splenic injury.

The principal manifestations of splenic rupture are abdominal pain (localized to the left upper quadrant but occasionally with radiation to the left shoulder) and shock or hypotension. Associated left lower rib fractures are frequent. Forty percent of patients with significant hemoperitoneum have no peritoneal signs.

The CT scan is a highly sensitive and specific test for detecting splenic injury; however, surgery should not be delayed for a CT scan in obvious cases.

Treatment

Treat shock with intravenous infusion of crystalloid solution followed by whole blood as soon as typing and cross-matching are done. Intravenous access should include at least one large-bore ($\geq$ 16-gauge) venous cutdown (Chapter 3).

Immediate laparotomy is necessary to control hemorrhage. Splenectomy is required in 40–50% of cases; in the remainder, surgical repair can save the spleen. Minor injuries to the spleen documented by a CT scan and with minimal blood loss can be managed nonoperatively. These patients require hospitalization, close observation, and a repeat CT scan in 8–12 hours.

Disposition

Hospitalize all patients with suspected or documented splenic rupture.

RENAL HEMATOMA OR LACERATION (See also Chapter 20.)

Hematuria is usually present, and evidence of flank contusion or penetrating injury may be present as well. Intravenous urography, CT scan with intravenous contrast medium, or renal angiography is helpful in confirming the diagnosis. Further management is outlined in Chapter 20.

LIVER INJURY

Blunt trauma may cause an intrahepatic hematoma or liver fracture. Penetrating trauma commonly causes lacerations.

Diagnosis

There may be no symptoms or only right upper quadrant pain and tenderness. Blood loss may be severe, leading to hypotension or shock. The CT scan is a sensitive and specific diagnostic test, but it should be reserved for investigation of hemodynamically stable patients with equivocal findings.

Treatment

Treat shock (as above and Chapter 3).

Immediate laparotomy is mandatory to control hemorrhage. Although some liver hematomas and lacerations will not require surgery to control bleeding, an aggressive operative approach produces a better overall outcome.

Disposition

Hospitalize all patients with liver injury.

GASTRIC INJURY

Diagnosis

The stomach is rarely injured by blunt trauma, but penetrating gastric injuries are common and are usually found in pairs (entry and exit wounds).

Treatment

Treat shock as outlined for splenic rupture (above), and institute nasogastric suction. Immediate laparotomy is necessary to control hemorrhage and reduce peritoneal soilage.

Antimicrobial prophylaxis is usually administered. A cephalosporin (eg, cefazolin, 50–70 mg/kg/d intramuscularly or intravenously in 2–3 divided doses) is commonly used, although other antibiotics are also satisfactory.

Disposition

Hospitalize all cases of gastric disruption (perforation, etc). Patients with intramural hematoma—if the condition is accurately diagnosed in the emergency department—need not be hospitalized if there is no gastric outlet obstruction.

DUODENAL TRAUMA

Diagnosis

Duodenal injuries may follow blunt or penetrating trauma. The diagnosis is often difficult, since early symptoms and signs may be minimal; the physician must be alert to the possibility of such injuries in appropriate circumstances. Perform an upper gastrointestinal tract x-ray series using water-soluble contrast medium in patients with a history of blunt epigastric trauma. Dye extravasation indicates rupture. CT scan is useful, especially when swallowed contrast medium is used.

Treatment

Treat shock as outlined above for splenic rupture, and institute nasogastric suction. Immediate laparotomy is necessary for patients with duodenal perforation; the mortality rate is nearly 100% if operation is delayed 24 hours or more.

Antimicrobial prophylaxis is usually given (see Gastric Injury, above).

Disposition

Hospitalize all patients with clinically demonstrable duodenal injury.

INTESTINAL TRAUMA

Diagnosis

The small intestine is the organ most commonly injured following penetrating abdominal trauma; injury is uncommon after blunt trauma. In contrast to colonic injury, peritonitis is often delayed and is associated with less obvious symptoms. Free air may be seen on plain films of the abdomen with the patient upright; however, there are *no* sensitive or specific diagnostic measures. Since only subtle findings may be noted initially, the physician must remain alert to the possibility of this diagnosis.

Treatment

Treat shock (as above and Chapter 3), and start antimicrobial prophylaxis (Table 19–1).

Immediate laparotomy is indicated to minimize peritoneal soilage and control hemorrhage.

Disposition

Hospitalize all patients with perforation of the small intestine.

COLONIC TRAUMA

Diagnosis

Injuries to the large bowel are more serious than those to the small bowel, because there are more intraluminal bacteria, the concentration of particulate matter is greater, and the blood supply to the organ is less abundant. In contrast to small bowel injury, colonic injury usually causes obvious peritonitis of rapid onset, unless the spillage is retroperitoneal. Colonic injury should be suspected in all cases of obvious penetrating wounds of the abdomen and in intrarectal injuries, often sustained during sexual play.

Treatment

Treat shock (as above and Chapter 3), and start antimicrobial prophylaxis (Table 19–1).

Immediate laparotomy is mandatory to control hemorrhage and reduce fecal soilage of the peritoneal cavity.

Disposition

Hospitalize all cases of colonic perforation.

PANCREATIC TRAUMA

Diagnosis

Injury to the pancreas is uncommon and difficult to diagnose, since symptoms and signs are nonspecific and may be minimal initially. Pancreatic trauma most commonly occurs following blunt trauma to the epigastrium in which the pancreas is crushed against the spine. Persistently elevated serum amylase levels suggest pancreatic trauma, but this sign is not always present. CT scan is the most sensitive noninvasive diagnostic procedure.

Treatment

Treat shock (as above and Chapter 3).

Immediate laparotomy is mandatory for debridement. The mortality rate increases linearly with time if operation is delayed and is 80% after 24 hours if injury to the pancreatic ducts has occurred.

Disposition

Hospitalize all patients with clinically evident pancreatic trauma, since serious illness may occur.

REFERENCES

Blaisdell FW, Trunkey DD: *Abdominal Trauma*. Vol 1 of: *Trauma Management*. Thieme-Stratton, 1982.

Cogbill TH et al: Severe hepatic trauma: A multi-center experience with 1335 liver injuries. J Trauma 1988;28:1433.

Daum GS et al: Dipstick evaluation of hematuria in abdominal trauma. Am J Clin Pathol 1988;89:538.

Demetriades D et al: Penetrating injuries of the diaphragm. Br J Surg 1988;75:824.

Fabian TC et al: A prospective study of 91 patients undergoing both computed tomography and peritoneal lavage following blunt abdominal trauma. J Trauma 1986;26:602.

Fischer RP, Miller-Crochett P, Reed RL II: Gastrointestinal disruption: The hazard of nonoperative management in adults with blunt trauma. J Trauma 1988;28:1445.

Freeark RJ: Blunt torso trauma. Surg Clin North Am 1977;57:1317.

Gomez GA et al: Diagnostic peritoneal lavage in the management of blunt abdominal trauma: A reassessment. J Trauma 1987;27:1.

Howell HS, Bartizal JF, Freeark RJ: Blunt trauma involving the colon and rectum. J Trauma 1976;16:624.

Kazarian KK et al: Stab wounds of the abdomen: An analysis of 500 patients. Arch Surg 1971;102:465.

Kearey PA Jr et al: Computed tomography and diagnostic peritoneal lavage in blunt abdominal trauma: Their combined role. Arch Surg 1989;124:344.

Klein S et al: Hematuria following blunt abdominal trauma: The utility of intravenous pyelography. Arch Surg 1988;123:1173.

Moore EE, Marx JA: Penetrating abdominal wounds: Rationale for exploratory laparotomy. JAMA 1985;253:2705.

Nance FC et al: Surgical judgment in the management of penetrating wounds of the abdomen: Experience with 2212 patients. Ann Surg 1974;179:639.

Nichols RL et al: Risk of infection after penetrating abdominal trauma. N Engl J Med 1984;311:1065.

Pearl RA et al: Splenic injury: A 5-year update with improved results and changing criteria for conservative management. J Pediatr Surg 1989;24:121.

Pelligra R, Sandberg EC: Control of intractable abdominal bleeding by external counterpressure. JAMA 1979;241:708.

Robertson HD et al: Management of rectal trauma. Surg Gynecol Obstet 1982;154:161.

Shorr RM et al: Selective management of abdominal stab wounds: Importance of the physical examination. Arch Surg 1988;123:1141.

Smego DR, Richardson JD, Flint LM: Determinants of outcome in pancreatic trauma. J Trauma 1985;25:771.

Sykes LN et al: Wound ballistics: An update. Contemp Surg 1986;29:23.

Trunkey DD et al: Management of pelvic fractures in blunt trauma injury. J Trauma 1974;14:912.

Weigelt JA, Kingman RG: Complications of negative laparotomy for trauma. Am J Surg 1988;156:544.

Genitourinary Trauma

20

Sharron L. Mee, MD, & Jack W. McAninch, MD

EMERGENCY DIAGNOSIS & MANAGEMENT

Urinary and genital injury occurs in 10–15% of all cases of abdominal trauma. Since injuries to other organ systems are often more obvious, the emergency department physician must be aware of the potential for urologic injuries and perform the appropriate diagnostic evaluations early. Clues to possible genitourinary tract injury include (1) obvious direct injury to the genitalia, (2) blunt or penetrating trauma near the genitourinary tract, (3) hematuria, (4) pelvic fracture, and (5) unsuccessful attempt to pass a urinary catheter. The physician must look for concurrent injuries elsewhere and treat them. (See Chapter 4.)

Immediate Treatment
A. Establish Airway: Intubate if necessary (Chapter 46).

B. Ensure Adequate Ventilation: Identify and treat pneumothorax and tension pneumothorax (Chapter 18). Provide oxygen at 6–10 L/min by mask or nasal cannula.

C. Assess Circulation: Control gross external hemorrhage, check vital signs, and assess for the presence of shock (Chapter 3).

D. Perform Brief Neurologic Examination: Check pupillary size and reactivity. Determine level of consciousness.

E. Begin Treatment for Shock, If Present:

1. Insert 2 or more large-bore ($\geq$ 16-gauge) intravenous catheters.

2. Rapidly administer 1–2 L crystalloid solution.

3. Obtain laboratory specimens for blood typing and cross-matching, complete blood count, serum electrolyte and amylase determinations, and arterial blood gas analysis.

4. Initiate cardiac monitoring.

5. Insert a nasogastric tube.

6. Inspect for signs of urethral injury (blood at the meatus, perineal hematoma, prostate displacement). If no signs of urethral injury are seen, insert a urinary catheter. If the catheter passes easily, obtain a urine sample and examine it for hematuria (urine dipstick test and microscopic urinalysis). If blood is present at the meatus or other signs of urethral injury exist, bladder catheterization should not be attempted until urethral injury is ruled out by retrograde urethrography. Further evaluation for injury to the kidneys, ureters, and bladder should be performed.

In the unstable patient with abdominal trauma, intravenous contrast medium (2 mL/kg) should be injected as soon as possible after insertion of intravenous catheters for x-ray diagnosis of renal or ureteral injury while the patient is still in the trauma unit.

A thorough history should be obtained, including a description of the cause of injury and, in cases of penetrating trauma, the type of weapon. High-velocity projectiles cause extensive tissue damage that may not be initially apparent.

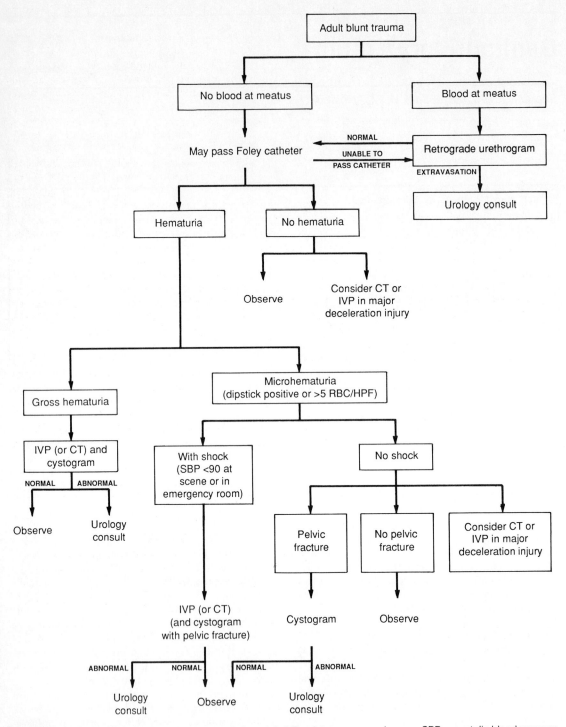

Figure 20–1. Algorithm for staging blunt trauma in the adult. IVP = intravenous pyelogram; SBP = systolic blood pressure. (Reproduced, with permission, from Tanagho EA, McAninch JW: *Smith's General Urology,* 13th ed. Appleton & Lange, 1992.)

A systematic physical examination provides information to guide further urologic evaluation. Fractures of the lower ribs are often associated with renal injuries and pelvic fractures with bladder and urethral injuries. Diffuse abdominal pain may indicate intraperitoneal bladder rupture or retroperitoneal hematoma. An abdominal bruit may suggest a renal vascular injury. Perineal hematoma, a dislocated prostate on rectal examination, and blood at the urethral meatus are associated with urethral injury. Scrotal contusions and hematomas require evaluation for possible testicular rupture.

Special Examinations

When injury to the genitourinary tract is suspected on the basis of history or physical examination, further diagnostic studies are required to establish the extent. Figs 20–1, 20–2, and 20–3 set forth recommended studies and indications for urologic consultation. In genitourinary system injuries, noted differences exist among adult blunt trauma, penetrating trauma, and pediatric blunt trauma.

A. Catheterization: Before placing a urethral catheter, the physician should carefully inspect the urethral meatus for blood. Blood at the meatus indicates urethral injury and requires analysis by retrograde urethrography. If no blood is present, a 16–18F catheter can be carefully passed into the bladder to obtain urine for analysis. Sterile technique and generous amounts of intraurethral lubricant should be used to prevent iatrogenic injury. Gross or microscopic hematuria indicates urologic trauma; however, the degree of hematuria does not correlate with the extent of injury.

Significance of hematuria: In the unstable patient, positive results for hemoglobin on the urine dipstick test require immediate urologic investigation even before results of formal microscopic urinalysis are available. However, not all adult patients sustaining blunt trauma require full imaging evaluation of the kidney (Fig 20–1). Mee et al (1989) have made the following recommendations based on findings in over 1000 blunt renal trauma injuries: patients with gross hematuria or microscopic hematuria with shock (systolic blood pressure < 90 mm Hg) should undergo radiographic assessment; patients with microscopic hematuria without shock need not. However, should physical examination or associated injuries prompt reasonable suspicion of a renal injury, renal imaging should be undertaken. This is especially true of patients with rapid deceleration trauma, who may have renal injury without the presence of hematuria.

All patients who sustain penetrating injuries and have more than 5 red blood cells per high-power field on microanalysis, positive hemoglobin on dipstick analysis, or injuries in a site that makes urinary injury likely should undergo full staging of the injury.

Pediatric patients with blunt trauma and more than 5 red blood cells per high-power field, positive hemoglobin on dipstick analysis, or a strong suspicion of injury should undergo complete staging (Fig 20–3).

B. Excretory Urography: In the unstable patient, 150 mL (2 mL/kg) of intravenous contrast me-

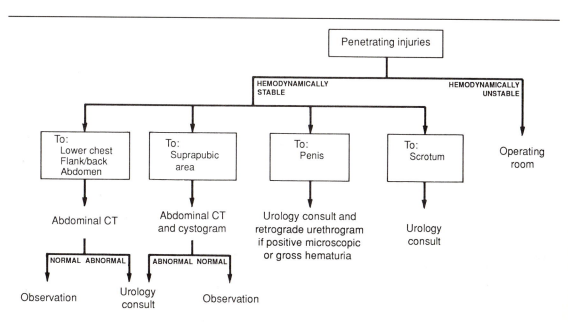

Figure 20–2. Algorithm for staging penetrating trauma in the adult. (Reproduced, with permission, from Tanagho EA, McAninch JW: *Smith's General Urology,* 13th ed. Appleton & Lange, 1992.)

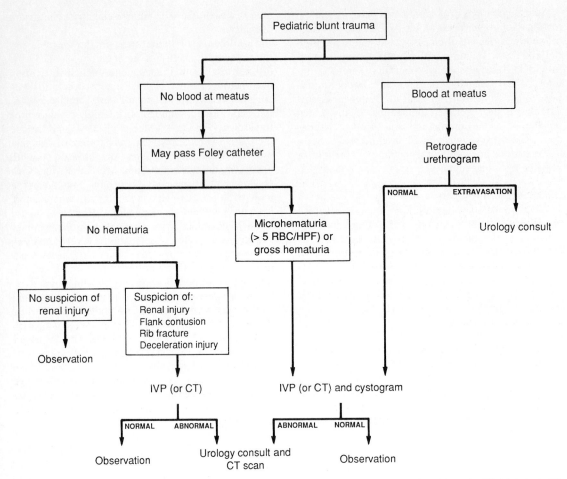

Figure 20–3. Algorithm for staging blunt trauma in children. (Reproduced, with permission, from Tanagho EA, McAninch JW: *Smith's General Urology,* 13th ed. Appleton & Lange, 1992.)

dium can be rapidly injected immediately after intravenous catheters have been inserted. Plain abdominal films permit visualization of the kidneys as well as any fractures of the ribs, vertebrae, or pelvis. Excretory urography provides valuable information about bilateral renal function and the extent of upper urinary tract injury and can be accomplished without undue delay before emergency surgery that might be required. Hemodynamically stable patients should undergo more deliberate and complete excretory urographic evaluation. Nephrotomograms may be obtained for more definitive diagnosis.

C. Retrograde Urethrography: When urethral injury is suspected (eg, scrotal hematoma, blood at the meatus, high-riding prostate), retrograde urethrography should be performed before any catheter is passed. A small (12F) balloon catheter can be inserted into the urethral meatus, 3 mL of water placed in the balloon to hold the catheter in place, and 20 mL of water-soluble contrast medium injected to outline the urethra. Extravasation of contrast medium into

the deep bulbar area indicates anterior urethral disruption, whereas retropubic extravasation is indicative of posterior urethral disruption.

D. Retrograde Cystography: Bladder evaluation is required in the presence of gross or microscopic hematuria associated with pelvic fractures or lower abdominal penetrating injury. Contrast material (300–350 mL) is instilled through a urethral catheter until the bladder is fully distended. A film is taken with the bladder full and a second drainage film obtained after complete emptying. These films will indicate intra- or extraperitoneal extravasation as well as the extent of the surrounding pelvic hematoma.

E. CT Scan: CT scans clearly demonstrate the extent and size of parenchymal lacerations and perirenal hematomas. They can detect urinary extravasation of contrast dye (Fig 20–4) and distinguish between major and minor injuries. CT scan is noninvasive and 3-dimensional and can accurately assess associated abdominal injury. It is particularly useful

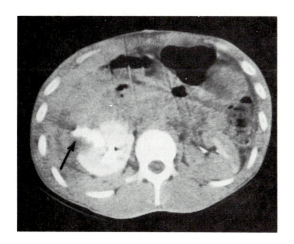

Figure 20–4. CT scan detects urinary extravasation of contrast dye (arrow), indicating laceration in right kidney following knife stab wound. CT scan also shows large right retroperitoneal hematoma (line). (Reproduced, with permission, from Tanagho EA, McAninch JW: *Smith's General Urology,* 13th ed. Appleton & Lange, 1992.)

for rapid diagnosis in patients with multiple injuries and for further urologic evaluation when excretory urography fails to provide definitive results.

F. Arteriography: Arteriography may help define suspected renal arterial injuries and parenchymal lacerations. In pelvic fractures, it is also useful to de-

tect and localize persistent bleeding that might result in embolization.

RENAL INJURIES

Renal injuries are the most common injuries of the urinary system. Although well protected by heavy lumbar muscles, ribs, vertebral bodies, and viscera, the kidneys have unusual mobility; consequently, parenchymal damage and vascular injuries due to stretch on the vessels easily occur (Fig 20–5). Minimal trauma may cause renal injury in kidneys with a preexisting pathologic condition such as tumor or hydronephrosis.

Blunt traumatic injuries caused by automobile accidents, falls, or blows to the abdomen account for 80% of renal injuries seen in urban hospitals and up to 95% of such injuries in rural hospitals. Rapid deceleration injuries sustained in high-speed vehicular collisions or falls can result in major renal vascular injury. Penetrating injuries, usually from gunshot or stab wounds, account for 20% of renal injuries in an urban setting. The extent of injury cannot be judged on the basis of hematuria or the appearance of the entrance or exit wound.

Microscopic or gross hematuria after abdominal trauma indicates urologic injury; however, gross hematuria may occur in minor renal trauma and mild hematuria in major trauma.

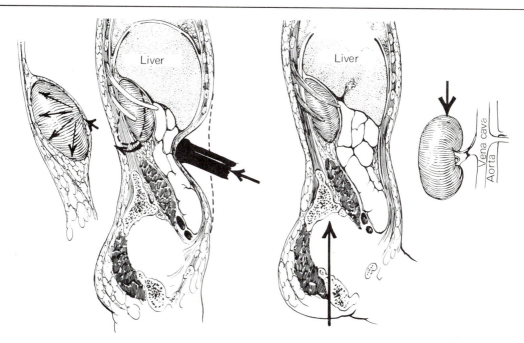

Figure 20–5. Mechanisms of renal injury. *Left:* Direct blow to abdomen. Smaller drawing shows force of blow radiating from the renal hilum. *Right:* Falling on buttocks from a height (contrecoup of kidney). Smaller drawing shows direction of force exerted upon the kidney from above. Tear of renal pedicle. (Reproduced, with permission, from Tanagho EA, McAninch JW: *Smith's General Urology,* 13th ed. Appleton & Lange, 1992.)

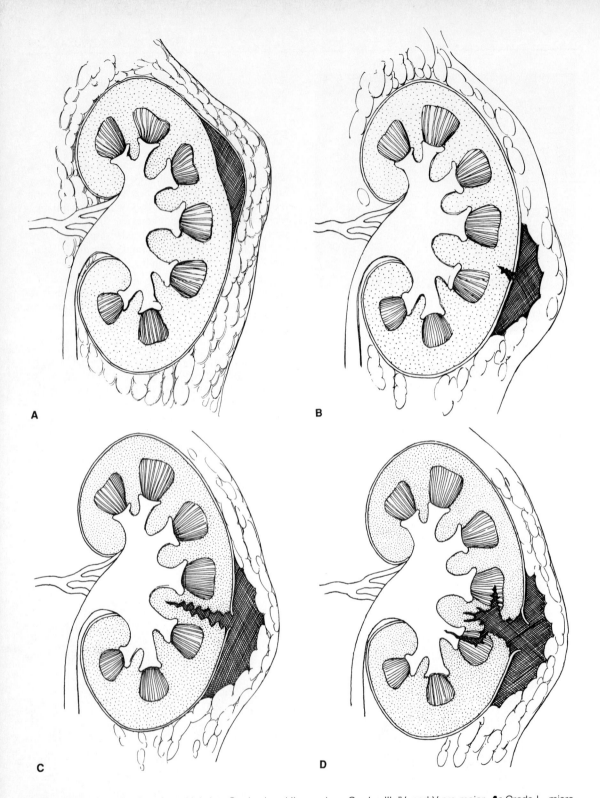

Figure 20–6. Classification of renal injuries. Grades I and II are minor. Grades III, IV, and V are major. **A:** Grade I—microscopic or gross hematuria; normal findings on radiographic studies; contusion or contained subcapsular hematoma without parenchymal laceration. **B:** Grade II—nonexpanding, confined perirenal hematoma or cortical laceration less than 1 cm deep without urinary extravasation. **C:** Grade III—parenchymal laceration extending less than 1 cm into the cortex without urinary extravasation. **D:** Grade IV—parenchymal laceration extending through the corticomedullary junction and into the collecting system. A laceration at a segmental vessel may also be present. **E:** Grade IV—thrombosis of a segmental renal artery without a parenchymal laceration. Note the corresponding parenchymal ischemia. **F:** Grade V—thrombosis of the main renal artery. The inset shows the intimal tear and distal thrombosis. **G:** Grade V—multiple major lacerations, resulting in a "shattered" kidney. **H:** Grade V—avulsion of the main renal artery and/or vein. (Reproduced, with permission, from Tanagho EA, McAninch JW: *Smith's General Urology,* 13th ed. Appleton & Lange, 1992.)

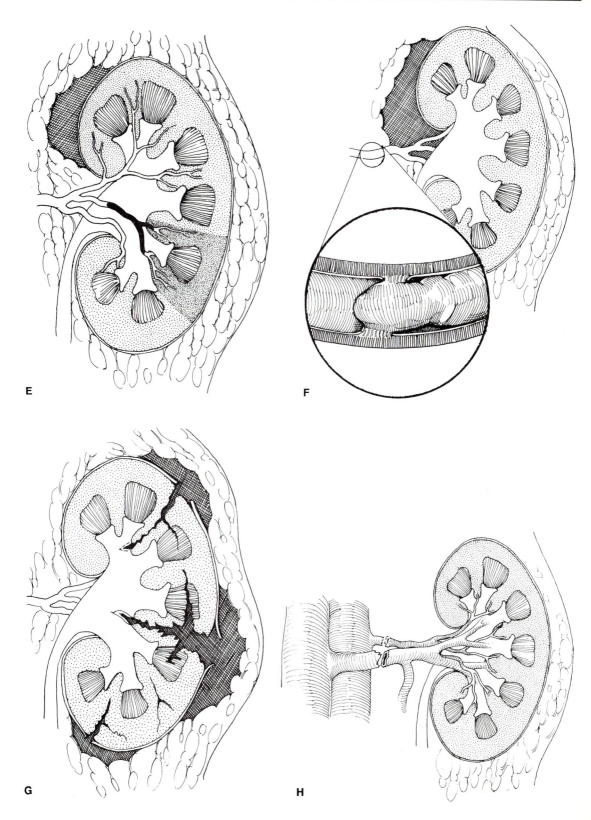

E

F

G

H

Figure 20–6. (*Cont.*)

Diagnosis

A. Symptoms and Signs: Pain may be localized to one flank or over the abdomen, but visceral injury or pelvic fracture may obscure symptoms of renal injury. Nausea and vomiting, flank ecchymosis, or lower rib fractures may be noted. There is usually visible evidence of abdominal trauma. Extensive blood loss and shock may result from retroperitoneal bleeding.

A palpable mass may indicate retroperitoneal hematoma or urinoma. If the retroperitoneum has been torn, hemoperitoneum will cause diffuse abdominal tenderness and ileus.

B. Laboratory Findings: Microscopic or gross hematuria is usually present in cases of significant blunt renal trauma but may be absent in vascular injuries caused by rapid deceleration or penetrating trauma. Serial hematocrit determinations should be obtained to assess ongoing retroperitoneal hemorrhage.

C. Staging and X-ray Findings: Staging of renal injury begins with excretory urography. Patients with gross or microscopic hematuria (> 5 red blood cells per high-power field or positive results on dipstick testing) and those thought to have renal injury should receive 150 mL (2 mL/kg) of intravenous contrast medium in addition to fluid administered for resuscitation (more hemodynamically stable patients can undergo routine study). Indications for study are clearly defined in algorithms (Figs 20–1, 20–2, and 20–3). The initial film after injection will not only identify bony fractures, free intraperitoneal air, and displaced bowel but also establish the presence or absence of both kidneys and define the renal outlines, the collecting systems, and the ureters. Nephrotomography is indicated when the urogram does not fully define the extent of injury. Adequate staging of 85% of renal injuries can be achieved by using excretory urography combined with tomography (Fig 20–6).

1. Minor renal trauma (85% of cases)–Renal contusions, subcapsular hematomas, and superficial cortical lacerations are considered minor trauma. These injuries usually lessen or delay excretion of contrast medium dye in the affected kidney.

2. Major renal trauma (15% of cases)–Deep corticomedullary lacerations may extend into the collecting system, resulting in extravasation of urine in the perirenal space. Large retroperitoneal and perinephric hematomas may accompany these deep lacerations. Extravasation of dye, an obscured renal outline, and a shift in the normal position and axis of the affected kidney are associated radiographic signs (Fig 20–7).

3. Vascular injuries (1% of all blunt trauma cases)–Vascular injuries include total avulsion of the renal artery and vein, partial avulsion of the segmental branches of these vessels, and main renal artery or segmental artery thrombosis without avulsion.

Lack of excretion of contrast medium on excretory urography suggests a main renal artery injury, severe

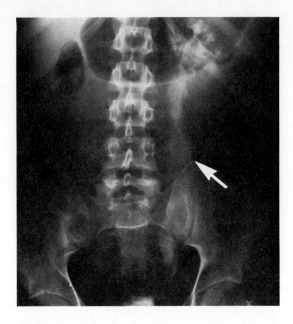

Figure 20–7. Blunt renal trauma to left kidney demonstrating extravasation (at arrow) on excretory urography. (Reproduced, with permission, from Tanagho EA, McAninch JW: *Smith's General Urology,* 13th ed. Appleton & Lange, 1992.)

contusion causing vascular spasm, or absence of the kidney. Further evaluation with CT scan or arteriography is required. Should the results of urography be abnormal or inconclusive and the patient stable, additional staging studies should be performed. CT scan provides excellent information regarding renal injuries: it defines the depth and extent of lacerations; demonstrates extravasation with great sensitivity; clearly depicts the size and extent of retroperitoneal hematoma; and detects arterial injury. Arteriography, which defines arterial injuries and renal lacerations, can be used when CT scan is unavailable or not definitive (Fig 20–8). Radionuclide renal scanning is used in staging renal trauma but is not readily available in the emergency setting and is not as sensitive as either CT scan or arteriography. Sonography at present is nonspecific and does not provide sufficient diagnostic information.

Treatment

Patients with microscopic hematuria and minor injuries (contusions and superficial parenchymal lacerations) defined by appropriate staging may be managed conservatively and discharged home with arrangements made for urologic follow-up care. Patients with gross hematuria and minor injuries should be hospitalized and placed at strict bed rest until the hematuria has resolved. Vascular injuries and major renal injuries associated with extensive extravasation or an expanding or pulsatile hematoma require operative intervention. Penetrating injuries from gunshot

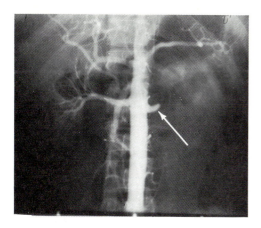

Figure 20–8. Arteriogram following blunt abdominal trauma shows typical findings of acute renal artery thrombosis (arrow) of left kidney. (Reproduced, with permission, from Tanagho EA, McAninch JW: *Smith's General Urology,* 13th ed. Appleton & Lange, 1992.)

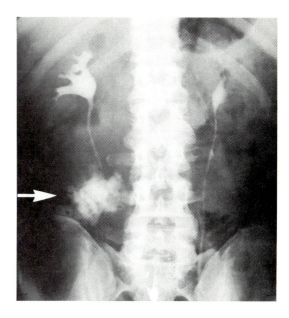

Figure 20–9. Stab wound of right ureter shows extravasation (arrow) on intravenous urogram. (Reproduced, with permission, from Tanagho EA, McAninch JW: *Smith's General Urology,* 13th ed. Appleton & Lange, 1992.)

and stab wounds require surgical exploration unless thorough evaluation (CT scan or arteriography) demonstrates only minor parenchymal injury without extravasation of contrast medium.

URETERAL INJURIES

The ureter is rarely injured. Gunshot and stab wounds are the most common cause of ureteral injury due to external trauma. Rapid deceleration injuries can avulse the ureter from the ureteropelvic junction. Complications arising from failure to recognize ureteral injury include urinomas, abscess, fistula formation, and hydronephrosis.

Diagnosis
A. Symptoms and Signs: Diagnosis of ureteral injury is made mainly on the basis of suspicion. Physical findings are nonspecific and are usually related to associated intra-abdominal injuries; microhematuria is present in 90% of cases. Gunshot wounds to the abdomen and stab wounds to the lumbar or flank area may cause ureteral injury, and they require diagnostic evaluation.

B. X-Ray Findings: Excretory urography should be performed whenever a penetrating injury occurs over the course of the ureter (Fig 20–9). Injection of 150 mL (2 mL/kg) of intravenous contrast medium during initial resuscitation efforts permits prompt visualization of the urinary tract. The urogram may only reveal faint extravasation of contrast medium, mild ureteral dilatation proximal to the injury, or mild hydronephrosis. When the results of urography are equivocal, a retrograde ureterogram should be obtained in the stable patient.

Treatment
All patients with suspected or documented ureteral injuries require urologic consultation. Prompt surgical exploration with ureteral repair is necessary.

BLADDER INJURIES

Rupture of the bladder most commonly occurs in association with blunt trauma and pelvic fracture (Fig 20–10). The bladder or urethra is ruptured in about 15% of pelvic fractures (usually due to automobile and pedestrian accidents). Extraperitoneal rupture (75%) is often due to perforation from bony fragments; intraperitoneal rupture (25%) may occur in the absence of pelvic fractures if the bladder is distended during a direct blow to the lower abdomen. Bladder rupture must be suspected in inebriated patients subjected to lower abdominal trauma, even if presenting symptoms are minimal.

Diagnosis
A. Symptoms and Signs: Pelvic fracture and gross hematuria will be present in over 90% of patients with rupture of the bladder. Hemodynamic instability is commonly due to extensive blood loss from disruption of pelvic vessels and associated injuries. Signs of an acute abdomen indicate intraperitoneal rupture. Evidence of lower abdominal injury resulting from gunshot or stab wounds should lead the physician to suspect bladder injury (Fig 20–1).

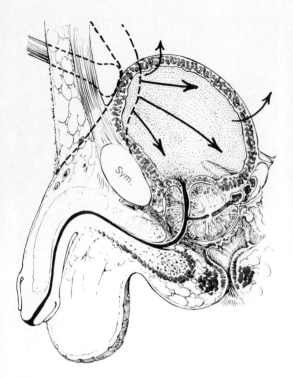

Figure 20–10. Mechanism of vesical injury. A direct blow over the full bladder causes increased intravesical pressure. If the bladder ruptures, it will usually rupture into the peritoneal cavity. (Reproduced, with permission, from Tanagho EA, McAninch JW: *Smith's General* Urology, 13th ed. Appleton & Lange, 1992.)

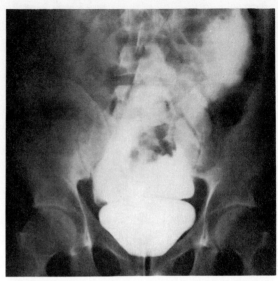

Figure 20–11. Cystography in a 26-year-old man who sustained a physical assault revealed gross intraperitoneal and extraperitoneal extravasation of contrast medium. (Reproduced, with permission, from Mee SL, McAninch JW, Federle MP: Computerized tomography in bladder rupture: Diagnostic limitations. J Urol 1987;137:207.)

B. Laboratory Findings: Obtain a urine sample by urethral catheterization unless there is blood at the urethral meatus. Bloody urethral discharge indicates urethral injury, in which case urethrography should be performed promptly. Examine the urine for blood; gross hematuria is common, microscopic hematuria less so. Urine should also be cultured for pathogenic organisms.

C. Imaging: A plain abdominal film demonstrates associated pelvic fractures. Retrograde cystography should then be performed in the presence of gross or microscopic hematuria associated with pelvic fracture or lower abdominal penetrating injury. Completely distend the bladder with 300–350 mL of contrast material, and obtain a film of the lower abdomen. After the bladder has been completely emptied, take a drainage film to demonstrate areas of extraperitoneal extravasation that may have been obscured on the filling film (15% of cases). When it is properly performed, this technique is nearly 100% accurate in detecting bladder rupture.

CT scan can detect bladder rupture through the presence of intraperitoneal fluid and extravasation of contrast dye from the bladder (Fig 20–11). However,

CT scan cannot reliably rule out bladder rupture in the absence of these findings.

An excretory urogram is indicated for all patients with trauma-induced hematuria, since abdominal trauma may have injured the kidneys and ureters as well as the bladder.

Treatment

Treat shock and hemorrhage first. Obtain urologic consultation when bladder rupture is suspected. Early operative repair with suprapubic drainage of the bladder is successful and associated with minimal complications.

URETHRAL INJURIES

Urethral injuries are uncommon and occur most often in men secondary to blunt trauma. Injuries to the posterior urethra are associated with pelvic fracture in 95% of cases. Trauma to the anterior urethra commonly occurs with straddle injuries. Stricture formation, impotence, incontinence, and chronic urinary tract infection are potential severe complications of urethral injuries.

Patients occasionally present to the emergency department with hematuria following the introduction of a foreign object into the urethra or following a urologic procedure performed during the previous several days (eg, transurethral prostatectomy, bladder

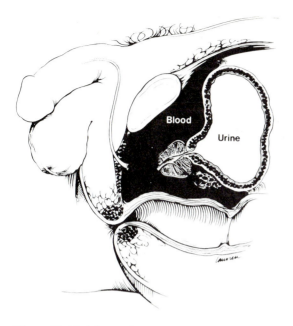

Figure 20–12. Injury to the posterior (membranous) urethra. The prostate has been avulsed from the membranous urethra secondary to fracture of the pelvis. Extravasation occurs above the triangular ligament and is periprostatic and perivesical. (Reproduced, with permission, from Tanagho EA, McAninch JW: *Smith's General Urology,* 13th ed. Appleton & Lange, 1992.)

mucosal biopsy). An accurate history of the event or procedure should be obtained so that the nature of the urinary tract injury can be anticipated. When hematuria follows the introduction of a foreign object, no attempt should be made to pass a urethral catheter until retrograde urethrography has been performed. Bleeding following a urologic procedure may respond to bladder irrigation through a 2-way urethral catheter. In both cases, urologic consultation is indicated.

1. POSTERIOR URETHRA

The posterior urethra, consisting of the prostatic and membranous portions, is most commonly injured during blunt trauma associated with pelvic fractures. The urethra is usually sheared off proximal to the urogenital diaphragm. The prostate is then displaced superiorly by the developing hematoma (Fig 20–12).

Diagnosis
A. Symptoms and Signs: The patient usually complains of inability to urinate and abdominal pain. Blood at the meatus is the most important sign of urethral injury. Retrograde urethrography is indicated before attempts to pass a catheter are made, since such attempts may convert a partial disruption to a complete disruption or cause infection of the periprostatic hematoma.

Suprapubic tenderness and pelvic fracture are noted on physical examination. Rectal examination may reveal superior displacement of the prostate and a large pelvic hematoma; however, superior prostatic displacement will not occur if the puboprostatic ligaments remain intact or if the disruption is complete.

B. X-Ray Findings: Extravasation of contrast material superior to the urogenital diaphragm on retrograde urethrography confirms the diagnosis of posterior urethral laceration (Fig 20–13).

Treatment
Obtain urologic consultation (Fig 20–1). Avoid urethral catheterization. Initial management should consist of suprapubic cystostomy to provide urinary drainage.

2. ANTERIOR URETHRA

The anterior urethra consists of the portion distal to the urogenital diaphragm. Lacerations and contusions can result from straddle injuries or instrumentation (Fig 20–14).

Diagnosis
A. Symptoms and Signs: The patient usually reports a fall and perineal pain. Sudden perineal swelling may have occurred after voiding. Blood at the meatus indicates urethral injury. If Buck's fascia remains intact, urinary extravasation will be confined to the penile shaft and perineum; with rupture of Buck's fascia, blood and urine may extend along the abdominal wall confined only by Scarpa's fascia. Rectal examination reveals a normal prostate.

B. X-Ray Findings: All suspected urethral injuries should be evaluated by retrograde urethrography, which will demonstrate the location and extent of injury.

Treatment
A. Contusions: If the patient can urinate without pain or bleeding, he may be discharged and treated at home with sitz baths. Urologic follow-up care within a week is advisable.

B. Laceration: Avoid catheterization. Bleeding in the perineum from the corpus spongiosum can usually be controlled with direct pressure over the site of injury. Obtain urologic consultation, and perform suprapubic cystostomy.

EXTERNAL GENITAL INJURIES

1. PENILE RUPTURE

Blunt trauma to the erect penis can rupture the tunica albuginea surrounding the corpora cavernosa.

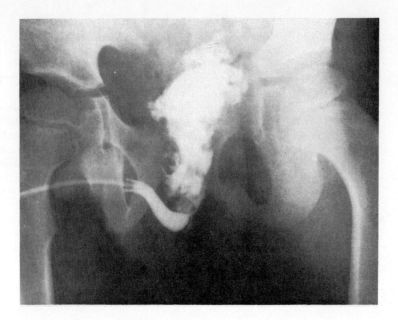

Figure 20–13. Ruptured prostatomembranous urethra shows free extravasation of contrast medium on urethrogram. No contrast medium is seen entering the prostatic urethra. (Reproduced, with permission, from Tanagho EA, McAninch JW: *Smith's General Urology,* 13th ed. Appleton & Lange, 1992.)

This uncommon injury requires immediate diagnosis and treatment.

Diagnosis

A. Symptoms and Signs: The patient usually reports a loud cracking sound while engaging in sexual intercourse; immediate detumescence and pain follow. A hematoma develops along the penile shaft. The axis of the penis may be deviated, and the fracture is occasionally palpable.

B. X-Ray Findings: Retrograde urethrography should be performed, since urethral laceration occurs in 20% of cases.

Treatment

Prompt surgical repair is required.

2. TESTICULAR TRAUMA

Blunt trauma to the scrotum may result in testicular rupture and in large hematoceles.

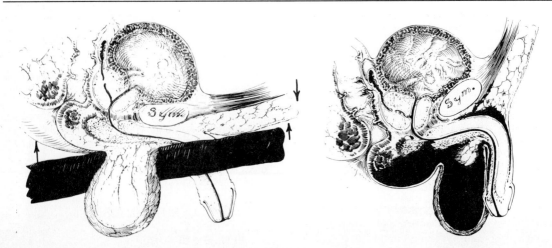

Figure 20–14. Injury to the bulbous urethra. *Left:* Mechanism: Usually a perineal blow or fall astride an object; crushing of urethra against inferior edge of pubic symphysis. *Right:* Extravasation of blood and urine enclosed within Colles' fascia. (Reproduced, with permission, from Tanagho EA, McAninch JW: *Smith's General Urology,* 13th ed. Appleton & Lange, 1992.)

Diagnosis

A. Symptoms and Signs: Pain and nausea and vomiting often accompany testicular injury. Scrotal ecchymosis and large hematomas may make testicular examination difficult.

B. Imaging: Sonography is highly sensitive in diagnosing testicular rupture. Testicular scanning may also suggest rupture, but it is more time-consuming and appears to be less reliable than sonography.

Treatment

Testicular rupture and penetrating injuries to the testicle should be surgically explored and repaired. If testicular rupture is ruled out, scrotal hematomas can be treated conservatively with elevation of the scrotum and sitz baths. Very large scrotal hematomas may require surgical drainage to minimize adverse effects.

3. GENITAL SKIN LOSS

Major skin loss to the penis and scrotum can occur from avulsion injuries, burns, and gunshot or stab wounds. Gangrene and urethral injury can be caused by obstructive rings placed at the base of the penis (during sexual play or as a punishment for enuresis in a child). Possible associated urethral damage should be investigated by urethrography. Superficial lacerations may be debrided and primarily repaired in the emergency department. Avulsion injuries or gangrene, however, require immediate surgical debridement and eventual reconstructive procedures.

REFERENCES

Emergency Diagnosis & Management

Breaux CW et al: The first two years' experience with major trauma at a pediatric trauma center. J Trauma 1990;30:37.

Carroll PR, McAninch JW: Staging of renal trauma. Urol Clin North Am 1989;16:193.

Grüssner R et al: Sonography versus peritoneal lavage in blunt abdominal trauma. J Trauma 1989;29:242.

Jacobs DG et al: Peritoneal lavage white count: A reassessment. J Trauma 1990;30:607.

Renal Injuries

Bretan PN Jr et al: Computerized tomographic staging of renal trauma: 85 consecutive cases. J Urol 1986;136:561.

Carroll PR et al: Renovascular trauma: Risk assessment, surgical management, and outcome. J Trauma 1990;30:547.

Cass AS: Renovascular injuries from external trauma: Diagnosis, treatment, and outcome. Urol Clin North Am 1989;16:213.

Hardeman SW et al: Urinary tract trauma: Identifying those patients who require radiological diagnostic studies. J Urol 1987;138:99.

McAninch JW, Carroll PR: Renal exploration after trauma: Indications and reconstructive techniques. Urol Clin North Am 1989;16:203.

Mee SL et al: Radiographic assessment of renal trauma: 10-year prospective study of patient selection. J Urol 1989;141:1095.

Moore EE et al: Organ injury scaling: Spleen, liver, and kidney. J Trauma 1989;29:1664.

Peterson NE: Complications of renal trauma. Urol Clin North Am 1989;16:221.

Peterson NE: Fate of functionless posttraumatic renal segment. Urology 1986;27:237.

Ureteral Injuries

Guerriero WG: Ureteral injury. Urol Clin North Am 1989;16:237.

Presti JC Jr, Carroll PR, McAninch JW: Ureteral and renal pelvic injuries from external trauma: Diagnosis and management. J Trauma 1989;29:370.

Rober PE, Smith JB, Pierce JM Jr: Gunshot injuries of the ureter. J Trauma 1990;30:83.

Bladder Injuries

Cass AS: Diagnostic studies in bladder rupture: Indications and techniques. Urol Clin North Am 1989;16:267.

Corriere JN Jr, Sandler CM: Mechanisms of injury, patterns of extravasation and management of extraperitoneal bladder rupture due to blunt trauma. J Urol 1988;139:43.

Mee SL, McAninch JW, Federle MP: Computerized tomography in bladder rupture: Diagnostic limitations. J Urol 1987;137:207.

Peters PC: Intraperitoneal rupture of the bladder. Urol Clin North Am 1989;16:279.

Urethral Injuries

Devine CJ Jr, Jordan GH, Devine PC: Primary realignment of the disrupted prostatomembranous urethra. Urol Clin North Am 1989;16:291.

Marshall FF: Endoscopic reconstruction of traumatic urethral transections. Urol Clin North Am 1989;16:313.

McAninch JW: Pubectomy in repair of membranous urethral stricture. Urol Clin North Am 1989;16:297.

Pierce JM Jr: Disruptions of the anterior urethra. Urol Clin North Am 1989;16:329.

Webster GD: Perineal repair of membranous urethral stricture. Urol Clin North Am 1989;16:303.

External Genital Injuries

Fournier GR Jr, Laing FC, McAninch JW: Scrotal ultrasonography in the management of testicular trauma. Urol Clin North Am 1989;16:377.

Jordon GH, Gilbert DA: Management of amputation injuries of the male genitalia. Urol Clin North Am 1989;16:359.

Kratzik CH et al: Has ultrasound influenced the therapy concept of blunt scrotal trauma? J Urol 1989;142:1243.

McAninch JW: Management of genital skin loss. Urol Clin North Am 1989;16:387.

McDougal WS: Scrotal reconstruction using thigh pedicle flaps. J Urol 1983;129:757.

Nicolaisen GS et al: Rupture of corpus cavernosum: Surgical management. J Urol 1983;130:917.

Vertebral Column & Spinal Cord Trauma

21

Henry M. Bartkowski, MD, PhD

IMMEDIATE MANAGEMENT OF THE PATIENT WITH SUSPECTED SPINAL INJURY

Suspect Spinal Cord Injury

People with blunt head injury or multiple injuries from blunt or penetrating trauma should be assumed to have cervical or thoracolumbar spine injuries until proved otherwise, unless they are fully alert and have no neck pain or palpable tenderness and no major injuries that might be distracting.

Immobilize Vertebral Spine

Immobilization of the vertebral spine is essential to prevent further injury to the spinal cord.

A. Supine Position: Optimal immobilization is obtained by placing the patient supine (face up) on a firm, flat surface (eg, rigid, long spine board) without a pillow and with lateral motion of the neck restricted by a rigid cervical collar (Philadelphia), lateral neck rolls connected with tape across the forehead, or traction. Traction is the most effective method and may be achieved immediately with a halter as shown in Fig 21–1. Skeletal traction with a 3-kg (7-lb) weight on a rope off the end of the bed provides the best means of emergency splinting and traction.

B. Lateral Position: If the patient cannot lie supine for any reason (eg, vomiting), the lateral position with the neck in neutral position is acceptable. The neutral position should be maintained throughout resuscitation procedures, physical examination, and x-ray evaluation by means of traction on the head, either by hand or with halter traction or tongs.

C. Technique for Moving the Patient: If the patient must be moved, the head should be held in traction in the neutral position and the head and trunk lifted or rolled as one unit (logroll).

Establish Airway, & Maintain Ventilation (See also Chapter 1.)

Airway obstruction may be manifested by gurgling or stertorous respirations, ineffective respiration (chest movement without movement of air), apnea, or cyanosis. High cervical cord transection (above C2 or C3) results in apnea due to intercostal muscle and diaphragmatic paralysis; cervical cord transection (above C6) or injury at a lower level may still result in respiratory failure because of intercostal muscle weakness or paralysis.

Note: Neck alignment and immobility must be maintained during attempts to establish adequate ventilation.

A. General Measures:

1. Using a tonsil tip sucker, clear mouth and upper airway of obvious foreign material.

2. Position the head in neutral position, avoiding motion of the cervical spine.

3. Insert nasal or oropharyngeal airway.

4. Provide supplemental oxygen, 10 L/min, by nasal prongs or mask if the patient is breathing, or support respiration with bag-mask combination (with supplemental oxygen) if hypoventilation is suspected.

5. Measure arterial blood gases as soon as possi-

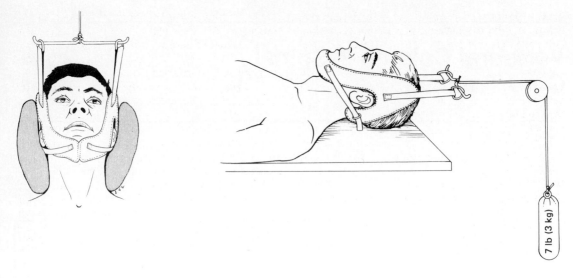

Figure 21–1. Halter traction.

ble to assess adequacy of ventilation, and monitor oxygen saturation using pulse oximetry, if available. Since intercostal muscles are often ineffective in patients with cervical spinal cord lesions in whom ventilatory efforts are provided by the diaphragm alone, such patients may tire easily, becoming progressively hypoxemic and hypercapnic. Repeated arterial blood gas measurements are therefore essential to monitor any changes in ventilatory status.

B. Endotracheal Intubation: If the measures described above fail to provide adequate ventilation or if hypoventilation or apnea is present, perform endotracheal intubation (Chapter 46). Endotracheal intubation should also be considered for airway control in the unconscious or obtunded patient with depressed gag and cough reflexes even if ventilation is adequate. If neck injury is accompanied by tracheal laceration, the trachea may be intubated directly through the wound.

Nasotracheal intubation is usually safer than orotracheal intubation in the patient with spinal injury, since the neck need not be extended. However, this method is technically more difficult. If nasotracheal intubation fails, orotracheal intubation with axial traction may be performed, preferably using a flexible fiberoptic bronchoscope to enable the tube to be passed into the trachea under direct vision. However, oral intubation, even with careful axial traction, allows significant subluxation in the injured cervical spine. Alternative means of intubation include nasotracheal intubation over a fiberoptic laryngoscope, "blind" orotracheal intubation using a lighted stylet, digital intubation, and retrograde intubation over a guide wire placed through the cricothyroid membrane (Chapter 2).

C. Cricothyrotomy: Rarely, in a patient with se-

vere craniofacial trauma who has distorted normal anatomic relationships, it may be impossible to establish an orotracheal or nasotracheal airway. Also, conventional means of intubation are sometimes unsuccessful in the otherwise normal patient. In such cases, direct intubation of the trachea through cricothyrotomy or tracheostomy is indicated (Chapter 46).

D. Suctioning of Secretions: Patients with weak intercostal or diaphragmatic muscles cannot produce a strong cough and are therefore predisposed to progressive airway obstruction without any change in neurologic deficit. Frequent suctioning should be performed. An endotracheal airway may be required for patients with voluminous secretions.

Treat Pneumothorax & Tension Pneumothorax

See Chapter 18.

Establish Satisfactory Circulation

A. Cardiac Arrest: If no pulse is detected, begin CPR (Chapter 1).

B. Shock or Hypotension: (See Chapter 3.) Shock (cool, pale skin; hypotension; abnormal mentation) or hypotension (systolic blood pressure < 90 mm Hg in an adult) may be due either to poor sympathetic tone below the level of the spinal cord lesion or to hypovolemia from other injuries. In most instances, hypovolemia is the cause.

1. Poor sympathetic tone–Keep the patient supine and horizontal. Blood pressure in the normovolemic patient with spinal injury is usually normal as long as the patient is supine, since minimal sympathetic tone is required in this position.

2. Hypovolemia–(See Chapter 3.) Insert 2 or more large-bore (≥ 16-gauge) intravenous catheters in an upper extremity; obtain blood for hematocrit, typing and cross-matching, electrolyte determinations, and renal function tests; and begin intravenous infusion of crystalloid solution to support blood pressure. Up to 3 L of crystalloid solution may be given before whole blood is required. *Caution:* Exercise care in fluid replacement, since patients with spinal cord injuries are at greater risk of heart failure than normal individuals.

If hypotension or shock is not quickly corrected by these methods, search for bleeding from other injuries (Chapter 4). Use of a pneumatic antishock (eg, MAST) garment for temporary control of hypotension is permissible, since its application does not significantly affect spinal cord function.

C. Normal Blood Pressure: Avoid excess fluid administration, which may increase spinal cord swelling or precipitate heart failure.

D. Hypertension: Although hypertension is rarely caused by spinal cord injury itself, the resulting bladder or bowel distention and subsequent autonomic discharge of the mass reflex may cause hypertension. More likely causes such as severe head injury or drug ingestion should be ruled out before hypertension is attributed to an injured spinal cord.

Minimize Neurologic Injury

A. Reduce Spinal Cord Swelling: Corticosteroids are useful in early treatment of spinal cord injury, but only if begun within the first 8 hours after injury. Give methylprednisolone, 30 mg/kg as an intravenous bolus, followed by a maintenance infusion of 5.4 mg/kg/h for 24 hours. Neurosurgical consultation should be obtained as soon as possible.

B. Give Antibiotics for Penetrating Injuries: Patients with penetrating spinal cord injury (eg, gunshot wound) should receive prophylactic antimicrobials. Nafcillin, 200 mg/kg/d intravenously in 4–6 divided doses, is widely recommended.

Treat Complications

A. Urinary Incontinence or Retention: Bladder dysfunction after spinal trauma may not be noted by the patient because of loss of sensation below the lesion. An indwelling catheter should be inserted in all cases of verified spinal trauma to prevent urinary retention and to aid in monitoring urine output.

B. Ileus: Paralytic ileus and gastric atony are common after spinal trauma. The patient should be given nothing by mouth, and a nasogastric tube should be inserted and connected to intermittent low-pressure suction.

Additional Measures

A patient with spinal cord injury is in need of the same resuscitative measures customarily employed in major trauma.

A. Insert an intravenous catheter, and administer fluids, blood, and nutrients as required.

B. Perform a baseline laboratory evaluation, including CBC with platelet estimate, coagulation panel, serum electrolyte concentrations, renal function tests, blood glucose concentration, and blood typing and cross-matching.

C. Treat other injuries. Evaluate and treat head injury and life-threatening conditions (eg, tension pneumothorax, cardiac tamponade, hemorrhagic shock) that take precedence over definitive treatment of vertebral and spinal cord trauma (Chapter 4). Maintain axial traction and skeletal stability during resuscitation and treatment. If feasible, obtain cervical spine x-rays (posteroanterior and lateral) when the patient's condition permits. Even if no fractures are apparent, the spine may be unstable due to severe ligamentous injury. Therefore, axial traction and skeletal alignment should be maintained if possible.

FURTHER EVALUATION OF THE PATIENT WITH SPINAL INJURY

History

Patients with spinal cord injuries can usually provide an accurate history of the injury, eg, auto collisions often result in cervical spine injuries that are frequently associated with head injuries; people who fall from heights often land on their feet and sustain fractures of the feet, hips, thoracolumbar spine, etc.

Complaints of back or neck pain should arouse a suspicion of spine injury. Stretching of the neck muscles, larynx, or esophagus in a hyperextension injury similar to whiplash may cause neck muscle pain and tenderness, hoarseness, or dysphagia. However, the absence of spinal pain does not eliminate the possibility of spinal injury, especially if the patient is under the influence of alcohol or other mind-altering drugs. Spinal injury should be considered in any patient with blunt head injury, a neurologic deficit anatomically consistent with a spinal level, or a penetrating injury to the neck, chest, or abdomen.

General Physical Examination

A brief general physical examination should precede specific assessment of neurologic function.

A. Obtain complete vital signs, including core temperature.

B. Carefully examine the head, chest, heart, abdomen, and extremities for other abnormalities. Remember that patients with spinal cord injuries may show few if any signs or symptoms of coexisting major injury because of anesthesia below the level of the lesion. Pain, guarding, rebound tenderness, and other signs may be absent despite the presence of fractured ribs, hemothorax, hemoperitoneum, peritonitis, and other major injuries. Examination of the genitals, rectum, and perineum may reveal priapism or abnormal rectal sphincter tone or perineal sensation suggestive of spinal cord injury. Diligent, repeated examinations and laboratory tests (eg, CBC with differential, peritoneal lavage) are necessary to detect unsuspected injury.

C. Gently but thoroughly examine the neck and spine for deformity, edema, ecchymosis, muscle spasm, or tenderness indicating possible vertebral fracture; a palpable defect in the posterior neck ligaments may be the only clue to major spinal injury.

Neurologic Examination

The emergency department neurologic examination for spinal trauma must be more thorough than that for head injury, although repetition and consistency in format and procedure are still important. Neurologic examination assesses the following functions:

A. Mentation: The spectrum of mentation includes all levels of consciousness ranging from alert to comatose.

1. An **alert** patient demonstrates an immediate and appropriate response to all external stimuli.

2. A patient in **coma** fails to respond normally to any external stimuli, including deep pain.

3. Gradation between these extremes is best described by specific responses to specific questions or sensory stimuli, eg, "Patient is sleepy but arouses to loud voice. Knows name and location, but not time or reason for being in the hospital." Avoid vague terms to describe states of consciousness (eg, obtunded, semicoma, semistupor, lethargy) in individual patients, since these terms may be subjective and less reliable, particularly when repeated examinations are performed by different people.

B. Motor Function: (See Tables 21–1 to 21–3.) Movement of extremities should be carefully assessed and graded as follows:

1. Normal movement means that the patient moves all extremities spontaneously, purposefully (ie, in response to specific commands), and with full strength and range of motion.

2. Paralysis denotes no movement of the extremity or muscle group, either spontaneously or in response to painful stimuli. (Stimuli should be applied both directly to the extremity and to the trunk, since failure to move may be secondary to hypesthesia of the extremity.) Failure to move at all, either spontaneously or in response to an unpleasant stimulus, may indicate paralysis due to a structural lesion (eg, fracture) or metabolic causes (eg, drug overdose). Often, failure to respond is simply due to an inadequately painful stimulus.

3. Gradation between these extremes should be described precisely, eg, "Patient extends right arm and leg, flexes left arm, and extends left leg in re-

sponse to supraorbital pressure." Avoid broad descriptive terms such as "paraparesis" or "decerebrate posturing." Grade muscle strength from 0 (no movement) to 5 (full strength).

4. Hysterical paralysis rarely enters into the differential diagnosis of paralysis associated with trauma. See Chapter 10 for distinguishing features.

C. Sensation: (See Figs 21–2 and 21–3 and Table 21–4.) Test as many sensory functions as possible in a patient with suspected spinal cord injury (in contrast to the more simple examination required for head trauma). Loss of some or all sensory functions below the lesion permits its precise anatomic localization. Perianal sensation should be tested; its presence eliminates the possibility of complete spinal cord transection and implies an improved prognosis.

1. Position, vibration, and light touch–The dorsal columns can be tested by determining response to vibration, light touch, and changes in position.

2. Pain and temperature–The ventral columns are tested by evaluating sensitivity to pain (pinprick) and temperature (Fig 21–4).

3. Impaired mentation–When mentation is impaired, a pinprick or deep painful stimulation may be the only reliable sensory test.

D. Brain Stem Reflexes: Brain stem reflexes are usually intact except in the case of high cervical spinal cord injury, when nystagmus (midgrain, pons), facial hypalgesia (spinal nucleus of the trigeminal nerve), and hypoventilation (phrenic nerve, intercostals) may be present. *Note: The presence of brain stem signs should not be attributed to spinal cord injury until an intracranial lesion has been excluded.*

E. Spinal Reflexes: Tendon jerks and plantar responses are usually absent below the level of an acute complete spinal cord transection (Table 21–5); asymmetry is also common. Spasticity or increased tone in muscle groups may occur with partial spinal cord injuries. Anal sphincter tone (reflex and voluntary) becomes flaccid following complete spinal cord transection. Priapism occurring soon after injury suggests immediate complete spinal cord lesion. Onset at a later time may indicate that the lesion has progressed from an incomplete to a complete stage. Sweating and skin vasomotor tone are absent below the level of a spinal cord lesion.

The bulbocavernosus reflex is dependent on an intact S1 and S2 spinal reflex. If the bulbocavernosus reflex is preserved in the presence of complete perineal sensory loss and flaccid paralysis of the lower extremities, it indicates that the period of spinal shock has passed and that the neurologic deficit is due to a lesion above the S1 segment. Absence of the bulbocavernosus reflex may indicate either the presence of spinal shock or a spinal cord lesion including the S1 and S2 segments. Spinal shock usually resolves within 24 hours and is accompanied by return of the bulbocavernosus reflex if the S1 and S2

Table 21–1. Segmental motor innervation: Upper extremity.[1]

Region	Muscle	C4	C5	C6	C7	C8	T1
Shoulder	Supraspinatus	X	X	X			
	Teres minor	X	X				
	Deltoid		X	X			
	Infraspinatus	X	X	X			
	Subscapularis		X	X	X		
	Teres major		X	X			
Arm	Biceps		X	X			
	Brachialis		X	X			
	Coracobrachialis		X	X	X		
	Triceps brachialis			X	X	X	
	Anconeus				X	X	
Forearm	Supinator longus		X	X			
	Supinator brevis		X	X			
	Extensor carpi radialis			X	X		
	Pronator teres			X	X		
	Flexor carpi radialis			X	X		
	Flexor pollicis longus				X	X	X
	Abductor pollicis longus				X	X	
	Extensor pollicis brevis				X	X	
	Extensor pollicis longus			X	X	X	
	Extensor digitorum longus			X	X	X	
	Extensor indicis proprius			X	X	X	
	Extensor carpi ulnaris			X	X	X	
	Extensor digiti quinti			X	X	X	
Hand	Flexor digitorum sublimis				X	X	X
	Flexor digitorum profundus				X	X	X
	Pronator quadratus				X	X	X
	Flexor carpi ulnaris				X	X	X
	Palmaris longus				X	X	
	Abductor pollicis brevis				X	X	X
	Flexor pollicis brevis				X	X	
	Opponens pollicis					X	X
	Flexor digiti quinti				X	X	
	Opponens digiti quinti				X	X	
	Adductor pollicis					X	X
	Palmaris brevis					X	X
	Adductor digiti quinti					X	X
	Lumbricales					X	X
	Interossei					X	X

[1]Reproduced, with permission, from Chusid JG: *Correlative Neuroanatomy & Functional Neurology,* 19th ed. Lange, 1985.

Table 21–2. Segmental motor innervation: Lower extremity.[1]

	L1	L2	L3	L4	L5	S1	S2
Hip		Iliopsoas					
				Tensor fasciae latae			
				Gluteus medius			
				Gluteus minimus			
				Quadratus femoris			
				Gemellus inferior			
				Gemellus superior			
				Gluteus maximus			
					Obturator internus		
					Piriformis		
Thigh		Sartorius					
		Pectineus					
		Adductor longus					
			Quadriceps femoris				
		Gracilis					
		Adductor brevis					
			Obturator externus				
			Adductor magnus				
			Adductor minimus				
				Semitendinosus			
				Semimembranosus			
					Biceps femoris		
Leg				Tibialis anticus			
				Extensor hallucis longus			
				Popliteus			
				Plantaris			
				Extensor digitorum longus			
					Soleus		
					Gastrocnemius		
					Peroneus longus		
					Peroneus brevis		
					Tibialis posterior		
					Flexor digitorum longus		
					Flexor hallucis longus		
Foot				Extensor hallucis brevis			
				Extensor digitorum brevis			
					Flexor digitorum brevis		
					Abductor hallucis		
					Flexor hallucis brevis		
					Lumbricales		
						Adductor hallucis	
						Adductor digiti quinti	
						Flexor digiti quinti	
						Opponens digiti quinti	
						Quadratus plantaris	
						Interossei	

Table 21–3. Motor function chart.[1]

Action to Be Tested	Muscle	Cord Segment	Nerves	Plexus
Shoulder Girdle and Upper Extremity				
Flexion of neck	Deep neck muscles (stemocleidomastoid and trapezius also participate)	C1–4	Cervical	Cervical
Extension of neck				
Rotation of neck				
Lateral bending of neck				
Elevation of upper thorax	Scaleni	C3–5	Phrenic	
Inspiration	Diaphragm			
Adduction of arm from behind to front	Pectoralis major and minor	C5–8, T1	Pectoral (thoracic; from medial and lateral cords of plexus)	Brachial
Forward thrust of shoulder	Seratus anterior	C5–7	Long thoracic	
Elevation of scapula	Levator scapulae	C3–5	Dorsal scapular	
Medial adduction and elevation of scapula	Rhomboids	C4, 5		
Abduction of arm	Supraspinatus	C4–6	Suprascapular	
Lateral rotation of arm	Infraspinatus	C4–6		
Medial rotation of arm	Latissimus dorsi, teres major, and subscapularis	C5–8	Subscapular (from posterior cord of plexus)	
Adduction of arm from front to back				
Abduction of arm	Deltoid	C5, 6	Axillary (from posterior cord of plexus)	
Lateral rotation of arm	Teres minor	C4, 5		
Flexion of forearm	Biceps brachii	C5, 6	Musculocutaneous (from lateral cord of plexus)	
Supination of forearm				
Adduction of arm	Coracobrachialis	C5–7		
Flexion of forearm				
Flexion of forearm	Brachialis	C5, 6		
Ulnar flexion of hand	Flexor carpi ulnaris	C7, 8; T1	Ulnar (from medial cord of plexus)	
Flexion of all fingers but thumb	Flexor digitorum profundus (ulnar portion)	C7, 8; T1		
Adduction of metacarpal of thumb	Adductor pollicis	C8, T1		
Abduction of little finger	Abductor digiti quinti	C8, T1		
Opposition of little finger	Opponens digiti quinti	C7, 8; T1		
Flexion of little finger	Flexor digiti quinti	C7, 8; T1		
Flexion of proximal phalanx, extension of 2 distal phalanges, adduction and abduction of fingers	Interossei	C8, T1		
Pronation of forearm	Pronator teres	C6, 7	Median (C6, 7 from lateral cord of plexus; C8, T1 from medial cord of plexus)	
Radial flexion of hand	Flexor carpi radialis	C6, 7		
Flexion of hand	Palmaris longus	C7, 8; T1		
Flexion of middle phalanx of index, middle, ring, or little finger	Flexor digitorum superficialis	C7, 8; T1		
Flexion of hand				
Flexion of terminal phalanx of thumb	Flexor pollicis longus	C7, 8; T1		
Flexion of terminal phalanx of index or middle finger	Flexor digitorum profundus (radial portion)	C7, 8; T1		
Flexion of hand				

(*continued*)

Table 21–3. Motor function chart.[1] (continued)

Action to Be Tested	Muscle	Cord Segment	Nerves	Plexus
Shoulder Girdle and Upper Extremity (cont.)				
Abduction of metacarpal of thumb	Abductor pollicis brevis	C7, 8; T1	Median (C7, 8 from lateral cord of plexus; C8, T1 from medial cord of plexus)	Brachial
Flexion of proximal phalanx of thumb	Flexor pollicis brevis	C7, 8; T1		
Opposition of metacarpal of thumb	Opponens pollicis	C8, T1		
Flexion of proximal phalanx and extension of the 2 distal phalanges of index, middle, ring, or little finger	Lumbricales (the 2 lateral)	C8, T1		
	Lumbricales (the 2 medial)	C8, T1	Ulnar	
Extension of forearm	Triceps brachii and anconeus	C6–8	Radial (from posterior cord of plexus)	
Flexion of forearm	Brachioradialis	C5, 6		
Radial extension of hand	Extensor carpi radialis	C6–8		
Extension of phalanges of index, middle, ring, or little finger	Extensor digitorum	C7–8		
Extension of hand				
Extension of phalanges of little finger	Extensor digiti quinti proprius	C6–8		
Extension of hand				
Ulnar extension of hand	Extensor carpi ulnaris	C6–8		
Supination of forearm	Supinator	C5–7	Radial (from posterior cord of plexus)	
Abduction of metacarpal of thumb	Abductor pollicis longus	C7, 8; T1		
Radial extension of hand				
Extension of thumb	Extensor pollicis brevis	C7, 8		
Radial extension of hand	Extensor pollicis longus	C6–8		
Extension of index finger	Extensor indicis proprius	C6–8		
Extension of hand				
Trunk and Thorax				
Elevation of ribs	Thoracic, abdominal, and back	T1–L3	Thoracic and posterior lumbosacral branches	Brachial
Depression of ribs				
Contraction of abdomen				
Anteroflexion of trunk				
Lateral flexion of trunk				
Hip Girdle and Lower Extremity				
Flexion of hip	Iliopsoas	L1–3	Femoral	Lumbar
Flexion of hip (and eversion of thigh	Sartorius	L2, 3		
Extension of leg	Quadriceps femoris	L2–4		
Adduction of thigh	Pectineus	L2, 3	Obturator	
	Adductor longus	L2, 3		
	Adductor brevis	L2–4		
	Adductor magnus	L3, 4		
	Gracilis	L2–4		
Adduction of thigh	Obturator externus	L3, 4		
Lateral rotation of thigh				

(continued)

Table 21–3. Motor function chart.[1] (continued)

Action to Be Tested	Muscle	Cord Segment	Nerves	Plexus
Hip Girdle and Lower Extremity (cont.)				
Abduction of thigh	Gluteus medius and minimus	L4, 5; S1	Superior gluteal	Sacral
Medial rotation of thigh				
Flexion of thigh	Tensor fasciae latae	L4, 5		
Lateral rotation of thigh	Piriformis	S1, 2	. . .	
Abduction of thigh	Gluteus maximus	L4, 5: S1, 2	Inferior gluteal	
Lateral rotation of thigh	Obturator internus	L5, S1	Muscular branches from sacral plexus	
	Gemelli	L4, 5; S1		
	Quadratus femoris	L4, 5; S1		
Flexion of leg (assist in extension of thigh)	Biceps femoris	L4, 5; S1, 2	Sciatic (trunk)	Sacral
	Semitendinosus	L4, 5; S1		
	Semimembranosus	L4, 5; S1		
Dorsal flexion of foot	Tibialis anterior	L4, 5	Deep peroneal	
Supination of foot				
Extension of toes 2–5	Extensor digitorum lingus	L4, 5; S1		
Dorsal flexion of foot				
Extension of great toe	Extensor hallucis longus	L4, 5; S1		
Dorsal flexion of foot				
Extension of great toe and the 3 medial toes	Extensor digitorum brevis	L4, 5; S1		
Plantar flexion of foot in pronation	Peroneus longus and brevis	L5, S1	Superficial peroneal	
	Gastrocnemius	L5, S1, 2	Tibial	
Plantar flexion of foot in supination	Tibialis posterior and triceps surae	L5, S1		
Plantar flexion of foot in supination	Flexor digitorum longus	S1, 2		
Flexion of terminal phalanx of toes II–V				
Plantar flexion of foot in supination	Flexor hallucis longus	L5, S1, 2		
Flexion of terminal phalanx of great toe				
Flexion of middle phalanx of toes II–V	Flexor digitorum brevis	L5, S1		
Flexion of proximal phalanx of great toe	Flexor hallucis brevis	L5, S1, 2		
Spreading and closing of toes	Small muscles of foot	S1, 2		
Flexion of proximal phalanx of toes				
Voluntary control of pelvic floor	Perineal and sphincters	S2–4	Pudendal	

[1]Modified from JC McKinley. Reproduced, with permission, from de Groot J: *Correlative Neuroanatomy*, 21st ed. Appleton & Lange, 1991.

segments are not directly involved in the spinal cord lesion.

Spinal Cord Syndromes

A. Complete Spinal Cord Lesion: The absence of sacral sparing (perianal sensation, rectal sphincter tone) indicates a complete spinal cord lesion, with recovery unlikely if the condition persists longer than 24 hours. Sacral sparing suggests an improved prognosis.

B. Partial Spinal Cord Lesions:

1. Brown-Séquard lesion–This is usually caused by penetrating injuries resulting in hemisection of the spinal cord. The findings include loss of distal ipsilateral position and vibration sense, distal ipsilateral motor loss and vasomotor paralysis, distal loss of pain and temperature sense below T12 on the *contralateral* side (including the genitals and perineum).

2. Central cord syndrome–This is usually due

PERIPHERAL DISTRIBUTION

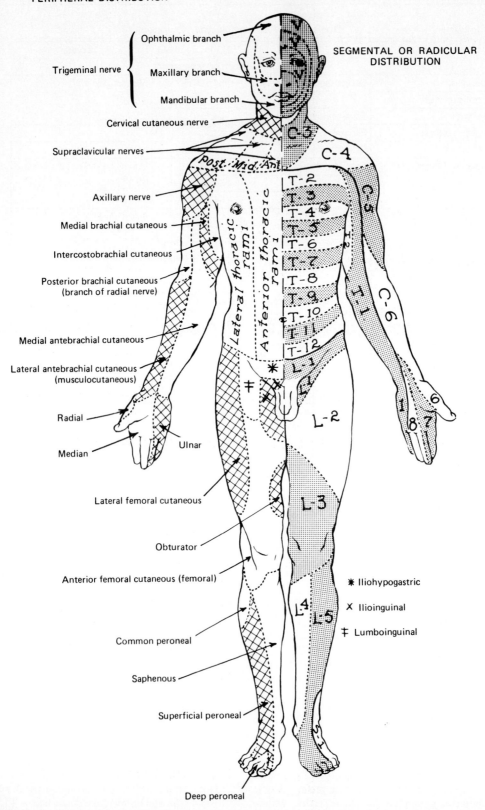

SEGMENTAL OR RADICULAR DISTRIBUTION

Trigeminal nerve
- Ophthalmic branch
- Maxillary branch
- Mandibular branch

Cervical cutaneous nerve

Supraclavicular nerves

Axillary nerve

Medial brachial cutaneous

Intercostobrachial cutaneous

Posterior brachial cutaneous (branch of radial nerve)

Medial antebrachial cutaneous

Lateral antebrachial cutaneous (musculocutaneous)

Radial

Median

Ulnar

Lateral femoral cutaneous

Obturator

Anterior femoral cutaneous (femoral)

Common peroneal

Saphenous

Superficial peroneal

Deep peroneal

✱ Iliohypogastric
✗ Ilioinguinal
‡ Lumboinguinal

Figure 21–2. Cutaneous innervation. (Reproduced, with permission, from Chusid JG: *Correlative Neuroanatomy & Functional Neurology,* 19th ed. Lange, 1985.)

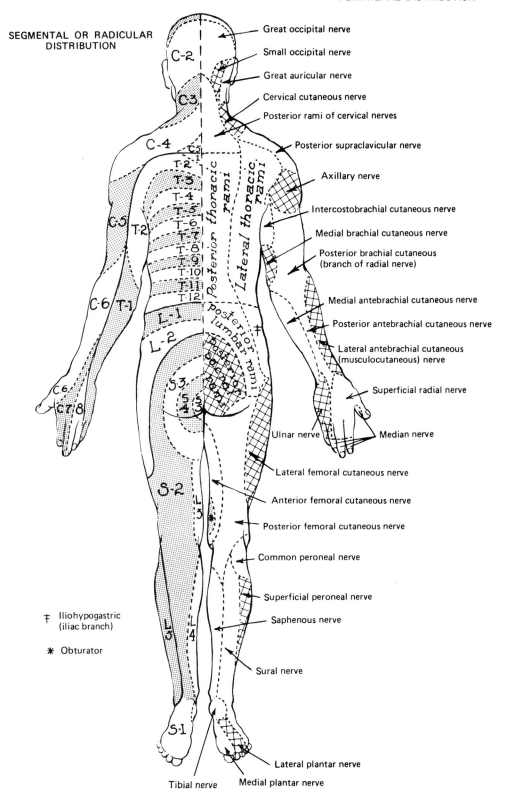

SEGMENTAL OR RADICULAR DISTRIBUTION

Great occipital nerve
Small occipital nerve
Great auricular nerve
Cervical cutaneous nerve
Posterior rami of cervical nerves
Posterior supraclavicular nerve
Axillary nerve
Intercostobrachial cutaneous nerve
Medial brachial cutaneous nerve
Posterior brachial cutaneous (branch of radial nerve)
Medial antebrachial cutaneous nerve
Posterior antebrachial cutaneous nerve
Lateral antebrachial cutaneous (musculocutaneous) nerve
Superficial radial nerve
Ulnar nerve
Median nerve
Lateral femoral cutaneous nerve
Anterior femoral cutaneous nerve
Posterior femoral cutaneous nerve
Common peroneal nerve
Superficial peroneal nerve
Saphenous nerve
Sural nerve
Lateral plantar nerve
Medial plantar nerve
Tibial nerve

Posterior thoracic rami
Lateral thoracic rami
Posterior lumbar rami

‡ Iliohypogastric (iliac branch)

* Obturator

Figure 21–3. Cutaneous innervation. (Reproduced, with permission, from Chusid JG: *Correlative Neuroanatomy & Functional Neurology,* 19th ed. Lange, 1985.)

Table 21–4. Commonly used landmarks for testing dermatomal sensation.

Location	Dermatome
Second rib	C4–T2
Nipple	T4
Lower rib border	T7–8
Umbilicus	T10
Inguinal ligament	T12–L1

to cervical hyperextension, involving the central gray matter and the central parts of the lateral spinothalamic tracts. Quadriplegia may result, with minimal sacral sparing. The upper extremities are more involved than are the lower extremities.

3. Anterior cord syndrome–This results from cervical hyperflexion injuries. Position and vibration (posterior column functions) are preserved, but motor function, temperature, and pain sensation are lost bilaterally below the lesion.

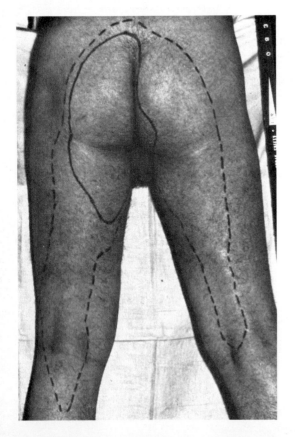

Figure 21–4. Sensory impairment in man with cauda equina syndrome after fracture of L1 vertebra. (Solid line = touch; broken = pain.) (Reproduced, with permission, from Chusid JG: *Correlative Neuroanatomy & Functional Neurology*, 19th ed. Lange, 1985.)

Reexamination

Neurologic examination is helpful only if it is repeated often enough to establish a diagnosis, suggest further diagnostic steps, or clearly establish a trend in neurologic function. The results of each examination may be seen as a point on a curve showing neurologic function with time. If successive examinations indicate improvement, further specialized testing may not be necessary. Failure to improve—verified by repeated examinations—indicates that additional studies are necessary, as does progressive deterioration from a baseline established by examination done on arrival in the emergency department. It is particularly important to note progressive neurologic dysfunction if injury involves the cervical spinal cord, since respiratory failure may result.

Laboratory Examination

Baseline studies required for all patients with suspected spinal cord injury include the following: CBC, urinalysis (specimen obtained by bladder catheterization), blood glucose concentration, serum electrolyte determinations, and renal function tests. Arterial blood gas measurements are necessary if ventilation is impaired or potentially threatened. *Note:* Lumbar puncture and examination of the cerebrospinal fluid are *not* helpful in the management of spinal trauma and should *not* be performed unless meningitis is suspected.

X-Ray Examination

Careful and correct interpretation of x-ray films is critically important in treatment of spinal cord injury. Most spine abnormalities, eg, minor facet fractures and nondisplaced fractures, are more easily recognized by a radiologist, whose help should be sought in all cases. *Note: Normal spine x-rays do not exclude the presence of spinal cord injury.* Central cord syndrome (central hemorrhage) and spontaneously reduced dislocations can be associated with normal x-rays, as can ligamentous tears resulting from flexion-extension injuries (whiplash). A thorough physical examination and a careful repeated neurologic evaluation are therefore essential in all cases.

A. Chest and Skull: X-rays of the chest and skull should be obtained when indicated.

B. Cervical Spine: Anteroposterior and lateral views of the cervical spine extending from C1 to T1 and an odontoid (open mouth) view are required if cervical cord injury is suspected. The lateral cervical spine view alone is only 79% sensitive in detecting cervical spine injuries. If the segments from C6 to T1 are not visible, a "swimmer's" view should be obtained by having the patient supine, with one upper extremity abducted and extended (arm raised above head) and the opposite upper extremity adducted and extended (arm kept at side of body). The shoulder of the adducted and extended extremity is then depressed by having a person stand at the foot of the bed

Table 21–5. Summary of reflexes.[1]

Reflexes	Afferent Nerve	Center	Efferent Nerve
Superficial Reflexes			
Corneal	Cranial V	Pons	Cranial VII
Nasal (sneeze)	Cranial V	Brain stem and upper cord	Cranials V, VII, IX, X, and spinal nerves of expiration
Pharyngeal and uvular	Cranial IX	Medulla	Cranial X
Upper abdominal	T7, 8, 9, 10	T7, 8, 9, 10	T7, 8, 9, 10
Lower abdominal	T10, 11, 12	T10, 11, 12	T10, 11, 12
Cremasteric	Femoral	L1	Genitofemoral
Plantar	Tibial	S1, 2	Tibial
Anal	Pudendal	S4, 5	Pudendal
Deep Reflexes			
Jaw	Cranial V	Pons	Cranial V
Biceps	Musculocutaneous	C5, 6	Musculocutaneous
Triceps	Radial	C6, 7	Radial
Periosteoradial	Radial	C6, 7, 8	Radial
Wrist (flexion)	Median	C6, 7, 8	Median
Wrist (extension)	Radial	C7, 8	Radial
Patellar	Femoral	L2, 3, 4	Femoral
Achilles	Tibial	S1, 2	Tibial
Visceral Reflexes			
Light	Cranial II	Midbrain	Cranial III
Accommodation	Cranial II	Occipital cortex	Cranial III
Ciliospinal	A sensory nerve	T1, 2	Cervical sympathetics
Oculocardiac	Cranial V	Medulla	Cranial X
Carotid sinus	Cranial IX	Medulla	Cranial X
Bulbocavernosus	Pudendal	S2, 3, 4	Pelvic autonomic
Bladder and rectal	Pudendal	S2, 3, 4	Pudendal and autonomics

[1]Reproduced, with permission, from deGroot J: *Correlative Neuroanatomy*, 21st ed. Appleton & Lange, 1991.

and pull on the patient's hand. The x-ray is shot upward through the axilla of the abducted, extended extremity. Oblique views increase the sensitivity of the cervical spine series and should be obtained in all patients with suspected cervical spine injury. Standard oblique views require neck rotation; this can be avoided by performing a "trauma oblique" view, which is a modification of the oblique view. The trauma oblique view is obtained by aiming the x-ray beam at a 60-degree angle to the plane of the table with the patient supine (and immobilized).

Special x-ray studies must be performed if all of the cervical vertebrae cannot be seen adequately with these techniques (see below).

Flexion-extension films of the cervical spine are indicated only if stability of the spine remains questionable after plain films and tomograms have been carefully reviewed. These films require an awake, cooperative patient who can flex and extend the neck on command without assistance but with a physician in attendance. If it is uncertain whether the spine is stable, proceed on the assumption that it is not.

C. Thoracic and Lumbosacral Spine: X-rays of the thoracic and lumbosacral spine should be performed when a thoracic cord or cauda equina injury is suspected, when a trauma victim is complaining of thoracic or lumbar back pain, or when an adequate spinal examination cannot be performed (eg, due to obtundation) on a victim of major multiple trauma.

D. Special Studies:

1. CT scan–If a body scanner is available, the CT scan is the easiest and perhaps the best method of looking for vertebral column and spinal cord injury. It may be combined with myelography for better visualization of the relationships between the spinal cord and the vertebral canal.

2. Tomography–Tomograms provide excellent detail of the spine, but they are more difficult to interpret (and no easier to perform) than CT scans.

3. Myelography–The decision to perform myelography should be made by a neurosurgeon. Myelography can be done safely by keeping the patient supine with the neck in neutral position while injecting contrast medium into the lumbar sac or the lateral

C1–2 interspace. Although myelography is helpful in evaluating patency of the spinal canal, it should only be done if noninvasive x-ray studies and the clinical situation indicate the need to do so.

Hospitalization

Hospitalization is required in patients with neurologic deficit, an unstable or potentially unstable vertebral column (with or without fracture), fractures or subluxation of vertebral bodies, or severe pain requiring parenteral analgesics for relief.

Patients with uncomplicated fractures (ie, linear and undisplaced) of the transverse processes, sacrum, and coccyx and with normal results on neurologic evaluation and x-ray do not require hospitalization. Provide symptomatic therapy as needed.

EMERGENCY TREATMENT OF SPECIFIC SPINAL INJURIES

VERTEBRAL FRACTURES WITHOUT SPINAL CORD INJURY

Diagnosis

In vertebral fractures without spinal cord injury, there is focal pain and tenderness over the vertebral column. Coughing or axial percussion of the head or feet may also cause pain that is referred to the fractured vertebral body. X-rays show fractures that may be in the vertebral body, the transverse processes, or the spinous processes. Coexisting dislocation or instability may be present. *The neurologic examination is normal.*

Treatment

Immobilize the patient on a firm surface (eg, rigid spine board), and use tape and lateral restraints (sandbags) or traction. Administer analgesia as needed.

Disposition

The only patients who do *not* require hospitalization are those with mildly symptomatic or asymptomatic, linear, undisplaced, stable fractures of the spinous or transverse processes, or similar fractures of the sacrum or coccyx. Such patients may be provided with analgesics and a cervical collar for immobilization (if fractures are in the cervical vertebrae). A return visit should be scheduled within 1 week.

All other patients should be hospitalized—specifically, those with displaced or unstable fractures; fractures of cervical, thoracic, or lumbar vertebral bodies; open fractures; and multiple fractures.

SPINAL CORD INJURY WITH OR WITHOUT VERTEBRAL FRACTURES

Diagnosis

Spinal cord injury with or without vertebral fractures is associated with neurologic symptoms and neurologic deficit. Findings are consistent with injury to the spinal cord (eg, sensory deficit ending circumferentially at T8). Bony injury to the vertebrae demonstrable on x-ray may or may not be apparent, since severe flexion-extension injuries and bony instability from ligamentous tears may cause serious or even fatal spinal cord injury without radiologically demonstrable abnormalities.

Treatment

A. Check the airway, gag reflex, and adequacy of ventilation, since high cervical cord lesions may cause death from respiratory insufficiency. Provide ventilatory support with a bag-mask combination or endotracheal intubation, if necessary.

B. Stabilize the vertebral column, using firm support and lateral restraints (sandbags) or traction (cervical halter or tongs) to minimize further injury to the spinal cord.

C. Correct hypotension by administering intravenous crystalloid solutions or placing the patient in a pneumatic antishock (eg, MAST) garment.

D. Insert an indwelling urinary catheter and a nasogastric tube. Give nothing by mouth.

E. Spinal cord swelling may be reduced by administering corticosteroids; however, the success of this treatment has not been proved. Give dexamethasone, 20 mg intravenously initially, then 10 mg intravenously every 6 hours for 7 days.

F. Obtain emergency neurosurgical consultation.

Disposition

All patients with neurologic deficit caused by spinal cord injury must be hospitalized.

WHIPLASH (HYPEREXTENSION) INJURIES
(Cervical Spine Sprain)

Diagnosis

Patients with whiplash have a history of abrupt hyperextension of the neck (usually from a motor vehicle accident), usually without loss of consciousness. Injury from hyperflexion often occurs as well. Symptoms such as neck pain or muscle spasm, headache, hoarseness, and dysphagia often do not appear until 12–24 hours after injury. Neck pain may be referred to the arms or chest. Physical examination may show tenderness of anterior neck muscles and limited range of motion. Specifically, there is no evidence of neurologic deficit. By definition, whiplash does not cause fractures that are evident on cervical x-rays, although severe injuries may rupture the anterior disk fibers and result in widened disk spaces. X-rays are usually normal but may show reversal of the normal cervical lordosis.

Treatment

Treatment consists of a cervical collar, heat, and analgesics (narcotics are often required). Muscle relaxants may be indicated. Bed rest may be necessary for several days to 1 week.

Disposition

Hospitalization is rarely required. Refer the patient to a primary-care physician or to an orthopedist.

REFERENCES

Bartkowski HM, Pitts LH: Neurologic injury. In: *Current Therapy of Trauma 1983–1984*. Trunkey DD, Lewis FR (editors). Mosby, 1984.

Bayless P, Ray VG: Incidence of cervical spine injuries in association with blunt head trauma. Am J Emerg Med 1989;7:139.

Bracken MB et al: Randomized controlled trial of methylprednisolone or naloxone in the treatment of acute spinal cord injury: Results of the Second National Acute Spinal Cord Injury Study. N Engl J Med 1990;322:1405.

Guthkelch AN, Fleisher AS: Patterns of cervical spine injury and their associated lesions. West J Med 1987;147:428.

Harris JH Jr: *The Radiology of Acute Cervical Spine Trauma*. Williams & Wilkins, 1978.

O'Malley KF, Ross SE: The incidence of injury to the cervical spine in patients with craniocerebral injury. J Trauma 1988;28:1476.

Rhee KJ et al: Oral intubation in the multiply injured patient: The risk of exacerbating spinal cord damage. Ann Emerg Med 1990;19:511.

Ringenberg BJ et al: Rational ordering of cervical spine radiographs following trauma. Ann Emerg Med 1988;17:792.

Roberge RJ et al: Selective application of cervical spine radiology in alert victims of blunt trauma: A prospective study. J Trauma 1988;28:784.

Ross SE et al: Clearing the cervical spine: Initial radiologic evaluation. J Trauma 1987;27:1055.

Yashon D: Spinal Injury. Appleton-Century-Crofts, 1978.

Yealy DM, Paris PM: Recent advances in airway management. Emerg Med Clin North Am 1989;7:83.

22

Orthopedic Emergencies

Peter G. Trafton, MD

IMMEDIATE MANAGEMENT OF LIFE-THREATENING PROBLEMS

MONITOR PATIENT & TREAT SHOCK
(See also Chapter 4.)

Patients who arrive in the emergency department with orthopedic injuries may also have major or multiple injuries to other systems. The presence of such injuries should be ruled out by appropriate examinations or laboratory studies. The initial approach should always be systematic and follow priorities as described in Chapter 3.

Assess Severity & Give Immediate Necessary Care
A. Ensure Adequate Airway: Intubate if necessary (Chapter 46), taking precautions to protect the cervical spine if cervical spine injury is suspected.

B. Undress the Patient: Strip all clothing from the patient, and quickly examine the entire body for obvious injuries. Do not remove embedded penetrating objects, since they may be blocking injured blood vessels and thus serving a useful hemostatic function.

C. Measure and Record Vital Signs: If blood pressure is normal in the supine position, determine blood pressure and pulse with the patient sitting up. (**Caution:** Do not let the patient sit up if neck or spine injury is suspected. See Chapter 21.) Postural hypotension or tachycardia usually indicates hypovolemia.

D. Evaluate and Treat for Shock: Look for signs of shock, eg, altered sensorium; cold, clammy skin; ashen pallor; arterial hypotension; weak and rapid pulse; air hunger; thirst.

Auscultate the chest for breath sounds, and verify adequacy of ventilation. Both blunt and penetrating injuries of the upper abdomen may involve the thorax (eg, pneumothorax or hemothorax, cardiac tamponade).

Treat shock or impending shock (supine hypotension). (See Chapter 3 for more detailed discussion.) Briefly—

1. Place patient supine.

2. Insert one or more large-bore (≥ 16-gauge) intravenous catheters or venous cutdowns.

3. Obtain blood for CBC, serum creatinine, electrolyte, and amylase measurements, and blood glucose determinations.

4. Type and cross-match for 6 units of whole blood or packed red blood cells.

5. Immediately begin a rapid infusion of crystalloid solution, and carefully monitor blood pressure. If more than 3 L of crystalloid solution is required to maintain adequate blood pressure in a trauma victim, cross-matched, type-specific, or universal donor whole blood (in that order of preference) should be substituted and given at comparable rates of infusion. Immediate surgical consultation is essential.

6. Administer oxygen, 5 L/min, by mask or nasal prongs.

7. Measure arterial blood gases: poor tissue perfusion will be reflected as metabolic acidosis and poor ventilation by hypoxemia and hypercapnia.

8. Insert a Foley catheter to monitor urine output, but first obtain a urethrogram if there is meatal blood or prostatic dislocation.

9. Insert a nasogastric tube to empty the stomach and evaluate bleeding.

Blood Loss

Pelvic disruptions, fractures of the femur, and multiple fractures of other long bones may cause hypovolemic shock and life-threatening blood loss (often occult). Table 22–1 sets forth blood loss associated with typical *closed* fractures.

Physical Examination

Inspect the entire body for signs of injury. Ask the patient who is able to cooperate to identify all painful areas, and pay special attention to these regions during evaluation. If head or neck injury is suspected, immobilize the head with sandbags and tape, or equivalent, and obtain cervical spine x-rays before moving the patient (see below and Chapter 21). Examine the chest, heart, abdomen, and bony pelvis. Examine all 4 extremities even if they are apparently uninjured. A seemingly normal extremity should be palpated to check for tenderness and should be put through a full range of motion. Stability of collateral ligaments is readily assessed by stressing joints in the varus and valgus directions. Check distal pulses.

Neurologic Examination

Perform a neurologic screening examination to assess level of consciousness, pupillary equality and reaction to light, muscle strength, sensation, and reflexes (Chapter 16).

X-Ray Examination

Obtain a cross-table lateral x-ray of the cervical spine plus anteroposterior and odontoid views and supine anteroposterior x-rays of the chest and pelvis. Include anteroposterior and lateral views of the entire spine if the patient reports pain in these regions or if pain response is altered by unconsciousness, intoxication, or other factors. X-rays of other areas should be obtained as indicated by history and examination.

SUSPECT & PREVENT POTENTIAL SPINE INJURIES

Spinal cord damage may or may not occur when injury to bone or ligament causes instability of the spine. Irreversible spinal cord damage can result from improper movement or positioning of a patient with an unstable spine. Many cases of spinal cord injury have significant potential for recovery that can be maximized by proper immobilization of the spine; this potential may be lost through careless handling.

Intoxicated injured patients or patients who have sustained any of the following are at risk for spinal injury: **(1)** head or facial injuries, **(2)** multiple trauma, **(3)** falls from a height, **(4)** high-energy motor vehicle accidents, or **(5)** gunshot wounds.

Preventive Measures (See Chapter 21 for details.)

A. Do not flex or rotate any part of the spine, and be particularly careful in handling the neck and head.

B. Keep the patient supine on a firm, padded surface.

C. Protect the neck with a rigid cervical collar (eg, Philadelphia collar) and with sandbags on both sides of the head (or equivalent); use adhesive tape to join the bags and secure them to the forehead.

D. Obtain x-rays of the entire spine in unconscious patients who have sustained significant trauma; a cross-table lateral cervical spine x-ray alone may miss important injuries. Remember that *apparently* normal results on x-rays do not rule out the possibility of ligamentous disruption with resulting instability. If spinal instability is suspected, protect the spine until the patient is able to cooperate and perform active flexion and extension maneuvers for x-rays under the supervision of the physician.

Table 22–1. Potential blood loss from closed fractures.

Site	Amount (in L)
Pelvis	1–5+
Fermur	1–4
Spine	1–2
Leg	0.5–1
Arm	0.5–0.75

FURTHER EVALUATION OF SUSPECTED ORTHOPEDIC INJURIES

History

Obtain as much information as possible from the patient and any witnesses about the details of the injury. Ask about all sites of pain and about loss of motor or sensory function. Inquire about preexisting musculoskeletal problems, especially those related to the injured areas. Ask about illnesses, operations, current medications, drug allergies, bleeding tendencies, and time of last food or drink.

Physical Examination

A. Inspect the front and back of all extremities for deformity (angulation, shortening, and abnormal rotation), swelling, ecchymosis, abrasion, and laceration.

B. Palpate extremities, pelvis, and spinous processes for tenderness, swelling, and deformity. Be alert for crepitus, but do not move an obvious fracture unnecessarily.

C. Examine all joints for swelling, deformity, instability, and loss of normal motion.

D. Confirm and document the presence of all peripheral pulses, and test motor and sensory function of each major peripheral nerve (Table 22–2).

X-Ray Examination

Splint injured parts before obtaining x-rays (see Essential Emergency Department Treatment, below). Monitor vital signs, prevent inappropriate manipulation, and make sure that x-ray studies are adequate. Both anteroposterior and lateral views are required. Include the joints above the below the injury in x-rays. Obtain x-rays of any area with tenderness, swelling, or deformity. Similar x-rays of the uninjured limb for comparison can be helpful, especially for assessment of growth plate injuries in children.

The physician caring for the patient must be sure to examine x-rays personally and not leave interpretation to the radiologist. After splinting is done, radiographs of extremities may be deferred, if necessary, to expedite life- or limb-saving treatment, including transfer to a trauma center.

Table 21–2. Screening tests for peripheral nerve function.

Nerve	Motor Test	Area of Sensation
Axillary (C5, 6)	Shoulder abduction	Lateral shoulder
Musculocutaneous (C5, 6)	Elbow flexion	Lateral forearm
Radial (C6–8)	Thumb extension	Dorsal web space between thumb and index finger
Median (C5–T1 or C6–T1) Branches to hand	Palpable contraction of thenar muscles	Palm of radial 3 digits
Forearm motor branch (anterior interosseous)	Thumb interphalangeal flexion	...
Ulnar (C7–T1)	Index finger abduction	Little finger
Femoral (L2, 3, 4)	Knee extension	Medial knee, medial calf
Obturator (L2, 3, 4)	Hip adduction	Medial thigh (variable)
Superior gluteal (L5)	Hip abduction	...
Inferior gluteal (S1)	Hip extension	...
Sciatic Tibial (L4, 5; S1–3) (posterior compartments)	Toe and ankle plantar flexion	Sole of foot
Peroneal (L4, 5, S1, 2) Deep branch (anterior compartment)	Toe dorsiflexion	Dorsal web, great and second toes
Superficial branch (lateral compartment)	Foot eversion	Rest of dorsum of foot

EMERGENCY TREATMENT OF SPECIFIC LIMB-THREATENING PROBLEMS

ARTERIAL INJURY
(See also Chapter 32.)

A pale, cold, painful, pulseless limb is typical of arterial injury; however, sensory loss may be the only early indication of vascular compromise. Occasionally, appearance of clinical findings and development of ischemia are delayed (eg, late thrombosis following an intimal tear of the popliteal artery). Suspect and look for arterial injury whenever an injury involves or approaches an artery. Early detailed arteriography is the best method for identifying arterial injury but may only delay limb-saving treatment when ischemia is obvious. A vascular surgeon should be consulted promptly in all cases of suspected arterial injury, and all of these patients require hospitalization.

TRAUMATIC AMPUTATION & REPLANTATION

Diagnosis

Possible replantation should be considered in patients with traumatic amputations. The more distal the injury, the greater the chance for successful replantation of the amputated part. Replantation is also more likely to succeed if the patient is a child and if the amputation is relatively clean, with little or no crushing or avulsion. The emergency physician must know in advance how to arrange immediate referral to the nearest replantation team and should always consult by telephone with a team member before admitting or transferring the patient.

Treatment

Treat shock, if present (Chapter 3). Use elevation of the amputation stump and a sterile compression dressing to control hemorrhage; use a tourniquet only if these methods are unsuccessful. Give tetanus prophylaxis (Chapter 24) and intravenous antibiotics as described under Treat Open Fracture, below.

Do not explore the amputated stump. Preserve the amputated part by wrapping it in sterile dressings moistened with Ringer's irrigation or normal saline and sealing it in a clean dry container (eg, plastic bag) stored at 4 °C (39.2 °F) (eg, refrigerator or ice water). Do not place the amputated part directly on ice or freeze it.

Disposition

Hospitalize or transfer the patient immediately, as directed by the replantation team.

COMPARTMENT SYNDROME

Increased interstitial pressure within a closed fascial compartment can obstruct microcirculation to the nerves and muscles lying within the involved space and cause tissue necrosis, which becomes irreversible after 4–6 hours. Such increased pressure results from hemorrhage or edema associated with acute injury (eg, fracture or contusion), sustained external pressure on a limb (eg, unconscious drug overdose victims who have lain in one position for a number of hours), or muscular overexertion (rare). Constricting casts, dressings, and splints can also increase compartmental pressure. Even marginally elevated compartment pressures can produce irreversible tissue damage if they persist long enough.

Diagnosis

Compartment syndrome usually develops several hours after injury (often after hospitalization) but may be seen in the emergency department, especially in patients who arrive some time after injury has occurred. *Compartment syndrome should be suspected in any unconscious patient with a swollen limb.*

A. Symptoms and Signs: Severe ischemic pain is the most prominent finding in the alert patient with acute compartment syndrome. Skin perfusion and arterial pulses are usually normal, since the pressure in the affected compartment need be elevated only enough to occlude capillary flow in the subfascial tissue. The entire involved compartment is tensely swollen.

Peripheral nerves are sensitive to ischemia, and progressive loss of sensory and motor function—often preceded by paresthesia—is a reliable early sign of compartment syndrome. It is important to test the function of each peripheral nerve in the extremity to avoid overlooking a problem that affects only one compartment (Table 22–2). Normal sensory and motor function of local nerves is extremely rare if a significant compartment syndrome is present at the time of examination.

Passive stretch of ischemic muscle is painful and is another sign of compartment syndrome. Local injury can cause stretch pain without ischemia, however.

B. Repeated Examination: It is advisable to hospitalize patients with displaced fractures or severe contusions of the leg or forearm, because repeated examinations are required to check for developing compartment syndrome. If motor and sensory functions cannot be tested because the patient is unconscious or has an associated nerve injury, it is wise to measure tissue pressure in all compartments that might be affected (consult an orthopedist).

Treatment

Release any constricting casts, splints, or dressings. Fasciotomy is effective treatment for compartment syndrome only if performed within a few hours after onset.

Disposition

Hospitalize the patient for observation, and *immediately* consult an orthopedist for clinical assessment, consideration of tissue pressure measurements, and possible fasciotomy.

OPEN FRACTURES

Any break in the skin that communicates with the hematoma and injured tissue surrounding a fracture permits bacterial contamination of the wound, which has markedly impaired resistance to infection. Gas gangrene, tetanus, acute pyogenic infection, and chronic posttraumatic osteomyelitis are potential sequelae of open fracture, even if the wound is only a puncture. Open pelvic fractures are especially dangerous, with a death rate approaching 50%. Penetrating wounds of joints should be treated in the same way as open fractures, since they also carry a significant risk of infection.

Diagnosis

When in doubt, assume that any nearby wound communicates with the fracture. Probing and limited exploration of wounds in the emergency department cannot reliably rule out open fracture.

The elasticity of the skin may conceal the fact that a spike of bone protruding from the fracture may have been contaminated during injury. Circumferential inspection of a fractured limb is necessary to avoid missing an open fracture. Careful rectal and vaginal examinations are mandatory for patients with pelvic fractures to identify lacerations produced by bone fragments.

Note: Fractures caused by gunshot wounds are open fractures and should be treated as such. Although some open fractures caused by low-velocity missiles can be treated without formal debridement, a surgeon experienced in treatment of fractures should promptly evaluate such a patient to make certain that fracture and soft tissue wounds are suitable for nonsurgical management.

Nerve, blood vessel, and muscle-tendon injuries should be carefully sought and treated in any patient with open fracture. The possibility of remote injuries must always be remembered.

Treatment

Prompt surgical debridement is required. While the patient is in the emergency department, apply a sterile dressing and splint, and give tetanus prophylaxis (Chapter 24) and intravenous antibiotics (p 322).

Disposition

Hospitalize the patient immediately, and obtain orthopedic consultation.

BATTERED CHILD SYNDROME
(See also Chapter 42.)

Young children with fractures or other injuries may be victims of child abuse. Among children under 3 years of age, one-third of fractures are due to abuse. Such children who are discharged from the emergency department without appropriate parental counseling have a 50% risk of further injury and a death rate of 10%.

Child abuse occurs in all socioeconomic classes. The physician should keep in mind that injuries may have been caused by someone other than the concerned parent who brings the child to the emergency department.

Diagnosis

The possibility of child abuse must be considered whenever an injured child is evaluated. Child abuse is suggested by injuries in children under 3 years of age, vague history, injuries more severe than those expected on the basis of the description of the "accident," and evidence of repeated trauma (records of recurring emergency department visits, multiple skin and head lesions, and x-rays or a bone scan showing fractures of long bones, ribs, skull, often in various stages of healing).

Treatment

Diagnose and treat specific injuries as described below. Document findings clearly in the medical record. Include a full account of the events surrounding the injury as related by those who brought the child to the emergency department.

Disposition

Obtain immediate pediatric consultation. Hospitalize the child if abuse is strongly suspected or confirmed. By law in the USA, the physician *must* make a report to the appropriate child welfare agency if child abuse is suspected.

ESSENTIAL EMERGENCY DEPARTMENT TREATMENT

CORRECT DEFORMITY

Correct severe or moderate deformity due to fracture or dislocation as soon as possible to minimize soft tissue damage by relieving skin tension and compression or excessive stretching of nerves, arteries, or veins. If pain is severe and no contraindication exists, intravenous narcotics (eg, morphine, 3–5 mg) may be given slowly as needed. Do not forcibly correct deformity close to or involving a joint without x-ray confirmation of the diagnosis and technical expertise in the appropriate reduction maneuvers.

Most angulated fractures can be aligned satisfactorily with firm but gentle manual traction along the axis of the injured bone, with attention directed to correcting rotational deformity (Fig 22–1). While one person holds the injured limb in gentle traction, another inspects the posterior surfaces and then applies a splint. If complete correct is difficult to attain, splint the limb in the best position that can be safely achieved, and obtain immediate consultation if neurovascular function or integrity of the skin is compromised.

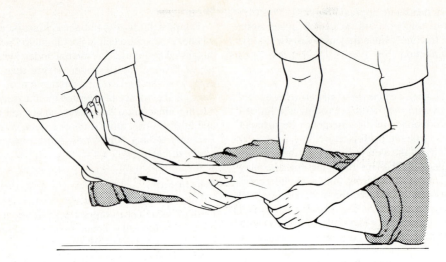

Figure 22–1. Technique of manual traction to align an angulated fracture and correct deformity.

TREAT OPEN FRACTURE

Control associated bleeding with ample sterile pressure dressings and splints as described below. If debridement will be delayed more than a few hours, consider copious irrigation of the wound with sterile Ringer's irrigation or saline and application of iodophor solution (eg, povidone-iodine) to dressings.

Give appropriate tetanus prophylaxis (Chapter 24). Give antistaphylococcal antimicrobials parenterally (eg, cefazolin, 20 mg/kg intravenously every 8 hours). For more severe wounds, gram-negative coverage is appropriate as well (eg, add gentamicin, 1 mg/kg every 8 hours, or substitute ceftriaxone, 1 g every 12 hours). Give nothing by mouth, to prepare the patient for surgery.

Obtain immediate orthopedic consultation. Debridement and irrigation by an experienced fracture surgeon in a well-prepared operating room are required in all cases of open fracture.

Be alert for wounds adjacent to presumably closed fractures. Bacterial colonization will occur within a few hours even on superficial skin abrasions. If underlying bone or ligament injuries require surgery, this must be performed at once, before bacterial colonization of abrasions can occur, or it must be postponed until the abrasions have healed completely. Such delays for skin healing may compromise the ultimate results of treatment.

SPLINT EACH INJURED AREA

Splint injuries as soon as possible (definitely before moving the patient from the emergency department or obtaining x-rays). The injured extremity should be elevated slightly above the heart to minimize swelling without impairing perfusion.

Intravenous administration of a narcotic analgesic (eg, morphine, 3–5 mg intravenously every hour) provides prompt pain relief for splinting, x-rays, and movement of the patient. Coexisting head or abdominal injuries may contraindicate the use of narcotic analgesics.

Splinting is an improvisational art. It requires correction of gross deformity and application of well-padded rigid or semirigid supports that do not constrict the injured area. Well-padded plaster slabs, held in place with loose bias-cut stockinet, are most adaptable. Commercially fabricated splints, circumferential pneumatic splints (inflated just enough to support the limb), and even cardboard or thickly folded newspapers can be used effectively in most body regions, although traction splints are advisable for the femur.

Splint elbow injuries and hip dislocations in moderate flexion (30–60 degrees). Most other injuries can be splinted in a neutral position.

Splints should generally include joints above and below the site of injury (eg, immobilize the shoulder and wrist if the elbow is injured).

Open fractures with protruding bone ends can often be splinted most effectively if the bone is allowed to retract into the wound when the limb is realigned. Inform the operating surgeon that protruding bone has been reduced back into the wound.

Splinting techniques for various areas follow.

Cervical Spine

Use a combination of a rigid cervical collar and lateral neck rolls or sand bags, with adhesive tape across the forehead, or an equivalent immobilizing device. When an unstable injury is present, application of skeletal traction using Gardner-Wells tongs should be considered. Directions for application are attached to the tongs. Povidone-iodine is applied liberally to the hair and scalp just above the ears. Lidocaine 1% is infiltrated into the area down to bone, and the tongs are positioned 1 cm above the ears, in line with the external auditory meati. The pins are advanced into the skull until the appropriate pressure is indicated. Traction is applied via an appropriate pulley or by passing a rope over the end of the stretcher. The weight applied depends on the level of injury. Too much force may overdistract an injury of the upper cervical spine. Generally, 3 kg (7 lb) is adequate for upper (occiput through C-2) cervical spine injuries, with up to 7–9 kg (15–20 lb) for lower cervical spine injuries. Consultation and x-ray monitoring of alignment in traction are necessary.

Shoulder

Use a sling and swathe (Fig 22–2) for shoulder injuries unless shoulder dislocation prevents positioning of the arm across the chest.

Humerus

Use a padded U splint (Fig 22–3) with a sling and swathe for injuries to the shaft of the humerus.

Elbow & Forearm

Use a padded posterior splint (Fig 22–4) with sling and swathe for injuries to the elbow and forearm.

Wrist & Hand

Use a padded volar splint for wrist injuries (Fig 22–5), and elevate the limb above the level of the heart. Note that the usual sling does not provide this level of elevation. (See Fig 22–17 if the thumb must be splinted and Fig 22–18 for finger splinting.)

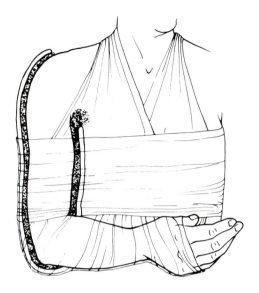

Figure 22–3. U splint with sling and swathe for immobilization of humeral fractures. Make sure that the axilla is well padded.

Thoracolumbar Spine & Pelvis

Keep the patient supine on a firm padded surface, and use the logrolling technique as required. Use traction with an ankle hitch (supplied with a splint such as that in Fig 22–6) and a 4.5- to 6.8-kg (10- to 15-lb) weight over the foot of the bed if there is proximal displacement of half of the pelvis. Convert this

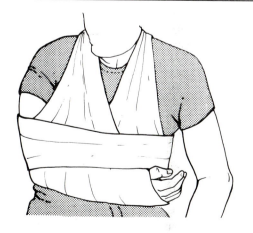

arm and shoulder injuries.

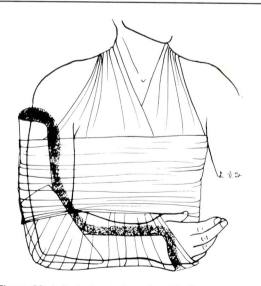

Figure 22–4. Posterior plaster splint with sling and swathe for immobilization of elbow or forearm injuries. Abundant cast padding is first wrapped around the arm. The posterior plaster must be reinforced medially and laterally to the elbow, but neither padding nor plaster should constrict the antecubital fossa.

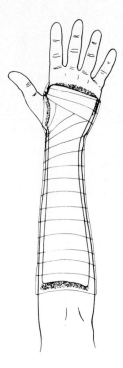

Figure 22–5. Volar splint for immobilization of wrist injuries.

temporary splinting to skeletal traction as soon as possible.

Hip & Femur

Dislocations of the hip produce a flexion deformity that should *not* be corrected during splinting. If flexion deformity is present, use pillows or folded linen or blankets to support the leg as it lies. For additional stability during transport, add adhesive tape restraints. Fractures can be splinted for several hours with a fixed traction splint using a standard Thomas splint or a commercially available device (Fig 22–6). Skeletal traction is required for continuing immobilization of unstable femur fractures, although skin traction is often used with a light weight for hip fractures in the elderly.

Knee

Highly unstable fractures and dislocations of the knee may require a traction splint (Fig 22–6). Most other knee injuries can be immobilized with well-padded plaster slabs from groin to ankle or a commercially available "knee immobilizer." Padding behind the knee maintains 10–15 degrees of flexion (Fig 22–7) when the knee is splinted.

Tibia

Splints must control both foot and knee in tibial injury. Equally satisfactory are a traction splint with just enough tension to provide stability, well-padded plaster slabs from groin to toes, or a prefabricated or improvised splint that achieves the same objectives.

Ankle

If fracture of the ankle is rotationally unstable, splint from the upper thigh to the toes (see Ankle Joint Injuries, below). Otherwise, apply plaster that has been shaped into a U over ample padding (Fig 22–8).

Foot

A pillow splint is excellent for inpatient care (Fig 22–9). If the patient is ambulatory, however, a posterior plaster slab is added to the previously described U splint, with ample padding for the foot (Fig 22–10).

Note: Elevation of the injured limb is advisable. The use of crutches and instructions to avoid weight bearing are an essential part of the early outpatient treatment of musculoskeletal injuries of the lower extremity.

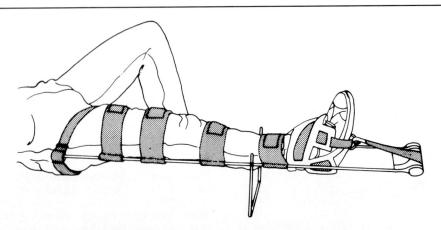

Figure 22–6. Thomas traction splint for fractures of the femur.

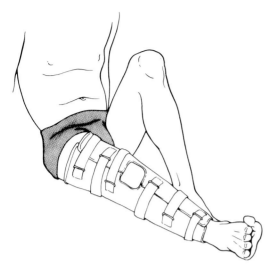

Figure 22–7. Splint for immobilization of knee injuries. The injured knee should be splinted in slight flexion using padding behind the knee.

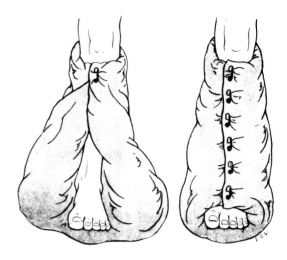

Figure 22–9. Pillow splint for temporary immobilization of ankle or foot injuries in patients confined to bed. (Reproduced, with permission, from Way LW [editor]: *Current Surgical Diagnosis & Treatment,* 9th ed. Appleton & Lange, 1991.)

Dislocations

Reduce all joint dislocations as soon as possible, but only after examination and x-ray have confirmed the nature of the injury and the neurovascular status of the limb. Examine the limb immediately after reduction to assess stability. Does dislocation readily recur? If so, special precautions are necessary to maintain joint alignment. X-rays are mandatory after manipulation to confirm that reduction is complete and that there are no other injuries. Obtain immediate orthopedic consultation and assistance for treating dislocations that are not easily reduced or that require special expertise (see specific injuries, below).

Fractures With Skin Damage

Skin damage (abrasions, lacerations) near fractures suggests open fracture. Even minor skin injuries are

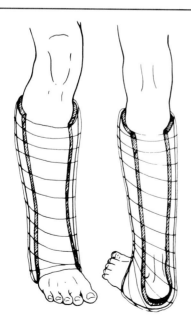

Figure 22–8. U-shaped plaster splint and padding for immobilization of ankle injuries.

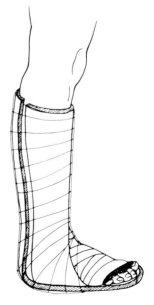

Figure 22–10. Combined U splint and posterior-plantar plaster slab with padding for ambulatory (non-weight-bearing) patient with foot injuries.

significant, because they rapidly become colonized by bacteria and necessitate postponement of fracture surgery until they have healed. Since fracture surgery may frequently be performed during the first few hours after injury, immediate orthopedic evaluation is required whenever skin damage is noted in the region of a fracture that may need operation.

PROVIDE ANALGESIA

Bone and joint injuries are often very painful. Therefore, narcotic analgesia is an important part of emergency treatment. Several key points must be remembered: **(1)** Pain may be a sign of serious, progressive injury, especially ischemia due to arterial occlusion, compartment syndrome, or even an excessively tight cast. **(2)** Analgesia may interfere with discovery of an associated injury, especially those of the brain or abdomen. **(3)** Analgesia may dangerously depress respiratory function. **(4)** Pain is usually relieved significantly after reduction of a dislocation or after adequate splinting of a fracture. **(5)** Response to narcotic analgesics may be increased in the elderly, the intoxicated, the hypersensitive, and the premedicated (especially with a benzodiazepine) patient.

When painful manipulation is necessary, analgesia is usually best provided by giving small amounts of intravenous narcotic (eg, morphine sulfate, 2–10 mg titrated slowly over 4–5 minutes, with smaller doses for elderly individuals). An intravenous line should first be established and maintained. Naloxone (Narcan, others) should be immediately available for administration to counteract intravenous narcotic overdoses (0.4 mg intravenously every 2–3 minutes as needed). The antagonistic effect of naloxone does not last as long as the depressant effects of narcotics. Therefore, continued observation and perhaps retreatment are required. Fluid administration may be needed to counteract hypotension. Ventilation and oxygenation may also be required. Provisions for both must be immediately available.

Premedication with a benzodiazepine is often recommended and employed for suitable patients but should be recognized as increasing the risk of complications. Unlike the case for narcotics, a specific antidote does not exist for these agents, which should be used sparingly and as an *adjunct* to narcotics. Remember that relief of pain, rather than sedation or amnesia, is the desired effect. Midazolam (Versed) is occasionally advocated. It is a short-acting benzodiazepine that can be given intravenously (2–2.5 mg initially, then titrating to slurred speech slowly over 2–3 minutes, usually no more than 0.1–0.15 mg/kg, or significantly less if narcotics also will be used). Midazolam potentiates narcotics. It is a *general anesthetic* in large enough amounts. It is risky in the elderly and must be used with great care.

A mixture of nitrous oxide and oxygen gases, with a demand regulator as part of a proprietary administration system (Nitronox) has been used effectively as the sole analgesic for children. However, it is contraindicated for intoxicated patients and those who have also received parenteral narcotics, which severely limits its safety for most injured emergency department patients.

A sterile solution of local anesthetic (eg, lidocaine 1% without epinephrine to a maximum of 1 mg/kg) can be injected directly into a fracture hematoma to provide analgesia during manipulative reduction of a fracture, especially those of the distal radius. Such a **hematoma block** is rarely needed for application of a splint, may result in significant systemic absorption with toxicity, and is best deferred to an experienced orthopedic surgeon. Local anesthetic infiltration or peripheral nerve blockade can provide helpful relief of pain for treatment of peripheral fractures, dislocations, and wounds. Training, experience, and thorough preliminary neurovascular examination are essential.

When parenteral narcotic analgesics are required in the emergency department for skeletal injuries, intravenous narcotics (eg, morphine sulfate, titrated slowly up to 2–10 mg, which may need to be repeated after about an hour) should be the mainstay. Continued evaluation of the patient is necessary to identify pain that may indicate a complication of injury or treatment as well as to identify overmedication. For more stable and less uncomfortable patients, an intramuscular narcotic injection may be appropriate.

If outpatient management has been chosen for a skeletal injury, pain should be controlled by splinting the injury, followed by rest, elevation, and ice packs. If these measures are insufficient, oral analgesics may be added. Generally, a nonnarcotic agent (eg, acetaminophen, 650 mg orally every 4 hours; aspirin, 650 mg orally every 4–6 hours; or ibuprofen, 400 mg orally every 6 hours) is used first. For more painful injuries, it may be necessary to substitute codeine compound, 30–60 mg orally every 3–4 hours as needed; hydrocodone compound, 5–10 mg orally every 3–4 hours as needed; or oxycodone compound, 5–10 mg orally every 6 hours as needed (for a few days only). These agents may be used in the emergency department *if* oral medication is appropriate.

Each emergency department should establish appropriate local protocols for analgesia use and precautions in collaboration with the orthopedic surgery and anesthesiology consultant staff.

GENERAL CONSIDERATIONS IN TREATMENT OF MUSCULOSKELETAL INJURIES

DEFINITION OF COMMON ORTHOPEDIC TERMS

Fracture

A fracture is a broken or crushed bone that is usually evident on x-rays but is sometimes manifested initially only by localized tenderness.

A. Major Types:

1. Closed fracture–The skin is not broken, and there is no wound communicating with the fracture site.

2. Open fracture–Skin and underlying tissue injuries permit communication between wound and fracture site.

3. Articular fracture–Articular fractures involve joint surfaces and may be associated with ligament injuries and with complete or partial dislocations. They may be open or closed.

B. Variations:

1. Undisplaced–An undisplaced fracture is a hairline fracture without loss of normal anatomic configuration. This configuration must be present on both anteroposterior and lateral x-rays, because superimposed shadows on a single view can make a fracture appear undisplaced when it is not.

2. Displaced–A displaced fracture is one in which separation of fracture fragments has occurred, with loss of anatomic configuration.

3. Angulated–In an angulated fracture, bending or angular deformity may result from separation of fracture fragments or from asymmetric impaction of cancellous bone fragments.

4. Comminuted–A comminuted fracture is one in which the involved bone is broken into more than 2 pieces.

5. Avulsed–An avulsion fracture is one composed of bone fragment (usually near joints) pulled off by attached ligaments or tendons. These fractures are often inappropriately called "chip" fractures. They should be recognized instead as indications of serious ligament or tendon injuries rather than as inconsequential defects analogous to chips on the rim of a teacup.

Dislocation

Dislocation denotes a disruption of the normal relationships between articular surfaces. Dislocation should be suspected whenever a joint is deformed or does not move in the normal fashion. Note that x-rays are necessary to confirm the diagnosis. Damage to the joint capsule and other ligaments often occurs with dislocation, so that joint instability may be noted after reduction. Incomplete dislocations are often called **subluxations.**

Sprain

A sprain is a complete or partial tear of ligaments occurring either within the ligaments themselves or when they are torn off at their attachment to bone. Although some authorities use the word "sprain" to denote only partial tears, the word as used here denotes complete tears also. Although x-rays are advisable, physical examination, not x-ray studies, is the key to diagnosis of sprains (ligaments are radiolucent). Swelling and tenderness over a ligament and pain when it is stretched suggest a sprain. Excessive motion of the joint when the ligament is stressed confirms the diagnosis. Stability is compared with that of the contralateral joint. Sprains are graded on the basis of the following criteria:

(1) Grade I–Minor incomplete tear. The ligament is tender and painful, but there is no laxity (excessive varus-valgus or anterior-posterior mobility when stress is applied). Swelling and ecchymosis are usually minimal.

(2) Grade II–Significant incomplete tear. On physical examination, there is laxity but also a convincing end point beyond which no further opening of the joint occurs. Swelling and ecchymosis may be moderate to severe and associated with moderate to extreme tenderness.

(3) Grade III–Total failure of the ligament involved. No end point is felt when stress is applied to the ligament during examination of the joint. Pain and muscle spasm can often mask a grade III sprain, so that the diagnosis is easily missed.

Note: If the joint cannot be stressed adequately enough to demonstrate a firm end point or to document opening, the patient must be referred to a specialist for evaluation within 1–2 days.

Strain

A strain is partial disruption of a musculotendinous unit short of complete rupture. A strain may be caused by overuse or by acute injury, when a muscle contracts against an overwhelming force. Local tenderness and pain with use are present. Although weakness usually accompanies the pain, the action of the injured muscle should be unimpaired (eg, ability to extend the knee against gravity).

Tendon Rupture

Rupture of a tendon—including its avulsion from bone, with or without a small attached fragment—results in weakness or loss of ability to produce a characteristic motion. Physical examination must therefore test specifically for function of tendons in an injured area.

GROWTH PLATE INJURIES

Whenever a child sustains trauma near the end of a long bone, injury to the epiphyseal growth plate (also called the physis) should be considered. The growth plate is readily injured because it is weaker than ossified bone or ligament. Some ligaments and tendons attach to bony apophyses that are attached to the metaphysis by a cartilaginous growth plate (eg, medial humeral epicondyle). Avulsion of such apophyses may leave no evidence on x-ray other than displacement. The Salter-Harris system is commonly used to classify growth plate injuries (Fig 22–11). Classification is not as important as recognition in providing appropriate treatment in the emergency department.

Diagnosis

A. Symptoms and Signs: Tenderness and swelling localized to the region of the physis suggest a growth plate fracture even if x-rays do not show damage. The radiolucent growth cartilage may be minimally displaced or—even though totally disrupted—may have been aligned anatomically at the moment of x-ray exposure.

B. X-Ray Findings: X-ray signs of growth plate injuries can be subtle, with complete absence of typical fracture lines. The following are common signs of injury:

1. Appearance different from that of an identical view of the uninjured side obtained for purposes of comparison. (Although comparative x-rays are not required for all cases, they are helpful if the diagnosis is uncertain.)

2. Widening or asymmetry of the growth plate.

3. Displacement of the epiphysis on a single view, especially the lateral view of the distal radius or distal tibia.

4. Hemarthrosis or rotational malalignment

when the entire epiphyseal region is unossified, as in the elbow of a very young child.

5. Fractures through the growth plate revealed by x-rays taken while angular stress is applied to this region. Such stress x-rays should always be obtained before the diagnosis of ligamentous disruption is made in a child.

6. A triangular metaphyseal fracture fragment based on the growth plate (Thurston-Holland sign).

C. Severe Injuries to the Growth Plate Without Obvious X-Ray Findings:

1. Compression injuries (eg, falling from a height and landing on a foot, crushing the distal tibial physis) may substantially affect bone growth. The region is stable on examination, with only swelling and tenderness as clues to significant injury.

2. Avulsion of the perichondrial ring (eg, result of lawn mower injuries to the medial side of the ankle) is also associated with disturbances of bone growth. Even though x-rays show no skeletal damage, such injuries should be recognized as more than just loss of skin and subcutaneous tissue.

Treatment & Disposition

Displaced fractures involving a growth plate or an adjacent articular surface require orthopedic consultation before the child is discharged from the emergency department.

Splint the injury, and consult an orthopedist. Give nothing by mouth in case surgery is required.

If it is *certain* that a growth plate injury is undisplaced, splint the limb, and arrange for orthopedic follow-up within 3 days. Injuries to the distal femoral or distal humeral epiphysis are exceptions and require orthopedic consultation before the child can be discharged from the emergency department.

In some cases, x-rays appear normal, yet the child refuses to use the extremity. Even though the exami-

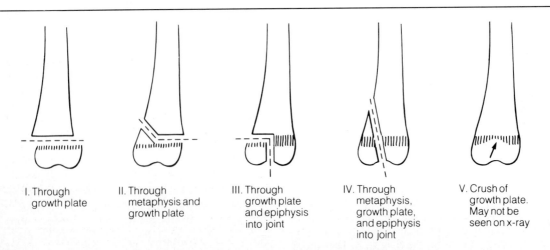

Figure 22–11. Salter-Harris classification of growth plate injuries.

I. Through growth plate

II. Through metaphysis and growth plate

III. Through growth plate and epiphysis into joint

IV. Through metaphysis, growth plate, and epiphysis into joint

V. Crush of growth plate. May not be seen on x-ray

nation may not disclose a specific point of maximal tenderness, the child should be presumed to have a possible undisplaced growth plate injury. Splinting and orthopedic consultation are required.

EXAMINATION & EVALUATION

Initial Evaluation

Accurate diagnosis, not definitive treatment is the primary role of the emergency department in the care of musculoskeletal injuries. Although musculoskeletal injuries are rarely life-threatening, they may be associated with other injuries that are. Certain injuries that threaten survival of the limb require urgent operation to reduce the risk of amputation. Other injuries of muscles, bones, and joints may cause permanent disability that can be minimized with timely appropriate care. Even seemingly trivial injuries may have adverse results if proper care is not provided early.

Aftercare

The purpose of follow-up care is to make sure that corrective measures are instituted promptly if complications develop. Since continuing observation and care are important in musculoskeletal injury, few patients can receive complete treatment in a single visit to the emergency department. Therefore, arrangements for suitable aftercare must be part of the emergency treatment. Details necessarily vary with the patient, the nature of the injuries, the training and experience of the emergency physician, the preferences of the orthopedic consultant, and local practices. There is no substitute for a close working relationship between emergency physician and consultant. The physician with sufficient training and experience in the management of musculoskeletal injuries may begin definitive care of some disorders in the emergency department without benefit of orthopedic consultation, but such treatment should be within the limits of the individual's competence.

Complications

The following indicate problems during treatment of extremity injuries that require immediate evaluation and usually urgent consultation and treatment:

(1) Increasing pain or swelling.

(2) Decreasing motor or sensory function.

(3) Localized pain, pressure, or rubbing under a cast or splint.

(4) Lack of full active motion of proximal and distal joints (eg, finger or shoulder motion should not be impaired during cast treatment for a wrist fracture). Both joint flexibility and motor function must be regularly assessed.

(5) Loss of alignment of a reduced or previously undisplaced injury, as shown by follow-up physical examination or by x-rays in the splint or cast.

DISPOSITION & DISCHARGE INSTRUCTIONS

Before discharging the patient from the emergency department, the physician should review postreduction x-rays and provide the patient with written and oral instructions that include a follow-up appointment, a list of symptoms and signs indicating the need for more urgent attention, information on where to obtain further emergency care if necessary, and activities permitted, including whether weight bearing is allowed and whether elevation of the injured part is needed.

Adequate analgesia must be provided. If more than 30–60 mg of a codeine compound every 3 hours is needed for pain relief, the patient should return to the emergency department, since hospitalization is probably required. Consider providing an anti-inflammatory drug if bursitis, tendinitis, or another inflammatory process is present. Aspirin (650–975 mg every 4–6 hours) or another nonsteroidal anti-inflammatory agent (eg, ibuprofen, 400 mg 4 times daily) may be used.

Consider splitting and loosening a circumferential cast, including padding, if it is applied over injuries that are likely to be associated with significant swelling.

EMERGENCY TREATMENT OF SPECIFIC MUSCULOSKELETAL INJURIES

SHOULDER GIRDLE

1. STERNOCLAVICULAR JOINT INJURY*

Diagnosis

Sternoclavicular joint injury is associated with a history of anteroposterior or transverse crushing injury to the upper chest. Local pain, tenderness, and swelling are noted. If the sternoclavicular joint is dislocated, the medial clavicle is either more prominent (if dislocation is anterior) or less prominent (if dislocation is posterior) than it is on the uninjured side. Posterior dislocation is rare but can cause serious respiratory or vascular compromise by narrowing the superior mediastinum. The diagnosis is confirmed by

---

*The term "joint injury" refers to dislocation, ligamentous rupture or sprain, or articular fracture. The text discusses each type of injury in detail if differentiation is important for proper emergency care.

CT scan or cephalic tilt x-ray taken with the patient supine and the x-ray beam angled cephalad at 40 degrees from the vertical. The film is placed under the patient's head, so that the sternoclavicular joints are projected upon it (see Fractures and Dislocations of the Shoulder in Rockwood and Green reference).

Treatment

Apply a sling and swathe (Fig 22–2). Observe the patient for development of respiratory and vascular problems.

Disposition

Obtain immediate orthopedic consultation for urgent closed reduction of posterior displacement. Hospitalization is advisable because of the potential for serious internal injuries. Seek consultation for anterior dislocation before the patient leaves the emergency department.

2. CLAVICULAR FRACTURE

Diagnosis

Fracture of the clavicle is caused by an indirect or direct blow to the shoulder. Tenderness and swelling are noted, and deformity is clearly seen on x-ray (anteroposterior and occasionally apical lordotic views). Confirm the function of all upper extremity nerves (Table 22–2) to rule out brachial plexus injury. Confirm that upper extremity pulses are palpable and that swelling and venous congestion are absent to rule out associated vascular injury.

Treatment

Use a sling and a figure-of-eight bandage (Fig 22–12) or commercially prepared equivalent.

Disposition

Unless complications are noted, arrange orthopedic referral within 3–5 days. A figure-of-eight bandage that is too tight may cause swelling or neuropathy; the patient should be warned about these problems and instructed to loosen the bandage if needed.

3. ACROMIOCLAVICULAR JOINT INJURY

Diagnosis

Acromioclavicular joint injury is associated with a history of a fall onto the shoulder with subsequent local pain. Tenderness, swelling, and often deformity, with prominence of the distal clavicle, are seen.

X-rays (anteroposterior and tangential scapular views) may show fracture or upward displacement of the distal clavicle, which is accentuated by hanging a 4.5-kg (10-lb) weight from each wrist and obtaining a single anteroposterior view showing both acromioclavicular joints. Acromioclavicular joint injuries are graded in severity as follows:

(1) Grade I–Minimal tear of the acromioclavicular ligament or displacement of the joint.

(2) Grade II–Significant damage to the acromioclavicular ligaments without increase in the coracoclavicular distance on weight-bearing radiographs.

(3) Grade III–Complete tear of both the acromioclavicular and coracoclavicular ligaments, with evident increase in the coracoclavicular distance on plain and weight-bearing views.

Treatment

Apply a sling and swathe (Fig 22–2).

Disposition

Arrange for orthopedic referral within 3–5 days. If skin abrasion or grade III injury is present, obtain immediate orthopedic consultation. Surgery is sometimes recommended for grade III injuries.

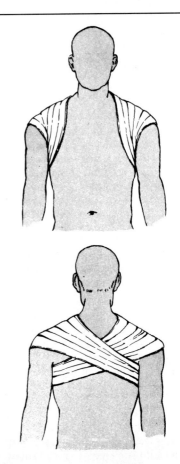

Figure 22–12. Figure-of-eight bandage for immobilization of a fractured clavicle. (Reproduced, with permission, from Way LW [editor]: *Current Surgical Diagnosis & Treatment,* 9th ed. Appleton & Lange, 1991.)

4. SCAPULAR FRACTURE

Diagnosis

Fracture of the scapula is caused by a direct blow to the area. Tenderness and limited painful motion of the shoulder are found.

X-ray (anteroposterior and tangential scapular views) confirms the diagnosis. Assess shoulder joint alignment, and look for fracture involving the glenoid process (the articular surface for the humerus) on x-ray. Other, potentially serious injuries (chest, abdomen, etc) may be associated.

Treatment

Apply a sling and swathe (Fig 22–2).

Disposition

The patient should be referred to an orthopedist within 3–5 days unless the shoulder joint is involved, in which case prompt consultation for possible earlier treatment is required (especially if the joint is incongruent or the skin abraded).

SHOULDER JOINT INJURY

1. DISLOCATION

Diagnosis

There is a history of injury that displaces the shoulder joint. Anterior dislocation usually results from abduction and external rotation of the arm. Posterior dislocation is most often caused by seizures.

A. Symptoms and Signs: Patients have pain, tenderness, loss of normal shoulder motion, and deformity, which may not be recognized unless both shoulders are uncovered and examined simultaneously. Assess neurovascular function, noting especially sensation in the lateral shoulder area, which is diminished with axillary nerve injury.

1. Anterior dislocation—Anterior dislocation is more common than posterior dislocation and is characterized by more apparent deformity. The arm on the affected side is held by the opposite hand in slight abduction. The acromion is prominent, and the shoulder looks "squared-off." Look for an associated fracture of the humeral tuberosities.

2. Posterior dislocation—Posterior dislocation of the shoulder joint is rare and is frequently missed during initial evaluation. The arm on the affected side is held adducted against the chest and internally rotated. The posterior surface of the shoulder is more prominent than that of the normal side. *A shoulder that does not externally rotate beyond the neutral position is assumed to have sustained posterior dislocation until it is proved otherwise.* Appearance of the injured joint on an anteroposterior view x-ray is easily confused with that of a normal shoulder. The tan-

gential scapular or axillary lateral view shows the posterior position of the humeral head.

B. X-Ray Findings: Anteroposterior and lateral x-rays are essential for evaluating any acutely injured shoulder (Fig 22–13). An axillary lateral x-ray, taken with the arm flexed forward on a foam pad and abducted as far as the patient allows, is necessary to exclude a posterior dislocation and confirm the relationship of humeral head to glenoid.

Treatment

A. Reduction: Immediate closed reduction using adequate analgesia is generally successful. Sustained traction along the dislocated humerus with countertraction on the thorax with a sheet is a safe and effective reduction maneuver (Fig 22–14). The goal is to decrease reflex muscle spasm by intravenous administration of narcotics and continuous traction. Once the spasm is overcome, reduction will occur easily or can be encouraged by gently guiding the humeral head onto the glenoid process while traction is maintained. A similar approach using traction applied to the adducted humerus will reduce posterior dislocations of the shoulder, although relatively greater muscle spasm may make reduction more difficult than that of anterior dislocation.

Morphine, 3–5 mg intravenously followed by additional 3- to 5-mg increments every 5–15 minutes as needed, is recommended until an adequate analgesic effect has been obtained. Morphine has the advantage of permitting reversal of respiratory depression with naloxone, if required, after the shoulder is reduced.

B. Postreduction Care: After reduction, apply a sling and swathe (Fig 22–2); reevaluate the patient's neurovascular status; and confirm successful reduction with adequate x-rays. It is important to watch patients carefully after reduction, because they may be excessively sedated by analgesia once the pain of dislocation has been relieved.

Disposition

Obtain immediate orthopedic consultation if reduction cannot be achieved. Otherwise, discharge the patient after arranging for orthopedic consultation within 3–5 days to determine the length of immobilization and the rehabilitation program.

2. ROTATOR CUFF TEAR

A tear of the tendinous cuff formed by the subscapularis, supraspinatus, infraspinatus, and teres minor muscles produces shoulder pain and weakness. Small attritional tears may develop without any specific injury. Larger acute tears may be produced by falls on the arm, especially in middle-aged or older people.

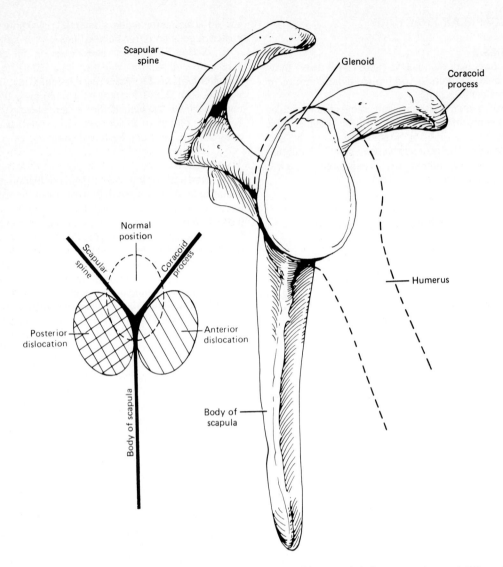

Figure 22–13. Sketch of view on tangential lateral x-ray shows the body of the scapula in its narrowest aspect. If the patient is poorly positioned, the medial and lateral borders are not superimposed. Normally, the humeral head shadow lies directly over that of the glenoid, which may be hard to see. The position of the glenoid is indicated by the confluence of the scapular spine, the body of the scapula, and the coracoid process. A dislocated humeral head lies anterior or posterior to this point.

Diagnosis

The patient complains of shoulder pain and tenderness and is unable to abduct the arm or hold it abducted against gravity. X-rays usually show no abnormalities but should be obtained to rule out other injury.

Treatment

Apply a sling and swathe (Fig 22–2), and provide oral analgesia.

Significant shoulder disability can be minimized by early rehabilitation measures emphasizing passive range of motion exercises. Larger tears should be repaired surgically for maximal recovery of strength.

Disposition

The patient should see an orthopedist within 3–5 days.

3. ACUTE BURSITIS OR TENDINITIS

Diagnosis

Inflammation of the rotator cuff tendon or of the overlying subdeltoid bursa can produce severe shoulder pain of acute or gradual onset, occasionally following overuse. Acute calcific tendinitis is severely painful, and the shoulder may appear swollen and inflamed. Progressive shoulder stiffness will develop if

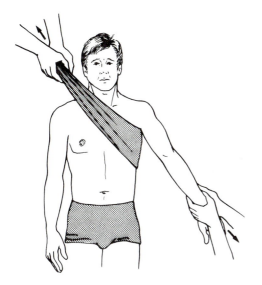

Figure 22–14. Method of producing traction on dislocated humerus and countertraction on thorax for reduction of shoulder dislocation.

the shoulder is immobilized without proper attention to rehabilitation measures. Tenderness and pain occur with motion, especially through the arc from 60 to 120 degrees of abduction.

Consider the possibility of septic bursitis or septic arthritis, particularly if the patient has other chronic medical problems. If fluid is present in either the subdeltoid bursa or the shoulder joint, it should be aspirated for staining with Gram's stain, culture, and cell count to rule out infection. Such fluid is not obvious on physical examination, so that aspiration must be attempted if infection is suspected.

X-rays (anteroposterior, in internal and external rotation, and axillary lateral views) usually show no abnormalities unless calcific deposits are present (most often near the greater tuberosity).

Treatment

Apply a sling and swathe (Fig 22–2). Provide analgesia and anti-inflammatory medication. Local injection of corticosteroids often provides striking relief. Start shoulder range of motion exercises promptly if symptoms are only mild or moderate or if referral to an orthopedist must be delayed for several days. The best initial exercise is the "pendulum," in which the patient bends 90 degrees at the waist and gently swings the affected arm in as large a circle as possible. This should be done for a minute or so several times a day.

Disposition

Obtain prompt orthopedic consultation if pain is severe or infection is suspected on the basis of syno-

vial fluid analysis. Otherwise, discharge the patient, and arrange for orthopedic referral within 3–5 days.

4. PROXIMAL HUMERAL FRACTURE

Undisplaced fractures of the proximal humerus can generally be managed with splinting of the injured area followed as soon as possible by progressive rehabilitation exercises. Displaced fractures frequently require surgical treatment. It is important not to miss a dislocation of the shoulder (glenohumeral) joint that may be associated with fracture.

Diagnosis

Symptoms and signs include pain, tenderness, loss of ability to move the arm, and progressive swelling and ecchymosis. Examine distal pulses and peripheral sensory and motor function to assess the integrity of the neurovascular system. X-rays (anteroposterior and tangential scapular lateral views) demonstrate fracture. Check for comminution or displacement, and demonstrate the relationship of the humeral head to the glenoid process with an axillary lateral, or equivalent, view. For undisplaced fractures, anteroposterior views in internal and external rotation may be required to confirm the diagnosis.

Treatment

Apply a sling and swathe (Fig 22–2), and provide analgesia.

Disposition

If the fracture is undisplaced, refer the patient to an orthopedist within 3–5 days. If the humeral head is dislocated, the fracture is displaced, or a neurovascular deficit exists, obtain immediate orthopedic consultation.

ARM, ELBOW, & FOREARM INJURIES

1. HUMERAL SHAFT FRACTURE

Diagnosis

Humeral shaft fracture is characterized by pain, tenderness, deformity, and progressive local swelling and ecchymosis. Check the patient's neurovascular status—especially function of the radial nerve (Table 22–2). X-rays (anteroposterior and tangential scapular lateral views of the entire humerus) show the fracture and define displacement, angulation, or comminution.

Treatment

Immobilize the humerus with a plaster U splint that has ample padding, especially over the axillary end of the splint, the humeral epicondyles, and the ulnar nerve (Fig 22–3). Additionally, a sling and swathe are required to splint the injured arm to the chest (Fig 22–2). Provide analgesia.

Disposition

Immediate consultation with an orthopedist is required if neurologic deficit is noted or develops during treatment. Refer the patient to an orthopedist within 1–3 days.

2. ELBOW REGION INJURY

Some elbow injuries are easy to diagnose, whereas others are difficult, especially if they occur in children, in whom the cartilaginous structure of the distal humerus has not fully ossified. Precise physical localization of tenderness must be compared with x-ray findings. Early consultation with an orthopedist is advisable if the diagnosis is uncertain.

Diagnosis

A. Symptoms and Signs: Swelling, deformity, and limited elbow motion—either on flexion-extension or on supination-pronation—suggest significant elbow injury. Neurologic and vascular damage may occur with displaced elbow injuries, after which compartment syndrome of the forearm may develop over several hours. It is therefore mandatory to assess motor and sensory function of the ulnar, median, and radial nerves and to palpate for presence of pulses at the wrist.

If skin abrasions are present, any surgery that is required should be performed early, before bacteria colonize the abrasion. If more than 8–12 hours have elapsed since injury, it may be advisable to delay necessary surgery until the abrasion is fully healed; the delay may compromise repair of the skeletal injury.

B. X-Ray Findings: X-rays should be examined carefully for signs of dislocation, fracture lines with or without displacement, abnormally shaped bone that might reveal an undisplaced fracture, and any difference in identical films of the uninjured side. Such comparative x-rays are especially helpful in evaluating elbow injuries in children. Fluid (usually blood) resulting from elbow injury and accumulating posterior to the distal humerus may lift periarticular fat away from the bone, producing the so-called "positive fat pad sign." In contrast, visible fat anterior to the distal humerus is a normal finding, except when joint capsule distention causes it to appear triangular. This so-called "sail sign" also suggests an occult fracture. The shaft and head of the radius normally point at the capitellum humeri on all views. The trochlea should lie congruently in its fossa in the proximal ulna. More information on elbow disorders may be found in the references listed at the end of this chapter.

Treatment

A. Fractures of the Elbow: Fractures of the distal humerus with displacement should be splinted with the arm bent at an angle of about 45 degrees. The limb should then be elevated. Immediate consultation with an orthopedist is required for closed or possibly open reduction because there may be progressive swelling with compromise of neurovascular function.

Fractures of the olecranon process usually require surgery, which should be performed within 6–8 hours if skin around the fracture is abraded, a frequent occurrence with elbow injuries. Olecranon fractures associated with complete or partial dislocations on the elbow also require immediate consultation.

Fractures of the head or neck of the radius, undisplaced fractures of the distal humerus, and uncomplicated fractures of the olecranon may be splinted in neutral position (Fig 22–4). Refer the patient to an orthopedist within 1–3 days. Associated complete or partial dislocation, neurologic or vascular injuries, and compartment syndromes require immediate orthopedic consultation.

B. Elbow Dislocations: Closed reduction of elbow dislocations is usually possible, although it becomes more difficult if delayed. Adequate analgesia (morphine, 3–5 mg intravenously, with additional 3- to 5-mg doses as needed) is necessary unless reduction is done soon after injury.

The method of reduction is as follows (Fig 22–15):

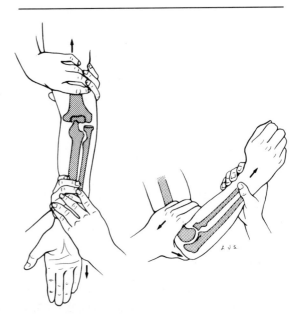

Figure 22–15. Reduction of posterior elbow dislocation by applying manual traction on the forearm while an assistant stabilizes the humerus. If radial or lateral displacement is present, it must be corrected before reduction is completed by flexion of the elbow.

An assistant provides counteraction by stabilizing the humerus while the operator holds the patient's forearm. The operator then keeps the patient's elbow flexed 40–60 degrees and pulls the forearm away from the humerus, with the force in the long axis of the humerus, producing distraction (separation of joint surfaces) of the elbow. Medial or lateral displacement is then corrected as necessary. Then, while the force on the elbow is steadily increased, the forearm is displaced anteriorly. Flex the elbow once the coronoid process clears the distal humerus. After reduction, confirm that the elbow joint has a full range of motion and stability, and splint the joint in 90–110 degrees of flexion. Obtain anteroposterior and lateral x-rays to confirm reduction. Repeat neurovascular examination. Support the splinted arm with a sling and swathe (Fig 22–4). Orthopedic referral is necessary.

C. Subluxation of the Radial Head ("Nursemaid's Elbow," "Pulled Elbow"): This injury occurs in children, usually in those under 7 years of age, and may represent as many as 25% of elbow injuries in this age group. The mechanism of injury is a sudden pull on the child's arm with the elbow extended and pronated. Initial pain is brief, but the child resists moving and using the affected arm. Examination reveals well-localized tenderness over the radial head, and pain occurs with attempted supination or elbow flexion. The elbow is not swollen or deformed. Even though the results are usually normal, x-rays must be obtained to rule out other injuries. Undisplaced fractures elsewhere in the upper extremity may have a similar presentation, so the entire arm and shoulder should be checked for tenderness.

Once the diagnosis is apparent, reduction is accomplished by supinating the forearm while the elbow is stabilized with the operator's opposite hand; the stabilizing hand should feel for a characteristic snap as the radial head is restored to its normal position proximal to the annular ligament. If supination fails to achieve reduction, the elbow should then be flexed as far as possible, often against some resistance, to produce the snap signifying reduction. Reduction is usually painful, but if it is successful, the child will be comfortable within a few minutes and will use the arm normally. Immobilization is not needed for the first or second such injury, but parents should be warned to avoid pulling the child by the arm.

If reduction is not achieved, the diagnosis may be incorrect, and an orthopedist should be consulted before the child is discharged from the emergency department. Orthopedic consultation is also advisable for recurrent subluxations but is not necessary after a completely successful reduction.

Disposition

Early follow-up for supervised rehabilitation is essential even in undisplaced elbow injuries. Displaced distal humerus fractures, unreduced or unstable dislocations, and elbow injuries that compromise neurologic or vascular function require immediate orthopedic consultation and usually hospital treatment.

Patients with undisplaced, uncomplicated injuries that have been appropriately splinted may be referred within 1–3 days to an orthopedist for confirmation of the diagnosis and plans for rehabilitation.

3. FOREARM FRACTURES

Diagnosis

Forearm fractures are associated with a history of a fall on an outstretched arm or a direct blow to the forearm, followed by local pain and tenderness. Deformity and abnormal mobility of the shaft of the radius or ulna (or both) may be present. Tenderness or deformity of the wrist or elbow suggests associated articular injury. There may be open wounds or abrasions.

The physician should assess function of the radial, median, and ulnar nerves (Table 22–2) and check for compartment syndrome affecting flexors, extensors, or both (p 320).

X-rays (anteroposterior and lateral) must include elbow and wrist joints, which may be dislocated, especially if a displaced fracture involves only one forearm bone. In a Monteggia fracture, the ulna is broken and the head of the radius is dislocated at the elbow. In a Galeazzi fracture, the radius is broken and the distal radioulnar joint is disrupted at the wrist.

Treatment

Splint the limb as shown in Fig 22–4. Prescribe analgesia as needed.

Disposition

Patients with dislocations, open fractures, closed fractures with abrasions of overlying skin, or injuries with associated compartment syndromes require immediate orthopedic consultation. If significant deformity is not substantially corrected by provisional reduction and application of a splint, progressive swelling may be severe.

Most displaced fractures of the forearm in adults require open reduction and internal fixation, and arrangements should be made for orthopedic consultation within 24 hours. Hospitalization is usually advisable.

Forearm fractures in children are almost always treated with closed reduction, which should generally be performed as soon as possible. Orthopedic evaluation is therefore required before the child is discharged from the emergency department.

Patients with undisplaced, uncomplicated forearm fractures that have been properly splinted may be referred for orthopedic consultation within 3 days.

WRIST JOINT INJURIES

Diagnosis

The wrist is usually injured by falling on an outstretched hand. Pain, swelling, tenderness, and deformity with limited or painful motion are common. Because the median and ulnar nerves can be affected by wrist injury, their motor and sensory function must be carefully assessed. Good x-rays are essential for accurate diagnosis.

A. Fractures of the Distal Radius: Colles' fracture is the most common type of fracture of the distal radius. Dorsal displacement and shortening occur. Comminution may involve the radiocarpal and distal radioulnar joints. Fractures of the distal radius sustained by young adults with normal bone are usually severe and may require more aggressive early treatment than does a typical Colles fracture through the osteoporotic bone in an elderly patient. Palmar displacement of a fracture of the distal radius (Smith's fracture) occasionally occurs and requires different definitive treatment, although preliminary management in the emergency department is similar to that of Colles' fracture.

Fractures of the distal radius in children frequently involve the cartilaginous growth plate and may be difficult to recognize on x-rays. Suspect growth plate fracture whenever tenderness in the appropriate area is noted, even if x-rays show no apparent abnormality.

B. Fracture-Dislocations: Fractures with associated dislocation of the radiocarpal (wrist) joint may be diagnosed by loss of the normal alignment of the carpus with the radius. Anterior or posterior displacement is seen on the lateral view, along with a displaced fracture of either the palmar or the dorsal lip of the articular surface of the radius.

C. Carpal Dislocations: Carpal dislocations are frequently overlooked in the emergency department despite symptoms and signs of injury. Fractures are absent or difficult to detect, and the deformity is subtle on anteroposterior x-ray. The key to diagnosis is a true lateral x-ray. The lunate must articulate with the distal radius and the capitate with the lunate (Fig 22–16).

Dislocations may displace the lunate anteriorly or (rarely) posteriorly. The most common dislocation is the perilunate, with the capitate displaced from the concave surface of the distal lunate. A displaced scaphoid fracture is frequently present. Carpal fractures may be associated with dislocations or may be isolated injuries with or without displacement. Small "chip" fractures may be a sign of serious injury to the ligaments of the wrist.

D. Scaphoid Fractures: Fractures of the scaphoid (carpal navicular) are notoriously difficult to see on x-rays (anteroposterior in neutral as well as ulnar and radial deviation, lateral, and navicular oblique). Tenderness in the anatomic snuffbox, between the extensor tendons of the thumb, suggests scaphoid fracture even if x-rays do not show a fracture line. A patient with snuffbox tenderness should be placed in a thumb spica splint (Fig 22–17) for 10–14 days, after which x-rays should be repeated, because resorption of bone makes any fracture line more obvious after time has elapsed following injury.

E. Carpometacarpal Joint Fractures: Fractures and fracture-dislocations of the carpometacarpal region are common. Tenderness is usually well localized, but swelling rapidly masks deformity. Bennett's fracture is a fracture of the base of the thumb metacarpal with dislocation of the thumb carpometacarpal joint. Reduction is difficult to maintain with a cast, so the injury often requires surgery.

An analogous injury occurs on the ulnar side of the wrist with fracture-dislocation of the fifth or fourth

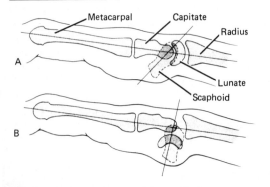
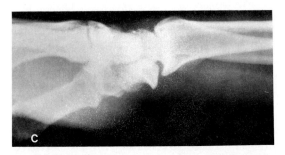

Figure 22–16. A: Normal anatomy of the wrist. Note that the proximal end of the capitate rests in the lunate concavity. A straight line drawn through the metacarpal and capitate into the radius should bisect the lunate. The scaphoid makes an angle of 45 degrees with the long axis of the radius. **B:** Lunate dislocation. Lunate dislocates volarly. The angle between the scaphoid and the long axis of the radius is 90 degrees instead of the normal angle of 45 degrees. **C:** X-ray of volar dislocation of lunate. (Reproduced, with permission, from Way LW [editor]: *Current Surgical Diagnosis & Treatment,* 9th ed. Appleton & Lange, 1991.)

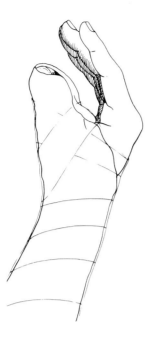

Figure 22–17. Thumb spica splint: a slab of plaster applied over adequate padding and secured with a loose elastic bandage.

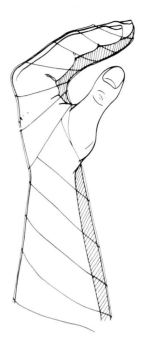

Figure 22–18. Volar wrist and hand splint for immobilization of metacarpal shaft fractures and wrist injuries. A plaster slab is applied over adequate padding and secured with a loose elastic bandage.

and fifth carpometacarpal joints. Signs are subtle on routine anteroposterior and lateral x-rays. Dorsal displacement of the base of the metacarpals is easily recognized on an oblique film with the x-ray beam tangent to the dorsum of the ulnar metacarpals. Such an x-ray should be obtained whenever the base of the metacarpals on the ulnar side is swollen or tender.

Treatment

Thumb and scaphoid injuries require a thumb spica splint (Fig 22–17). Other wrist injuries can usually be immobilized satisfactorily with a volar wrist splint (Fig 22–5) or a volar wrist and hand splint (Fig 22–18). Remove any rings immediately.

Slings usually do not provide sufficient elevation for acute wrist and hand injuries, which should be kept above the level of the heart to prevent swelling. Begin active or passive range of motion exercises for fingers and shoulder. Prescribe analgesics as required.

Disposition

All dislocations and significantly displaced or open fractures require immediate orthopedic consultation. Patients with uncomplicated, undisplaced fractures and sprains may be referred for orthopedic follow-up within 3–5 days.

HAND INJURIES
(See also Chapter 23.)

Proper evaluation of hand injuries requires simultaneous consideration of the structure and function of all components of the hand (muscles, bones, nerves, arteries, etc). The close structural proximity of nerves, arteries, and bone increases the chance of associated lesions, and skeletal injuries of the hand cannot be treated without regard for maintenance of sensibility and mobility of the hand and integrity of the skin overlying the injury. The summary here of common fractures and joint injuries of the hand supplements Chapter 23, in which the anatomy and examination of the hand and soft tissue injuries are discussed in detail.

1. METACARPAL SHAFT FRACTURES

Diagnosis

Localized tenderness and swelling indicate a metacarpal fracture. Deformity may be absent or, if present, may be due to rotation, shortening, angulation, or a combination thereof. Anteroposterior and lateral x-rays demonstrate the injury. The lateral film must be examined closely for evidence of angulation. Rotational deformity must be assessed by physical examination, since it is poorly shown by x-rays. Rotational malalignment is evident when the metacarpophalangeal joints are fully flexed, in which position the fingers should be nearly parallel.

Crush injuries of the hand must be distinguished from those associated with less severe soft tissue trauma but deceptively similar x-rays. Crush injuries may require fasciotomy for compartment syndromes involving the intrinsic muscles of the hand and should be evaluated in the emergency department by an experienced surgeon.

Treatment

Reduce any deformity as much as possible, and support the injured limb with a volar wrist and hand splint (Fig 22–18). An ulnar gutter splint (Fig 22–19) is satisfactory if injury involves only the metacarpals of the fourth or fifth finger. As illustrated, the metacarpophalangeal joints should be flexed to nearly a right angle, and the interphalangeal joints should be comfortably extended. Elevate the limb, and provide appropriate analgesia. Remove any rings immediately.

Disposition

Although definitive treatment of properly splinted,

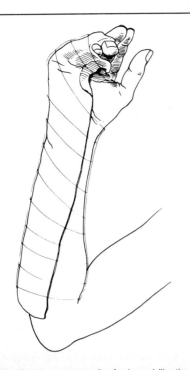

Figure 22–19. Ulnar gutter splint for immobilization of injuries to the metacarpals of the fourth and fifth fingers. A plaster slab is applied to the ulnar border of forearm and hand over adequate padding. It is secured with a loose elastic bandage.

uncomplicated metacarpal shaft fractures may usually be delayed safely for a few days, some orthopedists prefer to treat these injuries before significant swelling develops, so that early telephone consultation is helpful in arranging evaluation and treatment by a specialist.

A displaced fracture that has been reduced requires x-rays after a plaster cast has been applied. The x-rays should be carefully checked, because incomplete reduction is not acceptable.

Patients with undisplaced fractures, splinted as described, should be referred for follow-up by an orthopedist within 3–5 days.

2. METACARPAL NECK FRACTURES

Diagnosis

Metacarpal neck fractures—often called boxer's fractures—are common injuries that usually involve the fourth or fifth finger and are impacted, with angulation, the apex of which points dorsally. Local tenderness and swelling, difficulty in extending the finger, and loss of prominence of the knuckle are usually apparent. If such fractures are disimpacted and reduced, the deformity tends to recur because of comminution of the volar side of the fracture. Fortunately, disability is usually minimal in spite of angular deformity of the 2 mobile ulnar metacarpals.

Unless they are reduced anatomically, metacarpal neck fractures of the index and middle fingers are more likely to cause problems with hand function than are those of the fourth or fifth fingers.

Check for rotational deformity. When the metacarpophalangeal joints are fully flexed, the phalanges should be parallel if there is no rotational deformity. Suspect human bite (tooth) wound if there is a laceration dorsal to a metacarpophalangeal joint (see below, under Finger Metacarpophalangeal Joint Injuries, and also Chapter 23).

X-rays (anteroposterior, lateral, and oblique) demonstrate the site of injury, but the degree of angulation can be difficult to determine because of overlapping metacarpal shadows on the lateral view.

Treatment

Apply a volar wrist and hand splint (Fig 22–18) or ulnar gutter splint (Fig 22–19). Elevate the limb, and provide appropriate analgesia.

Disposition

Closed fractures may be referred for orthopedic evaluation within 3–5 days. Open fractures require consultation for urgent definitive therapy.

3. THUMB METACARPOPHALANGEAL JOINT INJURIES

Diagnosis

The metacarpophalangeal joint of the thumb is exposed to injury by any mechanism that wrenches the distal thumb. Dislocations are usually obvious. Ligamentous injuries are less obvious but must be identified early, since they can disable the thumb if treatment is inadequate.

Avulsion fractures may be a sign of ligamentous injuries and are occasionally large enough to disrupt the articular surface. Tenderness and swelling of the thumb metacarpophalangeal joint require anteroposterior and lateral x-rays of the involved *thumb,* because the usual views of the hand are not well positioned for showing the thumb.

If x-ray results are normal, confirm stability of the collateral joint ligaments by attempting to angulate the proximal phalanx radially (laterally) and medially relative to the metacarpal shaft (Fig 22–20). Grasp the proximal phalanx, and attempt to open the joint space on either side, first with the metacarpophalangeal joint extended and then with it flexed at 30 degrees. Feel for a convincing end point beyond which no laxity occurs, and compare laxity with that of the opposite thumb. Local or regional anesthesia is often required for adequate examination.

Tear of the ulnar collateral ligament of the thumb is an injury known as "gamekeeper's thumb." It is

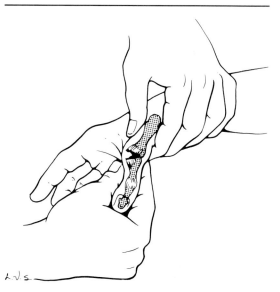

Figure 22–20. Stress examination of the thumb metacarpophalangeal collateral ligament. The ulnar side is more frequently injured. Test both sides in extension and 30 degrees of flexion. Compare the injured digit with the uninjured thumb. Feel for a firm end point and absence of excessive laxity.

also a common ski injury resulting from a fall on an outstretched hand that is holding a ski pole.

Thumb injuries may involve avulsion of tendons. Therefore, confirm active extension and flexion of the metacarpophalangeal and interphalangeal joints.

Treatment

Thumb metacarpophalangeal dislocations must be reduced promptly. Unlike finger metacarpophalangeal joint dislocations, those involving the thumb can usually be reduced with analgesia and distal traction but occasionally require open reduction because of displacement into the joint of the fibrocartilaginous plate that reinforces the volar portion of the joint capsule.

Do not attempt to correct extension deformity until normal length has been restored by traction. After a dislocation has been reduced, obtain x-rays with the joint in a splint or cast, and carefully check for instability of the ligaments.

If missed, an ulnar collateral ligament tear may result in disability. A complete tear usually requires operative repair. A thumb spica splint (Fig 22–17) is appropriate temporary immobilization for all injuries to the thumb.

Disposition

Patients with fractures and ligamentous injuries of the thumb should be referred to a specialist. Immediate consultation is required for open fractures, joint injuries, and unreduced dislocations. Unless skin damage is present, closed fractures and ligamentous injuries can be splinted and the patient referred for orthopedic consultation within 3 days.

4. FINGER METACARPOPHALANGEAL JOINT INJURIES

Diagnosis

Swelling, tenderness, and limitation of motion indicate an injury to the metacarpophalangeal joint (knuckle). Hyperextension deformity is typical of dislocation. Lacerations and puncture wounds over the dorsum of the knuckle should suggest the possibility of human bite wounds resulting from a blow to the mouth, and the patient must be asked specifically whether this has happened (Chapter 23).

Avulsion fractures of the base of the proximal phalanx indicate injuries to ligaments. If avulsion fractures disrupt more than one-fourth of the articular surface, open reduction may be required to restore the articular surface.

Metacarpophalangeal dislocations of the index or the little finger may be classified as simple or complex.

(1) Simple dislocations show marked hyperextension, and closed reduction is possible.

(2) Complex dislocations are only slightly hyperextended and show dimpling of the skin of the proximal volar flexion crease resulting from trapping of the fibrocartilaginous plate between the dislocated phalanx and the metacarpal head. These injuries require open reduction.

Anteroposterior, lateral, and oblique x-rays are required for all finger metacarpophalangeal joint injuries to confirm dislocations and rule out fractures.

Treatment

The severity of "fist-in-mouth" human bite wounds is easily underestimated, as they often appear superficial in spite of entry into the underlying metacarpophalangeal joint. Infections progress rapidly and are usually due to multiple organisms, including anaerobes. *All such injuries should be evaluated and treated by an experienced hand surgeon.* In general, hospitalization is necessary for administration of intravenous antibiotics (eg, cefazolin, 1 g intravenously every 8 hours, with either gentamicin, 80 mg every 8 hours, or aqueous penicillin G, 10 million units intravenously over 24 hours) and observation. Failure to respond in 24 hours or the earlier judgment of the hand surgeon may be indications for surgical exploration and debridement. Splinting, elevation, and tetanus prophylaxis should be provided initially.

Simple dislocations are reduced after adequate regional anesthesia by keeping the metacarpophalangeal joint hyperextended about 90 degrees, flexing the interphalangeal joints, and moving the base of the proximal phalanx distally over the metacarpal head before attempting to flex the metacarpophalangeal joint. Confirm reduction by fully flexing the injured digit and by taking x-rays after the hand and forearm (Figs 22–18 and 22–19) are splinted in flexed position.

Complex dislocations should be temporarily splinted (Fig 22–18) while arrangements are being made for open reduction in the operating room within a few hours.

Avulsion fractures should be splinted as shown in Fig 22–18.

Disposition

Open injuries and complex metacarpophalangeal joint dislocations require prompt examination by an orthopedist in the emergency department. Patients with closed fractures, sprains, and simple metacarpophalangeal dislocations that have been reduced and splinted properly should be referred to an orthopedist within 3 days.

5. PHALANGEAL SHAFT FRACTURES

Diagnosis

Phalangeal shaft fractures are characterized by tenderness, swelling, deformity, and instability. Examine the patient carefully for rotational deformity, which is best demonstrated by the lack of relative alignment of the fingernails. In the normal hand, although the proximal phalanges appear nearly parallel, the fingers do converge, so that each points toward about the same spot at the base of the thenar eminence.

Anteroposterior and lateral x-rays confirm fractures but fail to detect malrotation. X-rays should also be obtained after splinting to confirm proper reduction.

Treatment

Align the fracture as well as possible, and apply a wrist and hand splint that includes the injured finger to a point just short of its tip. Generally, an adjacent normal finger should be included in the splint. Transverse fractures of the proximal phalanx frequently angulate with the apex of the fracture on the palmar side, but this can be controlled by increasing metacarpophalangeal flexion. Elevate the limb, and provide appropriate analgesia.

Disposition

Displaced phalangeal fractures require open or closed reduction performed by an experienced surgeon. Unless there is skin damage or neurovascular compromise, other phalangeal fractures that can be aligned as well as possible by splinting (confirmed by x-ray) should be seen by a specialist within 3 days if x-rays after splinting show satisfactory alignment. If significant angulation or shortening persists after splinting and reduction, obtain consultation before the patient leaves the emergency department.

6. PROXIMAL INTERPHALANGEAL JOINT INJURIES

Diagnosis

The proximal interphalangeal joint is commonly injured. Because this joint is crucial for normal finger function, disabling loss of motion is likely unless scrupulous attention is paid to treatment and subsequent rehabilitation. Tenderness, swelling, and in some cases deformity are the signs of injury.

Evaluate the following aspects of the joint, using regional anesthesia if necessary: (**1**) joint instability (sideways bending and hyperextension), (**2**) extensor function (full extension against resistance), (**3**) function of the flexor digitorum superficialis (active flexion of the proximal interphalangeal joint while the other 3 fingers are held in full extension), and (**4**) function of the flexor digitorum profundus (active flexion of the distal interphalangeal joint against resistance).

Dislocations are commonly dorsal (ie, middle phalanx displaced dorsally to the proximal phalanx). Palmar dislocation is rare but important, because it causes avulsion of the central slip of the extensor aponeurosis from its attachment to the base of the middle phalanx, with subsequent boutonniére deformity (see Fig 23–13). Forceful dislocations occasionally rupture the skin and require urgent surgery to prevent infection. Anteroposterior and lateral x-rays confirm the direction and presence of dislocation and exclude fracture-dislocation.

Sprains involve the collateral ligaments (radial or ulnar) of the volar fibrocartilaginous plate. Instability indicates ligament rupture. X-rays obtained while stress is applied to the joint may be used to demonstrate collateral ligament injuries.

Acute closed disruptions of the central slip of the extensor aponeurosis appear similar to joint injuries. Maximal tenderness is middorsal. The typical boutonniére deformity develops slowly (days to weeks), since the lateral bands of the extensor tendon must displace toward the palmar side of the digit; however, active proximal interphalangeal joint extension is weak and incomplete immediately after injury.

Treatment

Dislocations and fracture-dislocations require immediate reduction, followed by tests for stability and tendon function as described above. Digital nerve block (after sensory examination) (Chapter 46) often aids reduction and permits adequate assessment of stability. Postreduction x-rays are needed to confirm that reduction is successful and maintained.

Unstable ligament injuries, including those noted after reduction of a dislocation, should be protected with a wrist and hand splint and examined within 3 days by an orthopedic or hand surgeon. Surgery may be advisable.

Stable ligament injuries are splinted by taping the proximal and middle phalanges to an adjacent uninjured finger without constricting the injured finger. This technique of "buddy-taping" permits protected active mobilization of the injured joint.

Palmar proximal interphalangeal dislocations and other closed disruptions of the central slip of the extensor tendon are reduced and splinted with the proximal interphalangeal joint in full extension. In this case, the other finger joints are *not* splinted.

Disposition

Careful follow-up is essential for proximal interphalangeal joint injuries. Too much or too little immobilization, splinting in an incorrect position, or delay of necessary surgery can result in permanent disability. Consultation is therefore advisable. Unreduced dislocations require immediate referral. If joint alignment is satisfactory on x-ray and if proper splints have been applied, patients with uncomplicated proximal interphalangeal joint injuries can be referred for evaluation within 3 days.

7. DISTAL INTERPHALANGEAL JOINT INJURIES

Diagnosis

Distal interphalangeal joint injuries are characterized by tenderness, swelling, deformity, and loss of motion and are often the result of a blow to the fingertip. As with proximal interphalangeal joint injuries, stability and tendon function must be assessed by specific tests (see Diagnosis in previous section on proximal interphalangeal joint injuries). The commonest injury is a "mallet finger" (see Fig 23–12), with flexion of the distal interphalangeal joint. Anteroposterior and lateral x-rays are essential for diagnosis.

Simple mallet finger injuries with uncomplicated disruption of the tendon or a small dorsal avulsion of the extensor tendon at the point of insertion must be distinguished from more extensive injuries that involve palmar subluxation of the distal phalanx. Avulsion of the flexor digitorum profundus tendon from its palmar insertion on the distal phalanx causes local tenderness and inability to flex the distal interphalangeal joint.

Treatment & Disposition

See Chapter 23 for details of treatment of fingertip injuries and mallet finger. If fracture-subluxation or avulsion of the flexor digitorum profundus tendon is present, apply a wrist and hand splint, and arrange for repair by a specialist within 3 days.

PELVIC RING INJURIES

Undisplaced pelvic ring fractures usually result from falls by old people with osteoporosis. More severe pelvic injuries that may have a similar appearance on x-ray are caused by high-energy trauma, eg, motor vehicle collisions or falls from a height. These fractures are serious injuries because of life-threatening hemorrhage and associated head, thoracic, abdominal, vascular, and genitourinary injury, in addition to the skeletal injury. Posttraumatic respiratory failure is a common complication.

Diagnosis

Assess the patient for shock and visceral or genitourinary injury as in any multiply injured patient (Chapter 4). Check for posterior tenderness in the region of the sacroiliac joint. Perform pelvic and rectal examinations, and assess peripheral pulses and the function of peripheral nerves (Table 22–2).

Pain, tenderness, and especially mobility of the iliac bones can be assessed by grasping their anterior portions and alternatively compressing them together and then spreading them apart (Fig 22–21).

Proximal displacement of one hemipelvis (Mal-

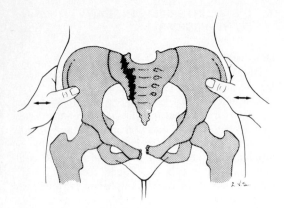

Figure 22–21. Compression-distraction test for stability of the pelvic ring. If the iliac crests can be pressed together or pulled apart, the pelvis is unstable. With more severe instability, one hemipelvis may be displaced proximally.

gaigne's injury) causes apparent shortening of the leg.

Anteroposterior x-ray of the pelvis is required in patients with multiple trauma, in those with pelvic pain or tenderness or injuries above and below the pelvis, and in those with femoral fractures. Although grossly displaced pelvic fractures and injuries to the pubic rami are easy to recognize, posterior disruptions of the pelvic ring are often hard to distinguish regardless of whether they are due to dislocations of the sacroiliac joint or to fractures of the ilium or sacrum. CT views of the posterior pelvis aid definitive management of pelvic ring injuries. They should not be allowed to delay more urgent treatment.

If urethral bleeding is present, obtain a urethrogram before attempting to insert a Foley catheter. A cystogram is usually required to exclude bladder rupture (Chapter 20). Patients with pelvic injuries must be closely monitored for hypovolemic shock while x-rays are being obtained.

Treatment

Monitor the patient, and treat for hemorrhagic shock (Chapter 3). Splint the pelvis by keeping the patient recumbent on a firm padded surface and using the logrolling technique as necessary. If shortening of the limb is present, use 2.3–3.6 kg (5–8 lb) of traction with an ankle hitch. This should be promptly replaced with skeletal traction or external skeletal fixation. MAST garment or early external fixation may help control life-threatening hemorrhage.

Disposition

Patients with pelvic injuries resulting from high-energy trauma require immediate evaluation in the emergency department by a general surgeon, an orthopedist, and a urologist, if necessary. Prompt external fixation can greatly aid the treatment of hemodynamically unstable patients with mechanically unstable pelvic ring fractures. Patients with pelvic injuries resulting from low-energy trauma should also be hospitalized and monitored closely, with frequent recording of vital signs. The need for orthopedic consultation is less urgent in these patients, although an orthopedist should still be consulted within 1 day.

HIP JOINT INJURIES

Hip injuries in young people with normal bones are usually caused by high-energy trauma, eg, motor vehicle or pedestrian accidents or falls from a height. Patients who have sustained high-energy trauma are more likely to have multiple injuries. In elderly patients with osteoporosis, hip fractures may be caused by relatively minor trauma, such as a simple fall to the floor from a standing position.

Fractures of the acetabulum, dislocations of the hip, and fractures of the proximal femur result from blunt trauma delivered to the hip, either locally or along the femur, as occurs when an automobile passenger's knee strikes the dashboard in a head-on collision. Such an accident may damage both the knee joint and the hip. Fractures of the hip may cause severe internal bleeding, and all such patients should be carefully monitored for shock. Confirm neurologic function of the lower extremity (Table 22–2). Sciatic nerve injuries are not infrequent, particularly those involving the peroneal portion of the sciatic nerve.

Diagnosis

A. Symptoms and Signs: Groin pain that is increased by hip motion is characteristic of hip joint injuries. Rotational deformity and true shortening of the leg are present with displaced injuries but may be slight or absent if there is no displacement. In some cases, the only signs of an undisplaced fracture of the proximal femur are pain at the extremes of motion or when the examiner strikes the heel of the patient's extended leg.

B. X-Ray Findings: *Note:* Patients with hip injuries must be closely monitored while x-rays are being taken. To avoid missing an undisplaced fracture of the hip, x-rays must include an anteroposterior view of the whole pelvis taken with the legs internally rotated for a true anteroposterior view of the proximal femurs. A cross-table lateral (Smith-Petersen) view of the hip is essential in evaluating proximal femoral injuries, but it provides a poor view of the acetabulum.

Occasionally, posterior fracture-dislocation of the hip joint is hard to recognize because displacement is directly posterior, without proximal migration. This injury is evident on an oblique view with the pelvis rotated 45 degrees, so the involved hip is lifted off the table.

Complete x-ray evaluation of an acetabular fracture also requires both right and left oblique (45-degree, Judet) views. A CT scan provides valuable information about hip dislocations and fractures of the acetabulum. It should not be allowed to delay urgent treatment, however.

C. Classification of Hip Injuries:

1. Hip dislocations–These are usually posterior but may be anterior; either type may be associated with fractures of the acetabulum or femoral head. Central (medial) dislocation may occur when the femoral head is driven medially toward the pelvis and through the acetabulum. A relatively fixed deformity may be obvious: Posterior dislocation is characterized by mild flexion, internal rotation, and adduction; anterior dislocation by greater flexion than in posterior dislocation, external rotation, and abduction. Hip dislocations must be recognized, because they require urgent treatment. Some posterior fracture dislocations have relatively subtle abnormalities on anteroposterior radiographs, so that additional views are advisable if an injury is questioned.

2. Femoral neck fractures–Such fractures may be impacted, with valgus deformity; undisplaced; or displaced partially or completely. These fractures, which are within the hip joint, are associated with less severe bleeding than extracapsular fractures but pose a greater risk to the hip joint.

3. Intertrochanteric fractures–These fractures are characterized by fracture lines running across the metaphyseal region from the greater to the lesser trochanter. Comminution, displacement, or both may be present.

4. Subtrochanteric fractures–These extend into the proximal femoral shaft below the lesser trochanter and are usually caused by high-energy blunt trauma.

Treatment

Monitor the patient, and treat for hemorrhagic shock (Chapter 3).

A. Dislocation: Splint the hip in the position of deformity with pillows, etc. Dislocated hips require urgent reduction to avoid the increased risk of avascular necrosis of the femoral head associated with reductions delayed more than a few hours.

If emergency surgery is required for associated injury, reduce the dislocated hip after muscle relaxation is achieved by general anesthesia. Although closed reduction with analgesia and sedation can be accomplished in the emergency department, management in the operating room is preferable, since additional damage to the articular cartilage can occur when reduction is attempted with inadequate muscle relaxation. Allis's technique (Fig 22–22) is generally satisfactory for reduction of posterior hip dislocations. In a stable patient with an isolated injury, Stimson's technique, the same maneuver with the patient prone, may be used.

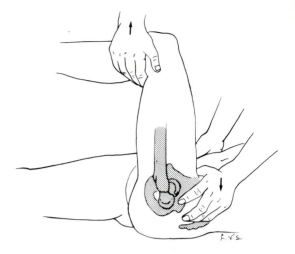

Figure 22–22. Allis's technique for reduction of posterior hip dislocation. Both hip and knee are flexed 90 degrees. An assistant stabilizes the pelvis while the operator pulls the femur anteriorly, rotating it slightly internally and externally to aid reduction, which is achieved mainly by deliberate, steady traction.

If reduction is performed in the emergency department, it is essential to assess hip stability by flexing the joint to see whether dislocation recurs. Traction is sometimes necessary to prevent acute redislocation. Postreduction x-rays must be carefully examined to ensure that a bone fragment is not interposed between the femoral head and the acetabulum. A postreduction CT scan is advisable.

B. Fracture: Splint the lower extremity with a traction device as shown in Fig 22–6. Femoral neck fractures in the young (< age 50) should be operated on within a few hours after injury to decrease the risk of avascular necrosis. For such patients, preoperative preparations should be made urgently. For older patients, a period of traction generally precedes operation on displaced hip fractures.

Disposition

Hospitalization is required for all hip fractures and dislocations. Obtain prompt orthopedic consultation.

FEMORAL SHAFT FRACTURES

Femoral fractures are usually caused by direct blows, twisting forces applied to the leg, or gunshot wounds. Such fractures are often the result of high-energy trauma associated with multiple injuries or significant blood loss. Injury to the femoral artery or sciatic nerve and other neurovascular damage may occur. Posttraumatic respiratory failure occurs occasionally, more often in the multiply injured. Its frequency can be reduced by adequate resuscitation and urgent fracture fixation.

Diagnosis

Pain, tenderness, shortening or angular deformity, and progressive swelling are present. Be sure to examine the skin, peripheral nerves, and pulses. Anteroposterior and lateral x-rays confirm the diagnosis. An anteroposterior x-ray of the pelvis is essential to check for associated hip joint injuries. Although the ipsilateral knee is difficult to examine, the physician must check for localized tenderness and swelling, which suggest injury to this joint, a common occurrence when fractures involve both the femur and the tibia of the same limb.

Treatment

Monitor the patient, insert a large-bore intravenous catheter, and treat for hemorrhagic shock (Chapter 3). Apply a Thomas (or equivalent) traction splint (Fig 22–6). Skeletal traction with 7- to 10-kg (15- to 25-lb) force is required for adequate control of most displaced femur fractures in young adults.

Disposition

Hospitalize the patient, and obtain immediate orthopedic consultation.

KNEE JOINT INJURIES

Knee injuries are common emergency department problems. Although exact diagnosis may be difficult, significant ligamentous disruptions must be identified early, to permit optimal treatment. "Waiting to see how it does" is not an acceptable emergency department approach to knee injury.

Fresh knee injuries with swelling, limited motion, limp, and especially laxity of the ligaments or severe pain preventing adequate stress testing should be examined by an orthopedist within 1–3 days. Even if nonoperative treatment is chosen, a carefully supervised rehabilitation program, started promptly, improves the outcome of all but the most minor knee injuries.

History, physical examination, and standard x-rays are the mainstays of diagnosis. Arthroscopy and MRI are often helpful. Neither should be recommended until the patient has been evaluated by an orthopedic surgeon.

1. PENETRATING WOUNDS OF THE KNEE

The knee is often exposed to penetrating injuries. Since its joint cavity extends at least 5 cm (2 in) proximal to the patella in adults, the possibility of knee joint injury should be considered for all penetrating trauma of the distal thigh. A sewing needle lost in a shag rug may penetrate a crawling child's knee to be broken off inside or be withdrawn intact, leaving no explanation for subsequent pyogenic arthritis.

Diagnosis

Any wound close to the knee should suggest penetration of the knee joint. Effusion may or may not be present. Penetration is confirmed by anteroposterior and lateral x-rays that show air in the joint, although this finding is not always present. Look also for foreign material and osteocartilaginous fracture fragments when examining x-rays of the injury.

The diagnosis may also be confirmed by distending the joint with an injection of sterile saline (perhaps tinted with a few drops of methylene blue dye). The solution is injected into the joint cavity through uninjured tissue, using any standard approach normally employed for arthrocentesis (Chapter 46). If the fluid leaks through the wound, the joint is open. Probing a wound to see if it enters the joint is of limited value and may further contaminate the area.

Treatment

Apply a sterile dressing, and splint the knee in slight flexion (Fig 22–7). Give tetanus prophylaxis as necessary (Chapter 46). Start antibiotics (eg, cefazolin, 1 g in adults, 20 mg/kg in children, intravenously every 6 hours). Penetrating wounds of the knee joint require surgical treatment. Aspirate effusion fluid, and send a sample to the laboratory for staining with Gram's stain, cell count, and culture and sensitivity tests. Although hematogenous septic arthritis of the knee can often be treated without surgery, infection that occurs after a penetrating wound requires arthrotomy. After a specimen of fluid has been sent for culture, begin antibiotics based on results of Gram-stained smear, and obtain prompt orthopedic consultation for emergency arthrotomy.

Disposition

Hospitalization and orthopedic consultation are required.

2. KNEE DISLOCATION

Diagnosis

Gross instability or deformity on physical examination or x-ray indicates that the femorotibial joint has been dislocated. Do not confuse this injury with patellar dislocation (see below). Evaluate neurovascular status distal to the injury. Even if pedal pulses are present, a femoral arteriogram is advisable because of the high incidence of intimal tears resulting from stretch injuries of the popliteal artery (see Fig 32–1). Such tears may cause delayed thrombosis and subsequent limb loss (Chapter 32). An arteriogram is not necessary if ischemia is obvious and is contraindicated if it will delay revascularization.

Treatment

Reduce gross deformity by applying traction to the tibia and manipulating it as needed to align it with the femur. Apply a traction splint with just enough force to maintain alignment.

Disposition

Hospitalize the patient for observation and possible surgery, and obtain immediate consultation from an orthopedist and a vascular surgeon.

3. KNEE LIGAMENT INJURY

Diagnosis

Severe ligamentous injuries resulting in gross instability in multiple planes should be considered the equivalent of knee dislocation. Lesser degrees of ligamentous disruption often permit walking, albeit with a painful limp, limited motion, and a sensation of the knee giving way. If the knee capsule is torn, effusion may be minimal, but swelling usually develops within the surrounding tissues over several hours. Tenderness generally extends along an injured collateral ligament proximal or distal to the joint.

Active and passive range of motion must be confirmed. Check to see that the patient is able to lift the leg off the bed while maintaining knee extension (straight leg raising) to confirm quadriceps mechanism integrity.

Sideways (varus-valgus) and anteroposterior stability of the injured knee must be compared with that of the uninjured knee, which should be examined first. With the patient supine, lift the heels, and check to see if extension is full but not excessive. Both in full extension and in 30 degrees of flexion, confirm stability in the varus and valgus positions. Instability in extension suggests posterior capsule and cruciate ligament damage. Sideways instability felt only when the knee is flexed suggests damage to a collateral ligament (Fig 22–23).

Posterior displacement of the tibia on the femur produced by gravity when the knee and hip are flexed is a significant sign of posterior cruciate injury, even if the tibia on the injured side falls only a few millimeters more posterior than the one on the normal side (Fig 22–24).

Anterior displacement can be difficult to demonstrate. Lachman's test is more sensitive than the traditional "anterior drawer" test, which is performed with the knee flexed 90 or more degrees. Lachman's test is done with the knee flexed 15–20 degrees. The proximal tibia is grasped in one hand and the distal femur in the other. *Any* increased forward mobility of the tibia relative to the femur, compared with the uninjured knee, indicates significant damage to the anterior cruciate ligament (Fig 22–25). A knee with an acutely ruptured anterior cruciate ligament may be completely stable on examination, but the physician

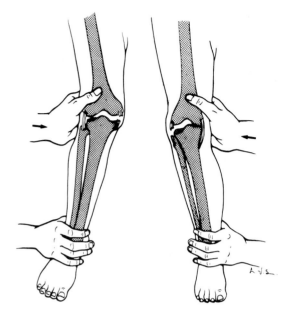

Figure 22–23. Valgus and varus stress tests for rupture of the medial and lateral collateral ligaments of the knee. More laxity than in the uninjured knee or lack of a firm end point constitutes a positive test. Pain and muscle guarding may make interpretation difficult.

should remember that this injury is the commonest cause of acute hemarthrosis in a stable knee. Definitive diagnosis of rupture of the anterior cruciate ligament in an apparently stable knee usually requires arthroscopic examination. Tests for rotational instability (pivot shift, jerk, Losee, etc) are difficult to perform and interpret in the painful, acutely injured knee.

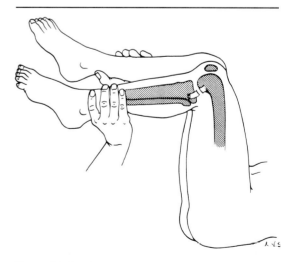

Figure 22–24. Rupture of the posterior cruciate ligament is a likely diagnosis when the tibia of the injured knee sags posteriorly below the distal femur when the legs are held flexed 90 degrees at the hip and knee.

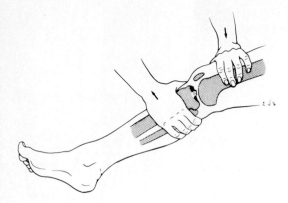

Figure 22–25. Lachman's test for rupture of the anterior cruciate ligament. Attempt to pull the tibia forward relative to the femur while the knee is slightly flexed. Any increase in laxity compared to the uninjured knee signifies injury.

Obtain anteroposterior and lateral x-rays of the knee in all cases of suspected injuries to knee ligaments to check for associated fractures.

Treatment & Disposition

A. Severe Ligamentous Injury: Severe ligamentous injury with gross instability is treated as knee dislocation (see above). Complete tears of the ligaments of the knee may require surgery. If skin abrasions are present, obtain immediate orthopedic consultation so that necessary surgery can be performed before significant bacterial contamination occurs. Neurovascular injury (suspected or confirmed) also requires consultation. Patients with neurologic or vascular injury require hospitalization.

B. Lesser Degrees of Ligamentous Injury: If skin and neurovascular status are undamaged and if injury to the ligaments is less severe, splint the knee as shown in Fig 22–7. Provide crutches for ambulation without weight bearing on the injured knee. Control pain with a codeine compound or equivalent unless tense hemarthrosis develops, in which case sterile aspiration of the joint with an 18-gauge needle usually helps relieve pain. A gentle compression dressing may then be applied to the knee underneath the splint. Make arrangements for orthopedic consultation within 24 hours.

Note: In the absence of painful distention of the joint, there is no need to aspirate an acutely injured knee unless there is a possibility of infection or other type of inflammatory arthritis, for which analysis of joint fluid is mandatory.

4. INTRA-ARTICULAR FRACTURE

Diagnosis

Pain, bony tenderness, and swelling or effusion with or without deformity and instability suggest intra-articular fracture, which may involve the patella, distal femur, or tibial plateau.

X-rays are required to confirm the diagnosis. A cross-table lateral view often shows a layer of fat floating on the hemarthrosis. An intercondylar notch view of the femoral condyles or "sunrise" view of the patella may demonstrate osteochondral fractures not seen on anteroposterior and lateral views. Oblique views may also help identify and evaluate fractures of the tibial plateau.

Examine the skin carefully, since urgent orthopedic surgical consultation is required when abrasions are present.

Patellar fractures often result in disruption of the musculotendinous unit of the quadriceps, which is confirmed by lack of active knee extension against gravity and by displacement of fracture fragments on x-ray films, especially on the lateral view. Quadriceps rupture may also occur through the tendinous region proximal to the patella or through the patellar ligament distally.

Intra-articular fractures of the femur and tibia may cause disruption of articular surfaces, ligamentous avulsions, or both. *Caution:* Tibial plateau fractures may be subtle and are easily missed if local tenderness is not elicited with care.

Treatment

If the femorotibial joint is unstable or if similar instability is caused by a fracture just above or below the knee joint, treat the injury as a knee dislocation (see above). If the femorotibial joint is stable, treat the injury as a ligamentous injury (see above).

Disposition

Obtain prompt orthopedic consultation in all cases. The patient may require hospitalization for surgical treatment. Even minor-appearing fractures should be evaluated by an orthopedist within 3 days.

5. PATELLAR DISLOCATION

Diagnosis

Occasionally, the patella is still dislocated when the patient seeks treatment in the emergency department; more commonly, spontaneous reduction has occurred, and the diagnosis is made only by careful history taking and examination with the possibility of patellar dislocation kept in mind.

There is a history of the knee suddenly "going out of joint" or "dislocating" with weight bearing and perhaps twisting of the affected leg. The episode may be the first occurrence of dislocation or a recurrent problem.

The injury is obvious if the patella is still dislocated, but otherwise there is only medial parapatellar tenderness, apprehension, or even recurrence of dislocation when the examiner attempts to displace the patella laterally. Patellar dislocation often causes progressive hemarthrosis, especially if it is the first occurrence. Confirm the ability to "straight leg raise." X-rays may show small fracture fragments adjacent to the medial or lateral side of the patella.

Treatment

If the patella is still dislocated, reduce it by fully extending the knee, flexing the hip, and manually displacing the patella medially onto the articular surface of the femur. Aspirate a tense hemarthrosis. Splint the knee in extension (Fig 22–7). Provide crutches. Some weight bearing may be allowed if the knee is well splinted. Give oral analgesics (eg, codeine compound) as needed.

Disposition

For uncomplicated patellar dislocations, refer the patient to an orthopedist within 3 days. If abrasions are present, the patient should be seen by an orthopedist within a few hours. Early surgery is occasionally advisable for first-time patellar dislocations and must be performed promptly if there are skin abrasions that may become colonized by bacteria.

6. HEMARTHROSIS

Diagnosis

Fluid that rapidly accumulates within the knee joint after injury is almost always due to bleeding into the joint and usually indicates significant structural injury, commonly a tear of the anterior cruciate ligament or peripheral detachment of a meniscus. In both cases, the joint may be stable and x-rays may show no deformity.

Caution: Avoid the nonspecific diagnosis of "traumatic hemarthrosis" or "traumatic effusion" for knee injuries. Specific early diagnosis and appropriate treatment may prevent development of chronic knee problems.

Knee x-rays should be obtained, including anteroposterior, lateral, and patellar ("sunrise") views. A "tunnel" view will help in visualizing the intercondylar notch of the femur.

Arthrocentesis is not necessary unless a tense, painful effusion exists. Follow strict sterile technique.

Treatment & Disposition

Hemarthrosis of the knee should be considered an indication of a significant knee injury. Immediate

treatment should be the same as that outlined for ligament injuries, above.

7. MENISCUS INJURIES

Meniscus tears are common knee injuries that are difficult to diagnose clinically. Tears may be asymptomatic, may be only painful, or may interfere with knee motion or stability, depending on location and extent. The causative injury may be rotational stress applied to a loaded, flexed knee and may seem rather trivial.

A meniscus tear should be suspected when the patient presents with knee pain, limping, and difficulty moving the joint. Examination typically shows one or more of the following: lack of full passive extension ("locking," especially if relieved by manipulation), joint line tenderness, effusion, pain provoked by internal or external rotation of the flexed leg (especially with the patient prone and the tibia pressed against the femur). Usually, there is no significant varus-valgus instability. Signs of acute or chronic anterior cruciate laxity may, however, be present. X-rays are negative. McMurray's test, producing a "clunk" or pain at the joint line by extending the flexed knee, is difficult to perform and interpret in acutely injured, painful knees.

Definitive diagnosis and usually treatment as well are obtained by arthroscopy. Patients with suspected meniscal lesions should be referred for orthopedic evaluation and consideration of arthroscopy early, because of the potential damage to the articular surface that results from continued use of a knee with a significant meniscal tear and because of the rapid return to satisfactory function that this ambulatory procedure usually provides. Crutches, rest, a knee immobilizer, and analgesia as needed are provided pending orthopedic evaluation.

TIBIAL SHAFT FRACTURES

The tibia is the most frequently fractured long bone and may be broken by direct blows, missile wounds, crushing injuries, and indirect twisting forces. The fibula is often fractured as well. Open fractures of the tibia are more frequent than those of any other bone and are often major problems when there is loss of overlying skin. Compartment syndromes and associated neurovascular injuries are common complications. Prompt and effective emergency department management of patients with tibial fractures can help to decrease the risks of infection, nonunion, tissue necrosis, and amputation.

Diagnosis

Localized tenderness, swelling, and deformity are usually obvious with tibial fractures. Check the area around the fracture for breaks in the skin, and confirm the presence of peripheral pulses and nerve function (Table 22–2). Anteroposterior and lateral x-rays should confirm the presence of fracture, although if it is undisplaced, oblique views may be required.

Treatment

Correct gross deformity, and splint the limb, including the knee and foot. A traction splint (Fig 22–6) applied with just enough tension to stabilize the leg is usually sufficient. Elevate the injured limb slightly above the level of the heart. Provide analgesia (p 326). Observe the patient closely for signs of compartment syndrome.

Disposition

Hospitalization is almost always advisable. Orthopedic consultation should usually be obtained promptly in every case but may be delayed for several hours if no complications are present and the limb is satisfactorily splinted.

ISOLATED FIBULAR SHAFT FRACTURES

Diagnosis

Localized tenderness is easily elicited in isolated fractures of the fibular shaft. Anteroposterior and lateral x-rays should demonstrate the injury, but oblique views may be required. With fibular fractures, it is crucial to make sure that there are no associated injuries. Compartment syndromes may develop after direct blows to the fibular region. Fibular shaft fractures are frequently associated with damage to the knee or ankle, so both of these joints must be carefully checked for ligamentous injuries or other fractures. Occasionally, the common peroneal nerve is injured by the same force that fractures the fibula, so its function must be carefully tested (Table 22–2).

Treatment

If fibular injury is isolated, with no associated injury, apply a compression dressing with gentle pressure; provide crutches for partial weight bearing, and advise rest with elevation of the limb above the level of the heart for the first 2 days after injury. Discuss the danger signs of compartment syndrome with the patient. Provide oral analgesia (codeine compound or equivalent), and arrange for orthopedic consultation in 3–5 days.

Disposition

Hospitalize the patient if pain is severe, if compromise of neurovascular structure or function has occurred, or if the patient would be unable to return without delay to the hospital if such problems developed. Otherwise, outpatient care is sufficient.

ANKLE JOINT INJURIES

Evaluation of ankle injuries is difficult, because the stability of this joint depends on the combined integrity of multiple bones and ligaments. Together the tibia and fibula form a socket for the talus called the ankle mortise. Dorsiflexion and plantar flexion occur within the mortise, but normally, no sideways mobility or tilting occurs. The crucial relationship is that between the talus and the tibia. The lateral malleolus (distal fibula) maintains the proper relationship of these bones as long as it is intact and is securely attached to the distal tibia by the syndesmosis (distal tibiofibular ligaments). The medial side of the ankle joint is stabilized by the deltoid ligament and its tibial attachment, the medial malleolus. Injuries of these structures tend to occur in combinations, with involvement of ligaments as well as or instead of malleolar fractures. This is easy to identify when there is gross disruption of ankle joint congruity, eg, a fracture-dislocation (Fig 22–26), but may be much more subtle.

The ultimate outcome of ankle injury depends upon reestablishing and maintaining normal joint relationships during the healing period.

Diagnosis

Fracture-dislocations should be obvious, with gross deformity, and complete talar displacement evident on the lateral x-ray. Less severe ankle injuries require careful evaluation to avoid confusion of stable undisplaced injuries with those that appear satisfactorily aligned but may displace if inadequately treated. Physical findings (ligamentous tenderness

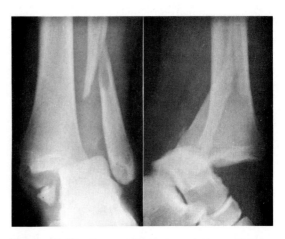

Figure 22–26. Fracture-dislocation of the ankle. Anteroposterior (left) and lateral (right) x-ray views of closed fracture of the lower fibular shaft and medial malleolus with dislocation of the inferior tibiofibular and ankle joints in a 35-year-old man. (Reproduced, with permission, from Way LW [editor]: *Current Surgical Diagnosis & Treatment,* 9th ed. Appleton & Lange, 1991.)

and abnormal mobility), thorough inspection of x-rays, and knowledge of the patterns of typical ankle injuries are the keys to diagnosis.

Tenderness that is present both medially and laterally increases the likelihood of instability, but unilaterally tender ankles can also be unstable. The ability to slide the talus medially or laterally in the mortise confirms instability.

X-rays (anteroposterior, mortise, and lateral views) (Fig 22–27) are essential for evaluation of ankle trauma. Early follow-up of ankle injuries by an orthopedist is the safest way to avoid underestimating the severity of ankle injuries.

Diagnostic Significance of Talar Displacement

Lateral shift of the talus results from fractures of the lateral malleolus at or above the level of the syndesmosis and is associated with disruption of the syndesmosis and medial malleolar fracture or rupture of the deltoid ligament. Tenderness of the deltoid ligament and syndesmosis can be difficult to identify. Instability of the talus can be identified by manipulation, but this may be too painful.

Careful examination of a mortise view x-ray is required. This is a true anteroposterior view of the ankle joint, the axis of which runs approximately between the tips of the malleoli. Internal rotation of the ankle joint of approximately 15 degrees is sufficient to place the intermalleolar axis parallel to the x-ray film, which should show a radiolucent joint space of constant width above and on both sides of the talus. Widening of the space between the talus and an intact medial malleolus indicates a tear of the deltoid ligament. Widening of the space between the distal tibia and fibula indicates disruption of the syndesmosis.

Ankle Injuries in Children & Young People

Ankle injuries in children and teenagers often involve disruption of growth plates, since physeal cartilage is generally weaker than ligaments. Localization of tenderness to the growth plate region of the distal fibula or tibia, with less tenderness of adjacent soft tissues, suggests fracture of the physis. If the fracture is undisplaced, x-rays may appear normal. However, the limb should be splinted just as after any undisplaced fracture. Growth plate injuries require orthopedic consultation within 24 hours if there is any displacement, since rapid healing in young people may make delayed reduction impossible.

1. FRACTURES OF THE MALLEOLI

Diagnosis

In the absence of obvious deformity, palpation can be helpful. The lateral radiograph should also be inspected carefully for displacement of any lateral malleolus fracture, for a fracture of the posterior tibial lip ("posterior malleolus"), and for posterior subluxation or dislocation of the talus relative to the tibia. Tenderness well localized to the injured bone suggests an undisplaced fracture, which is usually visible on x-ray. On lateral view x-rays, look carefully at the lateral malleolus, since fractures of this bone are often nearly parallel to the anteroposterior plane and therefore hard to discern on that view.

If both malleoli are fractured or if the talus is shifted sideways from its normal position, the ankle is definitely unstable; however, it may be unstable even if only one malleolus is fractured (Fig 22–27). It is important to remember that some fractures of the proximal fibula are equivalent to displaced lateral malleolar fractures. Therefore, during examination of an injured ankle, it is essential to palpate the entire fibula and obtain x-rays of the entire bone if tenderness is present proximal to the ankle region.

Treatment

A. Stable Ankle Injuries: Undisplaced fractures of the medial or lateral malleolus should be immobilized in a U splint (Fig 22–8), protected from weight bearing with crutches, and elevated for a few days. Patients should be referred for orthopedic consultation within 3–5 days.

B. Unstable Ankle Injuries: Displaced fractures of one or both malleoli are unstable with regard to tilt, lateral displacement of the talus, and rotation. Look for shift of the talus as shown in Fig 22–27. Open fractures and skin abrasions are common and require prompt surgery and immediate orthopedic consultation. Deformity should be reduced promptly to mini-

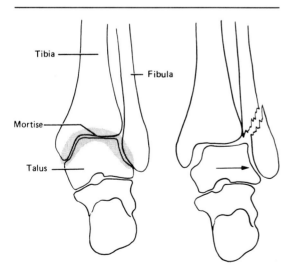

Figure 22–27. Fracture-dislocation of the ankle. Drawing of mortise view x-ray of the ankle showing displaced fracture of the lateral malleolus with lateral displacement of the talus, implying ruptured deltoid ligament.

mize swelling and to avoid necrosis of tightly stretched skin. Reduction usually requires internal rotation of the foot after traction has been established distally (Fig 22–28). Subsequent splinting must include the slightly flexed knee as well as the foot to control rotation of the ankle, and it requires a *long leg* cast or splints over adequate padding, applied while the ankle is held in reduction. Obtain x-rays after the leg has been placed in the cast or splint to confirm that the talus has been reduced to a position which is as anatomically normal as possible.

Disposition

If the ankle is dislocated or cannot be kept reduced (as shown by x-rays obtained promptly after application of the splint) or if there is an open fracture or skin abrasion, immediate orthopedic consultation is needed. Comminuted fractures of the distal tibia involving the transverse articular surface are serious injuries that also require immediate orthopedic evaluation and hospitalization.

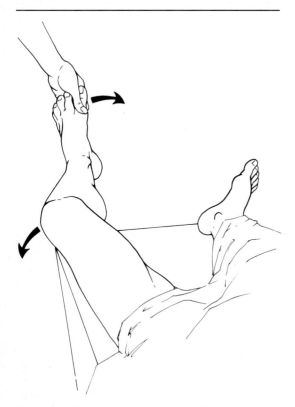

Figure 22–28. Technique of internal rotation of the foot for reduction of unstable external rotation ankle injuries. Hip and knee are flexed 45–60 degrees, and the hip is allowed to fall into external rotation, so that the knee points toward the wall of the room. The foot is grasped by the toes as illustrated and rotated internally, so that the toes point toward the ceiling. The leg must be held in this position while a long leg splint or cast is applied.

Unstable ankle injuries without significant displacement and without other complications need not be immediately examined by an orthopedist as long as adequate splinting has been achieved and alignment of the splinted joint has been confirmed by x-ray. Plans should be made for adequate monitoring and early follow-up. Hospitalization may be advisable. When in doubt, consult with an orthopedic surgeon. Some orthopedists advocate immediate internal fixation of ankle fractures before significant swelling occurs. If this treatment is chosen, the patient should be hospitalized and prepared for surgery at once.

Orthopedic consultation for patients with undisplaced fractures of either malleolus can be delayed for 3–5 days, as noted above.

2. LATERAL COLLATERAL LIGAMENT SPRAINS

Diagnosis

Common inversion injuries of the ankle cause sprains of the lateral collateral ligament complex of graded severity (p 327). Swelling can be diffuse distal to the lateral malleolus, but careful examination should localize maximal tenderness to the anterior fibulotalar ligament and possibly the fibulocalcaneal ligament.

X-rays of the ankle usually show no abnormalities but occasionally show extra-articular avulsion fractures, especially of the lateral malleolus, talus, and base of the fifth metatarsal (see below). Other x-ray findings following inversion ankle sprains are osteochondral fractures of the talus or more serious impaction-adduction fractures of the medial malleolus, both of which require early orthopedic consultation.

Rupture of the anterior fibulotalar ligament causes "anterior drawer" instability of the ankle joint, as shown by physical examination (Fig 22–29) or a lateral x-ray with appropriate stress applied to the joint. When the calcaneofibular portion of the lateral collateral ankle ligament is also ruptured, inversion instability is present but is masked by normal inversion of the subtalar joint. Stress x-rays can confirm excessive inversion between the talus and the tibia, but this examination is painful and may require anesthesia.

Results of physical examination that are inconsistent with findings associated with a lateral collateral ligament injury in a patient who complains of a "sprained ankle" should suggest the need for more thorough examination to search for bone or ligament injury elsewhere about the ankle, rupture of the Achilles tendon, or dislocation of the peroneal tendons from their normal position behind the lateral malleolus (see below).

Treatment

If lateral swelling and tenderness are more than just minimal or if the patient is unable to walk with-

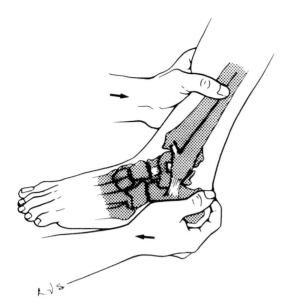

Figure 22–29. Anterior drawer test for ruptured anterior fibulotalar component of the lateral collateral ankle ligaments. Compare laxity (ability to displace the foot anteriorly) with that of the uninjured side.

out limping, apply a plaster U splint over adequate padding, and mold it into slight eversion. Additional immobilization can be obtained by adding a posterior splint (Fig 22–10).

Provide crutches, and advise elevation of the limb and avoidance of weight bearing. *Do not apply a cast to a recently sprained ankle,* because if swelling has not occurred, it will, and the cast may become too tight. On the other hand, a cast applied over significant swelling will rapidly become too loose.

Caution: Do not undertreat ankle sprains and thus risk chronic inversion instability and pain. It is usually simplest to immobilize and protect the joint for all but the most minor injuries, thereby overtreating some stable sprains of the lateral ankle ligament.

Minor sprains may be treated with a pneumatic U splint or equivalent and crutches, with activity and weight bearing gradually increasing over 2–3 weeks.

Disposition

Patients with presumably minor sprains may not need follow-up but should be instructed in protection of the limb until normal comfort, strength, and agility return. They should also be advised to seek follow-up care if pain and disability are severe or if recovery is delayed more than 2–3 weeks. Patients with severe sprains should be referred for orthopedic evaluation within 3–5 days.

TENDON PROBLEMS NEAR THE ANKLE

Pain, localized tenderness, and partial or complete loss of function are typical of tendon injuries. Swelling may be obvious or very slight. The patient often describes the injury in general terms, eg, "I sprained my ankle." Common injuries affecting tendons in this region are rupture, retinacular avulsion, and tendinitis or tenosynovitis.

1. TENDON RUPTURE

Diagnosis

Rupture most frequently involves the Achilles tendon, which should be palpated whenever a patient complains of ankle injury. Careful questioning reveals that the ankle "gave way" suddenly (often during a jump) and that a twisting motion was not the mechanism of injury. The rupture produces an audible "crack." The patient is usually 30–40 years old. Swelling may mask a palpable defect in the tendon.

Active ankle plantar flexion is present, since the long flexors of the toes, etc, are still intact. Weakness is evident, and walking on tiptoe is impossible. To confirm the diagnosis, have the patient kneel on a chair with the feet hanging free over the edge. Squeeze the relaxed calf, a maneuver that normally causes plantar flexion of the ankle. If the Achilles tendon is ruptured, plantar flexion on the injured side is much less than on the uninjured side (Fig 22–30).

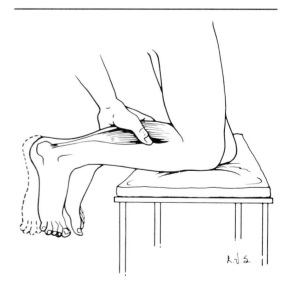

Figure 22–30. Test for Achilles tendon continuity. Squeeze the relaxed calf while observing the amount of ankle plantar flexion thus produced. If the tendon is ruptured, less motion occurs compared with that on the uninjured side.

Treatment & Disposition

Splint the ankle, provide crutches, and arrange orthopedic consultation within 3 days.

2. "PLANTARIS RUPTURE"

The so-called plantaris tendon rupture syndrome is almost always a partial tear of the gastrocnemius or soleus muscle. This common condition begins suddenly while running or jumping, with mid to lower third calf pain. Occasionally, a "pop" or sensation of tearing is noted. Tenderness is in the muscle belly rather than the Achilles tendon. Normal plantar flexion occurs with calf compression (see above). Active plantar flexion is strong but painful. Swelling and ecchymosis may develop, usually after a day or 2. Usually, only symptomatic treatment is needed with ice, elevation, gentle elastic bandage compression, and crutches or limited activity. Stretching and strengthening exercises are begun as soon as symptoms permit.

3. PERONEAL TENDON DISLOCATION

Diagnosis

Retinacular avulsion permits the peroneal tendons to be dislocated anteriorly, so that they lie obliquely across the lateral malleolus instead of behind its posterior edge, as is normal. Retinacular avulsion is a common skiing injury. The mechanism of injury is forceful contraction of the foot evertors against resistance.

Tenderness is present behind the malleolus, and dislocation of the tendons is palpable, especially with the foot in dorsiflexion, unless swelling is sufficient to mask it.

X-rays may show avulsion fracture of the posterior lip of the malleolus.

Treatment & Disposition

Splint the ankle, provide crutches, and arrange for orthopedic consultation within 3 days.

4. TENDINITIS & TENOSYNOVITIS

Diagnosis

Acute tenosynovitis is usually the result of overuse; rarely, it is due to infection, especially disseminated gonococcal infection or inflammatory disease (eg, Reiter's syndrome). Tenosynovitis can be disabling enough to interfere with normal walking and may prevent participation in the sport that initially caused the injury.

Tenderness is well localized to the involved portion of the tendon and its sheath. Crepitus may be manifest with motion, and swelling or erythema is often present. Pain occurs when the tendon is used to position the foot against resistance. However, good strength of the associated muscles is usually noted, particularly if testing does not produce much movement of the tendon within its sheath.

Treatment & Disposition

A. Mild Discomfort: Give oral anti-inflammatory drugs (eg, aspirin, 650 mg 4 times a day), and counsel the patient to avoid activity that causes pain. Stretching exercises should be started as symptoms subside, and a supervised rehabilitation program may be helpful.

B. Severe Discomfort: Discomfort severe enough to cause a noticeable limp requires a splint, crutches, and oral anti-inflammatory agents (eg, ibuprofen, 600 mg 3 times a day, or comparable nonsteroidal drug). Arrange for orthopedic consultation within 3 days.

If disseminated gonococcal infection is suspected, see Chapter 34 for guidelines for diagnosis and treatment.

FRACTURES & DISLOCATIONS OF THE TALUS

Diagnosis

Talar fractures are characterized by swelling, tenderness over the injury, and pain that is increased by ankle motion. Fractures of the talus associated with ankle or subtalar joint dislocations may be open fractures or may severely stretch the overlying skin, so that deformity is obvious. Check for skin abrasions, and assess distal neurovascular function.

X-rays should include an anteroposterior view of the foot in addition to the usual anteroposterior, lateral, and mortise views of the ankle. Look not only for common avulsion fractures but also for fractures of the neck of the talus, either undisplaced or with displacement of either the body or the head. Confirm the status of ankle, subtalar, and talonavicular joints. The body and head of the talus may also be fractured, with disruption of articular surfaces that is usually apparent on x-ray. Compare x-rays with those of the uninjured foot, and obtain orthopedic consultation if necessary.

Treatment & Disposition

Displaced talar fractures with damage of overlying skin or malalignment sufficient to cause skin tension are emergencies that require urgent orthopedic consultation and surgery. Dislocations of ankle, subtalar, and talonavicular joints are also emergencies that require urgent reduction to prevent progressive soft tissue damage. Splint the limb (Fig 22–9), elevate it, and follow the procedure for open fracture if a wound is present. Obtain orthopedic consultation immediately.

Undisplaced talar fractures and avulsion fractures may be treated initially like other stable ankle injuries. Patients should be referred for consultation within 3 days. Extreme swelling may occur with fractures of the talar body or neck, and hospitalization is usually advisable for these injuries.

FRACTURES OF THE CALCANEUS

Diagnosis
Most calcaneal fractures are the result of a fall, with force borne primarily by the patient's heels. Bilateral injuries are common, as are associated vertebral body compression or burst fractures.

The heel is painful, tender, and often widened, with decreased height. Swelling develops rapidly in all but the most minor injuries. The skin is occasionally disrupted by a calcaneal fracture and can also become necrotic later owing to extreme soft tissue swelling. Therefore, the condition of the skin at the time of initial examination must be carefully recorded. The back should be examined for tenderness and limited motion.

X-rays (lateral, axial, and anteroposterior views of the foot, sufficiently exposed to demonstrate the calcaneocuboid joint) demonstrate fractures of the calcaneus. Fracture lines may not be obvious, but the shape of the bone is altered by a significant fracture, so that the subtalar joint facets of the calcaneus may no longer be congruent with those of the talus. The normal obtuse angle formed by the body and tuberosity of the calcaneus may be flattened or even rendered concave. A CT scan helps define the injury and is advisable if open reduction is to be considered.

Obtain anteroposterior and lateral x-rays of the spine if the patient has back pain or local tenderness or if necessary to exclude a thoracolumbar spine injury.

Treatment
Apply a pillow splint (Fig 22–9). Elevate the foot. Provide analgesia as required. If the patient's general condition permits, morphine, 3–5 mg/h intravenously, may be required.

Disposition
All patients with significant fractures of the calcaneus should be hospitalized. Orthopedic consultation should be obtained promptly for patients with open fractures and for those with serious associated spinal fractures. Some surgeons recommend immediate open reduction and internal fixation for displaced calcaneal fractures if it can be carried out before soft tissue swelling is severe. If this is not being considered, orthopedic consultation is less urgent, but the patient should still be seen within 24 hours. Severe pain and tense swelling may indicate a compartment syndrome that requires immediate fasciotomy.

TARSOMETATARSAL JOINT INJURIES

The normally stable joint between the metatarsals and the tarsus (the medial 3 cuneiform bones and the cuboid bone laterally) may be disrupted in motor vehicle accidents and falls from a height.

Diagnosis
Signs of tarsometatarsal joint injuries are tenderness, swelling, and especially instability, elicited by grasping the forefoot in one hand and the heel in the other and demonstrating excessive motion in any plane, compared with the movement of the uninjured foot. Injury need not involve all metatarsals. Check carefully for distal neurovascular compromise.

X-rays may show little evidence of this severe injury, which is suggested by avulsion fractures of any of the medial 4 metatarsal bases. The second metatarsal normally lies between the first and third cuneiform bones like a tenon within its mortise. Therefore, a fracture of the base of the second metatarsal suggests disruption of the tarsometatarsal joint. Displacement of the metatarsals may be slight and is easier to recognize if x-rays of the uninjured foot are obtained for purposes of comparison. Oblique views may be helpful.

Treatment
Swelling progresses rapidly. Elevation of the limb, application of a pillow splint, and appropriate analgesia are required. Attempt to reduce severe deformity with distal traction on the forefoot.

Disposition
Immediate orthopedic consultation and hospitalization are advisable. Open reduction and internal fixation provide the best results for unstable tarsometatarsal joint injuries.

FRACTURE OF THE BASE OF THE FIFTH METATARSAL

Diagnosis
Fracture of the base of the fifth metatarsal is usually caused by an inversion injury that may also have sprained the lateral collateral ankle ligaments. Local tenderness and a fracture line seen on x-ray confirm the diagnosis.

Treatment & Disposition
Treatment and disposition are initially the same as

for lateral collateral ankle ligament sprain, although a walking cast may be required once swelling permits.

FRACTURE OF THE METATARSAL SHAFT

Diagnosis

It is important to determine the mechanism of injury in fracture of the metatarsal shaft. Crushing injuries or those caused by an object running over the foot tend to be only slightly displaced; however, there may be extensive soft tissue damage, with risk of delayed sloughing of much of the forefoot. The deformity associated with fracture may be masked by swelling.

Anteroposterior and lateral x-rays usually demonstrate metatarsal fractures, but oblique views may be required. The significance of fractures of the base of the metatarsals as described above should not be overlooked.

Fatigue fractures of metatarsal shafts ("march fractures") are relatively common. Patients have pain and point tenderness but do not always have a history of dramatically increased activity. X-rays usually show no abnormality when symptoms first develop. If taken more than 2 weeks later, x-rays show periosteal new bone formation and (occasionally) a fracture line. A bone scan will show increased radioisotope activity in the involved area before radiographic abnormalities occur.

Treatment

Splint the foot with a pillow or U splint with plantar slab (Figs 22–9 and 22–10). Crutches are required if the patient is discharged. Advise elevation of the limb and appropriate analgesia.

Disposition

Crush injuries, such as those incurred when the patient is run over by a motor vehicle, usually require hospitalization. Obtain prompt orthopedic consultation if neurovascular deficit or open fracture is present. Displaced fractures require orthopedic consultation before the patient is discharged from the emergency department, since reduction and fixation may be required. Hospitalization may be advised by the orthopedist. Patients with undisplaced fractures of the metatarsals may be discharged with arrangements made for orthopedic follow-up within 3–5 days after treatment has been given as outlined above.

FRACTURES & DISLOCATIONS OF THE TOES

Diagnosis

Crushing injuries and direct blows from "stubbing" are the usual causes of fractures and disloca-

tions of the toes. Be alert to the possibility of open injuries and of significant soft tissue damage from crushing injuries. Tenderness, swelling, and deformity are usually apparent. Anteroposterior and lateral x-rays should demonstrate fractures and dislocations of the toes, but the joints must be carefully examined, and oblique views may be required.

Treatment

A. Dislocations: Dislocations of the metatarsophalangeal or interphalangeal joints must be promptly reduced. Longitudinal traction on the toe should suffice, but local anesthesia may be required. Inject lidocaine (without epinephrine) into the web spaces adjacent to the digital nerves, which are located toward the plantar surface. Do not inject lidocaine into the toe itself. After reduction, confirm stability by stressing the joint. Splint the injury by taping the injured toe to its neighbor. Tape applied to an injured toe must allow room for swelling or should be removed if it later constricts the toe. Postreduction x-rays are needed to confirm reduction. A loose shoe with a stiff sole adds protection. This may be patient's own shoe (eg, hiking boot). Alternatives are thick-soled cast shoes and "postoperative" shoes with wooden soles. (Subungual hematomas are discussed in Chapter 23.)

B. Fractures: The great toe bears enough weight that special treatment is necessary if fracture occurs. Apply a temporary U splint with plantar slab that extends beyond the tip of the toe (Fig 22–10). Advise the use of crutches and avoidance of weight bearing. A short leg walking cast or "postoperative" wooden-soled shoe may be used later to permit ambulation without crutches.

Displaced fractures of the great toe may require internal fixation if the deformity cannot be corrected by closed techniques or if there is significant articular involvement. Orthopedic consultation is advised in these cases.

Closed fractures of the lesser toes are treated as described above for dislocations of the toes, with attention directed primarily to the maintenance of gross alignment.

Disposition

Open fractures and unreduced dislocations of the toes require immediate orthopedic consultation. Patients with other toe injuries may be referred for orthopedic follow-up in 3–5 days after treatment has been given as described above.

COMMON PITFALLS

Among the most common malpractice claims in emergency medicine are missed orthopedic injuries. Commonly missed are carpal bone injuries of the wrist (particularly scaphoid fractures), rotational deformity of metacarpal and phalangeal fractures, tendon injuries in the hand, radial head fractures, posterior dislocation of the shoulder, pubic ramus and femoral neck fractures in elderly patients, tarsometatarsal joint injuries, patellar tendon tears, and compartment syndromes. It is important to have a high index of suspicion with injuries to these areas, particularly if soft-tissue swelling or pain out of proportion to x-ray findings is present. Comparison films, immobilization, and repeat x-rays in 7–10 days may be of value. Orthopedic consultation or referral should be made when in doubt.

REFERENCES

Browner BD et al: *Skeletal Trauma.* Saunders, 1991.

Casteleyn PP, Handelberg F, Opdecam P: Traumatic hemarthrosis of the knee. J Bone Joint Surg [Br] 1988;70:404.

D'Ambrosia RD: *Musculoskeletal Disorders: Regional Examination and Differential Diagnosis.* Lippincott, 1977.

Feagin JA Jr: The office diagnosis and documentation of common knee problems. Clin Sports Med 1989;8:453.

Gersoff WK, Clancy WG Jr: Diagnosis of acute and chronic anterior cruciate ligament tears. Clin Sports Med 1988; 7:727.

Hoppenfeld S: *Physical Examination of the Spine and Extremities.* Appleton-Century-Crofts, 1976.

Keene JS: Diagnosis of undetected knee injuries: Interpreting subtle clinical and radiologic findings. (2 parts.) Postgrad Med 1989;85:153,161.

Lowenstein SR et al: Vertical trauma: Injuries to patients who fall and land on their feet. Ann Emerg Med 1989; 8:161.

Mackersie RC et al: Major skeletal injuries in the obtunded blunt trauma patient: A case for routine radiographic survey. J Trauma 1988;28:1450.

Manoli A II: Compartment syndromes of the foot: Current concepts. Foot Ankle 1990;10:340.

Moore MN: Orthopedic pitfalls in emergency medicine. South Med J 1988;8:371.

Moore RE III, Friedman RJ: Current concepts in pathophysiology and diagnosis of compartment syndromes. J Emerg Med 1989;7:657.

Rang M: *Children's Fractures,* 2nd ed. Lippincott, 1983.

Rockwood CA Jr, Green DP, Bucholz RW (editors): *Fractures,* 3rd ed. Lippincott, 1991.

Szabo RM, Manske D: Displaced fractures of the scaphoid. Clin Orthop 1988;230:30.

23

Hand Trauma

Eugene S. Kilgore, Jr., MD, FACS, & William L. Newmeyer, MD

Abbreviations Used in This Chapter

CM	Carpometacarpal
DIP	Distal interphalangeal
IP	Interphalangeal
LET	Lateral extensor tendon
MET	Middle extensor tendon
MP	Metacarpophalangeal
PIP	Proximal interphalangeal
TET	Terminal extensor tendon

EMERGENCY EVALUATION & TREATMENT

Hand injuries are common and frequently threaten the patient's livelihood and life-style, causing severe economic and social hardship. *The ultimate consequence of any hand injury depends upon the quality of early care.*

The nature and extent of hand injuries can almost always be assessed by the simple techniques of history, examination by one thoroughly familiar with the functional anatomy of the region, and an absolute minimum of laboratory tests. Hand injuries are seldom life-threatening, but significant disability is always a possibility. *It is far better to undertreat and refer* than to overtreat and cause avoidable iatrogenic injury or disability. A stepwise approach to problems of the hand (as outlined below) is recommended.

Note: (**1**) The course of recovery depends upon the quality of initial care. (**2**) To save a hand is to save an economic life.

Position the Patient

Except in the case of trivial injuries, the patient should first be supine on the examining table. The hand should be placed on a firm support that can be positioned against or attached to the table. Clothing around the arm should be removed to the shoulder. Lighting should be good, preferably wall- or ceiling-mounted.

Control Bleeding

Bleeding is controlled by direct pressure with sterile gauze packs, elevation, and, if necessary, an arterial tourniquet (eg, blood pressure cuff inflated above systolic blood pressure). *Do not use clamps unless all other measures fail.* "Blind" clamping of vessels can lead to further injury.

Obtain History

A. Current Injuries: The mechanism of injury should be ascertained by questioning the patient or others. An exact description of how the injury occurred will help determine the need for x-ray, antibiotics, urgent consultation, or no consultation. Specific questions about the following may be required:

1. Crush injury.
2. Torsion injury.
3. Lacerations and exactly what device caused them.
4. Circumstances surrounding open wounds—whether inflicted in a dirty (eg, sewer or barnyard) or clean (eg, kitchen) area.

B. Relevant Past History:

1. History of prior or existing hand or upper extremity injuries or disorders—Dupuytren's fasciitis, arthritis, and benign tumors are the most common nontraumatic problems noted.
2. Bleeding disorders likely to influence hemostasis (eg, hemophilia).
3. Factors that might impair wound healing (eg, use of corticosteroids).
4. Tetanus immunization status (Chapter 24).
5. Any allergies.
6. General state of health, medications, ongoing treatments.

Examine the Hand

· Examination of the hand is started while the history is being taken. In the event of an open wound, proper instruments and sutures must be made ready (p 362). Sterile technique is essential at all stages of the examination and early treatment of hand injuries. A sensory examination should be done with a fine needle before anesthesia is used. Before beginning active examination, anesthetize the injured area of the hand, and apply and inflate a tourniquet.

A. Anesthesia: Anesthesia must be used if a wound is to be explored or sutured. The preferred anesthetic is 1% lidocaine *without* epinephrine. Never use epinephrine with local anesthetics in hand injury, as it may constrict the vessels and interfere with blood flow.

1. Regional or digital block–(See Fig 23–1.) Block anesthesia is preferred and is administered before tourniquet inflation. Half-inch (1.5-cm) needles of 25, 27, or 30 gauge should be used with small volumes of plain 1% lidocaine. In a digital block, about 0.5–1 mL around each digital nerve is the correct amount. The injection should never render the tissues tense.

In blocking peripheral nerves, the surgeon must be familiar with the anatomy of nerve distribution and the surrounding tissues. To avoid intravascular injection, always aspirate before injecting the anesthetic agent.

2. Local infiltration–(See Fig 23–2.) Wounds can be infiltrated locally as long as the amount of anesthetic injected does not make the tissues tense.

Palmar view

Dorsal view

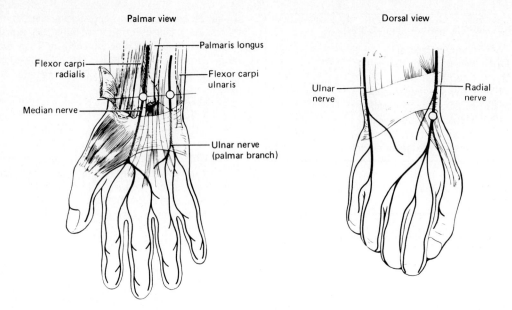

Figure 23–1. Nerve blocks at wrist. **Left:** Median and ulnar nerve block. **Right:** Radial nerve block. (Reproduced, with permission, from Dunphy JE, Way LW [editors]: *Current Surgical Diagnosis & Treatment,* 3rd ed. Lange, 1977.)

3. Amount of solution–Systemic toxicity from overdosage may occur when large areas are anesthetized. This can be avoided by calculating the number of milligrams of drug in the volume of solution that may be required and then limiting the volume of injection so as to avoid giving a toxic dose (see Table 24–1).

4. Inflamed areas–Anesthetic solutions should not be injected into inflamed areas unless these directly overlie an abscess that is to be drained. Such injections impair local tissue resistance to infection,

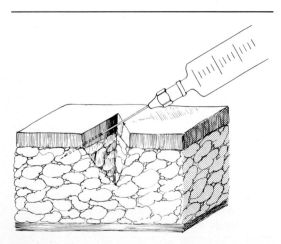

Figure 23–2. Injection of local anesthetic. (Reproduced, with permission, from Dunphy JE, Way LW [editors]: *Current Surgical Diagnosis & Treatment,* 5th ed. Lange, 1981.)

may result in rapid systemic absorption because of the increased vascularity of inflamed tissues, and may be ineffective if the local tissue pH is low enough to reduce the anesthetic agent's ionic dissociation, which is essential for anesthetic activity.

B. Application of Tourniquet: An arm tourniquet should *always* be in place on the arm when hand wounds are examined or treated. A blood pressure cuff can be used but should be inverted so that the tubes extend cephalad and out of the way. When the cuff is in place, it should be wrapped with cast padding to keep it from unwrapping when inflated.

When the anesthetic has taken effect and examination of the wound is about to start, the arm is elevated for 30 seconds and held there while the cuff is inflated to 275–300 mm Hg and the tubes clamped with Kelly clamps to prevent deflation. This is well tolerated by most patients for at least 15–20 minutes.

C. Examination Sequence: By dividing the examination into 4 distinct steps, much useful information can be gained rapidly.

1. Observe the posture of the hand lying supine and at rest upon the examining table. Any marked variation from the normal stance should alert the examiner to the possibility of deforming injury.

2. Observe active function of the various musculotendinous units and skeletal structures within the areas of injury (p 359).

3. Assess loss of sensibility by testing for sweat and for awareness of pain by using a fine needle in areas of suspected nerve injury. Two-point discrimination is a sensitive, objective measure of sensory deficit. This may be difficult to do accurately, and the character and location of a wound may be more helpful than sensory nerve testing in determining nerve injury. Sensory testing must be performed before application of a tourniquet and administration of anesthetics.

4. Inspect the wound, using a simple 2-power magnifying loupe. A tourniquet should be in place but should *not* be inflated until the anesthetic has become effective unless there is uncontrollable hemorrhage (see above). The examination must proceed concurrently with early treatment such as cleansing and debridement (Chapter 24) before definitive emergency treatment and suturing are done. *Note:* In handling and examining tissue, remember that removal of blood clots and careful manipulation of tissues to preserve the microcirculation are far more important in avoiding infection than the type of antiseptic wound preparation used.

EXAMINATION OF THE HAND & ASSESSMENT OF FUNCTION
(See Figs 23–3 and 23–4.)

The hand is a highly mobile organ of extraordinary sensibility and remarkable adaptability, but it can be rendered useless or worse than useless by injury causing permanent stiffness, pain, or loss of sensibility. Prevention of permanent damage requires a sound knowledge of functional hand anatomy.

Terminology
(See Fig 23–5.)

The hand and each finger have ulnar and radial sides and palmar and dorsal surfaces. There are 5 digits numbered and named as follows: I (thumb), II (index), III (long or middle), IV (ring), and V (small [little]). Commonly used abbreviations for the joints of the hand are shown in the box at the beginning of the chapter. Always specify which hand is injured, and note whether it is the dominant or nondominant hand.

Skin & Circulation

The skin of the palm sweats freely and is thick, tough, tethered by fascia, highly innervated, and well cushioned by fat. The dorsal skin, by contrast, is thin, very mobile, and less well supplied with sensory nerves. The arterial supply is mainly palmar. Venous and lymphatic drainage is mainly dorsal and can be impeded by dorsal injury, constriction, or taut skin.

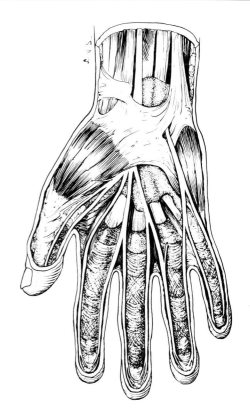

Figure 23–3. Palmar hand with skin removed reveals flexor tendons with their sheaths and the median and ulnar nerves with their terminal sensory branches. (Modified and reproduced, with permission, from Way LW [editor]: *Current Surgical Diagnosis & Treatment,* 9th ed. Appleton & Lange, 1991.)

Twelve Extrinsic Flexors
(See Fig 23–3.)

  A. Anatomy:

  1. There are 3 wrist flexors: the flexor carpi ulnaris (innervated by the ulnar nerve), the palmaris longus (median nerve), and the flexor carpi radialis (median nerve).

  2. There are 9 digital flexors (one for each IP joint).

  a. The flexor pollicis longus (innervated by the median nerve) flexes the thumb IP joint.

  b. A flexor digitorum superficialis (sublimis) moves each PIP joint (all median nerve). Each superficialis is generally able to contract independently, because the muscles are independent for each digit.

  c. A flexor digitorum profundus moves each DIP joint (median nerve to index and long fingers; ulnar nerve to ring and small fingers). The 3 ulnar profundi have a common muscle mass, and therefore one cannot contract and move one of these digit tips independently.

  B. Testing of Flexors:

  1. The flexor carpi radialis is tested by having the

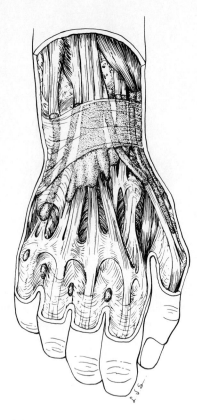

Figure 23–4. Cutaway view of the dorsal hand demonstrates that the extensor tendons are ensheathed only at wrist level. (Modified and reproduced, with permission, from Way LW [editor]: *Current Surgical Diagnosis & Treatment,* 9th ed. Appleton & Lange, 1991.)

patient flex the wrist; the flexor carpi ulnaris is tested by spreading the fingers. The palmaris longus is tested by having the patient spread the fingers while flexing the wrist.

2. The superficialis flexors are tested by holding 3 digits not being tested in full extension and directing the patient to flex the fourth one. PIP flexion indicates an intact superficialis to that finger.

3. The profundus flexors are tested by asking the patient to actively flex all of the fingers so that the distal pads of the fingers meet the distal palm.

4. The flexor pollicis longus is tested by having the patient actively flex the terminal phalanx of the thumb.

Twelve Extrinsic Extensors
(See Fig 23–4.)

All extensors are innervated by the radial nerve.

A. Anatomy:

1. Central wrist extensors–The extensor carpi radialis longus and extensor carpi radialis brevis insert into the bases of the second and third metacarpals, respectively.

2. Extensor and ulnar deviator–The extensor carpi ulnaris inserts into the base of the fifth metacarpal.

3. Abductor pollicis longus–The abductor pollicis longus deviates the wrist radially and stabilizes the base of the thumb (first metacarpal). It is tested by abducting the thumb radially.

4. Two thumb extensors–The extensor pollicis brevis acts mainly at the MP joint; the extensor pollicis longus acts at the IP joint in concert with the intrinsics but, unlike the intrinsics, can extend the joint with much force and can even hyperextend it.

5. Four finger extensors–An extensor digitorum communis to each finger forms the central slip (middle extensor tendon) of the extensor hood.

6. Index and small fingers–The index and small fingers have independent (proprius) extensor tendons as well. These extend these fingers when the long and ring fingers are flexed.

B. Testing of Extensors: Test the extensors by asking the patient to extend the fingers at the MP joint and to extend the IP joints. The latter is achieved by action of the extensor in conjunction with the intrinsic tendons in the extensor hood. The proprius tendons of the index and small fingers always lie ulnar to the extensor digitorum communis of each.

Twenty Intrinsic Muscles

A. Anatomy: Of 20 intrinsics, 15 are innervated by the ulnar nerve and 5 by the median nerve. In conjunction with the extensor tendon, they form the extensor hood mechanism, which is a proximally based triangular sheet of 3 interconnected tendons. The lateral margins ("lateral bands") are the small lateral extensor tendons (LETs) from the intrinsic muscles. The central large tendon ("central slip") from the extrinsic extensors is called the middle extensor tendon (MET), which inserts on the middle phalanx of each finger. The terminal extensor tendon (TET) is made up of a coalescence of METs and LETs into a very thin tendon that inserts on the distal phalanx. In the case of the thumb, which has only 2 phalanges, the equivalent of the MET is the extensor pollicis brevis; the equivalent of the TET is the extensor pollicis longus. The intrinsics flex the MP and extend the IP joints and abduct and adduct the digits. Working all together, they cup the palm.

B. Testing of Intrinsics:

1. Testing of thenar and hypothenar intrinsics–The thenar and hypothenar intrinsics act to pronate the thumb and little finger and thereby "cup" the palm. Have the patient make the distal fat pads of the thumb and small finger meet.

2. Testing of other intrinsics–Have the patient abduct and adduct the extended second through fifth digits; then flex these digits at the MP joints while extending the PIP and DIP joints.

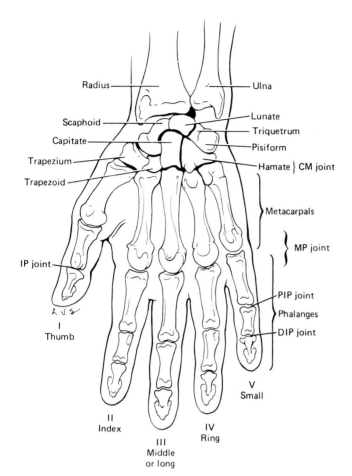

Figure 23–5. Terminology of bones and joints of the hand.

Examination of Nerve Injuries

The 3 major nerves to the hand are the radial, median, and ulnar nerves.

A. Radial Nerve: The radial nerve innervates all extensors.

1. Motor testing–Muscle testing is done by having the patient extend the wrist and digits (Fig 23–6C).

2. Sensory examination–The radial nerve gives off a sensory branch that provides sensibility for the dorsal-radial aspect of the hand (Fig 23–6A and B).

B. Median Nerve: The median nerve innervates 9 of 12 extrinsic flexors, the lumbricals to the index and long fingers, and the 3 muscles of the thenar eminence, which are mainly concerned with opposition.

1. Motor testing–

a. High median nerve–Testing for high median nerve injuries is done by flexing the DIP joint of the index finger and the IP joint of the thumb (Fig 23–7).

(1) Have the patient passively hold the fourth and fifth fingers fully flexed into the palm and follow this by full active flexion of the second and third fingers (Fig 23–7C).

(2) Have the patient flex the thumb to touch the distal palm at the base of the fifth finger (Fig 23–7D).

b. Low median nerve–To test for low median nerve loss (eg, at the wrist), have the patient pronate the thumb, pressing the distal fat pad of the thumb against that of the ring finger. Then feel for a firm, contracted abductor pollicis brevis alongside the thumb metacarpal.

2. Sensory examination–The median nerve provides sensibility to the radial two-thirds of the palm and the palmar surfaces of the thumb, the index and long fingers, the radial side of the ring finger, and the dorsal surface of the middle and distal phalanges of these fingers (Fig 23–7A and B). Because of the importance of this zone of sensibility, the median nerve is called the "eye of the hand."

C. Ulnar Nerve: The ulnar nerve innervates 15 of the 20 intrinsic muscles and only 3 extrinsic muscles.

1. Motor testing–The intrinsics are tested by any of the following maneuvers: With the palm flat on the table, have the patient abduct and adduct the fingers, cross the fingers, or forcefully move the pointed index finger in a radial direction.

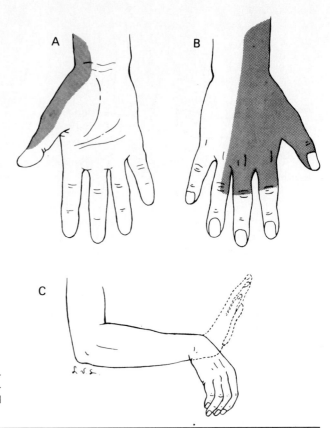

Figure 23–6. Palmar **(A)** and dorsal **(B)** areas of autogenous radial nerve sensibility. Loss of radial sensibility is not critical. A simple test for main trunk radial paresis is shown in **(C).**

The extrinsics are tested as follows: Forcefully flex the tips of the ring and small fingers to meet the distal palm to evaluate their profundi (Fig 23–8C); then forcefully spread the fingers apart and palpate for a tensed flexor carpi ulnaris tendon at the wrist.

2. Sensory examination–The ulnar nerve innervates the radial and ulnar halves of the pads of the small finger, the ulnar half of the pads of the ring finger, and the ulnar side of the hand (Fig 23–8A and B). The additional loss of sensibility on the dorsoulnar aspect of the body of the hand signifies a high lesion well proximal to the wrist.

X-Ray Examination

Any severe injury to the hand requires x-rays to detect fractures, dislocations, and opaque foreign material or gas. Special positions should be requested, depending on the site and direction of trauma. If there is any doubt about the normalcy of the skeleton, comparable views of the opposite side should be taken for comparison.

The Record

The history and physical examination, results of laboratory tests (CBC, urinalysis) and x-ray examinations, diagnosis, and treatment should be recorded in the emergency department chart. It is helpful to use a diagram of the hand for the immediate recording of some of the anatomic and functional data.

Instructions to the Patient

The patient should call in occasionally and should have a definite follow-up appointment (specific doctor, place, and time), usually within 2–4 days. Strict instructions should be given to keep the injured hand *up, dry, quiet, and free of constriction* by snug jewelry or clothing. Provide analgesics as needed. Appropriate antibiotics must be taken in the dose and for the duration prescribed.

EQUIPMENT & MATERIALS FOR TREATMENT

Instruments, Antiseptic Solutions, & Sutures

A. Needles: Suturing should be carefully done with fine-pointed and very sharp cutting needles (eg, Ethicon P-1, P-3).

B. Suturing Material: Fine (4-0, 5-0, or 6-0)

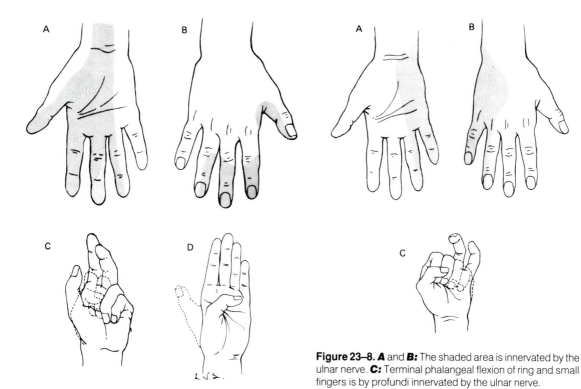

Figure 23–7. **A** and **B:** Autogenous median nerve sensibility is indicated by the shaded areas. The profundi of the index and long fingers **(C)** are innervated by the median nerve, as is the flexor pollicis longus **(D).**

Figure 23–8. **A** and **B:** The shaded area is innervated by the ulnar nerve. **C:** Terminal phalangeal flexion of ring and small fingers is by profundi innervated by the ulnar nerve.

monofilament polypropylene suture material is preferred for the skin closure. Only in infants and children should an absorbable suture such as 5-0 or 6-0 chromic or plain catgut be used.

C. Instruments: Fine plastic surgery forceps, retractors, clamps, and needle holders are required.

D. Skin and Wound Preparation: The skin around the wound may be sterilized as described in Chapter 24. Take care not to splash disinfectants in the wound itself. The hand and wound may be irrigated with normal saline or even tap water (hydrogen peroxide can be toxic and is less preferable). Avoid prolonged soaking.

Dressings, Splints, & Antibiotics

A. Inner Dressings:

1. Petrolatum-impregnated gauze followed by a surgical gauze sponge saturated with water (tap water or sterile saline solution) is applied over the wound as the "core" dressing. The wetness draws blood from the wound and prevents dead space. None of this goes circumferentially around the digit, hand, or forearm.

2. A foam pad such as a Reston pad with an adherent surface on one side (or comparable substitute) is then applied over the core dressing.

3. Soft elastic gauze (Kerlix, Kling) or cast padding to form a soft, well-padded dressing is applied over the foam pad and may go circumferentially around the part.

B. Splint or Circumferential Cast:

1. The wrist is the most important joint to splint for all major hand injuries, even if only one digit is injured.

2. Well-padded plaster as a splint or cast protects the hand.

3. For isolated pain-free dorsal injuries at the DIP or PIP joint, a tongue blade cut to the length of 2 phalanges and padded with gauze or foam rubber makes an excellent splint. If there is a wound over the joint, such a splint should be placed on the palmar side; if not, it is placed on the dorsum.

4. The most useful palmar splint consists of 10–12 layers of plaster cut to fit the involved digit or digits and extending halfway up the volar surface of the forearm. It is padded with a thin foam pad (eg, Reston) and held in place with a loosely wrapped roll of plaster of paris, bias-cut stockinet, or elastic bandage. The hand generally should be in the "position of function," ie, slight wrist extension and MP flexion, with the PIP and DIP joints in partial extension and the thumb web open (Fig 23–9). Modification must be applied to take tension off a specific wound.

C. Sling: No patient should leave the emergency department without a sling to hold the hand at the level of the heart or higher to promote venous and lymphatic drainage. Slings that hold the hand lower

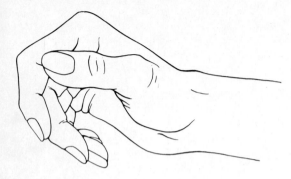

Figure 23–9. Position of function of the hand. Note graded flexion of fingers and slight dorsiflexion of wrist.

than the heart encourage the development of tissue edema. To avoid a tourniquet effect, the extremity should usually be outside of a sleeve.

D. Antibiotic Prophylaxis: For contaminated wounds, give antibiotics active against staphylococci or streptococci, eg, dicloxacillin, 250–500 mg orally 4 times daily. Cloxacillin, oxacillin, cephalexin, combined amoxicillin and clavulanate potassium (Augmentin), or erythromycin is also effective. Contaminated wounds may be irrigated with bacitracin.

MANAGEMENT OF SPECIFIC TYPES OF HAND INJURIES

LACERATIONS

1. SIMPLE CLEAN (TIDY) LACERATIONS

Small lacerations (superficial lacerations not extending into subcutaneous fat and not perpendicular to lines of skin tension) can be closed by use of sterile surgical tapes (eg, Steri-Strips). Splinting may help healing. Place the finger in a finger splint, or immobilize it with a padded tongue blade, taking care not to cause congestion or pressure on the wound. The patient should be seen in 2–3 days or may telephone in if healing is progressing uneventfully. In the interim, the patient should avoid wearing snug clothing or jewelry around the area and should keep the dressing dry. The hand should be kept at or above the level of the heart to prevent any throbbing pain.

2. MORE SEVERE CLEAN (TIDY) LACERATIONS

Diagnosis & Treatment

Use a tourniquet to obtain a bloodless field (p 358) so that deep structures can be carefully evaluated. Careful handling of tissues is essential.

Approximate the wound margins with everting sutures, either interrupted or (in the case of long wounds) continuous sutures. A horizontal running mattress suture is useful to evert skin edges on the hand (Fig 23–10).

Disposition

The patient should return within 2–4 days to the clinic or office for wound check. Telephone check-in often is satisfactory. Sutures are removed after 7–10 days.

3. DIRTY (UNTIDY) WOUNDS

Diagnosis & Treatment

Apply a tourniquet to evaluate dirty wounds. Cleanse first with tap water or sterile saline (hydrogen peroxide can be toxic, and other wound cleansers may be preferable). Debridement should be limited to devitalized tissue. Careful handling of tissues is essential. Do not sacrifice good tissue just because it is stained. Dirty wounds should never be closed under tension. If the edges cannot be easily approximated, the wound should be left open and a primary or delayed split-thickness skin graft applied. Potential dead space may be drained, utilizing a small Penrose drain left in place for 36–48 hours. Consider the need for local and systemic antibiotics and tetanus prophylaxis (Chapter 24).

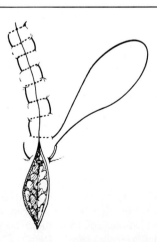

Figure 23–10. Continuous horizontal mattress suture.

Disposition

The patient should return in 1–3 days to the clinic or office for a wound check. Sutures are removed after 7–10 days.

FINGERTIP INJURIES

1. SLIGHT PAD LOSS

Diagnosis

If the area of loss is less than 1 cm^2 (⅜ in^2), healing by epithelization is satisfactory.

Treatment & Disposition

Cover with a small nonadhesive sterile dressing, and wrap the finger in a bulky dressing. Check the injury in 2–3 days.

2. EXTENSIVE PAD LOSS

Diagnosis

Extensive pad loss is loss of more than 1 cm^2 (⅜ in^2) of skin with or without fat and bone.

Treatment

If the amputated fingertip pad has been retained, is clean, and is in good condition, it may be reattached as a full-thickness skin graft provided that the undersurface is debrided of fat and bone. The avulsed skin should be sutured in place with a minimum number of sutures and with care taken not to create tension. A petrolatum-impregnated gauze dressing should be applied, followed by a soft, bulky dressing and forearm cast.

An alternative method that is more certain to be successful is a very thin onlay split-thickness skin graft, which serves well enough as a biologic dressing. The graft may be taken with a razor blade from the volar taut surface of the same forearm and should be thin enough so that the lettering on the razor blade may be read through it. The graft is placed on the wound *without sutures,* covered with bismuth tribromophenate gauze (Sigmaform, Xeroform) and wet gauze cut to fit the wound, and anchored with narrow strips of paper tape (Steri-Strips) or, preferably, strips of foam pad (Reston). It is helpful to paint the uninjured part of the digit with tincture of benzoin to make the tape or foam pad adhere well. The injured digit and an adjacent digit are incorporated in a well-padded soft dressing and a forearm cast. Dress the donor site of the graft with bismuth tribromophenate gauze. If the wound oozes or bleeds excessively, grafting should be delayed for 24–48 hours and a gentle compression dressing applied in the interim.

Disposition

If the pad loss is 2–3 cm^2 (¾–1 3/16 in^2), dress the wound and refer the patient to a hand specialist within 1–3 days. More extensive pad loss may require hospitalization and more elaborate surgery (eg, pedicle flap) for optimal results.

3. SUBUNGUAL HEMATOMA

Diagnosis

Hematoma from blunt trauma (eg, a hammer blow) rupturing subungual blood vessels is the most common nail and nail bed injury. An x-ray of the digit will rule out a fractured phalanx, an injury commonly associated with blunt trauma.

Treatment

One method for draining trapped blood is to heat a paper clip over an alcohol flame and touch it to the nail to quickly melt a hole. Alternatively, drilling the nail plate or undermining the tip of the nail to drain trapped blood relieves pressure and offers immediate relief. An effective method is to perform digital block (Chapter 24), and make a hole in the base of the nail with a No. 18 needle or fine dentist's drill rotated between the operator's fingers. Commercially available drills are also useful. Zinc oxide ointment under the dressing promotes drainage.

Disposition

The patient should return in 3–5 days to the clinic or office for wound check.

4. AVULSION OF NAIL

Diagnosis

Avulsion of the nail results from a force elevating the tip of the nail and ripping it off its bed, or downward crushing force sufficient to tear the base of the nail out of the eponychial sulcus, ripping open the nail bed and carrying the nail plate on a palmar-based pedicle flap.

Treatment

Nails avulsed at the base should be completely removed. If they are left in place, a badly lacerated nail bed that requires repair may inadvertently be overlooked. The unremoved nail also creates a dead space that promotes scarring and infection.

A. Removal of Nail: Anesthetize by digital block. Remove the avulsed nail by inserting a clamp under the distal attached portion of the nail and advancing it proximally, removing the nail by spreading the clamp. The exposed nail bed should be covered with sterile petrolatum gauze and a portion of the gauze tucked into the nail sulcus. A lacerated nail bed should be meticulously closed with 6-0 or 7-0 catgut on a fine ophthalmic needle.

B. Reattachment of Distal Torn Finger Flap:

If the distal portion of the finger has been torn off with the nail and has been left attached to the finger by a volar pedicle, the flap should be anatomically reduced and held with strips of paper tape (eg, Steri-Strips), or it should be sutured back in position with 6-0 catgut. Antibiotics should be administered.

C. Management of Fractures: Open fractures of the distal phalanx are reduced and held by soft tissue suturing. If the fracture is displaced, internal fixation with a Kirschner wire may be necessary.

Disposition

The patient should return in 2–3 days to the clinic or office for wound check and dressing change. Complicated problems should be referred to a hand surgeon and an immediate appointment made.

DISTAL EXTENSOR TENDON INJURIES*

1. LACERATION OF EXTENSOR TENDONS

Diagnosis

Dorsal finger and hand wounds frequently result in a partially or completely lacerated extensor tendon or extensor hood mechanism. The extent of injury can only be determined by adequate exposure and direct examination.

Treatment

If the tendon ends can be retrieved easily with minimal extension of the wound or by slight stretching of the skin, the tendon should be repaired in the emergency department by a simple figure-of-eight suture or a crisscross suture technique with 4-0, 5-0, or in infants, 6-0 nylon (Fig 23–11). A padded plaster fore-

---

*Flexor and proximal extensor tendon injuries are discussed with flexor tendon injuries on p 373.

arm cast is then applied with the digit and hand positioned so that the repair is relaxed as much as possible. No individual joint should be hyperextended, nor should all joints be simultaneously extended. The MP joint should not be immobilized in full extension, because contraction of collateral ligaments may result in fixation of the joint in extension. One or more neighboring fingers should always be immobilized with the injured digit.

Disposition

If the tendon ends are not easily retrieved, a hand surgeon should be notified immediately and arrangements made for repair as soon as possible.

The patient should return in 3–5 days for observation in 21 days for removal of the cast and skin sutures. In the interim, antibiotics should be administered locally in the wound and given systemically for 2–3 days (p 364).

2. MALLET FINGER

Diagnosis

Mallet finger is caused by laceration or avulsion of the extensor tendon at its insertion into the distal phalanx. A fracture, if present, requires an x-ray for diagnosis. Unopposed flexor tendon function causes flexion at the DIP joint and produces "mallet" deformity. A secondary swan-neck deformity may develop (Fig 23–12).

Treatment

A. Open Mallet Injuries: Open injuries are treated by tenorrhaphy and intramedullary fixation of the DIP joint by a hand surgeon. Give prophylactic antibiotics (p 364).

B. Closed Mallet Injuries: Closed injuries may be treated by continuous dorsal external padded splint fixation of the DIP joint in full extension for 6–8 weeks. During splint changes, the joint should be

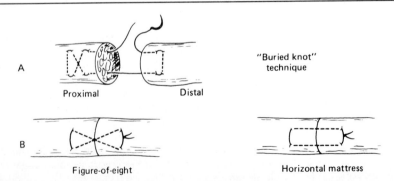

A

Proximal   Distal

"Buried knot" technique

B

Figure-of-eight

Horizontal mattress

Figure 23–11. Methods of tenorrhaphy. **A:** For large-caliber tendons. **B:** These suture techniques are best for thin tendons with limited separation of stumps (eg, digital extensors). (Reproduced, with permission, from Schrok TR [editor]: *Handbook of Surgery,* 7th ed. Jones Medical Publications, 1982.)

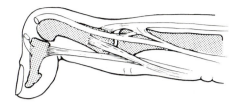

Figure 23–12. Mallet finger with swan-neck deformity. Rupture, laceration, or avulsion of the insertion of the extensor mechanism results in mallet finger. (Reproduced, with permission, from Way LW [editor]: *Current Surgical Diagnosis & Treatment,* 9th ed. Appleton & Lange, 1991.)

held up in extension. The digit should be kept dry to prevent maceration of the skin.

Disposition

The patient should return every 7–14 days to the clinic or office for check on progress and new splints.

3. BOUTONNIÈRE DEFORMITY

Diagnosis

In boutonnière (buttonhole) deformity, the distal joint is hyperextended and the PIP joint of the finger (the MP joint of the thumb) is flexed (Fig 23–13). Extensor hood integrity is lost at the apex of the PIP joint of the finger (MP joint of the thumb) as a result of laceration or blunt trauma to the dorsum of the joint. The deformity is rarely manifest immediately after trauma and comes on insidiously as a result of gradual stretching of the injured hood. The underlying head of the bone protrudes through the hood, pushing aside the MET (extensor pollicis brevis of the thumb), which recedes, and the LETs, which slip volarly to become flexors of the joint and hyperextensors of the distal joint.

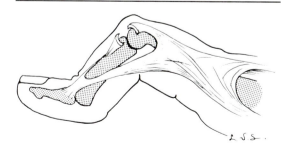

Figure 23–13. Boutonnière deformity. Avulsion or laceration of the central extensor mechanism results in a flexion deformity at the PIP joint and hyperextension at the DIP joint—the boutonnière, or buttonhole, deformity. (Reproduced, with permission, from Way LW [editor]: *Current Surgical Diagnosis & Treatment,* 9th ed. Appleton & Lange, 1991.)

Treatment

A. Open Injuries: Open injuries should be repaired (by a hand surgeon) as soon as possible with figure-of-eight nylon sutures and the joint splinted in full extension for 4 weeks with a palmar digital splint.

B. Closed Injuries: Closed injuries must be suspected if there is a history of a direct blow to the dorsum of the joint followed by swelling. Treatment consists of 4 weeks of PIP (thumb MP) splinting in extension to avoid boutonnière deformity, which rarely occurs if prompt treatment is provided.

Secondary reconstruction of this deformity is very difficult and may never restore full motion of the IP joints.

Disposition

Open injuries should be irrigated and covered and the patient sent to a hand surgeon at once. Patients with closed injuries should return in 7–10 days to the clinic or office for check of progress.

BONE & JOINT INJURIES

Bone and joint injuries are discussed in more detail in Chapter 22, but a few general principles are emphasized here.

Diagnosis

If there is any question of bone or joint injury on x-ray, obtaining added views in other planes and identical views of the opposite extremity or a follow-up view in 7–10 days may resolve the issue.

Treatment

A. Splinting: *The wrist joint is the principal joint governing movement and comfort of an immobilized fracture.* Therefore, it should be splinted initially. In addition, to splint one finger well, an adjacent finger should be splinted with it. The thumb may be immobilized alone. The preferred position should be that of wrist extension, functional finger flexion, and opposition of the thumb. If there is throbbing pain at any time, it must be relieved promptly (eg, split and spread the cast and dressing).

B. Stable Injuries: Stable dislocations or fractures can usually be treated in the emergency department by reduction and splinting, with appropriate anesthesia. *Force should never be used.* In lieu of force, open reduction is preferred.

C. Open or Unstable Injuries: Open or unstable injuries require a specialist's skill. The patient should be given a temporary splint and dressing and referred to a hand surgeon immediately. Give prophylactic antibiotics (p 364).

Disposition

Patients with closed, stable injuries should return in 24–72 hours for assessment of comfort and integrity of the cast. Patients with open joint injuries, unstable injuries, or injuries that cannot be reduced easily must be referred early to a specialist experienced in hand surgery.

INFECTIONS

Infections of the hand are frequently encountered in emergency departments. Nearly all infections result from neglect following trauma and are fostered by venous congestion and tissue edema.

Careful handling of tissue, elimination of dead space, immobilization and elevation of the arm immediately after injury, and avoidance of constriction by snug clothing or jewelry are far more important in preventing infection than any type of wound preparation or antibiotic prophylaxis. The objective of treatment of all infections is to reverse congestion and restore normal circulation. If there is a possibility of serious infection, immobilize the hand in a boxing glove cast. Applying zinc oxide ointment next to the skin in the inner (core) dressing promotes drainage by preventing drying, caking, and sealing off of the wound.

All existing or potential infections should be monitored closely—eg, hourly or daily depending on the severity.

Infections that may be treated in the emergency department include those of the nail folds, felons, simple abscesses, and cellulitis. Patients with other infections should be immediately referred.

1. PARONYCHIA & EPONYCHIA

Diagnosis

Inflammation leading to a collection of pus inside the nail fold is seen after trauma and often as a consequence of stress (Fig 23–14A). If neglected, it may extend around the entire nail margin and cause a floating nail. The usual cause is *Staphylococcus aureus*. Cultures are rarely necessary.

Treatment

Treatment consists of simple elevation of the nail fold with a No. 11 scalpel at the site of maximum tenderness or pus (Fig 23–14B). Generally, there is no pain if an abscess is already pointing and no blood is drawn with the scalpel. If the scalpel causes any pain, a digital block anesthetic should be administered. Use zinc oxide ointment under the dressing.

Antimicrobial agents are not indicated unless extensive cellulitis or lymphangitis is present.

Disposition

As with any hand infection, the patient should elevate the part and return in 2–3 days.

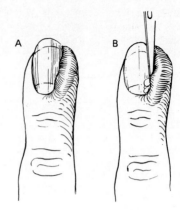

Figure 23–14. Incision and drainage of paronychia (Reproduced, with permission, from Way LW [editor]: *Current Surgical Diagnosis & Treatment,* 9th ed. Appleton & Lange, 1991.)

2. FELON

Diagnosis

A felon is an abscess of the distal fat pad of the digit. *S aureus* is the usual pathogen.

Treatment

After digital block anesthesia has been achieved, a felon should be drained where it points—usually in the mid pad—by a central longitudinal incision, care being taken not to cross the flexion crease of the distal joint (Fig 23–15). Classic teaching to the contrary, fishmouth and lateral incisions may do much harm to blood vessels and nerves and often do not adequately

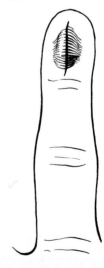

Figure 23–15. Incision of felon. (Reproduced, with permission, from Way LW [editor]: *Current Surgical Diagnosis & Treatment,* 9th ed. Appleton & Lange, 1991.)

treat the problem. Septa (fascial strands) do *not* have to be divided. Use zinc oxide under the dressing.

Antimicrobial agents and cultures are not indicated unless cellulitis or lymphangitis is present or there is involvement of flexor sheath or bone.

Disposition

The wound should be checked in 1–3 days to be certain pain is less and drainage is adequate.

3. SIMPLE ABSCESSES

Diagnosis & Treatment

Simple abscesses should be adequately incised and drained. Zinc oxide ointment should be used under the dressing. If involvement is extensive, keep the part elevated. Antimicrobial agents and cultures are not indicated unless cellulitis or lymphangitis is present.

Disposition

The patient should be checked in 1–2 days.

4. CELLULITIS
(Including Human & Animal Bites)

Diagnosis

Cellulitis may be an extremely severe infection; in the preantibiotic era, some cases were fatal. An ill patient with cellulitis and fever and leukocytosis should be hospitalized for parenteral antibiotic therapy and evaluated by a hand specialist for the need for incision to release tension and for drainage.

Treatment

Cellulitis is treated with appropriate splinting, elevation, and antibiotics.

A. Uncomplicated Cellulitis: Most cases of cellulitis are caused by group A streptococci. Penicillin V, 0.5 g orally 4 times daily for 5–7 days, is the drug of choice. Erythromycin, 0.5 g orally 4 times daily, may be used in the patient allergic to penicillin.

B. Following Animal Bites: Cellulitis caused by animal bites (especially by a cat) may be caused by *Pasteurella multocida.* Penicillin, 0.5 g orally 4 times daily for 5–7 days, is the drug of choice. Tetracycline, 0.5 g 4 times daily orally, should be substituted for penicillin in patients allergic to penicillin. Animal bites that penetrate a joint or tendon sheath or deep space require urgent prophylactic treatment (preferably by a hand surgeon). Immobilization of the whole hand and wrist in a boxing glove cast and support of the arm in a sling are essential early in treatment.

C. Following Abscess Formation: If the cellulitis begins as an abscess, examination of a Gram-stained smear of pus and culture of pus will aid in selection of antibiotics. *S aureus* is the usual patho-

gen, and either an oral penicillinase-resistant penicillin (eg, dicloxacillin, 0.5 g 4 times daily) or erythromycin (0.5 g orally 4 times daily) is suitable for therapy. Oral cephalosporins (cephalexin, etc) and clindamycin are rarely indicated.

D. Following Human Bites; Atypical Cellulitis: Cellulitis resulting from human bites (mixed anaerobes) or perhaps due to unusual pathogens (eg, *Haemophilus influenzae, Aeromonas hydrophila, Eikenella corrodens*)—or of unusual severity—should be treated in the hospital. Blood cultures should be obtained and the advancing edge of the cellulitis aspirated with a 25-gauge needle attached to a 3- to 5-mL syringe. The aspirate should be stained with Gram's stain and cultured for both aerobic and anaerobic organisms. While awaiting results of culture, give clindamycin, 30–40 mg/kg/d intravenously in 3 divided doses; plus gentamicin or tobramycin, 5 mg/kg/d intramuscularly or intravenously in 3 divided doses. A cephalosporin (eg, cefamandole, 100 mg/kg/d intravenously in 4 divided doses) may be substituted for the gentamicin or tobramycin.

Cellulitis due to human bites requires special care, particularly when a tooth has penetrated an MP or IP joint, a joint crease, or a tendon bursa. Hospitalization for administration of parenteral antibiotics is mandatory, and surgical drainage is often necessary. Consultation with a hand specialist should be obtained immediately.

Disposition

Hospitalization under the care of a hand specialist is required for severe cases (extensive cellulitis, involvement of tendons or joints, infections of the palmar space, systemic symptoms, or unusual pathogens) or if the patient is unreliable or unable to take oral antibiotics. Patients with cellulitis managed as outpatients should be seen every day and hospitalized if the process continues.

5. SUPPURATIVE TENOSYNOVITIS

Diagnosis

Suppurative tenosynovitis (nongonococcal) is characterized by swelling, erythema, and tenderness along the tendon sheath and, most importantly, exquisite pain on passive movement of the flexor tendon in the digit or the extensor tendon crossing the wrist. In flexor tenosynovitis, passive movement is definitely achieved by holding the fingernail alone and prying it dorsally to extend the distal joint. The infection may have occurred because of an open wound contiguous to the involved tendon.

Treatment & Disposition

In selected reliable patients with a confirmed diagnosis, outpatient therapy with close follow-up may be possible. Whenever there is inflammation with significant swelling, immediate hospitalization under the care of a hand specialist is required for open surgical drainage and parenteral antibiotic therapy. After obtaining appropriate specimens for culture, begin a cephalosporin (eg, cefazolin, 100 mg/kg/d in 3 divided doses) intravenously without waiting for the results of cultures. Immobilize the wrist and hand in a boxing glove cast, and support the arm in a sling until operation can be performed.

6. DISSEMINATED (HEMATOGENOUS) GONOCOCCAL INFECTION

The diagnosis and treatment of gonococcal infection are discussed in Chapter 34. In young adults, tenosynovitis is often caused by gonococcal infection. The tenosynovitis is not associated with an open wound near the involved tendon sheath but is frequently associated with pustular skin lesions typical of gonococcal infection. Hospitalization for intravenous antibiotic therapy is usually indicated. In selected reliable patients whose diagnosis is confirmed, outpatient therapy with close follow-up may be possible. See Chapter 34 for recommended treatment.

NONINFECTIOUS TENOSYNOVITIS OR MYOSITIS

Diagnosis
In noninfectious tenosynovitis or myositis, there is usually a history of sustained vigorous, repetitive effort to which the extremity is unaccustomed, eg, clipping shrubbery with a hand clipper. Pain and tenderness develop and may be accompanied by crepitation (tendinitis or myositis crepitans). The most common tendons affected are the extensors under the extensor retinaculum. The muscle involved is invariably the abductor pollicis longus.

Treatment
Treatment consists of immediate splinting and administration of anti-inflammatory agents (eg, aspirin). Reevaluate the patient in 24–48 hours. Glucocorticoids should not be injected if an infectious process is suspected.

Disposition
The patient should return or telephone in 1–3 days.

MINOR CONSTRICTIVE PROBLEMS

Diagnosis
The following 3 common constrictive problems are often seen in the emergency department. Only the first is usually a true emergency.

A. Carpal Tunnel Syndrome (Compression of the Median Nerve): Characterized by aching and numbness over the distribution of the median nerve (Fig 23–7), with sparing of the small finger. These symptoms often awaken the patient from sleep and may be elicited by full flexion of the wrist for 30 seconds (Phalen's maneuver). Tapping over the median nerve at the wrist crease may feel like an electric shock (Tinel's sign). This nerve compression may present as an emergency, with rapid onset of acute edema and progressive loss of feeling after trauma, inflammation, or allergy, and it requires urgent consultation with a hand specialist.

B. Stenosing Flexor Tenosynovitis (Trigger Thumb or Trigger Finger): Characterized by local tenderness over the proximal tendon pulley at the MP joint, with pain referred to the PIP joint and a snapping when the finger or thumb goes through an active range of motion.

C. De Quervain's Tenosynovitis of Tendons in the First Dorsal Compartment on the Radial Side of the Wrist: Characterized by pain and tenderness when these tendons are actively or passively stretched; specifically, when the fist is clenched over the thumb while the wrist is put into marked ulnar deviation (Finkelstein test).

Treatment
A. Corticosteroid-Lidocaine: Injection of a long-acting glucocorticoid (eg, triamcinolone) and 1% lidocaine into the synovial bursa at the site of involvement gives good temporary relief. In all 3 types of problems, the injection should be performed with a 25- or 27-gauge, 1.5-cm (½-in) needle, using amounts of solution appropriate to the given area. *Note:* The patient should be warned about immediate transient anesthesia and also about possible secondary skin depigmentation and fat atrophy at the injection site. To reduce the likelihood of these effects, dexamethasone may be substituted for triamcinolone.

1. Carpal tunnel syndrome–1 mL of glucocorticoid and 2–3 mL of lidocaine. *Never* inject into the substance of the median or ulnar nerves.

2. Flexor tenosynovitis–About 0.5 mL each of glucocorticoid and lidocaine. Inject into the synovial bursa through the tender flexor pulley at the base of the digit.

3. De Quervain's disease–About 0.5 mL each of glucocorticoid and lidocaine at the radial styloid process but avoiding the radial nerve.

B. Splinting: Injection therapy is occasionally augmented by splinting, particularly in the case of carpal tunnel syndrome. A light cock-up wrist splint worn during the hours of sleep may benefit those whose sleep is broken by their symptoms.

Disposition
The patient should return in 3–7 days for a check-

up, or sooner if needed. If the injection and splinting fail to provide relief, surgical release of the tight ligament or sheath may be required.

THERMAL INJURIES
(See also Chapter 37.)

1. FIRST-DEGREE BURNS

Diagnosis & Treatment
Simple burns (redness without blistering) are treated with cold tap water rinse and analgesia. Comfort may be augmented by a soft nonirritative wrap to protect and immobilize the part. Elevation and avoidance of constriction by snug garments are also advised.

Disposition
The patient should return or telephone after 1–2 days.

2. SECOND-DEGREE BURNS

Diagnosis & Treatment
Blisters signify partial-thickness (second-degree) burns, which always retain cutaneous sensation even though they are variable in depth. The blisters act as a good dressing and, unless bulky and friable, should be left intact until the serum is resorbed or they rupture spontaneously. Second-degree burns may be dressed with a bulky dressing and the hand splinted in the position of function. If blisters break, the remnant tissue should be debrided. On areas of second-degree burns not covered by intact blisters, silver sulfadiazine (Silvadene) may be added topically. Tetanus prophylaxis must be current (Chapter 24). In the case of burns caused by hot tar, the tar may be removed as described in Chapter 37.

Disposition
Patients with extensive burns or marked edema should be immediately referred to a hand specialist for evaluation and possible hospitalization. Patients with lesser involvement should be seen every 1–3 days for a dressing change, especially once blister debridement is started.

3. THIRD-DEGREE BURNS

Diagnosis & Treatment
Full-thickness (third-degree) burns require bulky loose sterile dressings with an anti-infective agent such as silver sulfadiazine. Appropriate elevation and splinting are also advised. Tetanus prophylaxis must be current (Chapter 24).

Disposition
If the burn is extensive (eg, > 1–2 cm^2 [$\frac{3}{8}$–$\frac{3}{4}$ in^2]) or is over the dorsum of a joint, refer the patient immediately to a hand specialist for decisions about the need for debridement and grafting.

4. ELECTRICAL BURNS
(See also Chapter 38.)

Burns from electricity are of 2 kinds: crossed circuit, producing arc heat; and conduction of high-voltage current within the tissues. Arc heat is often more frightening than extensively injurious to tissues. There is generally blackening of the skin owing to deposit of carbon. The burn may be anywhere from first-degree to third-degree in severity but is usually localized. The treatment of arc heat burns is the same as that of other thermal burns.

High-voltage conduction burns involve a point of entry and another point of exit. The deep tissues are often coagulated out of proportion to surface skin changes. Blood vessels and nerves are the pathways of conduction and therefore most vulnerable. Immediate irreversible ischemia and paralysis are common. Such cases require hospitalization under the care of a hand specialist for urgent fasciotomy where prophylactically indicated and for observation for systemic effects of shock. Appropriate debridement (even amputation), grafting, and reconstruction will follow. Extremity destruction is sometimes overwhelming.

If the electrical conduction pathway within the body is not limited to the hand but also involves other areas, consideration should be given to possible myocardial injury. An ECG and CK-MB measurement should be obtained. Cardiac monitoring is necessary if myocardial injury is suspected.

5. FROSTBITE
(See also Chapter 38.)

Exposure to cold may result in superficial or deep frostbite depending on the windchill factor and duration of exposure. Measures to prevent this vasoconstrictive disorder and the irreversible microvascular thrombotic events that lead to gangrene include the following: (**1**) avoiding exposure to wind, cold metal, snow, and ice by wearing protective gloves; (**2**) preserving total body heat by wearing suitable clothing and head gear and avoiding sweat-producing physical effort or alcohol consumption; (**3**) ensuring adequate caloric intake, high in fat and carbohydrate; and (**4**) refraining from smoking.

Superficial frostbite is limited to the skin. It exists when the discomfort of fingers exposed to cold is replaced by numbness. Reversal by warming is urgently required and is usually heralded by a warm tingling sensation.

Deep frostbite is signaled by pain and swelling of the entire hand, followed by extensive blister formation and dysesthesia. Deep frostbite requires hospitalization under the care of a hand specialist. Cryofibrinogenemia aggravates the problem and is worsened by the use of heparin, which facilitates precipitation of cryofibrinogen. Treatment consists of rest and warming the patient and the hands. Immersion in water at 37–40 °C (98.6–104 °F) for a short time (eg, 20 minutes) may be beneficial. Blisters must be debrided and dressed with sterile dressings. Sympathetic blockade should be considered.

FOREIGN BODIES

Fishhooks, splinters, and other objects may have barbs or barblike projections that prevent withdrawal from the wound in the normal retrograde way. Removal is possible by pushing the foreign body along the direction of entry and removing it via a counterincision where it presents under the tented skin. Nerve block or other anesthesia and tourniquet ischemia are necessary before extraction is attempted. Prophylactic antibiotics are often necessary.

Foreign bodies embedded in the hand may be difficult to locate and remove. The diagnosis is based on the history and examination, and x-rays are almost always useful in the case of glass or metal. If immediate accessibility and easy removal seem possible, an attempt can be made to remove the foreign body using regional anesthesia, a tourniquet, and sterile technique with loupe magnification. Typically, however, the discoloration of tissues by blood precludes the immediate search for a foreign body, which will be found much more easily after 3–4 weeks when phagocytosis has cleared the blood. Before starting the procedure, tell the patient that if search and removal prove at all difficult (eg, longer than 10–15 minutes), the procedure will be abandoned and referral made to a hand specialist.

Consider leaving an entry wound open by inserting a loose drain, dressing with zinc oxide ointment or wet gauze, and elevating and immobilizing the part. Give prophylactic local or systemic antibiotics and tetanus prophylaxis (Chapter 24). The patient can usually be assured that retrieval of small deep foreign bodies is not urgent, since they do not travel in the body, and that it is often contraindicated by the difficulty and risk of removal.

COMPLEX HAND INJURIES

Classification

Complex injuries include the following: amputations, serious tendon injuries, nerve injuries, high-

pressure injection injuries, closed compartment syndromes, mangling injuries, gunshot wounds, and wringer injuries.

Evaluation & Initial Management

In complex injuries, emphasis should be placed on early, rapid diagnosis and institution of supportive therapy. Many complex injuries require referral to a hand specialist immediately or early. In all cases, use conservative measures as outlined below.

A. Avoid Manipulation: Once the decision has been made to transfer or hospitalize, the part should not be handled, probed, manipulated, or otherwise disturbed unless absolutely necessary. Foreign material that can be easily lifted out should be removed. Protect with a sterile dressing and, if necessary, a loosely applied splint pending definitive management.

B. Prepare for Possible Urgent Surgery: If there is a reasonable likelihood of surgery within 8–10 hours, give nothing by mouth. An intravenous infusion should be started in the uninjured limb and laboratory work ordered.

C. Give Antibiotics: In the case of open or penetrating wounds, antibiotics should be given parenterally (preferably intravenously in the uninjured extremity) as soon as possible; the earlier they are started, the more effective they are. Give nafcillin, oxacillin, or cephalothin, 100–200 mg/kg/d intravenously in 4–6 divided doses; or cefazolin, 50–100 mg/kg/d intravenously or intramuscularly in 2–3 divided doses.

1. AMPUTATIONS

Amputations account for about 1% of hand injuries.

Diagnosis & Evaluation

The diagnosis of amputation is obvious on inspection of the part. Amputations are generally classified as partial (incompletely severed part) or complete.

Generally, tidy amputations at the level of the middle phalanx or the wrist or distal forearm have the best chance of functionally successful replantation. In the case of single-digit amputation, surgeons are much more inclined to favor replantation of a thumb than of a single finger. Discussions with the patient or relatives regarding the feasibility of replantation should be left to the hand surgeon.

Treatment & Disposition
A. Replantation Possible:
1. Place the amputated member in gauze moistened with saline and then place it in a sealed plastic bag or container that is maintained at 4 °C (eg, on wet ice). *Do not freeze the amputated part,* since this destroys its viability.

2. After starting appropriate supportive measures, transport the patient and the amputated part as rapidly as possible to the nearest microvascular facility. Be sure to telephone ahead before transfer so that the hand surgeon and operating room will be ready upon arrival of the patient.

B. Replantation Impossible: If the amputated member either is not recovered or is clearly not salvageable, appropriate in-house or emergency department surgery should be undertaken to close the stump. Except for the simple fingertip pad amputation discussed above, these injuries should almost always be referred to a hand specialist.

2. FLEXOR & PROXIMAL EXTENSOR TENDON INJURIES

Almost all flexor tendon injuries and those extensor injuries in which the proximal tendon has retracted out of reach are considered complex injuries. Management of easily accessible extensor tendon injuries is discussed on p 366.

Diagnosis
A crucial step in the emergency management of any flexor or proximal extensor tendon injury is to *suspect* that it may exist and make the proper diagnosis. Impairment of a partially divided tendon (sometimes subtotally or even totally divided) may be functionally masked at the outset, only to become evident hours, days, or weeks later.

In open injuries, tendon lacerations can often be diagnosed by the abnormal stance of the involved part of the hand and almost always by careful functional examination. If the diagnosis is not obvious but the location of the wound raises the possibility of tendon injury, direct examination of the wound is indicated. Visualization of flexors can be difficult anywhere, whereas visualization of extensors is difficult mainly when they lie proximal to the metacarpal necks.

Occasionally, the emergency physician will see a closed profundus tendon rupture. Such an injury almost always follows sudden violent stretch of the flexor, after which the patient is unable to flex the distal phalanx.

Treatment
Obtain immediate consultation with a hand specialist. Dress the wound after irrigation, and splint the wrist and hand. Remove jewelry and snug garments, and elevate the extremity until definitive treatment can be given. Flexor tendon repair may be delayed as long as 10 days without compromising the eventual outcome. If tendon repair is to be delayed, the wound should be sutured and appropriate antibiotics administered (eg, cephalothin, 1–2 g intravenously, followed by cephalexin, 500 mg orally 4 times daily for 3–5 days).

Disposition
Visualization of a lacerated tendon sheath is reason for referral unless the entire course of the tendon gliding beneath the laceration is observed to be intact. If in doubt, refer immediately, because neglected partial tendon lacerations can go on to rupture.

3. NERVE INJURIES

Diagnosis
Early diagnosis is crucial. The cause and nature of injury, the symptoms, or the location and depth of a laceration may suggest possible nerve injury. If careful motor, sweat, and sensory examination is performed and sometimes repeated more than once for the sake of consistency in appropriate cases (Figs 23–16 and 23–17), few significant nerve injuries will be missed.

Treatment
Appropriate dressing and splinting should be applied when indicated and the patient warned about injury to anesthetized skin until definitive treatment can be given.

Disposition
Refer the patient to a hand surgeon, and determine when the patient is to be transferred for definitive care.

4. HIGH-PRESSURE INJECTION INJURIES

Diagnosis
High-pressure jets of a variety of hot and cold fluids (grease, water, plastics, organic solvents) and gases are widely used in industry. Accidental penetration of the skin through a pinpoint portal of entry may result in devastating damage, even though the initial (postinjection) appearance of the hand or other body part is usually deceptively normal. This is because the foreign material spreads instantly along tissue planes and is widely distributed in the hand or other part. Spread of material up a flexor tendon sheath after penetration of a digital pad is quite common. An x-ray should be obtained, because some injected materials are radiopaque (eg, lead-based paint). When a chemical, inflammatory, or thermal response becomes manifest 4–12 hours after injury, extensive ischemia and tissue necrosis may be seen. The history is the most important clue to the severity of injury.

Treatment & Disposition
A. Give analgesics for pain if necessary, and splint the extremity in a sling for comfort.

B. Obtain x-rays.

C. Give nothing by mouth, and consult a hand

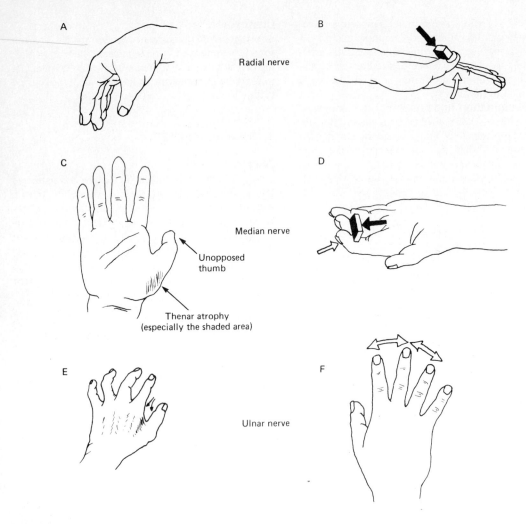

Figure 23–16. Assessing nerve injury. **A:** Wrist drop in radial injury. **B:** Forceful extension of thumb tip is lost in radial nerve injury. **C:** "Ape hand" deformity in median nerve injury. **D:** Forceful flexion of tip of index finger is lost in high median nerve injury. **E** and **F:** Thumb web atrophy and clawing of ring and small fingers, and loss of abduction and adduction in ulnar nerve injury. (Reproduced, with permission, from Schrock TR [editor]: *Handbook of Surgery,* 7th ed. Jones Medical Publications, 1982.)

surgeon immediately regarding referral. Prompt tetanus prophylaxis, systemic antibiotics, and decompressive surgery (eg, fasciotomy) must be arranged in most cases. Even so, the prognosis for maintaining circulation and salvaging function is often dismal.

5. CLOSED COMPARTMENT SYNDROMES

A compartment syndrome (eg, congestion progressing to various degrees of ischemia) can occur in any space of the digit, hand, forearm, or arm. It may involve a single space (eg, the distal pulp space of the digit) or multiple spaces (eg, extensor and flexor compartments of the forearm and intrinsic muscle compartments of the hand). Obstructed venous flow

leads to microvascular stagnation and death of muscle, fat, and nerves. Compartment syndrome may result from external compression (eg, a tight cast, prolonged pressure against an extremity of a comatose patient) or from internal swelling (eg, from severe bleeding, crush injury, burn, fracture, allergy, or infectious or noninfectious inflammatory reaction). The fate of a neglected case in which surgical decompression has not been performed is late fibrosis and severe functional impairment.

Diagnosis

The typical patient presents with a history of progressive severe pain (eg, throbbing) and a rock-hard compartment. When the whole forearm and hand are involved, there is hypoesthesia, reluctance or inabil-

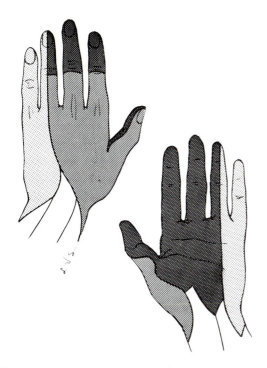

Figure 23–17. Sensory distribution in the hand. Dotted area, ulnar nerve; diagonal area, radial nerve; darker area, median nerve. (Reproduced, with permission, from Way LW [editor]: *Current Surgical Diagnosis & Treatment,* 9th ed. Appleton & Lange, 1991.)

ity to move the digits, and pain on passive extension of flexed digits. Pain perception may be lost as pressure on the nerves destroys their conducting ability.

Treatment

Treatment is supportive until definitive surgical decompression can be performed. Support the part in a sling, and give analgesics for pain.

Disposition

Urgent hospitalization for surgical decompression under the care of a hand specialist is indicated.

6. MANGLING INJURIES

Diagnosis

Mangling injuries include gunshot and blast wounds, severe open crush wounds, severe bites by large animals, and a large variety of ripping or tearing injuries. The common denominator is multitissue involvement, distortion, and general untidiness.

Treatment

Rapid initiation of supportive measures, loose

bulky sterile dressings and splinting, immediate administration of antibiotics (eg, cefazolin, 50–100 mg/kg/d intravenously or intramuscularly in 2–3 divided doses), and definitive surgical treatment are important to a successful outcome.

Disposition

All such injuries require immediate hospitalization and referral to a hand specialist for operative debridement and repair.

7. WRINGER INJURIES

Diagnosis

The extremity is caught and drawn between rollers, which may destroy circulation both by compression as well as speed of rotation. Such injuries may also avulse skin and other tissues, fracture or dislocate bones and joints, or cause major friction burns.

Treatment

Treatment is the same as for mangling injuries.

Disposition

Contact a hand specialist immediately, and arrange for referral.

**SPECIAL EMERGENCY
DEPARTMENT PROBLEMS**

1. REMOVAL OF RINGS

All rings, bracelets, wristwatches, and snug shirt-sleeves and coat-sleeves should be prophylactically removed whenever injury, surgery, infection, or other cause of acute swelling of any part of the hand exists. Failure to do so may lead to serious congestion and unnecessary complications.

A ring on a swollen finger can be removed in one of 3 ways:

A. Lubricate the skin with soap, and carefully slip the ring off.

B. Wrap the digit snugly with string from the distal tip to just below the ring, and in that way "milk" edema out of the digit so the ring can be removed over the string.

C. Cut the ring with a commercial ring cutter, spread it with 2 pairs of pliers, and remove it. This is the preferred method when there is significant digital injury or swelling distal to the ring.

2. SNAKEBITE

See Chapter 38 for treatment.

REFERENCES

American Society for Surgery of the Hand: *The Hand: Examination and Diagnosis,* 3rd ed. Churchill Livingstone, 1990.

American Society for Surgery of the Hand: *The Hand: Primary Care of Common Problems,* 2nd ed. Churchill Livingstone, 1990.

Beasley RW: *Hand Injuries.* Saunders, 1981.

Conolly WB, Kilgore ES: *Hand Injuries and Infections.* Year Book, 1979.

Flatt AE: *Minor Hand Injuries.* Mosby, 1963.

Hodgkins ML, Grady D: Carpal tunnel syndrome. West J Med 1988;148:217.

Kilgore ES, Graham WP III (editors): *The Hand: Surgical and Nonsurgical Management.* Lea & Febiger, 1977.

Kilgore ES, Newmeyer WL: Hand. Chapter 15 in: *Handbook of Surgery,* 7th ed. Schrock TR (editor). Jones Medical Publications, 1982.

Kilgore ES, Newmeyer WL: Hand emergencies. Chapter 57 in: *Quick Reference to Pediatric Emergencies,* 2nd ed. Pascoe DJ, Grossman M (editors). Lippincott, 1978.

Lampe EW: *Surgical Anatomy of the Hand.* CIBA Symposium 1969;21:No.3.

Lister G: *The Hand: Diagnosis and Indications.* Churchill Livingstone, 1977.

Lucas GL: Assessing the acutely injured hand. Resident Staff Physician (Aug) 1982;28:82.

Mann RJ: *Infections of the Hand.* Lea & Febiger, 1988.

Newmeyer WL: *Primary Care of Hand Injuries.* Lea & Febiger, 1979.

Rank BK, Wakefield AR, Hueston JT: *Surgery of Repair as Applied to Hand Injuries.* Williams & Wilkins, 1973.

Semple C: *The Primary Management of Hand Injuries.* Year Book, 1979.

Wound Care*

24

Robert L. Walton, MD, & W. Earle Matory, Jr., MD, FACS

EMERGENCY MANAGEMENT OF LIFE-THREATENING PROBLEMS

All patients with open wounds should be examined thoroughly for evidence of serious or life-threatening injuries that may not be obvious on initial presentation. Life-threatening conditions must be treated immediately. CPR must be instituted at once (Chapter 1). Adequate ventilatory status must be ensured and shock (Chapter 3) and hemorrhage treated prior to wound assessment. The possibility of internal bleeding must be kept in mind.

When facial and scalp injuries are present, look closely for evidence of intracranial or cervical spine injury. If cervical spine injury is suspected, immobilize the neck before performing radiologic evalua-

*With contributions by Steven H. Turkeltaub, MD, Scottsdale, Arizona.

tion. Serial neurologic examinations are crucial to the evaluation of any head injury.

HEMOSTASIS

Prior to wound closure, absolute hemostasis must be established to prevent hematoma formation and further blood volume depletion. This is accomplished by direct and indirect methods. It is preferable to employ indirect methods first in order to carefully assess the wound, avoid possible injury to important structures, and allow time for replacement of significant blood loss.

Indirect Hemostasis

Indirect methods of achieving hemostasis in the acute wound include elevation, pressure, application of vasoconstrictive agents, and chemical promoters of clotting. These methods are usually effective in the control of diffuse vascular oozing and lymph extravasation.

A. Elevation: Elevation of the injured part "above the level of the heart" is least damaging to the tissues and markedly diminishes capillary oozing. Caution is required in elderly patients with arteriosclerotic vascular disease, since elevation of the lower extremity may induce tissue hypoxia.

B. Pressure: Pressure can be utilized in various ways to effect hemostasis. Direct pressure over a vigorously bleeding wound is perhaps the most commonly utilized method for rapid control of blood loss. In extremity wounds, a proximally placed blood pressure cuff is frequently employed to control bleeding of distal wounds. In either case, take care to avoid the potential sequelae arising from excessive pressure.

Simple cutaneous lacerations are usually manifested by a diffuse capillary ooze that can be an annoying interference with inspection and repair. A simple pressure dressing applied to the wound for 20 minutes will usually control oozing. Ideally, pressure should not exceed capillary pressure (30 mm Hg) and should not impede vascular flow to distal parts. For proximal extremity wounds, pressure should be applied in graded fashion from the distal aspect of the extremity to the wound to avoid the "tourniquet" effect of the dressing. The graded pressure is accomplished with bulky dressings and elastic bandages. The capillary flow and sensibility of distal parts should be frequently assessed to avoid ischemic injury.

The use of tourniquets in extremity wounds should be reserved for isolated digital injuries or for complex injuries associated with excessive blood loss or requiring specialized examination. The tourniquet is placed proximal to the wound (usually the upper arm) and is inflated to 20–30 mm Hg above systolic pressure. Ischemia resulting from this maneuver can be tolerated by most patients for 15–20 minutes. How-

ever, the ischemia produces a reactive vasodilatation upon release of the tourniquet and may result in resumption of bloody oozing or hematoma formation.

C. Vasoconstriction: Epinephrine-containing solutions are frequently employed in acute wounds to control capillary oozing. Concentrations of 1:400,000–1:100,000 units are used for these purposes. After infiltration, a full 7 minutes is required for maximal vasoconstrictive effect. *Caution:* Epinephrine decreases local wound defense mechanisms and should not be used in contaminated wounds because of the increased risk of infection. Although it will not affect the viability of acute random cutaneous flaps, epinephrine can induce vasospasm that may lead to necrosis of tissues supplied by an "end-arterial circulation." For this reason, epinephrine is contraindicated in the management of wounds of the penis, of any digit, of the tip of the nose, or in any tissue with circulation compromised by the trauma.

D. Chemical Hemostatic Agents: Hemostatic agents such as Avitene, Gelfoam, or Surgicel should be avoided in the emergency department setting, since they have been shown to potentiate infections in contaminated wounds.

Topical bovine thrombin can cause an allergic or anaphylactic reaction, intravascular coagulation, or death.

Direct Hemostasis

Direct methods of hemostasis include ligation and electrocauterization of the cut vessel ends. Direct hemostasis should be employed for bleeding that cannot be controlled by indirect methods. An exception to this rule is injury to major vascular tributaries (ulnar, femoral, brachial artery, etc). Further injury to the cut vessel end resulting from attempts at direct hemostasis may preclude successful repair. In these situations, it is wise to apply firm pressure to the wound and consult a vascular surgeon.

A. Ligation: Simple tying or suture ligation is indicated for most vessels more than 2 mm ($\frac{1}{16}$ in) in external diameter. To avoid excessive tissue trauma, one must precisely identify and clamp the vessel end prior to ligation. Cut arteries usually require only simple tying. Veins, however, do not hold ligatures well, and suture ligation is preferable. Suture ligation may be performed by passing the suture needle through a portion of the vessel wall and then circumferentially tying the vessel. This method prevents slippage of the ligature. *Caution: Arteries and veins should not be ligated en masse, since this may predispose to arteriovenous fistula formation.* Absorbable sutures are preferred for tying and suture ligation in the acute wound. Synthetic absorbable sutures (polyglycolic acid [Dexon] and polyglactin [Vicryl]) are advantageous because of their low reactivity and high friction coefficients. Chromic catgut is also satisfactory.

B. Electrocautery: Damped electric current is

effective in coagulating small vessel ends. Monopolar cautery causes approximately 3 times as much tissue necrosis as bipolar coagulation. Pinpoint coagulation is preferred, with delivery of the least amount of current needed for vessel thrombosis. *Caution:* Some surgeons use undamped electric current for cutting tissues during debridement of the acute wound. Although quite effective in diminishing blood loss, cutting current inflicts significant thermal injury to the surrounding tissues and increases their susceptibility to infection. It is therefore not recommended for wound debridement or hemostasis.

C. Chemical Cautery: *Caution:* Silver nitrate and other caustics achieve hemostasis through tissue coagulation but are not recommended for wound hemostasis because of the amount of tissue necrosis they produce.

WOUND ASSESSMENT

HISTORY

A detailed, thorough history is essential for assessing the extent of injury and for organizing appropriate wound management.

Three basic questions are used to reconstruct the history of the injury.

When Did the Injury Occur?

The time of injury is important for determining the interval between injury and treatment. Most civilian injuries contain fewer than 10^5 bacteria per gram of tissue in the first 6 hours and are therefore relatively safe to close. After the first 6 hours, bacteria may proliferate and increase the risk of infection if the wound is surgically closed. Exceptions to the 6-hour limit vary depending on the degree of wound contamination, the mechanism of injury, and the location of the wound. As a rule, local tissue resistance is directly proportionate to blood supply. Facial lacerations may often be closed safely within 24 hours of injury, owing to the abundant blood supply in that area.

Where Did the Injury Occur?

What were the possible contaminants associated with the injury? Contact with feces, pus, saliva, or soil greatly increases the risk of infection and precludes primary closure.

How Did the Injury Occur?

The mechanism of injury and the type of instrument inflicting the wound influence subsequent management. Knowing the type of instrument that inflicted the wound will aid in assessing the extent of

injury as well as the need for further diagnostic studies. The degree of wound contamination depends in part of the state of cleanliness of the instrument inflicting the injury.

Types of Injuries

A. Lacerations: Lacerations cause minimal tissue injury and are relatively resistant to infection.

B. Puncture Wounds: Puncture wounds may become infected, especially if they are contaminated or if a foreign body is present.

C. Stretch Injuries: Stretch injuries can produce damage to blood vessels, nerves, ligaments, or tendons that is not visible superficially.

D. Compression or Crush Injuries: Compression or crush injuries result in the greatest amount of tissue necrosis. Hemorrhage into the soft tissues is common, resulting in ecchymosis and hematoma formation. The crushed tissue has a markedly impaired ability to heal and resist infection.

E. Bites: Bites are heavily contaminated and may require delayed closure.

Tetanus Immunization Status (See p 394.)

It is important to ascertain the tetanus immunization status of patients who have sustained open wounds. The date of the most recent booster shot should be determined.

Allergies

The existence of any allergies or adverse reactions should always be elicited before treatment is started. The patient should be specifically questioned about past problems with anesthetics, antibiotics, or analgesics, since this may remind the patient of a forgotten allergic or adverse reaction.

EXAMINATION

Careful inspection of the wound is imperative for proper management. Inspection should be conducted in an emergency care or surgical facility where adequate lighting and equipment are available. Sterile technique and gently handling of tissues are mandatory in order to avoid additional tissue injury or contamination.

Definitive wound evaluation requires a cooperative patient. In the unruly patient, it is perhaps wise to consider restraints, sedation, or local (see below) or general anesthesia—or even to postpone the examination, if possible, until more favorable conditions exist.

Assess Type & Extent of Injury

A. Is there loss of function in the injured part?

B. Are important underlying structures involved,

such as nerves, major blood vessels, ducts, ligaments, bones, or joints?

C. What is the level of contamination in the wound?

D. Are there any foreign bodies?

E. What is the viability of the injured parts? Are there any missing parts?

Examine for Avulsion Flaps

Avulsion flaps may result in a sizable amount of nonviable tissue that may not be apparent initially. Examination of the tissue with a fluorescent light after the administration of intravenous fluorescein (500 mg–1 g) is often helpful in determining the quality of vascular perfusion. Quantitative fluorescent analysis is occasionally used to gain a more precise measurement of tissue perfusion and viability (p 385).

Distally located flaps result in greater tissue destruction than proximally located flaps. Venous congestion is a sure sign of ultimate tissue death.

Amputated tissue may be reattached in some cases. The parts should be sealed in a dry, sterile container and cooled on ice. If replantation is considered a possibility, a microsurgeon or appropriate specialist should be consulted immediately.

Consider Location of Wound

A. Head and Neck: Deep injuries to the head and neck frequently involve important underlying structures (Chapters 17 and 32). These complex anatomic areas cannot be extensively debrided without major functional or cosmetic loss. Wound evaluation and repair are often best done in the operating room by a maxillofacial or general surgeon. The importance of serial evaluations of the central nervous system and cervical spine in the presence of major head and neck trauma cannot be overemphasized.

B. Chest and Abdomen: Wounds of the chest and abdomen must be evaluated for possible communication with a body cavity as well as internal organ injury (Chapters 18 and 19).

C. Extremities: Deep wounds in the extremities must be carefully examined and anatomic landmarks visualized. Pulse deficits or bruits may be present, and an arteriogram may be indicated in situations where the path of injury passes close to a major blood vessel (Chapter 32). Injuries to the extremities require detailed examination of nerve, tendon, and circulatory function (Chapter 23). Avoid extending the injury by inadvertent manipulation or haphazard probing. Make sure that no tourniquet is inadvertently left in place when a dressing is applied. Adequate lighting, exposure, and selection of instruments are mandatory. Most tendon and nerve repairs and all vascular repairs should be performed in an operating room.

Prepare for Definitive Care

After initial assessment, the wound should be covered with a sterile dressing until definitive management or further evaluation can be performed. Any x-rays should be obtained only after the wound has been protected from the possibility of additional contamination. If considerable delay in definitive evaluation and management is anticipated, the wound should be cleaned, conservatively debrided, and temporarily closed or covered. Extensive wounds—or minor ones involving major structures—are best evaluated and managed in the operating room.

ANESTHESIA

Preliminary Examination

A careful sensory and motor neurologic examination must be performed before administration of anesthetic.

Choice of Agent

Local and infiltrative anesthetics have varying attributes with regard to safety, potency, duration of action, and effects upon the local wound milieu (Table 24–1). Lidocaine is perhaps the safest local anesthetic, since allergic reactions are rare. The major problem with all local anesthetics is systemic absorption resulting in cardiovascular and central nervous system toxicity. For an adult, the maximum safe dose of 1% lidocaine without epinephrine is 5 mg/kg (do not exceed 300 mg); for 1% lidocaine with epinephrine, 7 mg/kg (do not exceed 500 mg). For children, the safety and efficacy of lidocaine and mepivacaine are known; child safety and efficacy of the other drugs in Table 24–1 are not known.

Topical Anesthesia

Topical anesthesia is especially useful in the management of small wounds in children who do not tolerate local infiltration. A commonly used combination solution is "TAC" (tetracaine, 5 mg/mL; adrenaline, 0.5 mg/mL; and cocaine, 50 mg/mL [*Note:* Various concentrations of cocaine have been used, as high as 118 mg/mL. However, lower doses provide nearly equivalent analgesia with less risk of cocaine toxicity]). To apply the solution, soak a gauze pad in it and place the pad directly over the wound for 5–10 minutes. Do not use over mucous membranes or areas with end-arterial circulation (fingers, toes, nose, penis). Anesthesia can often be judged by the appearance of blanching at the wound site. Use the minimal amount necessary, since cocaine toxicity may occur.

For abrasions or second-degree burns, application of a gauze pad soaked in 2% lidocaine solution may provide sufficient anesthesia for debridement and vigorous cleansing.

Inhalation Anesthesia

Inhalation anesthesia with nitrous oxide adminis-

Table 24–1. Drugs used for local anesthesia.[1]

	Cocaine	Procaine (Novocain)	Tetracaine[2] (Pontocaine)	Lidocaine (Xylocaine, Many Others)	Bupivacaine[2] (Marcaine, Sensoricaine)	Mepivacaine (Carbocaine)
Potency (compared to procaine)	3	1	10	2–3	9–12	1.5–2
Toxicity (compared to procaine)	4	1	10	1–1.5	4–6	1–1.5
Stability at sterilizing temperature	Unstable	Stable	Stable	Stable	Stable	Stable
Total maximum adult dose	100–200 mg	500 mg	50–100 mg	300 mg	175 mg	400 mg
Total maximum pediatric dose	...	...	...	4 mg/kg	...	5 mg/kg
Infiltration Concentration[3] Onset of action Duration	... ...	0.25–1% 5–15 min 45–60 min	0.05–0.1% 10–20 min 1½–3 h	0.5–1% 3–5 min 30–60 min	0.25% 5–10 min 1½–2 h	0.5% 5–10 min 1¼–2½ h
Nerve block Concentration[3] Onset of action Durartion	... ...	1–2% 5–15 min 45–60 min	0.1–0.2% 10–20 min 1½–3 h	1–2% 5–10 min 1–1½ h	0.25–0.5% 7–21 min 2–6 h	1–2% 5–10 min 1¼–2½ h

[1]Addition of vasopressor prolongs duration by 25–50%; exercise care when used topically, to avoid excessive systemic absorption.
[2]Not recommended for children.
[3]0.5% solution = 5 mg/mL; 1% solution = 10 mg/mL; 2% solution = 20 mg/mL.

tered by experienced personnel can be a useful adjunct, especially for children.

Local Infiltration

A. Method of Injection: Infiltration of a local anesthetic agent is performed gently near the edge of the wound or directly into the wound with a small (No. 25–30) needle (Fig 24–1). Pain associated with local infiltration is partly due to the stretching of sensitive nerve endings in the dermis and may also be due in part to the difference in acidity of some anesthetics (the pH of commercial preparations of lidocaine is 5.0–7.0). This can be overcome by using smaller amounts of more concentrated anesthetic solutions and slower infiltration rates or, in the case of lidocaine, by preparing it as a buffered solution (9 mL of 1% lidocaine, to which 1 mL of sodium bicarbonate solution, 44 meq/50 mL, is added). Restrict the dose of anesthetic to the least amount that will provide adequate anesthesia. This is particularly true for facial lacerations, where infiltration distorts important landmarks and makes precise matching of wound edges difficult. Infiltration of anesthetic directly into the wound is less painful but may spread infection in heavily contaminated wounds.

B. Epinephrine Hemostasis: Lidocaine and similar agents cause relaxation of spastic vessels, and bleeding may start again following local anesthesia. Addition of epinephrine overcomes this tendency and also prolongs the anesthetic effect. The concentration of epinephrine does not need to be higher than 1:400,000, and at least 7 minutes should be allowed for the full vasoconstrictive effect. Use a fresh vial of 1:1000 epinephrine, and dilute with plain 1% or 2% lidocaine. Premixed solutions of epinephrine-containing local anesthetics may lose their potency during prolonged storage.

Although epinephrine has been shown to have little adverse effect on survival of experimental cutaneous flaps, its use in patients with traumatically elevated skin flaps or in tissues with questionable viability is not recommended. Epinephrine should never be administered in areas where segmental blood supply is critical (eg, fingers and toes). Epinephrine is contraindicated in heavily contaminated wounds, since it severely compromises local wound defense mechanisms. The systemic side effects of

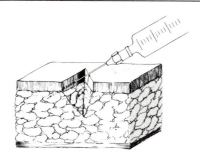

Figure 24–1. Injection of local anesthetic for wound closure (Reproduced, with permission from Dunphy JE, Way LW [editors]: *Current Surgical Diagnosis & Treatment,* 5th ed. Lange, 1981.)

epinephrine should be considered in patients with cardiovascular and peripheral vascular disease.

Regional Anesthesia

Regional anesthesia (sensory nerve blockade at a site proximal to the wound) is more difficult to achieve than local anesthesia, but it provides a larger anesthetic area and allows more extensive exploration and manipulation of the tissues. Since local wound anatomy is not distorted by regional block, more precise alignment of wound edges is possible. Onset of anesthesia is a function of the type of agent used and how close to the nerves the agent is injected. The duration of anesthesia can be prolonged with epinephrine (epinephrine should not be used for digital nerve blocks, however). Regional anesthesia is particularly applicable in extremity injuries complicated by heavy contamination or in extensive injury requiring long operating times for repair. It is also employed in those patients who are not good candidates for general anesthesia.

A. Examples: Examples of regional nerve blocks include axillary block; isolated ulnar, median, and radial nerve blocks; digital nerve blocks; trigeminal nerve blocks; sciatic and femoral nerve blocks; and spinal anesthesia. Digital, infraorbital, and submental blocks are commonly performed in the emergency department. Isolated ulnar, median, and radial nerve blocks should be performed only by an experienced physician.

B. Pitfalls: Pitfalls of regional anesthesia include difficulty in placing the anesthetic close to the supplying sensory nerve; loss of valuable time in waiting for its effects to take place; and risk of permanent injury to the nerve from direct infiltration of anesthetic into the nerve.

Common Regional Blocks for Hand Surgery

Several techniques for regional blocks in hand surgery are described below. Whatever the method used, a thorough understanding of anatomy is crucial. Avoid probing for paresthesias. Attempt to infiltrate the anesthetic without penetrating the nerve sheath, since this may cause injury to the nerve.

Use a 25- or 27-gauge needle; larger needles may cause significant nerve injury. Wait about 10 minutes for the full anesthetic effect in digital blocks and 20 minutes for wrist blocks.

A. Digital Block: The location of the common digital nerve bifurcation at the midpalmar crease is illustrated in Fig 24–2. Pierce the skin only once, and place 1 mL of 1% lidocaine next to the nerve bundle. Two injections are required to completely anesthetize the palmar surface of the finger. A dorsal or web space approach can also be made, in which case it should be noted that the bundle lies just volar to the line separating the palmar and the dorsal skin. When

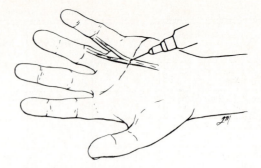

Figure 24–2. Digital block. Inject anesthetic into each side of the digit next to the neurovascular bundles at the mid-palmar crease.

the thumb is blocked, the mid volar location of the digital nerves must be taken into account.

B. Radial Nerve Block: The radial sensory nerve emerges beneath the brachioradialis tendon (Fig 24–3) about 6 cm (2⅜ in) above Lister's tubercle. Inject about 4 mL of lidocaine in a 2-cm (¾-in) wide band 4 cm (1⁹⁄₁₆ in) above Lister's tubercle.

C. Median Nerve Block: The median nerve at the wrist lies just radial and deep to the palmaris longus tendon and the transverse carpal ligament (Fig 24–4). The palmaris longus, when present, is easily identified by having the patient make a fist and flex the wrist. Insert the needle dorsally and distally between the palmaris longus and flexor carpi radialis, and inject 4 mL. The lidocaine can be milked into the carpal tunnel to achieve the maximum blocking effect.

D. Ulnar Nerve Block: The ulnar nerve and artery course just dorsal to the flexor carpi ulnaris at the wrist (Fig 24–5). Avoid inadvertent injection of anesthetic into the artery by aspirating as the needle is advanced. Inject 2 mL on the ulnar side of the flexor carpi ulnaris. An additional 2 mL should be injected on the radial side to achieve a total block.

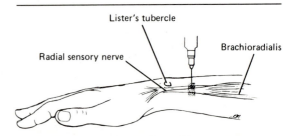

Figure 24–3. Radial nerve block, in which anesthetic is injected in a 2-cm (¾-in) wide band 4 cm (1⁹⁄₁₆) proximal to Lister's tubercule on the radial aspect of the forearm. (Modified and reproduced, with permission, from Newmeyer WL: *Care of Hand Injuries.* Lea & Febiger, 1979.)

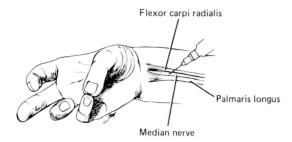

Flexor carpi radialis

Palmaris longus

Median nerve

Figure 24–4. Median nerve block. Inject anesthetic around the median nerve just proximal to the wrist. The nerve is located between the tendons of the palmaris longus and flexor carpi radialis. (Modified and reproduced, with permission, from Newmeyer WL: *Primary Care of Hand Injuries.* Lea & Febiger, 1979.)

Common Regional Blocks for Facial Surgery

A. Infraorbital Nerve Block: (See Fig 24–6.) The infraorbital foramen can be easily palpated along the anterior maxilla and lies along a line drawn between the pupil and the maxillary canine. Inject about 1–2 mL as the needle is advanced from a lateral to a medial direction. Avoid penetrating the nerve by being careful not to enter the foramen. An intraoral approach may also be used. Wait for symptoms of numbness of the upper lip. Infraorbital nerve block provides anesthesia of the cheek, upper lip, and parts of the nose.

B. Supraorbital Nerve Block: (See Fig 24–7.) The exit of the supraorbital nerve from the orbit is readily identified by palpating the supraorbital notch. Inject a total of 1–2 mL of anesthetic about 0.5 cm (3⁄16 in) above the orbital rim. Advance the needle from a lateral to a medial direction, and avoid penetrating the nerve. If both supraorbital and infratrochlear blocks are needed, the wheal should be extended medially toward the midline. Supraorbital block is helpful in anesthetizing the forehead.

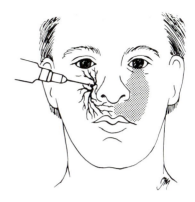

Figure 24–6. Infraorbital nerve block. Intraoral or percutaneous injection around the palpable infraorbital foramina will result in anesthesia within the stippled area.

CLEANING & DEBRIDEMENT

Hair Removal

Wounds in hairy areas are difficult to debride and suture, and hair in a wound acts as a foreign body, delaying healing and promoting infection. Shaving hair around wound edges facilitates management but invites wound infection if the infundibulum of the hair follicle is injured.

Contamination can be minimized by clipping the hair 1–2 mm (1⁄16 in) above the level of the skin. Depilatory agents and special razors equipped with recessed blades also allow safe removal of hair without infundibular injury.

Caution: Eyebrow and eyelash hair should never be removed, since removal destroys critical landmarks and makes accurate alignment of wound edges difficult. Misalignments may cause notch or step-off deformities in the brow line. Eyebrow hair also regrows slowly, creating a cosmetic problem.

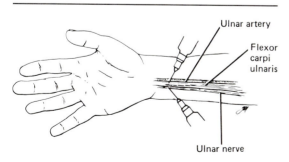

Ulnar artery

Flexor carpi ulnaris

Ulnar nerve

Figure 24–5. Ulnar nerve block. Inject anesthetic around the ulnar nerve just proximal to the wrist on either side of the flexor carpi ulnaris. (Modified and reproduced, with permission from Newmeyer WL: *Primary Care of Hand Injuries.* Lea & Febiger, 1979.)

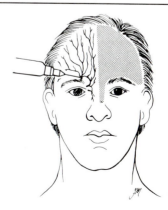

Figure 24–7. Supraorbital nerve block. Inject anesthetic slightly superior to the orbital ridge at the supraorbital notch. Stippling shows area of anesthesia from ipsilateral injection.

Mechanical Cleansing

As an adjunct to surgical debridement, mechanical cleansing of the wound by irrigation or scrubbing is quite effective. Soaps and detergents should not be used in the open wound in conjunction with mechanical cleansing.

A. Irrigation: To be effective, irrigating solutions must be delivered under pressure. The danger of tissue injury with high-pressure irrigation must be weighed against the benefits of decontamination.

Numerous devices are available for high-pressure irrigation, but the simplest and least expensive is syringe irrigation. A 35- or 50-mL syringe and a 19-gauge or blunt needle connected to a reservoir of irrigating fluid by a 3-way stopcock are most suitable. Bulb syringe irrigation has been shown to be no more effective in preventing wound infection than no irrigation at all.

Normal saline (or similar balanced crystalloid solution) is forcefully injected close to the wound surface and perpendicular to the surface of the skin. The amount of irrigant used depends upon the size of the wound and the suspected extent of contamination.

B. Mechanical Scrubbing:

1. Sponge—Mechanical scrubbing of the wound surface is usually best performed with a highly porous sponge. Sponges routinely used for hand washing work very nicely. Brushes and low-porosity sponges decrease the wound's resistance to infection.

2. Brush—"Abrasion tattooing," in which debris is embedded in the skin, requires vigorous scrubbing or dermabrasion to remove embedded debris. Soaps and detergents should not be used.

Skin & Wound Cleansers

The wound and surrounding skin should be cleansed to remove transient microflora, gross debris, coagulated blood, etc.

A. Normal Saline: In most instances, simply washing the open wound with saline under pressure (see above) removes most of the surface bacteria.

B. Nonionic Surfactant: The nonionic surfactant pluronic polyol F-68 has been shown to be effective as a wound cleansing agent without demon- strably impairing resistance to infection or wound healing.

C. Hydrogen Peroxide: The foaming action of hydrogen peroxide is frequently employed to remove particulate debris and recently clotted blood from wounds. *Caution:* For these purposes, dilute solutions of hydrogen peroxide (1% or less) must be used to reduce the potential for tissue injury associated with oxidation. In most cases, a less toxic means of wound cleansing may be preferred.

D. Ionic Soaps and Detergents: Ionic soaps and detergents (eg, pHisoHex) should *not* be used for wound cleansing, as they are extremely irritating to tissues and actually increase the potential for infection if used directly on the wound. They may be used for cleansing of intact skin surrounding the wound,

although they have not been shown to be superior to ordinary soap or other agents for this purpose. After application, they should be removed by thorough rinsing with water. Prolonged use of agents containing hexachlorophene (particularly in children) is associated with severe toxicity, including neurologic damage and even death.

E. Skin Disinfectants and Antimicrobials: These agents vary in their microbicidal effects in wounds. Most are irritating to normal tissues, and some may cause severe toxicity by their systemic absorption (chlorhexidine, antimicrobial powders, etc). Although a 1% solution of povidone-iodide is considered nontoxic, there is conflicting evidence regarding its efficacy in preventing wound infection. Tincture of iodine has actually been shown to potentiate wound infection, and its use can also result in elevation of blood iodine levels. Irrigation of wounds with antibiotic solutions is associated with a decreased rate of wound infection.

Debridement

Retained debris and devitalized tissue should be removed by surgical excision and mechanical cleansing. Mechanical debridement is discussed on p 391.

Surgical debridement consists of excising devitalized or severely contaminated tissues and irregular areas that interfere with wound closure. A stainless steel scalpel blade should be used for debridement.

A. Total Excision of the Wound: The simplest method of debridement is total excision of the wound, creating a surgically clean area. *Caution: Total excision is appropriate only for wounds that do not involve specialized structures (eg, injuries of the abdominal wall and thighs). In the hand and face, more selective debridement is indicated.*

1. Special gauze pack and closure—It is often helpful to pack the wound with gauze, close with sutures, and excise the entire mass as a tumor, leaving a cuff of normal tissue attached. Take care to avoid exposure of the gauze during dissection.

2. Vital staining—An alternative method of debridement is to stain the wound with a vital dye such as methylene blue, close, and excise the entire stained area.

B. Selective Debridement: In most situations, it is best to mechanically cleanse the wound (see above) and then perform selective debridement of all grossly nonviable tissue. A reliable laboratory test for tissue viability is not available, which means that viability must be assessed by careful inspection. Signs of tissue necrosis include gray or black color and lack of bleeding when the tissue is incised. All nonviable portions except certain fibrous tissue remnants should be removed. Mangled, irregular wound edges imply severe local tissue injury and should be sharply debrided. If, on initial or subsequent evaluation, it appears that adequate debridement would prevent tension-free simple closure, consult an experienced surgeon to manage the patient.

The potential viability of attached soft tissue parts depends on vascular supply as well as on the extent of injury. Venous effluent is the most critical component of vascularization. Traumatically elevated skin flaps should be assessed for capillary refill and the presence of venous congestion. Rapid capillary refill or cyanosis in the flap indicates venous obstruction. If there is a sharp demarcation between normal and abnormal perfusion of the flap, excision of the abnormal portion is indicated. If the area of perfusion is not well demarcated, the wound should be cleaned and closely observed. Consultation with a surgeon may be warranted.

Areas of questionable skin viability can be assessed by administering fluorescein intravenously and obtaining quantitative measurements using a fluorometer. This is the procedure of choice and is a more reliable predictor of tissue (flap) viability than the conventional Wood's lamp technique. Inject fluorescein, 2–4 mg/kg intravenously, and repeat within 20 minutes if necessary. *Caution:* Fluorescein dye may occasionally cause an allergic or anaphylactic reaction. Administer a test dose in all patients before giving the full amount.

Excision procedures on the face, particularly of specialized structures such as the ear or nose, require a conservative approach. The facial area has an abundant blood supply that enables tissues to survive on surprisingly small pedicles. In these cases, observation and expectant treatment are warranted. Surgical consultation should be obtained before any major debridement or debridement of a specialized part is performed.

C. Excised Tissue as Grafts: If conditions permit, excised tissue can serve as a graft. Even devascularized tissues should be retained if they serve an important function and can be made surgically clean. Examples include contaminated tendons, fascia, and dura, which can survive as free grafts if appropriate wound coverage is provided and they have been carefully decontaminated by vigorous irrigation with saline.

WOUND CLOSURE

After the wound has been examined, anesthetized, cleaned and debrided, and reexamined, the physician must decide whether or not to close it. Primary wound closure is preferable because of faster healing, less scarring, improved hemostasis, and better aesthetic and functional results. All foreign bodies should be removed to minimize the chance of infection.

Contraindications to Wound Closure

The following factors affect the risk of infection with wound closure and determine whether closure is justified.

A. Heavy Bacterial Colonization: (Over 10^5 organisms per gram of tissue.) Heavy bacterial contamination can only be determined with certainty by quantitative wound culture, which is seldom practical in the emergency department. Two alternative methods can be used in the emergency department to determine the level of bacterial contamination. In the first technique, the wound surface may be swabbed vigorously with a cotton swab and the material streaked on a microscope slide, stained with Gram's stain, and examined under $100 \times$ magnification. The presence of readily detectable bacteria and leukocytes indicates a high likelihood of heavy bacterial contamination.

A second method, the rapid slide technique, is more complex but more reliable. A biopsy specimen is obtained from a representative portion of the wound. In the laboratory, the specimen is homogenized; a 10% suspension is made in saline; and 50–100 μL of the material is placed on a microscope slide. After methanol fixation and staining with Gram's stain, the slide is examined under $400 \times$ magnification. The number of organisms per microscopic field is multiplied by 10^3 to determine the approximate number of bacteria per gram of tissue.

1. A prolonged interval (more than 6 hours) between injury and attempted closure is usually a contraindication to wound closure. In a generously vascularized area such as the face, wound closure may be attempted up to 24 hours after injury.

2. Heavily contaminated wounds (eg, bites) should be left open.

3. Active wound infection at the time of the emergency department visit contraindicates closure of the wound.

B. Major Tissue Defects: Closure is contraindicated (unless grafting is used) if the wound cannot be closed without excessive tension.

C. Other Factors: Closure is contraindicated if there are retained foreign bodies, devitalized tissue, or tissue with borderline adequate perfusion (high likelihood of infection).

Primary Closure
A. Objectives of Repair for Primary Wound Closure:
1. Precise alignment of injured parts to facilitate rapid healing, return of function, and a good cosmetic result.

2. Avoidance of tissue injury (excessive electrocautery, strangulating sutures, etc), hematoma formation, and wound tension.

B. Delayed Primary Closure: Contaminated wounds, if properly debrided, will gain resistance to infection if left open. After 48–96 hours, these wounds can then be closed with essentially no loss in wound healing time. Delayed primary closure should be considered in the case of wounds contaminated by feces, pus, a foreign body, or saliva in the case of bite wounds. Crush and blast injuries and avulsion injuries are markedly susceptible to infection and necrosis and should also be considered for delayed closure.

After initial debridement, the open wound is dressed with fine-mesh gauze and a sterile dressing. It is left undisturbed for the next 4 days unless unexplained fever develops. After this time, the wound is closed using sterile technique.

If delayed closure is elected, the patient should be hospitalized (for large or serious wounds) or seen daily on an outpatient basis.

1. SUTURE SELECTION

All sutures represent foreign bodies in the wound. For this reason, the smallest size and the least amount of suture that will achieve adequate tissue apposition should be employed. In contaminated wounds, sutures should not be used unless they are absolutely necessary to maintain alignment of tissue parts.

The choice of needle and suture size is generally dictated by the size and location of the wound and the desired precision of closure.

Atraumatic needles (round, tapered) are used for closing fascia, muscle, and subcutaneous tissues as well as for repairing lacerated vessels and nerves. Cutting needles are used primarily for dermal and epidermal closure, where the tough collagen fibers must be "cut" by the needle to allow easy passage of the suture.

Large-diameter suture materials (2-0, 3-0) are best for closing major fascial layers and tissues subjected to strong tensile forces (eg, knee and elbow wounds). The effective strength of a suture material is only as great as the strength of the tissue being sutured: fine sutures placed in wounds subject to mechanical stresses may result in disruption of the wound if the fine suture material pulls through the wound.

Generally, fine sutures are used in wounds (or their parts) requiring precise alignment; 5-0 and 6-0 sutures are preferred for closure of facial lacerations. Layered closure (fascia, dermis) of any wound allows placement of fine epidermal sutures anywhere on the body. The epidermis itself has little tensile strength, and sutures are placed in this layer only to achieve accurate alignment of wound edges.

Percutaneous closure of the epidermis and dermis in regions other than the face is best managed by the use of 3-0 or 4-0 suture material. Suture marks are the result of tension in the tied suture and the length of time the suture is left in place.

Absorbable Sutures

Absorbable sutures are biodegraded and lose their tensile strength in 2–6 weeks.

A. Gut Sutures: Sutures derived from sheep submucosa or beef serosa are digested by proteolytic enzymes in the wound. They are more rapidly degraded in the presence of infection. The knot-holding ability of plain gut is rather inconsistent; chromic gut seems to be better in this regard.

1. Plain gut–Plain gut incites an intense inflammatory reaction in the wound and loses its tensile strength within 2 weeks.

2. Chromic gut–Treatment of gut with chromium salts decreases its tissue reactivity and prolongs its survival to about double that of plain gut. In some studies, however, it has been shown to potentiate infection more than plain gut.

B. Synthetic Sutures: Polyglycolic acid (Dexon), polyglactin (Vicryl), and polydioxanone (PDS) produce minimal tissue reaction in the wound and are most commonly used for dermal and subcutaneous closures and vascular ligation.

1. Degradation–Polyglycolic acid and polyglactin are degraded by hydrolysis and lose 50% of their tensile strength in 14–20 days and about 90% by the fourth week (comparable to chromic catgut). Polydioxanone, a third-generation synthetic absorbable suture, loses 50% of its tensile strength in 5 weeks and 90% at 2 months.

2. Tying qualities–Although similar to silk in their handling characteristics, polyglycolic acid and polyglactin sutures do not hold knots quite as well. Polydioxanone looks, feels, and handles like monofilament nylon or polypropylene.

3. Use in acute wounds–Absorbable synthetic sutures are probably superior to gut sutures in acute wounds because of their low tissue reactivity and resistance to degradation in the presence of infection. The monofilament characteristics of polydioxanone make it almost the ideal synthetic absorbable suture.

Nonabsorbable Sutures

Nonabsorbable sutures are degraded very slowly or not at all in the tissues.

A. Silk: Silk sutures represent the most common type of natural fiber suture. Silk gradually loses its tensile strength and is classified as a slowly absorbable suture material. The tissue reactivity of silk is the greatest of all nonabsorbable sutures, and its use in acute wounds has generally been abandoned.

B. Stainless Steel and Metallic Clips or Staples: Stainless steel sutures and metallic clips have been employed for years because of their presumed inertness. These materials have been shown to increase infection rates significantly in contaminated wounds. The increase is probably due to the mechanical irritation resulting from their rigidity and not to corrosion. The stiffness of metallic sutures makes tying quite cumbersome.

Many types of disposable skin staple devices are available. The staple configurations vary but are primarily designed to approximate wound edges with minimal tissue trauma. Some staples actually project above the skin surface to avoid "staple marks." As with wound tapes, precise epidermal alignment is difficult to achieve with a skin staple, and these devices should not be employed for cosmetic skin closures. Because a stapled wound usually does not contain dermal sutures, its tensile strength is dependent upon the presence of the staple, and this must be kept in mind when considering staple closure of wounds subjected to increased tension (joint surfaces, mobile parts, etc). If early removal of the staple is contemplated, the wound should be supported by skin tapes until the wound gains sufficient tensile strength to withstand local biomechanical forces. The time required varies from 1 to 2 weeks depending on the wound's location.

C. Synthetic Sutures:

1. Dacron–Dacron is a polyester that elicits less tissue reaction than silk. Because of its high friction coefficient, it is difficult to handle as a suture. The friction injury imposed upon the tissues by Dacron can be overcome by coating it with Teflon.

2. Nylon–Nylon causes less tissue reactivity than Dacron, and its use in contaminated wounds results in lower wound infection rates.

a. Monofilament nylon sutures lose approximately 20% of their tensile strength within a year after placement in a wound. The monofilament form of nylon is quite stiff and does not hold knots well.

b. Multifilament nylon sutures completely lose their tensile strength in the wound after 6 months, but they are easier to tie than monofilament sutures.

3. Polypropylene and polyester–Polypropylene and polyester materials cause the least reactivity of all suture materials. They maintain their tensile strength indefinitely and are the suture material of choice of closure of contaminated wounds. These materials are used most commonly for fascia and skin closure. They are also advantageous in the repair of vascular, nerve, and tendon injuries. Because of their softer consistency, these materials generally hold knots better than nylon does.

2. WOUND TAPES

Sutureless closure of the acute wound provides maximum resistance to infection. Various tape materials have been used and have resulted in significantly diminished wound infection rates compared to those in suture closure. Tape closure is most advantageous in the contaminated wound but is also useful in superficial clean and tidy wounds, wounds in children, and wounds in obese patients.

Tape closure is inferior to suture closure in maintaining precise wound edge alignment and eversion,

requisites for cosmetically acceptable closure. However, tape closure is often used after early removal of sutures in order to minimize suture marks and to provide additional splinting of the wound until tensile strength is sufficient to resist local forces tending to pull the edges of the wound apart.

Attributes of Wound Tapes

A. Strength: To be effective, skin tapes must be strong enough to support the wound edges in close apposition until sufficient healing has occurred.

B. Adherence: The tapes must have excellent skin adherence and should not macerate the underlying skin surface. Removing all moisture and using a defatting agent (eg, acetone) enhances adhesiveness to the skin, and tapes so applied will adhere for up to 2 weeks. Although tincture of benzoin is occasionally used to increase adhesiveness and may indeed initially enhance tape adhesion, it is solubilized by skin oils and rapidly loses its effectiveness.

C. Types: Microporous, rayon-reinforced wound tapes satisfy the requirements for wound tapes quite well and are most often used today (eg, Steri-Strips; see Fig 24–8). Simple wound tapes can be fashioned from plain microporous 1.25-cm (½-in) paper tape and should be sterilized by applying iodine to the central area of the tape touching the wound.

Wound Tapes Over Deep Sutures

Suture closure in irregular lacerations and crush injuries allows for better approximation of skin edges than does tape closure. Moreover, tape only approximates the superficial portion of the wound, leaving

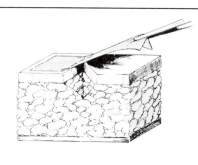

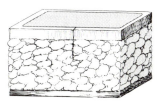

Figure 24–8. Epidermal closure with tape. **_Top:_** Gentle traction is applied on the Steri-Strip to approximate the edges. **_Bottom:_** Closure of wound. (Reproduced, with permission, from Dunphy JE, Way LW [editors]: *Current Surgical Diagnosis & Treatment,* 5th ed. Lange, 1981.)

the deeper wound layers more vulnerable to local biomechanical stresses and resulting in a weak, unsightly scar. In clean wounds, it is sometimes preferable to close the deeper layers with sutures and then approximate the superficial layers with tape.

3. WOUND STAPLES

Stainless steel wound staples (Ethicon, 3M, Deknatel, others) are occasionally used in the emergency department in selected cases. Wounds can be closed more quickly with staples than with sutures, especially long, linear lacerations. In some cases, when the costs of suture instrument sets, suture material, and labor are considered, stapling a wound may be considerably less costly. However, crushed or ischemic tissue may cause point necrosis and infection at the staple tip and produce a less cosmetically satisfactory result. Thus, staples should probably be limited to areas of less cosmetic importance, such as on the scalp or trunk.

4. CHOICE OF CLOSURE TECHNIQUE

The choice of an appropriate material for wound closure is based upon biologic and mechanical properties of the material and the characteristics of the wound. Decisions about layers to be closed are based upon several factors; the most important are stress, dead space, and skin approximation.

Fascia

In soft tissue wounds that do not involve the face, the strength of closure depends upon the fascia. Because fascia heals slowly, the suture material should be capable of maintaining its strength for a long time. Synthetic nonabsorbable sutures are best for this purpose.

Muscle & Fat

These tissues do not hold sutures well, and closure is performed primarily to obliterate dead space. Dead space results from traumatic tissue loss, debridement, or gaping of subcutaneous layers. Suturing of dead space invariably produces additional tissue trauma and necrosis and is contraindicated in the closure of contaminated wounds. When such suturing is performed, it should be accomplished with the fewest possible loosely placed sutures. Chromic gut or one of the synthetic absorbable sutures should be used for this purpose.

Skin

Skin closure may be accomplished by layers, full-thickness percutaneous sutures, skin tapes, or a combination of these methods. The type of skin closure method chosen depends on the forces tending to open the wound and how good a cosmetic result is desired. The width of the scar that will result from healing will be influenced by the local stresses of the surrounding tissues. The direction of maximum force of skin tension is usually parallel to the skin wrinkles. Wounds oriented in the same direction as local stresses are subjected to less tension during healing and consequently produce a less visible scar. Examples include transverse lacerations of the forehead and vertical lacerations of the upper lip. Wounds that cross lines of maximal skin stress will be subjected to increased tension during healing. These wounds frequently widen with time and have a tendency to form hypertrophic scars. Examples are transverse lacerations of the cheek and axial lacerations over the elbows.

The propensity of a scar to hypertrophy is also influenced by factors unrelated to its location or technique of closure. The tendency of children and adolescents to form hypertrophic scars is notorious and is probably influenced by elevated levels of growth hormone or other growth factors. Pregnant women have an increased incidence of hypertrophic scar formation that decreases with the resumption of normal menses after delivery; this tendency is often associated with a parallel increase in pigmentation coinciding with pregnancy. Some investigators have postulated that hypertrophic scars and pigmentation are under similar hormonal influences. An increased incidence of hypertrophic scar and keloid formation is also found in blacks and other dark-skinned races. These specific groups of patients will demonstrate an exaggerated scar formation response that can only be controlled by manipulation of the wound in ways beyond the technical aspects of closure. Not all patients in these groups will form hypertrophic scars, however, and it is impossible to predict which patients might, except perhaps in the case of those who have a history of hypertrophic scar formation. In these patients, precise wound closure using fine suture materials and atraumatic technique may lessen the degree of hypertrophic scarring that might otherwise result. Other methods of wound control include prolonged splinting, pressure bandages, corticosteroid therapy, and radiation therapy. In the acute wound, however, primary consideration is given to the location and orientation of the wound and its method of closure.

A. High-Stress Wounds: Layered wound closure is employed to support wounds subjected to high skin tensions. The dermis is approximated with interrupted sutures, usually absorbable synthetics (Fig 24–9A–C). These sutures should not involve the epidermis, because of the risk of epithelial cyst formation. The epidermal layers are then adjusted with fine nonabsorbable sutures or tapes (Fig 24–9D and E). This method of skin closure is commonly used for facial lacerations.

B. Low-Stress Wounds: Percutaneous sutures are used for most other sites. It is important to evert

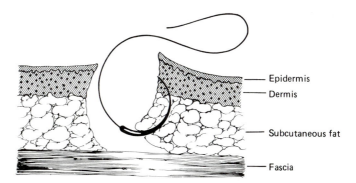

Epidermis
Dermis
Subcutaneous fat
Fascia

A. The strength of the closure lies in the dermis. Occasionally the subcutaneous fat is incorporated to obliterate dead space.

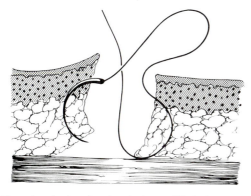

B. The suture is placed so that the knot will lie in the deepest part of the wound. Take care to avoid incorporating the epidermis with this suture, since epithelial cysts will form and result in suture extrusion.

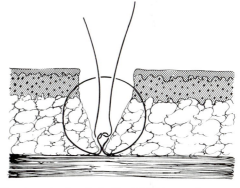

C. The dermal suture is tied just tightly enough to approximate the wound margins. Synthetic absorbable sutures are most commonly used for closure of the dermis.

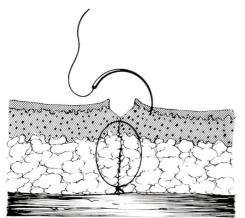

D. After the dermis is approximated, a fine "epidermal" suture is placed to align the wound edges. This suture adds little to the tensile strength of the wound closure.

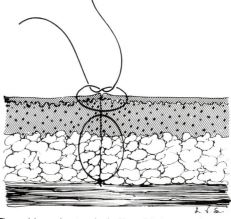

E. The epidermal suture is tied just tightly enough to approximate the epidermal edges of the wound. Since the strength of this closure lies in the dermis, the epidermal suture can be removed after 2–3 days. Skin tapes are often used to support the wound for an additional 7–10 days.

Figure 24–9. Layered cutaneous closure.

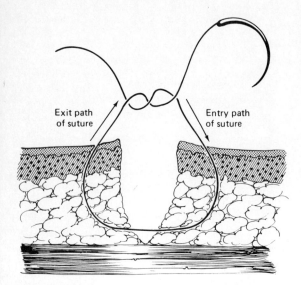

Exit path
of suture

Entry path
of suture

Figure 24–10. Percutaneous suture. Ideal placement of the suture everts the wound margins. This is accomplished by directing the needle away from the wound margin at the entrance point and toward the wound margin at the exit point. The path of a properly placed percutaneous suture will be wider at its base than at the skin entry and exit points.

the wound edges and to effect precise epidermal approximation to achieve the best results (Fig 24–10). Monofilament synthetic nonabsorbable sutures are the materials of choice for this type of closure. The size of suture material is not as important as the tightness of closure and the length of time the suture is left in place. These sutures should be removed by the seventh day to avoid epithelialization of the suture tracts. If additional support of the closure is required, as in wounds subjected to increased tension, skin tapes can be applied.

5. DRAINAGE OF THE WOUND

Drains constitute foreign bodies, produce tissue necrosis, serve as conduits for bacterial contamination of the wound, and are not very effective in preventing hematoma formation. If sound principles of management have been carefully followed, drains are usually unnecessary in the acute wound. If oozing cannot be controlled, it is preferable to delay wound closure. Drains, however, may be effective in evacuating pus and necrotic exudates that might be found in heavily contaminated or already infected wounds.

POSTOPERATIVE WOUND CARE & DRESSINGS

Postoperative wound care should provide an ideal environment for wound healing. This is accom-

plished primarily through the use of dressings. A dressing serves one or more of 7 different functions: protection, immobilization, control of edema (compression), absorption, debridement, delivery of topical medications (antibiotics), and cosmetic appearance.

Protection

Wounds closed by percutaneous sutures are susceptible to surface bacterial invasion for the first 48 hours after closure. During this time, the wound should be protected with sterile dressings or frequent suture line care.

A. Dressings: If dressings are used, nonadherent materials (Telfa, petrolatum-impregnated gauze, etc) are favored because removal is easy and does not disturb sutures or coated wound edges.

Petrolatum-impregnated dressings have been shown to decrease the rate of epithelialization in partial-thickness wounds. For this reason, ointment-impregnated dressings (bacitracin, combined neomycin sulfate and polymixin B sulfate [Neosporin], etc) or nonadherent occlusive dressings (Op-Site) are preferred for this particular type of wound.

Occlusive or semiocclusive polyurethane, methacrylate, silicone polymer, or gel dressings provide excellent protection, and most do not alter the rate of normal epithelialization. If the wound contains residual necrotic debris or significant levels of bacterial contamination, however, the risk of wound infection is increased with these dressings.

B. Undressed Wounds: Suture line care without a dressing is commonly employed for facial wounds and involves frequent meticulous cleansing with saline or dilute hydrogen peroxide solution. Cleansing removes the adherent coagulum from the suture-skin juncture, decreasing the likelihood of stitch abscess formation. After cleansing, the wound is dressed with an antibiotic cream or ointment (eg, bacitracin-neomycin).

C. Tape Dressings: Taped wounds are quite resistant to surface bacterial contamination. They usually require no protection other than that provided by the tape itself. These wounds should be checked frequently for wound drainage beneath the tape. Excessive drainage can cause maceration of the wound edge and thereby provide an excellent medium for bacterial proliferation.

Immobilization

Immobilization of the wound enhances resistance to infection and may accelerate healing.

A. Materials: Immobilization is accomplished with splints, bulky dressings, skin tapes, or combinations of these methods.

B. Duration of Immobilization: Ideally, immobilization of the wound should be continued until it is no longer vulnerable to infection and has gained sufficient strength to withstand the stresses of motion and skin tension. Wounds become resistant to infection within a week, but development of maximal strength requires about 6 weeks. Protracted immobilization will defeat its possible advantages, eg, may produce permanent joint contractures in elderly persons. The advantages of wound immobilization must be weighed against the undesirable consequences. Extended immobilization is advisable for wounds of the face or whenever a good cosmetic result is desired. Areas such as the jawline, chin, shoulder, and knee are subjected to more severe tissue stresses than are other areas and frequently require support for up to 3 months to achieve the best result. Extended wound support is also necessary in patients with neoplasms or immunodeficiency.

Control of Edema

Edema slows down the repair mechanisms and increases fibrous tissue proliferation. The wound with minimal edema will proceed to earlier complete healing and return of function. Peak wound edema occurs by 48 hours and gradually resolves over the next 4–6 days. Persistent tissue edema after 7 days suggests inflammation or infection. In most cases, a compression dressing is beneficial during the first week of wound healing. In wounds that are prone to hypertrophic scarring, edema persists locally for up to 2 years. In these wounds, continued pressure may be beneficial in controlling the extent of hypertrophic scarring. Custom-made elastic pressure garments are excellent adjuncts in this regard; otherwise, simple elastic bandages are equally effective.

A. Elevation: Elevation of the wound above the level of the heart is the simplest way to limit the amount of excess tissue fluid in the wound. In the ambulatory patient, the common triangular bandage sling or "yoke" sling serves these purposes well. Slings, like any other dressing, are only as good as patient compliance; instruction in their use is important if the goal is to be achieved.

B. Pressure Dressing: In certain situations, it is advantageous to apply pressure over the wound along with elevation by using bulky pressure dressings. *Caution:* (**1**) Compression dressings should not be used in crush injuries or in injuries that tend to develop into compartment syndromes, eg, severe injuries of the forearm or leg. (**2**) Continued pain or diminished sensitivity necessitates removal of the dressing and careful examination of the wound. (**3**) Although these dressings are often used to absorb bloody oozing at the operative site, they should not be employed as a substitute for diligent hemostasis.

1. Avoid constriction of proximal parts with these dressings, since venous and lymphatic congestion will occur as result of the tourniquet effect.

2. Bony prominences must be carefully padded, with generous use of bulk. To ensure uniform compression throughout and to avoid constriction and "pressure point" injury, smooth, even wrapping that avoids "lumps" is necessary when compression dressing is applied.

3. In managing hand wounds, it is important to place one or 2 layers of gauze between the fingers to prevent maceration by sweat. The toes and fingertips should be exposed so that the physician can assess sensibility and capillary refill.

4. Roller gauze or bias cut stockinet is preferred over elastic bandages, which are often too constricting. The finished dressing should be firm but not strangulating.

5. In extremity injuries, compression dressing should extend proximally from the most distal point. For example, a wound of the forearm requiring a compression dressing is managed by applying the dressing from the starting fingers to above the wound.

Absorption

The absorptive capabilities of a dressing are used to remove bloody and serous ooze from the wound or drainage site.

A. Closed Wounds: In closed wounds, dry dressings are preferable, since moist ones will cause maceration of the skin and invite bacterial invasion.

B. Open Wounds: In open wounds, it is preferable to apply moist dressings to the open wound surface and back them with dry dressings to achieve a "capillary effect." The exception to this principle is deep, tunnel-shaped wounds, where surface evaporation is limited, thus diminishing the capillary effect. These wounds are best managed by packing with dry gauze to achieve maximum absorption.

C. Materials: In all instances, absorptive dressings should be composed of fine-mesh gauze or spun fabric.

1. Cotton meshes and synthetic equivalents become incorporated into the wound as foreign bodies that incite tissue inflammation and cause subsequent bacterial proliferation.

2. Dextran polymers (eg, Debrisan wound-cleaning beads) have remarkable hygroscopic properties and serve well as absorbent dressings. They are quite effective in removing bacterial toxins and serous effluents from the wound surface. Wound healing is not significantly altered by their use.

Debridement
(See also p 384.)

A. Mechanical Debridement: Dressings are frequently used for mechanical debridement of the open wound.

The traditional wet-to-dry method utilizes avulsion of adherent tissues to remove devitalized remnants from the wound surface. Unfortunately, this method does not discriminate between viable and nonviable elements and reinjures the wound with each dressing change. Although painful and detrimental to wound healing, this method is effective in removing fine tenacious material from the wound surface. It should be discontinued as soon as the desired effect has been achieved.

The technique is as follows: Several layers of moist gauze are applied to the wound surface and allowed to dry. After about 4 hours, the adherent dressing is removed. Moistening the dry dressing before removal to loosen the dressing and lessen the pain of removal (as may be done by a sympathetic hospital attendant) defeats the purpose.

B. Enzymatic Debridement: An alternative to mechanical avulsion debridement is enzymatic debridement. Certain proteolytic enzymes are quite effective in removing particulate necrotic debris and fibrinous coagulum from the wound. A popular product is sutilains (Travase), which has been shown to cause little injury to the viable wound parts. This method of debridement requires dressing changes every 8–12 hours, and the patient should be closely monitored for early signs of infection. If cellulitis does develop, sutilains should be discontinued and the patient closely monitored for signs of invasive infection. Sutilains should not be used for longer than 48 hours at the same site, nor should it be used in areas larger than 10% of body surface area.

C. Saprophytic Debridement: Historically, it has been observed that housefly larvae (maggots) can ingest decaying human tissue and thrive. Saprophytic debridement apparently depends upon bacterial breakdown of necrotic tissue and assimilation of the organic components by the larvae. The process is quite effective and causes little or no discomfort. Viable tissue is not injured unless the bacterial population exceeds the host's resistance and causes an invasive infection.

Once advocated as alternative therapy in wound debridement, saprophytic debridement has fallen into disfavor primarily for aesthetic reasons. The emphasis on sanitation and sterility in contemporary medicine has precluded any realistic revival of this method of debridement. One may occasionally encounter a patient whose negligent wound care has resulted in larval infestation. Surprisingly, these wounds are usually quite clean and healthy-appearing.

Delivery of Topical Antibiotics

The most common medicaments used in a dressing are antibacterials. Topical antibacterials are employed to control bacteria that cannot be reached by systemic agents. They are *not* a substitute for adequate debridement.

A. Agents: Mafenide (Sulfamylon) and silver sulfadiazine (Silvadene) are most effective in this regard. These agents are also useful in partial-thickness injuries or marginally viable tissues (eg, abrasions, burns, crush injuries). By decreasing the potential for bacterial invasion, they diminish the likelihood of infection and the resulting tissue necrosis.

B. Adverse Reactions: Use of these agents must be monitored closely, since excessive amounts may cause acid-base imbalances (mafenide) or leukopenia (silver sulfadiazine). Both agents retard wound epithelialization and should be discontinued when the necrotic debris has been removed and wound bacterial counts are fewer than 10^5 organisms per gram of tissue.

Cosmetic Appearance

To the patient or casual observer, the sight of a wound is abhorrent and may be an occasion for adverse response. A dressing "hides" the wound and allows the patient to proceed with the process of rehabilitation without that distraction. In addition, a carefully applied, neat-appearing dressing reassures the patient that good wound care has been provided.

1. SPECIAL BIOLOGIC DRESSINGS

Acute wounds with extensive loss of skin are not often amenable to immediate closure by flaps or grafts. These defects favor bacterial invasion and may be associated with major losses of fluid, protein, and other metabolic essentials. Early closure may be impractical from the standpoint of patient tolerance or safety. In these situations, temporary skin substitutes may be beneficial. Biologic dressings duplicate all the protective functions of skin except permanence. Biologic dressings should be removed within 48 hours and fresh ones applied. Keeping the dressings on longer will increase their adherence and initiate rejection reactions that may be detrimental to wound healing. Homograft and amniotic membrane dressings are quite effective in reducing wound bacterial counts. In contaminated wounds, dressings should be changed every 24 hours.

A major pitfall of any biologic dressing is its inability to prevent bacterial proliferation in the presence of dead tissue or a foreign body. This drawback may constitute a relative contraindication to the use of a biologic dressing in the acute wound.

Natural Biologic Dressings

A. Pigskin: Many types of biologic dressings are available, but pigskin is most commonly used because it is readily available. It provides excellent protection and diminishes fluid losses, but it does not reduce bacterial populations in the wound. Effective reduction of bacterial counts requires a "take" of the biologic dressing to the wound surface.

B. Human Tissue: Human tissues are the only biologic dressings that will actually develop a blood supply from human wounds. For these purposes, homograft skin and human fetal membranes are quite advantageous. Cadaver skin is not readily available in most hospitals and is extremely expensive. Amniotic membranes are abundant and provide an excellent source of biologic dressings. If placed with their chorion side facing the wound, they will adhere much like a skin graft.

Synthetic Biologic Dressings

Over the past several years, synthetic dressings have been introduced that function somewhat like biologic dressings in their wound protection capabilities. Biobrane is a Silastic-collagen laminate that has been shown to have excellent adherence properties when applied to open wounds. When compared to human allograft, there is essentially no difference in pain relief, initial adherence, or the ability to keep bacterial counts in the wound below 10^5 organisms per gram of tissue. This and similar synthetics represent a significant advance in the materials used to temporarily cover the open wound. Further investigation is needed to determine their precise role in wound management.

2. POTENTIAL INFECTIONS & ANTIMICROBIALS

Antimicrobials are effective in preventing wound infection, particularly when the wound has fewer than 10^6 organisms per gram of tissue before treatment is started. Wounds with more than 10^6 organisms per gram of tissue often become infected despite antibiotic prophylaxis and should be left open. Systemic antibiotics, to be effective, must be started as soon as possible following injury, preferably within 4 hours. Topical antibiotics are commonly used to suppress bacterial growth, although their efficacy at preventing subsequent infection is probably low.

The likelihood of wound infection must be judged by the mechanism of injury, the level of contamination, the adequacy of debridement, and the general status of the patient.

Small inocula will result in infection if necrotic debris, foreign bodies, or altered tissue defense mechanisms (as occur in crush or contused wounds) are present. If adequate wound management must be delayed for any reason, then systemic antimicrobial prophylaxis should be considered.

Sharp lacerations are markedly resistant to infection and in most instances will not require chemoprophylaxis. Open wounds, by virtue of their inflammatory response and resistance to bacterial dissemination, rarely become infected unless the initial level of contamination is great and cannot be reduced by cleansing and debridement. Furthermore, the fibrinous coagulum in these wounds limits the possible effectiveness of systemic antimicrobials on bacterial contaminants, thus making their use impractical.

Deep wounds or those that involve poorly vascularized structures such as bone, tendon, ligament,

or fascia should be treated with systemic antibiotics prophylactically.

Oral mucosal lacerations rarely require systemic antibiotic prophylaxis, since the infection rate is low and randomized trials have not demonstrated a benefit from such treatment.

Grossly contaminated wounds such as those that come in contact with feces, pus, or saliva should not be closed. Systemic antimicrobial therapy is mandatory. The choice of drug is based on the suspected predominant pathogen (Table 24–2).

3. TETANUS PROPHYLAXIS

Tetanus prophylaxis is virtually 100% effective if used properly. Overutilization of tetanus toxoid may induce serious allergic reactions.

Investigate Previous Active Immunization

A history of standard primary immunization with tetanus toxoid (or DTP) followed by boosters every 10 years virtually guarantees immunity from tetanus. Nearly all individuals over age 2 in the USA have had primary immunization (3 doses at 4-week intervals followed by one booster), and this too nearly guarantees immunity. Even individuals with only 2 previous tetanus toxoid immunizations will develop antibody rapidly enough following a tetanus toxoid booster so that passive immunization will be unnecessary in most cases. Patients over 50 years of age, foreign-born patients, or patients unable to provide a history of tetanus immunization must be assumed to have incomplete immunization and should be treated according to Table 24–3.

Determine Risk of Tetanus

The risk of tetanus is greater with wounds that are heavily contaminated by soil or feces, those involving crush injury of surrounding tissue, and those

Table 24–2. Choice of antimicrobials for prevention of infection in specific types of wounds.[1]

Type of Wound	Antimicrobial of Choice	Adult Dose[2]
Human bite seen within 1–2 days	Penicillin or ampicillin (Alternative: erythromycin)	0.5–1 g 0.5 g
Human bite older than 2 days	Dicloxacillin (Alternative: erythromycin)	0.5 g 0.5 g
Animal bites	Ampicillin (pencillin for cat bites) (Alternative: tetracycline)	0.5 g 0.5 g
Other wounds	Dicloxacillin (Alternative: erythromycin)	0.5 g 0.5 g

[1]These recommendations apply only to wounds *without* evidence of infection at the time of examination.
[2]Four times daily orally for 3–5 days.

Table 24–3. Guide to tetanus prophylaxis in wound management.[1]

History of Tetanus Immunization (Doses)	Clean Minor Wounds		All Other Wounds	
	Td[2]	TIG[2]	Td[2]	TIG[2]
Uncertain	Yes	No	Yes	Yes
0–1	Yes	No	Yes	Yes
2	Yes	No	Yes	No[3]
3 or more	No[4]	No	No[4]	No

[1]Adapted from *MMWR* 1981;30:404.
[2]Td = tetanus and diphtheria toxoids, adult type, for persons over 7 years of age. DTP for children under 7 years of age. TIG = tetanus immune globulin.
[3]Unless wound is more than 24 hours old.
[4]Unless it has been more than 10 years since last dose.

coming to medical attention after a delay of more than 24 hours.

Select Active or Passive Immunizations

Table 24–3 shows the United States Public Health Service recommended tetanus immunization schedules. Td (tetanus toxoid combined with adult-dose diphtheria toxoid) is preferable to tetanus toxoid alone. If passive immunization is required, human tetanus immune globulin is preferred over horse serum. The recommended dose is 250–500 units intramuscularly. If equine tetanus antitoxin must be used, inquire about and test for horse serum allergy before administering. The usual dose is 3000–5000 units. If both Td and tetanus immune globulin or antitoxin are given, they should be administered in separate sites using separate syringes.

4. RABIES PROPHYLAXIS

Assess Risk of Rabies Exposure (See Fig 24–11.)

A. Species of Biting Animal: Carnivorous animals (especially skunks, foxes, badgers, bobcats, coyotes, raccoons, dogs and cats) and bats are more likely to be infected. Rabbits, squirrels, hamsters, guinea pigs, gerbils, chipmunks, rats, mice, and other rodents rarely transmit rabies in the USA.

B. Determine If Animal Is Rabid (If Possible): (*Note:* Behavior is *not* a reliable sign of the rabid state.) If examination of the brain for rabies is negative, it can be assumed that the saliva of that animal did not contain rabies virus.

1. Healthy domestic dogs and cats should be observed for 10 days by a veterinarian. If signs of rabies develop, the animal should be killed and its brain examined for rabies virus at the local public health laboratory.

2. Stray or unwanted dogs and cats that cause

bites should be killed immediately and examined for rabies.

3. Wild animals that cause bites should be killed immediately and the brain examined for rabies.

C. Circumstances of Biting Incident: *Unprovoked* attacks are more likely to mean that the animal is rabid. Bites from apparently healthy animals that are fighting or feeding or that have been picked up or petted should be considered *provoked* and so have a low likelihood of causing rabies.

D. Types of Exposure: Any penetration of skin by teeth is regarded as a bite. Nonbite exposure consists of contamination of scratches, abrasions, mucous membranes, or previous wounds with infected animal saliva.

E. Rabies Immunization Status of Animal: Vaccines are effective for cats and dogs, but are *not* effective in preventing rabies in other animals, especially wild animals that have been domesticated (eg, pet skunks, foxes).

F. Prevalence of Rabies in Region: Certain areas are devoid of rabies (eg, San Francisco, Great Britain). Some rural areas are considered at high risk for rabies (eg, Texas-Mexico border).

Management of Patients at High Risk

Provide tetanus prophylaxis (see above), and give antibiotics if indicated (see above). *Quickly* administer appropriate postexposure rabies prophylaxis (see Fig 24–11 and Tables 24–4 and 24–5).

Act quickly! The sooner antirabies measures are instituted, the more effective they are.

A. Wound Care: (This is the most important step.) Wash copiously with 20% green soap tincture and water. *Note:* Quaternary ammonium compounds and alcohol are no longer recommended.

B. Passive Immunization:

1. Rabies immune globulin USP–This neutralizing antibody should be given to all patients except those previously immunized who have documented antibody titers or those who have received preexposure human diploid cell rabies vaccine prophylaxis or a full course of human diploid cell rabies vaccine. Give 20 IU/kg at the onset of rabies therapy; rabies immune globulin can be given as late as the eighth day if necessary. Inject up to one-half the total dose in and around the wound and the remainder by deep intramuscular injection. Because rabies immune globulin may partially suppress the antibody response to duck embryo vaccine, no more than the recommended dose should be given.

2. Equine rabies immune globulin–This preparation should be used only when the human (USP) product is not available. Check for allergy to horse serum. The product contains 1000 IU/vial (about 5 mL). The dose is 40 IU/kg.

C. Active Immunization:

1. Human diploid cell rabies vaccine–Inacti-

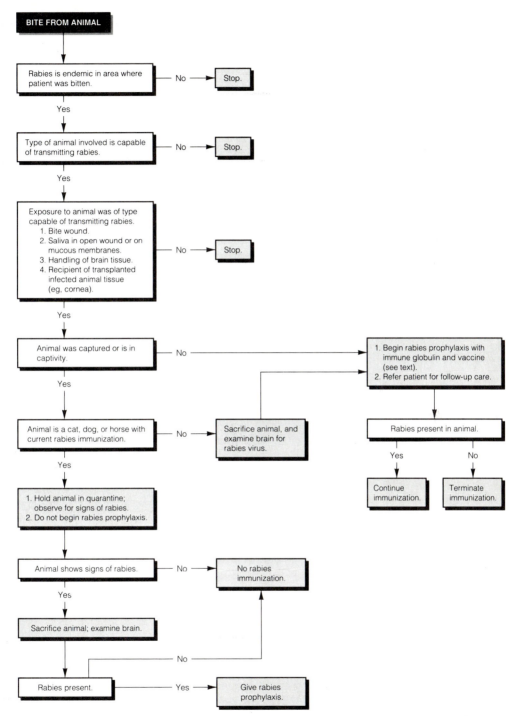

Figure 24–11. Algorithm for management of possible rabies exposure.

Table 24–4. Rabies postexposure prophylaxis guide.[1]

The following recommendations are only a guide. In applying them, take into account the species involved, the circumstances of the bite or other exposure, the vaccination status of the animal, and the presence of rabies in the region. Local or state public health officials should be consulted if questions arise about the need for rabies prophylaxis.

Animal Species	Condition of Animal at Time of Attack	Treatment of Exposed Person[2]
Domestic Dog and cat	Healthy and available for 10 days of observation.	None, unless animal develops rabies.[3]
	Rabid or suspected rabid.	RIG[4] and HDCV.[5]
	Unknown (escaped).	Consult public health officials. If treatment is indicated, give RIG[4] and HDCV.[5]
Wild Skunk, bat, fox, coyote, raccoon, bobcat, and other carnivores	Regard as rabid unless proved negative by laboratory tests.[6]	RIG[4] and HDCV.[5]
Other Livestock, rodents, and lagomorphs (rabbits and hares)	Consider individually. Local and state public health officials should be consulted on questions about the need for rabies prophylaxis. Bites of squirrels, hamsters, guinea pigs, gerbils, chipmunks, rats, mice, other rodents, rabbits, and hares almost never call for antirabies prophylaxis.	

[1]From *MMWR* 1980;29:265. Modified slightly.
[2]All bites and wounds should immediately be thoroughly cleansed with soap and water. If antirabies treatment is indicated, both rabies immune globulin (RIG) and human diploid cell rabies vaccine (HDCV) should be given as soon as possible, regardless of the interval from exposure.
[3]During the usual holding period of 10 days, begin treatment with RIG and vaccine (preferably with HDCV) at first sign of rabies in a dog or cat that has bitten someone. The symptomatic animal should be killed immediately and tested.
[4]If RIG is not available, use antirabies serum, equine (ARS). Do not use more than the recommended dosage.
[5]If HDCV is not available, use duck embryo vaccine (DEV) or other rabies vaccine. Local reactions to vaccines are common and do not contraindicate continuing treatment. Discontinue vaccine if fluorescent antibody tests of the animal are negative.
[6]The animal should be killed and tested as soon as possible. Holding for observation is not recommended.

vated virus vaccine prepared from rabies virus grown on human diploid fibroblasts has now been approved by the FDA for use in the USA and is the rabies vaccine of choice. This product has been 100% effective thus far (in over 1000 patients) in preventing rabies in persons bitten by animals known to be rabid. Antibody titers are 10 times higher than those achieved with duck embryo vaccine (see below), and the incidence of side effects has been much less.

Give five 1-mL doses intramuscularly on specified days. The first dose is given as soon as possible after the bite; subsequent doses are given on days 3, 7, 14, and 28. No booster dose is needed.

If preexposure human diploid cell rabies vaccine prophylaxis and adequate booster doses have been given (because of occupation as a veterinarian, for example), only two 1-mL intramuscular doses of human diploid cell rabies vaccine are needed, one as soon as possible after the bite and the other 3 days later. The full course of antirabies prophylaxis, including rabies immune globulin, should be given to those who have received a course of duck embryo vaccine but whose antibody titers have not been checked.

Routine serologic testing after treatment with human diploid cell rabies vaccine is no longer necessary unless the patient is immunocompromised or is taking corticosteroids. Those individuals taking steroids should discontinue the medication while receiving antirabies treatment.

2. Duck embryo vaccine–Duck embryo vaccine (rabies vaccine USP) is a killed virus vaccine prepared from embryonated duck eggs. In some areas, human diploid cell vaccine is not available, and it may be necessary to treat with duck embryo vaccine. It is given subcutaneously, preferably in the abdomen, in rotating sites. This vaccine is no longer being produced in the USA but may still be available in certain centers.

Give 21 (1-mL) injections (plus 2 boosters): one injection daily for 21 days, *or* 2 injections daily for 7 days, then one injection daily for 7 days. Two additional (1-mL) booster injections are necessary (rabies immune globulin decreases the antibody response). Give the first booster 10 days after injection No. 21 and the second booster 20 days after injection No. 21.

Determine antibody response at the time of the second booster (only 80–85% of patients have an antibody response at this time). If the antibody titer at the time of the second booster is inadequate, it is imperative to obtain human diploid cell-grown vaccine and give 3 injections on days 0 (the day that inadequate antibody titers are first identified), 7, and 14.

Adverse reactions: Local and mild systemic reactions occur in most patients but do not warrant cessation of therapy. Pain and erythema occur in all patients, fever and myalgias in 33%, adenopathy in 15%, and pruritus in 13%. Anaphylaxis and central nervous system reactions (transverse myelitis, neuropathy, encephalopathy) occur rarely but require

Table 24–5. Rabies immunization regimens.[1]

Preexposure

Preexposure rabies prophylaxis for persons with special risks of exposure to rabies, such as animal care and control personnel and selected laboratory workers, consists of immunization with either human diploid cell rabies vaccine (HDCV) or duck embryo vaccine (DEV), according to the following schedule, followed by a booster dose every 2 years.

Rabies Vaccine	Number of 1-mL Doses	Route of Administration	Intervals Between Doses	If No Antibody Response to Primary Series, Give:[2]
HDCV	3	Intramuscular	1 week between first and second: 2–3 weeks between second and third.[3]	1 booster dose.[3]
DEV	3 or 4	Subcutaneous	1 month between first and second; 6–7 months between second and third,[3] **or** 1 week between first, second, and third; 3 months between third and fourth.[3]	2 booster doses,[3] 1 week apart.

Postexposure

Postexposure rabies prophylaxis for persons exposed to rabies consists of the immediate, thorough cleansing of all wounds with soap and water, administration of rabies immune globulin (RIG) or, if RIG is not available, antirabies serum, equine (ARS), and the initiation of either HDCV or DEV, according to the following schedule.

Rabies Vaccine	Number of 1-mL Doses	Route of Administration	Intervals Between Doses	If No Antibody Response to Primary Series, Give:[2]
HDCV	5[4]	Intramuscular	Doses to be given on days 0, 3, 7, 14, and 28.	An additional booster dose.[5]
DEV	23	Subcutaneous	21 daily doses followed by a booster on day 31 and another on day 41.[3] **or** 2 daily doses in the first 7 days, followed by 7 daily doses. Then 1 booster on day 24 and another on day 34.[3]	3 doses of HDCV at weekly intervals.[3]

[1]From *MMWR* 1980;29:265. Modified slightly.
[2]If no antibody response is documented after the recommended additional booster dose(s), consult the state health department or CDC.
[3]Serum for rabies antibody testing should be collected 2–3 weeks after the last dose only in immunocompromised patients.
[4]The World Health Organization recommends a sixth dose 90 days after the first dose.
[5]An additional booster dose should be given only to immunocompromised patients.

cessation of duck embryo vaccine. Corticosteroids should be given only for life-threatening adverse reactions, since they can blunt the antibody response.

3. Other vaccines–Other inactivated vaccines (rabbit spinal cord, mouse grain, etc) are available outside the USA and are effective. Follow the manufacturer's instructions.

5. FOLLOW-UP CARE OF THE WOUND

After initial wound management, provisions must be made for follow-up and local wound care. The patient should be instructed in how to recognize signs and symptoms of wound complications. A specific appointment for return should be given before discharge from the emergency department. It is helpful to supply a printed list of danger signals and directions on care of the wound (Fig 24–12). A 24-hour call number should be provided.

Since every wound is unique, a patient form outlining wound care is inappropriate. Simple instructions giving specific details about wound care are useful in these situations. Patients want to know about limitations on activity, when they can bathe or shower, the type and frequency of dressing changes, when sutures will be removed, and precautions after suture removal.

The various changes that occur in a wound during the course of normal wound healing may cause anxiety, particularly in wounds of the face and other exposed areas. The patient should be told that thickening of the area surrounding a scar usually abates by 3 months. Redness of the scar usually persists for 3–6 months. The scar may assume various shades of blue depending upon the environmental conditions. If the patient is prone to develop hypertrophic scars or keloids, it is wise to mention this possibility (particularly in more heavily pigmented races, children, adolescents, and pregnant women and in wounds of the shoulders, anterior chest, elbows, and knees).

Itching of the scar is common and can be controlled by topical lactic acid preparations, menthol preparations (eg, Mentholatum, many others) or oral antihistamines. Massaging the scar will help soften it and enhance tissue pliability.

The fate of any wound as regards formation of a "good" or "bad" scar is unpredictable. It is best to advise the patient that the ultimate appearance of the scar will not be known for at least 9 months. Evaluation for possible scar revision should be delayed until after that time.

Your wound has been treated carefully by the attending physician, Dr _____. Every effort has been made to assure rapid healing. In some cases, because of the nature of the wound or other unforeseen problems, a complication might develop. If you should notice or experience any of the following danger signals, please contact our department as soon as possible (Phone: _____).

Wound Danger Signals

Persistent pain.
Sudden onset of severe pain.
Numbness or tingling of the fingertips or toes.
Fever, chills.
Bleeding from the wound.
Rapid swelling of the injured part.
Drainage from the wound.
Foul odor in dressing.
Redness surrounding the wound.
Red streaks on the arms or legs.

Figure 24–12. Sample printed list of danger signals and directions for patients being discharged from the emergency department.

6. SUTURE REMOVAL

The timing of suture removal depends upon many factors, such as location, type of wound closure, age, health, patient compliance, and presence of infection. Table 24–6 is a general guideline for suture removal in healthy adults with uncomplicated wounds. Modifications of these recommendations should be tailored to individual patients.

EMERGENCY TREATMENT OF SPECIFIC TYPES OF WOUNDS

FACIAL LACERATIONS

See Chapter 17.

Table 24–6. Timing of suture removal.

Location	Time (Days)
Eyelid	3
Cheek	3–5
Nose, forehead, neck	5
Ear, scalp	5–7
Arm, leg, hand, foot	7–10+
Chest, back, abdomen	7–10+

INTRAORAL LACERATIONS

Lacerations of the oral mucosa and tongue may not require closure if they are small. The rich blood supply promotes rapid healing, and cosmetic considerations are minimal. However, large or gaping wounds, through-and-through lacerations, and lacerations involving important deep structures, such as muscle or bone, require repair. In such wounds, after irrigation with saline, disrupted muscle should first be approximated with absorbable suture, (eg, 5-0 Vicryl) and the mucosa closed with absorbable suture (eg, 5-0 chromic gut or Vicryl). It is best to use the minimum number of sutures that will allow approximation of the wound edges.

Through-and-through lacerations of the lip merit special attention:

A. The wound should be irrigated thoroughly, inside and out. (A dry gauze roll between the lip and teeth will help prevent recontamination of the irrigated wound.)

B. The mucosal laceration is closed first with absorbable suture (eg, 5-0 chromic gut or Vicryl).

C. The wound is then reirrigated from the outside. The sutured mucosa will prevent reentry of saliva.

D. The orbicularis oris muscle, if disrupted, is approximated with absorbable suture (eg, 5-0 Vicryl).

E. The external skin is closed with interrupted sutures of 6-0 monofilament nylon. Extreme care must be taken to line up the opposing vermilion borders of the lip.

F. The adjacent teeth that produced the wound should be examined; they may be fractured or avulsed.

BLAST INJURIES

Assessment

Wounds resulting from high-velocity missiles and shotgun blasts are among the most severe encountered in civilian practice. Extensive tissue destruction is incurred locally, with loss or disruption of the wound parts to form a cavity. Sites distant from the point of impact may be injured as a result of shock waves transmitted through tissues. The extent of injury of these complex wounds is difficult to assess.

Treatment

A. Initial care is directed to hemostasis, cleansing, and minimal debridement. It is wise not to close primarily.

B. Repeated staged exploration at first presentation and then again 24 hours and 48 hours apart is used to remove necrotic or devitalized tissues.

C. Antibiotic prophylaxis is recommended. Cefazolin, 1 g intramuscularly or intravenously every 8 hours, is satisfactory.

D. The wounds are then closed secondarily, with priority given to reestablishment of bony relationships, followed by soft tissue coverage.

Disposition
Hospitalize all cases for management.

DEGLOVING INJURIES

Diagnosis
Separation of the skin and subcutaneous tissues from the underlying musculofascial planes constitutes a degloving injury. For flaps attached by a pedicle, the determinant of survival is their circulation.

Treatment
A. Grossly mangled, contaminated portions should be sharply debrided. Areas of venous congestion and demarcation should likewise be removed.

B. Areas of questionable viability are assessed with intravenous fluorescein as a marker of vascularity.

C. In extensive degloving injuries, it is often advantageous to completely remove the potentially nonviable but minimally injured parts and reapply them as free grafts after appropriate defatting and debridement.

D. For lesser injuries, the degloved segment should be cleansed, debrided, and carefully repositioned.

E. In all instances, the underlying soft tissue must be cleaned and appropriately managed.

F. The flap should then be sutured where it lies, without tension or stretching. These wounds often cannot be closed primarily.

G. A light compression dressing is employed to obliterate dead space.

H. Close monitoring of the reattached portions of the degloved skin is performed over the next 72 hours to assess tissue viability as well as infection.

I. Antimicrobial prophylaxis is helpful in preventing bacterial colonization in marginally viable flaps. Cefazolin, 1 g intravenously or intramuscularly every 8 hours, is satisfactory.

Disposition
All but trivial degloving injuries require hospitalization. Plastic surgical consultation is advisable.

AMPUTATIONS

Diagnosis
The greater the degree of ischemic injury resulting from interruption of blood flow, the less the chances for survival of the amputated part. Six hours is probably the longest time an amputated part can be deprived of its blood supply without cooling and still survive. Immediate cooling increases the tolerable ischemic time of the amputated part to 12–24 hours. This is particularly important when replantation must be delayed while the patient is transferred to a hospital where a surgical team skilled in replantation is available.

Contraindications to replantation are the presence of significant associated injuries that may be life-threatening, severe degloving or crush injuries of the amputated part, and major systemic disease.

Treatment
To ensure the most expeditious management, every emergency department should know the location of the nearest microvascular replantation center before arranging for patient transfer. Initial treatment is outlined below.

A. The amputated part should be gently cleansed of gross contaminants; dried; and placed in a clean, dry polyethylene bag. The bag is then placed in regular (wet) ice or in a refrigerator at 4 °C (about 40 °F).

B. Control hemorrhage by pressure or elevation or by tourniquet if these are not successful. The wound should be gently cleansed and covered with a sterile dressing.

C. Antimicrobial and tetanus prophylaxis should be considered in most instances. A parenteral cephalosporin is commonly employed for these purposes, eg, cefazolin, 1 g intramuscularly or intravenously every 8 hours.

D. Blood transfusion. Attention must be directed to the reestablishment of normal blood volume, as these injuries are occasionally associated with major blood loss.

Disposition
Immediately refer the patient to a facility where limb replantation can be done by experts in that procedure.

BITES

Most nonprimate mammalian bite wounds are minor, and only about 10% require suturing. The rare patient with major injuries sustained in an animal attack should be evaluated and treated as any other patient with severe trauma.

Meticulous wound care is the cornerstone of therapy for bite wounds and is the most important factor in preventing infection. The wound should be cleansed, debrided, and copiously irrigated (p 384). All bite wounds on the extremities should be treated aggressively with antibiotics and elevation and immobilization of the affected part.

Routine cultures in the absence of infection need not be obtained, since there is no useful correlation between positive cultures and wounds that later develop clinical signs of infection. If a wound yielding a positive culture does become infected, repeat cultures are likely to yield organisms different from the initial flora. Gram's stain of exudate may provide useful information about the infecting organism if it is positive; negative results on Gram-stained smears do not reliably rule out contamination.

Antimicrobial prophylaxis (Table 24–2) is recommended for all human and most cat bites but only in high-risk dog bites (below). The need for tetanus and rabies prophylaxis (Tables 24–3 and 24–4) should also be evaluated.

1. DOG BITES

Dog bites cause open wounds, often with tissue necrosis secondary to crush injury. Treat by prompt excisional debridement within 6 hours. If the extent of the wound or the length of time since injury precludes primary closure, the wounds should be irrigated, debrided, and left open or loosely sutured. Infection is unusual, and antimicrobial prophylaxis is not indicated in routine cases.

Dog bites associated with a high risk of infection are those of the hand, puncture wounds, and injuries more than 6–12 hours old. These wounds should be treated with vigorous local care and left unsutured. Antibiotic prophylaxis is recommended; a first-generation cephalosporin (eg, cephradine) or penicillinase-resistant penicillin (eg, dicloxacillin), 500 mg orally 4 times a day for 3–5 days, should be given. Low-risk bites do not require prophylactic antibiotics and may be sutured after appropriate wound care. Hospitalization is rarely indicated unless injuries are multiple or extensive or infection is present.

Infected bites should be cleansed and debrided (p 384) and the affected limb immobilized and elevated. A parenteral dose of a first-generation cephalosporin (eg, cefazolin, 1 g for adults, 8–17 mg/kg for children, intravenously or intramuscularly) should be administered in the emergency department and the patient discharged with oral antibiotics (same as those for prophylaxis, above) for 7–10 days. Patients should receive follow-up care within 1–2 days and be instructed to return earlier if their condition worsens. Patients with symptoms of sepsis should be hospitalized.

2. CAT BITES

Cat bites cause deep puncture wounds with little crush injury and are associated with a high risk of infection, mainly with *Pasteurella multocida*. Wounds caused by cat claws are considered equivalent to bites. Treatment includes local cleansing, debridement, and prophylactic antibiotics for all significant bites. Give penicillin VK, 500 mg orally in 4 divided doses for 5–7 days. Use tetracycline in patients allergic to penicillin.

Cat bite infections occurring within 24 hours are due to *P multocida* and should be treated with penicillin VK, as above. Consider parenteral administration of the first dose. Wounds becoming infected after 24 hours should be treated with a first-generation cephalosporin or penicillinase-resistant penicillin (see Dog Bites, above) for 7–10 days.

Hospitalization is rarely indicated unless infection is severe or involves the hand. Primary closure should not be performed except in low-risk, cosmetically disfiguring facial bites.

3. PRIMATE BITES

Adult human bites and bites by other higher primates are more serious than dog or cat bites. They are characterized by crush and tear injuries and are commonly located over the knuckles or the dorsum of the hand, frequently involving the tendons or joints. Inoculation of large numbers of bacteria from dental plaque also occurs. (Bites by children appear to carry a low risk of infection because of fewer mouth bacteria and less biting force.) Despite their rather innocuous initial appearance, these wounds are extremely dangerous, since they are prone to severe necrotizing infection.

Treatment & Disposition
A. Hospitalize patients with suspected tendon, joint, or cartilage involvement (eg, bites of the hand or ear) for vigorous irrigation, debridement, and parenteral antimicrobials (high-dose penicillin or clindamycin). Wounds of this type are never closed. Bites of other structures may be treated with vigorous irrigation and debridement in the emergency department, followed by antimicrobial prophylaxis (Table 24–2). The injured part should be elevated, immobilized, and checked frequently to assess the possible spread of infection. The patient should be reexamined within 6–18 hours and subsequently at 1- to 2-day intervals for a week.

B. Signs of necrotizing infection are progressive erythema, blistering, and frank necrosis. If these signs are already present at the time of initial evaluation, hospitalization is indicated for wide debridement of the involved parts and parenteral antimicrobial therapy.

PUNCTURE WOUNDS
(For needle sticks, see Fig 24–13.)

Puncture wounds are at risk of becoming infected, especially if dirty, contaminated, or containing foreign materials. Wounds associated with penetration through the soles of shoes (especially sneakers) often

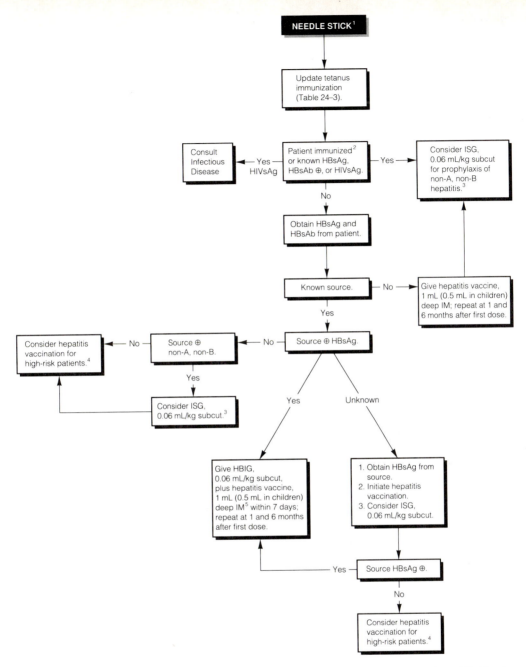

Figure 24–13. Algorithm for immunization in case of needle stick. (HBsAg = hepatitis B surface antigen; HBsAb = hepatitis B surface antibody; HIVsAg = HIV surface antigen; HBIG = hepatitis B immune globulin; ISG = immune serum globulin.)

---

[1]Needle stick wound from a needle used to flush intravenous tubing or to give medication through injection ports on intravenous tubing is at very low risk for transmission of hepatitis B infection. The wound should be cleaned and tetanus immunization updated as needed.

[2]Patients with at least 2 doses of hepatitis vaccine should have HBsAb level checked and, if low, should be treated as for nonimmunized state, with complete vaccination series. Patients (especially women) immunized via gluteal muscles should have HBsAb checked and be treated accordingly.

[3]Efficacy of ISG for prophylaxis of non-A, non-B hepatitis is uncertain.

[4]High-risk patients (HBsAg ⊕ and HBsAg⊖) include medical staff working in high-blood-exposure areas (eg, dialysis unit, emergency department, clinical and pathology laboratory, operating suite); staff of facilities for institutionalized persons; spouses of hemophiliacs and intravenous drug abusers; etc.

[5]Hepatitis vaccine should be given in the deltoid muscles, because buttock injection is associated with lower response rates, especially in women.

Note: If AIDS exposure is possible (source is an intravenous drug abuser, homosexual, transfusion recipient, etc), obtain human immunodeficiency virus (HIV) titer from source and from patient at time of exposure; if negative in patient, repeat at 3 and 6 months.

contain particles of debris and are particularly susceptible to infection. If joint capsule or bone is penetrated, septic arthritis and osteomyelitis can occur. *Pseudomonas* species are common pathogens.

All puncture wounds should be gently probed with forceps or a long (6.5-cm or 2.5-in), 22-gauge needle for the presence of foreign bodies; control pain as needed with 1% lidocaine anesthetic. Obtain soft-tissue x-rays of all wounds for which the history or mechanism of injury suggests retention of a foreign body (eg, broken glass, flying piece of metal), even if results of the wound probe are negative.

Treatment & Disposition

A. Irrigate wound with normal saline under pressure.

B. Cleanse with 1% povidone-iodine solution.

C. Probe gently and remove foreign materials. Local infiltration with 1% lidocaine and slight enlargement of the wound may be necessary for adequate exploration. Extensive dissection in the emergency department to search for small or deeply embedded objects is not recommended.

D. Ensure that tetanus prophylaxis is up to date (Table 24–3).

E. Treat dirty or deep wounds (especially those with possible joint or bone involvement) with pro-

phylactic antibiotics (adults, dicloxacillin or equivalent [erythromycin if patient is allergic to penicillin], 500 mg orally 4 times a day for 5–7 days; children, dicloxacillin, 25 mg/kg/d, erythromycin, 30–50 mg/kg/d, orally in divided doses every 6 hours). If penetration occurred through the sole of a sneaker (unless very superficial), consider prophylaxis against the high risk of *Pseudomonas* infection with antipseudomonal cephalosporin as a single parenteral dose (eg, ceftazidime, 1 g intramuscularly).

F. Instruct patients to elevate any involved extremity and, in foot injuries, to bear no weight for 3–5 days. Except in the case of superficial punctures, patients should be reexamined in 5–7 days or earlier if increased pain, redness, red streaking, or pus is noted.

G. Patients with pain persisting longer than 5–7 days or with an abnormal erythrocyte sedimentation rate may have osteomyelitis. In either case, obtain x-rays of the affected area and, if normal, consider limited bone scan of the area. Refer patients with osteomyelitis to the specialist appropriate to the area of involvement.

H. Retained foreign bodies in critical areas (eg, eye) require urgent specialty consultation. Refer patients with possible retained foreign bodies in noncritical areas for outpatient surgical removal in 2–3 weeks.

REFERENCES

Alvarez OM, Mertz PM, Eaglstein WH: The effect of occlusive dressings on collagen synthesis and re-epithelialization in superficial wounds. J Surg Res 1983;35:142.

Anderson AB et al: Local anesthesia in pediatric patients: Topical versus lidocaine. Ann Emerg Med 1990;19:519.

Bahamanyan M et al: Successful protection of humans exposed to rabies infection: Postexposure treatment with the new human diploid cell rabies vaccine and serum. JAMA 1976;236:2751.

Bartfield JM et al: Buffered versus plain lidocaine as a local anesthetic for simple lacerations.

Brand DA et al: Adequacy of antitetanus prophylaxis in six hospital emergency rooms. N Engl J Med 1983;309:636.

Callaham ML: Treatment of common dog bites: Infection risk factors. JACEP 1978;7:83.

Chact LA: Dogbite injuries in children. S Afr Med J 1975;49:718.

Chambers GH, Payne JF: Treatment of dog bite wounds. Minn Med 1969;52:427.

Collins TR, Burridge MJ: Rabies prophylaxis. Am Fam Physician (March) 1984;29:295.

Cooper WP et al: Quantitative wound cultures in upper extremity trauma. J Trauma 1982;22:112.

Dire DJ, Welsh AP: A comparison of wound irrigation solutions used in the emergency department. Ann Emerg Med 1990;19:704.

Edlich RF et al: Physical and chemical configuration of sutures in the development of surgical infection. Ann Surg 1974;177:679.

Edlich RF et al: *Technical Factors in Wound Management.* Chirurgecon, 1977. (Part of the series *Fundamentals of Wound Management in Surgery.* Dunphy JE, Hunt TK [editors].)

Finch R: Skin and soft-tissue infections. Lancet 1988;1:164.

Fitzmaurice LS et al: TAC use and absorption of cocaine in a pediatric emergency department. Ann Emerg Med 1990;19:515.

Francis CP et al: *Pasteurella multocida:* Infections after domestic animal bites and scratches. JAMA 1975;233:42.

Fraser DW: Preventing tetanus in patients with wounds. (Editorial.) Ann Intern Med 1976;84:95.

Furste W: Four keys to 100 percent success in tetanus prophylaxis. Am J Surg 1974;128:616.

Graham WP, Calabretta AM, Miller SH: Dog bites. Am Fam Physician (Jan) 1977;15:132.

Hattwick MAW et al: Postexposure rabies prophylaxis with human rabies immune globulin. JAMA 1974;227:407.

Hawkins J, Paris PM, Stewart RD: Mammalian bites: Rational approach to management. Postgrad Med (June) 1983;73:52.

Heller MB: Management of bites: Dog, cat, human and snake. Resident Staff Physician (Feb) 1982;28:75.

Henderson DK (moderator): Infectious disease emergencies: The clostridial syndrome. (Specialty conference.) West J Med 1978;129:101.

Herrmann JB: Tensile strength and knot security of surgical suture materials. Am Surg 1971;37:209.

Immunization Practices Advisory Committee, CDC: Diphtheria, tetanus, and pertussis: Guidelines for vaccine prophylaxis and other preventive measures. Ann Intern Med 1981;95:723.

Jones RC, Shires GT; Principles in the management of wounds. In: *Principles of Surgery.* Schwartz S1 (editor). McGraw-Hill, 1974.

Kilgore ES, Graham WP III: *The Hand.* Lea & Febiger, 1977.

Lindsey D, Nava C, Marti M: Effectiveness of penicillin irrigation in control of infections in sutured lacerations. J Trauma 1982;22:186.

Mertz PM, Eaglstein WH: The effect of a semiocclusive dressing on the microbial population in superficial wounds. Arch Surg 1984;119:287.

Miller A, Nathanson N: Rabies: Recent advances in pathogenesis and control. Ann Neurol 1977;2:511.

Moloney GE: The effect of human tissues on the tensile strength of implanted nylon sutures. Br J Surg 1961;68:528.

Newmeyer WL: *Primary Care of Hand Injuries.* Lea & Febiger, 1979.

Nicholson KG et al: Immunization with human diploid cell strain of rabies vaccine: Two year results. J Infect Dis 1978;137:783.

Peacock EE, Van Winkle W: *Wound Repair.* Saunders, 1976.

Postlethwait RW: Long-term comparative study of nonabsorbable sutures. Ann Surg 1970;171:892.

Poulton TJ, Miris GR: Peripheral nerve blocks. Am Fam Physician (Nov) 1977;16:100.

Recommendations of the Public Health Service Advisory Committee on Immunization Practice: Diptheria and tetanus toxoids and pertussis vaccine. MMWR (Dec 9) 1977;26:401.

Recommendations of the Public Health Service Advisory Committee on Immunization Practice: Rabies. MMWR (June 13) 1980;29:265.

Robson MC: Disturbancese in wound healing. Ann Emerg Med 1988;17:1274.

Rodeheaver GT et al: Bactericidal activity and toxicity of iodine-containing solutions in wounds. Arch Surg 1982;117:181.

Rodeheaver GT et al: Wound cleansing by high pressure irrigation. Surg Gynecol Obstet 1975;141:357.

Scher KS, Coil JA Jr: Effects of oxidized cellulose and microfibrillar collagen on infection. Surgery 1982;91:301.

Swartz MR, Kunz LJ: *Pasteurella multocida* infection in man: Report of two cases. Meningitis and infected cat bite. N Engl J Med 1959;261:889.

Weinstein L: Tetanus, N Engl J Med 1973;289:1293.

Wolcott MW: Dressings. Chap 11, p 192, in: *Ambulatory Surgery and the Basics of Emergency Surgical Care.* Wolcott MW (editor). [Formerly *Ferguson's Surgery of the Ambulatory Patient.*] Lippincott, 1981.

Wong KC, Pace NL: Anesthesia for ambulatory surgery. Chap 3, p 12, in: *Ambulatory Surgery and the Basics of Emergency Surgical Care.* Wolcott MW (editor). [Formerly *Ferguson's Surgery of the Ambulatory Patient.*] Lippincott, 1981.

Zukin DD, Simon RR: *Emergency Wound Care: Principles and Practice.* Aspen Publications, 1987.

Eye Emergencies

25

Khalid F. Tabbara, MD

I. EMERGENCY EVALUATION OF IMPORTANT OCULAR SYMPTOMS

EVALUATION OF THE RED OR PAINFUL EYE
(See algorithm, p 407, and Table 25–1.)

Rule Out Trauma

Injury from penetrating or blunt trauma or thermal or chemical burn should be obvious from the history. Management in such cases is discussed on pp 418–423.

Rule Out Foreign Body

The presence of ocular foreign body is usually suggested by the history. Persons working with high-speed tools (drilling, etc) may have a metal chip embedded in the cornea which was not noticed immediately and which presents as eye pain or redness. After inspection of the cornea, conjunctiva, and fornices for foreign bodies, fluorescein should be placed in the conjunctival sac (p 425) and the cornea examined with a slit lamp.

Rule Out Radiation Exposure Keratitis

Ask the patient about exposure to intense ultraviolet light (eg, sunlight at high altitude, sunlamps) or arc lights (eg, welders). Such exposure is highly suggestive of radiation burn. Administer a topical anesthetic, stain with fluorescein, and perform slit lamp examination; the presence of superficial punctate keratitis with corneal staining confirms the diagnosis.

Test Visual Acuity

Test corrected visual acuity using an eye chart. Significantly decreased corrected visual acuity (eg, 6/30 [20/100] in a patient who normally has 6/6

Table 25–1. Differential diagnosis of unilateral acute redness and pain of the eye not associated with trauma.[1]

History and Clinical Findings	Conjunctivitis	Iritis[2]	Acute Glaucoma	Corneal Infection (Bacterial Ulcer)	Corneal Erosion
Incidence	Extremely common.	Common.	Common.	Common.	Common.
Onset	Insidious.	Insidious.	Sudden.	Slow.	Sudden.
Vision	Normal.	Slightly blurred.	Markedly blurred.	Usually blurred.	Blurred.
Pain	None to moderate.	Moderate.	Severe.	Moderate to severe.	Severe.
Photophobia	None to mild.	Severe.	Minimal.	Variable.	Moderate.
Nausea and vomiting	None.	None.	Occasional.	None.	None.
Discharge	Moderate to copious.	None.	None.	Watery.	Watery.
Ciliary injection	Absent.	Present; circumcorneal.	Present.	Present.	Present.
Conjunctival injection	Severe; diffuse in fornices.	Minimal.	Minimal, diffuse.	Moderate, diffuse.	Mild to moderate.
Cornea	Clear.	Usually clear.	Steamy.	Locally hazy.	Hazy.
Stain with fluorescein	Absent.	Absent.	Absent.	Present.	Present.
Hypopyon	Absent.	Occasional.	Absent.	Occasional.	Absent.
Pupil size	Normal.	Constricted.	Middilated, fixed, and irregular.	Normal.	Normal or constricted.
Intraocular pressure	Normal.	Normal.	Elevated.	Normal.	Normal.
Gram-stained smear	Variable; depending on cause.	No organisms.	No organisms.	Organisms in scrapings from ulcers.	No organisms.
Pupillary light response	Normal.	Poor.	None.	Normal.	Poor to normal.

[1]The most helpful findings are shaded.
[2]Acute anterior uveitis.

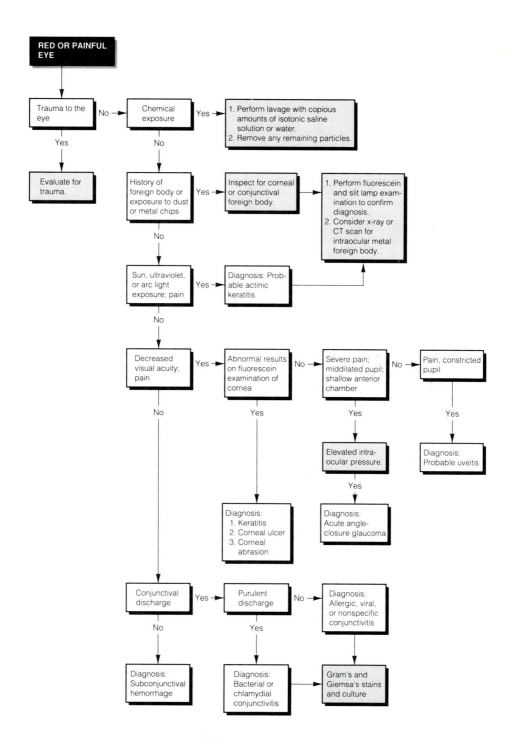

RED OR PAINFUL EYE

Trauma to the eye — No → Chemical exposure — Yes → 1. Perform lavage with copious amounts of isotonic saline solution or water.
2. Remove any remaining particles.

Yes ↓

Evaluate for trauma.

Chemical exposure — No ↓

History of foreign body or exposure to dust or metal chips — Yes → Inspect for corneal or conjunctival foreign body. → 1. Perform fluorescein and slit lamp examination to confirm diagnosis.
2. Consider x-ray or CT scan for intraocular metal foreign body.

No ↓

Sun, ultraviolet, or arc light exposure; pain — Yes → Diagnosis: Probable actinic keratitis

No ↓

Decreased visual acuity; pain — Yes → Abnormal results on fluorescein examination of cornea — No → Severe pain; middilated pupil; shallow anterior chamber — No → Pain, constricted pupil

Yes ↓ (Abnormal results)

Diagnosis:
1. Keratitis
2. Corneal ulcer
3. Corneal abrasion

Yes ↓ (Severe pain)

Elevated intra-ocular pressure.

Yes ↓

Diagnosis: Acute angle-closure glaucoma

Yes ↓ (Pain, constricted pupil)

Diagnosis: Probable uveitis

No ↓ (Decreased visual acuity)

Conjunctival discharge — Yes → Purulent discharge — No → Diagnosis: Allergic, viral, or nonspecific conjunctivitis

No ↓ (Conjunctival discharge)

Diagnosis: Subconjunctival hemorrhage

Yes ↓ (Purulent discharge)

Diagnosis: Bacterial or chlamydial conjunctivitis → Gram's and Giemsa's stains and culture

[20/20] vision) generally indicates disease of the eyeball or visual pathway. Rarely, individuals with severe bacterial conjunctivitis have slightly decreased visual acuity.

Look for Eye Pain or Redness With Decreased Visual Acuity

The principal differential diagnoses of decreased visual acuity with pain are corneal disease (ulcers, abrasions, erosions, keratitis), acute angle-closure glaucoma, and iritis. The main differentiating manifestations are listed in Table 25–1. Corneal disease may be diagnosed by slit lamp examination after staining with fluorescein. In **angle-closure glaucoma,** the cornea may be cloudy and the pupil is in the mid position or dilated, often irregular in shape, and displaced anteriorly (ie, shallow anterior chamber). There is severe eye pain. In **iritis,** the pupil is constricted and nondisplaced; pain is moderate.

Look for Subconjunctival Hemorrhage

Subconjunctival hemorrhage is often precipitated by violent coughing or vomiting; rarely, it may indicate systemic coagulopathy or systemic hypertension. The eye is not painful, and there is no conjunctival discharge. The palpebral conjunctiva is normal or minimally inflamed; there is blood under the bulbar conjunctiva.

Conjunctivitis

If there is conjunctival discharge and erythema, conjunctivitis is present. The clinical features of different types of conjunctivitis are set forth in Table 25–2. Bacterial conjunctivitis is generally characterized by moderate irritation ("scratchiness," "sand in the eye") and marked conjunctival hyperemia. There is a purulent discharge, which on the Gram-stained smear shows abundant polymorphonuclear neutrophil leukocytes (PMNs) and usually bacteria.

Disposition

Patients thought to have ocular conditions that may permanently decrease visual acuity (eg, acute angle-closure glaucoma) should be hospitalized. Patients with other conditions may be treated and discharged if close follow-up evaluation is ensured.

EVALUATION OF ACUTE UNILATERAL VISUAL LOSS
(See algorithm, p 409.)

Look for Trauma

Exclude trauma as a cause of visual loss. Both blunt and penetrating ocular injuries may result in blindness.

History & Examination

Obtain a history from the patient (rate of onset of visual loss; unilateral or bilateral; painful or painless; with or without redness). Ophthalmologic examination should emphasize visual acuity and visual field testing.

A. Inability to Visualize Retina: Cloudy media will completely obscure the retina (red reflex absent) or will make it impossible to visualize retinal landmarks such as the optic disk. Chronic causes of hazy media are common (eg, cataracts) and should not be confused with whatever is causing acute visual loss.

B. Abnormal Visual Fields: Grossly abnormal visual fields are usually caused by central nervous system disease and thus generally affect both eyes (not always to the same degree). The retinas are usually normal on ophthalmoscopic examination.

1. Hemianopia–Hemianopia is usually due to postchiasmal neurologic disorders, in which case

Table 25–2. Differential diagnosis of conjunctivitis.

Clinical Features	Bacterial	Chlamydial	Viral	Allergic	Irritant
Onset	Acute.	Acute or subacute.	Acute or subacute.	Recurrent.	Acute.
Pain	Moderate.	Mild to moderate.	Mild to moderate.	None.	None to mild.
Discharge	Copious, purulent.	Moderate, purulent.	Moderate, seropurulent.	Moderate, clear.	Minimal, clear.
Gram-stained smear	PMNs, bacteria.	PMNs, monocytes, no bacteria.	PMNs, monocytes, no bacteria.	Eosinophils present.	Negative.
Routine culture	Usually *Staphylococcus aureus,* pneumococci.	Negative.	Negative.	Negative.	Negative.
Special culture	. . .	*Chlamydia.*	Adenoviruses; occasionally enteroviruses; rarely others.	Negative.	Negative.
Preauricular adenopathy	Common.	Common.	Common.	No.	Rare.

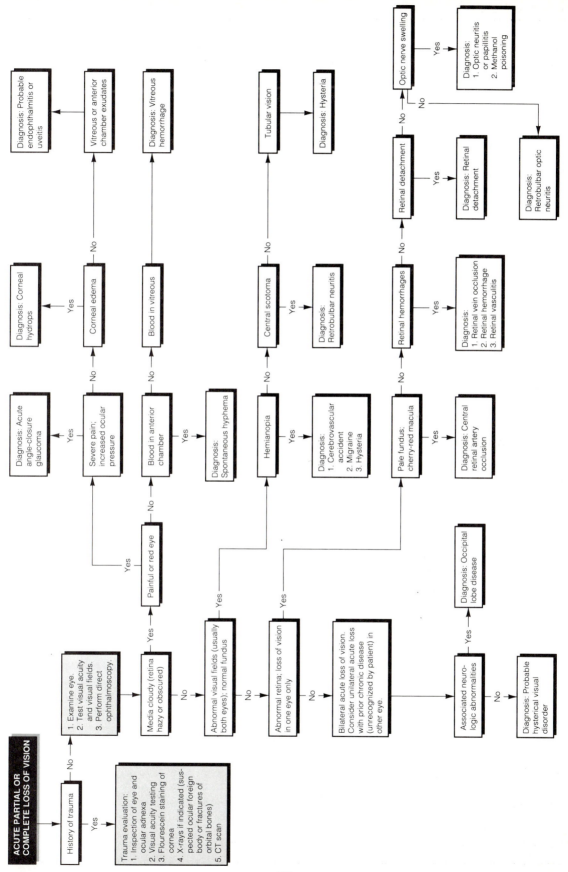

other acute neurologic lesions are present as well. Rarely, it is hysterical in origin.

2. Central scotoma–A central scotoma indicates isolated macular involvement typical of retrobulbar neuritis and may or may not be associated with pain.

3. Tubular vision–Tubular vision not in conformity with the laws of optics is characteristic of hysteria.

C. Abnormal Retina: An abnormal retina, usually in the one eye with visual loss, is characteristic of several rare conditions with serious import.

1. Central retinal artery occlusion–In central retinal artery occlusion, the fundus is usually pale with a cherry-red fovea. *This is a therapeutic emergency!* (See below.)

2. Central retinal vein occlusion–Central retinal vein occlusion is associated with multiple widespread retinal hemorrhages.

3. Retinal hemorrhage–Retinal hemorrhage from other causes (eg, anticoagulation) may produce visual loss.

4. Retinal detachment–Retinal detachment produces visual loss preceded by visual flashes. If visual acuity is affected, detachment is large and easily visible on direct ophthalmoscopy; however, small detachments may require indirect ophthalmoscopy for visualization. Flashes of light may also occur in patients with migraine or as a result of posterior vitreous detachment.

Differential Diagnosis

Causes of acute visual loss are listed below and discussed on subsequent pages.

A. Acute Angle-Closure Glaucoma: Acute angle-closure glaucoma causes corneal edema, but the more striking findings are eye pain; pupils fixed in mid position or dilated, often with irregular margins; a shallow anterior chamber angle (Fig 25–1); and greatly increased intraocular pressure. *Acute angle-closure glaucoma is a medical emergency!* (See below.)

B. Corneal Edema: Severe corneal edema of diverse causes (abrasion, keratitis, etc) may cause visual loss with eye pain.

C. Hyphema: Hyphema will show blood in the anterior chamber on inspection.

D. Vitreous Hemorrhage: Vitreous hemorrhage causes painless visual loss, which is often total. The anterior chamber is clear. The red reflex is often absent.

E. Endophthalmitis: Endophthalmitis (intraocular infection) is a rare condition usually associated with eye pain and decreased visual acuity. Eye examination will disclose pus in the anterior chamber or vitreous.

Disposition

All patients with sudden visual loss due to ocular disease should be seen by an ophthalmologist before being discharged from the emergency department.

II. OCULAR CONDITIONS REQUIRING IMMEDIATE TREATMENT

ACUTE ANGLE-CLOSURE GLAUCOMA

Acute angle-closure glaucoma results from sudden increase in intraocular pressure owing to blockage of

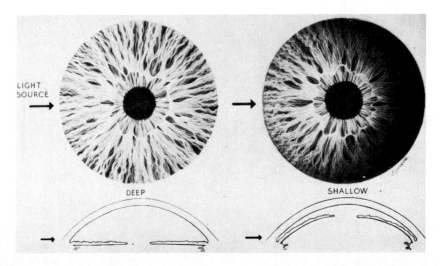

Figure 25–1. Estimation of depth of anterior chamber by oblique illumination. (Courtesy of R Shaffer.) (Reproduced, with permission, from Vaughan D, Asbury T, Tabbara KF: *General Ophthalmology,* 12th ed. Appleton & Lange, 1989.)

the outflow channels in the anterior chamber angle by the iris root. The sudden rise in intraocular pressure causes intraocular vascular insufficiency, which may lead to optic nerve or retinal ischemia. If the acute attack of angle-closure glaucoma is not managed promptly, permanent loss of vision may result.

Diagnosis

Acute angle-closure glaucoma is characterized by severe pain, halos around lights, blurred vision, photophobia, and nausea and vomiting. The affected eye is red, with a nonreactive middilated pupil (often with irregular margins), a hazy cornea, and a shallow anterior chamber angle. Intraocular pressure is usually markedly increased (see below for the technique of Schiotz tonometry). The patient may have hyperopia (farsightedness).

Differential Diagnosis
(See algorithm, p 409, and
Table 25–1.)

In **iridocyclitis,** intraocular pressure is normal and the pupil is small and constricted. In **conjunctivitis,** intraocular pressure is normal and the pupil is not affected. **Corneal ulcer** is diagnosed by fluorescein staining of the cornea.

Treatment

A. *Acute angle-closure glaucoma is an emergency!* Failure to provide prompt treatment may result in permanent blindness. Hospitalize the patient, and obtain ophthalmologic consultation for management on an urgent basis.

B. Reduce the intraocular pressure medically before surgery by one or more of the following means:

1. Glycerin, 1 g/kg body weight orally, in cold 50% solution mixed with chilled lemon juice.

2. Pilocarpine, 1–2% eye drops, 2 drops every 15 minutes for 2–3 hours.

3. Mannitol, 20%, 250–500 mL intravenously over 2–3 hours.

4. Acetazolamide, 500 mg orally or 250 mg intravenously.

C. Give sedation and analgesics as necessary to control pain and agitation.

Disposition

Acute angle-closure glaucoma calls for urgent referral to an ophthalmologist and hospitalization for initial medical treatment, followed by either surgery or laser therapy. Patients should undergo a peripheral iridectomy or laser iridotomy.

OCCLUSION OF CENTRAL
RETINAL ARTERY

Central retinal artery occlusion is most commonly embolic in origin (eg, carotid artery plaque, endocar-

dial vegetation). The retina is completely without blood as long as the artery is occluded, and visual receptors in the retina will degenerate within 30–60 minutes if blood flow is not restored.

Diagnosis

There is a typical history of sudden, complete, painless loss of vision in one eye, usually in an older person. Ophthalmoscopic examination discloses pallor of the optic disk, edema of the retina, cherry-red fovea, bloodless constricted arterioles that may be difficult to detect, and "boxcar" segmentation of blood in the retinal veins.

Treatment

Central retinal artery occlusion is an emergency! Note: If occlusion has persisted for over 1 hour without treatment, vision has most likely been permanently lost, and therapeutic measures will no longer be effective.

A. Surgical Decompression: *Note:* This procedure should be performed by an ophthalmologist. Within 30–60 minutes after onset (and after topical anesthesia), an anterior chamber paracentesis is performed with a 25- or 27-gauge needle attached to a 1-mL syringe. The needle is introduced at the limbus temporally and pointed toward 6 o'clock into the anterior chamber. The needle is kept parallel to the iris to avoid injury to the lens. Finally, 0.25 mL of anterior chamber fluid (aqueous) is aspirated and the needle removed.

B. Anticoagulants: There are some favorable reports on the use of anticoagulants in cases of partial occlusion of the central retinal artery or its branches. Give heparin, 10,000 units intravenously immediately; continue as needed (Chapter 33).

C. Other Measures: Gentle ocular massage may be performed. Rebreathing into an airtight bag may also be helpful in lowering blood pH and making patients less alkalotic. tPA may be given intravenously within 60 minutes after onset.

Disposition

All patients should be hospitalized on an urgent basis for treatment by an ophthalmologist.

ORBITAL CELLULITIS

Acute infection of the orbital tissues is commonly caused by *Streptococcus pneumoniae,* other streptococci, *Staphylococcus aureus,* and (chiefly in children) *Haemophilus influenzae.* Less frequently, certain fungi of the Phycomycetes group may cause orbital infections in diabetic patients (rhino-orbito-cerebral mucormycosis). Most causative organisms enter the orbit by direct extension from the paranasal sinuses (especially through the lamina papyracea of the ethmoid sinus) or through the vascular channels draining the periorbital tissues. Rarely, infection may spread to the cavernous sinus or meninges.

Diagnosis

There is a history of sinusitis or periorbital injury, pain in and around the eye, and sometimes reduced visual acuity. Examination discloses swelling and redness of the eyelids and periorbital tissues, chemosis of the conjunctiva, exophthalmos of varying degrees, and limitation of movement of the eye in all fields of gaze. Disk margins may be blurred, and fever is commonly present. There may be x-ray evidence of sinusitis. CT scan shows soft tissue orbital infiltration. The white cell count is elevated.

Differential Diagnosis

Orbital cellulitis must be differentiated from cavernous sinus thrombosis; the 2 diseases may occur together. Disorders not associated with periorbital cellulitis that must be differentiated include pseudotumor of the orbit, thyroid disease, and rhabdomyosarcoma (in children) or other tumors of the orbit.

Invasive infection due to fungi of the Phycomycetes group (*Mucor, Rhizopus,* and other genera) may present as rapidly progressive orbital cellulitis, often with cavernous sinus thrombosis as well. Consider this possibility if the patient is acidotic (diabetic ketoacidosis or renal failure) or immunosuppressed; examination often reveals coexisting maxillary sinusitis and palatal or nasal mucosal ulceration.

Treatment & Disposition

Obtain cultures of blood and periorbital tissue fluid. Begin cefuroxime, 100 mg/kg/d intravenously in 3 divided doses. Obtain urgent ophthalmologic consultation. All patients with orbital cellulitis should be hospitalized. CT scan of the orbit is obtained to rule out orbital abscess and intracranial involvement. Patients with orbital phycomycosis are given intravenous amphotericin B and may require surgical intervention for debridement of infected tissue. Neurosurgical consultation is required to rule out intracranial involvement.

CAVERNOUS SINUS THROMBOSIS

Cavernous sinus thrombosis is usually associated with orbital and ocular signs and symptoms. The disease results from hematogenous spread of infection from a distant focus or from extension from a throat, facial, paranasal sinus, or orbital infection. Cavernous sinus thrombosis starts as a unilateral infection and commonly spreads to involve the other cavernous sinus.

Diagnosis

The patient complains of chills, headache, lethargy, nausea, pain, and decreased vision. Fever, vomiting, and other systemic signs of infection are present. Ophthalmologic examination discloses unilateral or bilateral exophthalmos, absent pupillary reflexes, and papilledema. Involvement of the third, fourth, and sixth cranial nerves or of the ophthalmic branch of the fifth nerve leads to limitation of ocular involvement and decrease in corneal sensation.

Treatment & Disposition

A. Hospitalize the patient immediately, and send blood to the laboratory for culture and sensitivity studies. Ophthalmologic, neurologic, and medical consultation should be sought early. Obtain CT scan of the head and orbit.

B. Start an intravenous infusion of 5% dextrose in water for use in administering antibiotics by the intravenous route.

C. Start nafcillin, 200 mg/kg/d intravenously, in divided doses every 4 hours.

ENDOPHTHALMITIS

Endophthalmitis is acute microbial infection confined within the globe. Infection involving the sclera as well as other intraocular structures is called **panophthalmitis.** Infections of the globe can be exogenous or endogenous. Exogenous infection results from penetrating injury or may follow intraocular surgery or a ruptured corneal ulcer. Endogenous infection by the hematogenous route is less common and may be accompanied by fever and chills.

Diagnosis

The patient complains of pain, blurred vision, and photophobia. Examination discloses redness of the eye, chemosis of the conjunctiva, swelling of the eyelid, hypopyon (pus in the anterior chamber), and cloudy media (fundus hazily seen, or absent red reflex).

Treatment & Disposition

A. Hospitalize the patient immediately, and send blood (2 specimens) for culture and sensitivity studies. Urgent ophthalmologic consultation should be obtained. Give sedation and analgesics.

B. Start an intravenous infusion of 5% dextrose in half-normal saline for possible use in administering antibiotics by the intravenous route.

C. Apply an eye patch, and cover the eye. The patient may have to undergo anterior chamber tap and vitreous aspiration (by an ophthalmologist). Send specimens thus obtained for staining with Giemsa's and Gram's stains and for cultures on appropriate media.

D. Check stained smears of ocular fluid, and if no organisms are seen, give empiric subconjunctival and systemic antibiotics while results of culture are pending. Give methicillin, 100 mg; and gentamicin, 30 mg, both subconjunctivally (by an ophthalmologist); as well as nafcillin or oxacillin, 200 mg/kg/d in divided doses every 4 hours; and gentamicin, 5 mg/kg/d in divided doses every 8 hours.

RETINAL DETACHMENT

Detachment of the retina is actually separation of the neurosensory layer from the retinal pigment epithelium. Subretinal fluid accumulates under the neurosensory layer. Detachment may become bilateral in one-fourth of cases. Retinal detachment is more common in older people and in those who are highly myopic or aphakic. Hereditary factors may also play a role. Three types of primary retinal detachment are recognized: (1) rhegmatogenous detachment, from retinal holes or breaks; (2) exudative detachment, usually from inflammation; and (3) traction detachment, which occurs when vitreous bands pull on the retina. Minimal to moderate trauma to the eye may cause retinal detachment, but in such cases predisposing factors such as changes in the vitreous, retina, and choroid play an important role in pathogenesis. Severe trauma may cause retinal tears and detachment even if there are no predisposing factors.

Diagnosis

The patient complains of painless decrease in vision and may give a history of flashes of lights or sparks. Loss of vision may be described as a curtain in front of the eye or as cloudy or smoky. Central vision may not be affected if the macular area is not involved; this frequently causes a delay in seeking treatment. Patients in whom the macula is detached present to the emergency department with sudden deterioration of vision.

Intraocular pressure is normal or low as measured by Schiotz tonometry. The detached retina appears gray, with white folds and globular bullae. Round holes or horseshoe-shaped tears may be seen by indirect ophthalmoscopy in rhegmatogenous detachment. Vitreous bands or other changes may be seen in the traction type of detachment.

Differential Diagnosis

Primary retinal detachment should be differentiated from detachment secondary to other causes, eg, preeclampsia-eclampsia or tumors of the choroid.

Treatment & Disposition

The patient should be hospitalized at bed rest with both eyes patched. Early referral to an ophthalmologist should be arranged. If the macula is attached and central visual acuity is normal, the condition should be urgently treated by an ophthalmologist.

Retinal reattachment can only be accomplished by surgery, which is successful in about 80% of cases. If the macula is detached or threatened, operation should be scheduled on an urgent basis, since prolonged detachment of the macula results in permanent loss of central vision.

TOXIC CAUSES OF BLINDNESS

A wide variety of organic chemicals may lead to visual deterioration. Ingestion of chemicals that cause corneal or lenticular opacities usually leads to insidious onset of visual loss. Ingestion of compounds that cause damage to nervous tissue may lead to slow or rapid deterioration of vision. Exposure to toxic doses of methanol, halogenated hydrocarbons (eg, methyl chloride), arsenic, and lead may cause permanent visual damage. Acute or chronic administration of drugs such as ethambutol, Chloramphenicol, quinine, and salicylates may also cause optic neuritis and loss of vision.

Methanol Poisoning

By far the most common toxic cause of blindness is methanol (methyl alcohol). Ingestion of only a few milliliters may cause permanent blindness. Acute methanol poisoning causes nausea and vomiting and abdominal pain. Headache, dizziness, and delirium may occur. Loss of vision may be complete and sudden a few hours after drinking methanol or may occasionally be noted about 3 days after exposure. Pupillary reflexes are sluggish. Ophthalmoscopic examination shows swelling and hyperemia of the optic nerve head, distention of the veins, and peripapillary edema of the retina.

Hospitalize the patient immediately; see Chapter 39 for details of evaluation and treatment.

III. OTHER NONTRAUMATIC OCULAR EMERGENCIES

ACUTE DACRYOCYSTITIS

Acute infection of the lacrimal sac occurs in children as well as adults as a complication of nasolacrimal duct obstruction. The most frequently encountered causative organism is *S pneumoniae.*

Diagnosis

The patient complains of pain. There may be a history of tearing and discharge. Examination discloses swelling, redness, and tenderness over the lacrimal sac (Fig 25–2). The swelling is more prominent below the medial palpebral ligament.

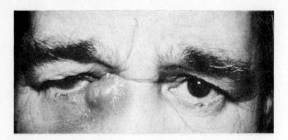

Figure 25–2. Acute dacryocystitis. (Reproduced, with permission, from Vaughan D, Asbury T, Tabbara KF: *General Ophthalmology*, 12th ed. Appleton & Lange, 1989.)

Pus should be collected by pressure applied over the lacrimal sac for Gram-stained smear and culture.

Treatment
A. Prescribe warm compresses 3–4 times daily.

B. Begin systemic antibiotic therapy with cefaclor or other first-generation cephalosporin, 20–25 mg/kg/d orally in 3–4 divided doses, until culture results are reported. Results of Gram-stained smears of purulent exudate may be helpful in guiding empiric therapy. Topical sulfacetamide, 10% eye drops, may be given every 2 hours, and erythromycin ophthalmic ointment, 0.5% (5 mg/g), at bedtime.

C. Massage of the nasolacrimal sac to express purulent discharge through the punctum is helpful in infants. The technique is to apply pressure over the lacrimal sac with a cotton-tipped stick (Q-Tip). Irrigation of the lacrimal sac with diluted antibiotics should be done by an ophthalmologist.

Disposition
The patient can be discharged to home care with a prescription for systemic antibiotics and instruction in how to apply warm local compresses. An ophthalmologist should be consulted for consideration of surgical correction. The patient should be seen again within 3–4 days.

ACUTE DACRYOADENITIS

Diagnosis
Infection and inflammation of the lacrimal gland is characterized by swelling, pain and tenderness, and redness over the upper temporal aspect of the upper eyelid.

Differential Diagnosis
Acute dacryoadenitis must be differentiated from viral infection (mumps), sarcoidosis, Sjögren's syndrome, tumors, leukemia, and lymphoma.

Treatment
Purulent bacterial infections should be treated in

the emergency department by incision and drainage of localized pus collections, antibiotics (eg, cefaclor, 20–25 mg/kg/d orally in 3–4 divided doses), topical warm compresses, and systemic analgesics.

Viral dacryoadenitis (mumps) is treated conservatively.

Disposition
The patient should be referred to an ophthalmologist for follow-up care.

ACUTE HORDEOLUM
(Sty)

Acute hordeolum is a common infection of the lid glands: the meibomian glands (internal hordeolum) and the glands of Zeis or Moll (external hordeolum). The most frequent causative organism is *S aureus.*

Diagnosis
Sty is characterized by pain and redness with variable swelling over the eyelid. A large hordeolum may rarely be associated with swelling of the preauricular lymph node on the affected side, fever, and leukocytosis.

Treatment
If pus is localized and pointing out to the skin or conjunctiva, a horizontal incision is made through the skin or a vertical incision through the conjunctiva. (This procedure should be performed by an ophthalmologist.)

Disposition
The patient can be discharged to continue treatment with warm compresses 3 times daily and topical antibiotic ointment (erythromycin or tetracycline) twice daily at home.

SPONTANEOUS SUBCONJUNCTIVAL HEMORRHAGE

Rupture of conjunctival or episcleral blood vessels may occur spontaneously or in association with minimal trauma, violent coughing, or retching. The possibility of blood dyscrasias and systemic hypertension must be investigated in recurrent subconjunctival hemorrhage.

Diagnosis
The conjunctiva suddenly becomes bright red in blotchy distribution. There is no pain, and vision is not affected. Severe cases may be characterized by chemosis and subconjunctival accumulation of blood clots. Check for hypertension, and obtain a complete blood count (CBC) with differential and coagulation panel (prothrombin time, partial thromboplastin time,

and platelet count) if hemorrhage recurs or if there is any other evidence of bleeding diathesis.

Treatment & Disposition

Treat with cold compresses within the first 12 hours after onset; later, with warm compresses for 10–15 minutes 3 times daily.

The patient can be discharged to private care or a clinic and should be seen within 2–3 days for follow-up examination and care if needed.

CONJUNCTIVITIS

Conjunctivitis is a frequent cause of red eye. It should be dealt with as an urgent medical problem until it is certain that the process is under control.

Causes of Acute Conjunctivitis

A. Infection: Bacterial, viral, parasitic, fungal, chlamydial.

B. Chemical Irritation: Chlorine gas, tear gas.

C. Allergy: Vernal keratoconjunctivitis, hay fever.

D. Skin Disorders: Stevens-Johnson syndrome, acne rosacea, Lyell's disease, Kawasaki's disease, psoriasis.

E. Systemic Disorders: Sjögren's syndrome, vitamin A deficiency.

Diagnosis
(See Table 25–2.)

The patient complains of a "scratchy" sensation or pain, with conjunctival discharge. One or both eyes may be affected. Adherence of the eyelids upon awakening is common in bacterial conjunctivitis.

Examination discloses conjunctival hyperemia, purulent or mucopurulent discharge, and variable degrees of lid swelling. Material should be taken from the conjunctival sac for smear (Gram's and Giemsa's stains) and for culture on blood and chocolate agar. Viral cultures may also be indicated.

Treatment

A. Instill topical decongestants (eg, phenylephrine, 1%; naphazoline, 0.1%), 1 drop in each eye 3–4 times daily.

B. Until laboratory reports are received, prescribe topical sulfacetamide, 10% eye drops, or ciprofloxacin, 0.3% eyedrops (an alternative to ciprofloxacin is ofloxacin), 4 times daily; and erythromycin or tetracycline ophthalmic ointment at bedtime for suspected bacterial conjunctivitis.

C. For suspected chlamydial infection (eg, history of urethritis), prescribe topical and systemic tetracycline or erythromycin. Give 0.5 g 4 times a day for 21 days (adult dose). Doxycycline, 100 mg twice a day, may be substituted for tetracycline.

Disposition

Discharge to home care with instructions to return in a few days. Patients who do not respond to treatment should be referred to an ophthalmologist.

BACTERIAL CORNEAL ULCER

Corneal infections may be due to bacteria, viruses, chlamydiae, or fungi. The conjunctiva may or may not be involved. Bacterial corneal ulcers are especially serious, since rapid perforation of the cornea and loss of aqueous humor may occur; bacterial endophthalmitis may occur if bacterial ulcers are not properly treated.

Diagnosis of Bacterial
Corneal Ulcers

The patient complains of pain and photophobia, blurring of vision, and eye irritation. Examination discloses conjunctival hyperemia and chemosis, corneal ulceration, or whitish-yellowish infiltration. The examination is facilitated by fluorescein staining and inspection with ultraviolet light. Hypopyon (pus in the anterior chamber) may be present. Scrapings from the cornea should be taken for culture and staining with Gram's and Giemsa's stains.

Differential Diagnosis

See Table 25–1.

Treatment

Management of bacterial corneal infections causing corneal ulcers must be instituted as early as possible until laboratory reports are received.

A. Treat gram-negative bacillary infection with topical gentamicin, 15 mg/mL fortified eye drops, instilled half-hourly during the day and every 2 hours during the night; and with gentamicin ointment, 3 times daily. An alternative antibiotic is topical ciprofloxacin.

B. Treat infection caused by gram-positive cocci every half hour with alternating doses of topical fortified gentamicin, 15 mg/mL, and topical fortified cefazolin, 50 mg/mL.

C. Specific antibiotics should be injected subconjunctivally (by an ophthalmologist) when the results of bacteriologic examinations are available.

D. Specific antibiotic therapy should be given whenever the causative agent is identified.

Disposition

If possible, the patient should be seen by an ophthalmologist before discharge from the emergency department. Hospitalization may be necessary, especially if hypopyon is present.

VIRAL KERATOCONJUNCTIVITIS

Viral keratoconjunctivitis is an acute conjunctivitis and keratitis caused most frequently by adenovirus (types 8 and 19).

Diagnosis

The patient complains of redness of the eye associated with tearing and moderate pain. The onset is often in one eye only, and this eye is more severely affected. Sensitivity to light (photophobia) may be noted 5–14 days after onset. Examination discloses swelling of the eyelids and bulbar conjunctival hyperemia, with follicles noted over the palpebral conjunctiva. A pseudomembrane may be noted over the palpebral conjunctiva. A tender preauricular lymph node can be palpated. Subconjunctival hemorrhage may occur within 48 hours. Corneal epithelial keratitis accompanies the conjunctivitis, but subepithelial opacities are not seen until 5–14 days after onset of symptoms.

In adults, the disease is confined to the external eye. Children may have fever, pharyngitis, and diarrhea (pharyngoconjunctival fever). Staining of conjunctival scrapings with Giemsa's stain demonstrates a predominantly mononuclear inflammatory reaction. When pseudomembranes occur, PMNs may be seen. Culture for adenovirus is usually positive in the first 2 weeks after onset. Chlamydial conjunctivitis should always be considered in the differential diagnosis.

Treatment

Treatment is symptomatic. Topical decongestants such as naphazoline, 0.1%, may be helpful. Dark glasses may relieve photophobia. If the diagnosis is uncertain, send material for culture for bacteria, and start sulfacetamide, 10% eye drops, 4 times daily; and tetracycline, 1% (10 mg/g) ointment twice daily, while awaiting laboratory results.

Since epidemics have been caused by spread of the viral agent by physicians and nurses, handwashing between examinations and complete sterilization of tonometer footplates are mandatory preventive measures.

Disposition

The patient should be discharged with instructions to seek a medical appointment in 2–3 days. Patients should take care to avoid spread of virus from ocular secretions to other family members, and they should preferably stay home from work for a few days to avoid spread of infection.

ACUTE HYDROPS OF THE CORNEA

Acute hydrops of the cornea may occur in patients with keratoconus who develop rupture of Descemet's membrane, with resulting infiltration of the corneal stroma by aqueous humor. This may occur suddenly, resulting in corneal clouding.

Diagnosis

The typical presentation is of sudden, painless, marked decrease in visual acuity in a patient with keratoconus. There may be mild eye irritation, and the cornea is cloudy as a result of corneal edema. The patient usually has keratoconus in the other eye. Bacterial or viral keratitis must be ruled out.

Treatment

A. Hypertonic eye drops, eg, sodium chloride, 2% or 5% solution, should be instilled 4 times daily for 1 week.

B. Apply a stream of hot air twice daily by hair dryer to speed dehydration of the cornea.

C. Patch the eye when there are epithelial defects.

Disposition

Refer the patient to an ophthalmologist within a few days.

HYPHEMA

Hyphema (blood in the anterior chamber) is usually caused by nonperforating trauma to the eye. In rare instances, hyphema may occur spontaneously as a complication of an ocular or systemic disorder.

Diagnosis

Hyphema is characterized by sudden decrease in visual acuity. If the intraocular pressure is elevated, there may be pain in the eye with or without headache.

The whole anterior chamber may be filled with blood, or a blood level may be seen. The conjunctiva is hyperemic with perilimbal injection.

Treatment

A. Elevate the patient's head 60 degrees.

B. Sedate the patient, and cover both eyes.

C. If intraocular pressure is elevated, give acetazolamide, 250 mg orally every 6 hours; or other carbonic anhydrase inhibitors (eg, methazolamide, 50 mg orally 2–3 times a day).

D. Intravenous mannitol, 20%, 250–500 mL over 2–3 hours, should be given if hyphema is total (filling the anterior chamber).

E. Recently, intracameral injection (performed by an ophthalmologist) of 25 μg of tPA has been shown to expedite the resorption of blood clots in the anterior chamber.

Disposition

Acute care by an ophthalmologist, including examination of the optic nerve head, is essential. The patient should be admitted to the hospital and examined daily.

Operative evacuation of nonabsorbed blood clots may be required. Recurrence of bleeding on the third to fifth days following injury is not uncommon.

UVEITIS
(Iritis & Iridocyclitis)

The uvea consists of the iris, ciliary body, and choroid. Anterior uveitis is inflammation of the iris and ciliary body, or iridocyclitis. Inflammation of all 3 structures is called panuveitis.

Diagnosis
(See Table 25–1.)

The patient complains of blurred vision, photophobia, and headache or ocular pain. Ciliary injection may be present around the limbus, and conjunctival injection may be minimal. Intraocular pressure may be elevated. There is no conjunctival discharge.

Treatment

A. Instill prednisolone acetate, 1% eye drops, 5 times daily. More frequent applications may be required in certain severe cases of anterior uveitis.

B. Instill a cycloplegic mydriatic agent, such as tropicamide or cyclopentolate, 1% eye drops, 1 drop every 10 minutes 4 times (the effect persists for 24 hours).

C. If intraocular pressure is elevated, give acetazolamide, 250 mg orally every 6 hours.

Disposition

Patients with uveitis should be seen the next day for follow-up care. Continuing care should be by an ophthalmologist. The cause of uveitis should be investigated.

VITREOUS HEMORRHAGE

Spontaneous hemorrhage into the vitreous body may result from local factors in the eye (eg, retinal tears, tumors, inflammation, venous occlusion, retinal detachment) or from associated systemic disorders (eg, hematopoietic diseases, diabetes mellitus, hypertension) (Table 25–3). Blood in the vitreous body clots rapidly, and removal of red blood cells is retarded because of the network of collagen fibers and hyaluronic acid.

Diagnosis

Vitreous hemorrhage is characterized by sudden, painless loss or deterioration of vision in the affected eye. The eye is not red. The red reflex of the fundus is hazy or faint or becomes black. Details of the retina and optic nerve are obscured by the cloudy vitreous.

Treatment & Disposition

A. The patient should be hospitalized at bed rest with both eyes patched and the head elevated 45 degrees.

B. An ophthalmologist should investigate the cause of vitreous hemorrhage. Partial or total vitrectomy may have to be considered later if absorption of blood does not occur or if vitreous clouding occurs secondary to organization of the blood clot. Photocoagulation of the neovascular network (ie, new blood vessel formation, as occurs in diabetic or sickle cell retinopathy), when present, may be considered in some cases as a prophylactic measure.

C. Recent studies have shown that intravitreal injection of 25 µg of tPA may be considered in selected patients with traumatic vitreous hemorrhage.

RETINAL HEMORRHAGE

Retinal hemorrhage may be due to trauma, local ocular disease, or systemic disorders (Table 25–4). Hemorrhages may occur in superficial or deep layers of the retina or in the preretinal or subhyaloid space.

Diagnosis

The patient may complain of sudden decrease in vision when hemorrhage occurs in the macular or

Table 25–3. Some known causes of spotaneous vitreous hemorrhage not associated with trauma.

Diabetic retinopathy
Retinal tear
Posterior vitreous detachment
Retinal vein occlusion
Retinal detachment
Sickle cell disease
Ocular toxocariasis
Hypertension

Table 25–4. Systemic conditions associated with retinal hemorrhage.

Hypertension
Atherosclerosis
Diabetes mellitus
Hemoglobinopathies, eg, sickle cell disease
Anemia
Subacute infective endocarditis
Leukemia, lymphoma
Hyperviscosity syndromes
Cancer (rarely) (breast, eye, etc)
Giant cell arteritis, Takayasu's arteritis
Infections, eg, cytomegalovirus
Autoimmune disease, eg, lupus erythematosus, polyarteritis
    nodosa
Intracranial tumor
Anticoagulation

paramacular area. Small peripheral retinal hemorrhages cause no symptoms.

Superficial retinal hemorrhages occurring in the nerve fiber layer are bright red and flame-shaped on ophthalmoscopic examination. Deep retinal hemorrhages are round and have a dark red color. Subhyaloid hemorrhage occurs in the space between the vitreous body and the internal limiting membrane and may have a boat-shaped appearance.

A neovascular network may rupture and cause retinal or vitreous hemorrhage.

Treatment & Disposition

Treatment depends on the cause; there is no specific treatment. The patient should be referred to an ophthalmologist for further care, eg, photocoagulation of new vessels associated with local or systemic conditions (eg, diabetes) to prevent recurrences.

CENTRAL RETINAL VEIN OCCLUSION

Central retinal vein occlusion occurs most frequently in elderly patients with glaucoma or hypertension. The incidence is increased also in diabetes mellitus, autoimmune diseases, Waldenström's macroglobulinemia, cryoglobulinemia, sickle cell disease, polycythemia vera, and leukemia.

Diagnosis

The patient complains of sudden painless loss of vision in one eye. Ophthalmoscopy reveals dilated and tortuous veins, retinal and macular edema, multiple or diffuse retinal hemorrhages, and attenuated arterioles.

Treatment & Disposition

There is no specific therapy. The patient should be referred to an ophthalmologist within 24 hours for assessment of possible glaucoma or associated systemic disease. If local predisposing factors such as glaucoma are ruled out, patients with occlusion should have a complete medical evaluation.

OPTIC NEURITIS

Optic neuritis may be due to a wide variety of causes, including demyelinating diseases, systemic infections, nutritional and metabolic disorders, exposure to toxic substances (arsenic, methanol, lead, tobacco), vascular insufficiency, and local extension of infection from intraocular structures, sinuses, or meninges. The term includes retrobulbar neuritis (inflammation of the optic nerve posterior to the globe), in which there are by definition no ophthalmoscopic findings.

Diagnosis

The patient complains of decreased vision in one eye and sometimes pain on moving the eye. The pupillary reflex is sluggish. Ophthalmoscopic examination in optic neuritis shows hyperemia of the optic nerve head (may not be present in retrobulbar neuritis), congestion of the large veins, blurring of the disk margin, peripapillary retinal edema, and flame-shaped hemorrhages near the optic nerve head. Visual field testing discloses a central scotoma.

Differential Diagnosis

Optic neuritis should be differentiated from papilledema, in which the pupillary reflexes are intact, the nerve head is more markedly elevated, and no central scotoma is detected on visual field testing although the blind spot is enlarged. Papilledema is usually bilateral and associated with increased intracranial pressure. Vision is unaffected.

Treatment & Disposition

Treatment depends on the cause. Systemic corticosteroids may be helpful in cases associated with demyelinating disease.

The patient should be referred to an ophthalmologist or neurologist for further care within 1–2 days.

IV. OCULAR BURNS & TRAUMA

OCULAR BURNS

Apart from the history, the diagnosis of chemical burns is usually based on the presence of swollen eyelids with marked conjunctival hyperemia and chemosis. The limbus may show patchy blanched areas with conjunctival sloughing, especially in the interpalpebral area. There is usually corneal haze and diffuse edema, with wide areas of epithelial cell loss and corneal ulcerations. Corneal ulcerations can be better visualized with blue light following instillation of fluorescein.

ALKALI BURNS

Diagnosis

Alkali burns (especially particulate alkali such as lime) are very serious, because even after apparent removal of the offending agent, lodgment of tiny particles within the cul-de-sac may continue and cause progressive damage to the eye.

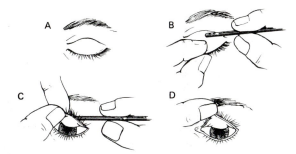

Figure 25–3. Eversion of the upper lid. **A:** The patient looks downward. **B:** The fingers pull the lid down, and a rod is placed on the upper tarsal border. **C:** The lid is pulled up over the rod. **D:** The lid is everted. (Redrawn and reproduced, with permission, from Liebman SD, Gellis SS [editors]: *The Pediatrician's Ophthalmology.* Mosby, 1966.)

Treatment

A. Instill a topical anesthetic *immediately* (proparacaine, 0.5%; or tetracaine, 0.5%), and then copiously irrigate the eye with isotonic saline solution or water for at least 5–10 minutes. A lid retractor may be useful.

B. Double eversion of the eyelids (Fig 25–3) should be performed to look for and remove material lodged in the cul-de-sac. Solid particles of alkali should be removed with forceps or a moist cotton applicator. After particles have been removed, irrigate again.

C. *Do not attempt to neutralize the alkali with acid, since the heat generated by the chemical reaction may cause further injury.*

D. Instill topical mydriatic eye drops, eg, atropine, 1%; or homatropine, 5%.

E. Instill antibiotic ointment (eg, gentamicin ointment, 0.3%).

F. Obtain some of the patient's own serum and have it available in a sterile bottle to be instilled as eye drops.

G. Parenteral narcotic analgesia is often required for pain relief, eg, morphine, 10 mg subcutaneously.

Disposition

Hospitalize the patient, and obtain immediate ophthalmologic consultation.

ACID BURNS

Diagnosis

Acid burns as a rule cause damage more rapidly but are generally less serious than alkali burns, because they do not cause progressive destruction of ocular tissues (as do alkali burns).

Treatment

A. Immediately after exposure, irrigate the eyes copiously with sterile isotonic saline solution, or tap water.

B. Topical anesthetic (proparacaine, 0.5%) may be instilled to minimize pain during irrigation.

C. *Do not attempt to neutralize the acid with alkali.*

D. Parenteral or oral narcotic analgesics may be necessary.

E. Patch the eye if corneal defects are present.

Disposition

Hospitalize all patients with severe acid burns, and obtain immediate ophthalmologic consultation.

THERMAL BURNS

Diagnosis

Injury due to thermal burns of the eyelids, cornea, and conjunctiva may range from minimal to extensive.

Superficial corneal burns have a good prognosis, though corneal ulcers may occur as a result of loss of corneal epithelium.

Thermal burns of the skin of the eyelids may be first-, second-, or third-degree. Conjunctival hyperemia is noted. The cornea may show diffuse necrosis of the exposed corneal epithelium in the interpalpebral area. Corneal haze due to corneal edema is frequently seen in thermal burns of the cornea and may lead to decrease in vision.

Treatment

The treatment of ocular burns is similar to the treatment of burns occurring elsewhere on the body (Chapter 37).

A. Provide systemic analgesia (morphine or equivalent is usually required).

B. Instill proparacaine, 0.5%; or tetracaine, 0.5%, to minimize pain during manipulation.

C. In cases of corneal burns, instill eye drops (atropine, 1%; or homatropine, 5%).

D. Patch the eye.

Disposition

Hospitalize patients with severe burns for local care and administration of systemic analgesia. Obtain ophthalmologic consultation.

BURNS DUE TO ULTRAVIOLET RADIATION

Destruction of the corneal epithelium by ultraviolet light is known as actinic keratitis, "snow blindness," and welder's arc burn (flash burn), depending on the source of ultraviolet radiation.

Diagnosis

The patient complains of pain and gives a history of exposure to ultraviolet light 6–12 hours earlier (eg, skiing, sunlamp). Examination discloses tearing, conjunctival hyperemia, and corneal haziness. There may be a superficial punctate keratitis, in which case punctate staining of the cornea is seen with fluorescein and with magnification (eg, slit lamp). Exposure to a welder's arc without protective filters produces keratitis similar to that resulting from ultraviolet radiation.

Treatment

A. Topical anesthetic should be instilled during the eye examination only. *Do not* give the patient a topical anesthetic to use at home.

B. Instill homatropine, 5% eye drops.

C. Instill gentamicin, 0.3% ointment, and apply a firm eye bandage. Recovery occurs within 12–36 hours.

D. Provide systemic analgesics for pain (aspirin and codeine or equivalent).

Disposition

Patients with severe burns should be hospitalized. All other patients should be seen for follow-up the next day (by an ophthalmologist, if possible).

MECHANICAL TRAUMA TO THE EYE

Ocular trauma may be classified as penetrating or nonpenetrating. Trauma can lead to serious damage and loss of vision. Eye injuries are common in spite of the protection afforded by the bony orbit and the cushioning effect of orbital fat. More widespread use of safety goggles would prevent most serious injuries to the eye.

Evaluation

Obtain a history of the injury from the patient or someone who knows what happened. Measure and record visual acuity with and without eyeglasses and through a pinhole aperture. Inspect the eyelids, conjunctiva, cornea, anterior chamber, pupils, lens, vitreous, and fundus for breaks in tissue and hemorrhage. Search for corneal lesion (abrasions, etc) by instilling fluorescein dye and examining the eye using a light with a light blue filter.

X-ray examination (orbital soft tissue film with contact lens localizer) or CT scan may be indicated to rule out radiopaque foreign bodies and to look for fractures of orbital bones.

Treatment & Disposition

Hospitalize patients with severe injuries, and consult an ophthalmologist immediately. Avoid causing further damage by manipulation. For more detailed discussion of treatment and disposition, see below under the specific type of injury.

A. For severe pain, photophobia, or foreign body sensation, instill a topical anesthetic, eg, proparacaine, 0.5%, 1–2 drops once or twice. Systemic analgesics may be required as well.

B. Cover the eye with a patch or eye shield.

C. For penetrating injuries, keep a sterile eye pad over the injured eye to minimize contamination.

PENETRATING OR PERFORATING INJURIES

Penetrating or perforating ocular injuries require immediate careful attention and prompt surgical repair to prevent possible loss of the eye.

Many facial injuries, especially those occurring in automobile accidents, are associated with penetrating ocular trauma. Some injuries may be concealed and inapparent because of eyelid swelling or because the patient's other injuries have dominated the attentions of the emergency department team. Such injuries, if not promptly attended to and adequately managed by an ophthalmologist, may lead to loss of vision.

Evaluation

Obtain and record a description of how the injury occurred. Examine the eye and ocular adnexa, including vision testing if the patient's condition permits. *Do not* apply pressure on the globe.

X-ray examination or CT scan is indicated to rule out intraocular radiopaque foreign body and to look for fractures of orbital bones.

Diagnosis

Penetrating injuries are those that cause disruption of the outer coats of the eye (sclera, cornea) without interrupting the anatomic continuity of that layer, thus preventing prolapse or loss of ocular contents. **Perforating injuries** are those resulting in complete anatomic disruption (laceration) of the sclera or cornea. Such wounds may or may not be associated with prolapse of uveal structures. Wounds of the sclera or cornea are often associated with intraocular or intraorbital foreign bodies.

Treatment

The objectives of emergency management of ocular penetrating or perforating injuries are to relieve pain, preserve or restore vision, and achieve a good cosmetic result. *Avoid needless examination.*

A. Relieve pain with morphine, 2–4 mg intravenously or subcutaneously; or meperidine, 50–75 mg intramuscularly, as needed. A sedative (eg, diazepam, 5–10 mg orally) may be required as well.

B. Cover the eye with sterile gauze or an eye pad. Patch the uninjured eye also to minimize ocular movements.

C. *Do not* manipulate the eye, instill eye drops, or apply antibiotic treatment.

D. Give tetanus prophylaxis if needed (Chapter 24).

E. Prohibit oral intake until the patient is examined by an ophthalmologist, since urgent surgery may be required. Provide hydration with intravenous fluids (eg, 5% dextrose in half-normal saline given at a rate of 125 mL/h for an adult).

F. Give parenteral antibiotics directed against gram-negative and gram-positive organisms (eg, cefazolin, 100 mg/kg/d intravenously or intramuscularly in divided doses every 8 hours; and gentamicin, 40 mg intramuscularly every 8 hours. Do not mix these 2 antibiotics in the same syringe).

G. Give antiemetic agents to prevent further injury. A useful drug for this purpose is chlorpromazine, 25–50 mg by deep intramuscular injection every 4–6 hours, or 10–25 mg orally every 4–6 hours as needed.

Disposition

The patient should be seen by an ophthalmologist for management of severe injuries, investigation of intraocular foreign bodies, and immediate surgical repair as required. Prompt repair of uveal prolapse decreases the risk of sympathetic ophthalmia in the uninjured eye. Delay in management of corneal lacerations may increase the risk of surgical and postoperative complications.

BLUNT TRAUMA TO THE EYE, ADNEXA, & ORBIT

Contusions of the eyeball and ocular adnexa result from blunt trauma. The outcome of such an injury cannot always be determined, and the extent of damage may not be obvious upon superficial examination. Careful eye examination is needed, along with x-ray examination or CT scan when indicated.

Types of Injury

A. Eyelids: Ecchymosis (see below), swelling, laceration, abrasions.

B. Conjunctiva: Subconjunctival hemorrhages, laceration of the conjunctiva.

C. Cornea: Edema, laceration, rupture.

D. Anterior Chamber: Hyphema, recession of angle, secondary glaucoma.

E. Iris: Iridodialysis, iridoplegia, rupture of iris sphincter, iris prolapse through corneal or scleral lacerations, iris atrophy (later).

F. Ciliary Body: Hyposecretion of aqueous humor, ciliary body prolapse through scleral lacerations.

G. Lens: Dislocation, cataract (later).

H. Vitreous: Hemorrhage, prolapse.

I. Ciliary Muscle: Paralysis or spasm.

Treatment & Disposition

A. Injury severe enough to cause intraocular hemorrhage (eg, vitreous hemorrhage or hyphema) involves the danger of delayed secondary hemorrhage from a damaged uveal vessel, which may cause intractable glaucoma and permanent damage to the eyeball. In such cases, hospitalize the patient at bed rest for 4 or 5 days with the injured eye bandaged to minimize the chance of further bleeding. Secondary hemorrhage rarely occurs after 72 hours.

B. Except for rupture of the eyeball itself, contusions do not usually require immediate definitive treatment. Apply an eye shield if the globe has been perforated.

C. Use atropine, 1% eye drops, twice daily. Acetazolamide, mannitol, or other systemic agents may be necessary to lower intraocular pressure.

D. Give analgesics, eg, acetaminophen with codeine (30 mg); morphine, 2–4 mg intravenously or subcutaneously; or meperidine 50–75 mg intramuscularly, as needed for pain.

E. Refer all patients to an ophthalmologist.

1. ECCHYMOSIS OF THE EYELIDS (Black Eye)

Diagnosis

Blood in the periorbital tissues may occur from direct trauma or a blow to adjacent areas (eg, nose). The loose subcutaneous tissue around the eye permits blood to spread extensively. The diagnosis is usually obvious. Always rule out trauma to the eye itself (hyphema, blowout fracture, or retinal detachment).

Treatment

Apply cold compresses to decrease swelling and help stop bleeding. Twenty-four hours later, apply hot compresses to accelerate absorption of the hematoma. Exclude more serious ocular injury by careful examination.

Disposition

If the eye itself is uninjured, no follow-up contact is necessary.

2. LACERATIONS OF THE EYELIDS

Diagnosis

Lacerations or other wounds of the eyelids may be

associated with serious ocular injuries not apparent at first examination—lacrimal system, levator muscle, optic nerve, etc. A meticulous search for such injuries is mandatory in every patient with eyelid lacerations.

Treatment & Disposition

Patients with lacerations of the eyelids require suturing and then complete ophthalmologic evaluation. Lacerations involving the tarsal plate, the upper eyelid, or medial canthal area should be repaired by an ophthalmologist.

3. ORBITAL HEMORRHAGE

Diagnosis

Exophthalmos and subconjunctival hemorrhage in a patient with a history of blunt trauma to the face suggest rupture of orbital blood vessels. There may be conjunctival chemosis or ecchymosis of the eyelids.

Treatment & Disposition

Apply cold compresses, and obtain urgent ophthalmologic consultation. Hospitalize for observation if severe injury has occurred.

4. FRACTURE OF THE ETHMOID BONE

The ethmoid bone is part of the medial wall of the orbit. Fracture of the ethmoid bone most frequently occurs with blunt trauma to the orbit.

Diagnosis

Fracture of the ethmoid bone is manifested by subcutaneous emphysema of the eyelids. There may or may not be ecchymosis of the eyelids. X-ray reveals air in the orbit. Fractures of other orbital bones should be ruled out by tomography.

Treatment

Fractures of the ethmoid bone usually do not require operative reduction.

A. Provide analgesia as needed, eg, morphine, 5–10 mg subcutaneously or intravenously; or acetaminophen with codeine (30 mg) orally.

B. Apply cold compresses.

C. Give a systemic antibiotic, eg, amoxicillin, 500 mg orally every 6 hours.

D. Instruct the patient to avoid sneezing or blowing the nose.

Disposition

Refer the patient to an ophthalmologist within 1–2 days.

5. BLOWOUT FRACTURES OF THE FLOOR OF THE ORBIT

Diagnosis

Blowout fracture may be associated with enophthalmos and hypotropia (visual axis of the injured eye is displaced downward in comparison to that of the sound eye), diplopia in the primary position or in upward gaze, limitation of ocular movement in upward gaze, and decreased or absent sensation over the maxilla. X-ray (tomography) or CT scan of the orbit shows orbital floor displacement.

Treatment

A. Provide analgesia as needed, eg, morphine, 2–5 mg intravenously or subcutaneously; or acetaminophen with codeine (30 mg) orally; and sedation with diazepam, 5 mg orally.

B. Apply a topical antibiotic ointment such as gentamicin, 0.3%.

C. Apply cold compresses and a sterile eye patch.

Disposition

Hospitalize the patient, and seek early consultation with an ophthalmologist and otolaryngologist because of possible fractures of the maxilla or zygoma. Obtain x-ray or CT scan of the orbit.

6. CORNEAL ABRASIONS

Diagnosis

The patient complains of pain, photophobia, and blurring of vision. There is usually a history of trivial trauma. Patients with severe pain and blepharospasm may require proparacaine, 0.5%, instilled in the eye to facilitate eye examination. In severe cases, the eye is red and the corneal surface is irregular and loses its normal luster. Staining with fluorescein reveals a defect in the corneal epithelium. Always rule out infection or perforation of the globe.

Treatment

A. Irrigate the eye gently with sterile saline solution to remove debris and loose foreign bodies.

B. In severe cases, instill 2 drops of either atropine, 1%, or homatropine, 5%, to relax the ciliary muscle and relieve pain.

C. Instill ophthalmic antibiotic ointment (eg, polymyxin B–bacitracin). *Caution:* Do not use ointment containing corticosteroids.

D. Apply a firm (not tight) eye bandage.

E. Provide analgesia as needed, eg, acetaminophen with codeine (30 mg) orally.

F. Avoid giving the patient topical anesthetics, which may lead to irreversible corneal damage.

Disposition

Patients with severe bilateral corneal abrasions

should be hospitalized. Refer other patients for daily outpatient follow-up care. Ophthalmologic consultation should be obtained for corneal abrasions that fail to resolve in 48–72 hours.

7. CORNEAL & CONJUNCTIVAL FOREIGN BODIES

Diagnosis

There may be a history of working with high-speed tempered steel tools (eg, drilling), or there may be no history of trauma to the eye and the patient may even be unaware of a foreign body in the eye. In most cases, however, the patient complains of a foreign body sensation in the eye or under the eyelid, or just irritation in the eye. A corneal foreign body can be seen with the aid of a loupe and well-focused diffuse light. Conjunctival foreign bodies often become embedded in the conjunctiva under the upper eyelid. The lid must be everted (Fig 25–3) to facilitate inspection and removal.

Sterile fluorescein should be instilled to visualize minute foreign bodies not readily visible with the naked eye or loupe. Rule out intraocular foreign body (in certain cases, soft tissue x-ray or CT scan may be required for this purpose).

Treatment

A. Some loose foreign bodies can be removed with a moist cotton applicator.

B. Foreign bodies superficially embedded can be removed with the tip of a hypodermic needle or blunt spud. Anesthetize the cornea first with proparacaine or tetracaine solution, 0.5%.

C. Instill ophthalmic antibiotic ointment (gentamicin, 0.3%; or sulfacetamide, 10%).

D. Cover the injured eye with a patch left on overnight.

Disposition

After the foreign body has been removed, the patient should be seen again in 24 hours to make certain that infection has not occurred.

Refer the patient to an ophthalmologist if foreign bodies are deeply embedded in the cornea, since they may have to be removed in the operating room under magnification.

V. EQUIPMENT & SUPPLIES

Basic Equipment

A great many specialized instruments have been devised for the investigation of eye disorders. Most emergency conditions can be diagnosed with the aid of a few relatively simple instruments. The following should be available in the emergency department:

A. Hand flashlight with fresh batteries.

B. Binocular loupe.

C. Ophthalmoscope (preferably with lens that has a blue filter).

D. Visual acuity chart (Snellen).

E. Tonometer.

F. Pinhole and occluder.

G. Eye shield (plastic or metal) and tape.

Basic Medications

A. Local Anesthetics: Proparacaine, 0.5%; or tetracaine, 0.5%.

B. Dyes: Sterile fluorescein papers, rose bengal solution.

C. Mydriatics: Tropicamide ophthalmic solution, 0.5% or 1%, is a satisfactory mydriatic when the examiner wishes to obtain a clearer view of the lens, vitreous, or ocular fundus. Eye drops (atropine, 1%; or homatropine, 5%) may be used in patients with iritis.

D. Miotics: Pilocarpine, 1% or 2%.

E. Antibacterial Agents: Tetracycline, 1% ophthalmic ointment; polymyxin B–bacitracin ophthalmic ointment; sulfacetamide, 10% ophthalmic solution or ointment; or gentamicin, 0.3% ointment (Table 25–5).

VI. COMMON TECHNIQUES FOR TREATMENT OF OCULAR DISORDERS

Eversion of the Upper Eyelid (See Fig 25–3.)

The patient is instructed to look down. Grasp the eyelashes at the outer margin of the lid with the thumb and forefinger of one hand, and gently and slowly draw the lid downward and outward. Using a cotton-tipped applicator, press against the upper edge of the tarsus over the center of the lid while turning the lid margin rapidly outward and upward over the applicator. With the lashes thus held against the upper orbital rim, the exposed palpebral conjunctiva can be inspected closely. After the examination is completed and the foreign body removed (if possible), when the patient looks up, the lid returns to its normal position.

Eye Drops

The patient should sit with both eyes open and looking up. Pull down slightly on the lower lid, and place 2 drops in the lower cul-de-sac. The patient is then asked to look down while finger contact on the lower lid is maintained. Do not let the patient squeeze

Table 25–5. Ocular antimicrobial therapy.[1]

Drug	Topical[2]	Subconjunctival[2]	Systemic[2] (Intravenous Unless Otherwise Indicated)
Amikacin	10 mg/mL	25 mg/0.5 mL/dose	. . .
Amphotericin B	1.5–3 mg/mL	50 µg/0.5 mL/dose every other day	. . .
Ampicillin	. . .	. . .	150–200 mg/kg body wt/d in 4 doses
Bacitracin	10,000 units/mL	. . .	. . .
Carbenicillin	4 mg/mL	125 mg/0.5 mL/dose	100–200 mg/kg body wt/d in 4 doses
Cefazolin	50 mg/mL	100 mg/0.5 mL/dose	15 mg/kg body wt/d in 4 doses
Cephaloridine	. . .	100 mg/0.5 mL/dose	. . .
Chloramphenicol	5 mg/mL	. . .	. . .
Erythromycin	5 mg/g (ointment)	100 mg/0.5 mL/dose	Oral: first dose 1 g; then 0.5 g every 6 hours
Flucytosine	1% solution	. . .	Oral: 50–150 mg/kg body wt/d in 4 doses
Gentamicin	3–10 mg/mL	20 mg/0.5 mL/dose	. . .
Methicillin	. . .	100 mg/mL; dose: 0.5–1 mL	. . .
Miconazole	1% solution or 2% ointment	5 mg/0.5 mL/dose	. . .
Nafcillin	. . .	. . .	1 g every 4–6 hours
Natamycin (pimaricin)	5% suspension	. . .	. . .
Nystatin	100,000 units/g (ointment)	. . .	. . .
Penicillin G	100,000–20,000 units/mL	1 million units/mL/dose	40,000–50,000 units/kg body wt/d in 4 doses or continuously
Polymyxin B	10,000–25,000 units/mL	10,000 units/mL/dose	. . .
Rifampin	1% ointment	. . .	Oral: 600 mg/d
Sodium sulfacetamide	10–15% solution	. . .	. . .
Sulfonamides	. . .	. . .	Oral: 70 mg/kg body wt/d in 4 doses, or 4 g, whichever is less
Tetracycline	5 mg/mL	. . .	Oral: 1.5 g/d in 4 doses for patients under 70 kg; 2 g/d if over 70 kg
Tobramycin	3–5 mg/mL	20 mg/0.5 mL/dose	. . .
Vancomycin	50 mg/mL	100 mg/mL; dose: 0.25 mL	. . .
Zinc sulfate	0.5 mg/mL	. . .	. . .

[1]Modified and reproduced, with permission, from Vaughan D, Asbury T: *General Ophthalmology,* 11th ed. Appleton & Lange, 1986.
[2]Treatment schedule: Topical: Every hour during day, every 2 hours during night, for 5 days. Subconjunctival: One injection daily for 4 days unless otherwise stated; in exceptionally severe cases, initial dose sometimes repeated after 12 hours. Systemic, intravenous, or oral: One dose daily for 5 days.

the eye shut. Do not touch the eye or the eyelid with the applicator; likewise, do not instill eye drops with the dropper held far away from the eye.

Ointments

Ointments are instilled in the same way as liquids. While the patient is looking up, lift out the lower lid to trap the medication in the conjunctival sac. The lids should be kept closed for at least 1 minute to allow the ointment to melt. Tubes of ointments may be warmed with warm water before the ointment is instilled in the lower fornix.

Eye Bandages

Eye bandages should be applied firmly enough to hold the lid fairly securely against the cornea. A single patch consisting of gauze-covered cotton is usually sufficient. A wraparound head bandage is seldom necessary. Tape is passed across the bandage from the cheek to the forehead. If more pressure is desired, use 2 or 3 patches.

Warm Compresses

Use a clean towel or washcloth soaked in hot tap water well below the temperature that will burn the thin skin covering the eyelids. Warm compresses are usually applied to the area for 15 minutes 4 times a day. The therapeutic rationale is to increase blood flow to the affected area and decrease pain and inflammation.

Removal of Superficial
Corneal Foreign Body

The main considerations are good illumination, magnification, anesthesia, proper positioning of the patient, and sterile technique. If possible, the patient's visual acuity should be recorded first.

The patient may be sitting or supine. A loupe should be used unless a slit lamp is available. (A loupe must be used if the patient is supine.) An assistant should direct a strong flashlight into the eye at an oblique angle. The examiner may then see the corneal foreign body and remove it with a wet cotton applicator. If this is not successful, the foreign body may be removed with a metal spud while the lids are held apart with the other hand to prevent blinking. An antibacterial ointment is instilled after the foreign body has been removed.

Most patients are more comfortable with a patch on the eye after removal of a foreign body.

Note: It is essential to see the patient the next day to be certain infection has not occurred and healing is under way.

Home Medication

At home, the same techniques should be used as described above except that drops should be instilled with the patient lying supine. Experienced patients (eg, those with glaucoma) are usually quite skillful in self-administration of eye drops.

Schiotz Tonometry

Tonometry is the determination of intraocular pressure using a special instrument that measures the amount of corneal indentation produced by a given weight. Tonometry readings should be taken on any patient suspected of having increased intraocular pressure.

A. Precautions: Tonometry should be done with great caution on patients with corneal ulcers. It is extremely important to clean the tonometer before each use by carefully wiping the footplate with a cotton swab moistened with sterile solution (be sure it is dry before using) and to sterilize the instrument once a day (dry heat). The tonometer should be sterilized by flame or in a hot air tonometer sterilizer after use on an inflamed eye.

Corneal abrasions are rarely caused by Schiotz tonometry. Epidemic keratoconjunctivitis can be spread by tonometry, and this can be prevented if the tonometer is cleaned before each use and the principle of handwashing between patients is meticulously observed.

B. Technique: Anesthetic solution (tetracaine, 0.5%; or proparacaine, 0.5%) is instilled into each eye. The patient lies supine and is asked to stare at a spot on the ceiling with both eyes or at a finger held directly in the line of gaze overhead. The lids are held open without applying pressure on the globe. The tonometer is then placed on the corneal surface of each eye and the scale reading taken from the tonometer. The intraocular pressure is determined by referring to a chart that converts the scale reading to millimeters of mercury. If the scale reading is 4 or less, the 7.5-g and 10-g weights are added separately to gain further information concerning the intraocular pressure. Normal intraocular pressure is 12–20 mm Hg.

C. Interpretation of Abnormalities: If the intraocular pressure is 20–30 mm Hg or more, further investigation is indicated to determine whether or not glaucoma is present. Tonometry is an effective screening device to select patients for glaucoma testing. Visual field testing and ophthalmoscopic examination should be done and tonometry repeated several times at different hours of the day or on different days before a diagnosis of glaucoma is warranted. If the pressure remains high on successive readings and there is a visual field defect or cupping of the optic disks, the diagnosis of glaucoma is established. In borderline cases, tonography may be helpful in establishing the presence or absence of glaucoma.

Corneal Staining

Corneal staining consists of instillation of fluorescein or other dyes (eg, rose bengal) into the conjunctival sac to outline irregularities of the corneal surface. Staining is indicated in corneal trauma or other corneal disorders (eg, herpes simplex keratitis) when examination with a loupe or slit lamp in the absence of a stain has not been satisfactory.

A. Precautions: Because the corneal epithelium—the chief barrier to corneal infection—is usually interrupted when corneal staining is indicated, be certain that whatever dye is used (particularly fluorescein) is sterile.

B. Equipment and Materials: *Note:* Fluorescein must be sterile. Fluorescein papers or sterile individual dropper units are safest. Fluorescein solution from a dropper bottle may be used, but there is a substantial risk of contamination.

C. Technique: The individually wrapped fluorescein paper is wetted with sterile saline or touched to the wet conjunctiva so that a thin film of fluorescein spreads over the corneal surface. Any irregularity in the cornea is stained by the fluorescein and is thus more easily visualized using a light with a blue filter.

D. Normal and Abnormal Findings: If there is no superficial corneal irregularity, a uniform film of dye covers the cornea. If the corneal surface has been altered, the affected area absorbs more of the dye and will stain a deeper green. It is customary to sketch the staining area on the patient's record for later comparison to show the progress of healing.

Estimation of Anterior Chamber Depth
(See Fig 25–1.)

Using a hand flashlight, shine the light obliquely and parallel to the plane of the iris across the cornea and anterior chamber. A normal anterior chamber will be fully illuminated. With a shallow anterior chamber (as in angle-closure glaucoma), the anteriorly displaced iris will cast a shadow.

VII. COMMON PITFALLS TO BE AVOIDED IN THE MANAGEMENT OF OCULAR DISORDERS

Dangers in the Use of Local Anesthetics

Unsupervised self-administration of local anesthetics is dangerous, because the patient may further injure an anesthetized eye without knowing it. Furthermore, most anesthetics delay healing. This is particularly true of butacaine, which also elicits a high incidence of allergic responses. Therefore, patients should not be given local anesthetics to take home. Eye pain should be controlled by systemic analgesics and an eye patch when indicated.

Errors in Diagnosis

The most common mistaken ophthalmologic diagnosis is conjunctivitis when the correct diagnosis should be iritis (anterior uveitis), glaucoma, or corneal ulcer (especially herpes simplex ulcer). The differentiation between iritis and acute glaucoma may be difficult also.

Misuse of Atropine

Atropine must never be used in routine diagnosis. It causes cycloplegia (paralysis of the ciliary muscle) of about 14 days' duration and can precipitate an attack of glaucoma if the patient has a narrow anterior chamber angle.

Dangers of Local Corticosteroid Therapy

Local ophthalmologic corticosteroid preparations, eg, prednisolone, are often used for their anti-inflammatory effect on the conjunctiva, cornea, and iris. Although it is true that a patient with conjunctivitis, corneal inflammation, or iritis can be made more comfortable with topical corticosteroids, it must be stressed that the corticosteroids are associated with 4 very serious complications when used in the eye: herpes simplex keratitis, open-angle glaucoma, cataract formation, and fungal infection. The most common complications are herpes simplex keratitis and glaucoma. Corticosteroids enhance the pathogenicity of herpes simplex virus, apparently by increasing the destructive effect of collagenase on the collagen of the cornea. This is evidenced by the fact that perforation of the cornea occasionally occurs when corticosteroids are used during the more active stage of herpes simplex corneal infection. Corneal perforation was a rare complication of dendritic keratitis before corticosteroids came into general use. In the treatment of any corneal inflammation, particularly if the corneal epithelium is not intact, the prolonged use of corticosteroids is sometimes complicated by fungal infection, and this may lead to loss of the eye. Topical corticosteroids can cause or aggravate open-angle glaucoma and, less commonly, can produce cataracts.

For these reasons, although the corticosteroids are valuable in the treatment of ocular disease, any patient on whom they are being used should be watched carefully for the development of complications. Corticosteroids should not be used unless specifically indicated, eg, in iritis, certain types of keratitis, and acute allergic disorders, and patients using prescribed topical corticosteroids should always see an ophthalmologist for follow-up examination.

Use of Contaminated Eye Medications

The external coats of the eye, including the sclera and the corneal epithelium, are resistant to infection. However, once the corneal epithelium or sclera is broken by trauma, the tissues become markedly susceptible to bacterial infection. For this reason, ophthalmic solutions that may be used in injured eyes must be prepared with the same degree of caution as fluids intended for intravenous administration.

Sterile, single-use disposable units of the common ophthalmic solutions should be used whenever liquid medication is instilled into an injured eye. For routine use in intact eyes, nearly all eye medications are now available in small plastic containers. It is safe to use these provided they are not kept a long time after opening (eg, > 1 month) and are not contaminated accidentally.

Overtreatment

Some patients with chronic conjunctivitis or keratitis may be made worse by overtreatment with topical medications.

REFERENCES

Bron AF et al: Ofloxacin compared with chloramphenicol in the management of external ocular infection. Brit J Ophthalmol 1991;75:675.

Cinotti AA: *Handbook of Ophthalmologic Emergencies,* 3rd ed. Med Exam Pub, 1985.

Friedberg MA, Rapuano CJ: *Wills Eye Hospital Office and Emergency Diagnosis and Treatment of Eye Disease.* Lippincott, 1990.

Gardiner PA: Accidents and first aid. (ABC of Ophthalmology Series.) Br Med J 1978;2:1347.

Hollwich F: Ophthalmology, 2nd ed. (traslated and adopted by F.C. Blodi) Georg Thieme Verlag and Thieme — Stratton Inc. 1985.

Howard GR, Vukich J, Fiscella RG et al: Intraocular tissue plasminogen activator in a rabbit model of traumatic hyphema. Arch Ophthalmol 1991;109:272.

Jamieson M: Loss of vision. Br Med J 1984;288:1523.

Kearns P: Traumatic hyphema: a retrospective study of 314 cases. Brit J Ophthalmol 1991;75:137.

Penna EP, Tabbara KF: Oxybuprocaine keratopathy: A preventable disease. Br J Ophthalmol 1986;70:202.

Roper-Hall MJ: *Eye Emergencies.* Churchill-Livingstone, 1987.

Schechter RJ: Mixing fortified antibiotic eye drops. Am J Ophthalmol 1991;112:459.

Smolin G, Tabbara KF, Whitcher J: *Handbook of Infectious Diseases of the Eye.* Williams & Wilkins, 1984.

Tabbara KF, Hyndiuk RA: *Infections of the Eye.* Little Brown, 1986.

Vaughan D, Asbury T, Tabbara KF: *General Ophthalmology,* 12th ed. Appleton & Lange, 1989.

26 ENT Emergencies: Disorders of the Ears, Nose, Sinuses, Oropharynx, & Teeth

Thomas A. Tami, MD, Roger L. Crumley, MD, & John Mills, MD

I. IMMEDIATE MANAGEMENT OF POTENTIALLY LIFE-THREATENING PROBLEMS

EPISTAXIS

Diagnosis & Treatment

A. General Measures: Calm the patient, and have the patient or (preferably) an assistant firmly pinch the patient's entire nose until initial evaluation is completed. This action usually blocks the bleeding site and stops anterior nosebleeds. The sitting position is preferable to recumbency unless hypotension or shock is present, because it reduces nasal arterial pressures and the risk of aspiration of blood.

1. Recognize and treat shock–Look for evidence of shock: feeble pulse; cool, pale skin; disordered mentation; etc. If there is a history or objective evidence of profuse bleeding, check for hypovolemia by measuring the patient's blood pressure and pulse in the supine, sitting, and standing positions. If there is evidence of significant blood loss, treat for hypovolemic shock. Insert a large-bore ($\geq$ 16-gauge) intravenous catheter. Draw blood for typing and cross-matching, hematocrit, hemoglobin concentration, clotting factor tests (prothrombin time, partial thromboplastin time, platelet estimate), and renal function tests (blood urea nitrogen and serum creatinine). Begin rapid intravenous infusion of crystalloid solutions (eg, normal saline or lactated Ringer's injection) to support blood pressure until whole blood can be typed and cross-matched.

Other diagnostic or therapeutic measures for hypovolemic shock may be necessary (Chapter 3).

2. Look for underlying cause–Ask about systemic factors that predispose to nosebleeds, such as hypertension, bleeding diathesis, anticoagulant or aspirin therapy, or hematologic disease. Measure blood pressure (hypertension) and hematocrit (polycythe-mia vera), and screen for clotting factor deficiency with prothrombin time and partial thromboplastin time determinations and a platelet count.

If systemic factors that predispose to epistaxis are present, they should be treated simultaneously. Lower the blood pressure until it is in the normal range (Chapter 28), and treat clotting defects with appropriate measures, if possible (Chapter 33).

B. Control of Hemorrhage:

1. Determine site of bleeding–Maintain the patient in the sitting position, using an ENT chair if available. Use a bright light source (headlight or head mirror), a nasal speculum, and an adequate suction device to determine the site of bleeding. Systematically examine the lateral and medial walls of the nasal cavity, and search for bleeding points.

2. Stop the bleeding–The site of bleeding tends to vary with the age of the patient, as described below.

a. Children–Nasal bleeding often originates in Kiesselbach's area, located anteriorly on the nasal septum and well supplied with blood, since its blood supply comes from several vessels. Bleeding can often be stopped by the application of a topical vasoconstrictor such as phenylephrine (2% Neo-Synephrine spray, others) or cocaine (4% spray or solution). If bleeding continues, it can be stopped by electrical cautery, silver nitrate cautery (Fig 26–1), or packing that is tightly pressed against the bleeding point.

To perform cautery, use silver nitrate-tipped sticks or an electrocautery device set at the coagulation setting. Cauterize under direct vision and only over the bleeding site. ***Caution:*** Do not cauterize a wide area of nasal mucosa, and do not cauterize both sides of the nasal septum, since septal necrosis may result. Electrical cautery is particularly dangerous in this regard.

To place an anterior pack, insert a continuous strip of petrolatum-impregnated gauze into the anterior nares, and firmly pack it in with forceps to fill all spaces. Cut off the strip when the packing is complete, and hold the gauze in place with tape. Pinching the nose gently (to further stem bleeding) may also be

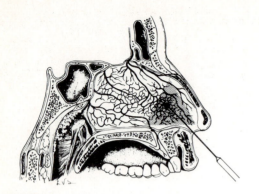

Figure 26–1. Cauterization of bleeding point in Kiesselbach's area. (Reproduced, with permission, from Way LW [editor]: *Current Surgical Diagnosis & Treatment,* 9th ed. Appleton & Lange, 1991.)

helpful. Leave the nasal pack in place for 48 hours, and refer the patient to an otolaryngologist or clinic within 24–48 hours. See Chapter 46 for further details.

b. Adults–Nosebleeds originate in the septum but usually more posteriorly than Kiesselbach's area. Bleeding can be stopped by placing long pledgets saturated with 4–5% cocaine in the nasal passages for 3–5 minutes. (*Caution:* Cocaine dosage should never exceed 200 mg [2 mL of 10% solution, 5 mL of 4% solution, and so forth].) This measure may shrink the mucosa covering the nasal conchae and improve visibility while providing vasoconstriction of the bleeding vessels. Bright lighting and suction usually reveal the bleeding point, although in occasional patients, bleeding is too profuse to permit localization. These patients usually require nasal packing on the side of the bleeding (see above). If bleeding continues, pack the other nostril as well. If the entire nasal chamber is filled with nasal packing and bleeding persists posteriorly, a posterior pack is necessary (Chapter 46).

c. Elderly patients–Older patients often present the most difficult problem in nasal bleeding. The source of bleeding is usually high and in the posterior part of the nose, often the lateral wall. It cannot be visualized by conventional rhinoscopy using an anterior approach. Calcified arteriosclerotic vessels are often responsible for the bleeding, and because of their inelasticity and ineffective vasospasm, bleeding is usually profuse and difficult to stop.

The quickest way to stop bleeding in a patient with suspected posterior epistaxis is to first place a posterior pack in the nasopharynx (Chapter 46) and then pack the nasal chamber anteriorly on both sides until bleeding is no longer seen either anteriorly or posteriorly. If bleeding recurs in the first few days after treatment or when the pack is removed (usually 5 days after insertion), surgery for arterial ligation is indicated. If the bleeding site cannot be seen but results

in anterior hemorrhage, the physician may try bilateral anterior packing (see above). The occasional patient in whom this technique successfully stops bleeding will be spared the necessity for hospitalization (required after placement of posterior packs).

Disposition

A posterior pack or balloon catheter should be left in place for 5 days, during which time the patient must be hospitalized. Patients with an anterior nasal pack need not be hospitalized but should be seen again in 1–2 days. Patients with epistaxis controlled by cauterization do not require follow-up.

NASAL DISCHARGE

Diagnosis

Causes of nasal discharge are set forth in Table 26–1. Nasal discharge is most often a trivial symptom related to allergy, vasomotor rhinitis, or a viral upper respiratory tract infection; however, more serious causes such as cerebrospinal fluid rhinorrhea or for-

Table 26–1. Causes of nasal discharge.

	Diagnostic clues
Potential emergencies	
Cerebrospinal fluid rhinorrhea	History of head trauma; high glucose level usually found in discharge (false-positive results may occur).
Foreign body	Primarily seen in children; unilateral airflow obstruction; object is evident on examination.
Sinusitis	Purulent discharge. Sinuses tender; abnormal sinus x-rays. Often a history of sinus infections.
Tumor	Primarily seen in adults; often unilateral airflow obstruction and blood-tinged discharge; tumor usually evident on rhinoscopy.
Chemical exposure	History of exposure to irritants; short-lived symptoms.
Group A streptococcal infection	Usually occurs in infants. Seropurulent discharge; culture shows many group A streptococci.
Nonemergencies	
Allergy	History of allergic rhinitis; pale, boggy mucosa; eosinophils in nasal secretions.
Viral upper respiratory tract infection	Red, swollen nasal mucosa; other symptoms of upper respiratory tract infection.
Vasomotor rhinitis	Relatively normal or slightly atrophic nasal mucosa. Symptoms are chronic.
Rhinitis medicamentosa	History of use of intranasal medication, usually decongestants. Red, swollen nasal mucosa.

eign body should be excluded by history and physical examination.

Ask about previous head trauma, sinusitis, allergy, or recent exposure to chemicals (irritating gases such as chlorine or ammonia; nasal decongestants). If head trauma has occurred, proceed as outlined in Chapter 16. Ask about symptoms of viral upper respiratory tract infection. Record temperature and other vital signs. Palpate and transilluminate the frontal and maxillary sinuses for signs of tenderness or swelling (see Sinusitis, below). Examine the nasal airway for signs of unilateral obstruction, perform rhinoscopy to evaluate the mucosa and look for possible foreign bodies or tumors, and obtain sinus x-rays.

Treatment & Disposition

Patients with suspected acute cerebrospinal fluid rhinorrhea should be hospitalized and evaluated by a neurologist or neurosurgeon. Nasal foreign bodies should be removed (see below); if the obstruction is thought to be due to tumor, urgent referral to an otolaryngologist is required. Rhinitis caused by medication or chemicals should be managed by discontinuing exposure to the offending material; referral is rarely indicated. If sinusitis is suspected, obtain sinus x-rays, and treat as described below. Rhinitis due to allergy or viral upper respiratory tract infection can be treated symptomatically.

Infants under 6 months of age with group A streptococcal infections may have serous nasal discharge rather than pharyngitis as the principal finding. Cultures for group A streptococci are indicated when purulent nasal discharge associated with fever occurs in this age group. Empiric antimicrobial therapy may be indicated depending on the local incidence of streptococcal disease and poststreptococcal complications and on the parents' willingness or ability to return with the patient for follow-up. The recommended treatment is benzathine penicillin G, 1.2 million units intramuscularly (one dose only).

NASAL OBSTRUCTION

The causes of nasal obstruction are shown in Table 26–2. Most of these conditions may be diagnosed from the history and direct inspection of the nasal cavity. Remove any foreign bodies (see Nasal Foreign Bodies, below). Drain septal hematomas and abscesses immediately, and start antimicrobial therapy, if indicated. Other conditions causing nasal obstruction should be treated symptomatically and the patient referred for definitive treatment.

Table 26–2. Causes of nasal obstruction.

	Diagnostic Clues
Choanal atresia	Rare; occurs only in newborns; fatal if not recognized (attempt to pass nasal catheter).
Foreign body	Primarily seen in children; acute unilateral airflow obstruction; object is usually evident on rhinoscopy.
Septal hematoma or abscess	Evident on rhinoscopy. Confirm by aspiration or drainage.
Tumor	Primarily seen in adults. Gradually progressive airflow obstruction, usually unilateral; nasal discharge (often bloodstained) common; tumor usually evident on rhinoscopy.
Deviated septum	Chronic unilateral airflow obstruction; evident on rhinoscopy.
Allergy	History of allergy; pale boggy mucosa. Bilateral. Eosinophils in nasal secretions.
Viral rhinitis	Other symptoms of viral infection; red, swollen mucosa. Bilateral.
Vasomotor rhinitis	Chronic condition; relatively normal mucosa; rarely causes complete obstruction.

PAIN IN THE EAR
(See Table 26–3.)

Diagnosis

Patients with ear pain should be asked about a history of swimming (otitis externa), trauma (chondritis), or ear disease that might be related to the present symptoms.

Inspect the pinna for chondritis. Palpate and gently tug on it to elicit pain that would indicate otitis externa. Using an otoscope, look carefully at the external auditory canal and at the tympanic membrane, and inspect its landmarks. Test the patient's hearing in both ears and in each ear separately. Examine other facial structures (teeth, temporomandibular joint, etc) to see whether the ear pain is being referred from some other area.

X-rays may be helpful if referred pain is suspected (dental abscesses, temporomandibular joint disease, etc).

Treatment & Disposition

For treatment and disposition, see under the specific conditions. If there is no apparent cause for the pain, urgent referral to an otolaryngologist is indicated.

SUDDEN DEAFNESS
(See Table 26–4.)

Diagnosis

A. History: Inquire about acoustic trauma (exposure to noise such as construction work, jet planes,

Table 26–3. Diagnostic clues to the cause of ear pain (otalgia).

	History	Physical Examination	Comments
External otitis	Recent swimming and previous attacks common. Discharge from ear.	Pain on movement of pinna. Purulent matter in external ear canal. Normal hearing.	If patient is elderly or diabetic, consider malignant otitis externa.
Infected sebaceous cyst	Pain without discharge.	Pain on movement of pinna. Cyst or abscess in ear canal or near pinna.	Relief of pain when drainage occurs (spontaneous or induced).
Chondritis and perichondritis	Trauma in some. If idiopathic, may have nasal or laryngeal involvement.	Tender, swollen pinna. May be bilateral.	
Suppurative otitis media and myringitis	Pain *inside* ear. Previous attacks, antecedent upper respiratory tract infection, and hearing loss common.	Fever common. Tympanic membrane red and bulbing, with landmarks obscured; may be perforated. Decreased hearing universal with otitis media.	Seen chiefly in children. Bullous myringitis most commonly associated with *Mycoplasma pneumoniae* infection.
Mastoiditis	Pain *posterior* to ear. Coexisting or antecedent otitis media common.	Tenderness of mastoid. May have slight pain on movement of pinna.	CT scan of mastoids preferable; mastoid x-rays may be helpful.
Referred ear pain	Source of pain may be teeth, larynx, tonsil, pharynx, or temporomandibular joint.	Ear examination is normal; may have minimal pain on movement of pinna.	Dental disease, pharyngitis, tonsillitis, parapharyngeal abscess, and temporomandibular arthritis are common causes.

rock bands, or guns) sustained without ear protection; barotrauma (diving, flying, etc); and direct mechanical trauma to the ear or head that might cause temporal bone fracture or disruption of the ossicles. Ask about associated vertigo or tinnitus and use of any ototoxic drugs.

B. Examination: First, determine the degree of hearing loss and whether it is unilateral or bilateral. Test hearing by determining whether the patient can hear a watch ticking or fingers rubbing together. If the patient cannot hear these soft noises, test speech comprehension by progressively increasing the volume of speech. The ear not being tested can be "masked" by occluding the ear canal with a finger placed over

Table 26–4. Diagnostic clues to the cause of sudden hearing loss or tinnitus.

Type of Hearing Loss	Cause	Proportion of Patients With Unilateral Disease	Diagnostic Clues
Conductive Air conduction ≤ bone conduction	Obstructed external ear canal	Most	Cerumen, hematoma, or foreign body in canal.
	Perforated tympanic membrane	Most	Perforation seen on examination.
	Dislocated ossicle	Most	Usually history of trauma; ossicle missing on examination.
	Otitis media (any type)	Some	Pain with pyogenic otitis; no pain with serous and secretory forms. Appearance of tympanic membrane helpful. Immobility of tympanic membrane diagnostic.
Sensorineural Air conduction > bone conduction	Acoustic trauma	Few	History of prolonged exposure to loud noise (eg, rock musician).
	Barotrauma	Few	History of diving (especially scuba), etc.
	Head trauma	Most	History of trauma. Fracture of temporal bone often present; can be demonstrated on appropriate x-rays or CT scan.
	Ototoxic drugs	Few	Especially furosemide, ethacrynic acid, aminoglycosides.
	Vascular insufficiency	Some	History of vascular disease elsewhere.
	Meniere's disease	Some	Vertigo in association with decreased hearing. Often episodic.
	Acoustic neuroma	Most	Tinnitus and mild hearing loss common.
	Other[1]	Variable	Depends on cause.

[1]A number of conditions (especially presbycusis) produce *gradual* hearing loss that is erroneously perceived by the patient as sudden in onset.

the tragus; vibrating the finger produces white sound that masks speech comprehension in that ear.

Next, determine whether hearing loss is conductive or sensorineural (Table 26–5). Use a 250- to 1000-Hz tuning fork (≥ 500 Hz is preferable) to perform the Weber and Rinne tests. In the Weber test, the stem of the vibrating tuning fork is firmly placed against the center of the patient's forehead; in unilateral hearing loss, lateralization occurs, as shown in Table 26–5. In the Rinne test, the stem of the vibrating tuning fork is placed first on the mastoid process (bone conduction) and then the tines of the fork are held immediately lateral to the external ear (air conduction). The differences in perception for bone conduction and for air conduction are compared (Table 26–5).

Examine the patient for nystagmus or unsteadiness of gait, either of which suggests vestibular involvement. Look for obstructions in the external ear canal and for perforations in the tympanic membrane (Fig 26–2) and ossicular disruption.

Laboratory testing is usually not helpful in emergency department evaluation of the patient with acute hearing loss.

Treatment & Disposition

For treatment and disposition, see under specific conditions (eg, cholesteatoma, perforation of the eardrum). Numerous agents have been used to reverse sudden neurosensory hearing loss. Some evidence supports the use of corticosteroids, eg, prednisone, especially for moderate losses. A tapering 10-day course, starting with 60 mg, is a reasonable regimen. These patients should be referred for formal audiometric evaluation and examination by an otolaryngologist.

TINNITUS

All of the conditions that may produce sensorineural hearing loss may also cause tinnitus, and many pa-

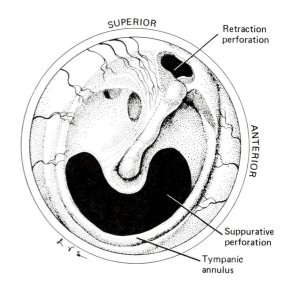

Figure 26–2. Drawing of right tympanic membrane as viewed through an otoscope, showing location of landmarks and common sites of perforation.

tients with tinnitus also have significant hearing loss. The primary importance of tinnitus is that it is a symptom alerting the physician to the possibility of significant sensorineural hearing loss that must be evaluated by audiologic testing and mastoid CT scan or x-rays if it is of recent onset. Acoustic neuroma must be ruled out as well, but this requires further tests that must be ordered by an otolaryngologist.

Tinnitus is such a common disorder that the need for further investigation is often difficult to determine. In general, tinnitus that is pulsatile, unilateral, or changing in character deserves further study. Pulsatile tinnitus often results from vascular causes such as aneurysms, arteriovenous malformations, or glomus tumors, all of which are potentially serious. When tinnitus is unilateral, a unilateral hearing loss (neurosensory or conductive) often is present and should be formally evaluated by an otolaryngologist. Tinnitus that is fluctuating or increasing often represents an active otologic condition and should also be thoroughly evaluated by an otolaryngologist.

Tinnitus due to mild salicylate toxicity should resolve a few hours after the dose is decreased or discontinued. See Chapter 39 for evaluation of more severe salicylate toxicity.

VERTIGO

Pathologic processes involving the central nervous system or inner ear may cause vertigo. In the patient having symptoms of vertigo for the first time, it is important to distinguish peripheral vertigo (caused by lesions of the vestibular nerve and inner ear) from

Table 26–5. Differentiating factors of sensorineural and conductive hearing loss.[1]

Feature	Conductive Hearing Loss	Sensorineural Hearing Loss
Patient's speech	Normal	Loud
Effect of noisy environment	Hears well	Hears poorly
Speech discrimination	Good	Poor
Comprehension of speech on telephone	Good	Poor
Weber test lateralization	To diseased ear	To good ear
Rinne test	Air conduction ≤ bone conduction	Air conduction > bone conduction

[1]Modified and reproduced, with permission, from Krupp MA, Chatton MJ, Werdegar D (editors): *Current Medical Diagnosis & Treatment 1985*. Lange, 1985.

central vertigo (caused by lesions of the central nervous system) (Table 26–6). True vertigo (a sensation that the surroundings are spinning around the patient) must be distinguished from nonspecific lightheadedness, since both are often called "dizziness" by the patient. Since true vertigo is associated with conditions that may cause death or serious disability, rapid evaluation is critical. The physician must look for signs of brain stem or cerebellar infarct (associated cerebellar or cranial nerve abnormalities on neurologic examination) or suppurative labyrinthitis (otorrhea, visible cholesteatoma, or perforation of the tympanic membrane seen on otoscopic examination).

Hospitalization is required if brain stem or cerebellar infarct or suppurative labyrinthitis is suspected or if the patient has severe symptoms, with accompanying nausea and vomiting. Most acute vertiginous episodes may be treated effectively with diazepam, 2–10 mg intravenously; adjust the dose according to the severity of symptoms. Otherwise, treat symptoms (see Meniere's Disease, below), and refer to an otolaryngologist or primary-care physician for evaluation within a few days.

FACIAL NERVE PARALYSIS

Sudden paralysis of the facial nerve is commonly seen in the emergency department. Although often referred to immediately as "Bell's palsy," this designation should only be given after a thorough search for other possible causes has been exhausted (Table 26–7). Although the etiology of true Bell's palsy is unknown, evidence suggests a viral cause. As is the case for other viral neuropathies, other cranial neuropathies can be associated with Bell's palsy.

Diagnosis

Since Bell's palsy typically has a sudden onset (hours to several days), a history indicating that the

Table 26–7. Causes of facial paralysis.

Inflammatory
  Acute otitis media
  Mastoiditis
  Herpes zoster (Ramsay Hunt syndrome)
Metabolic
  Diabetes mellitus
Primary neurologic disorders
  Multiple sclerosis
  Other dimyelinating diseases
  Stroke
Traumatic
  Temporal bone fracture
  Facial laceration
  Iatrogenic (Postmastoid or Parotid surgery)
Neoplastic
  Parotid tumor
  Ear tumor
  Acoustic neuroma
  Primary facial nerve neuroma
Idiopathic (Bell's palsy)

paralysis has been progressive over weeks or months should immediately raise the suspicion of other causes. The paralysis can commonly be preceded or accompanied by pain in the ear and postauricular region. The history should also emphasize other neurologic symptoms, hearing loss, tinnitus, otorrhea, recent viral infections, prior ear infections or ear surgery, and head trauma.

On physical examination, facial paralysis can be either partial or complete, and this should be well documented at the time of the initial evaluation. A full neurologic examination with special attention to the cranial nerves is also imperative. A careful otologic evaluation must be included to rule out infectious or neoplastic causes, and the parotid gland and neck should be carefully palpated for suspicious masses. Since eye closure is often a major difficulty for patients with facial nerve paralysis, a careful eye examination is essential to look for early evidence of keratitis or corneal ulceration.

Table 26–6. Causes and differentiation of central and peripheral vertigo.

	Central Vertigo (Central Nervous System Lesion)	Peripheral Vertigo (Inner Ear Lesion)
Nystagmus	Usually absent (vertical nystagmus may occur in central nervous system lesions without vertigo).	Usually present: horizontal or horizontal-rotatory, with constant direction.
Hearing loss	Rare.	Usually present.
Response to caloric testing	Often normal.	Usually shows abnormal function on involved side.
Other neurologic signs or symptoms	Usually present unless vertigo is due to drug toxicity.	Should not be present (eighth cranial nerve symptoms only).
Other symptoms	Rare.	Nausea and vomiting and sweating common.
Etiology	Drug toxicity. Cerebellar stroke. Brain stem stroke or ischemia.	Meniere's disease. Viral labyrinthitis. Benign paroxysmal postural vertigo. Acoustic neuroma. Suppurative labyrinthitis.

Treatment & Disposition

Bell's palsy is usually self-limited and completely resolves in 80–90% of cases. Although resolution is occasionally incomplete or is associated with synkinesis (mass facial motion), when this occurs a diagnosis other than Bell's palsy should be suspected. Resolution usually begins several weeks after onset; however, it is not unusual for several months to pass before recovery is complete.

Although the role of corticosteroids in the management of Bell's palsy is still controversial, their use in its acute management is becoming more widespread. Whether corticosteroid therapy accelerates improvement or simply provides symptomatic relief from the discomfort occasionally associated with this disorder is unclear. Since short-burst corticosteroids have few adverse effects in otherwise healthy patients (except in diabetics), their use in this situation can be justified.

Caring for the potentially unprotected eye is another important management issue. Poor eye closure is often accompanied by decreased lacrimation (often associated with facial palsy, since the lacrimal gland is innervated by the facial nerve). This combination can produce disastrous corneal complications if the eye is not given proper attention. Frequent moisturization with artificial tears as well as generous lubrication during sleep can help prevent corneal drying. Moisture chambers are also available that, when properly worn, can prevent drying of the eye. Taping the eye closed is fraught with potential problems if done incorrectly and is often best avoided.

Although most cases of Bell's palsy can be managed without subspecialty consultation, otolaryngologic or ophthalmologic referral is often prudent to ensure adequate evaluation and assist in monitoring both the return of facial function and the corneal status. Bell's palsy is a poorly understood but dramatic event in the life of patients. Continued reassurance emphasizing the need for patience is an essential part of caring for the patient.

SORE THROAT
**(See Table 26–8
and also Chapter 34.)**

When evaluating the patient who complains of a sore throat, first determine whether the airway is threatened. *Do not perform oropharyngeal examination in patients with severe pharyngeal pain associated with severe odynophagia (pain on swallowing), trismus, drooling, or dyspnea* until a lateral soft tissue x-ray (or CT scan) of the neck has been obtained to differentiate epiglottitis from pharyngeal abscesses, Ludwig's angina, or other more benign causes of pharyngitis. Examining the posterior pharynx of a patient with epiglottitis may precipitate sudden total airway obstruction. Patients with Ludwig's angina or

pharyngeal abscesses may likewise develop airway obstruction, although it is usually more gradual in onset.

Equipment for intubation, cricothyrotomy, or tracheostomy should be immediately at hand, and the patient must never be left unattended. If x-rays must be obtained outside the emergency department, the equipment necessary for intubation and personnel proficient in its use must accompany the patient.

Diagnosis

In patients without epiglottitis, carefully examine the oropharynx and neck, avoiding unnecessary manipulation. Tonsillar and peritonsillar abscesses are obvious on inspection. CT scan or lateral soft tissue x-rays of the neck are diagnostic for epiglottitis and parapharyngeal and retropharyngeal abscesses, and they are the best means of delineating the extent of Ludwig's angina. The history and physical examination of the oropharynx usually provide clues to other causes of pharyngitis (Table 26–8). For further details of diagnosis and treatment, see under the specific conditions (eg, pharyngeal and retropharyngeal abscesses, Ludwig's angina).

Treatment & Disposition

Patients with epiglottitis, Ludwig's angina, or large abscesses around the pharynx should be hospitalized for immediate otolaryngologic consultation and airway care. Patients with epiglottitis should have an endotracheal tube inserted only under direct vision in the operating room (tracheostomy is indicated only if the patient cannot be intubated). Patients with Ludwig's angina and abscesses should be carefully observed for development of airway obstruction. Start antibiotics and other treatments as discussed under the specific conditions and in Table 26–8.

II. EMERGENCY TREATMENT OF SPECIFIC DISORDERS

EXTERNAL EAR

EXTERNAL OTITIS

Diagnosis

The most common ear infection in adults is external otitis (swimmer's ear). This infection is initially a dermatitis of the skin over the conchal cartilage that progresses to frank infection. It is usually caused by staphylococci or *Pseudomonas aeruginosa*. Infection

Table 26–8. Diagnosis and treatment of conditions causing sore throat.

	Helpful Diagnostic Findings	Treatment
Epiglottitis	High fever, severe pain, hoarse voice, drooling, painful and difficult swallowing, dyspnea. Emergency lateral soft tissue x-ray of neck or CT scan is usually diagnostic. *Do not examine pharynx without equipment for intubation at hand.*	Obtain emergency ENT consultation for airway management. Obtain blood culture; begin antibiotics (cefuroxime, 100 mg/kg/d intravenously; or chloramphenicol, 100 mg/kg/d orally or intravenously).
Ludwig's angina	High fever, severe pain, elevated and retracted tongue, thickened floor of mouth. May have airway obstruction. Lateral soft tissue x-ray or CT scan confirmatory.	Hospitalize. Give penicillin G, 200,000 units/kg/d intravenously. Obtain ENT consultation.
Abscess (peritonsillar, parapharyngeal, retropharyngeal)	Severe pain, hoarseness, drooling, difficulty in swallowing, dyspnea. Lateral soft tissue x-ray often diagnostic in retropharyngeal abscess.	Hospitalize. Obtain ENT consultation. Consider incision and drainage. Give penicillin G, 200,000 units/kg/d intravenously.
Group A streptococcal infection	Fever, exudate, adenopathy common. Throat culture showing group A β streptococci is diagnostic.	Give penicillin or erythromycin (Chapter 34).
Infectious mononucleosis	Fever, exudate; often diffuse lymphadenopathy with splenomegaly. Heterophil antibodies present after 8–10 days of symptoms.	Symptomatic. Prednisone orally for severe symptoms.
Herpes simplex infection	Multiple oral and perioral ulcers and vesicles. Positive culture, antigen, or Tzanck test.	Intravenous or oral acyclovir, depending on severity (Chapter 34).
Acute necrotizing ulcerative gingivostomatitis (trench mouth; Vincent's angina)	Gray, ulcerated gingiva. Pharynx may be normal or covered with ulcerated lesions.	Give penicillin V or erythromycin. Peroxide mouthwashes. Refer to dentist.
Diphtheria	Fever; tenacious gray pharyngeal membrane. May have early neuritis or carditis. Culture for *Corynebacterium diphtheriae* is positive. Patient usually very ill.	Hospitalize. Give antitoxin and either erythromycin or penicillin G.
Gonorrhea	Often asymptomatic. Suspect if there is a history of oral-genital contact. Culture for *Neisseria gonorrhoeae* on selective medium (eg, Thayer-Martin).	Treat for gonorrhea (Chapter 34).
Tuberculosis	Usually associated with far-advanced pulmonary tuberculosis. Smear and culture for *Mycobacterium tuberculosis*.	Hospitalize for treatment of tuberculosis. Institute infection control precautions (single room, mask for patient, etc).

often follows exposure to water. Trauma associated with cleaning the ear may also precipitate the disease. Swelling and purulent discharge from the external auditory canal in a patient with tenderness elicited by movement of the pinna confirm the diagnosis.

Treatment

A small cotton wick should be placed in the ear canal to conduct topical medication toward the medial end of the ear canal. Combined steroid and antibiotic otic preparations, eg, Cortisporin-Otic or Pyocidin-Otic; and acetic acid, 2%, in aluminum acetate solution (Otic Domeboro), are both effective. The medication should be continued for 7–10 days. Systemic antibiotics are not necessary.

Disposition

The patient should be seen daily until improvement occurs. If conditions predisposing to malignant otitis externa are present (diabetes, advanced age), otolaryngologic consultation within 1–2 days is advisable.

MALIGNANT EXTERNAL OTITIS

Diagnosis

Malignant external otitis is an invasive variant of otitis externa that pursues a fulminant course and may result in osteomyelitis of the base of the skull and death. It usually occurs in elderly diabetic patients and is secondary to infection with *P aeruginosa*. Facial paralysis; neuropathy of cranial nerves IX, X, and XI; or the presence of granulation tissue or exposed bone in the ear canal suggests malignant external otitis.

Treatment & Disposition

Emergency hospitalization and consultation with specialists in otolaryngology and infectious diseases are required.

CHONDRITIS & PERICHONDRITIS

Diagnosis

Chondritis or perichondritis of the external ear may follow contusion or laceration of the auricle (including ear piercing for earrings) or secondary infection of an auricular hematoma, or it may result from spread of infection from other sites on the pinna. In perichondritis (infection of auricular soft tissue overlying the cartilage), the ear is red, hot, tender, and diffusely swollen, but with normal anatomy. If infection has extended to involve the auricular cartilage (chondritis), there will be gross deformity of the external ear as well.

Treatment & Disposition

Perichondritis usually responds to hot soaks and antimicrobials (eg, dicloxacillin, 500 mg orally 4 times daily for adults, 40 mg/kg/d orally in 4 divided doses for children). The patient should be seen in 1–2 days to ensure that recovery is progressing satisfactorily.

Patients with chondritis require examination by an otolaryngologist and head and neck surgeon and hospitalization for administration of antistaphylococcal antimicrobials (eg, nafcillin or equivalent, 150 mg/kg/d intravenously in 4–6 divided doses). Incision and drainage is indicated if localized fluctuance over the auricle suggests abscess.

SEBACEOUS CYST WITH CELLULITIS

Diagnosis

The external ear, particularly the postauricular aspect, is a frequent site of sebaceous cyst formation. These cysts are often infected and cause extreme pain and tenderness on movement of the pinna.

Treatment & Disposition

Incise and drain the cyst, and start antibiotic therapy (eg, dicloxacillin, 40 mg/kg/d orally in 4 divided doses [up to 500 mg 4 times daily for adults]). Following resolution of the acute infection, the sebaceous cyst should be removed in its entirety to prevent recurrence. Refer the patient to an otolaryngologist for subsequent definitive excision.

FROSTBITE OF THE AURICLE
(See also Chapter 38.)

Diagnosis

There is a recent history of exposure to cold. The involved auricle is white and anesthetic in frostbite. Blisters occur in severe cases.

Treatment & Disposition

Rapid rewarming of the auricular area with luke-warm (about 40–42 °C [104–107.6 °F]) saline compresses gives the best result. The ear should be protected with a gentle compression bandage, consisting of soft cotton fluff and wraparound roller gauze, until the extent of devitalized tissue can be determined. The patient should be told that the auricle will probably be deformed and that the ear will be more than normally susceptible to frostbite in the future. Refer the patient to an otolaryngologist or primary-care physician for follow-up within 2–3 days. Patients with extensive or severe frostbite of the auricle should be hospitalized. See Chapter 38 for further details.

IMPACTED CERUMEN

Diagnosis

The patient commonly reports a history of diminished hearing or a "plugged" ear and, less commonly, of ear pain. The diagnosis is obvious on examination of the ear canal.

Treatment & Disposition

Removal of impacted cerumen may be difficult. The method used depends on the type of cerumen involved.

A. Hard, dried wax is best removed by gentle irrigation of the ear canal with tap water at body temperature. Excessively cold or hot water causes vertigo, as occurs in the caloric test. Impacted hard wax can be softened for easier removal if the patient uses mineral oil or carbamide (urea) peroxide, 6.5%, in anhydrous glycerin (Debrox) for 7 days, or the wax can be softened and removed in the office by using *m*-cresyl acetate (Cresylate) on a cotton-tipped applicator.

B. Soft, moist cerumen is best removed by using a large Frazier suction tip through the ear speculum. A cerumen curet is helpful. Removal of cerumen must be performed gently, since the bony part of the ear canal is sensitive to touch.

FOREIGN BODIES IN THE EAR

Diagnosis

Foreign bodies in the ear canal cause various symptoms (primarily pain, discharge, or decreased hearing); the diagnosis is obvious on examination.

Treatment & Disposition

In small children, general anesthesia is sometimes indicated to ensure atraumatic removal of the foreign body. In older children and adults, a trial of local anesthesia and suction or manipulation with forceps is appropriate. Local anesthesia of the ear canal can be obtained by injecting lidocaine, 1%, mixed with a 1:100,000 solution of aqueous epinephrine beneath the skin of the ear canal using a 27- or 30-gauge needle and a tuberculin syringe. It is best to wait 3–5 minutes after injection before beginning any manipulation. Live insects in the ear canal should be immobilized with a few drops of topical anesthetic (eg, lidocaine) or mineral oil and then removed with a large metal suction tip.

After the foreign body has been successfully removed, patients do not require further care unless trauma to the canal is present, in which case treatment for external otitis should be started and follow-up as an outpatient arranged within 4–5 days.

EARDRUM & MIDDLE EAR

PERFORATIONS OF THE EARDRUM
(See Fig 26–2.)

Diagnosis

When perforation of the eardrum is a diagnostic possibility, ask carefully about a history of early or recent trauma, including explosions or direct trauma to the ear (eg, boxing of the ears). Tympanic membrane perforation with severe vertigo or complete hearing loss is an otologic emergency, because it indicates that the inner ear is involved. Traumatic or suppurative injury to the inner ear may be reversible with prompt surgery. Depending on the cause, perforation of the eardrum may be asymptomatic or may be associated with pain, hearing loss, or discharge from the ear.

When examining the tympanic membrane for perforation, use the largest possible speculum that the ear canal can accommodate. If it is not clear whether the eardrum has been perforated, use a pneumatic otoscope. Many clear areas in the eardrum resemble perforations when in fact they are healed perforations in which the middle fibrous layer has not regenerated. These areas resemble thin cellophane on examination with a pneumatic otoscope. A white cheesy substance visible through the perforation is a sign of cholesteatoma. Suppurative perforations may be associated with a purulent exudate coming from the middle ear.

Treatment & Disposition

Treatment and disposition depend on the specific condition.

A. Perforation With Severe Vertigo or Complete Hearing Loss: Involvement of the inner ear is likely if perforation of the membrane is associated with severe vertigo or complete hearing loss. Hospitalize the patient, and obtain emergency otolaryngologic consultation for possible decompressive surgery.

B. Cholesteatoma: A white cheesy substance is visible through the perforation. Temporal bone CT scan or x-rays show destruction of the mastoid area. If vertigo is present, cholesteatoma is an otologic emergency (see Suppurative Labyrinthitis & Perilabyrinthitis, below). If there is no vertigo, refer the patient to an otolaryngologist for elective surgery.

C. Traumatic Perforation: If acute traumatic perforation extends over more than 50% of the eardrum, surgical debridement and tympanoplastic repair in the operating room are indicated. The ear surgeon can also remove portions of squamous epithelium that may have spread to the mucosa of the middle ear. These bits of skin may cause cholesteatoma if they are not removed. Cooperative patients with smaller traumatic perforations of the eardrum may be examined every 3–4 days. Such perforations normally heal by themselves if left alone.

D. Suppurative Perforation: Suppurative perforation results when pus in the middle ear caused by otitis media ruptures through the tympanic membrane. Suppurative perforation is commonly located in the inferior portion of the tympanic membrane and has a kidney bean shape (Fig 26–2). Palpate the mastoid process; if it is tender, obtain mastoid CT scan or x-rays to determine whether suppurative mastoiditis has developed. Treat otitis media (see below), and refer the patient to an otolaryngologist or primary-care physician within 2–3 days for inspection of the eardrum to make sure the perforation is not extensive and that healing is progressing. If the perforation has not healed after 3 months, the patient should be referred for myringoplasty (graft repair of the perforation).

E. Retraction Perforation: Retraction perforation is seen in the upper portion of the eardrum superior to the mallear folds (Fig 26–2). Retraction perforation is almost always associated with bony erosion by cholesteatoma, and patients should be referred to an otolaryngologist within 2–3 days. Obtain mastoid CT scan or x-rays before the patient is referred, and treat complications (otitis media, mastoiditis) if present.

BULLOUS MYRINGITIS

Diagnosis

Bullous myringitis is inflammation of the tympanic membrane without involvement of the middle ear. It is usually due to viruses or *Mycoplasma pneumoniae*. Patients complain of severe pain. Examination shows tympanic membrane inflammation and bullae or hemorrhagic blebs. Hearing and mobility of the tympanic membrane are not affected.

Treatment & Disposition

Treatment is symptomatic unless *M pneumoniae* is thought to be the causative agent of infection, in which case erythromycin or tetracycline should be given.

ACUTE SUPPURATIVE OTITIS MEDIA

Diagnosis

Acute suppurative otitis media is a common infection of the middle ear cavity, especially in children. It often accompanies or follows a viral upper respiratory tract infection and is thought to be due in part to swelling and obstruction of the auditory (eustachian) tube. Common causative organisms are the pneumococcus and *Haemophilus influenzae;* the latter is seen primarily in children under 6 years of age.

Ear pain with erythema or bulging of the tympanic membrane confirms the diagnosis. In younger children, especially those with *H influenzae* infection, ear pain and systemic signs of acute infection may be less prominent, and immobility of the eardrum may be the only finding.

Treatment & Disposition

The treatment of choice is amoxicillin, 500 mg orally 3 times daily (for children, 30 mg/kg/d orally in 3 divided doses) or ampicillin, 500 mg orally 4 times daily (for children, 50 mg/kg/d orally in 4 divided doses). If infection due to ampicillin-resistant *H influenzae* is suspected, give trimethoprim-sulfamethoxazole (Bactrim, Septra), 8–10 mg/kg (trimethoprim) and 40–50 mg/kg (sulfamethoxazole) orally every 12 hours; or cefaclor (Ceclor), 40 mg/kg/d orally in 3–4 divided doses.

Infection may subside more quickly if a topical vasoconstrictor such as phenylephrine (eg, Neo-Synephrine, 0.25%), as nose drops or nasal spray, is used as well as an oral decongestant (eg, pseudoephedrine [Sudafed, others]; phenylpropanolamine in combination with phenylephrine and brompheniramine [Dimetapp, others]; or chlorpheniramine [Ornade, others]).

After antimicrobial therapy has been started, the patient should be seen within 2–3 days to determine whether recovery is progressing satisfactorily. If tympanic membrane perforation occurs during acute infection, the patient should be examined every 2 weeks until the perforation heals.

SEROUS OTITIS MEDIA

Diagnosis

Serous otitis media is caused by a collection of low-viscosity fluid in the middle ear space and follows obstruction of the auditory tube. It is often caused by viral upper respiratory tract infection. Ear congestion with hearing loss is the most common complaint. Consider carcinoma of the nasopharynx as a potential cause in middle-aged and elderly patients and particularly in patients of Chinese origin. Occasionally, a splashing sensation is felt in the ear when the head is moved. Examination of the tympanic membrane reveals a dull, amber-colored, immobile eardrum, often with a visible fluid level. Results in the Rinne test are abnormal, with bone conduction greater than air conduction.

Treatment & Disposition

A. If serous otitis media occurs secondary to upper respiratory tract infection, prescribe a decongestant for 2 weeks, with weekly follow-up examination. If fluid fails to disappear, referral to an otolaryngologist for possible myringotomy and insertion of a ventilating tube is indicated.

B. In middle-aged or elderly patients with serous otitis media, failure of fluid to disappear after 3 weeks requires referral to an otolaryngologist.

SECRETORY OTITIS MEDIA

Diagnosis

Secretory otitis media usually occurs in children who have had one or more bouts of acute suppurative otitis media. The middle ear responds to antecedent infection by producing mucinous gluelike material. Secretory otitis media, like serous otitis media, is not painful, and the only symptom is conductive hearing loss. If the child is old enough to respond appropriately, the Rinne tuning fork test confirms the diagnosis in the presence of an immobile tympanic membrane.

Treatment & Disposition

Although management includes a trial of decongestant therapy, it is often ineffective in treating the persistent effusion. A 3- to 4-week trial of antibiotic therapy often results in resolution. When the effusion persists despite these measures, referral to an otolaryngologist is necessary for consideration of myringotomy tube placement.

CHRONIC SUPPURATIVE OTITIS MEDIA

Diagnosis

The term chronic suppurative otitis media refers to chronic perforation of the tympanic membrane. Mastoid CT scan or x-rays should be obtained in every case to detect mastoiditis or cholesteatoma.

Treatment & Disposition

If mastoid CT scan or x-rays reveal cholesteatoma with destruction of bone, mastoidectomy is necessary. Because chronic perforation of the eardrum with cholesteatoma may be associated with several life-threatening intracranial complications (eg, brain abscess), all patients require immediate hospitalization and consultation with an ear specialist.

If there is no discharge through the perforation (indicating that there is no infection of the middle ear or mastoid), myringoplasty may be performed by an otologic surgeon to repair perforation and restore hearing.

COMPLICATIONS OF OTITIS MEDIA

Intracranial Abscess

Brain abscess, subdural abscess, or epidural abscess may be caused by spread of infection from cholesteatoma of the middle ear. The wall between the middle ear and the dura of the middle cranial fossa is bony but paper-thin. A cholesteatoma may erode through it, carrying purulent material to and beyond the dura of the temporal lobe of the brain. If the abscess is extradural (epidural), there may be only localizing neurologic signs in addition to purulent otorrhea. If the abscess has passed through the dura (subdural abscess), cerebrospinal fluid examination shows inflammatory cells. Coexisting meningitis (otogenic meningitis) may be present with the physical findings that are usually associated with meningitis. Patients with abscess of the temporal lobe may have aphasia, visual field defects, or other focal neurologic signs.

Immediate hospitalization is required for evaluation and possible surgery.

Otogenic Meningitis

Otogenic meningitis may follow uncomplicated acute suppurative otitis media but is more frequently associated with a chronic suppurative process. Patients with large cholesteatomas may have recurrent attacks of meningitis.

The patient should receive intravenous antimicrobials for 24–48 hours before surgical removal of the cholesteatoma is undertaken. See Chapter 34 for details of treatment.

Septic Lateral Sinus Thrombosis

Septic lateral sinus thrombosis is a serious illness that may be accompanied by a classic "picket fence" fever denoting intermittent invasion of the bloodstream by bacteria from the infected thrombus in the jugular vein. Septic lateral sinus thrombosis may or may not be associated with meningitis or cerebellar abscess. The diagnosis should be suspected when high, spiking fevers occur in a patient with purulent material draining from the ear.

Treatment includes immediate hospitalization for administration of intravenous antibiotics, mastoidectomy, and surgical removal of the infected thrombus from the involved sinus.

Facial Paralysis

Damage to the facial nerve from infections, tumors, or cholesteatoma of the middle ear is common, because the facial nerve passes through bone near the middle ear.

Hospitalize the patient for evaluation and possible surgery.

Petrous Apicitis (Gradenigo's Syndrome)

The 3 classic symptoms of petrous apicitis are purulent otorrhea, retro-orbital pain, and abducens nerve palsy. In this disease, infection extends medially in the temporal bone to break through and deposit epidural pus in the area of the trigeminal ganglion and sixth cranial nerve.

Immediate hospitalization is required for administration of intravenous antibiotics before mastoidectomy.

INNER EAR

MENIERE'S DISEASE (Paroxysmal Labyrinthine Vertigo)

Diagnosis

Meniere's disease causes vertigo that occurs in episodes lasting not less than 30 minutes and not longer than 24 hours. The spells of vertigo are intense, so that nausea and vomiting and diaphoresis are almost always seen during an attack. A feeling of pressure in the ear, tinnitus, and sensorineural hearing loss also occur. Meniere's disease often occurs in men past middle age. There is no definitive diagnostic test. Other causes of vertigo and hearing loss must be excluded (Table 26–6).

Treatment & Disposition

For the acute vertiginous episode, give diazepam, 5 mg intravenously over 5 minutes, for rapid symptomatic relief. Place the patient on a low-salt diet, and arrange for referral to an otolaryngologist. Some patients benefit from either antihistamines (eg, dimenhydrinate, 50–100 mg orally 3–4 times daily) or nicotinic acid, 50–150 mg orally 3–4 times daily. Hospitalization is rarely necessary, and then only for relief of symptoms.

VIRAL LABYRINTHITIS (Vestibular Neuronitis)

Diagnosis

Viral labyrinthitis differs from most other causes of vertigo originating in the inner ear in that hearing is normal. Nystagmus usually occurs in all directions of gaze, and the associated nausea and vomiting may be severe. Vertigo is usually incapacitating. Attacks last longer than in Meniere's disease—often 5 or 6 days—but recurrence is uncommon. The patient is usually left with a diminished response to the caloric test in the involved ear.

Treatment & Disposition

Hospitalization is often required for patients with severe symptoms. Diazepam, 5 mg intravenously over 5 minutes, may help relieve symptoms. Meclizine, 25–50 mg orally 3 times daily, also may alleviate symptoms.

BENIGN PAROXYSMAL POSTURAL VERTIGO

Diagnosis

Benign paroxysmal postural vertigo may occur after head trauma or may be idiopathic. Vertigo characteristically follows turning of the head to one particular side, usually with the patient supine. If this maneuver is repeated, vertigo does not recur after the second movement. Hearing is usually normal.

Treatment & Disposition

No specific treatment is known. The patient should be reassured that symptoms usually resolve after 4–5 months. If symptoms worsen or persist, the patient should return for further evaluation. Meclizine, 25–50 mg orally 3 times daily, may alleviate symptoms.

ACOUSTIC NEUROMA

Acoustic neuroma causes vertigo, unsteadiness during walking, and light-headedness. Tinnitus and hearing loss occur frequently. Significant vertigo that interferes with daily activities and lasts longer than 3 weeks should arouse a suspicion of acoustic neuroma. X-rays may show enlargement of the internal auditory canal. Definitive diagnosis is usually made by CT scan.

The patient should be referred to an otolaryngologist for evaluation.

SUPPURATIVE LABYRINTHITIS & PERILABYRINTHITIS

Diagnosis

In suppurative labyrinthitis and perilabyrinthitis, the inner ear is damaged by nearby infection in the temporal bone. Usually, a cholesteatoma has eroded parts of the temporal bone adjacent to the inner ear, and the contiguous infection causes an inflammatory reaction in the perilymph of the inner ear. Patients often have poor hearing and intermittent vertigo. If cholesteatoma or perforation of the tympanic membrane is visible, the **fistula test** is often diagnostic: Using a pneumatic otoscope, induce positive pressure

in the ear canal. In such patients, the eyes deviate to the opposite side (away from the affected ear), and the patient experiences vertigo until positive pressure is relieved; in normal subjects, no vertigo or eye deviation occurs. Mastoid CT scan or x-rays show erosion of the mastoid air cells in the temporal bone.

Treatment & Disposition

Hospitalize the patient immediately, and obtain otolaryngologic consultation. Begin intravenous antibiotics (eg, cefuroxime, 100 mg/kg/d intravenously in 3 divided doses), and prepare the patient for emergency mastoidectomy within 48 hours to prevent further inner ear damage.

MASTOID

MASTOIDITIS

The mastoid air cell system is in contiguity with the middle ear space. As a result, acute suppurative otitis media is typically associated with an acute suppurative process of the mastoid air space. Usually, when infection in the middle ear subsides, disease in the mastoid subsides also. Occasionally, however, infection smolders in the mastoid after the otitis media has cleared, a condition known as acute coalescent mastoiditis.

Diagnosis

Symptoms and signs include tenderness over the mastoid tip, fever, and, in some cases, sagging of the posterosuperior ear canal as seen through the otoscope. Mastoid CT scan or x-ray shows opacification of the mastoid with destruction of the intercellular septa, although x-ray findings are not discernible until 2 weeks after onset of the mastoid infection. Fluid in the mastoid air cells without septal destruction is not usually interpreted as mastoiditis.

Treatment & Disposition

Urgent hospitalization for administration of parenteral antibiotics (eg, cefuroxime, 100 mg/kg/d intravenously in 3 divided doses, pending results of culture) and mastoidectomy are required.

CHOLESTEATOMA

Cholesteatoma is a collection of desquamated epithelial cells resulting from growth of squamous epithelium into the middle ear. Cholesteatoma behaves like a benign tumor in that it compresses and erodes adjacent structures as it grows. It occurs most frequently as a result of peripheral perforations of the tympanic membrane that may be minute.

Diagnosis

Suspect cholesteatoma in any patient with painless chronic otorrhea and perforation of the tympanic membrane (ie, chronic otitis media). Examination usually discloses conductive hearing loss, and in many patients, the cholesteatoma can be visualized through or behind the tympanic membrane as a white, cheesy mass. Obtain mastoid CT scan or x-rays in every case of suspected cholesteatoma to look for bony erosion and superimposed mastoiditis.

Treatment & Disposition

No emergency treatment is indicated for the cholesteatoma itself, though therapy for complications (mastoiditis, etc) should be started. The patient should be seen by an otolaryngologist within a few days.

SINUSES

SINUSITIS

Sinusitis is most commonly due to bacterial infection of the sinus cavity that is exacerbated by obstruction of sinus drainage (eg, because of viral infection). Other conditions causing sinusitis or paving the way for bacterial infections include viral upper respiratory tract infections, allergies, polyps, and tumors in or near the sinuses.

Diagnosis

Sinus pain and tenderness are characteristic of acute sinusitis. There may also be swelling over the affected sinus and purulent nasal discharge. Systemic symptoms of infection are common. Specific symptoms depend on which sinus is involved (Table 26–9). Sinus x-rays (Figs 26–3 and 26–4) should be ordered in all cases. The physician should consider the possibility of tumor or, in frontal sinusitis, a mucopyocele in all patients with sinusitis. Sinus x-rays in these cases show a mass lesion eroding bone.

Culture (for bacteriologic diagnosis of sinusitis) is useful only if the specimen is obtained by direct aspiration of sinus contents, usually performed by an otolaryngologist. Culture of purulent nasal discharge is useless, since false-negative and false-positive results may occur. Therefore, unless the patient is sufficiently ill to warrant sinus puncture or surgical drainage, treatment must be empiric. The usual pathogens are pneumococci, streptococci, and *H influenzae*.

Table 26–9. Clinical findings in acute sinusitis.[1]

Sinus	Symptoms and Signs	X-Ray Signs
Maxillary	Pain and tenderness of upper teeth and cheek overlying affected sinus.	Upright Waters view shows air-fluid level or thickened mucosa. Affected sinus is opacified when compared with contralateral sinus or orbit.
Ethmoid	Central facial pain and tenderness (glabella, root of nose). Often occurs in association with maxillary sinusitis.	Base and lateral views show loss of bony septa and opacification.
Frontal	Frontal sinus pain and tenderness. Rule out mucopyocele (see text).	Caldwell, lateral Waters views show air-fluid levels, loss of "scalloped" pattern, or sinus opacification.
Sphenoid	Poorly localized pain in mastoid, occipital, or parietal regions.	Base and lateral views show opacification, air-fluid levels.

[1]If erosion of bone is seen on sinus films, a tumor, mucopyocele, or (rarely) osteomyelitis should be suspected.

Treatment

Amoxicillin, 30 mg/kg/d orally in 3 divided doses (up to 500 mg 3 times daily) for 10 days, is the drug of choice. Trimethoprim-sulfamethoxazole, 8–10 mg/kg/d (trimethoprim) in 2 divided doses, may be substituted in patients allergic to penicillin. In cases resistant to these standard antibiotics, amoxicillin with clavulanate or cefuroxime axetil offer good oral alternatives with broader spectra and beta-lactamase resistance. Cefuroxime, 100 mg/kg/d intravenously in 3 divided doses, may be used for hospitalized patients while results of culture are pending. Prescribe an oral decongestant (eg, pseudoephedrine, 30–60 mg every 4–6 hours). Nasal decongestant sprays should be provided as well; however, because of the potential rebound phenomenon associated with these sprays, their use should be limited to no more than 4–5 days of continual use.

Take follow-up x-rays in 2 weeks to confirm that sinusitis has resolved in patients who show improvement. Any sinus infection that becomes chronic requires surgical drainage.

Disposition

Severely ill patients with systemic symptoms such as high fever and rigors or pain requiring parenteral narcotics for relief should be hospitalized immediately for administration of parenteral antibiotics, since decompressive surgery may be necessary. Patients with systemic symptoms (fever, etc) who fail to improve following a few days of outpatient therapy should also be hospitalized. Patients with a persistent air-fluid level after 2 weeks of treatment should be

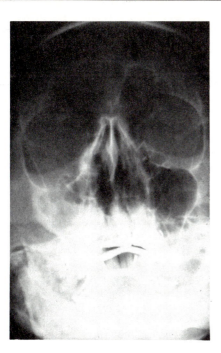

Figure 26–3. Acute maxillary sinusitis. Upright Waters view showing opacification of right maxillary sinus and normally aerated left side.

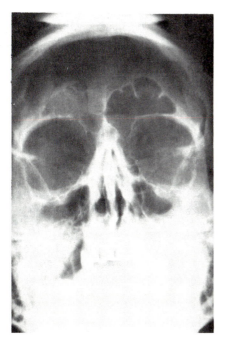

Figure 26–4. Acute frontal sinusitis. Waters view showing air-fluid level in left frontal sinus. Right frontal sinus does not have normal aeration because of prior surgery (space was filled with fat).

referred to an otolaryngologist for irrigation of the antra or surgery.

COMPLICATIONS OF SINUSITIS

As is the case for otitis media, intracranial complications can occasionally accompany sinusitis.

Osteomyelitis of the Frontal Bone

This complication of frontal sinusitis, also known as Pott's puffy tumor, typically presents with erythema, edema, tenderness, and doughy swelling of the forehead. Treatment usually consists of surgical removal of infected bone and administration of long-term parenteral antibiotics. A high index of suspicion must be maintained for other intracranial complications such as epidural or brain abscess.

Meningitis

Although meningitis can be associated with infections of any of the paranasal sinuses, it is most frequently reported in association with sphenoid sinusitis. Since partial antibiotic treatment can often mask the typical signs and symptoms of meningitis, patients may initially present with only mild headache, retro-orbital pain, or subtle changes in sensorium. A thorough physical and neurologic examination and a high index of suspicion are essential to the diagnosis. When suspected, CT scan (to rule out space-occupying intracranial lesions) followed by lumbar puncture can establish the diagnosis and guide definitive antibiotic therapy.

Epidural Abscess

Usually associated with frontal sinusitis and osteomyelitis of the posterior table of the frontal sinus, this condition is characterized by headaches and spiking fevers. When suspected, diagnostic evaluation with CT scan should be performed. Depending on the size of the abscess and the associated clinical picture, these abscesses can be managed either surgically or medically.

Subdural Empyema

This intracranial complication usually is associated with frontal sinusitis and consists of a collection of pus between the dura and leptomeninges. The clinical course is usually fulminant. Although initially intense headaches may be the only symptom, there is usually a rapid progression to nuchal rigidity, an altered level of consciousness, hemiparesis, hemiplegia, and seizures. CT scanning is crucial to localizing the infection and determining its site of origin. Subdural empyema is a true neurosurgical emergency requiring early craniotomy and drainage.

Brain Abscess

Although treatable, brain abscess frequently

causes substantial morbidity because of its often initial silent nature. The clinical presentation ranges from mild headaches and subtle personality changes to partial paralysis or complete obtundation. CT scanning is necessary to establish the diagnosis and initiate therapy. Delay in diagnosis, brainstem herniation, and multiple abscesses all have deleterious effects on ultimate outcome.

Orbital Cellulitis & Abscess

Orbital complications of sinusitis almost always are associated with ethmoid infections. When the initial presentation is the periorbital infection, its paranasal sinus origin frequently is overlooked. Although mild edema, erythema, tenderness, and pain on eye movement may be the only findings, spread of infection into the retrobulbar region can result in proptosis, ophthalmoplegia, and ultimately blindness. Extension of the orbital infection into the cavernous sinus also can occur, resulting in cavernous sinus thrombosis. Early recognition of a potential orbital complication of sinusitis is essential to early diagnosis and intervention.

NOSE

NASAL FOREIGN BODIES

Diagnosis

Impacted foreign bodies are seen almost exclusively in children or mentally incompetent patients, and there is frequently a history of the object (peanut, seed, etc) having been inserted into the nose. The patient may be asymptomatic or may present with nasal discharge, nasal obstruction, or even sinusitis. The foreign body causes unilateral airway obstruction (the patient can breathe out of one side of the nose but not the other) and is usually evident on rhinoscopy. The principal differential diagnosis is tumor, which is seen primarily in older children (angiofibroma) and in adults (especially of Chinese descent).

Treatment & Disposition

Spray the nasal chamber with 5% cocaine, and attempt to remove the object using a nasal speculum, good lighting, Adson forceps, and strong suction. Restrain the child firmly in order to avoid pushing the object farther into the nasal passage. Rarely, the object cannot be removed with ease, in which case immediate otolaryngologic consultation should be sought, since general anesthesia may be required for removal. After the object has been removed, the patient may be discharged without further follow-up

unless removal has caused extensive trauma to the nasal mucosa.

NASAL POLYPS

Diagnosis

There are 2 types of nasal polyps. **Allergic polyps** are pale yellow, with a glistening surface. Most patients with allergic polyps give a history of allergic symptoms, eg, sneezing, itching, nasal obstruction, and watery rhinorrhea, all of which are seasonal. **Inflammatory polyps** (secondary to chronic infection) are pink and have a more fleshy appearance than allergic polyps. They are more likely to be found in patients with chronic sinus infections who show fewer allergic symptoms.

Both kinds of polyps cause nasal obstruction and may be responsible for sinusitis by obstructing outflow of the protective blanket of mucus from the sinuses into the nasal chamber. Polyps usually start to grow in the ethmoid sinuses and progress to occlude the ostium of the maxillary sinuses.

Sinus x-rays should always be taken to document the extent of sinus involvement in patients with nasal polyposis. Involved sinuses reveal thickening of the lining membrane or complete opacification.

Treatment & Disposition

Refer the patient to an otolaryngologist for evaluation and treatment.

PHARYNX & HYPOPHARYNX

TONSILLAR & PERITONSILLAR ABSCESSES & CELLULITIS

Tonsillar abscesses may follow episodes of pharyngitis or tonsillitis, though they are observed much less frequently now than in the past. Abscesses within the tonsil itself are rare; much more common are peritonsillar abscesses (quinsy), in which pus moves into the peritonsillar fascial planes, usually the supratonsillar fossa. The infection is usually caused by streptococci and other components of normal mouth flora.

Diagnosis

Most cases begin with an attack of pharyngitis or tonsillitis. The initial symptoms of pharyngitis then worsen. Fever rises, pain becomes severe, and trismus and dysphagia develop. Occasionally, pain on swallowing is so severe that the patient may drool. The patient's mouth may be kept partially open because of trismus. Dyspnea occurs in some patients if the abscess causes significant obstruction of the airway.

Caution: If severe pain, trismus, drooling, or dyspnea is present, rule out epiglottitis with an emergency lateral soft tissue x-ray of the neck taken before examination of the oropharynx is attempted.

The patient appears anxious and shows signs of systemic infection. If the abscess is in the supratonsillar fossa (the most common location), the tonsils themselves are not markedly enlarged, but the soft palate on one side is edematous and swollen, the uvula shows deviation away from the affected side, and the tonsil is displaced inferomedially by the abscess (Fig 26–5). Gentle palpation of the peritonsillar and tonsillar tissues intraorally reveals swelling or fluctuance.

Treatment & Disposition

A. Mild or Early Cases: For patients without drooling, dyspnea, fluctuant abscess, or severe pain or signs of infection, give penicillin V or erythromycin, 500 mg orally 4 times a day (proportionately lower doses in children), with daily follow-up.

B. Moderate Cases: Although incision and drainage to manage peritonsillar abscess has been the standard for many years, outpatient treatment of moderately ill patients using needle aspiration and antibiotics has become more widely accepted. Several prospective studies evaluating the safety and efficacy of this alternative generally found an approximately 80% success rate. Failures consist of patients who ultimately require other, traditional methods of management such as surgical drainage or acute tonsillectomy. With good lighting, adequate topical anesthesia, an understanding of the anatomy of peritonsillar abscess, and proper training, permucosal needle aspiration can be successfully performed in most emergency departments (Fig 26–6).

C. Severe Cases: Patients with severe pain or signs of infection, drooling, dyspnea, or marked distortion of oropharyngeal structures must be hospitalized for administration of intravenous antibiotics (see recommendations for treatment of Ludwig's angina, below). Consultation with an otolaryngologist may be necessary for possible drainage of the abscess.

PARAPHARYNGEAL & RETROPHARYNGEAL ABSCESSES
(See Fig 26–7.)

Diagnosis

Symptoms associated with parapharyngeal and retropharyngeal abscess are similar to but often less severe than those seen with tonsillar abscesses, although dyspnea is more common as a presenting symptom. Retropharyngeal abscesses may follow oropharyngeal or neck trauma.

Physical examination may show bulging of the lateral or posterior pharyngeal wall. A lateral soft tissue x-ray of the neck is the most helpful diagnostic measure and shows anterior displacement of the trachea or posterior pharyngeal wall by the abscess (Fig 26–7). This x-ray view also shows epiglottitis, if present.

Treatment & Disposition

Immediate hospitalization is required for administration of intravenous antibiotics (see treatment recommendations for Ludwig's angina, below) and urgent otolaryngologic consultation regarding surgical drainage.

EPIGLOTTITIS*

Infection of the epiglottis and surrounding soft tissue is usually due to bacteria (especially *H influenzae*) and is most commonly seen in young children. *Epiglottitis is an immediate threat to life, since complete upper airway obstruction may occur suddenly at any time and may be precipitated by improper examination.*

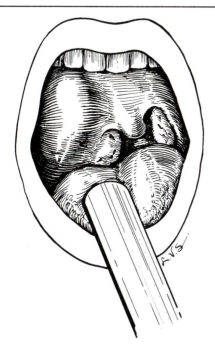

Figure 26–5. Appearance of the oral cavity with peritonsillar abscess located in the right supratonsillar fossa. The soft palate is swollen, and the uvula is displaced inferiorly and medially.

---

*Moses Grossman, MD, has contributed material for this section.

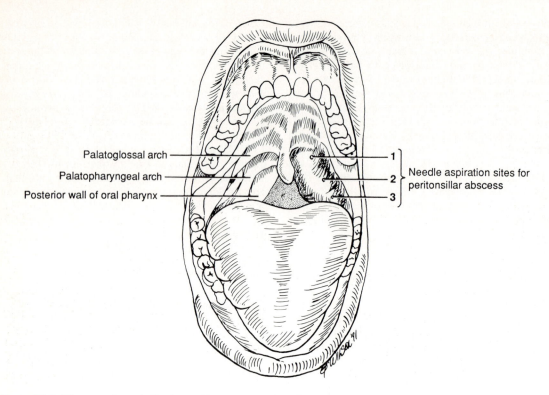

Palatoglossal arch
Palatopharyngeal arch
Posterior wall of oral pharynx

1
2
3
} Needle aspiration sites for peritonsillar abscess

Figure 26–6. When needle aspiration is used to manage peritonsillar abscess, aspiration should be attempted at each of these 3 anatomic locations.

Diagnosis

Symptoms are similar to those of tonsillar and pharyngeal abscesses: pharyngeal pain, trismus, and dysphagia. Odynophagia (pain on swallowing) is characteristic. Dyspnea or stridor occurs in some patients. On examination, the patient appears anxious and prefers the sitting position; fever and other signs of systemic infection are common. The mouth is held slightly open with the neck slightly extended, and drooling is common. *Do not examine the neck or mouth if epiglottitis is suspected*. Obtain a lateral soft tissue x-ray or a CT scan of the neck, with the patient in the sitting position. Both reveal a swollen epiglottis that is displaced posteriorly (Fig 26–8).

Treatment & Disposition

Hospitalization and immediate consultation with an otolaryngologist and an anesthesiologist about airway management are required. Administration of parenteral antibiotics is also required. Some controversy exists about airway management.

Children are at high risk of abrupt airway obstruction, so that orotracheal or nasotracheal intubation should be performed as soon as possible in the operating room. Tracheostomy is rarely indicated without first attempting intubation. *Note:* Total airway obstruction may be precipitated by such attempts; therefore, an otolaryngologist should be standing by with appropriate instruments to perform immediate tracheostomy if attempts at intubation fail.

In adults, airway obstruction is less common, and the physician may choose to observe the patient closely in an intensive care unit until the epiglottic inflammation has subsided. However, intubation is greatly preferred to observation, since the epiglottis may be safely examined with a flexible fiberoptic bronchoscope passed through the nose, and the patient may be intubated by passing the bronchoscope into the trachea and then passing an endotracheal tube over the bronchoscope. (This technique is usually not possible in infants and small children.)

H influenzae, pneumococci, and *S aureus* (occasionally) are common causes of epiglottitis; therefore, either cefuroxime, 100 mg/kg/d intravenously in 3 divided doses; or chloramphenicol, 100 mg/kg/d intravenously, is appropriate. Because bacteremia is common, blood should be drawn for culture before therapy is started.

CROUP*
(Laryngotracheobronchitis)

Croup is an infection of the airway that involves

---

*Moses Grossman, MD, has contributed material for this section.

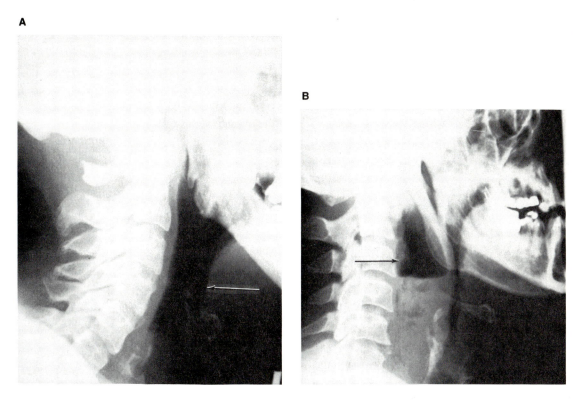

Figure 26–7. A: Normal lateral x-ray of the neck of an adult, using soft tissue technique. Note minimal soft tissue between cervical vertebrae and airway, patent airway, and normal size of epiglottis (arrow). **B:** Retropharyngeal abscess in an adult. The trachea is displaced anteriorly by the abscess (arrow), which contains an air-fluid level and gas from anaerobic bacteria.

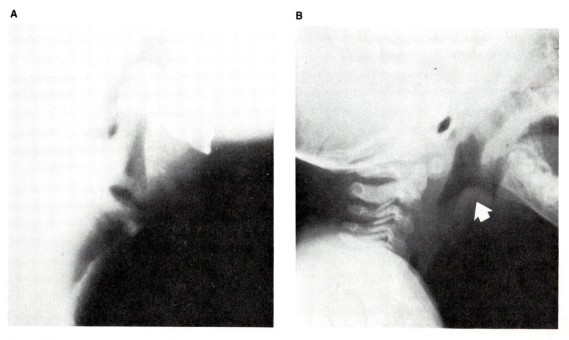

Figure 26–8. A: Epiglottitis in an adult man. Note markedly swollen epiglottis (arrow) and narrowed airway (line). **B:** Epiglottitis in an 11-month-old child. Note enlarged epiglottis (arrow) and obstructed airway.

the larynx and subglottic areas, although in many patients the trachea and large airways are also affected. It is almost always caused by viruses, usually parainfluenzavirus types 1–3. The disease is most common in children from 3 months to 3 years of age but may occur at any age. Because the airway is narrow in children, life-threatening airway obstruction tends to occur only in this age group.

Diagnosis

Croup is characterized by gradually progressive laryngitis and upper airway obstruction manifested by hoarseness, "barking seal" cough, and inspiratory airway obstruction (stridor). These symptoms are usually worse at night or when the child is agitated. Other manifestations of respiratory infection may be present, eg, fever, rhinitis, pharyngitis, and signs of pneumonia, atelectasis, or lower airway obstruction (wheezing).

The diagnosis may be established in most cases on clinical grounds alone. Since circumstances that irritate the child also frequently worsen airway obstruction, unnecessary and especially invasive laboratory studies should be avoided. Anteroposterior or lateral soft tissue neck x-rays show subglottic narrowing (Fig 26–9), thus confirming the diagnosis and excluding retropharyngeal abscess, foreign body, or epiglottitis, all of which may mimic croup. Arterial blood gas measurements may be needed as a guide to the adequacy of ventilation in seriously ill patients.

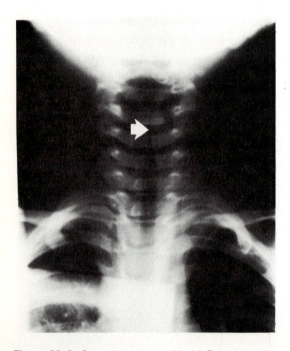

Figure 26–9. Croup in a 4-year-old girl. Posteroanterior neck film showing marked subglottic narrowing of airway (arrow).

Assessment of severity of disease is based on the degree of stridor, the presence of suprasternal and xiphoid retractions, the presence of cyanosis, and the level of consciousness.

Treatment

Disturb the child as little as possible. Minimize handling and invasive laboratory tests. Keep the child with the parent, if possible, and in a quiet place. Observe the child closely for signs of respiratory failure. Transcutaneous oximetry or arterial blood gas measurements are required if respiratory failure is suspected. Administer a cold water aerosol (the mainstay of therapy). Provide adequate hydration, intravenously if necessary. Sedation is contraindicated. *Note:* Severe restlessness should suggest hypoxemia and is an indication for arterial blood gas analysis. Antibiotics are not indicated unless a bacterial illness coexists (rare).

In severe croup, temporary improvement of stridor may be obtained with the use of aerosolized racemic epinephrine, 2.25%, diluted 1:4 in normal saline and administered by intermittent positive pressure. Corticosteroids may be beneficial in certain cases if used in high enough dosage (eg, dexamethasone, 0.5–1 mg/kg intramuscularly as a single dose). A laryngoscope and an appropriate-sized endotracheal tube (see Table 1–3) should be readily available in case of emergency; however, intubation or tracheostomy is seldom necessary, since life-threatening airway obstruction is uncommon.

Disposition

Hospitalization is indicated if severe inspiratory airway obstruction (intercostal, suprasternal, or clavicular retraction; cyanosis; obtundation; or hypercapnia) persists after initial treatment. Hospitalization is also required if the child's situation at home is not conducive to proper therapy or close observation or if the child lives far from a hospital and transport is not readily available. Hospitalize the child if the cause of airway obstruction is not clear and the diagnosis is uncertain.

Patients who do not require hospitalization may be discharged to home care with written instructions about treatment and the need to call or return for care if the child's condition worsens.

LUDWIG'S ANGINA

Ludwig's angina is a cellulitis of the sublingual and submandibular areas that is usually caused by normal mouth flora. It occurs most often in patients with poor dental hygiene or after dental procedures. Ludwig's angina can be life-threatening, since death may occur from airway obstruction or sepsis, including extension of the infection into the mediastinum.

Diagnosis

Ludwig's angina is characterized by submandibular pain and swelling, often followed by trismus and dysphagia; dyspnea is a late symptom. The sublingual and submandibular tissues are markedly swollen, often with a "woody" induration. The tongue is pushed superiorly and posteriorly and may protrude from the mouth. The anterior and lateral neck is also swollen and indurated, giving a characteristic "bull-necked" appearance. The patient often shows signs of systemic infection. Soft tissue films or CT scans of the neck are helpful in assessing airway patency.

Treatment & Disposition

Immediate hospitalization is required for administration of intravenous antibiotics: aqueous penicillin G, 300,000 units/kg/d in 4–6 divided doses; or clindamycin, 30 mg/kg/d in 3 divided doses, for patients who are allergic to penicillin. Obtain immediate otolaryngologic consultation to ensure an adequate airway. Airway management may require nasopharyngeal or endotracheal intubation, and tracheostomy is sometimes necessary. Surgical drainage may be necessary if pus accumulates.

TEETH

An adequate examination is mandatory, including teeth, gingiva, and surrounding soft tissues. Teeth can be referred to by number, beginning with the right upper wisdom tooth and proceeding right to left across the top (1–16), then left to right across the bottom (17–32), including missing teeth.

PAINFUL TOOTH

Diagnosis

A painful tooth is usually due to caries with inflammation of the pulp space or periapical and apical root abscess. The patient complains of pain on chewing or other motion of the tooth. Tapping or moving the affected tooth reproduces or worsens the pain and localizes it (with application of heat or cold, pain may be felt in more than one tooth).

Treatment & Disposition

Provide analgesia. Be aware that some drug abusers may be using feigned or real caries as a means of

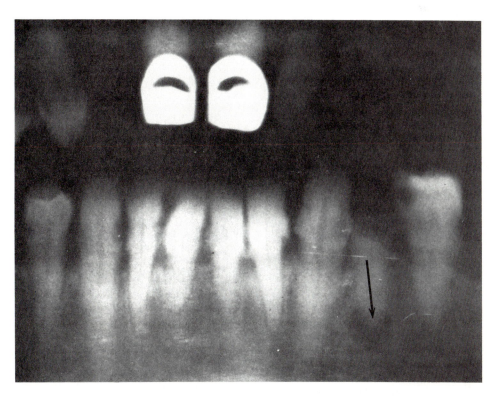

Figure 26–10. A typical apical abscess is easily diagnosed when an area of hyperlucency is identified at the apex of the tooth root (arrow).

obtaining narcotics. If an open carious lesion is visible, clove oil applied to the affected tooth may offer some relief. Refer the patient to a dentist for x-rays and definitive treatment.

PERIAPICAL & APICAL ABSCESSES

Diagnosis

Periapical and apical abscesses are basically carious teeth in which the infection in the pulp space has enlarged and extended around the apex of the tooth in the gingival socket. Patients experience severe tooth pain, usually continuous, and often have systemic symptoms of fever and malaise as well. Bacteremia occurs occasionally.

Examination shows a tender tooth; fluctuance of the surrounding gingiva is present in some cases. Systemic symptoms (eg, fever) are common. If the upper molars or premolars are involved, maxillary sinusitis may be present. If available, dental radiographs help establish this diagnosis. Typical radiographic findings of a periapical abscess are demonstrated on a panoramic x-ray in Fig 26–10.

Treatment & Disposition

If systemic symptoms are present, the patient should be hospitalized for administration of parenteral antibiotics (see Ludwig's angina, above) and emergency drainage of the abscess, which is usually accomplished by extraction. A fluctuant gingival abscess should be promptly incised and drained. Patients with minimal systemic symptoms can be discharged to outpatient status for a 24- to 36-hour period with analgesia and oral penicillin V (or erythromycin), 250–500 mg 4 times a day, and referred to a dentist within 1–2 days.

POSTEXTRACTION HEMORRHAGE

Occasionally, patients who have had dental surgery (usually extraction of molar teeth) hours to days beforehand develop bleeding from the tooth socket. Attempts to control bleeding by compression are useless. The tooth socket must be opened under local anesthesia and the bleeding site examined under direct vision. Bleeding in the bony tooth socket may be controlled with bone wax, whereas bleeding sites in the gingiva must be directly sutured or closed by electrocoagulation.

REFERENCES

Ballenger JJ: *Diseases of the Nose, Throat, & Ear,* 12th ed. Lea & Febiger, 1977.

Bluestone CD: Modern management of otitis media. Pediatr Clin North Am 1989;36(6):1371.

Cole RR, Jahrsdoerfer RA: Sudden hearing loss: An update. Am J Otol 1988;9:211.

Converse JM: *Surgical Treatment of Facial Injuries,* 3rd ed. Williams & Wilkins, 1974.

Crumley R: Common problems of the ear, nose, and throat. Prim Care 1982;9:2.

Cummings CW et al: *Otolaryngology—Head and Neck Surgery.* (4 vols.) Mosby, 1986.

DeWeese DD, Saunders WH: *Textbook of Otolaryngology,* 6th ed. Mosby, 1982.

Dingman RO, Natvig P: *Surgery of Facial Fractures.* Saunders, 1964.

Epperly TD, Wood TC: New trends in the management of peritonsillar abscess. Am Fam Physician 1990;42:102.

Gates J: *Current Therapy in Otolaryngology—Head and Neck Surgery.* Mosby, 1982.

Gerrish SP et al: Adult epiglottitis. Br J Med 1987;295:1183.

Grossman M, Dieckman RA: *Pediatric Emergency Medicine.* Lippincott, 1991.

Healy GB: Current concepts in otolaryngology: Hearing loss and vertigo secondary to head injury. N Engl J Med 1982;306:1029.

Hughes GB: Practical management of Bell's palsy. Otolaryngol Head Neck Surg 1990;102:658.

Kirchner JA: Current concepts in otolaryngology: Epistaxis. N Engl J Med 1982;307:1126.

McDonald TJ, Neel HB III: ENT for nonspecialists: External otitis. (Symposium.) Postgrad Med (May) 1975;57:95.

Paparella MM: Differential diagnosis of hearing loss. Laryngoscope 1978;88:952.

Parker GS et al: Intracranial complications of sinusitis. South Med J 1989;82:563.

Walike JW: Management of acute ear infection. Otolaryngol Clin North Am 1979;12:439.

Pulmonary Emergencies 27

John Mills, MD, & John M. Luce, MD

IMMEDIATE MANAGEMENT OF LIFE-THREATENING PROBLEMS
(See also Chapter 5.)

HEMOPTYSIS

Hemoptysis is a common condition with diverse causes (Table 27–1). It is usually a sign of relatively benign disorders such as bronchitis or posterior epistaxis, but it may also be due to serious illness such as lung cancer or tuberculosis. The amount of bleeding is usually small, being limited to blood-streaked sputum or a few teaspoonfuls of gross blood. On rare occasions, massive hemoptysis may cause serious complication or death. The severity of hemoptysis does not correlate with the severity of the underlying disease; serious illness such as lung cancer may be associated with minimal hemoptysis, and vice versa.

1. MASSIVE HEMOPTYSIS

Diagnosis
Patients who are coughing up large amounts (≥ 100 mL/h) of blood when seen in the emergency department or who have simultaneous respiratory distress are at serious risk of death from asphyxiation or exsanguination. This life-threatening emergency requires rapid and simultaneous implementation of diagnostic and therapeutic measures.

Treatment
A. Maintain Ventilation:
1. Begin oxygen, 5–10 L/min.
2. Keep the patient in a slightly head-down position (for postural drainage).
3. Maintain airway by vigorously suctioning out coughed-up blood. Do not suppress cough with narcotics or other sedating drugs.
4. Endotracheal intubation may be necessary to control the airway. Intubation will also cure hemop-

Table 27–1. Conditions causing hemoptysis.

Pulmonary hemoptysis
  Pulmonary parenchymal disease
    Bronchitis
    Bronchiectasis
    Tuberculosis
    Lung abscess
    Pneumonia
    Fungal infection of old cavities (eg, aspergilloma)
    Lung parasites (ascariasis, schistosomiasis, etc)
    Pulmonary neoplasms
    Pulmonary infarction
    Trauma (Chapter 18)
    Arteriovenous malformations
    Pulmonary vasculitis
    Goodpasture's syndrome
  Extrapulmonary disease
    Thrombocytopenia
    Other coagulopathies
    Heart failure
    Mitral stenosis
Nonpulmonary hemoptysis
  Aspiration of blood from nasal, oropharyngeal, gastrointestinal, or other bleeding site
Pseudohemoptysis
  Production of red-tinged sputum not due to blood

tysis secondary to an oropharyngeal or nasal source of bleeding.

5. The hemithorax suspected of being the source of the bleeding should be kept dependent.

B. Maintain Circulation:

1. Insert a large-bore intravenous catheter (≥ 16-gauge).

2. Draw blood for CBC, clotting studies (prothrombin time, partial thromboplastin time, and platelet count), and typing and cross-matching. Obtain 4 units of whole blood as an initial order.

3. Begin infusion of crystalloid solutions (eg, normal saline, acetated or lactated Ringer's injection).

4. Assess intravascular volume. Look for signs of hypovolemic shock (pale, cool skin; altered mentation), and measure the blood pressure and pulse with the patient in the supine position and also when sitting and standing if normal while supine.

5. Treat shock or hypotension with rapid infusion of crystalloid solutions (up to 3 L), followed by whole blood as needed (Chapter 3). A urinary catheter should be inserted for monitoring of urinary output if shock is present.

C. Monitor adequacy of ventilatory efforts and circulation by measurement of arterial blood gases and pH. Pulse oximetry, which measures the saturation of hemoglobin by oxygen, provides a guide to the oxygenation of arterial blood. However, the technique is not accurate in severely hypoxemic patients whose arterial saturation is below 90%. In addition, it provides no information about the arterial CO_2 tension. Pulse oximetry is most helpful when the measured saturation is normal or near normal.

D. Obtain a history, if possible, of previous pul-

monary or other conditions that might explain the hemoptysis (see Table 27–1 and next section).

E. Briefly examine the chest and abdomen for any obvious abnormality.

F. Obtain chest x-ray.

Disposition

A. Urgent thoracic surgical or radiologic consultation and hospitalization are required.

B. Emergency bronchoscopy and surgery are frequently required for management. The 2 main values of bronchoscopy are that (**1**) it shows where bleeding originates, so that the side with the affected lung can be kept dependent, and (**2**) it helps guide surgery. Massive hemoptysis is one situation in which rigid (as opposed to flexible fiberoptic) bronchoscopy may be preferred, because the larger lumen of the rigid bronchoscope permits better suctioning of blood. In desperate cases, selective intubation of one main stem bronchus may be required to prevent bleeding into the contralateral normal lung prior to operation.

An alternative approach is selective arteriography of the branch or branches of the bronchial artery that supplies the bleeding site, followed by embolization (with Gelfoam or other substance) of the vessel. Arteriography can be performed with or without bronchoscopy. This radiologic approach is becoming more popular and (if available) may replace surgery in the management of acute hemoptysis.

2. ACTIVE, MODERATE HEMOPTYSIS

Diagnosis

If the patient has active hemoptysis consisting only of moderate amounts of bloody sputum or small volumes (< 20 mL) of gross blood, management may proceed in a more leisurely and orderly fashion. The goal is to differentiate pulmonary bleeding due to intrinsic pulmonary disorders from that due to extrapulmonary disease (eg, coagulopathy) and to exclude nonpulmonary bleeding as a cause of hemoptysis (Table 27–1).

A. History:

1. Inquire about preexisting conditions known to be associated with hemoptysis.

2. Ask about otolaryngologic, cardiac, or pulmonary symptoms that might help localize the bleeding. For example, a history of recent localized chest pain or acute bronchitis should lead to an investigation of these areas as possible sites of bleeding.

3. Differentiating hemoptysis from hematemesis is occasionally difficult. Features suggesting that blood originated in the respiratory tract include frothy blood, absence of brown blood (hemoglobin altered by gastric acid), and association with coughing rather than vomiting. Because some of the sputum coughed up is swallowed, testing of stool and gastric aspirates for blood is not helpful in differentiating gastrointestinal from pulmonary bleeding.

B. Physical Examination:

1. Check vital signs, including pulse and blood pressure, supine, sitting, and standing to detect subtle degrees of volume depletion.

2. Examine the nose, mouth, posterior pharynx, and larynx, including indirect (or direct) laryngoscopy.

3. Examine neck, chest, heart, and lungs.

C. Laboratory and Special Examinations:

1. Obtain CBC and differential, arterial blood gas measurements, and coagulation panel (platelet count or estimate, prothrombin time, and partial thromboplastin time). Type and cross-match blood if anemia or hypotension is present.

2. If bloody sputum is being produced (either blood-tinged or frank blood), it should be stained with Gram's and Kinyoun's stains and examined microscopically; abundant leukocytes and bacteria in grossly bloody sputum indicate the presence of bacterial pneumonia or tuberculosis. If there is doubt about whether the red tinge is blood, a confirmatory chemical test for occult blood should be performed as well.

3. Chest x-ray should include erect posteroanterior and lateral films.

Treatment

A. Maintain Ventilation:

1. Provide supplementary oxygen initially (5–10 L/min); adjust or discontinue depending on results of blood gas analysis.

2. Maintain good pulmonary toilet; assist patient by percussion or suctioning as necessary. Do not suppress cough.

B. Maintain Circulation: Insert intravenous catheter ($\geq$ 16-gauge), and begin infusion of crystalloid solutions.

C. Treat Any Associated Conditions: Epistaxis, heart failure or other conditions may be causing or contributing to the hemoptysis.

Disposition

Hospitalize patients with hemoptysis if initial observation discloses severe disorders requiring prompt evaluation and treatment (eg, heart failure, tuberculosis). Most patients can be discharged and evaluated on an ambulatory basis, although hospitalization may be preferred for patients with active hemoptysis so that evaluation (eg, bronchoscopy or bronchial arteriography) may be performed. A follow-up appointment with an internist or other specialist should be made within 3–7 days.

3. MINIMAL HEMOPTYSIS & HEMOPTYSIS BY HISTORY ONLY

Diagnosis

Patients producing (or who report producing) only small amounts of blood-tinged or blood-flecked sputum generally should be evaluated in the same way as patients with active moderate hemoptysis (see above).

Treatment

A. No specific treatment for minimal hemoptysis need be instituted in the emergency department.

B. Coexisting conditions (bronchitis, pneumonia, etc) that may be causing or contributing to the hemoptysis should be treated.

Disposition

Hospitalize patients with minimal hemoptysis if initial observation discloses serious disorders requiring prompt evaluation and treatment (heart failure, tuberculosis). Most patients can be discharged and evaluated on an ambulatory basis. A follow-up appointment with an internist or other specialist should be made within 3–7 days.

PNEUMOTHORAX
(See also Chapters 5 and 18.)

Classification

Air may enter the pleural space either following puncture of the chest wall as a result of trauma (Chapter 18) or from rupture of lung parenchyma by congenital subpleural cysts, infection (bacterial pneumonia, tuberculosis), or overdistension (as noted below in the discussion of pneumomediastinum). In **simple pneumothorax,** entry of air into the pleural space ceases when pleural pressure equals atmospheric pressure, resulting in partial or total collapse of the lung on that side. In **tension pneumothorax,** air continues to enter (but not to leave) the pleural space during respiratory efforts, because the defect in the lung acts as a one-way valve, and pleural pressure becomes greater than atmospheric pressure. This usually shifts the mediastinum toward the contralateral uninvolved lung, compressing it and obstructing venous return to the heart. Death results from both decreased cardiac output and failure of gas exchange.

Diagnosis

A. Symptoms and Signs: Patients may be asymptomatic or may show mild to severe distress. In nontraumatic pneumothorax, patients generally present with some combination of chest pain, cough, and dyspnea. The symptoms may improve with time, even without resorption of pleural air. In asymptomatic patients, pneumothorax may be discovered on chest x-ray done for another reason. Occasionally, pneumothorax may occur in the course of a chronic illness (eg, asthma, emphysema) and confuse the clinical picture.

Percussion and auscultation reveal hyperresonance and decreased breath sounds on the affected side. In tension pneumothorax, the trachea may be shifted away from the collapsed side, neck veins may be distended, and tachycardia and hypotension may occur.

B. X-Ray and Laboratory Findings:
1. Posteroanterior chest x-ray will reveal all significant pneumothoraces except those localized to the anterior pleural space in supine patients, although detection may require an experienced radiologist. A posteroanterior chest film in expiration may enhance visualization of small pneumothoraces. Tension pneumothorax is usually (not always) associated with a mediastinal shift away from the pneumothorax.
2. Arterial blood pH, PO_2, and PCO_2 should be determined to assess the degree of respiratory insufficiency.

Treatment
A. Simple Pneumothorax: Tube thoracostomy should be performed in patients with severe dyspnea, respiratory distress, significant hypoxemia (arterial $PO_2 < 55$ mm Hg), complete collapse of one lung, progressive enlargement of the pneumothorax, bilateral pneumothoraces, or traumatic pneumothorax. A new technique for expanding the lung in uncomplicated pneumothorax involves aspirating the pleural air with a catheter connected to a Heimlich valve and then observing the patient for 6 hours in the emergency department. If reexpansion persists by chest x-ray at 6 hours, the patient may be discharged.
B. Tension Pneumothorax: Tube thoracostomy must be performed *immediately* after the diagnosis of tension pneumothorax is made (Chapter 46). Treatment may be initiated on the basis of a clinical diagnosis (ie, without x-ray) in the severely dyspneic or hypotensive patient. If there is a question about the diagnosis, thoracentesis with a 16-gauge needle (Chapter 46) may be used to confirm the presence of air under pressure in the pleural space while simultaneously providing some treatment.

Disposition
A. Hospitalization is indicated for patients who have received tube thoracostomy, including all patients with tension pneumothorax or bilateral pneumothoraces of any type. Patients whose lungs remain expanded after catheter aspiration and 6 hours of observation in the emergency department may be discharged with instructions to return if symptoms recur.
B. Patients with spontaneous, small to moderate-sized, unilateral, simple pneumothoraces of recent onset may be observed for a few days in the hospital without a chest tube to see if the condition is stable or improving.
C. Patients with stable, small, unilateral pneumo-

thoraces with no symptoms may be referred for follow-up on an outpatient basis. They should be seen within 1–2 days.

EMERGENCY MANAGEMENT OF SPECIFIC CONDITIONS

PNEUMOMEDIASTINUM & SUBCUTANEOUS EMPHYSEMA

Pneumomediastinum is commonly associated with pneumothorax. It occurs from rupture of an over-distended alveolus or a collection of such alveoli ("bleb") into the peribronchovascular interstitial space with dissection backward along the bronchi to the mediastinum. Since the mediastinal pleura is weaker than the pleura surrounding the lung, air may dissect into the mediastinum before entering the pleural space. Pneumomediastinum may occur without pneumothorax; air also may dissect through contiguous fascial planes into the neck and other soft tissues, causing subcutaneous emphysema. Occasional cases of pneumomediastinum are due to rupture of the esophagus (Boerhaave's syndrome), and this diagnosis should be considered if the patient is acutely ill and has a history of vomiting.

Diagnosis
Chest pain is a common symptom in pneumomediastinum. Diagnosis is made by hearing a mediastinal "crunch" on auscultation and seeing air in the mediastinum on chest x-ray. (These findings are also present in pyogenic mediastinitis, eg, following esophageal rupture.) Subcutaneous emphysema presents as soft tissue swelling, especially in the neck. A crackling sound is heard when the tissues are compressed.

Treatment & Disposition
No specific treatment is indicated unless there is esophageal rupture (Chapter 18). Associated conditions such as pneumothorax should be corrected. Analgesics may be required.

Hospitalization should be considered for severe cases (extensive spread of mediastinal air) or those complicated by other disorders (eg, mediastinitis) or for patients who require narcotics for pain relief.

PLEURODYNIA

Pleurodynia is an acute, self-limited, and benign (though uncomfortable) illness. Most cases occur in young adults and are thought to be caused by viruses, especially group B coxsackieviruses.

Diagnosis

Systemic symptoms are mild (low-grade fever, malaise), but pleuritic pain is severe (hence the name "devil's grip"). Examination may disclose low-grade fever and a pleural rub in some cases, although many patients have a normal examination. Chest x-ray usually shows no abnormalities, but there may be a small amount of pleural fluid, a small pulmonary infiltrate, or both. The leukocyte count and the erythrocyte sedimentation rate are usually normal or only minimally elevated. Viral pleuritis may sometimes be accompanied by pericarditis, which may be diagnosed by a friction rub upon auscultation or an enlarged cardiac silhouette on chest x-ray.

Treatment

No specific therapy is available. For symptomatic relief, indomethacin (Indocin), 25–50 mg 3 times daily orally, or similar nonsteroidal anti-inflammatory agents may be effective. Aspirin is said to be less effective. Narcotic analgesics may be needed.

Disposition

Hospitalization is necessary only for patients who require parenteral analgesics or who also have pericarditis.

PLEURAL EFFUSION

Pleural fluid may accumulate in the course of many diseases; in fact, virtually any condition affecting the structures within the thorax may be associated with pleural fluid. Depending on the cause, the pleural space may contain blood, lymph, serous fluid, or frank pus. Every patient with newly diagnosed pleural fluid requires prompt evaluation to determine the cause so that early and appropriate therapy can be given.

Diagnosis

A. Symptoms and Signs: The patient may complain of pleuritic or nonpleuritic chest pain or dyspnea. Chest examination discloses dullness, decreased breath sounds, and decreased tactile fremitus on the involved side. Egobronchophony is often present at the lung-fluid interface.

B. Imaging: Routine posteroanterior and lateral chest x-rays demonstrate pleural fluid in most cases (blunting of costophrenic angles, etc). Decubitus films are useful to differentiate pleural fluid from pleural scarring and to determine if the fluid is loculated or not. Bilateral decubitus films may be necessary to demonstrate fluid in the case of very small effusions. X-rays or CT scans may be helpful in differentiating effusions from lung abscess adjacent to the pleura.

Treatment

A. Oxygen: If dyspnea is present, obtain pulse oximetry or arterial blood gas measurements, and begin oxygen, 5 L/min, by mask or nasal prongs.

B. Thoracentesis: If chest examination or chest x-ray shows a massive fluid accumulation (ie, most of one hemithorax), prompt thoracentesis with removal of 500–1000 mL of fluid should be considered for relief of symptoms. Remove the fluid over 30–90 minutes to prevent pulmonary edema in the reinflated lung. Recovered fluid should be sent for cell count, determination of protein and glucose content, cytologic study, and cultures. If the patient is not in distress, thoracentesis should be deferred until after admission to the hospital.

Disposition

All patients with unexplained pleural fluid accumulations should be hospitalized for diagnosis and treatment. Stable patients with recurrent fluid of known cause (eg, metastatic cancer or heart failure) should be referred to their regular source of medical care or treated in the emergency department (eg, by thoracentesis) and discharged unless the underlying illness requires hospitalization.

ATELECTASIS

Collapse of alveoli and small airways in a portion of the lung may result from extrinsic compression (pneumothorax, hydrothorax, etc) or intrinsic abnormalities (hypoventilation, bronchial obstruction). Only intrinsic (resorption) atelectasis will be discussed here. In the emergency department, intrinsic atelectasis may be seen in conditions causing hypoventilation (secondary to drug overdose or severe pleuritic pain) or bronchial obstruction (asthma, foreign body, bronchial tumor, or aspiration).

Diagnosis

A. Symptoms and Signs: There are usually no findings other than those of the underlying disease, though patients with extensive atelectasis may experience chest pain, cough, or dyspnea. Physical findings may be absent but when present are nonspecific: dry crackles, decreased breath sounds, or dullness to percussion over the affected lung.

B. Laboratory and X-Ray Findings:
1. Chest x-ray shows areas of lung collapse. Coexisting signs may include depression or elevation of the hilum, elevation of a hemidiaphragm, or compensatory hyperinflation of other parts of the involved lung.
2. Arterial blood gases should be measured to as-

sess respiratory function; hypoxemia and hypocapnia may be present.

Treatment

Emergency treatment should include supplemental oxygen, chest physical therapy, control of airway secretions (eg, suctioning of a comatose patient), and treatment of underlying conditions (eg, aspiration of gastric contents, drug overdose).

Disposition

Almost all patients with atelectasis must be hospitalized for evaluation and treatment. The only exceptions are patients with chronic atelectasis of known cause who have failed to respond to vigorous therapy in the past (eg, carcinomatous bronchial obstruction) and those with very mild degrees of atelectasis (subsegmental) clearly due to self-limited disease (drug overdose, pleurisy).

PNEUMONIA & BRONCHITIS

Pneumonia and bronchitis (which may be difficult to differentiate from pneumonia clinically) are common emergency department problems that demand prompt diagnosis and treatment. Suspect pneumonia or bronchitis in the patient with fever, cough (particularly cough productive of purulent sputum), and leukocytosis.

Patients with HIV infection may present with bacterial pneumonia. Patients with AIDS frequently have pneumonia due to *Pneumocystis carinii, Mycobacterium tuberculosis,* or other pathogens. Such patients characteristically describe chronic fever, nonproductive cough, and weight loss. Leukocytosis is uncommon, suggesting that a bacterial process is present. Patients with pneumocystis pneumonia, despite fever, cough, dyspnea, and hypoxemia, may have a normal lung examination. The chest x-ray may show a diffuse heterogeneous infiltrate, or it may be normal. See Chapter 34 for details of evaluation and treatment.

PULMONARY ASPIRATION SYNDROME

Aspiration of gastric contents may produce lung injury by acid corrosion, bronchial obstruction with food particles, or induction of chemical pneumonitis that is later complicated by bacterial pneumonia. Aspiration of gastric acid (pH < 2) produces immediate pulmonary injury that pathophysiologically is a form of noncardiac pulmonary edema (see below). Aspiration of neutral gastric secretions admixed with food produces a more delayed injury; retained food particles may cause bronchial obstruction with atelectasis.

All of these conditions are included in the term pulmonary aspiration syndrome.

In contrast, **aspiration of oropharyngeal secretions,** especially in individuals with poor dental hygiene and large amounts of dental plaque, does cause bacterial pneumonia (so-called aspiration pneumonia). This necrotizing process may be acute or subacute in onset and commonly results in lung abscess.

Diagnosis

Pulmonary aspiration occurring in the hospital may occur during anesthesia, CPR, or other procedures. Community-acquired cases are usually associated with drug (including alcohol) intoxication, seizures, disorders of swallowing, or gastroesophageal sphincteric incompetence. Within minutes to hours after aspiration, the patient develops productive cough, dyspnea, fever, leukocytosis, and signs of consolidation, pulmonary rales, or dullness. Chest x-ray shows pulmonary infiltrate without a characteristic pattern, although dependent segments of the lung are more commonly involved.

Sputum shows abundant leukocytes but no bacteria (or scant normal flora) on microscopic examination. Cultures are sterile or show scant normal flora. Food particles may be present on gross examination of sputum.

Arterial blood gas and pH measurements must be made to assess ventilatory status. Pulse oximetry may suffice as a guide to arterial oxygenation if the saturation is high (> 90%).

Treatment

A. Provide respiratory support (eg, supplemental oxygen) as necessary on the basis of arterial blood gas measurements (or pulse oximetry) and clinical findings (Chapter 5).

B. Remove as much of the aspirated material as possible by oropharyngeal and tracheal suctioning.

C. Corticosteroids have not been demonstrated to be helpful and may increase susceptibility to infection.

D. Antibiotics should be given only if infection occurs and not as prophylaxis following an episode of aspiration.

Disposition

All patients should be hospitalized for observation and treatment as necessary.

NONCARDIAC PULMONARY EDEMA
(See Table 27–2.)

Pulmonary edema may be classified as cardiac (secondary to congestive heart failure) or noncardiac (adult respiratory distress syndrome), based on left atrial (pulmonary artery wedge) pressure measure-

Table 27–2. Noncardiac causes of pulmonary edema.

Drugs and poisons
  Heroin and other narcotics
  Salicylates
  Nitrofurantoin
  Hydrocarbons
Toxic gas inhalation
  "Smoke" (Chapter 37)
  Chlorine
  Oxides of nitrogen (silo-filler's disease)
  Ozone
  Phosgene
  Teflon (fluorine)
Miscellaneous causes
  Central nervous system disorders (trauma, seizures, etc)
  Near-drowning (Chapter 38)
  High altitude (Chapter 38)
  Major trauma
  Pulmonary contusion (Chapter 18)
  Uremia
  Shock (Chapter 3)
  Pancreatitis
  Intravascular coagulation
  Sepsis
  Fat embolism

ments. Cardiac pulmonary edema (Chapter 28) is due to increased left atrial pressure with fluid transudation and must be ruled out by careful examination; noncardiac pulmonary edema is secondary to injury of pulmonary capillaries with resulting leakage of fluid into the interstitial space and alveoli. Specific causes include sepsis, drugs, inhalation of smoke or toxic substance, near-drowning, burns, aspiration, pancreatitis, high altitude, and anemia.

Diagnosis

A. Symptoms and Signs: As a rule, the only symptoms are dyspnea and cough, although symptoms of the underlying disorder may be present as well. Some patients may have wheezing or cough productive of frothy or blood-tinged nonpurulent sputum. Rales are almost always present and are roughly proportionate to the severity of the illness.

B. Laboratory Findings: Hypoxemia is a universal finding, but arterial PCO_2 is variable. Early in the illness, most patients are hyperventilating and have hypocapnia. Later, with fatigue or a worsening clinical status, patients may become hypercapnic. In some cases (eg, narcotic-induced pulmonary edema), hypercapnia may be an early and consistent finding. Pulmonary arterial wedge pressure and left atrial pressures are not elevated in noncardiac pulmonary edema. Measurement of wedge pressure is usually necessary in the differential diagnosis of cardiac and noncardiac pulmonary edema and may also be helpful in the management of these conditions.

C. X-Ray Findings: Chest x-ray generally shows symmetric bilateral alveolar infiltrates, although variations are common, especially in individuals with underlying chronic lung disease. In early noncardiogenic pulmonary edema, chest x-ray may be normal.

Treatment

A. Provide Ventilatory Support:

1. Supplemental oxygen–Initially, provide high inspired oxygen concentrations (50–100%); when the results of pulse oximetry or arterial blood gases are available, adjust the rate of oxygen administration accordingly.

2. Intubation–Endotracheal intubation should be performed in patients who are obtunded or in whom arterial oxygenation and eucapnia cannot otherwise be maintained.

3. Mechanical ventilation–Mechanical ventilation, usually with positive end-expiratory pressure (PEEP), may be necessary to ensure adequate oxygenation and avoid oxygen toxicity.

B. Maintain Circulation: Avoid vigorous hydration or dehydration until cardiac output, central venous and pulmonary artery wedge pressures, and oxygen transport can be measured with a pulmonary artery catheter.

C. Give Specific Therapy: Provide specific therapy where applicable.

1. High-altitude pulmonary edema–Oxygen and urgent transportation to lower elevation.

2. Drug-induced pulmonary edema–Drug antagonists or removal (eg, charcoal hemoperfusion).

3. Uremic lung–Dialysis.

4. Sepsis–Antimicrobials (see Table 34–1).

Disposition

Hospitalize all patients for therapy. Very rarely, noncardiac pulmonary edema due to a specifically treatable condition (eg, high altitude, narcotics) will resolve rapidly and completely in a few hours, allowing the patient to be discharged from the emergency department.

ASTHMA

Asthma is characterized by periodic bronchospasm and hypersecretion of mucus with intervals of relative or complete good health. There are many causes, and many cases probably have more than one genetic mechanism. During attacks, bronchospasm and hypersecretion of mucus occur together (although one may predominate), resulting in expiratory airway obstruction and air trapping. Poorly ventilated areas of lung continue to be perfused by venous blood with consequent arterial hypoxemia, an early and constant finding in asthmatic attacks. Most patients with asthma are hypocapnic as a result of reflex hyperventilation; however, with progressive airway obstruction, fatigue, and increasing mismatching of ventilation and perfusion, patients may retain CO_2.

Conditions commonly associated with exacerbations of asthma are listed in Table 27–3. Some are remediable and should be specifically asked about when the history is recorded.

Table 27–3. Common precipitating factors in acute asthma.

Infection (especially upper respiratory tract viral infections)
Drugs (aspirin, nonsteroidal anti-inflammatory agents, food coloring)
Exercise
Emotional stress
Inhaled irritants (eg, air pollution, cigarette smoke)
Occupational exposure to dusts, gases, etc

Diagnosis

A. Symptoms and Signs: The principal findings in asthma are set forth below. Other allergic symptoms (rhinitis, sneezing, nasal obstruction, conjunctivitis), symptoms of purulent bronchitis or sinusitis, or chest pain may also be present.

Most patients complain of dyspnea and cough. Patients who have had many attacks may complain of "wheezing" or "asthma."

On inspection, most patients show some degree of respiratory distress and anxiety. Lack of apparent respiratory distress does not always mean the patient is having a mild attack, since severely ill patients may appear relatively comfortable owing to CO_2 retention. Tachycardia (heart rate > 120 beats/min in adults) may indicate a severe attack or previous sympathomimetic usage, or both. Pulsus paradoxus over 10 mm Hg is suggestive of intense respiratory effort and a more severe attack.

Most patients will have a prolonged expiratory phase of respiration and wheezing (often audible even without a stethoscope), usually with rhonchi and occasionally with rales. However, severe airway obstruction or hypercapnia may reduce airflow to the point where wheezing and breath sounds are inaudible.

Other points that should be noted on physical examination include cyanosis (usually indicating severe hypoxemia), sinus tenderness (sinusitis), flaring of nares, barrel chest (severe air trapping), unilateral decreased breath sounds or hyperresonance (pneumothorax), unilateral wheezing (foreign body or mucus plug), parasternal lift (right ventricular heave with acute cor pulmonale), use of accessory muscles of respiration, and abdominal distention (air swallowing with acute gastric dilatation).

B. Laboratory and Other Findings: Tests and procedures useful in the management of asthma are listed below in order of importance.

1. Spirometry—Although not useful in desperately ill patients (because of their inability to cooperate), spirometry is the single most useful method for judging severity and monitoring the response to therapy in cases of moderate severity. Common findings include markedly reduced airflows (decreased forced expiratory volume in 1 second [FEV_1] and peak expiratory flow rate [PEFR]) and air trapping (decreased vital capacity and increased total lung capacity, if measured). At least 3 measurements should be taken initially to familiarize the patient

with the test and to see if the patient is making sufficient effort.

2. Arterial blood gases—Blood gas determinations are a direct measure of cardiopulmonary function and should be part of the evaluation of every asthmatic patient sick enough to spend more than a brief time in the emergency department. The patient's symptoms and physical findings cannot be used to predict blood gas values. All patients with acute exacerbations of asthma will have hypoxemia (arterial PO_2 < 80 mm Hg)—even those with minimal bronchospasm undetectable by auscultation. A normal arterial PO_2 on room air suggests another diagnosis (eg, upper airway obstruction). Most patients are hypocapnic as a result of reflex hyperventilation.

Typical arterial blood gas measurements in a moderately ill patient would be as follows: PO_2, 67 mm Hg; PCO_2, 32 mm Hg; pH, 7.47. With progressively more severe illness, hypoxemia worsens and PCO_2 begins to rise. Thus, *a normal PCO_2 (35–45 mm Hg) during an attack generally indicates a very sick patient, and an elevated PCO_2 indicates a desperate situation.*

3. Pulse oximetry—Oxygen saturation may be depressed. However, in mild asthma exacerbations, hyperventilation may allow the PO_2 to be maintained despite an increasing alveolar to arterial oxygen gradient. Pulse oximetry is useful for monitoring but provides no information about PCO_2 and hence adequacy of ventilation.

4. Chest x-ray—In routine cases, chest x-ray is normal or shows mild thoracic hyperinflation. However, the x-ray may reveal complications of asthma—specifically, pneumothorax or atelectasis and plugging with mucus. Occasionally, clinically inapparent pneumonia will be found or another disease associated with wheezing (heart failure, pulmonary embolism, foreign body). Foreign bodies are an especially important cause of "asthma" in young children. Although the foreign body may not be visible on x-ray, the chest x-ray is virtually diagnostic if unilateral hyperinflation is present; the foreign object obstructs a main stem bronchus with a ball-valve effect.

5. ECG—The ECG usually reveals tachycardia. Frequent premature ventricular contractions or myocardial ischemia may result from asthma or be a sequela of its treatment and should be managed accordingly.

6. CBC and differential—Leukocytosis is common (especially in children) as a result of leukocyte demargination induced by endogenous and exogenous epinephrine, and it is not a reliable indicator of infection, although this is an unreliable finding that may vary depending on the laboratory. However, a shift to the left (to more immature leukocytes) is suggestive of infection. Marked eosinophilia occurs in some patients and suggests the need for early administration of corticosteroids. Eosinophilia does not indicate that asthma is due to allergy.

7. Electrolytes and tests of renal function–

Although seldom found, abnormalities disclosed by these tests may indicate dehydration or hypokalemia and thus have important implications for treatment (Chapter 36).

8. Microscopic examination of sputum–If sputum is being produced, it will usually show a few eosinophils and scant or no bacteria. Occasional patients (especially those with "infective asthma" or "asthmatic bronchitis") will have asthmatic episodes triggered by bacterial bronchitis.

Assessing Overall Severity of Attacks

Clinical findings are not reliable indicators of the severity of asthma. However, spirometric measurements are reliable and should be taken if feasible, even in patients with apparently mild attacks. Measurements of FEV_1 less than 1 L and PEFR less than 100 L/min indicate severe asthma. Other factors associated with severe asthma attacks are shown in Table 27–4. Obtundation and hypercapnia are the most serious prognostic signs.

Differential Diagnosis

In young patients with a long history of recurrent wheezing, there can be little doubt about the diagnosis. In the case of children, elderly patients, and patients with their first attack of "asthma," look carefully for other diseases causing bronchospasm. Illnesses other than asthma commonly associated with wheezing include the following:

A. Endobronchial Foreign Body: Aspiration of foreign bodies is particularly common in children. Suspect this diagnosis in a child with no history of wheezing, especially if the wheezing is unilateral or there is unilateral atelectasis. There is no response to bronchodilators. Since endobronchial foreign bodies are rarely radiopaque, bronchoscopy is usually necessary for diagnosis.

B. Pulmonary Edema: Some wheezing is common with cardiogenic pulmonary edema; it is perhaps less common in noncardiac types. "Cardiac asthma" probably is due to reflex bronchospasm and not to the compressive effect of fluid around the airways. The presence of rales and signs of heart failure (cardio-

Table 27–4. Factors associated with severe asthma attacks.

Duration more than 1 week
Persistence or progression of symptoms despite medication
Recent withdrawal of corticosteroid medication
History of respiratory failure
Fatigue when first seen
Cyanosis or severe hypoxemia
Pulsus paradoxus > 10 mm Hg
Barely audible breath sounds
Use of accessory muscles of respiration
Obtundation
Hypercapnia ($PCO_2 \geq 40$ mm Hg)
Complications (atelectasis, pneumothorax)

megaly, venous distention, gallop rhythms) rarely allows confusion in diagnosis, although these findings may be difficult to detect in a patient with coexistent chronic obstructive pulmonary disease. Pulmonary artery wedge pressure measurement may be required to decide difficult cases. Patients may respond to bronchodilators. Note that the diuretic action of aminophylline also may partially obscure the diagnosis.

C. Croup and Epiglottitis: Both of these conditions may cause upper airway obstruction, and in croup especially the onset may be gradual, mimicking asthma. The predominance of *inspiratory* obstruction over expiratory should suggest these diagnoses; soft tissue x-rays of the neck (posteroanterior and lateral) will also accurately differentiate these conditions from asthma.

D. Bronchitis or Bronchiolitis: Acute bronchitis in healthy individuals or acute exacerbations of chronic bronchitis may also be associated with wheezing. In children, viral pulmonary infections, especially those due to respiratory syncytial virus, may cause wheezing as well (bronchiolitis). The response to bronchodilators is variable.

E. Emphysema: Emphysema is associated with wheezing and air trapping but is due principally to airway collapse rather than bronchospasm. Although differentiation from asthma is usually easy on clinical grounds, enigmatic cases will require specialized pulmonary function tests. Response to bronchodilators is variable.

F. Parasitic Infection: Heavy infestation by certain parasites, especially filariae, may cause a syndrome of cough, wheezing, dyspnea, evanescent pulmonary infiltrates, and high eosinophilia. Suspect this diagnosis in individuals from endemic areas.

Treatment

Treatment should include respiratory support (supplemental oxygen or assisted ventilation) and measures to reduce bronchospasm, airway edema, hypersecretion of mucus, and airway plugging.

A. Respiratory Support:

1. Supplemental oxygen–Since patients with asthma who come to the emergency department may have unstable respiratory function, they should receive supplemental oxygen via nasal prongs (2–3 L/min). In most mild-to-moderate asthmatics, arterial blood gas measurements are not necessary, especially if the oxygen saturation by pulse oximetry is $\geq 90\%$ and PEFR is ≥ 100 L/min. In more severe attacks, an arterial blood gas reading should be obtained. If initial PO_2 is less than 60 mm Hg on room air, supplemental oxygen should be given and arterial blood gas measurements repeated 20–30 minutes later to make certain that PO_2 has risen satisfactorily and that CO_2 retention has not occurred. Patients who exhibit deterioration or increasing fatigue should have arterial blood gas determinations to detect hypercapnia.

2. Endotracheal intubation–"Immediate" endotracheal intubation for assisted ventilation is rarely needed in the emergency department. The only indication for this procedure is increasing obtundation, usually associated with severe hypercapnia ($PCO_2 \geq$ 55 mm Hg) and acidosis, where the risk of apnea is great (Chapter 5). For most other asthmatics, intubation should be considered only if arterial blood gas measurements worsen progressively despite therapy, as in any other form of respiratory failure. Intubation may be postponed until after a trial of intensive bronchodilator therapy even in patients with moderate CO_2 retention on admission to the emergency department, as long as they remain alert. However, such patients must be under continuous and reliable medical supervision with frequent monitoring of arterial blood gases.

B. Specific Therapy: Hypersecretion of mucus with subsequent plugging of airways is the most difficult problem to treat. Adequate but not excessive hydration by the oral or intravenous route and physical therapy (percussion, coughing, and possibly postural drainage) are probably beneficial and should be done in the emergency department. If dehydration is suspected on the basis of physical examination or laboratory tests, give lactated Ringer's injection or half-normal saline solution intravenously, 0.5–1 L/m², during the first 6 hours in the emergency department. Oral hydration is also effective and is useful in cooperative adults and children. *Caution:* Mist or aerosol therapy has not been shown to be helpful, and oral expectorants (eg, sodium iodide or glyceryl guaiacolate), positive pressure ventilation, bronchoscopy, and bronchial lavage are all potentially dangerous and should be avoided.

C. Drugs for Relief of Bronchospasm:

1. Sympathomimetics–Epinephrine, isoproterenol, and the relatively β_2-specific agonists isoetharine (Bronkosol, many others), metaproterenol (Alupent, Metaprel), albuterol (Proventil, Ventolin), and terbutaline (Brethine, others) are all effective. *Caution:* Sympathomimetics must be given in *decreased dosage* to older people (over age 50–60 years), those with coronary artery disease or a history of tachyarrhythmias, those who have recently been treated with these drugs, and those who show signs of toxicity (tremor, tachyarrhythmias, nervousness, myocardial ischemia).

a. Inhalation sympathomimetics–These are rapidly and reliably absorbed and are quite satisfactory for most asthma attacks.

(1) Isoproterenol, 0.5–1 mL of 1:200 solution in 3–5 mL of saline nebulized by compressed air or oxygen every 30–60 minutes.

(2) Metaproterenol (Alupent), 15 mg (0.3 mL of 5% solution) premixed in 2.2 mL of saline, given every 30–60 minutes by nebulizer.

(3) Albuterol (Proventil, Ventolin), 0.2–0.3 mL in 3 mL of normal saline, given every 30–60 minutes by nebulizer.

b. Parenteral sympathomimetics–These are necessary only for patients unable to cooperate with inhalation treatment, particularly small children. *Note:* Epinephrine in oil (Sus-Phrine) is erratically absorbed and should *not* be used for acutely ill patients.

(1) Terbutaline (Brethine), 0.25 mg (0.25 mL) can be given subcutaneously every 2–4 hours initially for 2 doses, then every 8 hours.

(2) Aqueous epinephrine, 1:1000, 0.1–0.5 mL subcutaneously every 30–90 minutes, may be repeated 3–4 times.

2. Corticosteroids–The mechanism of action of glucocorticoids in asthma is poorly understood, but these drugs probably work through their anti-inflammatory effects. The onset of action of corticosteroids is debated, but their effectiveness is not. Corticosteroids are useful for severe attacks, for patients who fail to respond to nebulizer therapy, and for patients who are presently taking or have recently discontinued corticosteroids.

a. Methylprednisolone–Give methylprednisolone sodium succinate (A-Methapred, Solu-Medrol, others), 1–1.5 mg/kg or 60–125 mg intravenously immediately; then give 20 mg intravenously every 4–6 hours until the attack is broken.

b. Other drugs–Prednisone orally in comparable doses is probably as effective as methylprednisolone. Other corticosteroids may be used also, with the possible exception of dexamethasone. *Note:* Corticosteroids should always be used in conjunction with other types of therapy.

3. Anticholinergics–Ipratropium bromide, an atropinelike compound, is available as a metered aerosol (Atrovent). It can be administered in doses of 2–6 puffs every 4–6 hours. Although most useful in patients with chronic bronchitis and emphysema, this drug may benefit asthmatic patients as well.

4. Magnesium sulfate–Magnesium sulfate ($MgSO_4$) has a bronchodilating effect that may be of benefit in asthma, and it has been increasingly reported in the literature and is used by some in clinical practice. Although its role in the treatment of asthma is under investigation, it has been safely administered to preeclamptic women for years. At present, it may be considered for treatment of life-threatening asthma that fails to respond to sympathomimetic bronchodilators. In adults, 1 g of $MgSO_4$ in 50 mL of normal saline or 5% dextrose in water is infused over 30 minutes. If necessary, an infusion of 1 g/h may be maintained. The effects of $MgSO_4$ are short-lived and abate after the infusion is discontinued. Blood pressure should be monitored and the infusion stopped if hypotension occurs. Deep tendon reflexes will be lost once serum magnesium concentrations reach 7–10 meq/L (normal concentrations are 1.5–2 meq/L); the infusion should be stopped if reflexes are lost. At magnesium concentrations of 10–15 meq/L, respiratory depression occurs, and at 30 meq/L, cardiac arrest may occur. However, the dose recommended for asthma is low (approximately one-fourth the dose used in preeclampsia), and side effects are unlikely.

5. Aminophylline–This moderately effective bronchodilator is the only theophylline derivative that can be given intravenously. The therapeutic ratio is low, with optimum blood levels being more than half of toxic levels. Its efficacy in the emergency setting has not been shown, whereas adverse effects (see below) are often encountered. Aminophylline is now considered a third-line drug after nebulized bronchodilators and intravenous corticosteroids. Aminophylline's mild diuretic effect may be helpful if wheezing is secondary to cardiogenic pulmonary edema.

If aminophylline is to be used, give a loading dose of 5–6 mg/kg intravenously in 100 mL of diluent over 30 minutes if the patient has not taken theophylline derivatives in the past 1–2 days; then continue with maintenance as shown in Table 27–5. The loading dose should be lower in patients who have been receiving theophyllines prior to arrival. Serum theophylline determinations are useful in long-term treatment of asthma but are not generally available (and have not been shown to be useful) in emergency management.

Oral or rectal administration is not recommended for emergency management because of slow and unreliable absorption, except in children to begin outpatient treatment. In this setting, aminophylline solution may be a convenient method for loading and is better tolerated and more rapidly absorbed than tablets.

Toxicity may be manifested by tachyarrhythmias, gastrointestinal upset (nausea and vomiting, cramps, diarrhea), and central nervous system irritability (nervousness, tremor, seizures).

Management of Asthmatic Attacks

A. Mild Attack: Take history, perform physical examination, and obtain spirometric measurement. Order chest x-ray, arterial blood gas determinations, or other studies based on findings.

Table 27–5. Maintenance doses of intravenous aminophylline.

Patient Category	Maintenance dose (mg/kg/h)	
	First 12 Hours	Subsequently[1]
Children	1	0.8
Young adults (smokers)	1	0.8
Young adults (nonsmokers)	0.7	0.5
Elderly patients	0.6	0.3
Patients with heart failure or liver failure	0.5	0.1–0.2

[1]If possible, subsequent infusion rates should be adjusted based on serum aminophylline levels (therapeutic range, 10–20 μg/mL).

1. Treatment–Give sympathomimetics such as metaproterenol (Alupent) by inhalation (preferable) or parenterally. Combine with oral hydration and perhaps oral aminophylline.

2. Disposition–If, after treatment, the FEV_1 is greater than 60% of the predicted value (or > 2.1 L in adults) or the PEFR is greater than 300 L/min, the patient may be given sympathomimetics and discharged for outpatient follow-up (to be seen within 1–2 days). If there is minimal or no improvement, proceed as for moderate attack.

B. Moderate Attack: Evaluate as above. Spirometry, pulse oximetry, and arterial blood gas determinations are essential. Chest x-ray, sputum examination, and other studies are often useful.

1. Treatment–

a. Begin oxygen, 2 L/min, by nasal prongs, and modify flow rate based on results of arterial blood gas measurements.

b. Establish an intravenous line, and start 5% dextrose in half-normal saline at a rate of 200 mL/h (for adults).

c. Give an initial dose of inhalation and parenteral sympathomimetics (eg, nebulized metaproterenol or subcutaneous epinephrine, 1:1000, 0.3–0.5 mL). If the patient fails to respond, begin corticosteroids. Consider inhaled ipratropium bromide, magnesium sulfate, or aminophylline, as discussed above.

d. If the patient is taking glucocorticoids or if they were recently discontinued, give intravenous glucocorticoids (methylprednisolone, 60–125 mg; hydrocortisone, 300 mg). Give other patients intravenous glucocorticoids (same doses as above) if the FEV_1 does not improve by 0.3 L (or PEFR by 60 L/min) 15–30 minutes after initial sympathomimetic therapy.

e. Reassess blood gases and clinical status in 15–30 minutes and again in 2–3 hours.

2. Disposition–Patients who do not dramatically improve (FEV_1 > 60%, PEFR > 300 L/min) within 2–3 hours almost invariably require hospitalization. Usually, patients should be discharged with their breathing as close as possible to baseline, and they should be able to ambulate without dyspnea or desaturation on pulse oximetry. Patients who remain dyspneic or uncomfortable should be admitted.

C. Severe and Catastrophic Attacks and Status Asthmaticus: Evaluate as for moderate attack.

1. Treatment–

a. Proceed as for moderate attack, except that glucocorticoids should be given intravenously immediately. Give methylprednisolone, 1–1.5 mg/kg, or 60–125 mg; or hydrocortisone, 300 mg.

b. Nebulized and parenteral sympathomimetics should be given (see above for dosages) while an intravenous catheter is inserted. Repeat nebulizer therapy every 15–30 minutes. Consider using ipratropium bromide (Atrovent) and magnesium sulfate. Intravenous aminophylline may also be started. ***Note:***

Epinephrine in oil (Sus-Phrine) is erratically absorbed and should not be used for acutely ill patients.

c. Pulse oximetry should be monitored continuously, and arterial blood gases should be reassessed within 10–20 minutes of initial therapy to make certain that deterioration is not occurring.

d. Obtain spirometric measurements if possible. Severely dyspneic patients may not be able to cooperate with FEV_1 measurements, but PEFR may be obtainable.

e. Assess the patient on admission and frequently thereafter for the presence of respiratory failure possibly requiring assisted ventilation.

2. Flowchart–A flowchart permits rapid review of the treatment given and the patient's response. The following should be recorded:

a. Date and time.

b. Temperature, pulse, respiration, pulsus paradoxus, and use of accessory muscles of respiration.

c. Wheezing (0–4+).

d. Arterial blood gas determinations (with carefully estimated FIO_2 [fraction of inspired oxygen] or O_2 flow rate).

e. FEV_1 (or PEFR).

f. Cumulative fluid administered.

g. Bronchodilators given (amount and time).

3. Disposition–Hospitalization is indicated for almost all patients with severe asthma. Very rarely, a previously untreated patient (or one with a self-limited cause of bronchospasm, such as inhalation of a provocative antigen) will present with a severe asthmatic attack and return to normal a few hours after initiation of vigorous therapy. Such patients may be considered for discharge from the emergency department. However, it must be remembered that asthmatics rarely if ever return to normal immediately following acute attacks. Even if they do not have a recurrence of asthma that brings them back to the emergency department—an all too common occurrence—their pulmonary function will be abnormal for days or weeks. Therefore, outpatient follow-up (within 5–7 days) is essential in management.

CHRONIC BRONCHITIS & EMPHYSEMA

Chronic bronchitis and emphysema often occur together, and both have a high correlation with smoking. These disorders are collectively known as **chronic obstructive pulmonary disease,** or COPD.

Chronic bronchitis is defined as daily cough for over 3 months of the year for 2 years in a row. Pathologically, there is mucous gland hypertrophy and hyperplasia, with leukocytic infiltration of bronchial mucosa. Chronic bronchitis is believed to contribute to production of emphysema in many patients.

Emphysema is defined as destruction of lung parenchyma with coalescence of alveoli. This may be proved pathologically or strongly suspected on the basis of pulmonary function tests; the clinical diagnosis is presumptive only. Increased lung compliance due to loss of lung parenchyma is associated with expiratory airway collapse and air trapping that may mimic bronchospasm. Change in compliance is also responsible for the barrel chest, overaerated lung fields, and flattened diaphragms seen on chest x-ray in these patients.

Diagnosis

A. Chronic Bronchitis: In addition to cough, chronic bronchitis is associated with dyspnea on exertion, wheezing, and rhonchi. Many patients are aware of their diagnosis from previous physician visits. They come to the emergency department during acute exacerbations manifested by increased volume and purulence of sputum and an increase in associated findings (eg, dyspnea, wheezing). Fever is unusual, and its presence should suggest complications such as pneumonia.

B. Emphysema: The only constant associated abnormality is dyspnea—initially present only on exertion, later present even at rest. Cough, sputum production, wheezing, barrel chest, use of accessory muscles of respiration, and other findings may or may not be present.

Evaluation of Patients With Chronic Bronchitis & Emphysema

A. History:

1. Present symptoms–Duration, severity, comparison with previous attacks (ie, more or less severe than usual).

2. Present medications–Identify precisely all medications being taken, with dosages and times of administration.

3. Past attacks of pulmonary disease–Severity, type of treatment, and results.

B. Physical Examination:

1. Obtain complete vital signs.

2. Assess degree of illness by observation and inspection.

3. Perform cardiac and pulmonary examinations, looking especially for heart failure and other complications of COPD (pneumonia, pneumothorax).

C. Laboratory Findings and Special Tests: The important laboratory tests are basically the same as those discussed in the section on asthma.

1. Arterial blood gas determinations– Arterial blood gas determinations are virtually mandatory for patients with chronic bronchitis or emphysema complaining of increased respiratory symptoms. Hypoxemia and diminished oxygen saturation on pulse oximetry are the only regular findings, but PCO_2 may be low, normal, or elevated. The significance of any given PCO_2 determination may be best evaluated by reference to arterial blood pH. Patients with chronic lung disease compensate for the acid load of chronic hypercapnia by bicarbonate retention, producing a relatively normal arterial blood pH. Thus, a markedly lowered arterial blood pH in conjunction with hypercapnia indicates that hypercapnia is probably of recent onset (within 1–2 days) or that the acidosis has a metabolic component. Knowledge of the patient's prior blood gas partial pressures and observation of mental status are also helpful in evaluating the significance of the arterial blood PCO_2.

2. Chest x-ray–This is most helpful in assessing possible complications of COPD, eg, pneumonia, atelectasis, pneumothorax, and heart failure.

3. ECG–Look for evidence of supraventricular and ventricular arrhythmias, myocardial ischemia, and cor pulmonale.

4. Gram-stained smears of sputum–Most patients with chronic bronchitis and emphysema have chronically infected airways, but the amount of sputum and the degree of purulence frequently increase during exacerbations. Examination of the Gram-stained smear will confirm the presence of significant infection (abundant PMNs) and may help in guiding antimicrobial therapy. Since virtually all exacerbations are caused by pneumococci or *Haemophilus influenzae,* empiric therapy without reference to the Gram-stained smear or culture may be satisfactory (below). Some patients with "pure" emphysema may not produce sputum.

5. Spirometry–Spirometry is useful in judging severity and monitoring response to treatment. Airway obstruction and reduced vital capacity are both seen.

6. CBC and differential–The white blood cell count is rarely helpful. It may be modestly elevated if the patient is receiving corticosteroids or has recently been taking sympathomimetic agents. In some patients, hemoglobin or hematocrit may show plethora sufficient to require phlebotomy (eg, hematocrit > 55%).

7. Serum electrolytes–Hypokalemia (often secondary to diuretics) and increased bicarbonate (secondary to chronic CO_2 retention or diuretic therapy) are common.

Treatment

A. Management of Respiratory Failure:

1. Oxygen–Begin oxygen at a rate of 1–2 L/min *(no more),* using nasal prongs, or increase FIO_2 to 24–28% using a Venturi mask. This slightly increased FIO_2 provides satisfactory oxygenation for most patients. Higher levels of FIO_2 may be associated with worsening hypercapnia or apnea. However, if a higher FIO_2 is required to achieve adequate arterial PO_2, oxygen should be given while the patient is closely monitored. Alternatively, intubation and mechanical ventilation should be considered.

2. Arterial blood gas measurements–Contin-uously monitor pulse oximetry, and repeat arterial blood gas measurements after 20–30 minutes to look for satisfactory improvement in oxygenation (arterial $PO_2 \geq 55$ mm Hg) without a significant increase in PCO_2 (an increase of 5–8 mm Hg is usually tolerable, especially if the pH is not too low initially and mental status is stable).

3. Bronchodilators–Although their effect may be marginal, bronchodilators and corticosteroids usually are tried in patients with acute exacerbations of COPD. The same dosages recommended for asthma are used (p 460).

4. Endotracheal intubation–Endotracheal intubation should be considered if the patient fails to improve or worsens with supplemental oxygen and other measures. Progressively falling arterial PO_2 or rising PCO_2, persistent metabolic acidosis, or worsening obtundation are all indications for intubation.

The best candidates for intubation and ventilatory support are patients with acute self-limiting conditions causing respiratory failure, eg, severe bronchitis, pneumothorax, or heart failure. Patients with relentlessly progressive chronic lung disease without a reversible component are poor candidates for assisted ventilation, since weaning them from the ventilator may well be impossible. In the emergency department, it may not be clear whether the patient's worsening respiratory failure is due to a reversible component, and under these circumstances, intubation and ventilatory support should be provided as needed.

5. Adjunctive measures–Other adjunctive measures such as adequate hydration and physical therapy (including postural drainage) may be helpful, particularly for patients producing large volumes of sputum.

B. Treatment of Infection: Patients with purulent sputum should receive antimicrobials, although the beneficial effect is apparently a small one. Ampicillin or amoxicillin, 0.5 g orally 4 times daily; tetracycline, 0.5 g orally 4 times daily; and trimethoprim-sulfamethoxazole (trimethoprim 80 mg, sulfamethoxazole 400 mg), 2 tablets twice daily, have all been shown to be effective. Ampicillin is somewhat easier to administer if parenteral therapy is required (1 g every 4 hours). If no sputum—or clear sputum without PMNs—is being produced, antimicrobial chemotherapy is probably unnecessary.

C. Treatment of Complications:

1. Heart failure is common and generally is best managed with oxygen and diuretics. Furosemide (Lasix), 20–40 intravenously, is the most useful agent in the emergency department setting. ***Caution:*** Digitalis glycosides should not be used acutely.

2. If plethora (hematocrit > 55%) is present, and particularly if it is associated with fluid overload from heart failure, therapeutic phlebotomy in the emergency department (250–500 mL) may be beneficial.

3. Atelectasis or significant pneumothorax should be treated if present.

Disposition

A. Indications for Hospitalization: Patients with progressive respiratory failure or those with reversible or treatable complications (heart failure, pneumonia, etc) should be hospitalized.

B. Indications for Discharge From the Emergency Department: Patients with stable respiratory failure, without a reversible component, even if severe in degree, may be discharged to their regular source of care. Patients with acute exacerbations of chronic bronchitis, if their ventilatory status is stable or only slightly worsened, may be discharged to follow-up within a few days.

CYSTIC FIBROSIS

Diagnosis

Cystic fibrosis is a generalized hereditary disease of apocrine glands associated with chronic bronchitis, chronic sinusitis, emphysema, and respiratory failure as well as pancreatic insufficiency, azoospermia, and increased sweat chloride levels. Clinically, these patients have a syndrome of chronic bronchitis and emphysema that develops at an early age (2–20 years), often with a history of the disease in relatives. In contrast to patients with chronic obstructive pulmonary disease, patients with cystic fibrosis have a high frequency of digital clubbing.

Treatment

A. Mobilization of mucus plugs by hydration and good pulmonary toilet is more important than bronchodilator therapy.

B. Most patients have chronic bronchitis or pneumonitis secondary to mucoid gram-negative bacilli (usually *Pseudomonas aeruginosa*) or staphylococci. Treatment should be initiated based on Gram-stained smear of sputum and culture. Combination therapy with an antipseudomonal penicillin (eg, ticarcillin, 300 mg/kg/d orally in 6 doses) and an aminoglycoside (eg, tobramycin, 6 mg/kg/d orally in 3 doses) is used frequently. Oral ciprofloxacin may be used for *P aeruginosa*. Some physicians regularly hospitalize patients with cystic fibrosis for administration of intravenous antibiotics.

Disposition

Hospitalization is required for evaluation and treatment of most patients with new respiratory symptoms.

ACUTE PULMONARY EMBOLISM & INFARCTION

A variety of clinical conditions (Table 27–6) may cause clots to form in the venous system that when dislodged will cause pulmonary emboli. Venous thrombosis may result from a generalized hypercoagulable state (eg, induced by prolonged use of birth control pills) or local stasis (eg, following fractures with casting, bed rest). Clots that cause clinically significant pulmonary embolism form most commonly in the iliofemoral and pelvic venous beds. Pulmonary embolization from veins of the distal lower extremities or from upper extremities is very rare.

When embolization occurs, the consequences and manifestations depend on the size of the embolism, the underlying cardiorespiratory status, and whether there is subsequent infarction of pulmonary tissue. With small- to medium-sized emboli, obstruction of a localized portion of the pulmonary vascular tree causes local atelectasis with resulting ventilation-perfusion ($\dot{V}/\dot{Q}$) abnormalities and hypoxemia. Reflex hyperventilation with resultant hypocapnia and tachycardia also occurs. With massive embolization (obstructing over 60% of the vascular bed), acute pulmonary hypertension, right heart strain, systemic hypotension, and shock may also occur. Fragmentation of large emboli with distal migration of clot or further embolization may result in stepwise changes in clinical status. Death may occur suddenly.

Diagnosis

A. Symptoms and Signs: The illness often begins abruptly, and there is almost always a predisposing underlying condition (Table 27–6). Dyspnea, cough, anxiety, and chest pain (retrosternal and oppressive or lateralized and pleuritic) occur in varying combinations. Hemoptysis may occur also. Syncope occurs only rarely.

Tachycardia and tachypnea are common. Low-grade fever, hypotension, cyanosis, signs of deep vein thrombosis, pleural friction rub, and signs of pulmonary consolidation may be present.

B. Laboratory Findings and Special Examinations: Because the symptoms and signs of pulmonary embolism are never diagnostic, precise diagnosis depends on laboratory tests.

1. Chest x-ray–Although the chest x-ray is ab-

Table 27–6. Conditions that predispose to pulmonary embolization.

Immobility (eg, bed rest)
Surgery
Fractures of large bones
Pregnancy and postpartum states
Use of oral contraceptives
Malignant neoplastic disease
Congestive heart failure
---

normal in most patients with pulmonary embolization with infarction, the abnormalities are often nonspecific (atelectasis, pleural effusions, small infiltrates, etc).

2. ECG–The ECG is usually normal (except for tachycardia) or shows nonspecific changes. In rare cases of massive embolization, there may be signs of myocardial ischemia (leading to the mistaken diagnosis of myocardial infarction) or of right heart strain.

3. Arterial blood gas measurements–Clinically significant pulmonary embolization is almost always associated with hypoxemia (arterial saturation < 90%, PO_2 < 80 mm Hg); however, this may be partially obscured by the reflex hyperventilation and hypocapnia that occur in most patients. Unfortunately, the combination of hypoxemia and hypocapnia is found also in a wide variety of other acute pulmonary conditions (pleurisy, pleural effusion, pneumonia, pulmonary edema, asthma) and is not specific for pulmonary embolism.

4. Radionuclide lung scans–In patients without known antecedent pulmonary disease, the perfusion radionuclide lung scan is a highly sensitive screening procedure for embolization. Almost all patients with emboli have an abnormal scan, and a normal scan therefore excludes significant embolization. However, a variety of other conditions can result in an abnormal perfusion scan (bronchospasm, bronchitis, emphysema), making a positive test very nonspecific.

The ventilation-perfusion ($\dot{V}/\dot{Q}$) scan has been preferred to a plain perfusion scan in the diagnosis of pulmonary embolism, since mismatches between ventilation and perfusion have been considered highly specific. For example, the finding of large segmental or subsegmental perfusion defects in areas of normal ventilation has been considered diagnostic for pulmonary embolism by many physicians. Studies suggest that large perfusion defects without matching ventilation abnormalities reflect a high probability of pulmonary embolism. However, the presence of small (less than segmental or subsegmental) perfusion defects with normal ventilation does not rule out pulmonary embolism, and the combination of small perfusion defects and matched ventilation abnormalities indicates neither a high nor a low probability of embolism. As a result, selective pulmonary angiography (into areas of perfusion abnormality identified on plain perfusion or $\dot{V}/\dot{Q}$ scans) is required in many, if not most, patients suspected of pulmonary embolism. Documentation of embolization by selective pulmonary angiography is required especially for patients in whom anticoagulation carries a high risk of side effects; for patients who will require long-term anticoagulation because of a persistent susceptibility to development of pulmonary embolism; for patients who will receive thrombolytic therapy; and for patients in whom a diagnosis of pulmonary embolization is unlikely on clinical grounds.

Treatment
A. Provide Respiratory Support:
1. Correct hypoxemia with oxygen, 5–10 L/min, by nasal prongs or mask.

2. If hypercapnia is present on admission, arterial blood gas measurements should be repeated within 15–20 minutes. Continuously monitor oxygen saturation by pulse oximetry.

3. Worsening hypercapnia with progressive obtundation is an indication for emergency intubation.

B. Start Anticoagulation Therapy:
Give a loading dose of heparin, 10,000 units intravenously, followed by continuous intravenous infusion of 1000–3000 units per hour. Monitor coagulation factors (eg, activated partial thromboplastin time), and keep them 1.5–2 times normal values. The dosage of heparin may be tapered as symptoms abate.

C. Consider Thrombolytic Therapy:
Although anticoagulation is sufficient treatment for most patients with pulmonary embolism, a few present with hemodynamic compromise or florid shock and may benefit from removal of clot from the pulmonary artery. Surgical embolectomy was once used, but chemical lysis of the clot is now preferred. Thrombolytic agents such as streptokinase, urokinase, and tissue plasminogen activator (tPA) achieve such lysis and may also prevent damage to the pulmonary vascular bed and to venous valves in the extremities, although authorities do not agree on the validity of these benefits. Thrombolytic therapy may be associated with severe bleeding and cannot be used in patients with recent trauma, cerebrovascular accident, or gastrointestinal tract hemorrhage. See p 470 for a list of contraindications to thrombolytic therapy. Thrombolytic agents *should not* be given simultaneously with heparin and should be given in the emergency department only if an intensive care unit is unavailable.

Before thrombolytic therapy is started, standard protocols require that heparin be discontinued and that the thrombin time, prothrombin time, or activated partial thromboplastin time be less than twice the normal value. Unless it is absolutely essential, *do not* insert central venous catheters (eg, central venous pressure monitors) in patients receiving thrombolytic therapy. If such catheters must be used, insert them into a peripheral vein, and advance them retrograde into a central vein; any bleeding at the insertion site may then be easily controlled. The loading dose of streptokinase is 250,000 units given intravenously over 20 minutes, followed by 100,000 units/h for 24 hours; give hydrocortisone, 100 mg, before the streptokinase to prevent allergic reactions. If urokinase—which is more expensive but less toxic than streptokinase—is used, give a loading dose of 4400 units/kg, and follow with an intravenous infusion of the same dose every hour for 24 hours. Although not yet approved in the USA for treatment of pulmonary embolism, tissue plasminogen activator (tPA), 100 mg given intravenously (50 mg/h), is effective and appears to cause clot lysis more rapidly than streptokinase. The thrombin time, prothrombin time, or activated partial thromboplastin time should be 1.5–2 times normal during thrombolytic therapy. Thrombolytic agents should be discontinued if significant bleeding occurs; the action of these drugs can be reversed with fresh-frozen plasma. Heparin treatment should be reinstituted after thrombolytic therapy has been completed.

D. Treat Pain: Give morphine or meperidine as required, preferably by the intravenous route. Monitor arterial blood gases carefully to prevent CO_2 retention.

E. Treat Shock: Dopamine, 2.5–7.5 µg/kg/min intravenously may be started in the emergency department if shock is present and before thrombolytic therapy (Chapter 3). Vigorous fluid therapy should be avoided until central monitoring (preferably with a pulmonary artery catheter) can be instituted. *Note:* Central monitoring should be avoided entirely or performed through a peripheral venous entry side if thrombolytic agents are used.

F. Surgical Treatment: Thoracotomy with removal of emboli may occasionally be lifesaving. Generally, this procedure is reserved for patients with massive emboli and refractory hypotension, despite resuscitation, and in patients for whom thrombolytic therapy is contraindicated. A Greenfield filter may be introduced to capture further emboli.

Disposition

Hospitalize all patients for continued anticoagulation and supportive care. Patients with large emboli and hemodynamic impairment should be monitored in the intensive care unit.

Patients in whom pulmonary embolism is strongly suspected should be hospitalized for treatment with anticoagulation (if there are no contraindications) until a definitive diagnosis can be made.

CHRONIC PULMONARY VASCULAR DISEASE

Chronic pulmonary vascular disease is a rare cause of chronic exertional dyspnea. The diagnosis may be suspected but cannot be made definitively in the emergency department, since it requires sophisticated pulmonary function testing. The disease is due to gradual obliteration of pulmonary vasculature due to frequent embolization (parasites, clot, or foreign material) or other unexplained processes. Early in the disease, pulmonary artery pressures and arterial blood gas measurements may be normal at rest, and exercise is required to induce significant abnormalities.

Diagnosis

The diagnosis should be suspected in all patients with chronic exertional dyspnea, cough, pleurisy, and possibly right heart strain. Even if arterial PO_2 is normal at rest, these patients should not be diagnosed as "hysterical" without pulmonary function testing, including measurement of diffusing capacity (which is decreased). Hypoxemia and hypocapnia are usually accentuated or induced by exercise, even with nearly normal lung mechanics.

Treatment

Administer supplemental oxygen if arterial PO_2 on room air is 65 mm Hg or less. If cor pulmonale is present, diuretic therapy may be initiated as well (furosemide [Lasix], 20–40 mg intravenously).

Disposition

Hospitalize patients with acute worsening of symptoms (including those with cor pulmonale) or progressive respiratory failure. Consultation with the patient's regular physician may be helpful in determining disposition.

INTERSTITIAL PULMONARY DISEASES

A variety of conditions may produce diffuse pulmonary interstitial inflammation and fibrosis, including drugs, pneumoconioses, collagen diseases, sarcoidosis, and illnesses of unknown cause with pathologic features involving chiefly the lungs (eg, idiopathic interstitial fibrosis). Aside from the pneumoconioses and sarcoidosis, these illnesses are relatively uncommon. The principal feature of all of them is that dyspnea begins gradually and seldom occurs acutely without a background of increasing shortness of breath. When dyspnea of acute onset does occur, it is often due to intercurrent illness (eg, pulmonary infection).

Diagnosis

Many patients with interstitial pulmonary disease will know their diagnosis; if not, it can seldom be made with certainty in the emergency department setting, since lung biopsy is often required.

A. Symptoms and Signs: Gradually increasing dyspnea, especially on exertion, is the only reliable symptom. Chest pain, cough, sputum production, and other symptoms may occur but are inconstant. Physical findings are variable, but dry crackles (rales) are common. Cyanosis and clubbing may be present as well.

B. Laboratory Findings: Chest x-ray usually shows interstitial infiltrates, although this may be a subtle finding. Other changes may be present depending on the disease process (eg, hilar adenopathy in sarcoidosis, conglomerate fibrosis in silicosis, etc). Arterial blood gas measurements in most patients show hypoxemia and hypocapnia, although hyperventilation may partially correct the former.

Treatment & Disposition

Provide respiratory support as needed, and treat intercurrent disease (infection, etc).

Hospitalize patients with respiratory failure or recent marked worsening of symptoms or those in whom acute infection is suspected. Refer all patients not already under care to a pulmonary disease specialist.

REFERENCES

Bell RC et al: Multiple organ system failure and infection in adult respiratory distress syndrome. Ann Intern Med 1983;99:293.

Braun SR et al: A comparison of the effect of ipratropium and albuterol in the treatment of chronic obstructive airway disease. Arch Intern Med 1989;149:544.

Conces DJ et al: Treatment of pneumothoraces utilizing small caliber chest tubes. Chest 1984;94:55.

Dereine JP, Fleury B, Pariente R: Acute respiratory failure of chronic obstructive pulmonary disease. Am Rev Respir Dis 1988;138:1006.

Dorinsky PM, Gadel JE: Mechanisms of multiple nonpulmonary organ failure in ARDS. Chest 1989;96:885.

Emerman CL et al: A randomized controlled trial of methylprednisolone in the emergency treatment of exacerbations of COPD. Chest 1989;95:563.

Fitzgerald JM, Hargreave FE: The assessment and management of acute life-threatening asthma. Chest 1989;95:888.

Gross NJ: Ipratropium bromide. N Engl J Med 1988;319:486.

Jones J et al: Continuous emergency department monitoring of arterial saturation in adult patients with respiratory distress. Ann Emerg Med 1988;17:463.

McNamara RM et al: Intravenous magnesium sulfate in the management of acute respiratory failure complicating asthma. Ann Emerg Med 1989;18:197.

Moser KM: Venous thromboembolism. Am Rev Respir Dis 1990;141:235.

Overton DJ, Bocka JJ: The alveolar-arterial oxygen gradient in patients with documented pulmonary embolism. Arch Intern Med 1988;148:1817.

Pingleton SK: Complications of acute respiratory failure. Am Rev Respir Dis 1988;133:1463.

Pistoksi M, Miniati M, Giuntini C: Pleural liquid and solute exchange. Am Rev Respir Dis 1989;140:825.

Stein LM, Cole RP: Early administration of corticosteroids in emergency room treatment of acute asthma. Ann Intern Med 1990;112:822.

Summers QA, Sarala RA: Nebulized ipratropium in the treatment of acute asthma. Chest 1990;87:425.

Vallee P et al: Sequential treatment of a simple pneumothorax. Ann Emerg Med 1988;17:936.

Vathernen AS et al: High-dose inhaled albuterol in severe chronic airflow limitation. Am Rev Respir Dis 1988;138:850.

Wiener-Kronish JP et al: Lack of association of pleural effusion with chronic pulmonary arterial and right atrial hypertension. Chest 1987;92:967.

28

Cardiac Emergencies*

Melvin D. Cheitlin, MD, & Joseph A. Abbott, MD

Immediate Management

Cardiac disease is usually manifested by symptoms of chest pain, dyspnea or respiratory distress, cardiac arrest or syncope, or shock. Because these symptoms are so commonly encountered in the emergency department and because they may result from disease in many organs other than the heart, they are discussed separately (Chapters 1, 3, 5, 6, and 11). Since almost any cardiac disease is at least potentially life-threatening, no attempt has been made in this chapter to categorize disorders on the basis of severity or to assign priorities in treatment.

---

*See also Chapter 29 for emergencies due to cardiac arrhythmias.

CORONARY ARTERY DISEASE

ACUTE MYOCARDIAL INFARCTION (Coronary Occlusion)

Myocardial infarction results when arterial blood flow to the myocardium is suddenly decreased or interrupted. It is usually due to atherosclerotic coronary artery disease with sudden occlusion by thrombus; vasculitis or emboli are less common causes. When patients with chest pain and ST segment elevation are studied by coronary angioplasty within several hours of onset, complete occlusion, most often with thrombus, is found in 80–90% of cases. Rarely, patients dying of myocardial infarction are found to have normal coronary arteries, and infarction in such cases is presumably due to spasm of a coronary artery or thrombosis with complete lysis. Cocaine use has been associated with acute myocardial infarction, probably as a result of coronary spasm with or without intravascular thrombus formation. In myocardial infarction, severely ischemic and infarcted muscle contracts and relaxes poorly or not at all; if infarction is extensive, decreased cardiac output with heart failure or shock may result. After myocardial infarction, the ventricle may become aneurysmal or may even rupture. If conducting tissue is ischemic or infarcted, conduction abnormalities may occur. The infarcted endocardium attracts platelets and fibrin that may form mural clots which can subsequently embolize. During acute myocardial infarction, the myocardium is electrically unstable, resulting in ventricular arrhythmias that are frequently life-threatening.

Upon occlusion of a coronary artery, necrosis occurs in a time-dependent course, proceeding from endocardium to epicardium. Necrosis is almost complete within 4–6 hours if no reperfusion occurs. When residual perfusion by collateral vessels is present or lysis of thrombus occurs—either spontaneously or as a result of therapy—there will be salvage of myocardium. The earlier the reperfusion, the more myocardium is salvaged.

Diagnosis

A. Symptoms and Signs: Most patients with myocardial infarction have chest discomfort that is typically substernal and may radiate to the neck or left arm. Occasionally, pain occurs in atypical areas such as the right arm, shoulders, back, or epigastrium. The pain is usually oppressive or squeezing in character and may be associated with anxiety, restlessness, nausea and vomiting, abdominal bloating, dyspnea, and diaphoresis. It commonly begins at rest, worsens gradually, and frequently persists for hours. Occasionally, myocardial infarction is painless—especially in elderly or diabetic patients—and is manifested by the acute onset of left heart failure, hypotension, or cardiac arrhythmias.

Physical findings vary, and none are specific or diagnostic of myocardial infarction. An S_4 gallop or at times an S_3 gallop may be present. Occasionally, an apical systolic murmur of mitral insufficiency due to papillary muscle and left ventricular dysfunction is present. In patients with uncomplicated myocardial infarction, there may be no abnormal findings on physical examination. When cardiopulmonary physical findings are present, they tend to reflect the presence of complications (see below).

B. Electrocardiographic Findings: The ECG shows signs of infarction (high-voltage T waves, elevated ST segments, abnormal Q waves, etc) in about half of patients. In the remainder, the initial ECG shows only nonspecific ST–T wave changes, or may be normal. Note that a normal ECG *does not* rule out the possibility of myocardial infarction. There is, however, increasing evidence (eg, Slater et al; see references) that a normal initial ECG predicts either that the discomfort is not due to myocardial ischemia, or that, if it is, the resulting clinical course will be benign.

C. Laboratory Findings: Serum AST (SGOT) and LDH levels are elevated if samples are taken at the proper time, but in the emergency department, the time elapsed between onset of infarction and measurement of enzyme level is frequently so short that levels may still be normal.

The serum CK-MB isoenzyme determination is the most sensitive and specific laboratory test for myocardial infarction now available: results are seldom abnormal in other diseases. Elevation of CK levels begins 6 hours after infarction, peaks at 18–24 hours, and usually returns to normal by the third day. Occasional patients have a typical clinical picture, normal CK isoenzyme levels, and the evolution on the ECG of ST–T changes consistent with a diagnosis of myocardial infarction. A diagnosis of myocardial infarction can be made in this instance despite the normal isoenzyme levels.

Differential Diagnosis

For a complete differential diagnosis of chest pain, see Chapter 6. Aortic dissection, pericarditis, and gastrointestinal disorders (eg, peptic ulcer disease, pancreatitis) must be excluded in patients being considered for thrombolytic therapy.

Note: The diagnosis of myocardial infarction is suggested by the history, and a decision to admit the patient to the coronary care unit immediately should be based on this information alone. Because of the relatively benign course of patients admitted with a good history suggesting myocardial infarction and a normal initial ECG, in some institutions these patients are admitted to a monitored intermediate care unit rather than a coronary care unit. No amount of laboratory data obtained in the emergency department will definitely rule out myocardial infarction.

Treatment

Note: Patients with a high probability of having acute myocardial infarction by history and physical examination should be considered immediately for eligibility for thrombolytic therapy (see below). The effectiveness of thrombolytic therapy in reducing mortality and myocardial damage depends on how early it is given after the onset of symptoms.

A. Immediate Measures:

1. Begin intravenous infusion of 5% dextrose in water through a secure intravenous catheter. Use microdrip infusion to minimize volume overload. Two to three peripheral venous lines should be started in patients treated with thrombolytic agents.

2. Give lidocaine, 1 mg/kg by intravenous injection over 5 minutes, followed by a continuous infusion of 2–4 mg/min if there are ventricular premature beats. Use smaller doses (1–2 mg/min) if heart failure is present.

3. Begin oxygen, 2–5 L/min, by nasal prongs or mask.

4. Start electrocardiographic monitoring, and obtain 2-lead ECG.

5. If chest pain is present, give nitroglycerin, 0.5 mg sublingually, or one puff delivered to the oral mucosa. Repeat if no effect in 5 minutes. If chest pain returns and systolic blood pressure is above 100 mm Hg, start intravenous nitroglycerin at 10 μg/min and increase by 5 μg/min every 3–5 minutes until there is a 10% fall in systolic blood pressure or chest pain is relieved. The systolic blood pressure should not drop below 90 mm Hg. There is some evidence that intravenous nitroglycerin given early in acute myocardial infarction can prevent remodeling of the ventricle and preserve ventricular function.

6. Give a narcotic analgesic (eg, morphine, 2–8 mg intravenously) if chest pain persists.

7. Give furosemide, 40 mg by intravenous bolus injections if the patient has pulmonary edema.

8. Give patient a 0.3-g aspirin tablet to chew.

9. In the absence of contraindications for beta-blockers (heart rate < 55/min, systolic blood pressure < 90 mm Hg, moist rales above the lower third of the lung fields, advanced atrioventricular block, or history of asthma), give 15 mg of metoprolol in three 5-mg intravenous injections at 2-minute intervals. This is followed by oral metoprolol, 50 mg twice a day on the first day in hospital and 100 mg twice daily thereafter.

B. Additional Measures:

1. Establish a laboratory test data base: CBC with differential, serum creatinine and electrolyte measurements, blood urea nitrogen determinations, enzyme levels (preferably CK isoenzymes and LDH with isoenzymes). Platelet count, prothrombin time, partial thromboplastin time, and blood for typing (and cross-matching if needed) should be sent for patients to be given thrombolytic therapy.

2. Monitor urine output.

C. Thrombolytic Therapy: If the duration of chest discomfort is at least 30 minutes and less than 4–6 hours and there are no contraindications, pharmacologic revascularization with intravenous streptokinase, tissue plasminogen activator (tPA), or anisoylated plasminogen-streptokinase activator complex (APSAC) should be begun in the emergency department.

1. Indications for pharmacologic revascularization–

a. ST segment elevation of at least 0.1 mV in 2 or more leads (II, III, aVF or V_1–V_6, I, aVL) suggests acute injury in the absence of left bundle branch block.

b. Both chest pain and ST elevation are not relieved by 2–3 sublingual nitroglycerin tablets or nifedipine, 5–10 mg, or both.

c. Patient is less than 75 years of age.

d. Patient is alert and oriented, or a family member or friend familiar with patient's medical history is present.

e. There are no contraindications to thrombolytic therapy or anticoagulation therapy (see below).

2. Contraindications to pharmacologic revascularization–

a. Absolute contraindications–

(1) History of any cerebrovascular event (eg, stroke, transient ischemic attack, intracranial neoplasm, arteriovenous malformation, aneurysm).

(2) Recent (within 2 months) cranial or spinal injury or trauma.

(3) Severe, uncontrolled arterial hypertension (diastolic blood pressure > 110 mm Hg or systolic blood pressure > 180 mm Hg).

(4) Known bleeding diathesis.

(5) Active, internal bleeding (eg, serious gastrointestinal bleeding) within the previous 10 days.

(6) Recent (within 10 days) trauma or major surgery at a noncompressible site (eg, coronary artery bypass surgery, organ biopsy, intra-abdominal surgery, obstetric delivery).

(7) Known or suspected pregnancy.

b. Relative contraindications–In the following conditions, the risks associated with thrombolytic therapy may be increased, and clinical judgment should be used in evaluating expected benefits:

(1) Recent (within 10 days) puncture of a noncompressible blood vessel.

(2) Poorly controlled hypertension of several years' duration.

(3) Diabetic hemorrhagic retinopathy or hemorrhagic ophthalmic condition.

(4) Current treatment with an anticoagulant with prothrombin time of greater than 15 seconds.

(5) Advanced liver or kidney disease.

(6) Any other condition associated with a predisposition to bleeding (eg, ulcerative colitis, polycystic kidneys, gastrointestinal arteriovenous malformation, vascular tumors).

(7) Recent serious trauma including prolonged (> 5 minutes) or traumatic external cardiac compression or traumatic endotracheal intubation.

(8) Active peptic ulcer disease.

(9) Known or strongly suspected left heart thrombus.

(10) Infective endocarditis.

3. Dosages–If indicated, the following dosage regimens are recommended:

a. Streptokinase, 1.5 million units in 250 mL of 5% dextrose in water, given intravenously over 20 minutes.

b. tPA, 60 mg intravenously in the first hour, of which 6–10 mg is administered as a bolus over the first 1–2 minutes; 20 mg over the second hour; and 20 mg over the third hour. Recently, a front-loading regimen of 100 mg administered over 90 minutes, 65 mg in the first 30 minutes and 35 mg over the next 60 minutes, has been recommended. If the patient weighs less than 65 kg, give 1.25 mg/kg.

c. APSAC, 30 mg intravenously infused slowly over 5 minutes.

d. Urokinase, given as a loading dose of 0.5 million units over a 10-minute period. This is followed by infusion doses of 1.6–4.5 million units over 18–24 hours.

There is excellent evidence that myocardial reperfusion salvages myocardium—resulting in better ventricular function than conventional management—and improves survival if reperfusion occurs within 6 hours after the onset of symptoms of myocardial infarction (Gruppo Italiano per lo Studio della Streptochinasi nell'Infarto miocardico [GISSI] trial; see references). Thrombolytic therapy may be beneficial in patients with persistent chest pain for up to 24 hours after onset of symptoms (ISIS-2; see references). tPA results in a higher percentage of vessel patency (60–80%) than does streptokinase (30–60%) within the first hour, although the incidence of reperfusion is high in both. After the first hour, the incidence of vessel patency is markedly higher with tPA. However, tPA is considerably more expensive than streptokinase. A recently reported trial (GISSI-2; see references) shows no difference in mortality or ventricular function between tPA and streptokinase, although heparin in this trial was given subcutaneously 12 hours after fibrinolytic therapy was given, which may have allowed a high reocclusion rate following the tPA. A comparison of streptokinase and tPA with intravenous heparin is under way.

4. Heparin–Intravenous heparin, 5000-unit bolus followed by 800–1000 units/h, should be given in a separate line as tPA is infusing because of the short half-life of tPA and because of the danger of recurring thrombosis. Heparin should be continued for 48 hours or longer, maintaining activated partial thromboplastin time at twice normal. The role of intravenous heparin after treatment with tPA has not been definitely determined, but studies are under way.

Heparin may also potentiate the effectiveness of streptokinase. The optimal time to begin heparin administration after streptokinase therapy is under study.

5. Monitoring–Patients given thrombolytic therapy should be transferred to an intensive care unit as soon as possible after initiation of treatment. Monitor the following:

a. Blood pressure every 15 minutes during infusion and every 30–60 minutes thereafter.

b. ECG rhythm strip for reperfusion arrhythmias and ST segment changes.

c. Bleeding complications and change in neuro-logic status. Avoid venous or arterial punctures and unnecessary trauma.

d. Twelve-lead ECG 4 hours after the start of therapy and as needed (eg, for recurrence of chest pain).

e. CK with isoenzymes 4 hours after initiation of treatment and at 4-hour intervals for 24 hours.

D. Angioplasty: If the onset of the chest discomfort is within 4–6 hours and thrombolysis is contraindicated, the chest pain and ST segment elevation are still present, and a catheterization laboratory and qualified team are available, immediate coronary arteriography with angioplasty of the occluded vessel often is recommended.

Disposition

Hospitalize all patients with clinical histories suggesting myocardial infarction, and start electrocardiographic monitoring (in a coronary care unit if possible). Patients with suspected myocardial infarction and normal initial ECGs may be admitted to a monitored intermediate care unit.

Some studies suggest that "low-risk" patients with myocardial infarction (without complications) may be treated at home with results as good as are achieved with hospitalization, but this has not been the practice in the USA. Patients are occasionally treated outside of the intensive care unit, however (eg, those with chronic noncardiac disease or a poor prognosis for other reasons).

COMPLICATIONS OF MYOCARDIAL INFARCTION

About 10–15% of patients reaching the hospital with myocardial infarction die during hospitalization. One or more complications occur in over half of all patients with myocardial infarction.

1. SHOCK (Cardiogenic Shock)

Shock complicating myocardial infarction may be caused by extensive myocardial infarction with decreased cardiac output (most common), inappropriate reflex peripheral vasodilatation, arrhythmias, hypovolemia, right ventricular infarction, and mechanical complications such as ruptured ventricular septum and severe mitral regurgitation. Free-wall myocardial rupture results in tamponade and shock.

Diagnosis

Hypotension accompanied by confusion, obtundation or restlessness, cool skin, oliguria, and metabolic acidosis suggests shock. Mild to moderate hypotension alone is common in myocardial infarction and does not itself indicate shock. Shock in myocardial infarction may be due to many causes (see Table 3–1), which may be difficult to differentiate noninvasively (Table 28–1).

Treatment

Use any or all of the following measures as necessary. (See also Chapter 3.)

A. Give oxygen, 5–10 L/min, by mask or nasal prongs.

B. Monitor central pressure with a Swan-Ganz pulmonary artery catheter (or, far less desirably, a central venous pressure catheter, since in acute myocardial infarction, left ventricular filling pressure can be markedly elevated with normal right ventricular filling pressure, and vice versa). Use an arterial line to measure blood pressure. If possible, the insertion of these catheters should be deferred until the patient has been hospitalized.

C. Give a fluid challenge (200 mL of saline intravenously over 20 minutes) if the patient is not in congestive heart failure (ie, no rales, no pulmonary edema on chest x-ray). Repeat as needed if congestive heart failure does not develop.

D. Correct arrhythmias (see below).

E. Insert a Foley catheter, and measure urine output hourly.

F. Give dopamine (or dobutamine), 2.5–20 µg/kg/min by continuous intravenous infusion (an infusion pump is best). Use the smallest effective dose, guided by hemodynamic response.

G. When shock is caused by inappropriate vasodilatation (rare), alpha-adrenergic drugs such as norepinephrine are useful.

H. There is some evidence that acute revascularization by percutaneous transluminal coronary angioplasty (PTCA) might be particularly effective in patients who develop cardiogenic shock early (within 3–6 hours) after onset of myocardial infarction. Coronary arteriography with the intent of performing PTCA acutely should be seriously considered in such patients.

Disposition

All patients with cardiogenic shock must be hospitalized, preferably in an intensive care unit. It is generally preferable to transfer the patient as quickly as possible to the coronary care unit after giving basic treatment—correcting arrhythmias, starting fluid challenge, starting dopamine infusion, starting thrombolytic therapy when indicated—rather than to attempt to insert more sophisticated monitoring lines, which then must be disconnected when the patient is transferred.

2. CONGESTIVE HEART FAILURE

Congestive heart failure is caused by extensive myocardial infarction, volume overload, arrhythmias, acute mitral regurgitation, or ventricular septal rupture.

Diagnosis

Symptoms and signs of congestive heart failure include dyspnea, anxiety, tachypnea, tachycardia, pulmonary rales or frank pulmonary edema, jugular venous distention, hypoxemia, and typical findings on chest x-ray (cardiomegaly, pulmonary vascular plethora, Kerley B lines, pleural effusion, or pulmonary infiltrates consistent with pulmonary edema). Wheezing may also be a sign of congestive heart failure (cardiac asthma). Suspect right ventricular infarction in inferior myocardial infarction if signs of right heart failure (right ventricular gallops, elevated central venous pressure, hepatomegaly, peripheral edema) are prominent in the absence of signs of left heart failure (dyspnea, rales, pulmonary congestion on chest x-ray).

Treatment

A. Give oxygen, 5–10 L/min, by mask or nasal prongs.

B. Obtain arterial blood gas measurements. Treat respiratory failure if present.

C. Give furosemide, 20–40 mg by intravenous bolus injection. Diuretics are contraindicated if right ventricular infarction is suspected.

Table 28–1. Differential diagnosis by hemodynamics of heart failure and hypotension after myocardial infarction.

Arterial Pressure	Central Venous Pressure	Pulmonary Arterial Wedge Pressure	Stroke Volume Index	Diagnosis	Treatment
→	→ or ↑	↑	→ or ↓	Heart failure	Diuretics; preload and afterload reduction.
→ or ↓	→ or ↓	↓	↓	Hypovolemia	Saline volume loading.
→ or ↓	↑	→ or ↓	→ or ↓	Pulmonary embolism Right ventricular myocardial infarction	Ventilation/perfusion scan; saline or dextran; volume loading; *no* diuretics.
↓	→ or ↑	↑	↓	Cardiogenic shock	Inotropic agents; diuretics; preload and afterload reduction if arterial pressure can be maintained; counterpulsation.

→ = Normal; ↓ = Decreased or low; ↑ = Elevated or high.

D. Give morphine, 2–8 mg intravenously.

E. Apply nitroglycerin ointment, 1.25–2.5 cm (½–1 in), under an occlusive dressing.

F. Give inhalation sympathomimetics (eg, metaproterenol, terbutaline, albuterol) every 30–60 minutes for bronchospasm.

Disposition

Treatment in the emergency department should be restricted (if possible) to giving oxygen and obtaining arterial blood gas measurements. Most patients are able to tolerate immediate transfer to the coronary care unit, where heart failure can be treated much more satisfactorily with monitoring of arterial and pulmonary wedge pressures and drugs to reduce cardiac preload and afterload.

3. ACUTE MITRAL REGURGITATION & VENTRICULAR SEPTAL RUPTURE

Mechanical failure of infarcted tissue (eg, rupture of the ventricular septum or of papillary muscle supporting the chordae tendineae) is a common cause of acute mitral regurgitation and ventricular septal rupture. Minimal-to-moderate mitral regurgitation is common after myocardial infarction as a result of papillary muscle and left ventricular wall dysfunction. Severe degrees of mitral regurgitation can result from marked ischemia with little or no infarction and can be completely reversed with revascularization.

Diagnosis

Abrupt, severe congestive heart failure with pansystolic regurgitation murmur suggests acute mitral regurgitation or ventricular septal rupture. Echocardiography with bubble study to detect a shunt, a Doppler study to detect mitral regurgitation or the abnormal velocity jet of a ventricular septal defect, or a radioisotope shunt study can strongly suggest the proper diagnosis. Although the diagnosis is frequently certain by those noninvasive techniques, the patient usually requires catheterization and coronary arteriography before surgical repair is considered.

Treatment

A. Immediate Measures: These measures must be instituted in an intensive care unit to be truly effective.

1. Treat heart failure with diuretics, morphine, and nitroglycerin ointment (usually of minimal effectiveness).

2. Afterload and preload reduction with nitroprusside and captopril is a useful temporizing measure, especially in acute mitral insufficiency.

3. Obtain urgent cardiologic and cardiac surgical consultation.

4. Intra-aortic balloon pumping is a useful temporizing measure while the patient is being prepared for surgery.

B. Follow-Up Measures: The only lifesaving treatment for most patients is emergency cardiac catheterization followed by surgery.

Disposition

Hospitalize all patients for treatment and surgery.

4. MYOCARDIAL RUPTURE

The chief cause of myocardial rupture is mechanical failure of an infarcted ventricular wall.

Diagnosis

Myocardial rupture is an uncommon cause of sudden death during acute myocardial infarction, since it is responsible for only about 5% of deaths. Myocardial rupture is suggested by abrupt onset of hypotension with increased venous pressure (ie, cardiac tamponade). Electromechanical dissociation often occurs. Pericardiocentesis yields frank blood.

Treatment & Disposition

A. Perform pericardiocentesis to confirm the diagnosis and to relieve tamponade (Chapter 46).

B. Obtain emergency cardiac surgical consultation for immediate cardiac surgery. This is successful in the few cases in which rupture has been minimal with slow intrapericardial hemorrhage.

5. SYSTEMIC OR PULMONARY EMBOLIZATION

Systemic or pulmonary embolization is commonly caused by intracardiac mural thrombosis or phlebothrombosis.

Diagnosis

The most common findings in pulmonary embolism are sudden unexplained dyspnea and tachycardia. Occasionally, pleuritic pain, signs of right heart strain, or abnormal chest x-ray may occur. Patients at greatest risk are those with thrombus visualized in the left or right ventricle by 2-dimensional echocardiography. The diagnosis may be confirmed by lung scan or arteriography (Chapter 27). Systemic embolization is suspected when symptoms and signs of arterial occlusion occur. The clinical picture depends on the artery occluded, eg, flank pain and hematuria with renal artery embolism; pallor, pain, and loss of pulse with brachial or femoral artery embolism; stroke with cerebral artery embolism.

Treatment & Disposition

A. Give oxygen, draw blood for determination of prothrombin and partial thromboplastin times, and then begin systemic anticoagulation with heparin, 5000–10,000 units by bolus intravenous injection, followed by 1000–3000 units/h by continuous intravenous infusion. Pericarditis is a relative contraindication to anticoagulation because of the risk of bleeding into the pericardial sac, with resulting cardiac tamponade. Heparin is also contraindicated in patients with recent stroke, active duodenal ulcer, or active bleeding that cannot be controlled by direct pressure. Even though it does not cross the placenta, heparin must be used with caution in pregnant patients, especially during the third trimester. (Acute myocardial infarction during pregnancy is quite rare.)

With a massive pulmonary embolism with right heart failure and/or shock, intravenous fibrinolysis with streptokinase, urokinase, or tPA has been recommended in similar doses to those given for acute myocardial infarction. Occasionally, mechanical disruption of the embolic thrombus by a catheter has been lifesaving.

B. Seek appropriate surgical consultation (with a thoracic, general, or vascular surgeon) for patients with persistent hypotension, contraindications to thrombolytic therapy, or systemic embolization who may benefit from surgical intervention (eg, angioplasty and embolectomy for a pulseless and ischemic extremity).

C. All patients should be hospitalized in the coronary care unit.

6. PERICARDITIS

When transmural myocardial infarction causes pericardial inflammation over the area of necrosis, pericarditis may occur within the first week. Pericarditis occurring more than 1 week after myocardial infarction may be the result of Dressler's syndrome, an autoimmune reaction.

Diagnosis
Pericarditis usually does not appear until 2–3 days after the onset of myocardial infarction. The appearance of a friction rub is often the only manifestation; pain and electrocardiographic changes are often absent. Frequently, a small pericardial effusion may be detected by echocardiography. If a pericardial friction rub is heard in the first 24 hours after onset, suspect pericarditis as a primary diagnosis rather than as being due to acute myocardial infarction.

Treatment
Treat pain with a nonsteroidal anti-inflammatory agent such as indomethacin, 25–50 mg orally 3 times a day. If pain is severe, give morphine, 2–4 mg intravenously every 5–10 minutes, and repeat as necessary.

Disposition
Hospitalize the patient in a coronary care unit for control of pain and monitoring for possible cardiac tamponade (rare).

ANGINA PECTORIS

Myocardial ischemia (with attendant angina pectoris) results from an imbalance between myocardial oxygen supply and demand. Clinical findings vary depending on the severity of ischemia and on the frequency, duration, and rapidity of onset of ischemic episodes. If the demand for myocardial blood flow exceeds the capacity of the obstructed coronary arterial tree to supply it, the discomfort (angina pectoris) lasts until the excessive demand for coronary flow is reduced.

Discomfort is more intense and lasts longer when there is a marked decrease in coronary blood flow, as occurs with sudden marked increase in coronary artery obstruction resulting from abrupt development of thrombus over an atherosclerotic plaque, embolization to a coronary artery, or sudden occlusion by coronary artery spasm. If myocardial necrosis then occurs, the condition is termed myocardial infarction; otherwise, the episode is one of acute coronary insufficiency, or "preinfarction" angina.

If obstruction is so severe that coronary blood flow is barely adequate to meet resting demands, even small increases in myocardial oxygen demand may cause angina. In addition, small aggregations of platelets on a ruptured plaque, spasm, or increased vasomotor tone can cause minor changes in the caliber of the severely obstructed coronary artery and precipitate angina.

Myocardial ischemia can exist in the absence of any chest discomfort. In patients with severe ischemia, 24-hour electrocardiographic monitoring shows that 80% of the episodes of ST segment depression lasting for a minute or more are present without angina (so-called silent ischemia). Painless myocardial infarction is not unusual in elderly or diabetic patients.

Diagnosis
A. Stable Angina (Angina of Effort): By definition, the pattern of discomfort, its frequency of occurrence, and precipitating factors have remained the same for 1 month or longer.

Discomfort is usually substernal but may originate in other areas, eg, elbow, forearm, shoulder, neck, interscapular region, or jaw, although substernal discomfort eventually occurs. It is usually precipitated by activities that increase myocardial oxygen consumption (eg, exercise, eating, or emotional upset); lasts longer than 1 minute and usually less than 15 minutes; and is usually relieved by rest or nitroglycerin. Pain that meets these criteria usually indicates the presence of fixed coronary obstruction. The most important feature suggesting the diagnosis of angina pectoris is discomfort precipitated by exercise or emotion.

B. Unstable Angina: Anginal pain that begins in a patient previously free of pain (ie, pain of less than 1 month's duration) is called new-onset angina. Unstable angina is that which has changed in pattern, becoming more frequent (crescendo angina) and longer lasting. It is precipitated by a lesser degree of activity and may respond less to rest and nitroglycerin than does stable angina. Angina that occurs at rest without any obvious precipitating factor (rest angina) is the most serious form of unstable angina.

Sudden changes in angina not associated with increased myocardial oxygen demand (eg, increased blood pressure or heart rate) are presumed to be caused by a change in the anatomy of the coronary artery, eg, new vessel obstruction caused by progression of heart disease, development of thrombus, or other factors such as platelet aggregation or coronary spasm.

C. Acute Coronary Insufficiency (Preinfarction Angina): Typical anginal pain that lasts for more than 15–20 minutes suggests a provisional diagnosis of possible myocardial infarction. The patient should be hospitalized for observation. If the ECG subsequently fails to show changes consistent with myocardial infarction and if serum levels of myocardial enzymes fail to rise (as they usually do in myocardial necrosis), the patient is said to have acute coronary insufficiency (preinfarction angina).

D. Atypical Angina, or Prinzmetal's (Variant), Angina: Prinzmetal's angina occurs as a result of sudden, reversible, severe coronary artery obstruction (coronary artery spasm). It may occur in patients with fixed atherosclerotic coronary lesions and less often in those with minimal or no fixed coronary obstruction. Chest discomfort usually occurs without a precipitating cause. It frequently occurs at rest or awakens the patient at night. The discomfort frequently lasts longer than the usual episode of angina and is often accompanied by ST segment elevation (current of injury) that is transient and reversed in minutes after administration of nitroglycerin. With lesser degrees of spasm, ST segment depression may occur. Ventricular ectopy and ventricular tachyarrhythmias may also occur.

Differential Diagnosis
See Chapter 6.

Treatment & Disposition
A. Stable Angina: Nitroglycerin, 0.3 mg sublingually, is the drug of choice when pain first starts. It may also be taken prophylactically several minutes before activities that regularly precipitate angina. Pain is usually relieved in 1–2 minutes. The dose may be increased to 0.4–0.6 mg if the smaller dose is ineffective. Nitroglycerin tablets deteriorate in about 6 months; headache and sublingual tingling are common side effects of active tablets. Other drugs, eg, isosorbide, beta-blocking drugs, and calcium channel–blocking drugs, are useful but are not usually started at the first visit unless angina occurs frequently or on mild exertion.

Patients with stable angina that has exhibited a set pattern of frequency and precipitating factors over 1 or more months do not require hospitalization and should be referred for evaluation on an outpatient basis.

B. Unstable Angina, Preinfarction Angina, Rest Angina, Prinzmetal's Angina:

1. Give oxygen, 5–10 L/min, by mask or nasal prongs.

2. Hospitalize the patient immediately in the coronary care unit, and obtain daily ECGs and myocardial enzyme determinations (LDH and CK isoenzymes) to detect possible myocardial infarction.

3. Give morphine, 2–3 mg intravenously every 5–10 minutes, to relieve prolonged pain. Monitor blood pressure.

4. Give isosorbide dinitrate, 5 mg sublingually every 2–3 hours, for continued pain. Observe the pulse rate and blood pressure response. If the pulse rate increases by no more than 10 beats/min and there is no drop in blood pressure, a higher dose can be tried, or the drug may be given more frequently. Nitroglycerin paste, 1.25 cm ($\frac{1}{2}$ in), applied to the skin under an occlusive dressing every 4 hours, or transdermal nitroglycerin patches may be substituted.

If angina persists, intravenous nitroglycerin can be started at 10 μg/min and increased by 5 μg/min every 3–6 minutes until control of angina or a 10% drop in systolic blood pressure occurs.

5. Add a beta-adrenergic blocking agent (eg, propranolol, 10 mg orally) if pain recurs. The dose can be increased to 20 mg every 6 hours if no adverse response (eg, excessive bradycardia, mental obtundation, or drop in blood pressure) occurs after 1 hour. If necessary, the dose of propranolol can be increased to 240–480 mg/d in divided doses every 4–6 hours.

6. Start aspirin, 0.3 g/d. Aspirin has been shown to reduce the incidence of myocardial infarction and death by about 50%.

7. Heparinization may also be helpful in these patients; give 5000 units intravenously followed by 800–1000 units/h, maintaining activated partial thromboplastin time at twice normal.

8. Propranolol is contraindicated if the history and ECG suggest variant (Prinzmetal's) angina. Intravenous nitroglycerin or calcium channel–blocking drugs (nifedipine, diltiazem, verapamil) are the drugs of choice.

9. If pain continues despite treatment with adequate amounts of nitrates, propranolol, and calcium channel–blocking drugs, consider coronary arteriography in preparation for emergency coronary artery bypass surgery. If acute myocardial infarction has occurred and pain continues despite optimal medical management, arteriography and surgery must again be considered. Percutaneous aortic balloon pumping may also be useful.

HEART FAILURE

Heart failure is the expected outcome of many cardiac diseases. The basic abnormality is inability of the heart to maintain cardiac output sufficient to meet systemic demands. Compensatory mechanisms include (1) dilatation of the ventricle to maintain normal stroke volume (Frank-Starling mechanism); (2) retention of sodium and water by the kidneys to maintain intravascular volume; (3) increased activity of the sympathetic nervous system, leading to tachycardia and increased systemic vascular resistance; and (4) increased serum renin and angiotensin, which stimulate aldosterone output and cause retention of sodium and water as well as increased systemic vascular resistance. Cardiac output is usually maintained at normal levels or below, but at the expense of increased ventricular volume and filling pressure. The increased ventricular filling or diastolic pressures result in increased pulmonary or systemic venous pressures, with consequent pulmonary or peripheral edema. Tissue and organ dysfunction may result from increased venous pressure, decreased cardiac output, and edema.

Recently, it has been recognized that heart failure may occur primarily because of diastolic dysfunction where the ventricle appears to be noncompliant; therefore, even with normal diastolic volumes the high filling pressure results in pulmonary congestion. This type of heart failure is seen in hypertension, especially in elderly patients, in hypertrophic cardiomyopathy, and in myocardial ischemia. In many patients, both systolic and diastolic dysfunction are present. An echocardiographic-Doppler study should be performed in all patients with congestive heart failure to help determine the cause of the failure and the degree of systolic and diastolic dysfunction. The echocardiographic-Doppler study need not be done in the emergency department or at the first visit.

Although the distinction between mild to moderate heart failure and severe heart failure is not absolute, it has practical therapeutic implications.

SEVERE HEART FAILURE, INCLUDING PULMONARY EDEMA

Diagnosis

Frank pulmonary edema may occur with severe left heart failure. Patients experience dyspnea at rest (Chapter 5) and in severe cases may be cyanotic and cough up frothy sputum. Peripheral edema may or may not be present; edema may be severe (anasarca) in severe right heart failure. Pulmonary edema may be accompanied by wheezing or pleural effusion and is confirmed by chest x-ray. Cardiomegaly and a loud S_3 sound are usually present. Loud rhonchi and rales may interfere with more detailed evaluation.

Arterial blood gas measurements show hypoxemia; pH and PCO_2 vary, but hypocapnia and metabolic acidosis are common. With exhaustion, hypercapnia may occur, in which case intubation and mechanical ventilation are required. Obtain an ECG to detect the presence of ischemia even though there are no findings specific for heart failure. The differential diagnosis is discussed in Chapters 5 and 6.

Of paramount importance is the establishment of the cause of the heart failure. Specific causes have specific therapies, eg, valve replacement for pulmonary edema from severe aortic stenosis, or lowering of blood pressure for hypertension.

Note: Acute myocardial infarction or ischemia must be considered in all patients with sudden onset of congestive heart failure.

Treatment

A. Begin oxygen, 1–2 L/min, by mask or nasal prongs while awaiting the results of blood gas measurements.

B. Place the patient in a sitting or semi-Fowler position.

C. Insert a peripheral intravenous catheter, and give 5% dextrose in water by microdrip infusion to keep the catheter patent.

D. Give morphine, 2–4 mg intravenously. Repeat every 20–30 minutes as needed for dyspnea, but stop if somnolence or hypercapnia supervenes.

E. Give furosemide, 40 mg as an intravenous bolus. If the patient fails to respond in 10 minutes, repeat the dose once.

F. If severe bronchospasm is present, give inhalation sympathomimetics (eg, metaproterenol, terbutaline, albuterol) in saline, nebulized by compressed air, every 30–60 minutes. If bronchospasm persists, give a loading dose of aminophylline, 6 mg/kg intravenously over 30 minutes, and follow with an infusion of 0.3–0.5 mg/kg/h. Use lower doses for older patients and those with liver and renal disease (see Table 27–5).

G. Rotating tourniquets are effective but are not needed now that potent diuretics are available.

H. In severe cases, start afterload and preload reduction with nitroprusside and hydralazine or captopril, but only in an intensive care unit. If the cardiac index remains low, give dobutamine, 2.5–20 µg/kg/min by infusion pump. If blood pressure is low (< 100 mm Hg systolic), dopamine, 2–20 µg/kg/min by infusion pump, is preferred.

I. Digitalis is rarely indicated acutely except in the treatment of a specific arrhythmia.

Disposition

Hospitalize all patients except those with frequent recurrent episodes of pulmonary edema caused by known stable cardiac disease. In these latter patients, a brief stay for treatment in the emergency department may be sufficient. Search for the reason behind the recurrent pulmonary edema, eg, noncompliance with regard to prescribed diet and medications, paroxysmal arrhythmias, institution of a medication with a negative inotropic effect (eg, disopyramide), pulmonary emboli, or complicating diseases.

MILD TO MODERATE HEART FAILURE

Diagnosis

A. Symptoms and Signs: Nocturnal cough or dyspnea, orthopnea, dyspnea on exertion, and ankle swelling are common. The patient is not in distress at rest. Cardiomegaly is almost always found and is usually associated with some symptom or sign of underlying cardiac disease (eg, angina or findings characteristic of aortic stenosis). Other important signs include increased venous pressure, hepatojugular reflux, pulmonary rales or pleural effusions, sacral or peripheral edema, and S_3 gallop.

Since hypertension is one of the commonest causes of heart failure, record the blood pressure reading in both arms with the patient supine and sitting.

B. X-Ray Findings: Chest x-ray may demonstrate cardiomegaly and pulmonary congestion.

C. Electrocardiographic and Laboratory Findings: Although there are no specific electrocardiographic or biochemical manifestations of heart failure, it is nonetheless helpful to obtain an ECG, serum electrolyte determinations, renal function tests, and blood urea nitrogen and serum creatinine measurements. When renal blood flow is decreased, a rise in blood urea nitrogen out of proportion to the rise in serum creatinine is common (prerenal azotemia).

Treatment

A. Provide the patient with instructions for a low-sodium (1–2 g/d) diet.

B. Prescribe a diuretic. A thiazide diuretic (eg, hydrochlorothiazide, 25 mg orally twice daily with potassium supplementation) should be sufficient initial therapy for most patients.

C. Do not start digitalis therapy in the emergency department unless symptoms other than uncomplicated mild heart failure require it (eg, atrial fibrillation with rapid ventricular response). Digitalis is contraindicated in atrial fibrillation with ventricular response above 220 beats/min or with wide QRS complexes, since preexcitation may be present. In these cases, intravenous procainamide or DC cardioversion is used.

D. Control hypertension if present (see below).

Disposition

By definition, hospitalization is not required for patients with mild to moderate heart failure per se, although it may be prudent to hospitalize some patients (eg, unreliable patients, those with other underlying illnesses). All patients should be referred for long-term care and should be seen again within 1 week or less after their visit to the emergency department. Most of these patients will be candidates for angiotensin-converting enzyme inhibitor therapy (eg, captopril or enalapril). These afterload-reducing drugs have been shown to prolong life in patients with moderate congestive heart failure.

HYPERTENSION & HYPERTENSIVE CRISIS

Diagnosis

For the purpose of *emergency* care, hypertensive disease may be divided into 4 categories.

A. Mild to Moderate Hypertension: Blood pressure of 200/120 mm Hg or less, with no acute symptoms or signs attributable to hypertension.

B. Severe Hypertension: Blood pressure greater than 200/120 mm Hg, without new symptoms or signs attributable to hypertension.

C. Accelerated (Malignant) Hypertension: Blood pressure greater than 200/120 mm Hg associated with significant end-organ damage (eg, papilledema, renal dysfunction).

D. Acute Hypertensive Crisis: Blood pressure frequently greater than 220/150 mm Hg, with severe manifestations of headache, visual disturbances, papilledema, retinal hemorrhages, encephalopathy, congestive heart failure, pulmonary edema, aortic dissection, or hemorrhagic stroke.

Treatment

A. Categories of Management:

1. Mild to moderate hypertension requires no immediate therapy in the emergency department. Confirm abnormal blood pressure by several readings taken over 30–60 minutes in both arms and with the patient in varying positions. Examine the heart, ocular fundi, and peripheral vessels, and draw blood for serum electrolyte measurements and renal function tests. The patient should be informed of the diagnosis. It is reasonable to start the patient on thiazide diuretics after blood has been drawn for electrolyte measurements.

Because arrhythmias are a possible complication of diuretic use, it has recently been suggested that beta-blockers be considered the first-line drugs in treatment of chronic hypertension. Other sympathetic blocking agents, such as prazosin and clonidine, are also used if the first-order drugs are not successful. Angiotensin-converting enzyme inhibitor (eg, captopril or enalapril), has been found to be the most effective drug in some patients with chronic hypertension. Enalapril is longer acting and needs to be given only once or twice daily.

2. Severe hypertension in itself is not an acute emergency, although the chances of ultimate sequelae—and therefore the increased urgency of the need for treatment—are greater than in moderate hypertension. If severe hypertension is discovered in an individual without previously known hypertension—and especially if blood pressures recorded in the past have been in the normal range—hospitalization should be seriously considered to allow rapid, complete evaluation and prompt control of hypertension.

3. Accelerated (malignant) hypertension requires hospitalization and initiation of antihypertensive therapy as soon as possible. Drug treatment protocols are discussed below.

4. Hypertensive crisis is an immediate threat to life, and effective treatment must be started immediately in the emergency department, followed by prompt hospitalization and continued antihypertensive therapy.

B. Drugs Used to Treat Severe Hypertension Acutely:

1. Drugs acting within minutes–

Caution: Avoid rapid, severe drops in blood pressure, since watershed cerebral infarction can occur. Blood pressure should be gradually lowered to the 160- to 180-mm Hg range acutely and only further lowered gradually over a period of days with oral therapy.

a. Nifedipine is a vasodilator that has been used successfully in a dose of 10–20 mg sublingually to lower blood pressure within minutes. It is the initial drug of choice in the treatment of severe hypertension.

b. Nitroprusside is a potent vasodilator. Give by continuous intravenous infusion at a rate of 2–20 μg/kg/min. This drug lowers blood pressure in seconds; stopping the infusion results in rapid return of blood pressure to the previous level. Hospitalization in an intensive care unit and intra-arterial pressure monitoring are usually required.

c. Diazoxide is a vasodilator that is seldom used now that nifedipine is available. If used, it can be given with a fair degree of safety without the need for monitoring in an intensive care unit. Previously recommended large doses (300 mg) given intravenously rapidly have caused severe hypotension. More controlled lowering of blood pressure can be achieved by giving boluses of 0.5–1 mg/kg over 10 seconds every 5–10 minutes until desired effect or a total of 10 mg/kg. Give 50 mg initially. Furosemide, 20–40 mg intravenously, should be given concurrently, since diazoxide causes sodium and fluid retention. Do not use diazoxide in patients with aortic dissection.

2. Drugs acting within hours–

a. Furosemide is a diuretic as well as a preload reduction agent. Give 20–40 mg by rapid intravenous injection. Placing the patient in the semi-Fowler position is helpful. This drug is frequently combined with one of the other drugs that acts within hours.

b. Hydralazine is a vasodilator. Give 5–10 mg intravenously every 15 minutes, or 5–20 mg intramuscularly every 2–4 hours. Because hydralazine increases aortic shear forces (dP/dT), it is contraindicated in patients with aortic dissection. Propranolol (1–5 mg intravenously) may have to be added to control tachycardia and decrease dP/dT.

c. Methyldopa is an adrenergic antagonist. Give 500 mg by slow intravenous infusion every 2–4 hours.

d. Clonidine is an alpha-adrenergic stimulant that acts predominantly on the central nervous system. Give 0.2 mg orally to start, and follow with 0.1 mg every hour until blood pressure is controlled or until a total dose of 0.7 mg has been given.

e. Angiotensin-converting enzyme inhibitor (captopril, enalapril) blocks conversion of angiotensin I to II and is an arteriolar and venous vasodilator. Initiate captopril at 6.25 mg 3 times daily and gradually increase up to 50–75 mg 3 times daily. Enalapril is a longer acting drug and need be given only twice a day starting at 5 mg.

f. Calcium channel blockers have varying degrees of negative inotropic effects. Give verapamil, 40 mg orally 3 times a day up to 80–160 mg 3 times a day, or with the long-acting preparation, 240 mg/d; diltiazem, 30–60 mg orally 4 times a day, or with the long-acting preparation, 60–120 mg twice daily; or oral nifedipine, 10–20 mg 3–4 times a day, or with the long-acting preparation, 30–60 mg/d.

Disposition

Patients with accelerated hypertension and hypertensive crisis require immediate hospitalization. Patients with severe hypertension should be hospitalized if there are complications (eg, heart failure). Patients with mild to moderate hypertension should be referred to a clinic or primary physician for follow-up evaluation and treatment within 1–2 weeks.

PERICARDITIS, PERICARDIAL EFFUSION, & CARDIAC TAMPONADE

PERICARDITIS & PERICARDIAL EFFUSION

Acute pericarditis may result from viral or bacterial infections (including tuberculosis), collagen vascular diseases (especially rheumatic fever and disseminated lupus erythematosus), uremia, penetrating and nonpenetrating trauma, or myocardial infarction, and it may develop after pericardiotomy or irradiation of the mediastinum. It also may be associated with neoplasm (especially lymphomas and Hodgkin's disease). Pericarditis may also develop from annular or myocardial abscesses due to infective endocarditis. Pericardial effusion, and even cardiac tamponade, may develop in patients with acquired immunodeficiency syndrome (AIDS). Occasionally, drugs such as hydralazine or procainamide can cause an immune-response pericarditis. Varying degrees of myocarditis usually accompany pericarditis and account for the electrocardiographic changes. It is important to make an accurate etiologic diagnosis of pericarditis, if possible, since the specific cause may dictate the type of treatment required.

Diagnosis

A. Symptoms and Signs: Fever and symptoms of the underlying disease may be present. Acute pericarditis usually causes persistent anterior chest pain that is frequently made worse by lying down and made better by sitting up and leaning forward. A pleuritic component is common. Radiation of pain to the neck, left shoulder, or arm occurs frequently.

1. Pericardial friction rub–The most common and most important diagnostic finding is pericardial friction rub with 2 or 3 components. The rub is frequently accentuated by having the patient breathe deeply or lean forward on hands and knees. A pericardial rub is absent in some cases, however.

2. Pleural friction rub–A pleural friction rub may be present as well.

3. Pericardial effusion–Pericardial effusion is rarely revealed on physical examination and is usually suspected on chest x-ray and confirmed by echocardiogram. With large effusions, heart sounds may be diminished, and pulmonary consolidation, rales at the base of the left lung, and dullness to percussion below the left scapula (Ewart's sign) may be present. Pericardial rub may lessen or disappear as pericardial effusion develops or may persist in the face of a large effusion. A rapidly accumulating effusion may cause cardiac tamponade (see below).

B. X-Ray and Other Examinations:

C. ECG–The ECG is usually abnormal in pericarditis, but the most common findings are nonspecific ST and T wave abnormalities. Initially, changes relatively specific for pericarditis are ST segment elevation in many leads (usually I, II, aVF, and V_2–V_6), with preservation of the normal concavity of the ST segment. Return of ST segments to the baseline on the ECG in a few days is followed by symmetric T wave inversion. Occasionally, the J junction elevation of ST segments seen as a normal variant may be confused with the electrocardiographic changes of pericarditis; however, in the normal variant, these changes do not evolve further. In pericarditis, moreover, the ST segment elevation is usually 25% or more of the T wave height in leads V_5 or V_6. Depression of the PR segment is highly indicative of pericarditis.

2. X-rays–No chest x-ray changes are specific for pericarditis. In some patients, hypoventilation resulting from pleuritic pain may be sufficiently severe to cause atelectasis. The chest x-ray is also an insensitive indicator of pericardial effusion, especially in the case of rapidly developing effusions that only minimally distend the pericardial sac. An enlarged cardiac silhouette with a "water-flask" contour may be seen in the case of large effusions that have developed gradually. At times, the presence of pericardial fluid may be suspected if a radiolucent line representing epicardial fat is seen on the lateral chest x-ray well inside the cardiac silhouette and separated from the sternum by pericardial fluid.

3. Echocardiography–Echocardiography is the most sensitive and specific noninvasive test for pericardial fluid and should be performed in all cases of suspected pericardial effusion or pericarditis.

Treatment

A. Begin electrocardiographic monitoring.

B. Monitor blood pressure every 5–15 minutes.

C. In patients with hemodynamic instability, insert a central venous pressure catheter (Chapter 46), and monitor central venous pressure to detect signs of possible cardiac tamponade (Table 28–2).

D. Draw blood for CBC, serum electrolyte measurements, and renal function tests.

Table 28–2. Classification of cardiac tamponade.

	Blood Pressure	Heart Rate	Pulsus Paradoxus[1]	Central Venous Pressures
Normal hemodynamics (ie, pericardial effusion without cardiac tamponade)	Normal	Normal to increased	Not present (≤ 10 mm Hg)	Normal
Compensated cardiac tamponade	Normal	Normal to increased	Present (> 10 mm Hg)	Increased
Decompensated cardiac tamponade	Decreased; shock may be present	Increased	Present (> 10 mm Hg)	Increased

[1]Normal is defined as ≤ 10 mm Hg.

E. Relieve pain with morphine, 2–4 mg intravenously every 5–10 minutes, until pain is relieved; repeat as needed.

F. Obtain an echocardiogram as soon as possible to look for signs of pericardial effusion.

G. Consider consultation with a cardiologist.

H. Consider pericardiocentesis (Chapter 46) to aid in etiologic diagnosis, especially if there are signs of infection (fever, etc) suggesting pyogenic pericarditis or possible malignant pericarditis. If indicated, pericardiocentesis should be performed in an intensive care unit, preferably with fluoroscopic guidance, or the operating room. Pericardiocentesis in the emergency department should only be done to relieve decompensated cardiac tamponade and not to assist in etiologic diagnosis.

Disposition

Hospitalize all patients with acute pericarditis (with or without effusion), preferably in an intensive care or monitored intermediate care unit. Young patients with pericarditis who have had symptoms of several days' duration, who are hemodynamically stable with normal laboratory tests, and who are reliable often can be discharged with close follow-up in 1–3 days.

CARDIAC TAMPONADE

Accumulation of fluid in the pericardial space faster than the pericardium can accommodate it by distention results in compression of the heart, or cardiac tamponade. Pathophysiologic changes similar to tamponade may also result from constrictive pericarditis, although they are much more slowly progressive than tamponade resulting from rapidly accumulating pericardial fluid. The principal result of cardiac tamponade is reduced diastolic filling of the ventricles, with resulting reduced cardiac output. Ultimately, shock and death supervene.

Diagnosis

A. Symptoms and Signs:

1. There may be coexisting or antecedent signs or symptoms of pericarditis or pericardial effusion or of the disease process causing effusion. However, some patients develop cardiac tamponade without coexisting findings.

2. Tachycardia and hypotension–If cardiac tamponade progresses so that central venous pressure rises higher than 18 mm Hg, right ventricular filling decreases, causing subsequent decreases first in right ventricular and then in left ventricular stroke volume. There is frequently a sharp drop in venous pressure during ventricular contraction, causing the marked *x* descent in jugular venous pulsations. Reflex tachycardia and increased systemic vascular resistance result to support systemic blood pressure. As cardiac

tamponade worsens, these compensations fail, resulting in a sharp drop in cardiac output and blood pressure (decompensated cardiac tamponade). Because death follows rapidly if decompensated tamponade is not relieved, even slight hypotension or tachycardia occurring in patients with suspected pericardial effusion must be carefully monitored.

3. Pulsus paradoxus–In the normal healthy individual, systolic blood pressure drops no more than 8–10 mm Hg on normal inspiration. This change is exaggerated in cardiac tamponade, and there may also be a decrease in palpable pulse volume on inspiration. Pulsus paradoxus is common in cardiac tamponade resulting from pericardial effusion but is less common in tamponade associated with constrictive pericarditis.

4. Kussmaul's sign–During inspiration in cardiac tamponade there may be an *increase* in estimated central venous pressure (eg, by observation of jugular venous pulsation) rather than the normal decrease.

B. X-Ray and Other Examinations:

1. Central venous pressure monitoring–Central venous pressure monitoring should be started as soon as possible in all patients with suspected cardiac tamponade. As intrapericardial pressure rises, central venous pressure also rises to maintain right ventricular filling (and cardiac output) at normal levels. With inspiration there may be an increase in central venous pressure, rather than the normal decrease.

2. Echocardiography–Echocardiography is the most sensitive and specific noninvasive test for the presence of pericardial fluid and should be performed as soon as possible in all patients with suspected cardiac tamponade. With cardiac tamponade, there is marked swinging of the heart and collapse of the right atrial and ventricular chamber on expiration.

3. X-rays–Findings on chest x-ray usually are not helpful in the diagnosis of cardiac tamponade. A sudden marked increase in apparent heart size should suggest the possibility of pericardial effusion.

4. ECG–In cardiac tamponade, the ECG may show electrical alternans either of the QRS complex alone or of the entire complex (P, QRS, and T waves). This finding is rare in pericardial effusion without tamponade.

C. Classification of Cardiac Tamponade: The severity of cardiac tamponade may be classified as set forth in Table 28–2.

Treatment

A. Decompensated Cardiac Tamponade: *Note: Decompensated cardiac tamponade is an immediate threat to life and requires urgent treatment.*

1. Give oxygen, 5–10 L/min, by mask or nasal prongs.

2. Insert a large-bore ($\geq$ 16-gauge) peripheral intravenous catheter, and infuse crystalloid solution to support blood pressure. In an adult, give 300–500 mL in 10–20 minutes, and then continue the infusion based on the blood pressure response.

3. Give isoproterenol, 2–4 μg/min intravenously; or dopamine, 2–20 μg/kg/min intravenously. Adjust dosage based on the blood pressure.

4. Perform *immediate* percutaneous pericardiocentesis (Chapter 46) *in patients with shock that persists despite the above treatment measures.* Do *not* wait for confirmatory central venous pressure measurements or echocardiography.

B. Compensated Cardiac Tamponade:

1. Give oxygen, as described above.

2. Monitor blood pressure every 5–15 minutes.

3. Start continuous electrocardiographic monitoring.

4. Insert a central venous pressure catheter, and monitor central venous pressure.

5. Insert a large-bore (≥ 16-gauge) peripheral intravenous catheter, and keep it patent with crystalloid solution.

6. Confirm the presence of pericardial fluid or (rarely) pericardial thickening by echocardiography within 1 hour.

7. *Caution:* Do not administer diuretics or preload reduction (eg, nitrates) to control venous plethora (hypotension will result). If administration of a general anesthetic is contemplated, perform pericardiocentesis to relieve tamponade first. Anesthesia will cause withdrawal of sympathetic support to the heart and venous bed and will result in severe hypotension.

Disposition

Hospitalize all patients with suspected or documented cardiac tamponade, preferably in an intensive care unit, and obtain urgent cardiologic and cardiothoracic surgical consultation.

MYOCARDITIS & CARDIOMYOPATHY

Many diseases affecting the myocardial muscle have heart failure as their ultimate outcome. Secondary cardiomyopathies may be classified as shown in Table 28–3.

In most patients, the cause is unknown. The commonest cause of acute myocardial injury and heart failure is coronary artery disease with ischemia or infarction, and this diagnostic possibility must be considered in every patient who has sudden onset of congestive heart failure.

Diagnosis

Symptoms and signs may mimic those of almost any form of heart disease. Chest pain is common.

Table 28–3. Classification of causes of secondary cardiomyopathy, with examples.

Infectious
  Viral disease (coxsackie B and arbovirus infections, poliomyelitis)
  Bacterial disease (diphtheria)
  Parasitic disease (Chagas' disease)
  Rickettsial disease (scrub typhus)
Immunologic
  Rheumatic fever
  Systemic lupus erythematosus
Toxic
  Alcohol
  Emetine
  Doxorubicin
Muscular
  Pseudohypertrophic muscular dystrophy
Metabolic
  Hyperthyroidism
  Hypothyroidism
  Beriberi
  Glycogen storage disease
Infiltrative
  Amyloidosis
  Hemochromatosis
Neoplastic
  Lymphoma
Physical
  Hyperthermia
Peripartum

Mild myocarditis or cardiomyopathy is frequently asymptomatic; severe cases are associated with heart failure, arrhythmias, and systemic embolization. Manifestations of the underlying disease (eg, Chagas' disease) may be prominent.

Electrocardiographic abnormalities are always present, although the changes are frequently nonspecific. A pattern characteristic of left ventricular hypertrophy may be present. Flat or inverted T waves are most common, often with low-voltage QRS complexes. Intraventricular conduction defects and bundle branch block, especially left bundle branch block, are also common.

In acute myocarditis, cardiac enzymes (CK, LDH, and AST [SGOT]) are elevated; this is not true in chronic myocarditis.

Treatment

Bed rest is widely recommended, and there is some evidence supporting its benefits. If the cause of the disease is known (eg, trichinosis, acute rheumatic fever), begin therapy recommended for the underlying disease. Complications of myocarditis include chest pain, arrhythmias, embolization, and heart failure; these should be treated appropriately.

Disposition

Hospitalization is indicated unless the condition is chronic and stable.

AORTIC ANEURYSMS & DISSECTIONS

See Chapter 32.

CONGENITAL HEART DISEASE

The differential diagnosis of congenital heart disease is beyond the scope of this book. The general principles of management are outlined below as a guide for emergency physicians.

Classification

Classification of congenital heart disease is based on the hemodynamic effects produced or on specific anatomic abnormalities. Obviously, individual lesions may combine attributes from 2 or more categories, eg, tricuspid atresia is both a right-to-left shunt (owing to interatrial communication) and an atretic lesion.

A. Left-to-Right Shunts: Interatrial septal defect, interventricular septal defect, patent ductus arteriosus.

B. Right-to-Left Shunts: Cyanotic heart disease, eg, transposition of the great vessels, tetralogy of Fallot, pulmonary atresia, tricuspid atresia.

C. Valvular Stenosis, Hypoplasia, and Atresia: Pulmonary valve and aortic valve stenosis, tricuspid atresia, pulmonary atresia, mitral and aortic atresia.

D. Abnormalities of Position: Dextrocardia, transposition of the great vessels, corrected transposition.

E. Abnormalities of Great Vessels: Coarctation of the aorta, patent ductus arteriosus, arterial rings.

Pathophysiology

Large left-to-right shunts cause increased blood flow through the lungs and volume overload of one or both ventricles. Right-to-left shunts cause systemic venous return to bypass the lungs and go directly into the arterial circulation. The resulting arterial desaturation (if severe) may cause cyanosis.

Valvular obstruction (aortic or pulmonary stenosis) and aortic obstruction (coarctation of the aorta) cause afterload abnormalities of the involved ventricles.

Vascular rings around the trachea and esophagus cause symptoms resulting from obstruction (eg, dyspnea, cough, dysphagia).

CYANOSIS

All infants (under 1 year of age) who have cyanotic heart disease are at risk for potential serious illness with sudden life-threatening complications. Lesions producing right-to-left shunts are frequently undetected until after the newborn period, because pulmonary blood flow is maintained by a patent ductus arteriosus. When the ductus arteriosus begins to close, cyanosis becomes manifest. If the ductus arteriosus is the major source of pulmonary blood flow—as may be the case in pulmonary atresia—the patient may become markedly cyanotic and die rapidly after the ductus arteriosus closes.

No matter how well these children do or how asymptomatic they appear, their entire ability to oxygenate blood may depend on the presence of a patent ductus arteriosus, which may close unpredictably at any time.

Diagnosis

Cyanosis is most apparent in highly vascularized areas with superficial capillaries, eg, lips, oral and conjunctival mucosa, and nail beds. With more severe hypoxemia and desaturation, other areas of skin may appear cyanotic. The diagnosis may be confirmed by arterial blood PO_2 measurements.

Treatment & Disposition

All infants with cyanosis (intermittent or constant) should be hospitalized for immediate evaluation by a pediatric cardiologist, since emergency catheterization and angiocardiography may be necessary. Frequently, definitive diagnosis can be made by 2-dimensional echocardiography, with and without Doppler ultrasound.

Older children with stable cyanotic heart disease do not require emergency hospitalization but should be referred for evaluation. If other signs of cardiac disease are present (heart failure, arrhythmias, etc), hospitalization or treatment is indicated as appropriate.

ANOXIC SPELLS

Diagnosis

Anoxic spells are common in patients with cyanotic heart disease and usually start after the infant is 3 months of age or older. They are rarely seen after age 4–5 years. The spells frequently start with the infant's becoming fussy and developing increasing cyanosis and tachypnea. The infant then suddenly goes limp. These spells often occur in the morning after a good night's rest or when the child becomes more active, usually during feeding or straining at stool, and they are associated with sudden marked increases in right-to-left shunting.

Treatment

Place the child in the knee-chest position, and quickly give morphine, 0.2 mg/kg intramuscularly or subcutaneously. Give 100% oxygen by face mask, and be prepared to perform immediate intubation. If pH is 7.1 or lower, give sodium bicarbonate, 1–2 meq/kg, intravenously to correct acidosis. If hypoglycemia is present or suspected, give 10% glucose solution intravenously at a rate of 5–10 mL/kg/h, and monitor blood glucose concentration.

In children with anoxic spells and tetralogy of Fallot, propranolol, 0.01 mg/kg slowly intravenously has been helpful. The dose may be repeated in 5 minutes.

Disposition

An unexplained episode of syncope, "limp spell," or convulsions in any child with known cyanotic heart disease should suggest anoxic spells. The child should be hospitalized immediately.

HEART FAILURE

Congestive heart failure in infancy is usually associated with large left-to-right shunts at the ventricular level (eg, ventricular septal defect) or arterial level (eg, patent ductus arteriosus). It may also be associated with obstructive lesions such as aortic stenosis, aortic or mitral atresia, and coarctation of the aorta. Rarely, the cause can be anomalous origin of the left coronary artery from the pulmonary artery. Congestive heart failure may occur in the infant with atrial tachycardia or atrial flutter with rapid ventricular response, with or without preexcitation syndromes. Underlying heart disease need not be present.

Diagnosis

Congestive heart failure in infants is manifested by dyspnea on exertion just as it is in adults. Because the most common strenuous activity in which an infant engages is feeding, an infant with congestive heart failure will have to stop and breathe at the end of each swallow. Difficulty in taking the entire bottle in the usual 15–20 minutes may therefore be the principal manifestation of heart failure. In addition, the baby may be sluggish and fussy and have a weak cry.

Physical findings in these infants are those of the underlying lesion as well as those associated with congestive heart failure, and they include the following:

A. Aortic Murmurs (eg, pulmonary stenosis and coarctation of the aorta): Systolic ejection murmurs are heard. They are frequently accompanied by ejection clicks. Patent ductus arteriosus or aortopulmonary windows are associated with continuous murmurs heard at the base of the heart. If stenosis is severe or if cardiac output is severely decreased, the murmur may not be loud.

B. Tachypnea and Tachycardia: Tachypnea and tachycardia are usually present.

C. Sweating: Because of the increased activity of the sympathetic nervous system in children with congestive heart failure, profuse sweating is frequent.

D. Biventricular Failure: Isolated left heart failure is unusual in infants. Biventricular failure with ventricular gallops, rales, hepatomegaly, and edema is more common.

E. Venous Distention: Because of the short neck in infants, venous distention frequently cannot be detected.

F. Hepatomegaly: Hepatomegaly may develop within a few hours after the onset of congestive heart failure and may resolve just as quickly with therapy.

Disposition

A. Immediate Hospitalization: Any infant or child with newly diagnosed congestive heart failure—especially if it is associated with a systolic ejection murmur—must be hospitalized for immediate evaluation. The murmur may be due to aortic stenosis, pulmonary stenosis, or coarctation of the aorta, each of which requires prompt diagnosis and treatment.

B. Outpatient Care: Children with mild congestive heart failure due to stable, previously diagnosed congenital heart disease may be managed on an outpatient basis. Diuretics and digitalis (in older infants and children) are frequently effective.

PULMONARY HYPERTENSION

The child with a large ventricular septal defect or patent ductus arteriosus can develop significant irreversible changes in the pulmonary vascular bed within 2 years and must therefore be evaluated as soon as the problem is discovered.

Linear growth and weight gain may be slow. After age 2 years, compensatory mechanisms that decrease the size of the left-to-right shunt are frequent, eg, increased pulmonary vascular resistance, decreased pulmonary blood flow because of decreasing size of the ventricular septal defect, or development of infundibular pulmonary stenosis because of hypertrophy of the crista supraventricularis.

Prompt referral to a pediatric cardiologist is indicated if previously undiagnosed ventricular septal defect or patent ductus arteriosus is detected.

COARCTATION OF THE AORTA

The diagnosis of coarctation of the aorta is made by finding femoral pulses that are decreased or absent when compared to brachial pulses. If femoral pulses are present but faint, blood pressure taken with a cuff of the appropriate size in the upper and lower extremities should show lower blood pressure in the legs than in the arm if coarctation of the aorta exists. Prompt referral to a cardiologist is indicated.

REFERENCES

General
Bone RC (editor): Medical emergencies. (Part 1.) Med Clin North Am 1986;70:727. [Entire issue.]

Fulton DR, Grodin EM: Pediatric cardiac emergencies. Emerg Med Clin North Am 1983;1:45.

Rackley CE (editor): Advances in critical care cardiology. (Symposium.) Cardiovasc Clin (March) 1986;16:3. [Entire issue.]

Ram CV (editor): Cardiovascular emergencies. (Symposium.) Cardiol Clin 1984;2:153.

Congenital Heart Disease
McNamara DG: Twenty-five years of progress in the medical treatment of pediatric and congenital heart disease. J Am Coll Cardiol 1983;1:264.

Acute Myocardial Infarction
AIMS Trial Study Group: Long-term effects of intravenous anistreplase in acute myocardial infarction: Final report of the AIMS study. Lancet 1990;335:427.

Becker RC, Alpert JS: Current management of acute myocardial infarction. Curr Probl Cardiol 1989;14:507.

Braunwald E, Hollingsworth C, Passamani E (editors): Surgery in the treatment of coronary artery disease. (Symposium.) Circulation 1985;72(Suppl 6):1. [Entire issue.]

Goldhaber SZ et al: Thrombolytic therapy of acute pulmonary embolism: Current status and future potential. J Am Coll Cardiol 1987;10:9613.

Gruppo Italiano per lo Studio della Streptochinasi nell'Infarto miocardio (GISSI): Effectiveness of intravenous thrombolytic treatment in acute myocardial infarction. Lancet 1986;1:397.

Gruppo Italiano per lo Studio della Streptochinasi nell'Infarto miocardio (GISSI-2): A factored randomised trial of alteplase versus streptokinase and heparin versus no heparin among 12,490 patients with acute myocardial infarction. Lancet 1990;336:65.

Jaffe AS: Complications of acute myocardial infarction. Cardiol Clin 1984;2:79.

Jugdutt BI, Warnica JW: Intravenous nitroglycerin therapy to limit myocardial infarct size, expansion, and complications. Circulation 1988;78:906.

Lamas GA et al: A simplified method to predict occurrence of complete heart block during acute myocardial infarction. Am J Cardiol 1986;57:1213.

Lee L et al: Multicenter registry of angioplasty therapy of cardiogenic shock: Initial and long-term survival. Circulation 1987;76(Suppl 1):1041.

Neuhaus K-L et al: Improved thrombolysis with a modified dose regimen of recombinant tissue-type plasminogen activator. J Am Coll Cardiol 1989;14:1566.

Rosenthal ME et al: Sudden cardiac death following acute myocardial infarction. Am Heart J 1985;109:865.

Second International Study of Infarct Survival Collaborative Group (ISIS-2): Randomised trial of intravenous streptokinase, oral aspirin, both, or neither among 17,187 cases of suspected acute myocardial infarction. Lancet 1988;2:349.

Slater DK et al: Outcome in suspected acute myocardial infarction with normal or minimally abnormal admission electrocardiographic findings. Am J Cardiol 1987;60:766.

TIMI Study Group: Comparison of invasive and conservative strategies after treatment with intravenous tissue plasminogen activator in acute myocardial infarction. N Engl J Med 1989;330:618.

Topol EJ et al: A randomized trial of immediate versus delayed elective angioplasty after intravenous tissue plasminogen activator in acute myocardial infarction. N Engl J Med 1987;317:581.

Vlietstra RE, Holmes DR Jr: PTCA in acute ischemic syndromes. Curr Probl Cardiol 1987;12:703.

Heart Failure
DiBianco R et al: A comparison of oral milrinone, digoxin, and their combination in the treatment of patients with chronic heart failure. N Engl J Med 1989;320:677.

Dougherty AH et al: Congestive heart failure with normal systolic function. Am J Cardiol 1984;54:779.

Katz AM: Changing strategies in the management of heart failure. J Am Coll Cardiol 1989;13:513.

Massie BM: New trends in the use of angiotensin converting enzyme inhibitors in chronic heart failure. Am J Med 1988;84(Suppl 4A):36.

Packer M: Vasodilator and inotropic drugs for the treatment of chronic heart failure: Distinguishing hype from hope. J Am Coll Cardiol 1988;12:1299.

Parmley WW: Pathophysiology and current therapy of congestive heart failure. J Am Coll Cardiol 1989;13:771.

Parmley WW, Ryden L: Congestive heart failure: Advances in treatment. (Symposium.) Am J Cardiol 1989;63:10.

Angina & Treatment
Conti CR, Hill JA, Mayfield WR: Unstable angina pectoris: Pathogenesis and management. Curr Probl Cardiol 1989;14:557.

Corwin S, Reiffel JA: Nitrate therapy for angina pectoris. Arch Intern Med 1985;145:538.

Flaherty JT: Parenteral nitroglycerin: Clinical usefulness and limitations. Cardiovasc Clin 1984;14:111.

Goldberg S (editor): Coronary artery spasm and thrombosis. (Symposium.) Cardiovasc Clin 1983;13:1. [Entire issue.]

Henry PD, Perez JE: Clinical pharmacology of calcium antagonists. Cardiovasc Clin 1984;14:93.

Munger TM, Oh JK: Unstable angina. Mayo Clin Proc 1990;65:384.

Shub C: Stable angina pectoris: Medical treatment. Mayo Clin Proc 1990;65:230.

Pericarditis & Tamponade

Hall IP: Purulent pericarditis. Postgrad Med J 1989;65: 444.

Shabetai R: Changing concepts of cardiac tamponade. Mod Concepts Cardiovasc Dis 1983;52:19.

Spodick DH: Pericarditis, pericardial effusion, cardiac tamponade, and constriction. Crit Care Clin 1989;6:455.

Starnbach GL: Pericarditis. Ann Emerg Med 1989;17: 214.

Hypertension

Calhoun DA, Oparil S: Treatment of hypertensive crisis. N Engl J Med 1990;323:1177.

Vidt DG (editor): The practical management of patients with severe hypertension and hypertensive emergencies. (Symposium.) Am Heart J 1986;111:205.

Aortic Dissection

Crawford ES: The diagnosis and management of aortic dissection. JAMA 1990;264:2537.

Miller DC: Acute dissection of the aorta: Continuing need for earlier diagnosis and treatment. Mod Concepts Cardiovasc Dis 1985;54:51.

Valvular Heart Disease

Cheitlin MD: The timing of surgery in mitral and aortic valve disease. Curr Probl Cardiol 1987;12:71.

Frankl WS, Brest AN (editors): Valvular heart disease: Comprehensive evaluation and management. (Symposium.) Cardiovasc Clin (Feb) 1986;16:1. [Entire issue.]

29 Cardiac Arrhythmias

Joseph A. Abbott, MD, & Melvin D. Cheitlin, MD

Assessment of cardiac arrhythmia can proceed at a leisurely pace if the patient is hemodynamically stable, ie, if there is no pulmonary edema, shock, or chest pain. Ideally, a full 12-lead ECG and rhythm strip should always be obtained. If the arrhythmia cannot be determined by a standard ECG (usually leads II, V_1, and V_2 are most useful), then esophageal leads, right atrial leads, or His bundle recordings may be necessary for definitive diagnosis and for determination of treatment. Examples of common arrhythmias are given in the appendix to this chapter. Algorithms for the management of tachyarrhythmias are presented on pp 487 and 489. In the emergency department, it is easier to make a precise diagnosis of bradyarrhythmias than of tachyarrhythmias. However, bradyarrhythmias are less common, the mechanisms of the disorder are less complex, and integration of the electrocardiographic diagnosis into a therapeutic decision is easier. The definitive treatment for a chronic, symptomatic bradyarrhythmia not precipitated by medication is always a pacemaker.

TACHYARRHYTHMIAS
(See algorithms, pp 487 and 489.)

Patients who present with shock, chest pain, or severe heart failure as a result of tachyarrhythmias can be treated immediately with synchronized cardioversion, starting at 50 J and increasing as needed. Various maneuvers (eg, carotid massage) to identify the arrhythmia should not be tried. All underlying conditions contributing to the genesis of the tachyarrhythmia should be identified and treated.

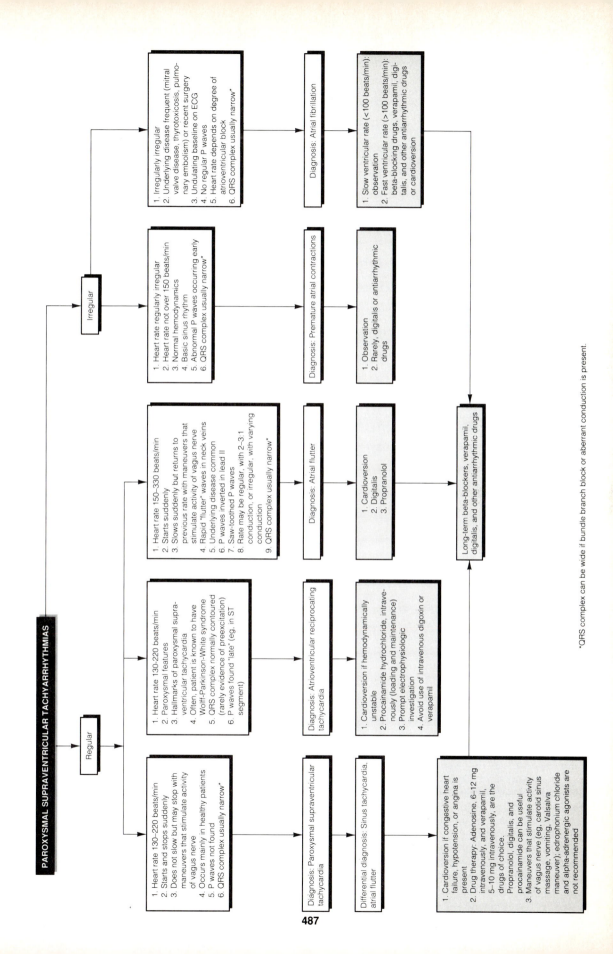

PAROXYSMAL SUPRAVENTRICULAR TACHYARRHYTHMIAS

Regular

Box 1
1. Heart rate 130-220 beats/min
2. Starts and stops suddenly
3. Does not slow but may stop with maneuvers that stimulate activity of vagus nerve
4. Occurs mainly in healthy patients
5. P waves not found
6. QRS complex usually narrow*

Diagnosis: Paroxysmal supraventricular tachycardia

Differential diagnosis: Sinus tachycardia, atrial flutter

1. Cardioversion if congestive heart failure, hypotension, or angina is present
2. Drug therapy: Adenosine, 6-12 mg intravenously, and verapamil, 5-10 mg intravenously, are the drugs of choice. Propranolol, digitalis, and procainamide can be useful
3. Maneuvers that stimulate activity of vagus nerve (eg, carotid sinus massage, vomiting, Valsalva maneuver); edrophonium chloride and alpha-adrenergic agonists are not recommended

Box 2
1. Heart rate 130-220 beats/min
2. Paroxysmal features
3. Hallmarks of paroxysmal supraventricular tachycardia
4. Often, patient is known to have Wolff-Parkinson-White syndrome
5. QRS complex normally contoured (rarely evidence of preexcitation)
6. P waves found "late" (eg, in ST segment)

Diagnosis: Atrioventricular reciprocating tachycardia

1. Cardioversion if hemodynamically unstable
2. Procainamide hydrochloride, intravenously (loading and maintenance)
3. Prompt electrophysiologic investigation
4. Avoid use of intravenous digoxin or verapamil

Box 3
1. Heart rate 150-330 beats/min
2. Starts suddenly
3. Slows suddenly but returns to previous rate with maneuvers that stimulate activity of vagus nerve
4. Rapid "flutter" waves in neck veins
5. Underlying disease common
6. P waves inverted in lead II
7. Saw-toothed P waves
8. Rate may be regular, with 2-3:1 conduction, or irregular, with varying conduction
9. QRS complex usually narrow*

Diagnosis: Atrial flutter

1. Cardioversion
2. Digitalis
3. Propranolol

Long-term beta-blockers, verapamil, digitalis, and other antiarrhythmic drugs

Irregular

Box 4
1. Heart rate regularly irregular
2. Heart rate not over 150 beats/min
3. Normal hemodynamics
4. Basic sinus rhythm
5. Abnormal P waves occurring early
6. QRS complex usually narrow*

Diagnosis: Premature atrial contractions

1. Observation
2. Rarely, digitalis or antiarrhythmic drugs

Box 5
1. Irregularly irregular
2. Underlying disease frequent (mitral valve disease, thyrotoxicosis, pulmonary embolism) or recent surgery
3. Undulating baseline on ECG
4. No regular P waves
5. Heart rate depends on degree of atrioventricular block
6. QRS complex usually narrow*

Diagnosis: Atrial fibrillation

1. Slow ventricular rate (<100 beats/min): observation
2. Fast ventricular rate (>100 beats/min): beta-blocking drugs, verapamil, digitalis, and other antiarrhythmic drugs or cardioversion

*QRS complex can be wide if bundle branch block or aberrant conduction is present.

487

SINUS TACHYCARDIA

Diagnosis
(See Appendix, Fig 29–2, p 503.)

Sinus tachycardia denotes a sinus rate over 100 beats/min. The rate is almost always under 160 beats/min, although healthy young adults may be able to develop sinus rates of 200 beats/min during strenuous exercise. Sinus tachycardia is a normal response to exercise and anxiety, and it also occurs in response to hypoxemia, anemia, hypovolemia, fever, myocardial infarction, congestive heart failure, hyperthyroidism, and pulmonary embolism and in association with the use of certain drugs.

Variations of the RR interval in the ECG are slight but characteristic of sinus tachycardia. Gradual slowing of the heart rate on carotid massage may help to differentiate sinus tachycardia from other supraventricular tachycardias.

Treatment & Disposition

Treat the underlying *cause* of sinus tachycardia. Treatment aimed at correcting the rapid rate itself may be harmful, especially if the sinus tachycardia is compensatory and supporting an adequate cardiac output. Disposition depends on the underlying condition.

PAROXYSMAL SUPRAVENTRICULAR TACHYCARDIA

Diagnosis
(See Appendix, Figs 29–5, 29–6, and 29–7, pp 504, 505, 506.)

Paroxysmal supraventricular tachycardia is characterized by abrupt onset of an atrial or atrioventricular junctional rate between 200 and 250 beats/min and is associated with 1:1 atrioventricular conduction. It is most commonly caused by atrioventricular node reentry. Symptomatically, it begins suddenly, is regular with little rate variation (< 1–2 beats/min) even over several hours, and terminates equally suddenly. Often, there is no underlying structural heart disease. Paroxysmal supraventricular tachycardia is a common presentation in Wolff-Parkinson-White syndrome (atrioventricular reciprocating tachycardia) and other variants of preexcitation syndromes. When ventricular aberration is absent and thus the QRS complex is narrow, the electrocardiographic diagnosis is straightforward. Often, location and timing of the P wave is not possible but, if accomplished, this marker greatly enhances the definition of the arrhythmia's mechanism and therefore ensures proper treatment.

Four mechanisms are responsible for paroxysmal supraventricular tachycardia. Three are types of reentry: (**1**) atrioventricular node reentry, the most common; (**2**) atrioventricular reciprocating tachycardia, which is usually due to a Kent accessory pathway; and (**3**) sinus node reentry. An ectopic atrial focus is another mechanism inciting paroxysmal supraventricular tachycardia. The differential diagnosis includes sinus tachycardia and atrial flutter. Sinus tachycardia is reviewed above. Classically, atrial flutter (see below) is associated with an atrial rate of about 300 beats/min and 2:1 atrioventricular block. The resultant ventricular rate is therefore about 150 beats/min. Note that ventricular tachycardia must always be excluded before making a diagnosis of supraventricular tachycardia with aberrant conduction. A common clinical error is to diagnose a broad QRS tachycardia as paroxysmal supraventricular tachycardia with aberration solely on the basis of hemodynamic stability.

Treatment
A. Hemodynamically Unstable Patients:

1. Synchronized DC cardioversion–In patients with shock, chest pain, or sudden-onset heart failure, or in patients with known Wolff-Parkinson-White syndrome (even if hemodynamically stable), immediate synchronized DC cardioversion is required. Administer sedation as necessary and as allowed by hemodynamic status. Begin DC shock at 50 J, increasing the dose by 50-J increments until sinus rhythm is achieved.

2. Other measures–Carotid sinus massage or adenosine, 6–12 mg rapid intravenous injection (adult dose), may be tried if cardioversion cannot be performed immediately. Verapamil, 5–10 mg intravenously, may also be used. *Note:* Verapamil is contraindicated in severe hypotension, in severe heart failure, or when paroxysmal supraventricular tachycardia is due to preexcitation, eg, in Wolff-Parkinson-White syndrome (see below). If pulmonary edema is mainly due to rapid ventricular response (as in mitral stenosis), then slowing of ventricular response with verapamil is useful.

B. Hemodynamically Stable Patients:

1. Vagal stimulation–Maneuvers that stimulate the vagus nerve, eg, carotid sinus massage, gagging, the Valsalva maneuver, or placing of the face in cold water, are at times effective. *Do not press against the patient's closed eyes to elicit a vagal response, since this has been reported to cause retinal detachment.*

Edrophonium chloride (Tensilon), a vagomimetic drug, 10 mg intravenously, may also be effective but may be associated with significant side effects such as hyperemesis and hypotension. With the availability of adenosine and verapamil, edrophonium is no longer recommended.

Raising the blood pressure with an **alpha-adrenergic agonist** stimulates the carotid baroreceptors and produces strong stimulation of the vagus nerve, which may convert the tachyarrhythmia to sinus rhythm. This maneuver can be dangerous, especially if the patient has atherosclerotic vascular disease, and it is no longer recommended.

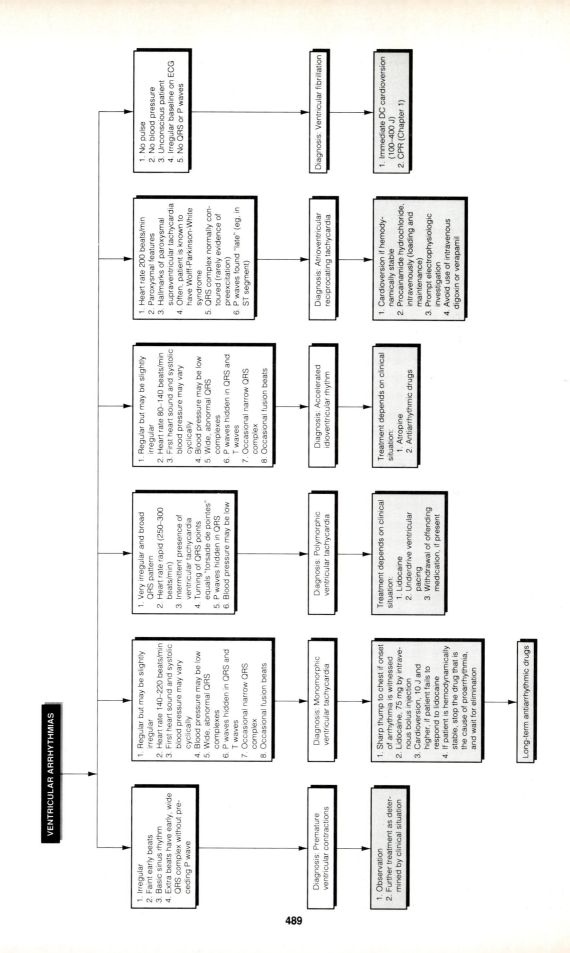

VENTRICULAR ARRHYTHMIAS

1. Irregular
2. Faint early beats
3. Basic sinus rhythm
4. Extra beats have early, wide QRS complex without preceding P wave

Diagnosis: Premature ventricular contractions

1. Observation
2. Further treatment as determined by clinical situation

---

1. Regular but may be slightly irregular
2. Heart rate 140–220 beats/min
3. First heart sound and systolic blood pressure may vary cyclically
4. Blood pressure may be low
5. Wide, abnormal QRS complexes
6. P waves hidden in QRS and T waves
7. Occasional narrow QRS complex
8. Occasional fusion beats

Diagnosis: Monomorphic ventricular tachycardia

1. Sharp thump to chest if onset of arrhythmia is witnessed
2. Lidocaine, 75 mg by intravenous bolus injection
3. Cardioversion, 10 J and higher, if patient fails to respond to lidocaine
4. If patient is hemodynamically stable, stop the drug that is the cause of proarrhythmia, and wait for elimination

Long-term antiarrhythmic drugs

---

1. Very irregular and broad QRS pattern
2. Heart rate rapid (250–300 beats/min)
3. Intermittent presence of ventricular tachycardia
4. Turning of QRS points equals "torsade de pointes"
5. P waves hidden in QRS
6. Blood pressure may be low

Diagnosis: Polymorphic ventricular tachycardia

Treatment depends on clinical situation:
1. Lidocaine
2. Underdrive ventricular pacing
3. Withdrawal of offending medication, if present

---

1. Regular but may be slightly irregular
2. Heart rate 80–140 beats/min
3. First heart sound and systolic blood pressure may vary cyclically
4. Blood pressure may be low
5. Wide, abnormal QRS complexes
6. P waves hidden in QRS and T waves
7. Occasional narrow QRS complex
8. Occasional fusion beats

Diagnosis: Accelerated idioventricular rhythm

Treatment depends on clinical situation:
1. Atropine
2. Antiarrhythmic drugs

---

1. Heart rate 200 beats/min
2. Paroxysmal features
3. Hallmarks of paroxysmal supraventricular tachycardia
4. Often, patient is known to have Wolff-Parkinson-White syndrome
5. QRS complex normally contoured (rarely evidence of preexcitation)
6. P waves found "late" (eg, in ST segment)

Diagnosis: Atrioventricular reciprocating tachycardia

1. Cardioversion if hemodynamically stable
2. Procainamide hydrochloride, intravenously (loading and maintenance)
3. Prompt electrophysiologic investigation
4. Avoid use of intravenous digoxin or verapamil

---

1. No pulse
2. No blood pressure
3. Unconscious patient
4. Irregular baseline on ECG
5. No QRS or P waves

Diagnosis: Ventricular fibrillation

1. Immediate DC cardioversion (100–400 J)
2. CPR (Chapter 1)

489

2. Adenosine—Adenosine (an endogenous nucleoside), 6–12 mg rapid bolus injection intravenously, is almost always effective in converting paroxysmal supraventricular tachycardia due to atrioventricular node reentry to sinus rhythm. The higher bolus dose may be repeated in 2 minutes if conversion has not occurred. *Note:* The success rate is similar to that of verapamil, but there is less chance of inducing or worsening hypotension. Thus, adenosine is a better pharmacologic selection than verapamil in a hemodynamically compromised patient. The onset of adenosine action is brisk, and the half-life of the medication (seconds) is the shortest of all antiarrhythmics. The drug is also effective in the treatment of paroxysmal supraventricular tachycardia due to atrioventricular reciprocating tachycardia, because it slows conduction in the atrioventricular node. It has no place in the treatment of other supraventricular rhythm disorders such as atrial flutter or fibrillation. The drug is antagonized by caffeine and theophylline and potentiated by dipyridamole. Coincident with the acute conversion of paroxysmal supraventricular tachycardia or transient sinus node depression or arrest, various degrees of heart block and even transient asystole may be induced. Flushing, hyperventilation, chest pain, or dyspnea are common but minor side effects. Care should be taken if the drug is administered to patients with pulmonary disease, because bronchospasm might be exacerbated or induced.

3. Verapamil—Verapamil (a calcium channel–blocking agent), 5–10 mg intravenously, is effective in converting paroxysmal supraventricular tachycardia to normal sinus rhythm. The dose may be repeated in 30 minutes but should not exceed 15 mg within 30 minutes. *Note:* Verapamil depresses myocardial function and should not be used if severe hypotension or left ventricular dysfunction is present or if paroxysmal supraventricular tachycardia is due to Wolff-Parkinson-White syndrome.

4. Other drugs—Propranolol, 2–5 mg intravenously; or digoxin, 0.5 mg intravenously, followed by 0.25 mg as often as every 2–4 hours; may also be effective. *Caution:* Do not give digoxin if a preexcitation phenomenon is suspected. Group I antiarrhythmics, such as procainamide hydrochloride and propafenone, intravenously, or flecainide, orally, are at times useful but should be considered second-line therapy for conversion of paroxysmal supraventricular tachycardia to sinus rhythm.

5. Synchronized DC cardioversion—DC cardioversion, 50 J, increased as needed, is the most effective therapy. Digitalis toxicity is a relative contraindication.

6. Overdrive pacing—Rapid atrial pacing requires the insertion, ideally under fluoroscopic guidance, of a contoured "J" transvenous pacemaker into the right atrial appendage. Catheter placement and the use of special very rapid overdrive (atrial rates up to 800 beats/min) or programmable pacing devices

with reversion algorithms to achieve overdrive or burst pacing should be supervised by a cardiologist familiar with this treatment and potential complications.

Disposition

Hospitalization is required if paroxysmal supraventricular tachycardia is complicated by shock or chest pain or if it is due to digitalis intoxication, a preexcitation syndrome, or a serious underlying disease that would in itself require hospitalization. Arrange follow-up care within a few days as for all other patients after conversion to normal sinus rhythm.

ATRIAL FLUTTER

Diagnosis
(See Appendix, Figs 29–8 and 29–9, pp 506 and 507.)

In atrial flutter, the atrial rate is usually 250–350 beats/min. This arrhythmia often develops in pulmonary disease or congestive heart failure. The ventricular rate is usually half the atrial rate (2:1 atrioventricular block); in the typical case, the atrial rate is 300 beats/min with a ventricular rate of 150 beats/min. Other degrees of atrioventricular block (3:1, 4:1, etc) may also occur. Regular and rapid atrial depolarization produces an undulating snakelike or saw-toothed baseline on the ECG. These flutter waves may not be apparent until the rate is slowed by carotid sinus massage. This maneuver increases the degree of atrioventricular block and slows the ventricular response, thus revealing the characteristic atrial complexes. Pure atrial flutter is rarely produced by digitalis intoxication.

Treatment

Cardioversion requiring as little as 25 J is the treatment of choice. (Atrial fibrillation usually requires more than 100 J.) Atrial flutter is inherently unstable and often reverts spontaneously without therapy to normal sinus rhythm or atrial fibrillation.

Although digitalis is been the classic drug of choice for atrial flutter, its use should be limited. Digitalization can convert atrial flutter to normal sinus rhythm but is mainly used to increase the degree of atrioventricular block and slow the ventricular rate. Invariably, so much digitalis is required to achieve the desired degree of atrioventricular block that digitalis toxicity develops. Initial use of DC countershock is therefore preferable. Intravenous administration of beta-blocking drugs or verapamil can also be used to achieve rapid increase in the degree of atrioventricular block in order to slow the ventricular response; these drugs may of themselves be successful in converting atrial flutter to a sinus rhythm. Very rapid atrial overdrive pacing has been used in special circumstances such as in postoperative patients. As noted above, this treatment requires familiarity with pacemaker lead placement and expertise with advanced pacing treatments.

Disposition

Hospitalization may be needed to correct the underlying disease state and to prevent recurrence.

ATRIAL FIBRILLATION

Diagnosis
(See Appendix, Fig 29–10, p 507.)

Atrial depolarization rates are faster than 350 beats/min, but atrial depolarization may be so rapid that distinct fibrillatory waves cannot be seen on the ECG. Atrial activity may intermittently appear to be regular (as in atrial flutter), or it may be very irregular. The ventricular response is always irregular. In some cases, atrial depolarizations may be of such low amplitude that they cannot be distinguished from atrial standstill. Atrial fibrillation is usually diagnosed on the basis of the typical irregular irregularity of the ventricular response, since atrial fibrillation is almost the only arrhythmia producing this pattern. Atrial fibrillation frequently occurs in acute myocardial infarction, pulmonary embolism, severe pulmonary disease, mitral valve disease, thyrotoxicosis, and potassium deficiency.

The differential diagnosis of atrial fibrillation includes multifocal atrial tachycardia (see Appendix, Fig 29–14, p 509) characterized by the following: 3 or more different types of P waves; varying PP, PR, and RR intervals; and a ventricular response usually faster than 120 beats/min. Multifocal atrial tachycardia is usually seen in elderly patients with chronic pulmonary disease, and it responds poorly to digitalis and other antiarrhythmic agents. Treatment of the underlying lung disease and normalization of blood gases (Chapter 27) are the most effective therapeutic measures. Verapamil, because it increases atrioventricular block and thus slows the ventricular response, is also an effective treatment option for this arrhythmia.

Atrial fibrillation may be associated with nonparoxysmal atrioventricular nodal reentrant tachycardia. The clue to the presence of nonparoxysmal atrioventricular nodal reentrant tachycardia is a regular ventricular rate and the presence of typical atrial fibrillatory waves. This arrhythmia, until otherwise ruled out, should be considered a complication of therapy for atrial fibrillation. The most common causes are digitalis intoxication, verapamil excess, or myocardial infarction. The mechanism of the arrhythmia is a combination of a complete atrioventricular block and a junctional rate that is faster than normal (> 60 beats/min).

Treatment

Although treatment depends mostly on the cause and hemodynamic effects of atrial fibrillation, emergency measures are relatively simple.

A. Severe Symptoms: If severe symptoms (angina, heart failure, or shock) are present, synchronized DC countershock (starting at 100 J) is the treatment of choice to restore sinus rhythm. Avoid cardioversion if digitalis toxicity is present. Systemic (including cerebral) emboli may complicate reversion to sinus rhythm, especially if atrial fibrillation has been present for over 24 hours.

B. Mild Symptoms: For mild symptoms, the goal of therapy is to slow the ventricular response. The preferred treatment approach is verapamil, 5–10 mg intravenously, or propranolol, 2–5 mg intravenously. Digitalis preparations have been used for years but in general are now less popular. However, if there is decreased left ventricular function, digoxin is still the drug of choice. Digoxin, 0.5 mg, is given intravenously, followed by 0.25 mg every 2–6 hours until the ventricular rate is ≤ 100 beats/min or until 1.25 mg of digoxin has been administered. *Caution:* Correct any hypokalemia before giving digitalislike preparations. If some RR intervals occur at a rate of 250 beats/min or faster, suspect preexcitation syndrome, and use intravenous procainamide or cardioversion.

Disposition

Hospitalization is required if the arrhythmia is new or if the patient has decreased cardiac output because of the rapid ventricular response.

PREEXCITATION ARRHYTHMIAS

Preexcitation arrhythmia may present as an episode of paroxysmal supraventricular tachycardia (atrioventricular reciprocating tachycardia, AVRT) or atrial fibrillation with an excessively rapid ventricular response.

Diagnosis
(See Appendix, Figs 29–6 and 29–7, pp 505 and 506.)

Wolff-Parkinson-White syndrome and its variants may be associated with both supraventricular and, less commonly, ventricular rhythm disturbances. In Wolff-Parkinson-White syndrome due to a Kent accessory pathway, the usual supraventricular arrhythmia is due to an orthodromic (impulse antegrade through atrioventricular node) atrioventricular reciprocating tachycardia, a subcategory of paroxysmal supraventricular tachycardia. The retrograde limb of the reentrant circuit is the accessory pathway. If aberrant ventricular conduction or fixed bundle branch block is absent, the contour of the QRS complex during the arrhythmia reveals no preexcitation (eg, absent delta wave) and the QRS complex is narrow. If the antegrade limb of the circuit is the accessory pathway and the retrograde limb is the atrioventricular node (antidromic tachycardia), a wide QRS complex is present and the tachycardia masquerades as ventricular tachycardia. With antidromic tachycardia, the ventricular response may be extremely rapid and can lead to ventricular fibrillation due to an R-on-T phenomenon. Drug therapy may precipitate this situation.

Treatment

A. DC Cardioversion: The safest treatment option for a patient with known Wolff-Parkinson-White syndrome, even when hemodynamically stable, is synchronized DC cardioversion starting at 50 J.

B. Procainamide: Intravenous procainamide hydrochloride should be initiated, 50–100 mg every 5 minutes to a total of 1000 mg, followed by a continuous infusion of 2–4 mg/min.

C. Other Antiarrhythmic Drugs: Beta-blockers (eg, propranolol or sotalol [investigational]) and group IC antiarrhythmics (eg, flecainide, 100 mg orally twice daily, increasing to a maximum dose of 150 mg twice daily) have, in general, proved both effective and well tolerated in patients with preexcitation syndrome without ventricular tachycardia or left ventricular dysfunction. Propafenone (group IC) 150 mg orally every 8 hours as a loading dose until the desired effect is reached, is an alternative approach. A maintenance propafenone dose of 300 mg twice a day is effective. Amiodarone is also effective but is associated with a significant incidence (up to 25%) of major toxic side effects related to the dose and the duration of therapy. Thus, amiodarone is not recommended for young patients who must be on long-term treatment.

Caution: Emergency treatment with intravenous digoxin has been associated with acceleration of ventricular rate or ventricular fibrillation and should be avoided. This is especially true in the patient with Wolff-Parkinson-White syndrome who has atrial fibrillation with a rapid ventricular response. Digoxin will increase block at the atrioventricular node and can then enhance conduction via the accessory pathway (antidromic tachycardia). Likewise, intravenous verapamil is contraindicated in the emergency treatment of the patient with known Wolff-Parkinson-White syndrome who has either atrioventricular reciprocating tachycardia or atrial fibrillation. Infusion of verapamil may cause vasodilatation and by lowering the systemic blood pressure result in a release of catecholamines. With catecholamines, the refractory periods of both the accessory pathway and the atrioventricular node are shortened, and a resultant acceleration of the ventricular rate may occur with an increased risk of ventricular fibrillation.

D. Invasive Electrophysiologic Study: This procedure is strongly recommended to lucidly and safely guide long-term treatment. Drug therapy not guided by electrophysiologic study may aggravate an otherwise "stable" arrhythmia. Invasive electrophysiologic study can also identify patients who should receive nonpharmacologic treatments (eg, pacemaker) and those who are candidates for surgical or transvenous catheter ablation of the accessory pathway.

Disposition

Hospitalization is indicated for patients with new-onset arrhythmia or those who are hemodynamically compromised. Patients with recurrent atrioventricular reciprocating tachycardia who respond promptly to treatment should have outpatient follow-up within a few days. Electrophysiologically guided treatment is strongly recommended for all patients, since even patients with "benign" paroxysmal supraventricular tachycardia are at risk for sudden death.

VENTRICULAR TACHYCARDIA

Ventricular tachycardia is a serious arrhythmia that often is not properly diagnosed even when obviously present. If hemodynamic compromise is severe (shock, severe heart failure, or coma), the diagnosis is rarely missed. However, when hemodynamic integrity is maintained, as when the ventricular tachycardia rate is relatively slow (< 200 beats/min) or atrial-to-ventricular synchrony is maintained, ventricular tachycardia is frequently misdiagnosed as paroxysmal supraventricular tachycardia with aberrant conduction. Proper diagnosis is essential, since ventricular tachycardia, no matter what the cause, is an arrhythmia that can rapidly degenerate into ventricular fibrillation and death.

Ventricular tachycardia occurs typically in patients with acute or chronic coronary artery disease. Because these patients already have poor left ventricular function and have lost the properly timed atrial contraction, hemodynamic deterioration is usual, even with relatively slow (< 200 beats/min) ventricular rates. Accelerated idioventricular rhythm ("slow" ventricular tachycardia) and polymorphic ventricular tachycardia (torsade de pointes) are 2 variations of this disorder (see below). Ventricular tachycardia induced by coronary artery spasm, catecholamine induction, or proarrhythmic effect of an antiarrhythmic drug must be considered in the differential diagnosis (see below).

Diagnosis
(See Appendix, Figs 29–29, 29–30, and 29–31, pp 515 and 516.)

Ventricular tachycardia often arises from a focus of irritability in the Purkinje fibers of the ventricle. The heart rate is usually 140–220 beats/min; rarely, it is as fast as 280 beats/min. Widened QRS complexes of a single contour (monomorphic) in association with atrioventricular dissociation, retrograde ventriculo-atrial Wenckebach block, fusion beats, and/or ventricular capture beats are the best electrocardiographic evidence of ventricular tachycardia, although the need for immediate therapy often favors acting on a presumptive rather than a precise diagnosis.

Documentation of the classic electrocardiographic criteria for ventricular tachycardia is sometimes important, especially if therapy for presumed ventricular tachycardia has proved ineffective. The criteria of Wellens and Kindwall are especially useful (Table 29–1). Ventricular tachycardia may be mimicked by supraventricular tachycardia associated with underlying bundle branch block, by aberrant conduction, or by Wolff-Parkinson-White syndrome or its variants. If lidocaine or other agents effective in the treatment of ventricular ectopic arrhythmias are used to treat supraventricular tachycardias with preexisting atrioventricular block, ventricular rates may actually *increase* as a result of accelerated atrioventricular conduction.

Treatment

Because of the risk of hemodynamic deterioration or degeneration into ventricular fibrillation, ventricular tachycardia is a serious emergency even in the asymptomatic patient with adequate cardiac output.

A. DC Cardioversion: The most rapidly effective treatment is synchronized DC cardioversion, which is contraindicated if digitalis intoxication is suspected. Ventricular arrhythmias will convert to sinus rhythm in about 80% of patients after a 50-J countershock; arrhythmias in the rest usually convert at higher energy levels (100–400 J).

B. Lidocaine: After DC cardioversion has been performed, give lidocaine, 1 mg/kg intravenous

bolus, followed by 2–4 mg/min continuous intravenous infusion, to prevent recurrence of the arrhythmia. In hemodynamically stable patients, lidocaine alone may be tried first. In patients with digitalis intoxication, intravenous lidocaine, phenytoin, or magnesium salts have also been reported useful.

C. Expectant Observation: An exception to the rule of vigorous antiarrhythmic therapy for ventricular tachycardia is the presence of a slow ventricular tachycardia (rate < 100 beats/min), also known as accelerated idioventricular rhythm (see Appendix, Fig 29–28, p 514). This arrhythmia is common in the early phases of myocardial infarction, causes little decrease in cardiac output, is self-limiting, and rarely degenerates into ventricular fibrillation. The authors recommend no treatment for this condition.

Disposition

Hospitalization is indicated for all patients with ventricular tachycardia, even if the arrhythmia reverts to sinus rhythm while the patient is in the emergency department. Patients with recurrent symptomatic ventricular tachycardia not associated with acute myocardial infarction should be hospitalized and considered for electrophysiologic study to reproduce the arrhythmia, to find the proper antiarrhythmic drug and dose that will prevent recurrence, and to determine whether a combination of automatic internal cardioverter defibrillator and antitachycardia pacemaker placement (p 499) or surgery is indicated.

PROARRHYTHMIC VENTRICULAR TACHYCARDIA

Diagnosis
(See Appendix, Fig 29–32, p 516.)

The possibility of a proarrhythmic response to or an arrhythmia exacerbation by an antiarrhythmic drug should be considered in the differential diagnosis of ventricular tachycardia. In the past, quinidine was a major culprit in drug-induced ventricular tachycardia; quinidine-induced ventricular tachycardia is often polymorphic (see below). With decreased use of quinidine, other type IC antiarrhythmic agents such as encainide, flecainide, and propafenone have assumed greater importance in this condition. Unlike quinidine-induced ventricular tachycardia, the type IC–induced ventricular arrhythmias are not heralded by prolongation of the QRS or QT interval. In encainide- and flecainide-induced ventricular tachycardias, the QRS has a monomorphic or even sine wave pattern and the ventricular rate is often relatively slow (< 150 beats/min). Patients with poor cardiac function may be at greatest risk. Flecainide-induced ventricular tachycardia may be precipitated by exercise. A similar condition has been described with amiodarone although polymorphous ventricular tachycardia may be more common with this medication (see below).

Table 29–1. ECG criteria for the diagnosis of ventricular tachycardia (VT).[1,2]

1. Atrioventricular dissociation indicates VT.
2. QRS width > 140 ms favors VT.
3. Left axis deviation > –30 degrees favors VT.
4. QRS configuration
   a. If RBBB shape:
      V_1: Monophasic or biphasic R wave pattern suggests VT.
      V_6: R to S ratio less than 1.0 suggests VT.
   b. If LBBB shape:
      V_1 or V_2: R wave in tachycardia < R wave in sinus suggests VT.
      V_1 or V_2: R wave > 30 ms suggests VT.
      V_1 or V_2: R wave onset to S nadir > 60 ms suggests VT.
      V_1 or V_2: notched S wave downstroke suggests VT.
      V_6: Q wave suggests VT.

[1]After Wellens and Kindwall (see References).
[2]The differential diagnoses of VT are a supraventricular tachycardia with preexisting bundle branch block, a rate-related ventricular aberration, or antegrade conduction over an accessory pathway. Note that these criteria may be violated if conduction-slowing antiarrhythmics (ie, type 1C and amiodarone) have been administered. VT = ventricular tachycardia, RBBB = right bundle branch block, LBBB = left bundle branch block, V_1 = precordial lead 1, V_2 = precordial lead 2, V_6 = precordial lead 6, ms = milliseconds.

Treatment

The goal of therapy is elimination of the offending agent rather than treatment of the rhythm disorder.

A. Urgent Treatment: Hemodynamic support with catecholamines may be required. DC cardioversion may be necessary if ventricular tachycardia is not hemodynamically tolerated, response to sympathomimetics is inadequate, or ventricular fibrillation develops. Life-threatening quinidine-induced ventricular arrhythmias require intravenous sodium bicarbonate administration to lower serum potassium levels in order to decrease intracellular potassium levels that had been elevated by quinidine blockade of potassium channels.

B. Expectant Observation: Vigorous intervention to a proarrhythmic ventricular tachycardia due to type IC agents or amiodarone has proved counterproductive. Additional drugs or cardioversion may seriously aggravate the ventricular tachycardia. Since ventricular rate associated with type IC proarrhythmic agents is often slow, the patient is usually hemodynamically stable. The therapy of choice in stable patients is hemodynamic support while awaiting clearance of the offending medication and eventual resolution of the arrhythmia.

Disposition

Hospitalization for rhythm and hemodynamic monitoring and possible urgent intervention is required during the drug clearance phase. Reevaluation of the patient's antiarrhythmic regimen is required before hospital discharge.

POLYMORPHIC VENTRICULAR TACHYCARDIA (Including Torsade de Pointes)

Diagnosis
(See Appendix, Fig 29–33, p 517.)

It is extremely important to accurately identify this type of ventricular tachycardia in order to correctly treat it and to prevent recurrence. Technically, any type of ventricular tachycardia not demonstrating monomorphism by ECG is classified as polymorphic ventricular tachycardia. There are many types and causes of polymorphic ventricular tachycardia. A spectrum of etiologies, involving both normal and abnormal cardiac structures, has been reported to cause this disorder. Drug induction is the most frequent cause. Torsade de pointes is but one type of polymorphic ventricular tachycardia. Electrocardiographic identification includes the ventricular tachycardia's intermittency (nonsustained ventricular tachycardia), a long QT interval when sinus rhythm is present, and a continuously varying ventricular tachycardia rate and morphology characterized by the ventricular tachycardia QRS "points," or spikes, changing polarity or "turning about" the ECG isoelectric baseline. A

premature ventricular complex occurring subsequent to a long compensatory pause frequently heralds this type of polymorphic ventricular tachycardia. This type of ventricular tachycardia is often present in the setting of an electrolyte disorder or sinus bradycardia. This arrhythmia is frequently due to a paradoxic response to conventional antiarrhythmic therapy and is also reported in patients taking amiodarone, sotalol (experimental), and phenothiazine or structurally similar psychotropic medications. Sudden fluctuation in electrolyte levels without frankly abnormal serum values may be responsible for the onset of the rhythm in patients who develop polymorphic ventricular tachycardia after years of remaining stable with conventional antiarrhythmic medications. *If it is drug-induced, do not treat the polymorphic ventricular tachycardia with the same or similar class of conventional antiarrhythmic drugs, which not only is ineffective but can also precipitate ventricular fibrillation and death.* Ischemic heart disease due to coronary artery spasm, acute myocardial infarction, and reperfusion arrhythmias may initiate nontorsade polymorphic ventricular tachycardia.

Treatment

Initial control of the arrhythmia is best accomplished by cessation of any offending agent or agents, infusion of lidocaine in therapeutic doses, and avoidance of other type I antiarrhythmics and bretylium. Phenytoin is ineffective. The treatment of choice is underdrive ventricular pacing using a temporary transvenous atrial or ventricular pacemaker set at modest pacing rates (90–110 beats/min). Overdrive pacing at rates above that of the polymorphic ventricular tachycardia is rarely necessary or desirable and can aggravate the condition. Cardiac pacing decreases the frequency and duration of polymorphic ventricular tachycardia. The patient can be gradually and completely weaned from pacer therapy by a decrease in the pacing rate over the next few days. Permanent cardiac pacing generally is not needed, but this depends on the cause of the condition. Treatment of acute quinidine-induced polymorphic ventricular tachycardia includes manipulation of the serum potassium level (see above). The treatment of reperfusion-induced polymorphic ventricular tachycardia may also require electrolyte manipulations. A comprehensive treatment plan may include nitrates, beta-blockers, or calcium channel blockers given independently or in combination, and placement of a permanent atrial or dual-chamber pacemaker and/or automatic internal cardioverter defibrillator. The treatment required depends on the cause, presentation, and clinical course of the polymorphic ventricular tachycardia in individual patients.

Disposition

Patients should be hospitalized in an intensive care setting for temporary underdrive pacing, correction of metabolic abnormalities, and evaluation of the underlying cause. This usually entails changes in medication and initiation of other types of antiarrhythmics. If the clinical course is benign, conventional medications may be successful in preventing recurrence (eg, beta-blockade for the exercise-induced variety). Aborted sudden death requires more aggressive management to prevent recurrence.

VENTRICULAR FIBRILLATION
(See also Chapter 1.)

Diagnosis
(See Appendix, Fig 29–34, p 517.)

Ventricular fibrillation causes absence of cardiac output and death within minutes. Urgent on-site diagnosis and treatment are mandatory. Initiation of cardiopulmonary resuscitation by bystanders and in-the-field defibrillation by emergency services personnel are associated with improved survival rates.

Treatment & Disposition

The treatment of choice is immediate DC countershock with 200 J initially, followed by a 400-J shock if the patient shows no response (Chapter 1). All patients who have been successfully resuscitated should be hospitalized in an intensive care unit. These patients should be considered for an electrophysiologic study before being discharged from the hospital.

BRADYARRHYTHMIAS

Marked slowing of the ventricular rate may be due to sinus node bradycardia or to sinus, atrioventricular, or intraventricular conduction defects. Slowing of the ventricular rate may be so profound as to cause cerebral dysfunction (Stokes-Adams attack) or cardiovascular collapse requiring CPR. The slow ventricular rate can reduce cardiac output and cause congestive heart failure and angina. Slow heart rates are remarkably well tolerated in many patients, however.

ATRIOVENTRICULAR BLOCK

Atrioventricular block is classified into 3 types based on electrocardiographic findings: first-degree atrioventricular block, in which the PR interval is abnormally long but no ventricular beats are "dropped"; second-degree atrioventricular block, in which some atrial beats are not conducted to the ventricle, ie, occasional beats are "dropped"; and third-degree atrio-

ventricular block (complete heart block), in which no atrial beats are conducted to the ventricle.

First-Degree Atrioventricular Block
(See Appendix, Fig 29–17, p 510.)

First-degree atrioventricular block is defined as prolongation of the PR interval beyond 0.22 second at normal heart rates. First-degree atrioventricular block is a common normal variant due to hypervagotonia that is often seen in athletes or young people in good physical condition. Digitalis and group I antiarrhythmic agents may produce first-degree atrioventricular block owing to excessive vagal stimulation, but first-degree atrioventricular block alone does not indicate drug intoxication.

No treatment is necessary.

Second-Degree Atrioventricular Block (Mobitz Type I)
(See Appendix, Figs 29–18 and 29–19, p 510.)

Second-degree atrioventricular block is more severe and more likely to be associated with disease, but it is also seen occasionally in normal people and in athletes with greater than normal vagal tone. In patients with acute myocardial infarction, second-degree atrioventricular block may precede the development of complete heart block.

A common type of second-degree heart block is known as Wenckebach heart block, or Mobitz type I second-degree atrioventricular block. In the Wenckebach type of heart block, the PR interval progressively increases with each heartbeat until the P wave does not conduct to the ventricle, and a dropped ventricular beat results. Classically, the atrial rate (ie, PP interval) remains constant, the PR interval lengthens, and the ventricular rate accelerates (RR interval shortens) until the dropped ventricular beat occurs, after which the PR interval shortens or resets and the entire cycle repeats itself. In the presence of 2:1 atrioventricular block (every other P wave is not conducted), the Mobitz I and Mobitz II mechanisms cannot be differentiated with a standard ECG.

Treatment is required only if the patient has symptoms from bradycardia or has unstable hemodynamics. The Wenckebach type of second-degree atrioventricular block usually does not progress to complete heart block, and in acute myocardial infarction (usually inferior infarction), it often responds to atropine. Furthermore, if complete atrioventricular block does occur, the escape pacemaker is usually located in the junctional tissue and is usually reliable and fast enough to maintain adequate cardiac output.

Hospitalization is necessary only for patients who have symptoms of bradycardia (rare in the absence of acute myocardial infarction) or those who have an underlying disease that requires hospitalization.

Second-Degree Atrioventricular Block (Mobitz Type II)
(See Appendix, Fig 29–20, p 511.)

In Mobitz type II second-degree atrioventricular block, the duration of the QRS complex may be normal or wide because of bundle branch block. In this type of second-degree atrioventricular block, the aberration is due to block below the junctional tissue, with the ventricular pacemaker located in the bundle branches or even the Purkinje fibers. PR intervals remain constant before the dropped beat.

Patients with Mobitz type II second-degree atrioventricular block often develop sudden third-degree, or complete, heart block with a Stokes-Adams attack. This type of second-degree atrioventricular block is common in patients with acute anterior myocardial infarction, and the prognosis is poor even with control of the arrhythmia by pacing, because the area of infarction involving the ventricular septum and anterior left ventricle is large, with resulting cardiac failure.

Hemodynamically unstable patients may be managed with atropine, 0.6 mg intravenously, which is usually not helpful; or isoproterenol, 2–20 μg/min by intravenous infusion pump, until a temporary transvenous pacemaker can be inserted. Insertion of a permanent ventricular demand pacemaker is usually required to control symptoms when second-degree atrioventricular block is chronic.

Third-Degree Atrioventricular Block (Complete Heart Block)
(See Appendix, Figs 29–21 and 29–22, pp 511 and 512.)

In complete heart block, the ventricular rate is independent of and slower than the atrial rate, with an idioventricular rhythm or an atrioventricular junctional rhythm pacing the ventricles. Any type of atrial rhythm may be present. With idioventricular rhythm, the ventricular rate is usually 25–40 beats/min, whereas with junctional rhythm, the heart rate may be nearly normal, ie, 50–60 beats/min.

Complete heart block may be congenital, in which case the lower pacemaker is usually junctional and the ventricular rate fast enough that patients are frequently asymptomatic and require no treatment. In patients with acquired complete heart block or with symptomatic congenital complete heart block, a permanent pacemaker should be inserted.

Treatment is as for sinoatrial block (see below).

SINUS BRADYCARDIA
(See Appendix, Fig 29–3, p 503.)

Sinus bradycardia occurs when the sinus rate is less than 60 beats/min. It is a normal finding in many athletes and young adults in good physical condition and in many elderly patients. It does not require treatment unless it is associated with cerebral symptoms related to decreased cardiac output.

Sinus bradycardia is also common in acute inferior myocardial infarction and requires treatment with atropine, 0.6 mg intravenously, if symptomatic hypotension or cerebral hypoperfusion occurs or if tachycardia caused by escape of an ectopic focus develops.

SINOATRIAL BLOCK
(See Appendix, Figs 29–15 and 29–16, p 509.)

Diagnosis

A. First-Degree Sinoatrial Block: First-degree sinoatrial block cannot be diagnosed by electrocardiography and requires invasive electrophysiologic studies for identification.

B. Second-Degree Sinoatrial Block: Second-degree sinoatrial block may take the form of a Wenckebach type of sinus heart rhythm with speeding up and then sudden lengthening of the PP interval; these irregularities are usually repetitive. Alternatively, there may be a single dropped sinus beat such that the long PP interval is a multiple of the normal sinus rate. Sinoatrial Wenckebach block must be differentiated from sinus arrhythmia. Sinoatrial block is not harmful in itself but may be a sign of symptomatic sinus node dysfunction. **Sinus pauses** occur when the sinus node fails to fire at the expected time or fires at intervals that are not a multiple of the normal PP interval. **Sinus node arrest** may be complete, with no atrial activity. The escape rhythm is usually a junctional rhythm, although occasionally an idioventricular escape rhythm occurs that may be too slow to maintain adequate cardiac output. Sinoatrial block and sinus node arrest can occur in patients with increased vagal tone, hyperkalemia, or sinus node ischemia, or they may occur for unknown reasons.

C. Sick Sinus Syndrome: Sinus node dysfunction of many types is included in so-called sick sinus syndrome (tachycardia-bradycardia syndrome). Patients may have sinus bradycardia, sinoatrial block, or sinus arrest. Ventricular and junctional escape rhythms may occur in conjunction with these supraventricular bradyarrhythmias. Manifestations of hypoperfusion (confusion, Stokes-Adams attacks, or frank cardiac arrest) may result from either slow or rapid ventricular responses. The ECG may be normal between attacks.

Treatment

A. Asymptomatic patients with normal peripheral perfusion do not require emergency department treatment.

B. Discontinue all drugs (propranolol, verapamil, sympatholytic agents such as methyldopa, reserpine) that may be causing bradyarrhythmias.

C. If symptoms or signs from bradyarrhythmia

are severe enough to require emergency treatment, give atropine, 0.6 mg intravenously, and repeat the dose if the patient fails to respond in 2–5 minutes, up to a total dose of 2 mg.

D. Isoproterenol, 2–20 µg/min by intravenous infusion pump, may be used to increase the ventricular rate until a pacemaker can be inserted.

E. A temporary transvenous pacemaker may be inserted if the patient can tolerate the delay inherent in its insertion.

F. If there is delay in placement of a transvenous pacemaker catheter and the situation is urgent, a transcutaneous pacemaker should be applied (Chapter 46). External pacing is usually quite uncomfortable and is best reserved for emergency situations. Survival using external transcutaneous pacing is low.

PACEMAKERS & PACEMAKER MALFUNCTION

In the majority of instances, permanent pacemakers are used to control an excessively slow heart rate, eg, in complete heart block or sinus node disease. However, the development of sophisticated microcircuitry has greatly expanded the potential for pacemaker application to include the control of tachyarrhythmias.

The prototype permanent pacemaker is the ventricular demand pacemaker (VVI) (Fig 29–35). One pacing lead goes to the ventricle, and the pacemaker is inhibited by any of the patient's own QRS beats. Today, most single-chamber demand ventricular pacemakers also have a rate-responsive (rate-adaptive) feature (VVI-R) that allows the pacemaker's ventricular rate to accelerate to meet metabolic needs, eg, rate acceleration with exercise (Fig 29–36). The typical demand atrial pacemaker (AAI) has one pacing lead going to the atrium, and the pacemaker is inhibited by any of the patient's own P waves. Rate-responsive features can be incorporated as well (AAI-R). Dual-chamber permanent pacemakers require leads to both the atrium and ventricle. This is done in an attempt to restore the normal atrioventricular sequence and thus facilitate the acceleration of the heart rate and cardiac output during exercise. This is an alternative method to achieve rate responsiveness. Dual-chamber pacemakers are often placed to prevent the "pacemaker syndrome" (see below). The most frequently placed permanent dual-chamber pacemakers are the VDD (atrial sense, ventricular pace, and ventricular inhibited), DVI (atrial and ventricular pace and ventricular inhibited), and DDD (pace and sense both atrium and ventricle). Dual-chamber permanent pacemakers are electronically

more complex than the VVI pacemakers, and interpretation of their ECGs requires more sophistication. Since patients often are unfamiliar with their pacemaker type and model, systematic analysis of the pacemaker ECG is mandatory to a logical decision regarding pacemaker malfunction. The ECG analysis method of Garson (see references) is recommended by the authors. A chest x-ray revealing the pacemaker housing and leads may allow identification of the manufacturer's identification and pacemaker model number.

A comprehensive review of pacemaker management is not the goal of this chapter. However, the reader should appreciate the complexity of problem solving. As an example, let us examine the strategy for troubleshooting a dual-chamber DDD pacemaker. Using the ECG, we must (**1**) measure the AV interval with the pacemaker in the DDD mode; (**2**) inspect the ECG for any variations in the ventricular QRS, which might be an indication of loss of atrial capture (atrial capture may be difficult to determine solely from inspection of the P waves); (**3**) reprogram the pacemaker (with the appropriate programming device) to each of its individual chamber modes to independently test atrial and ventricular sensing and pacing; (**4**) reprogram the pacemaker's atrial refractory period to a longer interval if retrograde atrial conduction is identified on the ECG, preventing an "endless loop" pacemaker-induced tachycardia; (**5**) with the pacemaker in the VVI mode, examine the patient for signs and symptoms of "pacemaker syndrome"; and (**6**) if the patient is stable, order a Holter monitor examination to obtain longer rhythm strips. It is also important to remember that more complex dual-chamber pacemakers do not last as long as single-rate VVI pacemakers, that with time atrial lead function is less stable than ventricular lead function, and that atrial fibrillation occurs in 20% of patients with atrial pacing leads, which could place the ventricular pacing rate at its upper rate limit and induce hemodynamic compromise. Antitachycardia pacemakers for nonpharmacologic termination of supraventricular tachycardia are also commercially available, and pacemakers for ventricular tachycardia cardioversion are in clinical trials. The complexity and sophistication of some of these latter devices are so great that the authors strongly recommend that any operator be completely familiar with the manufacturer's recommendations before reprogramming any modern device. Consultation with the manufacturer's representative is usually worthwhile.

Certain general principles regarding pacemaker technology remain constant. All pacemakers have an implanted power source that delivers a low-energy current to the ventricle, atrium, or both via a bipolar or unipolar electrode placed either transvenously or surgically into the right atrial appendage or ventricular apex. Direct surgical placement requires a thoracotomy and is usually done while performing other cardiac surgery. The epicardial electrodes are placed directly on the myocardial surfaces (eg, the ventricular electrodes are placed on the left ventricle). However, most pacemakers employ transvenous leads. Tined transvenous pacemaker leads can be identified by chest x-ray examination and are placed in defined positions such as the right ventricular apex for ventricular leads or the right atrial appendage for atrial leads. However, newer types of transvenous leads include active fixation permutations such as screw-in electrodes, which allow greater flexibility in lead placement. With this latter type of leads, positioning of transvenous ventricular and atrial leads is based on optimal sensing and pacing rather than on anatomic constraints. Since active fixation leads are often placed in positions other than the right ventricular apex (ventricular lead) or the atrial appendage (atrial lead), such lead positions (eg, midventricular septum or the lateral right atrial wall) might be erroneously interpreted from the chest x-ray as pacemaker lead displacement when, in fact, the lead is optimally placed.

Modern pacemakers rarely completely fail without some warning, especially if systematic follow-up and monitoring are regularly performed. Table 29–2 lists end-of-life indicators used by manufacturers to warn of the need for battery replacement. *Caution:* If cardioversion is necessary in a patient with a permanent pacemaker, make every attempt to keep the defibrillating paddles at least 10–15 cm (4–6 in) away from the pacemaker. It is preferable to use an anteroposterior position for the defibrillating paddles. At times, cardioversion will cause programmable pacemakers to go into a "fall-back" mode, in which the output rate is slower than desired. This situation is corrected by reprogramming the pacemaker.

Pacemaker Terminology

Pacemaker classification has been standardized by a letter coding system explained in Table 29–3.

Table 29–2. End-of-life indicators for permanent pacemakers.

Change to a specific rate
Gradually decreasing rate
Stepwise rate decrease
Change in magnet-mode rate only
Widening difference between magnet-mode and free-running rates
Telemetry of battery voltage
"Vario," cyclic function[1]
Sudden increase in pacer output intensity or stimulus duration or both.
Loss of sensing function

---

[1]Vario = Pacer cycles through beats of decremental output when magnet is applied. The number of beats cycled and not captured is a gross indicator of the margin of safety of the pacemaker output.

Types of Pacemakers in Common Use

Table 29–4 lists the more frequently encountered pacemaker feature combinations. A commonly placed pacemaker is the single ventricular lead, multiprogrammable, VVI device. This device prevents the rate from becoming too slow but does not allow the cardiac output to accelerate in response to physiologic needs. The introduction of atrial sensing and rate modulation (pacemaker rate adaption to metabolic needs) are attempts to overcome this constraint. Pacing with both single- or dual-chamber rate modulation devices is also available and includes devices such as an atrioventricular DDD-R pacemaker, which employs a combination of the patient's intrinsic atrial responses to metabolic needs (eg, acceleration and deceleration) and an independent physiologic sensor. However, about half of patients who need a pacemaker have disorders in which placement of a dual-chamber device is contraindicated (eg, fixed atrial fibrillation or flutter, giant and/or atonic atrial disease, or medical constraints such as debility). Single ventricular chamber rate modulation pacemakers responsive to physiologic responses are frequently employed in atrial disease states in which dual-chamber pacing is contraindicated.

A. Programmable (Demand) Pacemaker: The pacemaker recognizes spontaneous cardiac electrical activity and adjusts pacemaker-generated stimuli accordingly. The sensing rate is the native heart rate, below which pacemaker activity is triggered. Nonatrial sensing or rate modulation for electrical or physiologic factors (QT interval, ejection time, or cardiac volume) and metabolic or exercise sensing (respiration rate, muscle noise, temperature, blood pH, mixed venous saturation, and blood flow) are available.

B. Atrioventricular Dual-Chamber Pacemakers: This pacemaker recognizes atrial depolarization and stimulates the ventricle after an appropriate delay (Fig 29–37). Two electrodes are implanted, one in the atrium and the other in the ventricle. Rate modulation can be employed in these pacemakers as well (see above).

The advantage of this type of pacemaker is that it follows the atrial rate and therefore is capable of increasing or decreasing the rate in response to physiologic demand. It also preserves the "atrial kick" just before ventricular contraction that maximizes stroke volume. Versions of this pacemaker still occasionally are responsible for pacemaker-induced macro-reentry tachycardia ("endless loop" tachycardia). In general, redesign of these pacemakers and increased physician awareness of this complication have reduced the incidence of this arrhythmia.

C. External Programming: Advances in pacemaker technology have made available pacemakers in which rate, impulse strength and duration, and refractory period can be altered by externally applied signals to fine-tune the pacemaker, conserve battery

Table 29–3. A simplified generic code for pacemakers.[1]

Position	1	2	3	4	5
Catergory	Chamber(s) Paced	Chamber(s) Sensed.	Modes of Response(s)	Programmable Functions	Special Antitachyarrhythmia Functions
Letters used	V—Ventricle A—Atrium D—Double	V—Ventricle A—Atrium D—Double O—None	T—Triggered I—Inhibited D—Double[2] O—None R—Rate adaptive	P—Programmable (rate or output or both) M—Multiprogrammable C—Communicating O—None	B—Bursts N—Normal rate competition S—Scanning E—External A—Active antitachycardia fixation otherwise defined
Manufacturer's designation only	S—Single chamber	S—Single chamber			

[1]Data from: Bernstein AD et al: Report of the NASPE Mode Code Committee. PACE 1984;7:396.
[2]Triggered and inhibited response

life, and overcome problems such as increased refractoriness. These refinements and the increasing complexity of pacemaker technology have made electrocardiographic diagnosis of pacemaker failure much more difficult. (See Garson reference for a logical approach to pacemaker electrocardiographic interpretation.)

D. Antitachycardia Pacing: In general, antitachycardia pacemakers are of 2 varieties. One type, which is clinically available, has a lead in the atrium and is programmed to detect the onset of a reentrant paroxysmal supraventricular tachycardia or paroxysmal atrial flutter and to attempt one or more pacing perturbations for reversion. The other type, now in clinical trials, has a lead in the right ventricle and is programmed to detect the onset of ventricular tachycardia. This latter pacemaker delivers a series of pacing impulses to the ventricle and is designed to render the arrhythmia circuit refractory and so terminate the ventricular arrhythmia.

E. Automatic Internal Cardioverter Defibrillator: (See below.) Implantable automatic defibrillators have been developed for use in patients with recurrent ventricular tachycardia or ventricular fibrillation refractory to medical management. The patch and sensing electrodes are usually implanted via a thoracotomy or subxyphoid approach. The device is programmed to detect the development of a wide QRS, rapid-rate tachycardia or ventricular fibrillation. The cardioverter defibrillator delivers one or more internal electrical discharges of 25–35 J, thus terminating the ventricular tachycardia and defibrillating the patient.

Table 29–4. Examples of commonly used pacemakers and their ICHD[1] codes.

Simplified Generic Code	Description
VVO	Ventricular pacing, asynchronous; not programmable. There is one transvenous pacing lead going to the ventricle.
VVI	Ventricular pacing, asynchronous, inhibited (I) by sensing from the ventricle, and usually programable (ie, VVI-P) or multiprogrammable VVI-M). There is one lead going to the ventricle that both paces and senses. The pacemaker is inhibited by any of the patient's own QRS beats.
VVI-R	Similar to the VVI pacemaker but with rate responsiveness. Ventricular pacing, asynchronous, inhibited by sensing from the ventricle, and programmable. There is one pacing and sensing ventricular lead. In one type, the pacemaker case incorporates a piezoelectric sensor that responds to body movements (eg, exercise) and so increases the ventricular pacing rate. The R stands for rate-responsive or adaptive.
AAI	Demand atrial pacemaker that has one pacing and sensing lead implanted in the atrium. The pacemaker ensures a lower heart rate level. It is inhibited by any of the patient's own P waves, so that faster than lower limit rates allow for use of the patient's own sinus mechanism. Used in patients with sick sinus syndrome with the ability to accelerate their upper rates with exercise. Placement mandates intact atrioventricular conduction.
AAI-R	Same as the AAI pacemaker but like the VVI-R device has rate-responsive features incorporated into its rate-demand features, allowing an alternative method to increase the patient's atrial rate.
DVI	Dual-chamber atrial and ventricular pacing with ventricular sensing for pacemaker inhibition.
VDD	Ventricular pacing, atrial sensing, and ventricular sensing to inhibit the pacemaker discharge. This is a frequently placed permanent dual-chamber cardiac pacemaker.
DDD	Like the VDD device, this is a dual chamber, but it paces and senses both atrium and ventricle. This is also a frequently placed permanent dual-chamber cardiac pacemaker.

[1]ICHD = Intersociety Commission for Heart Disease Resources.

Definitive Diagnosis of
Pacemaker Dysfunction

Electrocardiography is the primary technique used for diagnosing pacemaker dysfunction. It is beyond the scope of this chapter to define the complexities of advanced pacemaker electrocardiography. However, a few general guidelines may be helpful: (1) Multi-programmability results in confusing ECGs. (2) The appropriate pacemaker manual should be reviewed for examples of ECGs that one might normally expect to find. (3) It may be necessary to discuss electrocardiographic findings with the manufacturer's representative. (4) The ECG should be interpreted in terms of pacing intervals rather than pacing rate. (5) The timing intervals of the paced and sensed events for both atrium and ventricle should be determined. (6) The goal is usually to determine if there is pacemaker malfunction or battery failure. (7) Surgical intervention may be needed for complete failure to pace or a runaway rate. (8) Other problems only suggest the need for action.

After the hemodynamic status has been stabilized and the patient is hospitalized (preferably with cardiac monitoring), elective procedures can be performed to identify the reason for pacemaker malfunction. For pacemakers in which rate, impulse strength, and duration can be externally adjusted, it is crucial to know all of the adjustments that have been made in order to be able to accurately diagnose pacemaker failure. *Caution:* The complexities of newer pacemakers make the diagnosis of pacemaker failure difficult. Common pacemaker problems include the following:

A. Complete Failure to Pace: Complete failure is often caused by a broken pacing wire or displacement of the wire from the myocardium. Complete battery failure is less likely (Fig 29–38). The ECG may not show the expected pacemaker artifact if the wire is broken. Polyurethane-coated pacemaker leads, placed in more than 100,000 patients, undergo spontaneous deterioration, and lead malfunction should always be suspected in these patients.

B. Failure to Capture: The ECG shows pacemaker artifacts, but these are not followed by QRS complexes. Failure to capture may be due to perforation of the ventricle or displacement of the pacing electrode from the myocardium as well as inadequate battery power or a rise in the pacing threshold. Some antiarrhythmic medications raise the cardiac pacing threshold.

C. Decreased Rate of Firing: If a fixed-rate pacemaker rate slows its rate in either the free running or the magnet mode (as shown by exact measurements of either the RR or pacing spike interval on an ECG), the commonest explanation is failing batteries, which may occur prematurely. Radiographic evaluation of battery function is a much less sensitive indicator than is lengthening of the RR interval. With the new lithium batteries, battery life is now 5–15 years.

D. Failure to Sense: If a demand ventricular pacemaker is competing with the native heart rate and not being inhibited following a native QRS, the pacemaker is not sensing the patient's spontaneous QRS and is operating at a fixed rate (Fig 29–39). This failure to pace on demand may be due to pacemaker dysfunction, partial dislodgment of the catheter tip from the myocardium, increase in the pacing threshold due to concomitant drug therapy, or endocardial fibrosis. Apparent failure to sense may not necessarily indicate failure of the unit and may occur if the refractory period is too short, if the sensing rate is faster than the pacing rate, or if right bundle branch block is present. Atrial lead sensing functions are less stable than ventricular (Fig 29–40). In a patient with a pacemaker who is in native underlying rhythm, the function of the pacemaker can be evaluated by an externally applied magnet that switches the implanted pacemaker into a fixed-rate nonsensing mode.

E. Pacemaker-Generated Tachycardia: "Endless-loop" pacemaker-induced or pacemaker-sustained tachycardia is now less commonly encountered. It is usually found in patients in whom DDD pacemakers have been placed to treat an excessively slow heart rate but whose atrioventricular node is still capable of retrograde conduction to the atrium. If the atrial refractory period of the pacer is short enough, there will be pacemaker sensing and subsequent atrial and ventricular discharge of the DDD device. Antegrade pacemaker discharge and retrograde atrial sensing may become rapid and sustained, simulating an accessory pathway, orthodromic atrioventricular reciprocating tachycardia. Treatment consists of disabling retrograde conduction or, what may be more practical, disabling atrial sensing. The pacemaker can be reprogrammed to a VVI mode, or the atrial refractory period can be lengthened, terminating the tachycardia.

F. Pacemaker Syndrome: This set of symptoms is usually related to the hemodynamic and electrophysiologic consequences of ventricular pacing, but it has also been documented to occur in single–atrial chamber pacemakers. The underlying defect is loss of atrioventricular synchrony, retrograde ventricular to atrial conduction, and loss of the rate response to activity or exercise. The symptoms may be mild or severe; the latter include shock, congestive failure, and chest pain. The definitive treatment for the ventricular-based pacemaker syndrome is to place a dual-chamber pacemaker.

Treatment of Acute Pacemaker
Failure to Pace

A. If the patient is hemodynamically unstable owing to an excessively slow pacemaker rate, as when the pacemaker impulse fails to capture the ventricle, initiate cardiac support with intravenous catecholamines. If possible, locate and use the appropriate pacemaker programmer to increase the output voltage (or current) of the pacemaker to its maximum in an effort to consistently capture the ventricle, or adjust the pacemaker rate to the desired level. If response to sympathomimetics is inadequate or if pacemaker reprogramming is unsuccessful, low-dose atropine sulfate (0.6 mg intravenously) can be used in an effort to accelerate the patient's intrinsic cardiac rate. If available, external cardiac pacing from the precordium can be attempted. "Blind" passage of a transvenous pacing lead into the ventricle using a balloon-tipped, "flow-directed" catheter can also be performed as an alternative source of cardiac pacing.

B. If the patient is hemodynamically stable, monitor the patient closely, and contact the patient's cardiologist, pacemaker implant surgeon, or internist for further assistance.

Disposition

Patients with pacemaker malfunction resulting in decreased cardiac output require immediate stabilization and hospitalization for cardiac monitoring and correction of the malfunction. Patients with early battery failure or slowing of pacing rate without other signs of cardiac dysfunction need to be hospitalized for urgent battery replacement.

AUTOMATIC INTERNAL CARDIOVERTER DEFIBRILLATOR

Automatic internal cardioverter defibrillators (AICDs) automatically detect and cardiovert, or defibrillate, malignant ventricular rhythms. In patients with the device, the incidence of sudden death from ventricular tachycardia or fibrillation has been dramatically reduced to less than 5% per year. Although the newer models of these devices have rate detection and output programmability, they are not pacemakers. It is anticipated that newer models currently being tested will incorporate antitachycardia and backup bradycardia pacing features.

Proper patient selection is crucial. Invasive and advanced electrophysiologic studies are needed to ensure proper application of these sophisticated devices. As their complexity increases, only centers experienced with various types of advanced pharmacologic and nonpharmacologic therapies should place these devices.

Surgical implantation via thoracotomy or subxyphoid approach is necessary to place the 2 ventricular patch output elements and the 2 screw-in ventricular sensing leads. These leads and patches have extensions that are connected to the automatic internal cardioverter defibrillator via subcutaneous tunnels; the device itself is placed in the abdominal wall (Fig 29–41).

This device is somewhat bulky and tends to mi-

grate if not well anchored. Elevations in sensing thresholds, as induced by the drugs amiodarone and possibly encainide and flecainide, may result in failure to discharge. Drug therapy, however, is often needed to suppress the frequency of the malignant arrhythmias or heart rate increases induced by exercise (eg, a beta-blocker). Battery life is shortened by frequent and repeated discharges.

The device can deliver up to 100 discharges over its life span of approximately 2–3 years. A system to detect the need for generator replacement is built into the device. Sensing and output settings can be altered by external programming. Telemetry functions are limited to frequency of discharge. Close patient follow-up is mandatory. *Caution:* A pacemaker magnet placed over the automatic internal cardioverter defibrillator may disable it. Even when the device is intentionally disabled, magnetic resonance imaging units may electromagnetically induce cardiac pacing and the pacing may be at excessively rapid rates (eg, ≥ 300 beats/min).

Definition of Automatic Internal Cardioverter Defibrillator Dysfunction

A. Failure to Successfully Perform Cardioversion or to Defibrillate: The newer automatic internal cardioverter defibrillator recycles 4 times if the original discharge fails to convert the arrhythmia to sinus rhythm. Thereafter, it will not discharge until after 30–40 seconds of sinus rhythm. Therefore, if the device does not successfully cardiovert or defibrillate and the patient is hemodynamically compromised, the usual measures for cardiopulmonary resuscitation and advanced life support must be initiated.

1. As with pacemakers, avoid placing defibrillator paddles on or near the automatic internal cardioverter defibrillator pack.

2. To determine if the sensing or ventricular patch electrodes are grossly malpositioned, take a 2-view chest x-ray. Note that some patients have an additional permanent pacemaker in place; it may be difficult to sort out the various leads.

3. At times, the automatic internal cardioverter defibrillator may sense only permanent pacemaker depolarizations and fail to sense an episode of ventricular fibrillation.

4. In-depth evaluation, possibly including repeat electrophysiologic studies, is usually required to determine the cause of failure to successfully cardiovert or defibrillate.

B. Inappropriate or Excessive Discharges: Rarely, a device may discharge when it is not needed. Usually, a supraventricular tachycardia is mistaken for ventricular arrhythmia, and the automatic internal cardioverter defibrillator responds accordingly. Sinus tachycardia or atrial fibrillation with a rapid ventricular response often is responsible. To correct for these inappropriate discharges, the older automatic internal cardioverter defibrillator devices could be deactivated by placing a donut magnet (the same as that used for pacemakers) on top of the power pack for 30 seconds. With magnet application, a beeping tone synchronous with the heartbeat is heard. When the beep becomes a steady tone, the magnet should be removed. The device, in its inactive mode, neither senses nor discharges. A newer model (Ventak 1550) is deactivated using radiofrequency telemetric communication. A magnet is still used for audible evaluation of sensing.

Treatment & Disposition

If there is failure to sense, discharge, or cardiovert, or if the automatic internal cardioverter defibrillator is deactivated, the patient should be stabilized and hospitalized. Further therapy depends on the type of dysfunction. The manufacturer's representative may be able to assist in the diagnosis and correction of a device malfunction.

APPENDIX: IDENTIFICATION OF ARRHYTHMIAS

This appendix gives sample ECGs for some common arrhythmias, ladder diagrams illustrating their

---

All figures with the exception of Figs 29–30, 29–31, 29–32, 29–33, 29–36, and 29–41 are reproduced, with permission, from Goldschlager N, Goldman MJ: *Principles of Clinical Electrocardiography,* 13th ed. Appleton & Lange, 1989 (or from the 11th edition of that text).

A = atrium; V = ventricular; AV = atrioventricular; SA = sinoatrial.

---

pathophysiology, and brief descriptions of how they may be recognized clinically.

SINUS MECHANISMS

Normal Sinus Rhythm
(See Fig 29–1.)
A. The heart rate is between 60 and 100 beats/min.

B. The P wave vector is normal (upright in leads II, aVF).

C. A slight variation in RR interval is characteristic (compared with atrial tachycardia).

Sinus Tachycardia
(See Fig 29–2.)
A. The heart rate is usually less than 160 beat/min; occasionally, it is between 160 and 220 beats/min.

B. Other characteristics of normal sinus rhythm are seen.

Sinus Bradycardia
(See Fig 29–3.)
A. The heart rate is less than 60 beats/min.

B. Other characteristics of normal sinus rhythm are seen.

Sinus Arrhythmia
(See Fig 29–4.)
A. A phasic variation in RR interval is synchronous with respiration.

B. Other characteristics of normal sinus rhythm are seen.

SUPRAVENTRICULAR TACHYCARDIAS

Atrial Tachycardias
(See Fig 29–5.)
A. P waves may or may not be visible; the P wave

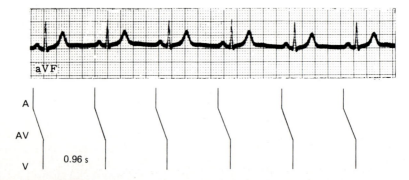

Figure 29–1. ECG showing normal sinus rhythm at a rate of 63 beats/min.

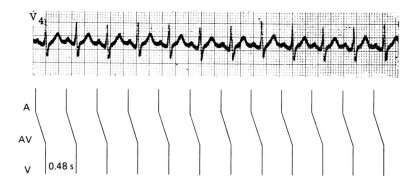

Figure 29–2. Sinus tachycardia at a rate of 125 beats/min. By definition, sinus tachycardia is present if there is sinus rhythm at a rate greater than 100 beats/min; the rate is usually less than 160 beats/min at rest. Note that there is a P wave before each QRS complex, that the P wave is upright in leads II and aVF, and that the PR interval is normal.

vector is frequently abnormal (flat or inverted in leads II, aVF).

B. If discernible, the PP interval should be absolutely regular and abnormally short. The atrial rate is usually less than 220 beats/min.

C. A QRS complex follows a P wave unless atrioventricular block is present. The P wave may be buried in the T wave.

D. Atrioventricular block may be seen, with a regular, repetitive relationship between the P wave and the QRS complex (eg, in 2:1 atrioventricular block, a QRS complex occurs after every other P wave).

Atrioventricular Nodal Reentrant Tachycardias
(See Figs 29–6 and 29–7A and B.)

A. Electrical activity originates in junctional tissue and spreads antegrade to the ventricle and retrograde to the atrium.

B. The rate is usually 120–200 beats/min.

C. P waves may precede or follow the QRS complex or be obscured by it. If P waves are present, the vector is usually abnormal (inverted in leads II, aVF). P waves that are difficult to see in standard ECG leads may be demonstrated with esophageal leads (Fig 29–7B).

D. The PR interval is shortened.

Atrial Flutter
(See Figs 29–8 and 29–9.)

A. Atrial activity produces a saw-toothed electrocardiographic pattern that is seen on all leads except where it is obscured by QRS or T waves.

B. The peak-to-peak rate is over 220 beats/min, usually 250–350 beats/min.

C. The predominant atrial wave is usually negative in lead II.

D. The QRS complex may occur in a pattern that is regular or "irregularly regular," with atrioventricular block, usually 2:1 but sometimes 3:2, 4:1, Wenckebach, etc (Fig 29–9).

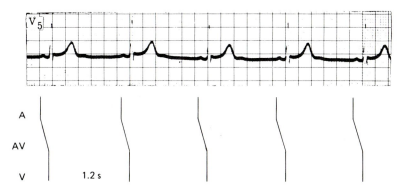

Figure 29–3. Sinus bradycardia at a rate of 50 beats/min. By definition, sinus bradycardia is present if there is sinus rhythm at a rate less than 60 beats/min. Note that there is a P wave before each QRS complex and that the PR interval is normal. In leads II and aVF, the P wave must be upright.

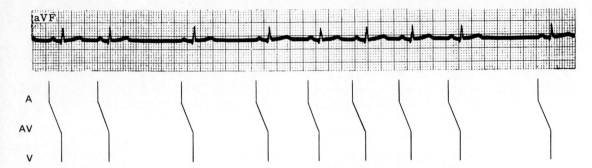

Figure 29–4. Sinus arrhythmia, which can be recognized by phasic variation in PP intervals; shortening with inspiration and lengthening (rate slowing) with expiration. Note normal P wave morphology and PR intervals, as occur with other sinus rhythms.

E. Atrial flutter may have 1:1 conduction at a rate of 300 beats/min with aberration (widening) of the QRS complex that can simulate ventricular tachycardia.

Atrial Fibrillation
(See Fig 29–10.)

A. Atrial activity is irregular and inconstant. The ECG may show very fine or very coarse activity. The degree of irregularity is variable, and at times atrial fibrillation may simulate atrial flutter.

B. The ventricular response is irregularly irregular (many different RR intervals without regular repetition).

Premature Atrial Contractions
(See Figs 29–11, 29–12, and 29–13.)

A. The P wave is premature, with shape and vector different from those of a sinus P wave. If it is early enough, the premature P wave may be obscured by the preceding T wave, as indicated by distortion of T wave morphology.

B. The premature P wave may be followed by a normal QRS or an aberrantly conducted QRS complex (usually of the right bundle branch block type).

If the premature atrial contraction is very early, it may not be followed by a QRS (blocked premature atrial contractions). This latter pattern may be mistaken for a sinus pause if the early P wave is not seen.

Multifocal Atrial Tachycardia
(Wandering Atrial Pacemaker or
Chaotic Atrial Rhythm)
(See Fig 29–14.)

A. Multifocal atrial tachycardia is an irregular atrial rhythm with 3 or more different types of P waves.

B. The PP, PR, and RR intervals vary. P waves are usually followed by a QRS wave. Early P waves may be followed by an aberrant QRS complex (of right bundle branch block configuration), or—if they are very early—they may be blocked (P wave without a following QRS wave).

PAUSES, BRADYCARDIAS, &
ATRIOVENTRICULAR BLOCK

Sinus Arrest
(See Fig 29–15.)

A. The PP interval is suddenly prolonged and not a regular multiple of the usual PP interval.

B. Escape beats (sinus, junctional, or ventricular) may occur.

Sinoatrial Block
(See Fig 29–16.)

A. The PP interval is abruptly prolonged.

B. The long PP interval is frequently a multiple of the usual PP interval (if there is 2:1 sinoatrial block). Alternatively, PP intervals may be regularly irregular if there is Wenckebach block originating in the sinoatrial node.

Atrioventricular Block:
First-Degree
(See Fig 29–17.)

First-degree atrioventricular block is manifested only by a PR interval longer than normal for the

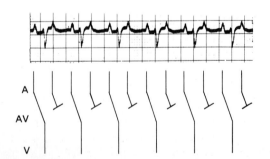

Figure 29–5. Paroxysmal supraventricular tachycardia with 2:1 atrioventricular block caused by digitalis toxicity. The atrial rate is 200 beats/min; the ventricular rate, 100 beats/min.

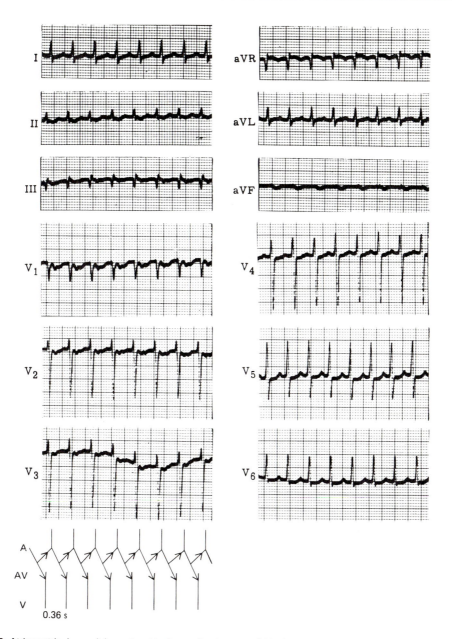

Figure 29–6. Atrioventricular nodal reentrant tachycardia at a rate of 188 beats/min as a result of a reentry mechanism.

patient's age and heart rate. For an adult with a heart rate between 80 and 100 beats/min, this is longer than 0.22 s.

Atrioventricular Block: Second-Degree (Mobitz Type I or Wenckebach) (See Figs 29–18 and 29–19.)

A. The P waves and PP intervals are regular, but periodically a P wave is not followed by a QRS wave.

B. In classic Wenckebach block there is a pro-gressive increase in the PR interval, resulting in a progressive shortening of RR intervals until a QRS complex is dropped. The PR interval then reverts to its shortest interval, and the sequence is repeated. The RR interval containing the dropped QRS is always shorter than twice the shortest RR interval without a dropped beat. The block can be 2:1, 3:2, 4:3, or other combinations (Figs 29–18 and 29–19).

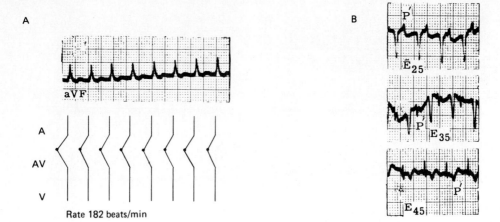

Figure 29–7. Atrioventricular nodal reentrant tachycardia at a rate of 182 beats/min. **A:** Lead aVF shows a poorly defined P wave following a QRS complex. **B:** Esophageal leads at a distance of 25, 35, and 45 cm (from the nose) show P after each QRS complex.

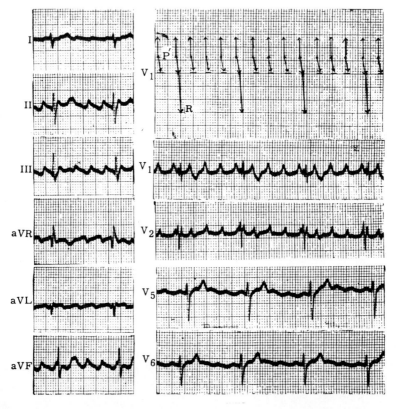

Figure 29–8. Atrial flutter at a rate of 250 beats/min with 4:1 atrioventricular block. Note the typical saw-toothed pattern of atrial activity.

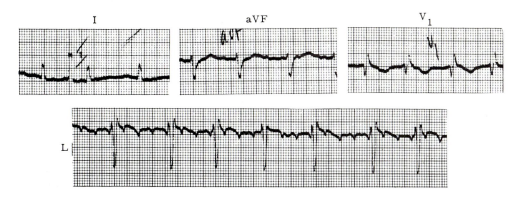

Figure 29–9. Atrial flutter, showing the value of Lewis leads. Standard ECG leads show an indeterminate type of atrial activity, but the Lewis lead (panel labeled with an L) shows atrial flutter with irregular ventricular response.

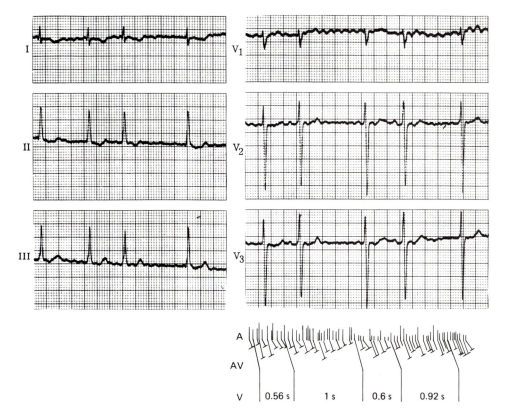

Figure 29–10. Atrial fibrillation. Ventricular response has been slowed by increasing atrioventricular block with digitalis glycosides.

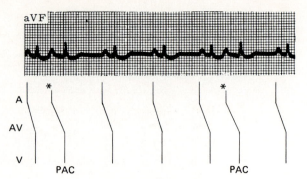

Figure 29–11. Premature atrial contractions (PAC) with 1:1 ventricular response. Note that the premature P wave distorts the preceding T wave.

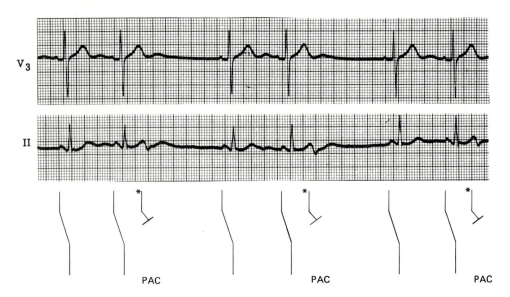

Figure 29–12. Premature atrial contractions (PAC) with blocked ventricular response. The QRS complex is dropped because premature atrial activity enters the atrioventricular node during the refractory period. Note that the premature P wave distorts the preceding T wave.

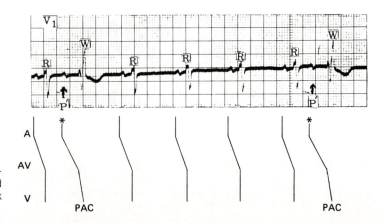

Figure 29–13. Premature atrial contractions (PAC) with an aberrantly conducted QRS complex (right bundle branch block pattern).

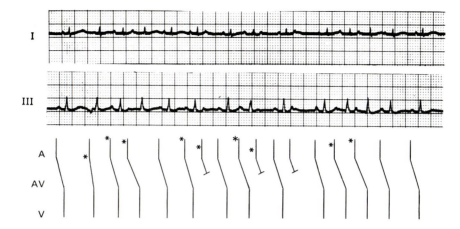

Figure 29–14. Multifocal atrial tachycardia at a rate of 140 beats/min. Note the varying P wave vectors and configurations (indicated diagrammatically by asterisks at various positions), varying PR and PP intervals, and resulting irregular ventricular rhythm. Some P waves are blocked.

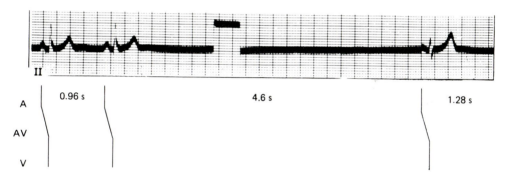

Figure 29–15. Sinus arrest (sudden increase in PP interval from the usual 0.96 s to 4.6 s) with sinus escape beat (recognized by different P wave morphology and PR interval) following carotid sinus massage.

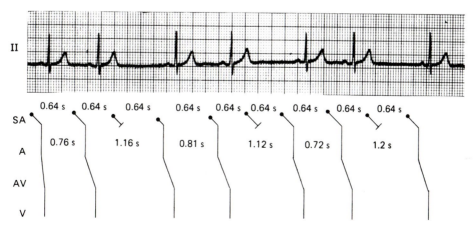

Figure 29–16. Sinus node exit block (3:2 Wenckebach type). Repetitively, 2 sinus-conducted beats are followed by a pause. All P waves are of the same form, the PR interval is constant, and no blocked atrial premature beats are evident. In this instance, the sinus node is firing regularly (but cannot be seen on the ECG). There is a progressive sinoatrial block with the result that every third sinoatrial discharge is not conducted.

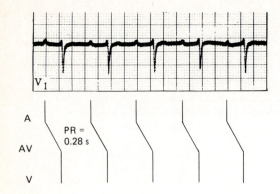

Figure 29–17. First-degree atrioventricular block. The PR interval is 0.28 s.

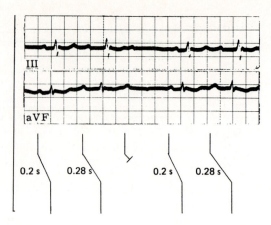

Figure 29–18. Second-degree atrioventricular block, Mobitz type I, demonstrating classic Wenckebach phenomenon. Note progressive lengthening of the PR interval until the QRS complex is omitted in a 3:2 ratio.

Atrioventricular Block: Second-Degree (Mobitz Type II) (See Fig 29–20.)

A. The P waves and PP intervals are regular, but (periodically) a P wave is not followed by a QRS wave.

B. The PR interval may be normal or prolonged.

C. Progressive prolongation of the PR interval before the QRS is dropped does not occur (Fig 29–20).

Atrioventricular Block: Complete (Third-Degree) (See Figs 29–21 and 29–22.)

A. The PP interval is constant and usually shorter (faster) than the RR interval. Any type of atrial rhythm may be present.

B. There is no temporal relationship between P waves and QRS waves (ie, they occur asynchronously).

C. The QRS complex may be normal or widened if bundle branch block is present or if the escape pacemaker is ventricular (Figs 29–21 and 29–22).

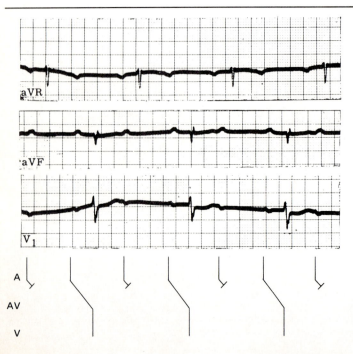

Figure 29–19. Second-degree atrioventricular block, Mobitz type I (Wenckebach). There is 2:1 atrioventricular conduction.

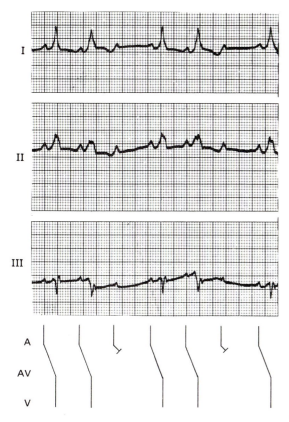

Figure 29–20. Second-degree atrioventricular block, Mobitz type II. There is 3:2 atrioventricular conduction with left bundle branch block. The PR interval is 0.16 s and is constant.

Atrioventricular Dissociation
(See Figs 29–23 and 29–24.)

A. The PP interval is constant but is frequently the same as or longer (slower) than the RR interval.

B. Periodically, there is no temporal relationship between P waves and QRS waves (dissociation); at other times, there is capture of the QRS or—by retrograde conduction (retrograde P wave)—the atrium can conduct when the impulse reaches the atrioventricular node at a time when the node is not refractory.

VENTRICULAR ARRHYTHMIAS

Premature Ventricular Contractions
(See Figs 29–25, 29–26, and 29–27.)

A. The QRS complex is premature, and either the P wave is absent or the PR interval is shortened.

B. The QRS morphology is widened and often bizarre (bundle branch block pattern, etc). If all the QRS complexes have the same configuration, they are called unifocal; if configuration varies, multifocal (variable coupling interval) or multiform (fixed coupling interval).

C. The R-PVC interval (coupling interval) may be constant for each premature ventricular contraction (coupled premature ventricular contractions) or may vary in duration.

D. When the PVC-PVC interval is constant (or a multiple of a constant interval) with a varying R-PVC interval, the premature ventricular contractions are said to be parasystolic (Fig 29–27).

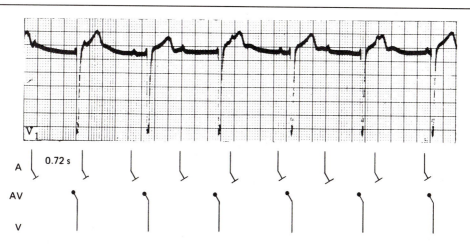

Figure 29–21. Complete atrioventricular block. The atrial rate is 83 beats/min; the ventricular rate, 54 beats/min. The QRS complex is narrow because the pacemaker is junctional and ventricular conduction is normal.

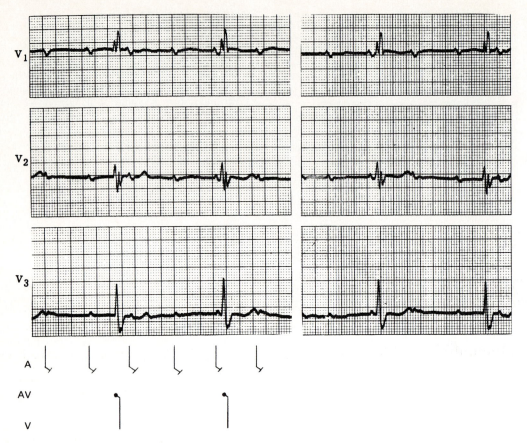

Figure 29–22. Complete atrioventricular block. The atrial rate is 88 beats/min; the ventricular rate, 37 beats/min. The QRS complex is widened because the pacemaker is venctricular (idioventricular rhythm).

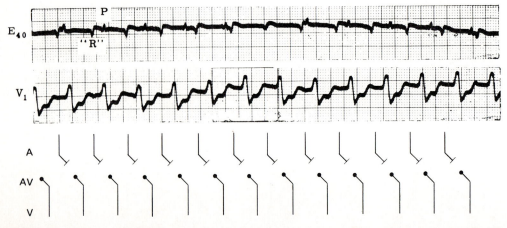

Figure 29–23. Atrioventricular dissociation. Tracings from esophageal (E_{40}) and precordial leads. Note that the atrial and ventricular rates are both 115 beats/min, but there are no capture beats.

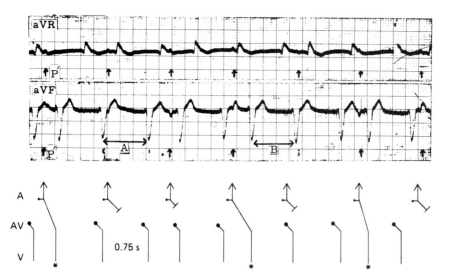

Figure 29–24. Atrioventricular dissociation. The atrial rate is 60 beats/min with an ectopic pacemaker (P wave inverted in lead aVF). There is a junctional rhythm at 85 beats/min with occasional capture beats (indicated by asterisks).

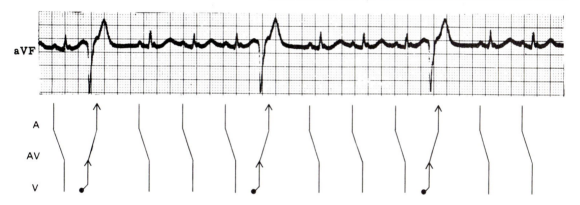

Figure 29–25. Premature ventricular contractions. This tracing illustrates coupled unifocal premature ventricular contractions (as shown by the constant R-PVC interval and the QRS morphology).

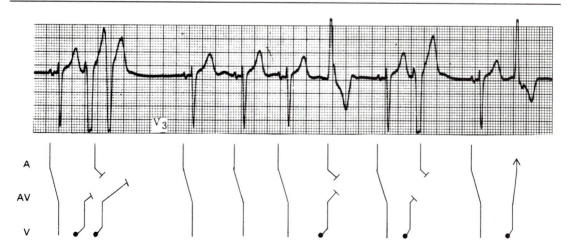

Figure 29–26. Premature ventricular contractions. There are multiform premature ventricular contractions (varying morphology but with fixed coupling interval).

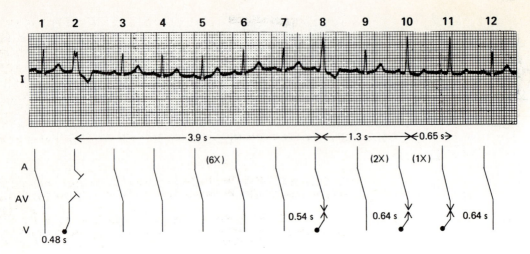

Figure 29–27. Premature ventricular contractions showing ventricular parasystole. On this tracing, beat 2 is a typical premature ventricular contraction. Beats 8, 10, and 11 are preceded by normal P waves, but the QRS morphology is a *fusion* of that of the premature ventricular contraction and a normal QRS complex *(fusion beat)*. Coupling intervals vary from 0.48 to 0.68 s. The PVC-PVC intervals are all multiples of 0.65 s (beats 2–8 = 3.9 s; beats 8–10 = 1.3 s; beats 10–11 = 0.65 s).

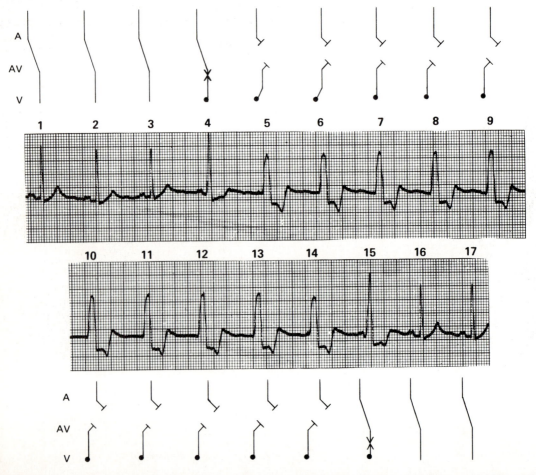

Figure 29–28. Accelerated idioventricular rhythm. Beats 5–14 show the wide QRS complexes (without P waves) characteristic of idioventricular rhythms. Beats 1–3, 16, and 17 are sinus beats, and beats 4 and 15 are fusion beats.

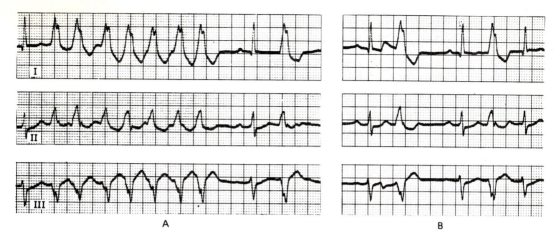

Figure 29–29. Ventricular tachycardia. **A:** Run of ventricular tachycardia after the first sinus beat. After 7 complexes, the tachycardia stops and a sinus beat occurs, followed by a premature ventricular contraction of the same configuration as the wide complex run of tachycardia. **B:** Later, in the same patient, premature ventricular contractions with the same configuration in bigeminy.

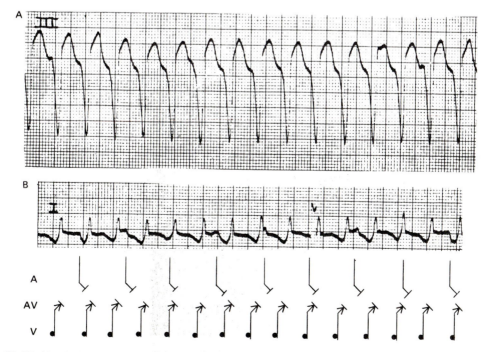

Figure 29–30. Ventricular tachycardia. **A:** Lead III. Wide QRS tachycardia at a rate of 150 beats/min. No distinct P waves can be seen. **B:** Lead I in same patient. P waves distort ST segments. The QRS complex is narrower in lead I than in lead III because part of the QRS complex is isoelectric in lead I. When the P waves—all of which are nonconducted—are plotted out, the atrial rate is 95 beats/min, and there is complete dissociation between atrial and ventricular depolarization.

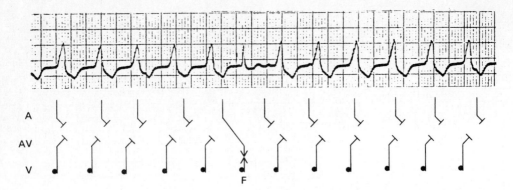

Figure 29–31. Ventricular tachycardia. There are wide, bizarre QRS complexes occurring at a rate of 130 beats/min. The single fusion beat (F) confirms the diagnosis.

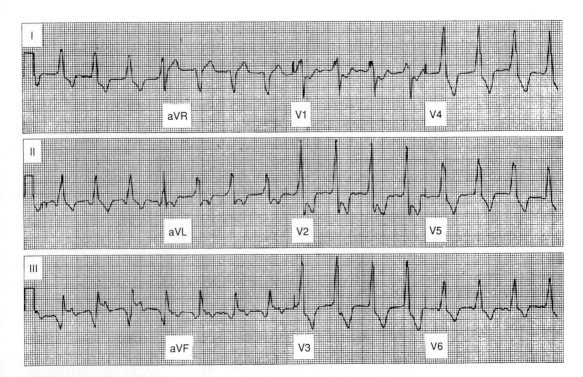

Figure 29–32. Twelve-lead ECG revealing a ventricular tachycardia with a monomorphic pattern due to a proarrhythmic response to a type IC antiarrhythmia. The ventricular tachycardia has a left bundle branch morphology (see Table 29–1 for diagnosis of ventricular tachycardia). There are retrograde P waves following each QRS. This excludes an atrial rhythm but not a junctional rhythm with retrograde conduction and a bundle branch block. Because the ventricular tachycardia rate was slow (90 beats/min), the patient was hemodynamically stable. Expectant observation allowed clearance of the antiarrhythmic medication and return of sinus rhythm.

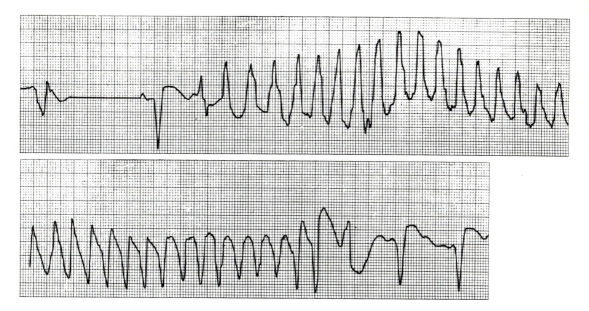

Figure 29–33. Polymorphic ventricular tachycardia (torsade de pointes). A long compensatory pause followed by a premature ventricular beat triggers the arrhythmia. The QRS spikes change polarity about the ECG baseline.

Idioventricular Rhythm
(See Fig 29–28.)
A. QRS complexes are wide, with bizarre configuration.

B. The heart rate is usually less than 50 beats/min. If the rate is over 50 beats/min, the rate is termed **accelerated idioventricular rhythm** (Fig 29–28).

C. Ventricular complexes may capture the atrium (inverted P wave in leads II, aVF), or they may be dissociated from atrial activity. If the basic sinus rate increases, the ventricle may be captured by a normal sinus pacemaker, and the idioventricular rhythm is suppressed.

Ventricular Tachycardia
(See Figs 29–29, 29–30, 29–31, and 29–32.)
A. QRS complexes are bizarre and wide; R is usually upright in lead V_1.

B. The QRS rate is usually between 100 and 140 beats/min (rarely as fast as 180 beats/min), with QRS complexes unrelated to P waves.

C. Capture beats may occur occasionally (a nar-

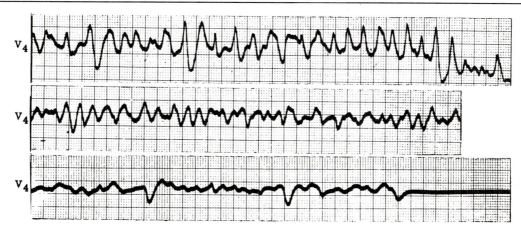

Figure 29–34. Ventricular fibrillation. There is rapid and irregular modulation of the baseline, without organized QRS complex activity.

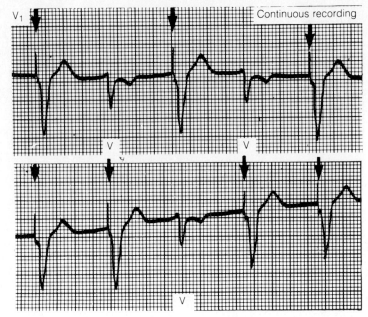

Figure 29–35. The generator has been programmed to pace at a ventricular rate of 75/min (interstimulus interval = 0.8 s), and output pulses are delivered 0.8 s after sensed spontaneous QRS complexes (V). When no spontaneous QRS complexes are sensed, ventricular pacing at the programmed rate occurs (arrows).

row QRS complex with associated P wave buried in the T wave of preceding beats). Fusion beats may also occur; the QRS is formed by depolarization from the atrium through the atrioventricular node and also from the ventricular pacemaker. The QRS is then a combination of the normal sinus QRS and the ventricular QRS.

Polymorphic Ventricular Tachycardia
(See Fig 29–33.)

A. The morphology and rate of QRS spikes vary continuously.

B. The QRS spikes change polarity or "turn about" the isoelectric baseline of the ECG.

C. The rhythm is usually initiated by a PVC occurring after a long compensatory pause.

Ventricular Fibrillation
(See Fig 29–34.)

A. There is irregular undulation of the baseline at variable rates (usually > 200 beats/min) without organized QRS activity.

B. Cardiac arrest is present in every instance.

PACEMAKER RHYTHMS

Ventricular-Inhibited Pacing (VVI)
(See Fig 29–35.)

A. There are occasional native heart beats (beats 2 and 3 in top panel and beat 3 in bottom panel).

B. The implanted pacemaker "senses" these na-tive beats and withholds a pacemaker beat in order to avoid competition between the ventricular beats.

C. The ventricle is otherwise paced at a rate of 75 beats/min.

Ventricular-Inhibited Pacing (VVI-R)
(See Fig 29–36.)

A. At rest, the pacemaker stimulates the ventricle to respond at a "normal resting" heart rate, ie, about 80 beats/min.

B. At exercise, the cardiac rate accelerates to ensure an increase in cardiac output. The cardiac rate is tachycardiac, ie, 113 beats/min.

C. A sensor responding to pectoral muscle motion and encased in the pacemaker can is responsible for this pacemaker rate acceleration.

Atrial & Ventricular Pacing in DDD Mode
(See Fig 29–37.)

A. The ventricle is continuously paced at a rate between 70 and 75 beats/min.

B. The atrium is intermittently paced. Beats 3, 4, and 5 in the top panel and beats 1, 2, and 3 in the bottom panel are atrial paced beats.

C. When the native atrial rate is faster than the atrial pacing rate threshold, the pacemaker senses the native atrial beats and withholds a pacemaker driven atrial beat in order to avoid competition between beats.

A. REST

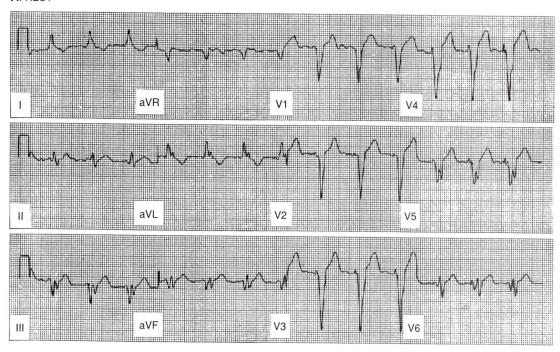

B. EXERCISE

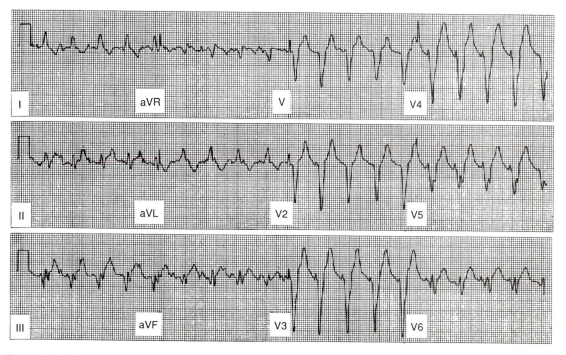

Figure 29–36. Twelve-lead ECGs of a VVI-R pacemaker with a transvenous lead pacing from the right ventricle and its response to treadmill exercise. **A:** The patient's ECG at rest when the resting pacemaker rate is 78 beats/min, its lower limit. **B:** At peak exercise, the pacemaker rate has increased to its upper rate limit of 113 beats/min. A piezoelectric sensor is enclosed in the pacemaker case that responds to chest wall motion due to exercise and accelerates the pacemaker rate in a stepwise fashion.

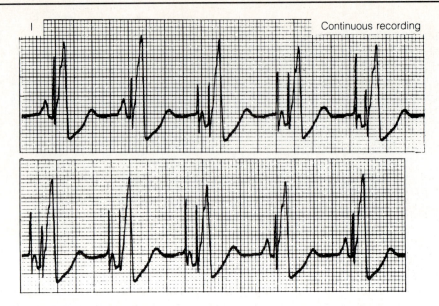

Figure 29–37. The first two P waves are sinus and inhibit the atrial pacing output circuit. The atrial rate then slows slightly, and the remaining P waves are paced at the programmed rate of 72/min. All QRS complexes are paced, since no spontaneous QRS complexes occur within the programmed atrioventricular interval of 0.14 s. Had a spontaneous QRS complex been stimulated by either a sinus or paced P wave, the ventricular output would have been inhibited.

PACEMAKER FAILURE

Failure to Capture
(See Fig 29–38.)

A. The ventricle is intermittently paced at a rate of about 80 beats/min (large arrows).

B. Frequently, the pacemaker discharges are not followed by a ventricular beat (beats 3 and 4 in both the upper and lower panels).

C. This failure to pace is due to either an absolute or relative weak ventricular pacemaker output stimulus.

Failure to Sense
(See Fig 29–39.)

A. The ventricle is paced at a rate of about 80 beats/min (large arrows).

B. Many pacemaker impulses are present when they should be absent (beats 2, 3, and 6 in the top panel and the last beat in the lower panel).

C. In this example, the ability not to pace is due to either an absolute or a relative weakness in ventricular pacemaker stimulus input.

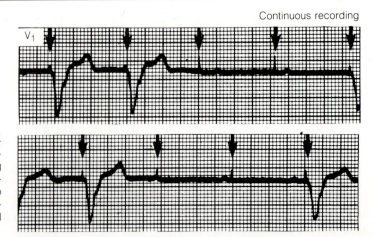

Figure 29–38. Intermittent failure to capture. Pacing artifacts are indicated by the arrows. Long pauses in paced rhythm, during which pacing artifacts occur but do not stimulate QRS complexes, indicate failure to pace. The problem could be due to generator failure or to an increase in the myocardial stimulation threshold.

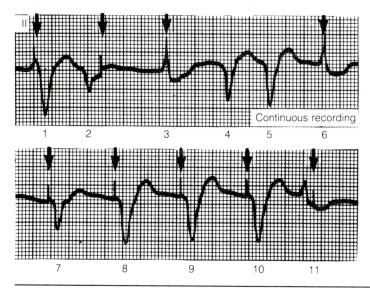

Figure 29–39. Intermittent "failure" to sense. Pacing stimuli are delivered earlier than expected (QRS complexes 2, 3, 6, and 11), indicating failure to sense those complexes, which is probably due to their poor signal quality. The delivery of pacing stimuli in the ventricular vulnerable period could result in repetitive ventricular rhythms.

"Pseudofailure"
(See Fig 29–40.)

A. The atrium is paced at a rate of about 80 beats/min.

B. The ventricle responds normally to these atrial beats, implying that the atrioventricular node and bundle branches successfully carry the intrinsic cardiac impulses. Because of this success, there is no need for the pacemaker to stimulate the ventricle.

C. Older ECG machines would reveal a constant amplitude of the bipolar pacemaker spike and allow inferences about the strength of the pacemaker's atrial output. Such inferential analysis (atrial output strength) is no longer possible since the introduction of the newer generation of digitally based ECG recording machines.

AUTOMATIC INTERNAL CARDIOVERTER DEFIBRILLATOR (AICD)

Chest X-Ray of AICD
(See Fig 29–41.)

A. As they do in this example, both large patches of the AICD should encompass the bulk of the ventricular muscle.

B. The AICD battery pack is too large to be placed in the chest wall and thus must be housed beneath the skin in the external wall of the abdomen.

C. The "screw-in" electrodes that allow sensing of the cardiac impulses and their character are placed into the external surface of the ventricular muscle at the time of surgical implantation.

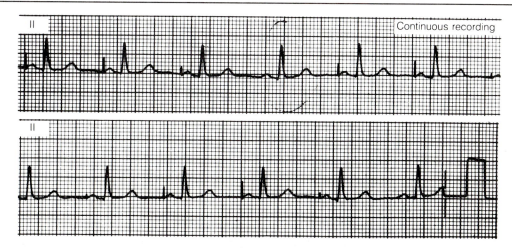

Figure 29–40. DDD pacing in which atrial pacing is followed by normally conducted QRS complexes, inhibiting ventricular output. Note the variation in amplitude of the output pulses, mimicking electrode fracture. Recording the ECG using analog equipment will clarify the issue.

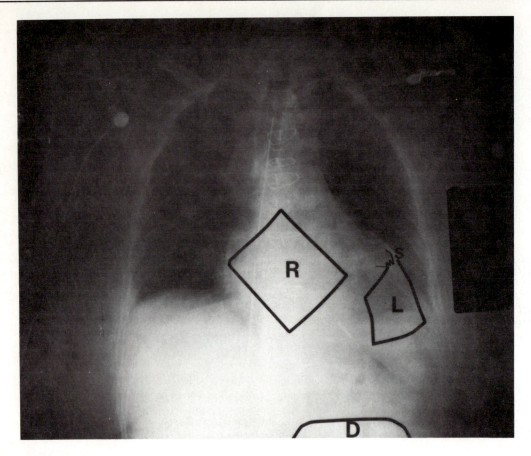

Figure 29–41. Chest x-ray (retouched for clarity) showing two AICD patches in a patient with an implanted cardioverter defibrillator. One patch is over the left ventricle (L), and one is over the right ventricle (R). The battery pack is partially seen in the abdomen (D), and one of 2 screw-in sensing electrodes (S) is identified. The patient had a sternal splitting thoracotomy to allow patches and sensing electrodes to be placed.

REFERENCES

Aktar M et al: Wide QRS complex tachycardia. Ann Intern Med 1988;109:905.

Anastasiou-Nana MI et al: Occurrence of exercise-induced and spontaneous wide complex tachycardia during therapy with flecainide for complex ventricular arrhythmias: A probable proarrhythmic effect. Am Heart J 1987;113:1071.

Cardiac Arrhythmia Suppression Trial (CAST) Preliminary Report: Effect of encainide and flecainide on mortality in a randomized trial of arrhythmia suppression after myocardial infarction. N Engl J Med 1989;321:406.

Den Dulk K et al: The Activitrax rate responsive pacemaker system. Am J Cardiol 1988;61:107.

DiMarco JP et al: Adenosine for paroxysmal supraventricular tachycardia: Dose ranging and comparison with verapamil. Ann Intern Med 1990;113:104.

Ewy GA: Urgent parenteral digoxin therapy: A requiem. J Am Coll Cardiol 1990;15:1248.

Funk-Brentano C et al: Medical intelligence: Propafenone. N Engl J Med 1990;322:518.

Furman S, Gross J: Dual-chamber pacemakers. Curr Probl Cardiol 1990;15:119.

Furman S et al: *A Practice of Cardiac Pacing,* 2nd ed. Futura, 1989.

Gabry M et al: Automatic implantable cardioverter defibrillators: Patient survival, battery longevity and shock delivery analysis. J Am Coll Cardiol 1987;9:1349.

Garson A: Stepwise approach to the unknown pacemaker ECG. Am Heart J 1990;119:924.

German LD, Ideker RE: Ventricular tachycardia: Mechanisms, diagnosis, and management. Med Clin North Am 1984;68:919.

Goldschlager N, Goldman MJ: *Principles of Clinical Electrocardiography,* 13th ed. Appleton & Lange, 1989.

Hoffman JR: Emergency department management of life-threatening arrhythmias. Emerg Med Clin North Am 1986;4:761.

Jackman WM et al: The long QT syndromes: A critical review, new observations and a unifying hypothesis. Prog Cardiovasc Dis 1988;31:115.

Josephson M et al: Differential diagnosis of supraventricular tachycardia. Cardiol Clin 1990;8:411.

Kerr CR et al: Sinus node dysfunction. Cardiol Clin 1983;1:187.

Kindwall KE et al: Electrocardiographic criteria for ventricular tachycardia in wide complex left bundle branch block tachycardias. Am J Cardiol 1988;61:1279.

Knowlton AA, Falk RH: External cardiac pacing during in-hospital cardiac arrest. Am J Cardiol 1986;57:1295.

Mattioni TA et al: The proarrhythmic effects of amiodarone. Prog Cardiovasc Dis 1989;31:439.

Nguyen PT, Scheinmen MM, Seger J: Polymorphous ventricular tachycardia: Clinical characterization, therapy, and the QT interval. Circulation 1986;74:340.

Proloid PJ et al: Aggravation of arrhythmia by antiarrhythmic drugs: Incidence and predictors. Am J Cardiol 1987;59:38E.

Rankin AC et al: Adenosine or adenosine triphosphate for supraventricular tachycardias? Comparative double-blind randomized study in patients with spontaneous or inducible arrhythmias. Am Heart J 1990;119:316.

Roden DM et al: Medical intelligence: Flecainide. N Engl J Med 1986;315:36.

Selzer A: Atrial fibrillation revisited. (Editorial.) N Engl J Med 1982;306:1044.

Symposium: Clinical Evaluation of Response to Antiarrhythmic Therapy. Am J Cardiol 1988;62:1. (Review.)

Torres V, Flowers D, Somberg JC: The arrhythmogenicity of antiarrhythmic agents. Am Heart J 1985;109:1090.

Troup PJ: Implantable cardioverters and defibrillators. Curr Probl Cardiol 1989;14:675.

Viskin S et al: Acute management of paroxysmal atrioventricular junctional reentrant supraventricular tachycardia: Pharmacologic strategies. Am Heart J 1990;120:180.

Waldo A: Mechanism of atrial fibrillation, atrial flutter, and ectopic atrial tachycardia: A brief review. Circulation 1987;75(Suppl III):37.

Wellens HJJ: The wide QRS tachycardia. Ann Intern Med 1986;104:879.

Wellens HJJ, Bar FWHM, Lie KI: The value of the electrocardiogram in the differential diagnosis of a tachycardia with a widened QRS complex. Am J Med 1978;64:27.

Wellens HJJ et al: The management of preexcitation syndromes. JAMA 1987;257:2325.

Winkle RA et al: Practical aspects of automatic cardioverter/defibrillator implantation. Am Heart J 1984;108:1335.

Wu D: Supraventricular tachycardias. JAMA 1983;249:3357.

Zipes DP (editor): Symposium on cardiac arrhythmias. (2 parts.) Med Clin North Am 1984;68:793, 1013.

30

Obstetric & Gynecologic Emergencies & Rape

Phillip J. Goldstein, MD

IMMEDIATE MANAGEMENT OF LIFE-THREATENING PROBLEMS

ABNORMAL VAGINAL BLEEDING
(See Table 30–1.)

Patients with active vaginal bleeding are at high risk of exsanguination and require immediate evaluation and treatment of other findings.

Emergency Evaluation & Treatment

A. Obtain vital signs with the patient supine.

1. Hypotension–Examine for hypotension or tachycardia due to depletion of intravascular volume. If blood pressure and pulse are normal in the supine position, measure them in the sitting position, and if still normal, in the standing position to detect more subtle volume depletion. Supine or postural hypotension indicates life-threatening hemorrhage.

2. Tachycardia–Tachycardia while the patient is resting or when she assumes the upright posture also may indicate probable vascular depletion.

B. Treat shock if present (Chapter 3). Briefly—

1. Insert at least one large-bore intravenous catheter ($\geq$ 16-gauge). A venous cutdown or central venous catheter may be preferable (Chapter 46) if peripheral venous access is not readily obtainable.

Table 30–1. Causes of abnormal vaginal bleeding.

Premenarcheal vaginal bleeding
  Menarche
  Tumor (vaginal, uterine)
  Genital trauma
  Foreign body
  Precocious puberty
  Hematuria
  Miscellaneous
Reproductive age bleeding
  Variations in normal cycle
    Hypermenorrhea (excessive bleeding at time of period)
    Polymenorrhea (menstrual periods < 21 days apart)
  Metrorrhagia (including ectopic)
    Abortion
    Pregnancy (including ectopic)
    Endocrine abnormality (idiopathic, estrogens, thyroid)
    Salpingitis
    Cervicitis
    Coagulopathy (factor VIII deficiency)
    Malignant neoplasm or polyps (cervical, vaginal, uterine)
    Ovarian cyst
    Myoma of uterus
    Trophoblastic tumor
  Miscellaneous (mittelschmerz)
Postmenopausal bleeding
  Carcinoma (cervical, uterine)
  Estrogen excess
  Atrophic vaginitis
  Cervical polyps
  Trauma
  Miscellaneous

2. Determine the amount of blood loss, and draw blood for the following:

a. Typing and cross-matching (reserve 4 units of fresh-frozen plasma and 2–4 units of packed red cells); whole blood may be used if it is readily available.

b. Platelet count, prothrombin time, and partial thromboplastin time to uncover any bleeding abnormality.

c. Hematocrit and CBC.

d. Renal function tests and measurement of serum electrolytes.

e. Arterial blood gas measurements and pH (useful in assessing adequacy of ventilation and perfusion).

f. If the patient is of childbearing age, obtain a serum or urinary monoclonal antibody pregnancy test.

3. Begin rapid infusion of crystalloid solution (Ringer's injection or normal saline), the rate depending on vital signs (eg, 200–1000 mL/h), to restore intravascular volume and maintain blood pressure until compatible blood becomes available for transfusion.

4. Infuse cross-matched blood as soon as possible. Give 2 or more units depending on vital signs.

C. Determine the cause of bleeding, and stop it. *The following measures should not be used in third-trimester pregnancy* (p 539):

1. Compression of uterus–Insert one hand in the vagina, elevate the uterus, and compress it against the abdominal wall and the other hand.

2. Culdocentesis–If there is a history of recent abnormal menstrual bleeding and if significant pelvic pain is present, culdocentesis is mandatory to rule out ectopic pregnancy (Fig 30–1).

D. If trauma has occurred, determine the extent of injury, and apply pressure to the bleeding site.

E. Obtain urgent gynecologic or surgical consultation.

Disposition

Patients with vaginal bleeding resulting in abnormal hemodynamics or anemia should be hospitalized.

PELVIC PAIN WITH OR WITHOUT BLEEDING
(See Table 30–2.)

Diagnosis

A. History: Obtain information about the following points:

1. Possible pregnancy (recent amenorrhea or abnormal period, intercourse without contraception, morning sickness, or tenderness of breasts of recent onset).

2. History of trauma, including rape or illegal abortion.

3. History of salpingitis.

4. History of ectopic pregnancy.

5. Duration of symptoms and relation to menses.

6. Type of pain (cramping or constant).

Table 30–2. Differential diagnosis of pelvic pain.

	History and Symptoms				Signs					Laboratory Findings		
	Relationship to Menstrual Period	Prior Salpingitis	Quality of Pain	Type of Vaginal Discharge	Fever	Cervix	Uterus	Adnexal Mass	Adnexal Tenderness	Culdocentesis	Urine Immunologic Pregnancy Test	Leukocytosis
Salpingitis	Accompanying or just after period.	+	Constant and severe.	Scant to purulent.	+	Tender with motion.	Tender.	None.	Usually bilateral.	Purulent.	–	++
Salpingitis plus tubo-ovarian abscess								+				Also, elevated erythrocyte sedimentation rate.
Incomplete abortion	Period of amenorrhea with recent spotting or frank blood.	±	Cramping and suprapubic.	Heavy blood clots.	–	Dilated.	Enlarged, tender.	None.	None.	Not indicated.	+ in 75%.	±
Septic abortion				Thick and bloody; foul-smelling.	+	Dilated, tender.	Enlarged, tender.	±	Bilateral.	Not indicated.	+ in 75%.	++
Ectopic pregnancy	Amenorrhea with recent spotting.	±	Intermittent; variable severity.	Scant but rarely none.	±	Slightly tender.	Normal to slightly enlarged.	+	Unilateral.	Nonclotting blood.	+ in 50%.	±
Ruptured ovarian cyst	Precedes period.	–	Sudden and severe.	None.	±	Normal.	Normal.	±	Unilateral.	Bloody fluid.	Indicated.	±
Mittelschmerz	Mid cycle.	–	Sudden.	Spotting.	–	Normal.	Normal.	None.	Unilateral.	Not indicated.	–	–
Torsion of ovarian tumor	None.	–	Intermittent; radiates to thigh.	None.	±	Slightly tender.	Slightly tender.	None.	Unilateral.	Not indicated.	–	–
Endometritis with or without IUD	Variable.	±	Cramping.	Scant or none.	+	Variable.	Slightly tender.	+ if tubal abscess.	Variable.	Not indicated.	±	±
Dysmenorrhea	Accompanies period.	±	Cramping.	Normal menses.	–	Normal.	Variable tenderness.	Negative.	Seldom.	Not indicated.	–	–
Appendicitis	None.	–	Periumbilical; cramping, progressing to constant right lower quadrant.	None.	±	Normal.	Normal.	None.	Unilateral. Right-sided.	Rarely purulent.	–	±

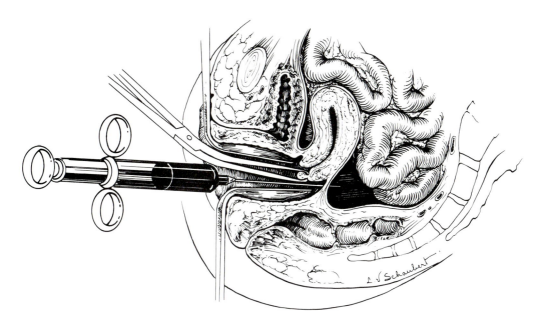

Figure 30–1. Technique of culdocentesis. With the patient in the lithotomy position, insert the largest possible vaginal speculum, and lock it in the open position. Disinfect the vaginal mucosa with povidone-iodine. Elevate and maintain tension on the cervix by caudal traction on a tenaculum. Insert an 18-gauge, 6.5-cm (2½-in) needle on a 20-mL syringe in the midline of the posterior fornix 1–1.5 cm (⅜–⅝ in) posterior to the cervix. Aspirate gently to obtain fluid present in the cul-de-sac. (Reproduced, with permission, from Pernoll ML [editor]: *Current Obstetric & Gynecologic Diagnosis & Treatment,* 7th ed. Appleton & Lange, 1991.)

7. Type and amount of vaginal bleeding or discharge.

8. Use of intrauterine contraceptive device.

B. Symptoms and Signs: Fever is often the first sign of infection, and pelvic warmth (from local inflammation) may be noted on bimanual examination. Pelvic organs are tender and engorged.

C. Laboratory Tests and Special Examinations:

1. The white cell count, differential, and erythrocyte sedimentation rate may reflect inflammation.

2. A pregnancy test is important if pain or bleeding is present (Table 30–3 and Fig 30–2). Qualitative monoclonal antibody tests of blood or urine are sensitive and may provide positive test results within 7 days of conception. They are also relatively inexpensive, easy to do, and can be performed in 5 minutes. When available, this is the preferred screening test for pregnancy. Quantitative blood tests are more sensitive but take 2–3 hours to perform and require expensive equipment and specially trained personnel. Tube tests are slightly more sensitive than slide tests but take 1–2 hours compared to 2–5 minutes for a slide test. These tests are performed using urine samples, and false-positive results may occur in the presence of psychotropic drugs, methadone, sperm, or proteinuria.

Table 30–3. Comparison of common pregnancy tests.

Type	Sensitivity (hCG in mIU/mL)	Specimen Required	Shortest Time From Last Menstrual Period to Positive Test (Days)	Time Needed to Perform Test
Slide	750–1500	Urine	38	25 minutes
Self-diagnostic (home pregnancy testing)	500–1500	Urine	38	1–2 hours
Tube	200–1000	Urine	30	1–2 hours
Radioreceptor assay	200	Blood	28–31	2–3 hours
Radioimmunoassay (quantitative)	5–40	Blood/urine	24	2–3 hours
Monoclonal antibody (qualitative)	25 (blood) 50 (urine)	Blood/urine	19–21	5 minutes

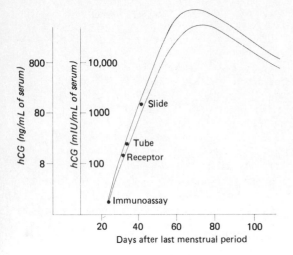

Figure 30–2. Serum hCG levels at various stages of pregnancy. The sensitivity of common assays for hCG (and the approximate time of pregnancy at which they would be positive) is also shown.

3. Obtain cervical swab cultures for gonococci and *Chlamydia* if infection is a possible diagnosis.

4. If culdocentesis shows nonclotting blood, ectopic pregnancy and ruptured ovarian cyst are possible diagnoses. Salpingitis or septic abortion is a possible diagnosis if purulent material is obtained. *Negative culdocentesis (no material obtained) does not exclude disease,* and the patient should be monitored for any signs of deterioration.

5. Laparoscopy or ultrasonography may be helpful when the diagnosis is uncertain.

Treatment & Disposition

If the diagnosis is uncertain but either ectopic pregnancy or septic abortion is a possibility, hospitalization or daily follow-up on an outpatient basis is mandatory.

EMERGENCY MANAGEMENT OF GYNECOLOGIC DISORDERS

Signs and symptoms of common pelvic disorders are listed in Table 30–4.

ECTOPIC PREGNANCY

Ectopic pregnancy is commonly encountered in the emergency department and may be difficult to diagnose. Since it is potentially life-threatening, it

Table 30–4. Clinical manifestations of common pelvic disorders.

Clinical Findings	Possible Causes
Bleeding	Trauma Postpartum hemorrhage Dysfunctional uterine bleeding Carcinoma
Pain	Salpingitis and tubo-ovarian abscess Ruptured ovarian cyst Torsion of tube and ovary Mittelschmerz Abdominal disorders (appendicitis, etc)
Pain and bleeding	Dysmenorrhea Endometriosis Endometritis
Pregnancy and bleeding	Placenta previa Ectopic pregnancy Spontaneous abortion Abruptio placentae
Pregnancy and pain	Ectopic pregnancy Degenerating fibroid (leiomyoma) Normal labor
Pregnancy with pain and bleeding	Labor with placenta previa Abruptio placentae Septic abortion Puerperal sepsis Ectopic pregnancy

should be suspected in any patient presenting with menstrual irregularities, vaginal bleeding, and pelvic or lower abdominal pain. The most common presenting complaint is vaginal bleeding, often scant at first, with crampy lower abdominal pain.

The incidence of ectopic pregnancy is increased in women using an intrauterine contraceptive device (IUD) and in those with a history of pelvic infection (eg, salpingitis), tubal surgery, and previous tubal pregnancies. About 98% of ectopic pregnancies are tubal.

Rupture of the uterine tube followed by free intraperitoneal bleeding from tubal vessels is the principal cause of illness and death.

Diagnosis

A. Symptoms and Signs: There is a history of the following: **(1)** amenorrhea or abnormal menses, followed by persistent vaginal bleeding; **(2)** pelvic pain following amenorrhea; and **(3)** intermittent pain (occasionally). Rupture of the uterine tube brings temporary relief of pain.

Symptoms of early pregnancy (eg, breast tenderness, nausea) may be present. Peritoneal pain is present after tubal rupture with bleeding into the peritoneum. Referred shoulder pain is occasionally present. Syncope or light-headedness may occur.

In the early stages of ectopic pregnancy, the results of pelvic examination may be normal. Symptoms, if present, may be completely nonspecific initially, because the tubal pregnancy producing them may be in the early stages of development. In advanced cases, a tender adnexal mass, enlarged uterus, or blood in the peritoneal cavity (eg, doughy cul-de-sac) may occur.

Obtain complete vital signs, including sitting and standing pulse and blood pressure measurements if normal in the supine position, to look for supine or orthostatic hypotension.

B. Laboratory Tests and Special Examinations:

1. Pregnancy test–The standard urine pregnancy tests are positive in only 50–75% of cases (Table 30–3). Radioimmunoassay for the β subunit of hCG is positive in more than 90% of cases, and with monoclonal antibody urinary pregnancy tests (eg, ICON), results are easily available. However, quantitative serum hCG determination, if available, is preferred over qualitative urine tests. In a normal intrauterine pregnancy in the first trimester, the β subunit of hCG should double every other day.

2. Ultrasonography–Vaginal ultrasound scan is useful in demonstrating an intrauterine gestational sac if present, virtually ruling out ectopic pregnancy. Occasionally, a mass can be seen in the adnexa or cul-de-sac, or products of conception can be visualized outside the uterine cavity, and ectopic pregnancy can be readily diagnosed. A small intrauterine sac ("pseudosac") may be seen, and ectopic pregnancy may still be a possibility. In very early pregnancy, the uterine cavity may appear empty.

3. Culdocentesis–Culdocentesis is the most useful procedure for demonstrating the presence of free blood in the pelvis (Fig 30–1). Culdocentesis may not demonstrate blood in some cases; on the other hand, blood may be recovered in rupture of a corpus luteum ovarian cyst occurring during *normal* intrauterine pregnancy.

4. Laparoscopy or laparotomy–Laparoscopy or laparotomy may be necessary to make a definitive diagnosis of ectopic pregnancy.

Treatment & Disposition

Treatment of possible or confirmed ectopic pregnancy and subsequent disposition vary with severity of symptoms.

A. Ectopic Pregnancy Highly Probable: Blood is found on culdocentesis, or ultrasound scan reveals empty uterine cavity and mass or products of conception in the adnexa or cul-de-sac. Pregnancy is confirmed by signs, symptoms, or positive pregnancy test, and the patient has pelvic tenderness or an adnexal mass.

1. Prevent or correct hemorrhagic shock by inserting a large-bore (≥ 16-gauge) intravenous catheter and infusing crystalloid solution for volume replacement. Type and cross-match for 2–3 units of whole blood. Insert a urinary (eg, Foley) catheter, and send urine for analysis.

2. Obtain emergency obstetric consultation, and prepare the patient for surgery. Obtain CBC; serum electrolyte, blood urea nitrogen, and creatinine determinations; coagulation profile; and other studies as required.

B. Ectopic Pregnancy Probable: Vaginal bleeding, pelvic pain, and tenderness without explanation are present in a woman of childbearing age. Pregnancy test results are positive or equivocal, but culdocentesis is negative.

1. Insert an intravenous catheter, and send blood for CBC and typing and cross-matching.

2. Obtain pelvic sonogram.

3. If ultrasonography cannot be performed or if the result is equivocal, obtain emergency obstetric consultation and consider hospitalizing the patient for observation.

C. Ectopic Pregnancy Possible: Vaginal bleeding or pelvic pain is present. Pregnancy is possible but unlikely. The results of physical examination and laboratory studies are normal. Ultrasonography cannot be readily obtained or the result is indeterminate.

1. Send blood for quantitative β–hCG.

2. Discharge the patient from the emergency department to outpatient care with a definite follow-up appointment for reevaluation within 1–2 days.

3. Give the patient *written* instructions explaining that ectopic pregnancy is a possible diagnosis and that she must be alert to the following symptoms, which would require that she return to the hospital immediately: (**1**) increased vaginal bleeding, (**2**) increased pelvic or abdominal pain, or (**3**) syncope.

4. Have the patient sign a statement saying that she has received such instructions.

SPONTANEOUS ABORTION

At least 20% of all pregnancies terminate in abortion, usually because of serious defects in the ovum. Half of abortions occur before the eighth week of gestation and another quarter before the 16th week.

Many of these early spontaneous abortions go unnoticed as a "delayed menstrual period." On the other hand, early spontaneous abortions are also a common cause of visits to the emergency department.

If the fetus dies but is not expelled, a "missed abortion" occurs. If this state persists for longer than 4–6 weeks, disseminated intravascular coagulation may occur.

Classification of Spontaneous Abortion

Symptoms and signs characterizing the various types of spontaneous abortion are described below.

A. Threatened Abortion:

1. Mild, transient uterine cramps with minimal transient vaginal bleeding are noted.

2. The cervix is long and closed.

3. Uterine size is compatible with the presumed length of pregnancy. Uterine size in centimeters measured from the top of the symphysis pubica to the top of the uterine fundus is a useful approximation of gestational age in weeks from 15–16 weeks through 32–33 weeks.

4. Symptoms of pregnancy continue, and the conceptus remains viable.

B. Inevitable Abortion:

1. Persistent uterine cramps and moderate vaginal bleeding are noted.

2. The cervical os is open (ie, a 0.5-cm [3/16-in] diameter sponge stick passes easily).

3. Passage of some or all of the products of conception is inevitable or is about to occur; ie, fetal or placental tissue is found in the vagina or protrudes through the cervical os, or the patient gives a history of passage of tissue.

4. Symptoms and signs of pregnancy disappear.

C. Incomplete Abortion:

1. Uterine cramps and vaginal bleeding are persistent and excessive.

2. Symptoms of pregnancy may disappear.

3. Products of conception are noted in the vagina, or the patient gives a history of passage of tissue.

D. Complete Abortion:

1. Uterine cramps markedly diminish or stop.

2. Vaginal bleeding ceases.

3. The entire conceptus is expelled.

4. Symptoms of pregnancy disappear.

E. Missed Abortion:

1. The products of conception are retained.

2. Symptoms and signs of pregnancy abate, and results of pregnancy tests change to negative.

3. Brownish vaginal discharge (rarely, frank bleeding) occurs.

4. Uterine cramps are rare.

5. Examination shows a small and irregularly softened uterus.

6. Ultrasonography fails to demonstrate a live fetus; ie, there is absence of fetal heart motion.

Diagnosis

A. Symptoms and Signs: Almost all patients have a history suggesting possible pregnancy:

1. Sexual intercourse without adequate contraception.

2. Period of amenorrhea.

3. Nausea and vomiting; breast tenderness.

4. Uterine cramps and vaginal bleeding.

5. Passage of fetal or placental tissue (in inevitable, incomplete, or complete abortion).

Caution: Pelvic examination should be performed on all patients with suspected abortion and on all pregnant patients with vaginal bleeding who have reached less than 20 weeks' gestation. Extreme care, however, must be exercised in examining patients in the second trimester; instruments should not be introduced into the cervical os. Beyond 20 weeks' gesta-

tion, pelvic examination should be done by an obstetrician because of the increasing risk of placenta previa.

B. Laboratory Tests and Special Examinations: Serum pregnancy test is positive. Urinary pregnancy test is positive in about 75% of cases. In the first trimester of pregnancy, a β–hCG level that does not double in 48 hours suggests fetal demise. Real-time ultrasonography, using abdominal or vaginal probes, can be diagnostic, eg, fetus without heartbeat or movement. Pathologic examination of tissue expelled by the uterus confirms passage of the products of conception.

Treatment & Disposition

Blood typing and antibody screening are required in all patients with abortion of any type. If patients are Rh-negative, give $Rh_o(D)$ immune globulin (Rho-GAM, many others), 1 vial, within 72 hours after any event in which fetal-maternal transfusion may occur, including abortion.

A. Threatened Abortion: Advise the patient to rest. Use analgesics and sedatives only if absolutely necessary, because of possible teratogenic effects. Do not use hormones, douches, or tampons. The patient should not engage in coitus. Ultrasound scan may reveal a gestational sac or evidence of fetal cardiac activity.

B. Incomplete or Inevitable Abortion: Hospitalize the patient if hypovolemia or anemia is present or if the pregnancy is past the first trimester. Treat hypovolemia if present. Perform suction curettage or dilation and curettage as the treatment of choice. An oxytocin drip, 20 IU of oxytocin in 1000 mL of crystalloid solution infused at a rate of 50–100 mL/h, may be tried as an alternative, but if it is unsuccessful in achieving evacuation of the uterus, cervical dilation and uterine evacuation by curettage must be performed.

C. Complete Abortion: The patient may be discharged to home care if vital signs and hematocrit are stable and if vaginal bleeding is clearly decreasing. If the diagnosis of complete abortion is certain or after surgical evacuation has been performed in the emergency department, give methylergonovine maleate (Methergine), 0.2 mg orally 3 times daily for 3 days, to help stop bleeding.

D. Missed Abortion (Retained Conceptus): Obtain CBC, differential, and coagulation panel (platelet count, prothrombin time, and partial thromboplastin time). Obtain disseminated intravascular coagulation screening tests if abnormal values are found. Hospitalize the patient, and prepare to perform dilation and curettage if there is evidence of infection or disseminated intravascular coagulation or if the products of conception have been retained more than 4 weeks.

Outpatient management of early missed abortion is possible if the patient is closely monitored for possible spontaneous abortion and if fibrinogen levels are measured weekly. Levels below 150 mg/dL call for evacuation of the uterus.

SEPTIC ABORTION

Septic abortion occurs after therapeutic abortion in 0.2% of procedures. Septic abortion may also arise as a result of nonsterile illegal abortion. The usual cause of sepsis is incomplete evacuation of the products of conception. Infection is usually due to mixed aerobic and anaerobic bacteria and is rapidly progressive, extending quickly through the myometrium and involving the adnexa and pelvic peritoneum. Septic pelvic thrombophlebitis with or without septic pulmonary embolization is an uncommon but devastating complication.

Diagnosis

A. Symptoms and Signs: Symptoms and signs are consistent with a history of recent pregnancy and induced abortion followed by pelvic pain and symptoms of infection. Repeated questioning in a private room by a physician who has gained the patient's confidence may be necessary to elicit a history of criminal abortion; in some cases, such a history is never obtained. Clinical findings include signs of infection (eg, fever, leukocytosis), diffuse pelvic tenderness, and profuse, foul vaginal discharge in most cases. Frank septic shock may be present.

B. Imaging Studies: Ultrasound or other imaging techniques (CT, MRI) may show retained intrauterine material, uterine emphysema, or intraperitoneal air from uterine perforation.

Treatment & Disposition

Evacuation of the uterine contents is crucial and is the mainstay of treatment. It should be preceded by broad-spectrum antibiotic therapy (see ¶E, below).

Note: Although antibiotic therapy alone is effective in the earliest stage of infection, many patients require emergency hysterectomy. Death may occur despite the best treatment.

A. Hospitalize the patient at once, and start general measures for septic shock (Chapters 3 and 34).

B. Obtain emergency surgical obstetric and gynecologic consultation.

C. Obtain samples of blood and uterine discharge for culture.

D. Draw blood for CBC, tests of hepatic and renal function, serum electrolyte determination, prothrombin time, partial thromboplastin time, platelet count, and disseminated intravascular coagulation screening tests if initial findings are abnormal.

E. After taking specimens for culture of aerobic and anaerobic organisms, give antibiotics, eg, clindamycin, 600 mg intravenously every 6 hours; plus gentamicin or tobramycin, 5 mg/kg/d intrave-

nously or intramuscularly in 3 divided doses. Monitor renal function and serum levels of gentamicin or tobramycin, adjusting subsequent doses in accordance with results. A third-generation cephalosporin (eg, moxalactam or cefoperazone, 2 g intravenously every 8 hours) may be substituted for tobramycin. Penicillin, 3–4 million units every 3–4 hours by intravenous infusion, may be added to the above regimen for broadened coverage (eg, against enterococci).

Alternative treatment regimens, which in the author's opinion are less satisfactory, include cefoxitin, 2 g intravenously every 4 hours; or chloramphenicol, 1 g intravenously every 6 hours.

CARCINOMA & OTHER TUMORS

Although gynecologic cancers seldom present as emergency situations, the emergency physician should be aware of the various presenting symptoms and risk factors associated with gynecologic cancers.

Carcinoma of the Vulva

Vulvar cancers are rarely sudden in onset and usually occur in women over 50 years of age. They are more common in women with a history of cervical dysplasia or cancer.

Patients seeking treatment for vulvar lesions in the emergency department should be advised to seek gynecologic consultation if any lesion initially thought to be due to infection or trauma fails to heal in a short time. Persistent unremitting vaginal pruritus is the single most common symptom of vulvar cancer and should never be dismissed as a frivolous complaint in the postmenopausal patient.

The greatest pitfall in diagnosis of any vulvar lesion is failure to perform biopsy of suspicious areas. Vulvar biopsy using the dermal punch method is easily accomplished even in the emergency department setting, and it should be performed whenever there is any doubt about the cause of a lesion or whenever it is uncertain whether the patient would return for further care.

Carcinoma of the Vagina

Vaginal cancers are rare. Bleeding is typically the presenting complaint. The patient is usually 50 years of age or older, but even teenagers have developed clear cell carcinoma—eg, girls whose mothers were treated with diethylstilbestrol during pregnancy.

The source of the vaginal bleeding must be identified, and a speculum should be used to carefully inspect the vaginal walls. Careful digital examination of the vaginal mucosa is critical to detect submucosal infiltration by the tumor.

Carcinoma of the Cervix

Vaginal bleeding is the most common symptom in

cervical cancer. Patients may be in their late 20s to (most commonly) early 40s. Patients often complain of persistent watery discharge. Speculum examination reveals a necrotic friable lesion on the cervix.

Uncontrollable bleeding from the cervix may be treated with applications of ferric subsulfate solution or vaginal packing. Manipulation should be kept to a minimum. Biopsy of the lesion at its margin with normal tissue usually confirms the diagnosis, but this procedure should be performed only in an operating room.

Carcinoma of the Endometrium

Postmenopausal bleeding is the most common symptom of endometrial carcinoma. Risk factors associated with endometrial carcinoma include ingestion of exogenous estrogens, obesity, infertility, Stein-Leventhal syndrome, and age over 50 years.

Diagnosis requires fractional dilation and curettage. An endometrial biopsy using a Pipelle catheter, if available, is simple to perform. The physician should not try to stop postmenopausal bleeding with administration of hormones (eg, estrogens or progesterone) without confirming the diagnosis beforehand with dilation and curettage performed as soon as possible after the bleeding episode (preferably within 1 month).

Carcinoma of the Ovaries

Patients with ovarian cancer may have abdominal distention from ascites, intestinal obstruction, or rarely, acute abdominal pain. The possibility of ovarian cancer should be considered in any woman with abdominal or pelvic symptoms. Definitive diagnosis requires surgical or gynecologic consultation for laparotomy or laparoscopy.

Other Tumors

Patients with gestational trophoblastic disease may present with heavy vaginal bleeding and symptoms similar to those of early miscarriage, but the following suggest trophoblastic disease: (1) heavy vaginal bleeding with or without passage of tissue, or great clusters of tissue aborted from the cervical os; (2) uterine size inappropriately large for dates; (3) profound anemia; and (4) history of molar pregnancy.

The diagnosis can be confirmed by ultrasound examination. Any patient presenting with neurologic signs and with a recent history of molar pregnancy or trophoblastic disease may have cerebral metastasis.

Central nervous system metastasis of trophoblastic disease represents a *true oncologic emergency,* since cerebral metastasis has the potential for cure as long as rapid growth or hemorrhage does not occur. Patients with trophoblastic disease should be hospitalized for gynecologic consultation and possible referral to a regional trophoblastic disease center, where help is readily available.

GENITAL TRAUMA

Genital trauma in women almost always occurs as a result of sexual activity, either forced (rape) or voluntary (foreign bodies introduced into the vagina in sexual play). Penile thrusts rarely produce trauma unless it is the first sexual experience.

Diagnosis

The most common presenting complaints are vaginal bleeding and pain or dyspareunia. Examination usually reveals bleeding from a tear in the genital mucosa or skin. Bleeding is rarely brisk enough to produce signs of hypovolemia, but if these are present, replace volume losses, and provide supportive care (Chapter 3). In prepubertal patients, general anesthesia may be required for adequate examination.

Treatment & Disposition

A. Determine whether rape has occurred, and proceed accordingly (p 534). Provide sedation or analgesia if necessary.

B. Treat hypovolemia if present.

C. Control vaginal bleeding temporarily with a vaginal pack or, if bleeding is from the external genitalia, with direct firm pressure (combined with an indwelling urinary catheter).

D. Hospitalize the patient if bleeding cannot be easily and definitively controlled, and obtain gynecologic consultation.

E. Small lesions at the introitus may be repaired in the emergency department under local anesthesia. However, small and seemingly minor vaginal tears may communicate with either the rectum or the peritoneum; consequently, such repairs are best performed by a gynecologist in an operating room with adequate anesthesia and good exposure.

RUPTURED OVARIAN CYST

Diagnosis

Ruptured ovarian cyst is associated with sudden, moderately severe pelvic or lower abdominal pain. There are no gastrointestinal symptoms. The patient is afebrile, and leukocytosis is variable. Tenderness is found over the affected ovary, and there are no masses. A pregnancy test should be obtained, since ectopic pregnancy is a possible diagnosis. Ultrasonography may show the presence of an ovarian cyst or free pelvic fluid and is useful to detect ectopic pregnancy. Culdocentesis may show blood or serosanguineous fluid.

Treatment & Disposition

The patient should be observed and may require hospitalization if the diagnosis is uncertain or if relief is required for severe pain. Surgery is rarely required.

TORSION OF OVARIAN TUMOR

Diagnosis

Torsion of ovarian tumor is associated with a history of attacks of cramps and pains in the lower abdomen and possibly in the flank. The symptoms, such as nausea, may be gradual, or they may occur suddenly if there is accompanying intraovarian bleeding. Discomfort is characterized by symptoms of pelvic mass, eg, painful defecation and dyspareunia. Ultrasonography may delineate the mass.

Treatment & Disposition

Hospitalize the patient, and obtain urgent gynecologic consultation. Pelvic ultrasonography may be a useful diagnostic tool, but laparoscopy is frequently required. Laparotomy is indicated if the diagnosis is confirmed or if the patient's condition deteriorates.

ENDOMETRIOSIS

Diagnosis

The patient with endometriosis gives a history of attacks of cramps and pains in the lower abdomen and possibly in the flank that are associated with menstruation. Symptoms may be gradual or sudden if there is accompanying bleeding. Acquired dysmenorrhea is most commonly due to endometriosis. Other symptoms include painful defecation and dyspareunia.

Treatment & Disposition

The patient should be referred for further gynecologic evaluation. Definitive diagnosis usually requires laparoscopy. Provide oral analgesia as needed.

DYSMENORRHEA

Diagnosis

Many women experience painful menstruation (dysmenorrhea). The pain is cramping in nature, may be debilitating, and is usually relieved by release of menstrual contents from the uterus. The pain occurs because of elaboration of excessive quantities of prostaglandins by the endometrium with subsequent increased uterine tone. It is *not* psychologic in origin.

Idiopathic dysmenorrhea usually begins at menarche and is probably more common than the acquired form. Acquired dysmenorrhea, occurring in the late teens and early 20s, may suggest endometriosis and is common in chronic pelvic inflammatory disease.

Treatment & Disposition

Both types of dysmenorrhea may be seen by the emergency physician and may be treated by aspirin; however, other prostaglandin inhibitors are more effective (eg, ibuprofen [Advil, many others], 400 mg orally every 6 hours; naproxen [Anaprox, Naprosyn], 250–275 mg orally every 6 hours; mefenamic acid [Ponstel], 250 mg orally every 6 hours). Local application of heat to the lower abdomen may be helpful as well.

MITTELSCHMERZ

Midcycle pain (mittelschmerz) is common in women with regular menstrual periods who are not taking birth control pills. These patients may commonly have midcycle spotting caused by an estrogen surge. There is no fever and no other abnormal bleeding such as that resulting from trauma to the cervix (eg, coitus, douching). Pain usually occurs over several cycles. There is no history of intermittent lower abdominal pain. Examination at the time of mittelschmerz may reveal some lower quadrant tenderness with or without rebound. Bimanual examination may show localized tenderness. A palpable ovary may be present, but a history of regular menses, lack of fever, and negative pregnancy tests confirm the diagnosis.

Mild analgesics and reassurance are usually adequate for these patients.

UTERINE PROLAPSE

Prolapse typically occurs because of muscular defects in the pelvic floor arising from childbirth.

Diagnosis

Uterine prolapse is characterized by variable symptoms of pelvic heaviness or a dragging sensation and lower back pain. Urinary retention of sudden onset may be a presenting complaint. Examination reveals a firm, muscular mass in the vagina or protruding from the vagina (procidentia) and having the shape and size of the uterus and cervix. Cystocele, rectocele, and enterocele are commonly associated with procidentia.

Treatment & Disposition

Acute *postpartum* prolapse is an emergency that requires immediate obstetric and gynecologic consultation. Patients with acute urinary retention or procidentia should have urgent gynecologic consultation. Patients with mild prolapse should be referred within 5–7 days for gynecologic evaluation and possible surgery.

SALPINGITIS & TUBO-OVARIAN ABSCESS

See Chapter 34.

RAPE (MEN & WOMEN)

Proper care of the alleged rape victim requires concern for the social and emotional consequences of the event as well as for the medical sequelae. The best care fulfills the requirements of the law while providing proper support and reassurance to the patient. The physician's responsibilities include the following:

A. Recognizing and managing life-threatening trauma (hemorrhagic shock, etc).

B. Obtaining informed written consent for physical examination, collection of evidence, photographic documentation, and treatment.

C. Shielding the alleged rape victim from other patients, bystanders, and visitors.

D. Accurately diagnosing and treating all physical injuries, both genital and nongenital.

E. Recording a detailed and explicit history of the event in the patient's own words.

F. Carefully collecting specimens for evidence, with accurate documentation and protection of the chain of evidence.

G. Providing psychologic support and follow-up.

H. Offering prophylaxis against pregnancy and sexually transmitted disease.

I. Avoiding a "diagnosis" of rape (it is not a medical diagnosis but a matter of jurisprudence). The physician should also avoid judgmental or conclusive language.

J. Being willing to testify in court.

Unless required to do so by statute, the emergency physician does not have a legal obligation to notify the police when treating a victim of alleged rape. Notifying the police is appropriate when the patient has consented (preferably in writing) to such notification. The physician may wish to refer the patient to a counseling organization that provides aid to victims of rape.

The responsibilities described above are usually best fulfilled by having teams experienced in working with rape victims perform the evaluation. They should follow an established written protocol and document all findings in writing.

1. MANAGEMENT OF THE FEMALE RAPE VICTIM

Diagnosis & Evaluation

A. Inform the police (with patient's consent).

B. Obtain written informed consent for examination.

C. Obtain and record the history in the patient's own words. Obtain answers to other specific questions (if they have not already been answered). Fig 30–3 is a sample rape evaluation form with the appropriate questions. Record the general appearance and demeanor of the victim, and note whether clothing is torn or stained.

D. Collect and label relevant evidence, and protect the chain of evidence.

1. Scrape under the fingernails, and also take trimmings from them.

2. Comb pubic hair, and look for loose hairs from the assailant.

3. Cut off a few pubic hairs and save them.

4. Collect any other loose hairs or dried blood.

5. Examine the perineum and other suspect areas with a Wood light (prostatic secretions are fluorescent even when dry).

6. Examine a saline wet mount of vaginal secretions for spermatozoa; record their number and motility.

7. Prepare 4 dried slides of vaginal contents (wash the vagina with saline if it is dry), and fix them with ether-alcohol.

8. Collect vaginal aspirate or washings into a screw-topped specimen tube for acid phosphatase determination (a positive reaction indicates the presence of prostatic fluid ejaculate).

9. Place a cotton swab of vaginal contents into a specimen tube (for typing of the blood group antigen in semen).

10. Obtain material from the cervix for culture for gonococci and *Chlamydia*.

11. Obtain urine for urinalysis (look for hematuria indicating genitourinary trauma).

12. Photograph all external lesions, but only with the patient's written consent.

13. If oral or rectal penetration has occurred, steps 5–9 should be repeated with specimens from those sites.

E. Perform a physical examination.

1. Thoroughly examine the patient for signs of trauma, discharge, or bleeding; record the results of the examination; and photograph all lesions (the last only with the patient's written consent).

2. Perform a pelvic examination.

a. Look carefully for signs of trauma to the external genitalia.

b. Note and record whether the hymen is intact and whether any hymenal tags are fresh (indicating trauma) or healed.

c. Using a warm, water-moistened speculum, carefully examine the vagina for lacerations. Rarely, peritoneal perforation may occur.

d. Evaluate the cervix for signs of preexisting pregnancy and trauma.

e. Examine the rectal area. If penetration has occurred, proctoscopy may be advisable.

F. Obtain blood for blood chemistry studies (if indicated), a serologic test for syphilis, blood typing (to compare the alleged assailant's type with that of the victim), and pregnancy testing.

Treatment

The physician should be empathic and concerned, never skeptical or judgmental. Comments and discussion should not be pursued in the presence of the patient.

A. Prevent sexually transmitted disease. Treatment for gonorrhea, *Chlamydia,* and syphilis (Chapter 34) should be offered but not forced upon the patient. Only about 3% of rapes result in gonorrhea, and only about 0.1% of cases result in syphilis. Follow-up cultures for *N gonorrhoeae* are essential. Perform a follow-up serologic test for syphilis 1 and 3 months after the rape.

B. Prevent pregnancy. Treatment for the prevention of pregnancy should be offered but not forced on the patient. Only about 1% of rapes result in pregnancy; the chances are much less if the victim is using an effective method of contraception. Give ethinyl estradiol, 200 µg, and norgestrel, 2 mg, orally over 12 hours in 2 divided doses (eg, Ovral, 2 tablets orally, repeating in 12 hours), to prevent implantation if it is certain that the patient is not already pregnant. The physician should advise the patient that nausea and vomiting may occur. Other possible regimens include diethylstilbestrol, 25 mg orally twice a day for 5 days; ethinyl estradiol, 5 mg/d orally for 5 days; or intravenous conjugated estrogens, 25 mg/d for 3 days. Explain that abortion can be made available at a later time.

Caution: Existing pregnancy is an absolute contraindication to the use of diethylstilbestrol, since this drug has been shown to cause birth defects. Warn the patient that this regimen may not be effective, and explain that a return visit within 1–2 weeks is essential to recheck a pregnancy test.

C. If the patient consents, report the incident to the proper authorities before the patient leaves the emergency department, since the police will want to question her. If the alleged victim is a child, the incident may be child abuse and should be reported to the appropriate child welfare authorities (Chapter 42).

D. Start rape counseling immediately, preferably directed by experienced personnel who are part of an established rape counseling program.

E. Arrange follow-up; a definite appointment (time, place, and physician or clinic) should be made.

2. MANAGEMENT OF THE MALE RAPE VICTIM

Diagnosis & Evaluation

A. Inform the police (with patient's consent).

B. Obtain written informed consent for examination.

C. Obtain and record the history as described above.

D. Collect and label relevant evidence, and protect the chain of evidence.

1. Scrape under the fingernails, and also take trimmings from them.

2. Collect any loose hairs or dried blood.

3. Using the techniques and preparations described in steps 5–9 under Management of the Female Rape Victim, examine samples of material from the mouth and rectum.

E. Perform a physical examination.

1. Thoroughly examine the patient for signs of trauma, discharge, or bleeding; record the results of the examination. Photograph all lesions, but only with the patient's consent.

2. Examine the mouth and the rectum for injuries. Proctoscopy may be advisable if penetration has occurred and if foreign objects were used, since peritoneal perforation may occur from rectal trauma.

F. Obtain blood for blood chemistry studies (if indicated), a serologic test for syphilis, and blood typing (to compare the alleged assailant's type with that of the victim).

Treatment

A. Offer treatment and preventive therapy for sexually transmitted disease, as described above and in Chapter 34.

B. If the patient consents, report the incident to the proper authorities before the patient leaves the emergency department, since the police will want to question him. If the alleged victim is a child, the incident may represent child abuse and should be reported to the appropriate child welfare authorities (Chapter 42).

C. Start rape counseling immediately, preferably directed by experienced personnel who are part of an established rape counseling center. The male victim of rape needs counseling just as much as the female victim of sexual assault.

INTRAUTERINE DEVICES

Problems With Intrauterine Devices (IUDs)

A. "Lost" IUD: In the emergency department, the most common problem relating to these devices is the "lost" IUD. The physician can check to see if the IUD is still properly placed by looking for the removal string protruding from the cervix (most women soon learn to feel for it with a finger). If no string can be found, the IUD may be located by uterine sonography or abdominal x-ray (for metallic IUDs). The IUD may be in an extrauterine position, in which case it should be removed surgically by laparoscopy or laparotomy, although this is usually not an emergency.

B. Emergency Removal of IUD:

1. Infection–The principal indication for removal of an IUD in the emergency department is in-

MEDICAL REPORT - SUSPECTED SEXUAL ASSAULT

PRINT OR TYPE   FORM 923   HOSPITAL

INSTRUCTIONS: Each physician and surgeon in a county hospital or in any other general acute care hospital who conducts a medical examination for evidence of sexual assault is required by law to complete this form where the patient has consented to be so examined. Each part of the form must be completed unless inapplicable. If the patient consents only to treatment complete only 1 A&B and IV B&C to the extent they are relevant to treatment and mail to police or sheriff after reporting the same information by phone to law enforcement. In filling out this form no civil or criminal liability attaches. Additionally, no confidentiality is breached in releasing this form to local law enforcement. Prior to commencement of the examination local law enforcement shall be notified by telephone.

I. GENERAL INFORMATION

A. PATIENT'S NAME   HOSPITAL ID NO.

B. ADDRESS   CITY   COUNTY   STATE   PHONE

C. AGE   BIRTHDATE   RACE (USE CODED SUB-GROUPS)   SEX   DATE AND TIME OF ARRIVAL   MODE OF TRANSPORTATION

D. ACCOMPANIED BY: NAME   ADDRESS   CITY   COUNTY   STATE   PHONE   RELATIONSHIP

E. OFFICER NO. 1   ID NO.   DEPARTMENT   PHONE

OFFICER NO.   ID NO.   DEPARTMENT   PHONE

II. PATIENT'S or PARENT'S or GUARDIAN'S CONSENT (Sign where indicated)

I UNDERSTAND THAT HOSPITALS AND PHYSICIANS ARE REQUIRED BY PENAL CODE SECTION 11160-11161 TO REPORT TO LAW ENFORCEMENT AUTHORITIES THE NAME AND WHEREABOUTS OF ANY PERSONS WHO ARE VICTIMS OF SEXUAL ASSAULT OR WHO HAVE SUFFERED INJURIES INFLICTED BY A DEADLY WEAPON OR IN VIOLATION OF A PENAL LAW AND THE TYPE AND EXTENT OF THOSE INJURIES. KNOWING THIS, I CONSENT TO INDICATED TREATMENT.

PATIENT OR PARENT OR GUARDIAN

I FURTHER UNDERSTAND THAT A SEPARATE MEDICAL EXAMINATION FOR EVIDENCE OF SEXUAL ASSAULT AT PUBLIC EXPENSE CAN, WITH MY CONSENT, BE CONDUCTED BY THE TREATING PHYSICIAN TO DISCOVER AND PRESERVE EVIDENCE OF THE ASSAULT. IF SO CONDUCTED, THE REPORT OF THE EXAMINATION AND ANY EVIDENCE OBTAINED WILL BE RELEASED TO LAW ENFORCEMENT. KNOWING THIS, I CONSENT TO A MEDICAL EXAMINATION FOR EVIDENCE OF SEXUAL ASSAULT.

PATIENT OR PARENT OR GUARDIAN

III. FINANCIAL RESPONSIBILITY OF LOCAL GOVERNMENT (Government Code Section 13961.5)

I HEREBY REQUEST A MEDICAL EXAMINATION & COLLECTION OF EVIDENCE FOR SUSPECTED SEXUAL ASSAULT OF THE ABOVE PATIENT AT PUBLIC EXPENSE.

OFFICER   ID NO.   DATE

IV. MEDICAL EXAMINATION

A. HISTORY ANSWER LINES 4-6 YES OR NO, OR EXPLAIN FOR EACH CATEGORY.

1. DATE AND TIME OF EXAM   DATE AND TIME OF ASSAULT

2. PHYSICAL SURROUNDINGS (BED, FIELD, CAR, ETC.)   IF PHYSICALLY RESTRAINED, HOW

3. PATIENT'S DESCRIPTION OF ASSAULT AND ASSOCIATED PAIN (PARAPHRASE)

NAME(S) AND NUMBER OF ASSAILANT(S)

WEAPON USED (GUN, KNIFE, ETC.)   IF FOREIGN OBJECT USED, WHAT AND WHERE

4. ACTS COMMITTED   COITUS   FELLATIO   CUNNILINGUS   SODOMY

5. DURING ASSAULT   VAGINAL PENETRATION (HOW)   EJACULATION: ☐ VAGINAL ☐ ORAL ☐ ANAL ☐ OTHER:

☐ ANAL PENETRATION (HOW)   ☐ CONDOM USED   ☐ VOMITED   ☐ LOSS OF CONSCIOUSNESS   ☐ OTHER:

6. AFTER ASSAULT   ☐ WIPED/WASHED   ☐ BATHED   ☐ DOUCHED   ☐ VOMITED   ☐ CHANGED CLOTHES   ☐ BRUSHED TEETH   ☐ DEFECATED

☐ OTHER:

7. MENSTRUAL HISTORY:

8. BP   PULSE   TEMP.   RESP.   KNOWN ALLERGIES

CURRENT MEDICATION   LAST TETANUS

B. GENERAL PHYSICAL 1. PATIENT'S GENERAL PHYSICAL APPEARANCE   HEIGHT   WEIGHT

61926-552 6-76 100M OSP

Figure 30–3. Rape evaluation form (California).

PATIENT'S NAME	HOSPITAL ID NO.	HOSPITAL

B. GENERAL PHYSICAL (Cont.) 2. LOCATE & DESCRIBE IN DETAIL ANY INJURIES OR FINDINGS (SPECULUM & BIMANUAL EXAM): TRAUMA, BRUISES, ERYTHEMA, EXCORIATIONS, LACERATIONS, WOUNDS, STAINS/FOREIGN MATERIALS ON BODY-MUCOID OR LIQUID MATERIAL, LOOSE HAIR, BLOOD, GRASS, DIRT, ETC.

TRACE OUTLINE USED & INDICATE LOCATION OF WOUNDS/LACERATIONS, USING 'X' FOR SUPERFICIAL, 'O' FOR DEEP; SHADE FOR BRUISES. WRITE OVER UNUSED OUTLINES. DESCRIBE IN DETAIL SHAPE OF BRUISES (ON ARMS OR OTHER EXTREMITIES) WHICH MAY INDICATE FORCE.

C. PELVIC IF A CHILD, PERFORM ONLY IF NECESSARY (SAME INSTRUCTIONS AS GENERAL PHYSICAL; IN ADDITION, NOTE PUBIC HAIR COMBINGS, DRIED SECRETIONS AND RECENT INJURIES TO HYMEN WHERE INDICATED.) TRACE AND MARK OUTLINE AS ABOVE.

FLUORESCENCE

VAGINAL	+	−
ORAL	+	−
RECTAL	+	−
OTHER	+	−

V. DIAGNOSTIC IMPRESSION OF TRAUMA AND INJURIES

VI. TREATMENT/DISPOSITION OF PATIENT

A. ☐ G C CULTURE ☐ VDRL ☐ PREGNANCY TEST ☐ POST COITAL ESTROGEN ☐ V.D. PRO-PHYLAXIS ☐ OTHER:

B. ORDERS:

MOTILE SPERM: ☐ PRESENCE ☐ ABSENCE ☐ NOT TAKEN

C. DISPOSITION: ☐ ADMIT TRANSFERRED TO

D. FOLLOW-UP WITHIN: ☐ MEDICAL ☐ STS ☐ PRIVATE MD ☐ OTHER

_____ _____ 48 _____ _____ _____ _____ _____ _____
HOURS DAYS HOURS DAYS HOURS DAYS HOURS DAYS

☐ RELEASED ACCOMPANIED BY: NAME ADDRESS RELATIONSHIP

VII. SPECIMENS

STAINS/FOREIGN MATERIALS (WHEN INDICATED)

LOOSE HAIR	_____	FINGERNAIL SCRAPINGS	_____
BLOOD	_____	DIRT OR GRAVEL	_____
THREADS	_____	VEGETATION	_____
GRASS	_____	CLOTHING	_____

DRIED SECRETIONS

	SLIDES	SWABS
VAGINAL	_____	_____
RECTAL	_____	_____
ORAL	_____	_____
ASPIRATES/WASHINGS	_____	_____
BITE MARKS	_____	_____
OTHER:		

PATIENT'S SAMPLES, TIME OF COLLECTION AT MD DISCRETION. _____

BLOOD	_____
HAIR FROM HEAD	_____
SALIVA	_____
HAIR FROM PUBIC AREA	_____

I HAVE RECEIVED THE INDICATED ITEMS AS EVIDENCE AND A COPY OF THIS REPORT.

OFFICER: _____ ID NO.: _____ DATE: _____

NURSE _____ SIGNATURE OF EXAMINING PHYSICIAN _____

61926-552 6-78 100M OSP

Figure 30–3 (cont'd). Rape evaluation form (California).

fection (salpingitis, endometritis, pyosalpinx, or pelvic peritonitis). The incidence of endometritis, salpingitis, and tubal abscess is increased in women using IUDs. Any of these conditions requires removal of the IUD so that infection can be completely cleared. If possible, the patient should be started on appropriate antibiotics *before the device is removed* in order to ensure adequate blood levels of the drug (see Salpingitis in Chapter 34).

2. Bleeding and pain–Persistent vaginal bleeding or pelvic pain usually requires removal of an IUD but not often on an emergency basis. Referral to the physician who inserted the device is preferable.

If referral is impractical, grasp the string of the IUD with a Kelly clamp or other long grasping forceps, and pull with gentle but increasing force until the IUD emerges from the uterus. *Do not jerk the string, since it may detach from the device and make removal more difficult.* If the string is not easily seen after manipulation with a speculum, use a special IUD remover to locate and grasp the string. Alternatively, explore the endocervix with a crochet hook; this generally frees the string so that it can be easily grasped and the device removed.

C. Serious But Rare Problems:

1. Perforation of the uterus–Perforation of the uterus is a probable diagnosis in patients with IUDs who have symptoms of endometritis, salpingitis, or peritonitis. Physical examination, an abdominal x-ray, and sonography show that the IUD is embedded in the uterine wall or actually free in the peritoneum. Emergency hospitalization is required.

2. Pregnancy with IUD in place–If pregnancy is a firm diagnosis or a strong possibility and an IUD is still in place, seek emergency obstetric consultation. Ectopic pregnancy is a distinct possibility in the pregnant patient with an IUD still in place.

DISORDERS OF THE VULVA & VAGINA

Vaginal and vulvar cancers and other lesions are discussed on p 531. Vaginitis, gonorrhea, genital herpesvirus infection, and genital abscesses are discussed in Chapter 34.

A WARNING ABOUT DISCONTINUING CONTRACEPTION

Treatment of gynecologic problems in the emergency department may require discontinuing the patient's current form of contraception. The emergency physician advising this course of action must warn the patient of the possibility of pregnancy and offer appropriate contraceptive advice. Discontinuation of oral contraceptives or IUD use because of

treatment in the emergency department should not be allowed to result in an unwanted pregnancy.

EMERGENCY MANAGEMENT OF OBSTETRIC DISORDERS

PREGNANCY

Diagnosis

The diagnosis and differential diagnosis of pregnancy are a critical skill in the emergency department, where many serious obstetric disorders, eg, abortion or ectopic implantation, may be seen.

A. Early Symptoms and Signs: Amenorrhea, nausea and vomiting, syncopal attacks, breast tenderness or tingling, and urinary symptoms (especially frequency) are early symptoms of pregnancy. Early signs of pregnancy include cervical cyanosis and softening, vaginal cyanosis, softening and enlargement of the uterus, and breast enlargement and tenderness. **Legal proof of pregnancy** requires evidence of fetal heart tones on auscultation, or demonstration of fetal parts or movement by palpation, x-ray, or ultrasonography; these are obviously late findings.

B. Laboratory Tests: Urinary immunodiagnostic tests for pregnancy may occasionally be negative until about the time of the second missed period. False-positive results are rare at any time, except with trophoblastic tumors. Serum monoclonal antibody tests and radioimmunoassay for the β subunit of hCG are highly specific and sensitive enough to diagnose pregnancy before the first missed period.

Trophoblastic tumors ranging from benign hydatidiform mole to choriocarcinoma can present as incomplete abortion or bleeding during the second trimester of pregnancy without evidence of fetal activity. Serum hCG is often high (false-positive pregnancy test).

Ectopic pregnancies and spontaneous abortions may cause false-negative results of urine immunologic pregnancy tests.

Differential Diagnosis of Pregnancy

The differential diagnosis of pregnancy includes disorders producing secondary amenorrhea (endocrinopathies, emotional stress, drugs, malnutrition, and menopause) and those producing abdominal or uterine enlargement (obesity, tumors, pseudopregnancy [pseudocyesis]).

DISCOMFORTS OF PREGNANCY

Pregnant women are subject to many discomforts, any of which may cause a visit to the emergency department. If drug therapy of these complaints is contemplated, only drugs generally recognized as safe in pregnancy should be used, and the patient should be informed of potential benefits and risks. Common problems include vomiting, backache, syncopal attacks, urinary symptoms (with and without demonstrable urinary tract infection), heartburn, constipation, hemorrhoids, varicose veins, leg swelling, and cramps. Rarely, pregnant women may have very severe abdominal pain localized to one or another quadrant. Round ligament pain may present this way. The pain tends to be fairly constant, not cramping. Temperature and white blood cell count are usually normal. Treatment consists of oral analgesics and bed rest.

Nausea and vomiting are common in the first trimester and usually occur in the morning. Persistent vomiting (hyperemesis gravidarum) with dehydration, elevated specific gravity of urine, ketonuria, and hemoconcentration may require hospitalization for parenteral hydration and nutrition. Symptomatic treatment of nausea and vomiting is preferred, eg, soda crackers immediately upon arising in the morning; small, frequent, low-fat meals.

HYPEREMESIS GRAVIDARUM

Diagnosis

Hyperemesis gravidarum is usually easily diagnosed. However, other causes of vomiting, such as infection, diabetes mellitus, or abdominal disorders, must be excluded.

A. Symptoms and Signs: Patients who are known to be pregnant or have symptoms and signs of pregnancy (see above) complain of persistent vomiting, often with postural dizziness, presyncope, weight loss, or other signs of dehydration. Hyperemesis gravidarum usually resolves early in the second trimester. Physical examination reveals signs of dehydration: hypotension or postural hypotension, tachycardia, dry mucous membranes, and collapsed neck veins. Patients are rarely in severe shock.

B. Laboratory Tests: The test for pregnancy usually is positive, although early in pregnancy urinary tests may be negative. Blood tests may show hemoconcentration, elevated BUN or creatinine, hypokalemia, or metabolic alkalosis. The urine usually appears concentrated with high specific gravity and ketonuria.

Treatment

A. Insert an 18-gauge intravenous catheter (a larger bore is rarely needed).

B. Draw blood for CBC, electrolytes, and renal function.

C. Infuse crystalloid solution containing glucose (eg, 0.9% saline with 5% dextrose) to correct hypovolemia. (Glucose administration will inhibit ketogenesis.) The amount and rate of administration depends on the severity of dehydration.

D. Replace potassium as needed.

E. If emesis persists, administer an antiemetic:

1. Prochlorperazine, 5–10 mg intravenously (or intramuscularly), or

2. Promethazine, 25 mg intravenously (or intramuscularly), or

3. Trimethobenzamide, 200 mg per rectum.

Caution: Because of the potential for adverse effects to the fetus from the administration of antiemetics, parental consent should be obtained and documented prior to administration of antiemetic agents.

Disposition

Patients with persistent vomiting or ketonuria should be hospitalized. Patients whose emesis is controlled and whose ketonuria resolves may be discharged with telephone follow-up in 1–2 days. Antiemetic tablets or suppositories may be prescribed for the patient to use only as needed.

THIRD-TRIMESTER BLEEDING

The most common causes of third-trimester bleeding are abruptio placentae, placenta previa, lower genital tract bleeding, or systemic coagulopathy. The least severe cause, lower genital tract bleeding, should be diagnosed only after the more severe conditions have been excluded systematically.

Third-trimester bleeding must be treated as a grave emergency threatening the life of both mother and fetus. Vaginal, rectal, or speculum examination must never be done in the emergency department, since it may initiate hemorrhage.

Diagnosis

A. Placental Disorders:

1. Abruptio placentae–Premature separation of the placenta from the endometrium is characterized by severe abdominal and pelvic pain and tenderness. The separation is associated with hemorrhage into the subplacental space (between the uterus and the placenta) and in most cases presents as vaginal bleeding (Fig 30–4A). In some cases, however, the subplacental hemorrhage may be concealed ("occult abruption") (Fig 30–4B). Preeclampsia-eclampsia is common, and disseminated intravascular coagulation may occur as well.

2. Placenta previa–A placenta implanted in the lower uterine wall usually causes painless bleeding in small volumes that occurs regularly over a short period of observation. Such seemingly small blood loss may produce a false sense of security, since sudden massive hemorrhage can occur at any time.

A

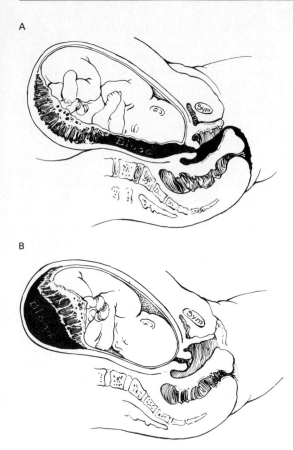

B

Figure 30–4. Types of premature separation of the placenta. **A:** Apparent bleeding. **B:** Concealed bleeding. (Redrawn and reproduced, with permission, from Beck AC, Rosenthal AH: *Obstetrical Practice,* 7th ed. Williams & Wilkins, 1957.)

B. Systemic Coagulopathies: Coagulation disorders are uncommon as the sole cause of third-trimester bleeding. Diagnosis is confirmed by routine coagulation studies.

Treatment

A. Obtain emergency obstetric consultation.

B. Evaluate the patient for hypovolemia (as shown by supine or postural hypotension), and correct, if present, with intravenous infusion of crystalloid solution or whole blood.

C. Insert a large-bore (≥ 16-gauge) intravenous catheter.

D. Draw blood for CBC, coagulation studies (prothrombin time, partial thromboplastin time, fibrinogen, and platelet count), and measurement of blood urea nitrogen and serum creatinine. Type and cross-match for 4 units of whole blood, preferably fresh.

E. Monitor fetal heart tones.

F. Obtain urine for urinalysis, and monitor urine output with an indwelling urinary catheter.

G. The pregnant patient should never be maintained for any length of time in the supine, recumbent position (see Trauma in Pregnancy, below).

Disposition

Hospitalize the patient immediately, and move her to a delivery unit as soon as possible. Fetal bradycardia increases the urgency of the need for cesarean section.

TOXEMIA OF PREGNANCY (Preeclampsia-Eclampsia)

Diagnosis

Preeclampsia-eclampsia describes a condition that covers a spectrum of symptoms and a continuum of severity. The condition is characterized by pregnancy-induced hypertension, by proteinuria, and when severe (eclampsia), by seizures. Symptoms of preeclampsia and eclampsia are so variable that a woman in the third trimester of pregnancy who comes to the emergency department with *any* complaint should have her blood pressure checked and urinalysis performed to detect early signs of preeclampsia-eclampsia.

A. Symptoms and Signs: Symptoms and signs are variable and may include headache, various visual symptoms, and vertigo. Nausea and vomiting and abdominal pain may occur. Especially alarming is pain in the right upper quadrant and epigastrium, "hepatic pain," which is due to compression of the swelling liver by its capsule. Nervousness, irritability, and even frank seizures may occur.

Hypertension or rising blood pressure relative to the patient's *normal* blood pressure is a significant sign. Note that blood pressure may not be sufficiently elevated to be "abnormal" because of the physiologic decline in blood pressure normally associated with pregnancy.

There is usually peripheral edema. Spasm of retinal arterioles and hemorrhage may occur. Hepatomegaly or hepatic tenderness (or both) may be present.

B. Laboratory Findings: Critical laboratory findings confirming the diagnosis of preeclampsia-eclampsia are decreased urine output, elevated blood urea nitrogen and serum creatinine levels, decreased creatine clearance, proteinuria, and evidence of disseminated intravascular coagulation.

Treatment & Disposition

Patients with suspected preeclampsia-eclampsia should be evaluated by an obstetrician before they are discharged from the emergency department.

A. Mild Preeclampsia: Mild preeclampsia is characterized by diastolic blood pressure under 105 mm Hg, trace to 1+ proteinuria, good urinary output, and absence of other symptoms. The patient should rest in bed at home. Provide sedation with barbiturates (eg, phenobarbital, 30–60 mg orally 3–4 times daily) as needed. The patient must be closely monitored (eg, twice weekly).

B. Moderate to Severe Eclampsia: Moderate to severe eclampsia is characterized by proteinuria greater than 2+, diastolic blood pressure greater than 105 mm Hg, seizures, anuria, or severe edema. Hospitalize patients who are more than mildly ill or who worsen on bed rest at home. It is better to err on the side of hospitalization, since eclampsia occurring out of the hospital greatly increases the chances of maternal or fetal death.

Treat hyperreflexia with magnesium sulfate, 2–4 g in 50 mL of 5% dextrose in water or in 5% dextrose in half-normal or normal saline given over 30 minutes as an intravenous loading dose, followed by 1 g/h, obtained by dissolving 20 g of magnesium sulfate in 1 L of 5% dextrose in water, by controlled intravenous infusion (infusion pump). The use of phenytoin is controversial.

Treat hypertension with intravenous hydralazine (Alazine, Apresoline), 20 mg in 50 mL of lactated Ringer's injection or 5% dextrose in water, infused at a rate of 1 mg every 2 minutes. An infusion pump should be used if possible. When blood pressure falls below 160/110 mm Hg, slow the infusion to a rate of about 1 mg/h, and adjust to maintain desired blood pressure. *Do not* reduce blood pressure to "normal" levels (120/80 mm Hg), since renal shutdown may result.

Insert a urinary (Foley) catheter. Monitor fluid intake and urinary output closely, and test urine for specific gravity and hematuria.

When neurologic and cardiovascular status is stable, transfer the patient to a hospital equipped to manage high-risk obstetric patients.

TRAUMA IN PREGNANCY

Trauma due to gunshot wounds, assault, or automobile accident may cause abruptio placentae, ruptured fetal membranes, or direct fetal trauma. Maternal coagulation profiles should be obtained in addition to standard laboratory tests, since pregnant patients are more at risk for disseminated intravascular coagulation. The fetal heart rate and uterine contractions should be followed for several hours by electronic fetal monitoring; diagnostic fetal ultrasound should also be performed. The patient should never be maintained in the supine position, which can cause compression of the inferior vena cava and aorta, leading to reduced cardiac output. The stretcher or table may be tilted to the left or a wedge (pillow) placed under the patient's right hip.

The Kleihauer-Betke test detects fetal blood cells in the maternal circulation and is a helpful means of quantifying fetal bleeding; it may help identify fetal hypovolemia before obvious fetal distress occurs.

Treat shock (Chapter 3), but if possible avoid drugs that cause uterine vasoconstriction (eg, most vasopressors); ephedrine is safe. X-rays and an antishock garment (eg, MAST) with the leg compartments inflated may be used in pregnant patients as necessary. If required, peritoneal lavage using the supraumbilical approach may be used.

LABOR & DELIVERY

In many hospitals, patients in active labor are seen initially in the emergency department. A calm and orderly approach to evaluation of these patients—as well as established policies for transfer of responsibility from emergency department staff to obstetric staff—is essential for proper management.

Evaluation
A. History: If records from prenatal visits are not available, ask the patient about recent or intercurrent illness and such risk factors as diabetes mellitus, valvular heart disease, or previous cesarean section delivery. Ask whether the membranes have ruptured. Determine parity. Estimate the due date and gestational age of the fetus.

B. Physical Examination:
1. Record complete maternal vital signs.
2. Perform brief physical examination of the mother.
3. Determine frequency and intensity of uterine contractions.
4. Check for vaginal discharge by speculum examination (blood or meconium). The presence of amniotic fluid may be detected by an alkaline reaction (yellow turning to blue) with Nitrazine paper.
5. Determine fetal position, and sketch it on an outline of the female figure.
6. Determine the fetal heart rate during and between uterine contractions.
7. Perform vaginal examination. *Note: Do not* perform digital examination if vaginal bleeding is present. Determine the presenting part and the degree of dilation and effacement of the cervix by speculum.

Diagnosis
Progressive labor is characterized by uterine contractions occurring every 3 minutes and dilation of the cervical os. Abnormal signs requiring urgent obstetric consultation include fetal bradycardia (< 100 beats/min) during or after uterine contractions, vaginal bleeding (on history or examination), transverse or breech presentations, and maternal illness (eg, eclampsia, coma, major trauma).

Treatment
A. Premature Birth: Infants under 36 weeks of gestational age are likely to require neonatal intensive care. If there is no such nursery in the facility

where the mother has sought treatment, consider transferring her to another facility. Children are better off being born in the site where the nursery exists than being transferred to the site after birth.

Give crystalloid solution, 1000 mL over 3–4 hours, and monitor cardiovascular status carefully. Consider use of subcutaneous terbutaline (0.25 mg) to inhibit labor for possible transfer. The dose may be repeated in an hour.

B. Routine Labor: When delivery is imminent, give nothing (or sips of clear fluids only) by mouth. Maintain or reinstate adequate hydration with intravenous fluids. Give analgesia if there are no contraindications. Notify the patient's obstetric care provider that she is in the hospital and in active labor.

C. Emergency Department Delivery: If the examiner determines that the presenting part is in vertex position and is near the vulva, it is probably better to allow the patient to deliver in the emergency department than to rush her into elevators and through corridors to the delivery unit.

1. Delivery– Analgesia (eg, meperidine, 50 mg intravenously or intramuscularly) may be given as needed to the mother with an uncomplicated term pregnancy. Delivery may be accomplished in either the lithotomy or the Sims position. Try to prepare a clean field (wash the vulva and perineum). Prevent sudden uncontrolled delivery of the fetal head.

Clear the infant's nasal passages and airway. If there is thick meconium staining of the amniotic fluid, be prepared to clear the airway *carefully* and immediately, ie, clear the nostrils with a suction bulb (or DeLee suction trap, if available) after the head is delivered but before the body is delivered. Check for the umbilical cord. The physician may need to intubate the infant *immediately,* before spontaneous respirations occur, and apply suction to the trachea.

Cut the umbilical cord after ligating it about 2–3 in (5–7.5 cm) from the infant's abdomen.

Deliver the placenta with *gentle* traction on the cord if it comes out easily. If the patient is not vigorously bleeding, the placenta may be left in place while the patient is sent to the delivery room for further measures, eg, suture of lacerations.

2. Postpartum measures– Dry and examine the infant, and resuscitate if necessary. *Keep the baby warm.*

Monitor the mother's blood pressure every 5 minutes for 15 minutes and then every 15 minutes for 1 hour. A sample of the infant's clotted cord blood should be sent for ABO and Rh typing and a serologic test for syphilis.

Disposition

Hospitalize the newborn infant for evaluation and supportive care.

POSTPARTUM HEMORRHAGE

Diagnosis

Rarely, a patient returns to the hospital a few days after delivery with brisk vaginal bleeding that may or may not be associated with hemorrhagic shock. The usual cause of postpartum hemorrhage is retention of the products of conception in the uterus. Other possible causes are subinvolution of the placental site, vaginal tears, or bleeding from an episiotomy.

Treatment & Disposition

A. Treat hemorrhagic shock if present (Chapter 3).

1. If bleeding is brisk, insert the fingers of one hand into the vagina, and compress the uterus against the abdominal wall.

2. Insert a large-bore (≥ 16-gauge) intravenous catheter, and start infusion of crystalloid solution, followed by whole blood if the hematocrit falls (Chapter 3).

3. Monitor vital signs and urinary output.

4. Draw blood for CBC, coagulation studies (prothrombin time, partial thromboplastin time, and platelet count), blood urea nitrogen, and serum creatinine.

5. Type and cross-match for 4 units of blood.

B. Obtain emergency obstetric and gynecologic consultation.

C. Methylergonovine, 0.2 mg intramuscularly, may be tried to help slow the bleeding. Methylergonovine should *not* be used if the patient has preeclampsia.

D. The definitive treatment is dilation and curettage, which may be performed in the emergency department using paracervical block anesthesia and suction evacuation of the uterus. An obstetrician should be in attendance, since postpartum surgery may result in uterine perforation.

E. Patients whose cause of bleeding is definitively treated and are otherwise stable can be discharged with close follow-up in 2–3 days. All other patients should be hospitalized and obstetric consultation obtained as needed.

PUERPERAL SEPSIS & ENDOMETRITIS

Diagnosis

Symptoms of puerperal sepsis in the early postpartum period are fever, peritoneal pain, and vaginal discharge. Examination reveals abdominal tenderness, exquisite uterine tenderness, and purulent lochia with leukocytes and bacteria on Gram's stain.

Treatment & Disposition

If there are signs of sepsis, obtain obstetric and gynecologic consultation, and hospitalize the patient immediately. Patients with minimal symptoms may be managed as outpatients. Obtain samples of blood and discharge for diagnostic culture and sensitivity testing. Start antibiotics in accordance with the following recommendations:

A. Severely Ill Patients: Give penicillin, 20–30 million units daily by continuous intravenous infusion (or bolus injection); and tobramycin or gentamicin, 1.7 mg/kg every 8 hours intravenously or intramuscularly. Before beginning treatment with gentamicin, obtain baseline serum creatinine levels; during treatment, obtain serum creatinine levels 1–2 times per week, and follow gentamicin peaks and troughs weekly. Clindamycin, 600–900 mg every 6–8 hours intravenously, may be added to the penicillin and gentamicin.

B. Mildly Ill Patients: Doxycycline, 100 mg orally twice daily (or tetracycline, 500 mg orally 4 times daily), or ampicillin, 500 mg orally 4 times daily for 10–14 days, may be used for outpatients. *Caution:* Do not use doxycycline or tetracycline if the patient is breast-feeding.

PUERPERAL MASTITIS

Postpartum infection of the breast is almost always due to infection with *Staphylococcus aureus.*

Diagnosis

The diagnosis of puerperal mastitis is based on systemic signs of infection, pain, and tenderness of the involved breast. Abscess formation may occur, and blood cultures are occasionally positive.

Treatment & Disposition
A. Mild Cases (Afebrile):
1. Apply warm compresses to the affected breast. The patient may continue to breast-feed.
2. Give cloxacillin, 500 mg orally 4 times daily. Clindamycin, 300 mg orally 4 times daily, may be substituted if the patient is allergic to penicillin.
B. Severe Cases (Suspected Abscess):
1. Hospitalize the patient, and obtain surgical consultation.
2. Give one of the following antistaphylococcal antibiotics:
a. Nafcillin or equivalent, 150 mg/kg/d intravenously.
b. Clindamycin, 450 mg intravenously every 8 hours; or erythromycin, 0.5 g intravenously every 6 hours. Either of these drugs may be substituted in patients allergic to penicillin.

REFERENCES

Barnes AB, Wennberg CN, Barnes BA: Ectopic pregnancy: Incidence and review of determinant factors. Obstet Gynecol Surv 1983;38:345.

Berkowitz RL, Couston DR, Mochizuki TK: *Handbook for Prescribing Medications During Pregnancy,* 2nd ed. Little, Brown, 1986.

Briggs GG, Freeman RK, Yaffe SJ: *Drugs in Pregnancy and Lactation.* Williams & Wilkins, 1990.

California Medical Association: Guidelines for interview and examination of alleged rape victims. West J Med 1975;123:420.

Cartwright P et al: Performance of a new enzyme-linked immunoassay urine pregnancy test for the detection of ectopic gestation. Ann Emerg Med 1986;15:1198.

Dingfelder JR: Primary dysmenorrhea treatment with prostaglandin inhibitors: A review. Am J Obstet Gynecol 1981;140:874.

Ectopic pregnancy. Chapter 26 in: Novak's *Textbook of Gynecology,* 19th ed. Jones HW Jr, Jones GS (editors). Williams & Wilkins, 1981.

Eschenbach DA: New concepts of obstetric and gynecologic infection. Arch Intern Med 1982;142:2039.

Gestational trophoblastic neoplasia: An invitational symposium. J Reprod Med 1981;26:179.

Goldstein SR et al: Very early pregnancy detection with endovaginal ultrasound. Obstet Gynecol 1988;72:200.

Hanlon JT et al: An evaluation of the sensitivity of five home pregnancy tests to known concentrations of human chorionic gonadotropin. Am J Obstet Gynecol 1982; 144:778.

Haycock GE: Emergency care of the pregnant traumatized patient. Emerg Clin North Am 1984;2:843.

Hayman CR et al: Rape in the District of Columbia. Am J Obstet Gynecol 1972;113:91.

Jenny C et al: Sexually transmitted diseases in victims of rape. N Engl J Med 1990;322:713.

Marrs RP, Mishell DR Jr: Placental trophic hormones. Clin Obstet Gynecol 1980;23:721.

Marshall BR, Hepper JK, Zirbel CC: Sporadic puerperal mastitis: An infection that need not interrupt lactation. JAMA 1975;233:1377.

Mead PB, Beecham JB, Maeck JV: Incidence of infections associated with the intrauterine contraceptive device in an isolated community. Am J Obstet Gynecol 1976; 125:79.

Obstetric hemorrhage. Chapter 21 in: *Williams Obstetrics,* 17th ed. Pritchard JA, MacDonald PC, Gant NF (editors). Appleton-Century-Crofts, 1985.

Ogle ME et al: Preeclampsia. Ann Emerg Med 1984;13:5.

Pearlman MD et al: Blunt trauma during pregnancy. N Engl J Med 1990;323:1609.

Robertson WH: A concentrated therapeutic regimen for vulvovaginal candidiasis. JAMA 1980;244:2549.

Romero R et al: The value of serial human chorionic gonadotropin testing as a diagnostic tool in ectopic pregnancy. Am J Obstet Gynecol 1985;66:357.

Stovall TG et al: Emergency department diagnosis of ectopic pregnancy. Ann Emerg Med 1990;19:1098.

Tintinalli J et al: Clinical findings and legal resolution in sexual assault. Ann Emerg Med 1985;14:447.

Weinstein LN: Current perspective on ectopic pregnancy: A review. Obstet Gynecol Surv 1985;40:259.

Woodling BA, Evans JR, Bradbury MD: Sexual assault: Rape and molestation. Clin Obstet Gynecol 1977; 20:509.

Genitourinary Emergencies

31

John Mills, MD, & Jack W. McAninch, MD

IMMEDIATE MANAGEMENT OF SERIOUS & LIFE-THREATENING CONDITIONS

OLIGURIA OR ANURIA

General Considerations

Decreased or absent urine output can occur from such widely diverse disease states as intravascular volume depletion or bladder outflow obstruction. In attempting to determine the cause of decreased urine output, it is helpful to categorize the mechanism as prerenal (eg, resulting from decreased or abnormal renal perfusion), renal (resulting from intrinsic renal disease), or postrenal (disease of the urinary collecting system distal to the renal parenchyma).

A. Prerenal Causes: Hypovolemia, sepsis, heart failure, etc.

B. Renal Causes: Glomerulonephritis, renal vein thrombosis, etc.

C. Postrenal Causes:

1. Supravesical obstruction–Supravesical obstruction rarely causes oliguria or anuria, since bilateral disease is required to produce decreased urine flow.

    a. Ureteral obstruction (usually tumor).

    b. Ureteropelvic or ureterovesical obstruction.

2. Intravesical and infravesical obstruction–Intravesical or infravesical obstruction is more common than supravesical obstruction (Table 31–1).

    a. Prostatic hypertrophy or carcinoma.

    b. Drugs with atropinic or adrenergic effects.

    c. Neurologic diseases.

    d. Bladder stones or tumors.

    e. Urethral strictures or valves.

Diagnosis

A. History:

1. Obstruction–Differentiate between reduced urine output (with normal or nearly normal voiding patterns) and oliguria associated with difficulty in voiding, feeling of incomplete voiding, diminished urinary stream, etc, which are suggestive of obstruction.

2. Other abnormalities–Ask about coexisting cardiac, pulmonary, renal, or other underlying dis-

Table 31-1. Diagnostic clues to the cause of bladder outlet obstruction.

Cause	Frequency of Occurrence	Results of History and Physical Examination	Laboratory Tests and Other Studies
Prostatic hypertrophy	Common.	Gradually increasing difficulty in voiding, often with abrupt worsening. Enlarged prostate on rectal examination is common.	Urethral catheterization may be difficult. Large amount of residual urine in bladder.
Urethral strictures or valves	Uncommon.	Often previous attacks of urethritis or urethral trauma. Onset may be gradual or abrupt.	Urethral catheterization often difficult. Large amounts of residual urine. Urethrogram or urethroscopy is diagnostic.
Bladder stones or tumor	Uncommon.	Hematuria is common. Obstruction may be intermittent.	Urethral catheter is passed without difficulty. Cystogram or cystoscopy is diagnostic.
Neuropathic bladder	Very uncommon.	Onset may be gradual and painless or abrupt and painful. Look for associated neurologic abnormalities (sacral dermatomal hypesthesia, poor rectal sphincter tone, neuralgic pain).	Urethral catheter passed without difficulty. Cystometrogram is diagnostic.
Traumatic urethral injury	Uncommon.	Male; history of trauma, prostatic dislocation, urethral bleeding.	*Do not pass catheter.* Retrograde urethrogram and percutaneous cystogram are diagnostic.

ease that might contribute to renal or prerenal oliguria.

3. Drugs–Ask if the patient is taking drugs (eg, antihistamines, sympathomimetics) that might cause problems in urination or be nephrotoxic.

B. Physical Examination:

1. Vital signs–Obtain complete vital signs, including temperature, blood pressure, and pulse, which should be measured with the patient both supine and sitting. Standing blood pressure should be measured to detect hypotension if blood pressure is normal in the supine and sitting positions. Correct volume depletion, if present (Chapter 3).

2. General examination–Perform a brief general physical examination, and look for signs of cardiac, pulmonary, renal, or hepatic disease that might be associated with oliguria of prerenal or renal origin. Look for other signs of dehydration, such as dry mucous membranes or poor skin turgor.

3. Distended bladder–Palpate the lower abdomen to determine whether there is a suprapubic mass consistent with a distended bladder. A distended bladder is manifested as a firm (but not hard) mass that is adjacent to the symphysis pubica and is dull to percussion. The diagnosis may be confirmed by passage of a Foley catheter, ultrasonography, radiologic studies (CT scan, abdominal x-ray), or, if necessary, percutaneous needle aspiration (Chapter 46).

4. Prostate examination–Examine the prostate. Perform a rectal examination, looking especially for masses, prostatic hypertrophy, prostatic tenderness, or prostatic dislocation (associated with trauma).

C. Detection of Bladder Outlet Obstruction: Bladder outlet obstruction (complete or partial) is strongly suggested by a palpable bladder in a patient who is unable to void or who has a feeble urinary stream or feeling of incomplete voiding. Whether lower abdominal pain is present depends on the rapidity of obstruction; acute obstruction causes rapid bladder distention and severe pain if sensation is intact.

Diagnostic features of some of the common causes of bladder outlet obstruction are set forth in Table 31–1.

Treatment

A. Serious Underlying Disease: If the patient is acutely ill or obviously in shock or has sepsis, heart failure, or other serious coexisting conditions that might cause prerenal oliguria, these disorders must be evaluated and treated before those of the urinary tract.

B. Distended Bladder (Presumed Bladder Outlet Obstruction):

1. Gain venous access. Insert an intravenous catheter, and draw blood for CBC, electrolyte determinations, and blood urea nitrogen and serum creatinine measurements. Leave the catheter in place to provide access for possible administration of intravenous fluids.

2. Drain the bladder.

a. Urethral catheter–Try to pass an indwelling urethral (Foley) catheter. if this maneuver succeeds, drain the bladder, record the volume of urine obtained, and send a urine specimen for culture and urinalysis. Gradual bladder drainage is not a proved method of decreasing bladder atony or mucosal hemorrhage. If bladder outlet obstruction is relieved by passage of a Foley catheter and is apparently due to a transient cause (eg, drugs), the catheter may be removed and the patient observed for ability to void after the effects of any drugs are presumed to have dissipated. In patients with fixed bladder outlet obstruction (eg, benign prostatic hypertrophy), leave the catheter in place, and obtain urologic consultation within 1–2 days.

b. Suprapubic catheter—If a urethral catheter cannot be passed and a urologist is not available for consultation within a few hours, insert a suprapubic catheter for temporary drainage (Chapter 46). A large (16-gauge) needle-clad catheter (eg, Intracath) will provide satisfactory emergency bladder drainage.

3. Treat cystitis and prostatitis, if present (see Dysuria, below).

4. Hospitalize patients who require an indwelling suprapubic catheter, those who have systemic symptoms (fever, chills), and those who need additional diagnosis and treatment (eg, for management of postobstructive diuresis, azotemia, sepsis, or electrolyte abnormalities).

C. Bladder Not Palpable; Patient Able to Void: If the patient can void on command but continues to complain of a poor urinary stream (or if this is observed directly) or if the patient experiences a feeling of incomplete voiding, partial bladder outlet obstruction is likely.

1. Draw blood for CBC, electrolyte determinations, and blood urea nitrogen and serum creatinine measurements. Send a urine specimen for urinalysis and culture.

2. Treat cystitis or prostatitis, if present.

3. If blood chemistry results and urinalysis are normal, schedule an excretory urogram, and refer the patient to a urologist. The presence of azotemia or electrolyte abnormalities indicates severe or longstanding obstructive uropathy, and the patient should be hospitalized.

D. Bladder Not Palpable; Patient Unable to Void: Consider the following in the differential diagnosis: (**1**) intrinsic renal disease, (**2**) occult prerenal disease (unlikely, since most causes would be obvious on brief physical examination), (**3**) occult bladder outlet obstruction, or (**4**) supravesical obstructive uropathy (rare).

1. Draw blood for CBC; serum glucose, electrolyte, calcium, and phosphorus measurements; and tests of renal and hepatic function.

2. Obtain chest and abdominal x-rays to help evaluate the size of the kidneys and bladder. Ultrasonography is the best noninvasive test for evaluating kidney and bladder size.

3. Ensure adequate hydration. In an adult without obvious volume overload (eg, pulmonary or peripheral edema), give 1–2 L of fluid orally or intravenously, and observe the patient for 1–2 hours. In an individual with normal kidneys, this amount should produce a brisk flow of urine.

4. If anuria persists despite adequate hydration and if the bladder is not distended, the cause of the anuria is likely to be proximal to the bladder (prerenal, renal, or, rarely, bilateral ureteral obstruction). Bladder catheterization, with strict adherence to sterile technique, should be performed to confirm the

lack of urine output. Hospitalize the patient for further evaluation.

Disposition

Hospitalization is required for patients with persistent unexplained anuria or severe oliguria (< 500 mL/d), those with systemic symptoms, those who require indwelling suprapubic catheters, and those with markedly abnormal electrolyte concentrations or renal function tests.

Patients with partial bladder outlet obstruction (ie, feeble urinary stream, with or without palpable bladder) should be referred to a urologist if renal function is normal or nearly normal.

Asymptomatic patients with an indwelling urethral catheter should be reexamined or referred to a urologist within 1–2 days.

SCROTAL PAIN
(See Table 31–2.)

Diagnosis

A. Trauma: Trauma commonly causes testicular or scrotal pain. Careful questioning may be required to elicit the circumstances under which the trauma occurred. See Chapter 20.

B. Viral Orchitis: Mumps virus and the enteroviruses may cause acute unilateral or bilateral orchitis. In orchitis due to mumps virus, there is usually associated parotitis.

C. Urolithiasis: Rarely, patients with urolithiasis present with pain localized mainly in the scrotum; however, in most cases, back or flank pain has preceded the scrotal pain, or there is a history of nephrolithiasis. In such cases, the testicle and epididymis are normal to palpation. Hematuria is an important diagnostic clue. The diagnosis may be confirmed by excretory urography.

D. Incarcerated Hernia: Inguinal hernias incarcerated in the scrotum may cause scrotal pain that may be confused with testicular pain. Bowel sounds are heard in the scrotum early in incarceration; if the hernia strangulates, bowel sounds are no longer audible. Intestinal hernia is almost always associated with clinical findings of intestinal obstruction (Chapter 7). Ultrasonography is diagnostic.

E. Testicular Torsion, Epididymitis, and Torsion of the Testicular Appendages: (See Table 31–2.) Because of the urgent necessity to diagnose and treat testicular torsion within 6 hours to prevent loss of the testis, testicular torsion must be promptly ruled out in all patients with scrotal pain. It may be difficult to distinguish from epididymitis or torsion of testicular appendages as edema and inflammation progress to involve the entire scrotal sac and contents.

1. Testicular torsion—Testicular torsion tends to occur in young men—it is uncommon in men over 25 years of age and rare in men over 30 years of age.

Table 31–2. Diagnostic clues to the cause of acute scrotal pain.

	History	Physical Examination	Urinalysis Results	Other Laboratory Studies	Treatment and Disposition
Trauma	History of injury.	Scrotal hematoma often present.	Variable; may have hematuria.	Sonogram.	Obtain urologic consultation (Chapter 20).
Urolithiasis	Antecedent flank or back pain; occasionally abdominal pain.	Testicle minimally tender or nontender.	Hematuria.	Stones on excretory urogram.	Obtain urologic consultation (p 553).
Viral (eg, mumps) orchitis	Gradual onset, coexisting mumps parotitis common.	Tender testicles (unilateral or bilateral); epididymis rarely involved.	Normal.	Viral cultures (throat, stool) if available; characteristic 4-fold rise in serum antibody titer.	Elevate and immobilize testicle (eg, with athletic supporter), give analgesics, and discharge for follow-up care.
Incarcerated hernia	Gradual onset; crampy pain.	Fluid rushes heard in scrotum (early); abdominal tenderness consistent with intestinal obstruction.	Normal.	Characteristically abnormal results on ultrasound studies; abdominal x-ray results often abnormal (intestinal obstruction).	Obtain general surgical consultation; hospitalize.
Epididymitis	Gradual onset; history of urethritis or urinary tract infection common; older men (> age 25 years).	Tender epididymis (often unilateral) with normal testicle early in course; pain relieved by elevating scrotum. If needed, use spermatic cord block (see text) to facilitate examination.	Leukocytes; bacteria in some cases (coexisting urinary tract infection).	Normal results on Doppler and ultrasound studies; radionuclide scan shows uptake in epididymis.	1. Prescribe bed rest and elevation of scrotum, with analgesics as needed. 2. Treat underlying urethritis or urinary tract infection with antimicrobials (Chapter 34). 3. Discharge all patients for follow-up care.
Testicular torsion	Abrupt onset (minutes to hours); history of testicular pain in some; boys and young men (< age 25 years).	Tender testicle, often elevated and horizontally displaced; normal epididymis (if palpable). Use spermatic cord block to facilitate examination.	Normal.	Characteristically abnormal results on Doppler examination and radionuclide scan.	Obtain emergency urologic consultation; hospitalize for surgery. Attempt manual detorsion (see text).
Torsion of testicular appendage	Abrupt onset.	Firm nodule with point tenderness on upper anterior pole of testis; testical normal.	Normal.	Transillumination may reveal affected appendage as black dot; normal results on Doppler ultrasound and radionuclide studies.	1. Prescribe bed rest and elevation, with analgesics as needed. 2. Surgery is often needed to relieve pain. 3. Obtain urologic follow-up care.

There is often a history of episodes of similar scrotal pain, representing torsion with spontaneous repositioning of the testicle. The pain is abrupt in onset, severe, unilateral, and often associated with nausea and vomiting. Tenderness is initially noted only in the testicle; however, with persistent torsion and the resulting testicular hypoxia, pain and tenderness spread to involve contiguous intrascrotal structures.

Examination early in the illness shows an elevated testicle that is apt to lie in the horizontal position. The epididymis may be felt in an abnormal position (eg, anteriorly) in the early stages. Later, the entire scrotal contents become swollen and tender, making examination virtually useless (the epididymis is no longer distinguishable from the testis by palpation).

2. Epididymitis–(See Chapter 34.) Epididymitis tends to occur in sexually active men over 20 years of age. There may be a history of urinary tract infection or urethritis. Pain begins gradually and is less severe than in testicular torsion. Prehn's sign may be helpful in differentiating between torsion and epididymitis: If pain is reduced when the scrotum is lifted over the symphysis pubica, the pain is due to epididymitis; if pain increases, the cause is probably torsion. Physical examination reveals a tender epididymis, often unilateral and often with erythema and edema of the scrotal skin. Early on, the testicle may be normal or minimally tender. However, as edema worsens, the epididymis becomes indistinguishable from the testicle on palpation, and a reactive hydrocele may develop, making it difficult to differentiate epididymitis from testicular torsion. Urinalysis or microscopic examination of urethral mucus will show leukocytes in most cases of epididymitis, indicating preceding urinary tract infection or urethritis.

3. Torsion of testicular appendages–Testicular appendages (appendices testes) are located on the upper anterior pole of the testes. Pain is usually sudden in onset and can be severe, with nausea and vomiting. Physical examination reveals a small, firm nodule in the upper anterior pole of the testis with point tenderness. The scrotal skin and testicle are usually normal and minimally tender. In advanced cases, marked edema and appearance of a reactive hydrocele may cause difficulty in ruling out testicular torsion.

4. Specialized diagnostic tests for differentiating torsion from epididymitis–These tests should not delay emergent urologic consultation and surgical treatment of patients with high probability of testicular torsion (ie, patients under 18 years of age with acute unilateral testicular pain and no signs or recent history of urinary tract infection).

a. Spermatic cord block–Anesthetizing the scrotal contents will facilitate accurate examination. Inject lidocaine without epinephrine (2%), 5–10 mL, around the spermatic cord at the external inguinal ring.

b. Doppler ultrasonic stethoscope–The Doppler ultrasonic stethoscope provides a simple and quick method of diagnosis. The testis to be examined is supported with one hand and the instrument is guided over the surface with the other hand. The testis is systematically auscultated, beginning behind the testis and directly over the testicular artery as it enters the testis. Absence of pulsatile sound from the painful testis is diagnostic of testicular torsion, although false-negative results can occur. Examination of the noninvolved testis serves as a control.

c. Radionuclide scan–In epididymitis, scanning of the scrotum after intravenous injection of technetium Tc 99m sodium pertechnate reveals increased scrotal uptake on the affected side, whereas torsion shows decreased uptake.

d. Ultrasonography–Ultrasonography can differentiate between swelling of the testis and swelling of the epididymis and show if there is an incarcerated hernia. Ultrasonography can also detect the presence of varicocele and testicular cysts and masses. Ultra-

sonography with color-flow imaging is a useful noninvasive test for diagnosing testicular torsion.

**Treatment & Disposition
(See Table 31–2.)**

If testicular torsion is present, obtain urgent urologic consultation, and prepare the patient for immediate surgery. Manual detorsion may be tried if the urologist will be delayed. Detorsion of the testicle (either manual or surgical) must be accomplished within 6 hours to save the testicle. Torsion causes the left testicle to rotate counterclockwise and the right one clockwise (Fig 31–1), and the affected testicle should be twisted in the opposite direction when detorsion is attempted. Since the testis affected by torsion is usually rotated a minimum of 360 degrees (one turn), the physician should initially attempt to untwist the testicle by counter-rotating it one turn. The testis will usually return to normal position of its own accord after this maneuver, even if it was originally twisted more than one complete revolution. Infiltrate the spermatic cord near the inguinal ring with lidocaine without epinephrine (2%), 5–10 mL, to facilitate the maneuver, and give analgesics as needed. *Regardless of the result of manual detorsion, emergency surgery is indicated* to perform detorsion—if necessary—and to secure the testicle. Without surgery, retorsion may occur at any time.

In patients with suspected epididymitis or orchitis,

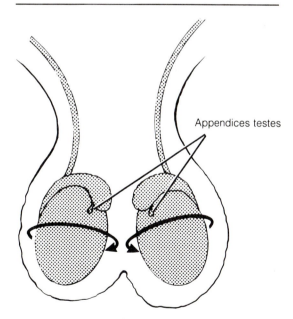

Figure 31–1. Torsion of the testicle. View of the testicles, epididymides, testicular appendages, and scrotum, showing direction of rotation of the testicles during torsion (as seen by the physician standing at the foot of the patient's bed and looking down at the patient). Manual detorsion should rotate the testicles in the opposite direction.

Appendices testes

urologic consultation should be sought if the diagnosis is in doubt. If epididymitis is present, see Chapter 34 for treatment.

Torsion of the testicular appendage (after testicular torsion is excluded) is managed with bed rest, scrotal elevation, analgesics, and follow-up care within 1–2 days. Surgical excision is often needed for adequate pain control.

PAINLESS SCROTAL MASS LESIONS
(See Table 31–3.)

Conditions causing painless (or relatively painless) scrotal swelling are not true emergencies, although testicular tumors are life-threatening and require urgent evaluation (within a few days).

Table 31–3 sets forth helpful diagnostic features of conditions associated with painless scrotal swelling. With the exception of patients who develop left-sided varicoceles before 30 years of age, patients with newly diagnosed testicular enlargement or mass lesions should be referred to a urologist.

DYSURIA

Cause

Common causes of dysuria and their associated clinical findings are given in Table 31–4. Urethral diverticula, urolithiasis, endocervical gonorrhea, balanitis, and urethral warts are uncommon causes of dysuria.

Diagnosis
A. Dysuria in Males:
1. **Urethritis**—In males, urethritis is a much more common cause of dysuria than is urinary tract infection. Attempt to express urethral discharge by milking the urethra, and send the material for culture and smear. If no discharge can be obtained, sample the anterior 2–3 cm (¾–1³⁄₁₆ in) of the urethra with a calcium alginate, Dacron, or cotton swab or wire loop, smear some of the urethral secretion obtained on a slide, and send the swab for culture for *Neisseria gonorrhoeae*. If facilities are available, also send a urethral swab in *Chlamydia* culture medium for culture and fluorescent antibody testing for *Chlamydia* infection. *Do not use a wood-handled cotton swab, since wood is toxic to the Chlamydia organism.* Smears should be stained with methylene blue or Gram stain and examined microscopically. The presence of more than 5 leukocytes per × 400 field indicates urethritis; the presence of intracellular diplococci (gram-negative if a Gram stain was done)—especially without other bacteria—indicates gono- coccal urethritis. See Chapter 34 for treatment of gonorrhea and nongonococcal urethritis.

Dysuria without evidence of urethral or urinary tract inflammation (< 5 white blood cells per × 100 field, negative culture) is rare in men and may represent low-grade infection. Treatment for urethritis is usually indicated.

2. **Prostatitis**—If no evidence of urethritis is found, obtain a midstream clean-voided urine specimen (supervise the patient so that it is collected properly). PMNs in the urine in the absence of urethritis are diagnostic of urinary tract inflammation. Prostatitis (either alone or associated with urinary tract infection) may be excluded by rectal examination and by fractionated urinalysis (3-glass test), including examination of expressed prostatic secretions. To perform the 3-glass test, prepare the patient as for a clean-voided urine specimen (retract the foreskin and cleanse the urethral meatus). Have 3 sterile containers available, labeled 1, 2, and 3. Have the patient void the first 10–15 mL of urine into the first glass, and then use the second glass for a midstream urine specimen. Have the patient stop voiding well before he feels that the bladder is empty. Then perform prostatic massage, and collect any prostatic secretions expressed. Have the patient void again, and collect the first 10–20 mL of urine in the third glass. Fraction No. 1 represents urethral urine; No. 2, bladder urine; and No. 3, prostatic secretions mixed with urine.

For further information on treatment, see Chapter 34.

Table 31–3. Diagnostic clues to the cause of common painless scrotal masses.

	History and Physical Examination	Other Diagnostic Studies
Varicocele	Usually asymptomatic mass; some patients have mild pain. Mass is separate from testis; feels like "bag of worms," especially in upright position. Size increased by Valsalva maneuver.	Not usually required, since physical examination is diagnostic. Ultrasonography also helpful in diagnosis of enigmatic cases.
Hydrocele	Gradually enlarging painless cystic mass that transilluminates. **Note:** Hydrocele may complicate tumor.	Aspiration yields clear fluid. Ultrasonography helpful in diagnosis.
Spermatocele	Asymptomatic mass separate from and superior to the testicle.	Aspiration reveals white cloudy fluid with immotile sperm. Ultrasonography also helpful in diagnosis.
Testicular tumor	Patient often a young adult. Asymptomatic enlargement of testis, rarely painful. Examination shows firm, nontender mass that does not transilluminate. Gynecomastia, virilization, or feminization occurs rarely.	Ultrasonography helpful in confirming mass lesion. Surgical exploration required for exact diagnosis of all testicular mass lesions.

Table 31–4. Diagnostic clues to common causes of dysuria.

Condition	Sex More Commonly Affected	History and Physical Examination	Diagnostic Studies
Urethritis	Men.	Dysuria, usually severe. Clear or purulent urethral discharge.	Leukocytes in urethral discharge or on urethral swab. Tests for gonococcal or chlamydial infection are often positive.
Prostatitis	Men only.	Pelvic pain and dysuria. Fever common. Tender, boggy prostate on examination.	Prostatic massage produces leukocytes and bacteria in urethral discharge or urine ("3-glass test").
Urethral stricture	Men.	Dysuria, may have split or reduced urinary stream.	Urethroscopy or urethrogram.
Urethral caruncle	Women (usually postmenopausal).	Mild dysuria; examination may show lesion.	Urethroscopy.
Dysuria-frequency syndrome (urethral syndrome)	Women only.	Dysuria and urgency. May have urethral discharge.	Pyuria; leukocytes in urethral discharge or on urethral swab.
Vaginitis	Women only.	External dysuria, vaginal discharge dyspareunia.	Vaginal smear or culture shows *Candida*, *Gardnerella vaginalis*, or *Trichomonas vaginalis*.
Genital herpes	Women.	History of herpes (if recurrent); vesicles and ulcers on external genitalia.	Positive results on tests for herpes simplex.
Urinary tract infection	Mainly women.	Dysuria, urgency, frequency; cloudy or foul-smelling urine. May have fever, flank or suprapubic tenderness.	Pyuria and bacteriuria; urine culture shows more than 10^3 bacteria/mL (often > 10^5/mL).
Urethral trauma	Either (mainly children).	History or evidence of genital manipulation or trauma.	Hematuria occasionally.
Psychogenic	Either.	No logical pattern to symptoms. Examination normal.	Normal results on urinalysis. No leukocytes on urethral swab. Tests for gonococcal and chlamydial infection negative.

3. Urinary tract infection–Leukocytes, usually with bacteria, are found on microscopic examination of a midstream urine specimen. Urine dip reagent strips that test for the presence of leukocyte esterase and nitrite are equivalent to the urine sediment analysis at detecting pyuria when both are positive. They are increasingly being used as a screening tool and may eliminate the need for microscopic examination. Culture usually shows bacteria of a single species (usually > 10^5 colony-forming units per milliliter but occasionally only 10^2–10^4, especially with certain organisms [eg, *Candida* species or enterococci]). *Note:* Urinary tract infection is unusual in men under 60 years of age unless there are associated urinary tract abnormalities or homosexual sexual activity.

4. Local causes–Inspect the penis and urethral meatus for balanitis and intrameatal pathologic structures (warts, herpetic ulcers) that are commonly associated with dysuria. Urethral strictures often cause dysuria, and observation of the urinary stream while the patient is voiding may confirm the diagnosis (split or intermittent stream).

B. Dysuria in Females:

1. Collection of urine–Obtain an uncontaminated urine specimen for microscopic analysis. Urine dip reagent strips that test for the presence of leukocyte esterase and nitrite are equivalent to the urine sediment analysis at detecting pyuria when both are positive.

They are increasingly being used as a screening tool and may eliminate the need for microscopic examination. Contamination of the specimen is usually indicated by the presence of squamous (vaginal) epithelial cells visible microscopically (eg, ≥ 5 cells per $\times$ 100 field); if these are seen, the specimen should be discarded, and another, uncontaminated specimen obtained. Proper collection techniques for adults are as follows:

a. Midstream clean-voided urine–This method of collection is satisfactory in most cases but requires a reasonably intelligent, coordinated, and well-motivated patient.

b. Catheterization–A small straight (9F) catheter should be used for quick "in and out" catheterization, since it is more comfortable than the 14–18F Foley type catheter. Contamination may occur.

c. Suprapubic aspiration–(See Chapter 46.) Suprapubic aspiration is useful in special situations (eg, for infants) and is associated with a very low contamination rate.

2. Clinical differentiation of causes of dysuria in women–

a. Dysuria-frequency syndrome (urethral syndrome) and urinary tract infection–Both these conditions are characterized by dysuria without vaginal symptoms (eg, discharge) and by pyuria (< 5 white cells per $\times$ 400 field). If bacteria are seen in the urinary sediment, urinary tract infection is a more likely diagnosis than urethral syndrome. Occasionally, women with dysuria-frequency syndrome may have no pyuria.

b. Local causes—If results on urinalysis are normal, if there are vaginal symptoms associated with dysuria, or if pain is felt outside the urinary tract ("external dysuria"), perform a pelvic examination to look for vaginitis (Chapter 34), genital herpes, or a urethral caruncle. Urethral caruncle is found in postmenopausal women and is a small, nontender red lesion resembling a strawberry on the dorsal aspect of the urethral meatus. In addition, it is helpful to culture endocervical mucus for gonococci, since gonococcal infection in women may be associated with dysuria.

Dysuria Associated With Hematuria in Either Sex

The presence of large numbers of erythrocytes (with PMNs) in the urine in either sex should suggest hemorrhagic cystitis, concomitant urolithiasis, or urethral manipulation (see Hematuria, below).

Treatment & Disposition

Treat the various causes of dysuria as follows:

A. Urinary Tract Infections: For treatment of cystitis, pyelonephritis, and urethral syndrome, see Chapter 34.

B. Gonorrhea: See Chapter 34.

C. Vaginitis: See Chapter 34.

D. Prostatitis: See Chapter 34.

E. Other Conditions: Patients with other conditions (eg, urethral stricture or diverticulum) should be referred to a urologist or gynecologist for evaluation.

HEMATURIA (Without Trauma)

Cause

Common causes of hematuria and their associated clinical findings are set forth in Table 31–5. See Chapter 20 for management of hematuria associated with trauma or genitourinary manipulation.

Renal vein thrombosis, renal arterial embolization, drug-induced (cyclophosphamide, penicillins) interstitial cystitis, or other conditions are uncommon causes of hematuria.

Diagnosis

A. History:

1. Hematuria associated with abdominal or flank pain and tenderness suggests urolithiasis or, less commonly, renal vascular disease.

2. Hematuria associated with dysuria and urinary urgency and frequency suggests hemorrhagic cystitis (either drug-induced, infectious, or idiopathic).

3. Systemic conditions associated with hematuria include idiopathic thrombocytopenic purpura, sickling hemoglobinopathies, or excessive ingestion of coumadin anticoagulants.

Table 31–5. Diagnostic clues to common causes of hematuria.

	History and Physical Findings	Diagnostic Studies
Trauma	History or evidence of local genital, abdominal (renal), or pelvic trauma or recent genitourinary instrumentation.	See Chapter 20.
Tumor	Often long-standing painless hematuria.	Excretory urogram reveals upper urinary tract tumors; cystogram or cystoscopy shows bladder tumor.
Urolithiasis	Intermittent hematuria usually associated with pain. Bladder stones may be painless but may be associated with intermittent urinary obstruction.	Excretory urography reveals ureteral stone, obstruction, or postobstructive hydroureter; cystoscopy or cystography shows bladder stones.
Infection (including tuberculosis)	Dysuria common.	Pyuria often present. Urine culture shows bacteria (usually $\geq 10^5$ colonies/mL).
Glomerulonephritis	May follow streptococcal infection; often associated with autoimmune diseases (eg, systemic lupus erythematosus). Gradual onset. Hypertension common.	Urinalysis shows leukocytes, red cell casts, and frequently proteinuria; blood urea nitrogen and serum creatinine elevated.
Prostatitis	Dysuria often present. Abnormal (large or tender) prostate.	Pyuria often present.
Urethral stricture, foreign body, or manipulation	Often painful. Local abnormality may be obvious on examination.	Urethroscopy reveals stricture or foreign body.
Sickling hemoglobinopathy or sickle cell trait	Intermittent hematuria that may be painless (trait) or painful (disease).	Urinalysis shows red blood cells and isosthenuria. Hemoglobin electrophoresis abnormal.
Bleeding diathesis	Painless hematuria. History of coagulation defect. Evidence of bleeding elsewhere (purpura, etc). Anticoagulant use.	Coagulation tests show thrombocytopenia, prolonged prothrombin time, etc (Chapter 33).

4. Bleeding from other perineal areas, especially menstrual flow, may be mistaken for hematuria.

B. Physical Examination:

1. Examine the external genitalia for local causes of hematuria (intraurethral trauma, etc).

2. Examine the abdomen, back, and pelvis for tenderness and evidence of trauma.

3. In males, perform a rectal examination for evaluation of the prostate after a urine specimen has been obtained.

C. Laboratory Examination:

1. Urinalysis–Perform urinalysis to confirm the diagnosis of hematuria. Carefully performed microscopic examination of a freshly voided midstream urine specimen is essential to the evaluation of hematuria; look especially for erythrocyte casts which suggest glomerulonephritis. In men, fractionated urinalysis (initial, midstream, and terminal specimens) is also helpful in localizing the source of hematuria.

2. Other laboratory tests–

a. Further laboratory testing (except possibly urine culture) is not usually needed for bacterial hemorrhagic cystitis.

b. Patients with urolithiasis should have baseline serum electrolyte determinations and renal function tests, especially prior to obtaining excretory urogram.

c. Patients in whom a bleeding disorder is suspected or the cause of hematuria is unknown should have the following laboratory examinations: CBC and differential; platelet estimate; determination of prothrombin and partial thromboplastin times; serum electrolyte determinations; and renal function tests.

D. Special Studies:

1. An excretory urogram may be necessary for evaluation of urolithiasis, trauma, tumors, and renal arterial or venous disease. In most cases, this x-ray should be obtained while the patient is still in the emergency department.

2. Cystoscopy is essential for evaluation of bladder or urethral hematuria due to tumors and other causes. It may also be helpful for localizing hematuria of the upper genitourinary tract to one side or the other. The need for cystoscopy should be determined by the consulting urologist.

3. Other studies such as radionuclide scans, CT scans, sonograms, or angiograms may be needed in special situations, but urologic consultation should be obtained before these are requested.

Treatment & Disposition

Treat the various causes of hematuria as follows:

A. Trauma: See Chapter 20.

B. Urinary Tract Infection: See Chapter 34.

C. Suspected Tumor: Refer the patient to a urologist for evaluation. Consider hospitalization in order to expedite diagnostic procedures.

D. Urolithiasis: See below.

E. Glomerulonephritis: Hospitalize the patient, and obtain consultation with a nephrologist.

F. Prostatitis: See Chapter 34.

G. Urethral Strictures and Foreign Bodies: Refer the patient to a urologist.

H. Unknown Cause: Patients with hematuria of unknown cause (especially gross hematuria) should be hospitalized for evaluation and treatment.

EMERGENCY TREATMENT OF SPECIFIC DISORDERS

UROLITHIASIS (Renal Colic)

Patients with stones in the urinary tract commonly present to the emergency department. Stones usually form in the renal pelvis, and symptoms occur either with passage of the stone into the ureter or as the result of infection, or both. Bladder stones are less common and may present with hematuria or intermittent urinary obstruction.

Diagnosis

A. Symptoms and Signs: The initial symptom is usually unilateral flank pain that rapidly becomes excruciating, radiating anteriorly to the ipsilateral lower quadrant of the abdomen or to the scrotum or labia. The pain may be so severe that the patient faints; occasionally, there is no pain, and the patient presents with complaints of hematuria. Eliciting a history of pain that shifts anteriorly and inferiorly from the flank as the stone moves distally in the urinary tract may be helpful in differentiating renal colic from other types of abdominal pain.

Some patients note gross hematuria. Nausea and vomiting are frequent. If complicating infection is present, there may also be signs and symptoms of pyelonephritis. Inquire about a history of similar attacks or a predisposing condition, eg, previous documented urolithiasis, gout, hypercalcemia.

Vital signs are usually normal in the absence of infection, although bradycardia from vagal hypertonicity or tachycardia from pain may be seen. Some degree of ileus is usually present. Tenderness over the affected kidney (costovertebral angle tenderness) and ureter can be elicited.

B. Laboratory Findings:

1. Hematuria (gross or microscopic) is present in most cases. Occasionally, a patient presents with pain and no hematuria.

2. Although a smear and culture of urine should be obtained as a matter of routine, bacteria will be present only if infection is superimposed.

3. Blood urea nitrogen and serum creatinine levels are usually normal. Serum calcium, phosphorus, and uric acid levels should also be obtained but are usually normal.

C. X-Ray Findings: (See Fig 31–2.) About 90% of renal stones are radiopaque. An excretory urogram is essential to verify that the opacity is indeed a stone within the urinary tract, and this study should be obtained within 24–48 hours in every patient with suspected urolithiasis. An excretory urogram is also helpful in evaluating renal function and determining the degree of obstruction to urinary flow. Hypertonicity of the iodinated dyes used in excretory urography may facilitate passage of ureteral stones. Patients with recurrent episodes of ureteral stones whose history and physical examination results are typical of urolithiasis may be managed without excretory urogram. *Caution:* Avoid excretory urograms in the following patients: **(1)** those with serum creatinine levels above 1.4 mg/dL, because of the increased risk of inducing renal failure; **(2)** those who may have multiple myeloma (elderly patients with proteinuria and elevated serum creatinine level), since acute renal failure may be precipitated; **(3)** those with documented allergy to iodine or iodinated dyes. If excretory urogram is necessary for diagnosis, premedicate the allergic patient one-half hour before the test with diphenhydramine (Benadryl, others), 50 mg intravenously, and methylprednisolone, 125 mg intravenously.

D. Ultrasound: Renal ultrasound can be a useful noninvasive diagnostic test that can often reveal urinary calculi and hydronephrosis, although it is not as sensitive as an excretory urogram, particularly for small stones. It may be of value in the patient with past allergic reactions to intravenous contrast media or in patients whose stones are radiolucent.

Treatment

About 90% of renal stones are passed spontaneously. Basic treatment is as follows:

A. Provide Analgesia: Begin analgesics as soon as the diagnosis has been established with reasonable certainty. Give morphine, 4–8 mg by slow intravenous injection, and repeat as needed. Ketorolac

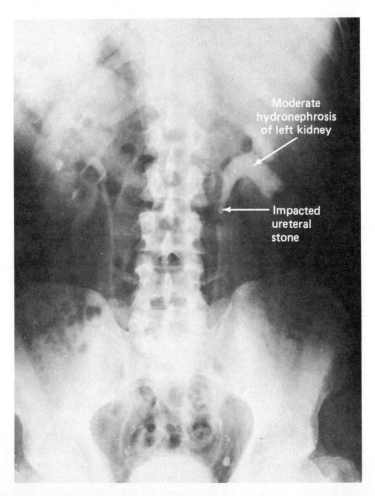

Figure 31–2. Stone in left upper ureter causing moderate obstruction. (Reproduced, with permission, from Tanagho EA, McAninch JW: *Smith's General Urology,* 13th ed. Appleton & Lange, 1992.)

(Toradol) is a new injectable nonsteroidal anti-inflammatory agent that is equipotent with mild narcotic analgesics. It is nonsedating and may be of value in patients who are suspected of drug seeking. The standard adult dose is 30–60 mg intramuscularly. If the patient is not ill enough to be hospitalized, give one of the following by mouth: **(1)** acetaminophen with codeine, 60 mg every 3–4 hours; **(2)** meperidine, 50 mg every 2–3 hours; or **(3)** oxycodone, 5 mg every 4–6 hours.

B. Ensure Adequate Hydration: Although authorities usually recommend drinking 2–3 L of fluid per day, this is probably of more value in preventing the formation of more stones than in facilitating passage of an existing stone.

C. Strain Urine: Patients with their first episode of urolithiasis or those who pass stones of unknown composition should strain their urine through a sieve, and the stone should be submitted for chemical analysis. The nets used to scoop up small tropical fish work well for this purpose.

Prevention

Specific preventive therapy can be recommended after the composition of the stone has been determined by chemical analysis.

Disposition

A. Patients with any of the following conditions require hospitalization:

1. Pain requiring parenteral analgesics.
2. Persistent vomiting or ileus.
3. Coexisting pyelonephritis.
4. Documented or suspected renal dysfunction (elevated blood urea nitrogen or serum creatinine levels, bilateral ureteral stones, oliguria or anuria, hydronephrosis).
5. Pain that persists for more than 2–3 days, suggesting persistent urinary obstruction.

B. Patients who do not require hospitalization should be referred to a urologist within 24–48 hours for further evaluation and treatment.

DISEASES OF THE MALE GENITOURINARY SYSTEM*

1. TORSION OF THE TESTICLE

Diagnosis

Torsion of the testicle usually occurs in boys or young men and is uncommon over age 20. There is abrupt onset of severe pain in the scrotum, followed by rapid swelling of the involved testicle and, subse-

---

*Diseases of the female genitourinary tract are discussed in Chapter 30.

quently, the scrotum. If the patient is examined early in the disease, the testicle is elevated and horizontally displaced. Nausea and vomiting may occur.

Epididymitis and orchitis may be confused with torsion of the testicle; helpful differentiating features are discussed in the section on scrotal pain and in Table 31–2. The diagnosis may be confirmed by Doppler ultrasound examination or radionuclide scanning.

Treatment & Disposition

A. Provide analgesia. Usually, parenteral narcotic analgesics are required (eg, morphine, 2–10 mg intravenously or intramuscularly, depending on the patient's size).

B. Prepare for surgery. Give nothing orally, obtain blood for CBC and renal function tests, and begin an intravenous infusion of 5% dextrose in half-normal saline.

C. Obtain immediate urologic or general surgical consultation. If a delay in surgery or urologic consultation is anticipated, attempt manual detorsion (p 549). Detorsion (manual or surgical) must be performed within 6 hours to prevent testicular infarction.

2. ORCHITIS

Orchitis is usually due to mumps virus, in which case coexisting parotitis is common. Other causes (eg, vasculitis) are rare. If the diagnosis is in doubt or specific treatment appears warranted, obtain urologic consultation. Otherwise, symptomatic relief may be achieved with recumbency and analgesics. Rarely, mumps orchitis results in sterility.

3. PRIAPISM

Diagnosis

Priapism is a rare disorder consisting of a prolonged, painful erection, unassociated with sexual stimulation. About 25% of cases are associated with leukemia, metastatic carcinoma, or sickling hemoglobinopathies. If the patient does not know whether he has these conditions, a CBC, differential, and sickling test should be performed. The cause is unclear in most patients.

Treatment

Administer ice-water enemas. The erection usually subsides spontaneously in 2–3 hours. Partial exchange transfusion (removal of approximately 1 L of blood and replacement with 4–5 units of packed red blood cells and normal saline as needed) may be effective, especially for patients with sickling hemoglobinopathies. Additional therapeutic measures that have been advocated (without proof of efficacy) include spinal anesthesia, needle aspiration of the corpora cavernosa, and irrigation of the corpora with anticoagulants. Generally, these procedures should be performed after the patient has been hospitalized. If these methods fail, operation is necessary.

Disposition

Hospitalize all patients with persistent priapism or those with serious underlying disease (sickling hemoglobinopathy, leukemia). Obtain urgent urologic consultation. Refer other patients to a urologist as soon as possible.

4. BALANITIS

Balanitis is bacterial or fungal infection of the space between the glans penis and the foreskin. It is manifested by pain and discharge from around the foreskin. Retraction of the foreskin reveals a purulent exudate over the glans, often with small superficial ulcerations. Gram-stained smears (culture is usually unnecessary) show PMNs and mixed bacterial flora.

Treatment consists of peroxide soaks 4 times a day and oral penicillin V (the potassium salt) or ampicillin, 500 mg orally 4 times a day. If phimosis or paraphimosis coexists, see the next section. Elective circumcision is usually indicated after one or more episodes of balanitis; refer the patient to a urologist.

5. PHIMOSIS & PARAPHIMOSIS

Phimosis is a fibrous constriction of the foreskin preventing retraction; it is often associated with

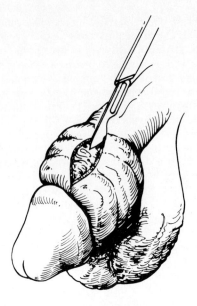

Figure 31–3. Method of performing a dorsal slit of the foreskin for balanitis with paraphimosis. An incision made through the tight band of skin as shown will relieve the paraphimosis.

balanitis. Phimosis *without* balanitis may be an indication for elective circumcision, but it is not an emergency. Surgical correction should not be attempted in the emergency department.

Paraphimosis occurs when the retracted foreskin develops a fixed constriction proximal to the glans. The penis distal to the constricting foreskin may become swollen and painful, or even gangrenous, and urinary retention may result. Attempt manual reduc-

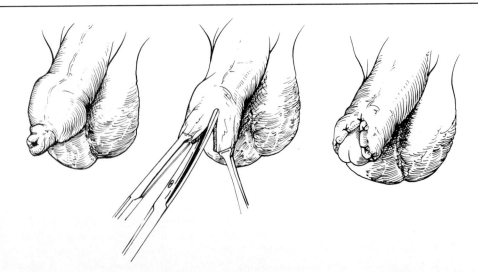

Figure 31–4. Method of performing a dorsal slit of the foreskin for phimosis.

tion: Squeeze the glans firmly for 5–10 minutes to reduce its size. Then move the prepuce distally while the glans is pushed proximally. If manual reduction is impossible, dorsal slit of the foreskin is necessary (Figs 31–3 and 31–4). Refer the patient to a urologist for elective circumcision.

REFERENCES

Abuelo JG: The diagnosis of hematuria. Arch Intern Med 1983;143:967.

Berger RE et al: Manifestations and therapy of acute epididymitis: Prospective study of 50 cases. J Urol 1979;121:750.

Bolann BJ, Sandberg S, Digranes A: Implications of probability analysis for interpreting results of leukocyte esterase and nitrite test strips. Clin Chem 1989;35:1663.

Carlson KJ, Mulley AG: Management of acute dysuria: A decision-analysis model of alternative strategies. Ann Intern Med 1985;102:244.

Coe FL, Brenner BM, Stein JH: *Nephrolithiasis.* Vol 5 of: *Contemporary Issues in Nephrology.* Churchill Livingstone, 1980.

Dans PE, Klaus B: Dysuria in women. Johns Hopkins Med J 1976;138:13.

Haynes BE, Bessen HA, Haynes VE: The diagnosis of testicular torsion. JAMA 1983;249:2522.

Hooton TM, Barnes RC: Urethritis in men. Infect Dis Clin North Am 1987;1:165.

Johnson JR, Stamm WE: Diagnosis and treatment of acute urinary tract infections. Infect Dis Clin North Am 1987;1:773.

Kleeman CR: Kidney stones. West J Med 1982;132:313.

Stamm WE et al: Causes of the acute urethral syndrome in women. N Engl J Med 1980;303:400.

Stamm WE et al: Diagnosis of coliform infections in acutely dysuric women. N Engl J Med 1982;307:463.

Stamm WE et al: Treatment of the acute urethral syndrome. N Engl J Med 1981;304:956.

Tanagho EA, McAninch JW (editors): *Smith's General Urology,* 13th ed. Appleton & Lange, 1992.

Vordermark JS II et al: The testicular scan: Use in diagnosis and management of acute epididymitis. JAMA 1981; 245:2512.

Wright JE: Torsion of the testis. Br J Surg 1977;64:274.

32

Vascular Emergencies

Carol A. Raviola, MD, & Donald D. Trunkey, MD

Most vascular emergencies are due either to disruption of the blood vessel wall with bleeding (eg, from penetrating trauma) or to occlusion of the blood vessel lumen (eg, by an embolus or thrombus). The major consequences of these events are blood loss or acute distal ischemia. If vascular injury is untreated, hypotension or tissue necrosis may occur.

I. VASCULAR EMERGENCIES DUE TO TRAUMA

IMMEDIATE MANAGEMENT OF LIFE-THREATENING VASCULARINJURIES

Maintain Airway & Treat Associated Injuries

See Chapters 1 and 5. Treat associated life-threatening head, thoracic, and abdominal injuries (Chapters 4, 16, 18, 19).

Stop Hemorrhage

A. Stop active bleeding from arterial or venous hemorrhage by gentle manual compression.

B. Avoid clamping the bleeding vessel, since this will cause further injury.

C. Avoid the use of tourniquets.

D. Do not remove embedded objects, since they may be preventing further bleeding.

Treat or Prevent Shock (See also Chapter 3.)

A. Insert 2 or more large-bore ($\geq$ 16-gauge) intravenous catheters or perform venous cutdowns. Two intravenous access sites are preferable if the patient is already in shock or is bleeding profusely.

B. While intravenous catheters are being inserted, draw blood for CBC, serum electrolyte, glucose, and creatinine measurements, and typing and cross-matching (reserve 6–8 units of packed red blood cells or whole blood).

C. Begin intravenous infusion of crystalloid solutions (eg, normal saline or acetated or lactated Ringer's injection) to support blood pressure. Up to 2–3 L of crystalloid solution may be given before whole blood must be administered.

D. Replace blood. The number of units administered depends on the severity of existing blood loss and on anticipated loss from projected surgery. Use fresh whole blood whenever possible.

Prevent Further Vascular & Nerve Injury

All fractures and joint dislocations associated with abnormal pulses should be carefully reduced and splinted to reduce further neurovascular damage. Control hemorrhage by pressure; avoid clamping vessels to stop hemorrhage. Consider arteriography.

Minimize Ischemia

Keep ischemic limbs horizontal. Do not use tourniquets.

Relieve Pain

Provide adequate analgesia; if necessary, give morphine, 5–15 mg intramuscularly or intravenously every 3–4 hours as needed.

Obtain Surgical Consultation

All documented or suspected vascular injuries should be examined promptly by a general or vascular surgeon before the patient is transferred from the emergency department. Delay may result in loss of function of the limb.

Hospitalize as Required

Hospitalize all patients with arterial or major venous injuries.

General Considerations

Acute vascular injury may result in either hemorrhage or tissue ischemia.

A. Arterial Injury:

1. Hemorrhage–Obvious external hemorrhage is present in many patients. Occult bleeding into soft tissue fascial planes, the retroperitoneum, pelvis, or body cavities may also occur.

2. Ischemia–Ischemia from arterial injury must be recognized and treated promptly, since increased tissue pressure and swelling from ischemia further compromise arterial perfusion, and prolonged ischemia results in irreversible tissue damage.

B. Venous Injury:

1. Hemorrhage–Obvious or occult bleeding usually occurs following venous injury. It is rarely life-threatening except in the case of central veins (eg, vena cava).

2. Ischemia–Tissue ischemia from venous trauma alone is rare, although venous obstruction may worsen preexisting tissue ischemia resulting from arterial injury.

C. Causes of Vascular Injury:

1. Penetrating trauma–Penetrating trauma is the most common cause of peripheral vascular injury and ranges in severity from innocuous simple puncture wounds to extensive wounds caused by high-velocity missiles.

2. Blunt trauma–Blunt trauma may also cause peripheral vascular injury. Contusions or crushing injuries of an artery may cause either transmural disruption with hemorrhage, or partial disruption of the artery and elevation of the intima from an intramural hematoma. Thrombosis of a segment of artery may also occur. Blunt trauma with posterior dislocation of the knee may cause disruption of the popliteal artery (Fig 32–1). Blunt trauma may also indirectly contribute to vascular occlusion by creating large hematomas near a blood vessel. Hematoma formation may lead to arterial spasm, distortion, or compartment syndromes, all of which may interfere with arterial flow.

3. Chemicals–Chemical injury to blood vessels is increasing in frequency. It is generally iatrogenic or associated with parenteral drug abuse. Intra-arterial injection of drugs that are chemically irritating to tissues (eg, barbiturates) causes occlusion of small peripheral vessels (p 575) (Fig 32–2). If occlusion is severe, all or part of the limb may be lost. Extravasation of intravenously administered chemicals may also cause associated arterial spasm or tissue necrosis. Barbiturates, phenytoin, vasopressors, and chemotherapeutic agents (eg, doxorubicin) are notable examples. High doses of certain intravenously administered vasopressors (eg, dopamine) can cause intense peripheral vasoconstriction with ultimate digital ischemic necrosis.

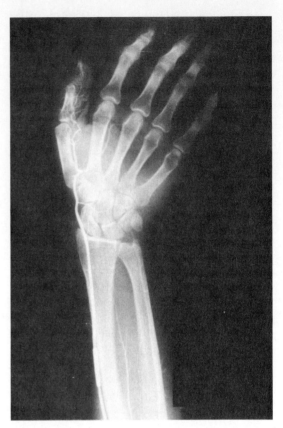

Figure 32–2. Intentional self-injection of pentobarbital into the right radial artery. The arteriogram shows fusiform dilatation of the radial artery in the forearm. The palmar arch had been thrombosed and does not fill with contrast medium, and there is severe vasospasm of the vessels to the second finger.

D. Sequelae: Late sequelae associated with major vascular injuries include false aneurysms and arteriovenous fistulas.

1. False aneurysms–False aneurysms result from walled-off disruptions of vessel walls. They enlarge over time, may compress adjacent veins or nerves, and may rupture without warning.

2. Fistulas–Fistulas may occur after adjacent arteries and veins are injured simultaneously, usually as a result of stab wounds or missile injury. The fistula may enlarge over time and cause increased cardiac output. If the fistula involves the blood supply to an extremity, dilated veins may be observed in that extremity. Turbulent blood flow through the fistula results in an obvious thrill or bruit. Fistulas may also compress adjacent nerves or impede collateral circulation, or they may rupture, causing a severe hemorrhage.

Principles of Diagnosis

A. Physical Examination: If there is a wound in

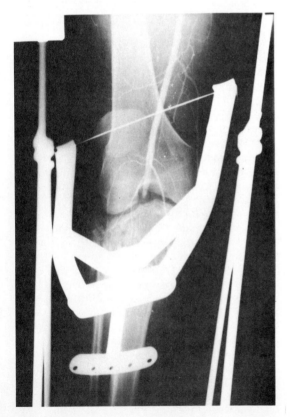

Figure 32–1. Arteriogram after posterior dislocation of the knee, showing injury to the popliteal artery. The diagnosis was confirmed at operation.

the vicinity of a major blood vessel, the physician must assume that vascular injury has occurred. The findings listed below may not appear for hours to days following a significant vascular injury, and *absence of these findings does not rule out the possibility of vascular injury.*

1. Signs–Clinical manifestations of vascular injury include an expanding or pulsating hematoma, to-and-fro or continuous murmurs of arteriovenous fistulas, a false aneurysm, loss of pulses, progressive swelling of the part, unexplained ischemia or dysfunction, and unilateral cool or pale extremities.

2. Pulses–The physician should perform a complete vascular examination unless treatment of other life-threatening injuries precludes it.

a. Palpation–Palpate all peripheral pulses: carotid, axillary, brachial, radial, femoral, popliteal, dorsalis pedis, and posterior tibial.

b. Doppler ultrasound examination–The presence of blood flow in a peripheral vessel can be detected using a standard pocket Doppler apparatus. Any assessment of the normality of this flow requires concomitant pressure measurements or wave form analysis.

3. Murmurs and bruits–Auscultation over injured areas should be performed to detect bruits or murmurs.

4. Neurologic function–The physician should also assess neurologic function. Paresthesia may be an early sign of developing vascular problems (eg, compartment syndrome).

B. Arteriography: Arteriography is the single best method of confirming suspected vascular injury. In addition, arteriography defines the nature and extent of injury and is essential to the surgeon contemplating corrective surgery. Specific indications for arteriography are set forth in Table 32–1.

Caution: Arteriography should *not* be performed in a patient whose condition is unstable and who needs emergency laparotomy or thoracotomy. The procedure should be delayed until after resuscitation and treatment of the life-threatening emergency, either in the emergency department or in the operating room.

Table 32–1. Indications for arteriography following trauma.

Neck injuries—zones I and III
Chest injuries
   Mediastinal widening on chest x-ray
   Deviation of trachea to the right
   Obscuring of aortic shadow
Abdominal injuries
   Nonvisualizing kidney on urography
   Bleeding pelvic fractures
All penetrating wounds of extremities in proximity to major vessels
Dislocation of the knee
All fractures associated with abnormal pulses

EMERGENCY MANAGEMENT OF SPECIFIC VASCULAR INJURIES

NECK INJURIES
(See also Chapter 17.)

Diagnosis

Arterial injury in the neck may cause hemorrhage or cerebral ischemia. The hemorrhage may be obvious or may be diverted into the thorax, causing hemothorax. Arterial injury with bleeding into the fascial planes of the neck may cause venous obstruction or airway obstruction. Concomitant injury of nonvascular structures (trachea, esophagus) is common.

Treatment

A. Emergency Measures: It is more difficult to control hemorrhage from vessels in the neck than from those in the extremities.

1. *Digital pressure is the only method that should be used.*

2. Avoid tourniquets and clamping.

3. Do not remove an embedded object, since it may be preventing hemorrhage.

B. Complications:

1. Air embolism–When large neck veins are injured, air embolism is a possible complication that can be prevented by keeping the patient supine and applying digital pressure to the injured vessel. If air embolism is believed to have occurred, the patient should be placed on the left side, head lower than feet, to trap air emboli in the right ventricle. Administer 100% oxygen.

2. Airway obstruction–Obstruction resulting from airway compression due to the expanding hematoma should be managed by endotracheal intubation.

C. Further Treatment Measures: Further management of vascular injuries of the neck depends on the zone of injury (Fig 32–3). All patients with zone I and zone III neck injuries should undergo arteriography as soon as vital signs are stable. Some surgeons recommend routine arteriography of zone II injuries as well.

1. Zone I (thoracic outlet) injuries–These injuries require arteriography because of the high incidence of associated vascular injury, which frequently requires surgical correction (Fig 32–4).

2. Zone II injuries–Surgical exploration is usually recommended if the injury penetrates beneath the platysma muscle, even if there are no local findings (Fig 32–5). Associated injuries to the venous system, trachea, or esophagus are not ruled out by negative findings on arteriography.

3. Zone III injuries–Arteriography should be performed in zone III injuries because the relation-

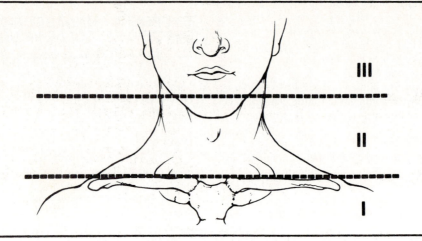

Figure 32–3. Zones of vascular injury in the neck.

ship of the blood vessels to the base of the skull often precludes distal control of hemorrhage at operation. Zone III vascular injuries are often best managed by nonsurgical techniques such as balloon tamponade or angiographic embolization of a vertebral artery injury in the intervertebral canal (Figs 32–6 and 32–7).

Disposition

Asymptomatic patients with mild neck injuries due to blunt trauma or penetrating injuries that do not cross the platysma muscle may be discharged from the emergency department. Hospitalize all other pa-

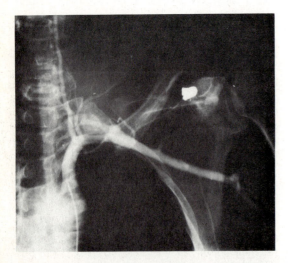

Figure 32–4. Zone I injury—Despite multiple gunshot wounds in the left parasternal area, distal pulses in the left arm were normal, and there were no thrills or bruits. The arteriogram shows a large false aneurysm of the left subclavian artery distal to the origin of the vertebral artery.

tients with neck injuries, and seek consultation with a general or vascular surgeon.

CHEST INJURIES
(See also Chapter 18.)

Diagnosis

Arterial or venous injury to the chest may result in hemothorax, apical hematoma, or widened mediastinum caused by contained rupture of blood vessels.

A. Patients with uncontained penetrating injuries of the great vessels rarely survive longer than a few minutes.

B. Hemorrhage resulting from blunt or decelerating force or from small penetrating wounds may be contained briefly in fascial planes. Lack of active bleeding at the site of injury should not be taken as a sign that the patient is in stable condition, since massive bleeding almost always recurs within a few hours.

C. Transfemoral retrograde aortic arch arteriography is mandatory in any patient who has suffered a rapid deceleration injury and has fracture of the first or second ribs or findings associated with traumatic rupture of the thoracic aorta (Table 32–2).

Table 32–2. X-ray findings associated with traumatic rupture of the thoracic aorta.

Left apical "cap" (fluid in the apical pleural space)
Widened mediastinum
Deviation of trachea to the right
Depression of left main stem bronchus
Obscuration of the aortic arch
Hemothorax

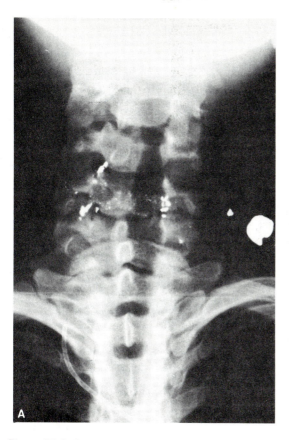 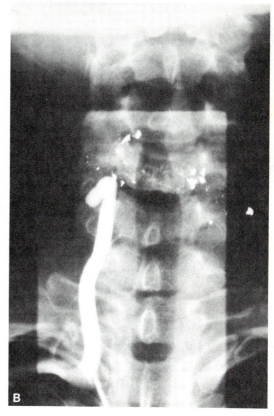

Figure 32–5. Zone II injury—***A:*** Hematoma in the right posterior neck caused by a low-velocity .38-caliber bullet passing through the right vertebral body of C5. ***B:*** Arteriogram shows a carotid-internal jugular arteriovenous fistula that was successfully corrected.

Treatment & Disposition

All patients with a widened mediastinum or documented thoracic aortic injury must be transported immediately to a hospital equipped to handle repair of the thoracic aorta, since most patients with ruptures contained in the fascial planes surrounding the aorta will die from exsanguination within 48 hours if they do not undergo operation. It is important to maintain intravascular volume with packed red blood cells, whole blood, or crystalloid solutions during transport. Occasionally, exsanguinating hemorrhage requires emergency thoracotomy for the control of bleeding.

PULMONARY VASCULAR INJURIES

Diagnosis

Most patients present with penetrating chest or abdominal trauma and rapidly expanding hemothorax, visible on chest x-ray. Rarely, blunt chest trauma is associated with pulmonary vascular injury.

Treatment & Disposition

Most patients can be managed with a chest tube that uses suction and allows the lung to reexpand and block the bleeding vessel. Continued massive bleeding requires prompt surgery. Consider the use of autotransfusion (Chapter 46). Prompt consultation with a general, vascular, or thoracic surgeon is required, since exsanguination can occur rapidly.

Hospitalization is indicated for all patients.

ABDOMINAL INJURIES
(See also Chapter 19.)

Diagnosis

Injuries to major vessels within the abdominal cavity present mainly as hemorrhagic shock that fails to respond to resuscitative efforts. Although arteriography is rarely required to diagnose vessel injury in the abdomen, it is useful both diagnostically and therapeutically in patients with severe pelvic trauma who have ongoing bleeding, since angiographic embolization can be effective treatment in certain injuries.

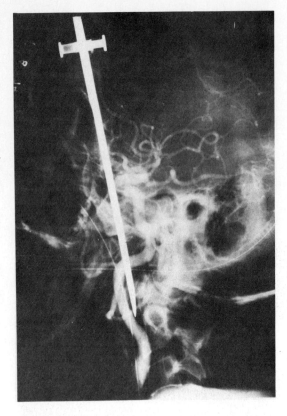

Figure 32–6. Zone III injury—Knife wound sustained by a 57-year-old man who was stabbed in the head. Bilateral carotid arteriograms, including this one of the left carotid, showed no injury. The patient recovered uneventfully after surgical removal of the knife.

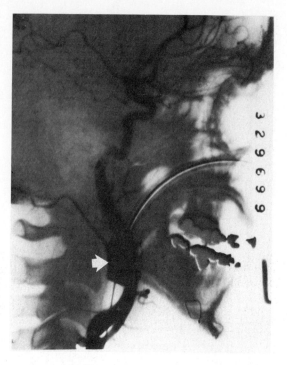

Figure 32–7. Zone III injury—Injury to the left internal carotid artery sustained by a 48-year-old man after a blow to the neck that resulted in a fractured mandible and right hemiparesis. Angiography showed a false aneurysm high in the artery (arrow) but failed to show a large surrounding hematoma that was causing marked anterior displacement of the artery. The hemiparesis resulted from emboli originating in the injured vessel.

Aortography is also useful in establishing the diagnosis of renovascular pedicle injury in trauma patients with nonvisualization of a kidney on urography (Chapter 20). CT scan may also be helpful.

Treatment & Disposition

Immediate operation is the only effective treatment for abdominal vascular injuries. Support blood pressure with infusion of intravenous fluids (colloid or crystalloid solutions) until surgery can be performed. Packed red blood cells or whole blood should be used as soon as available (Chapter 3).

A portable chest x-ray (upright, if possible) should be obtained before laparotomy to rule out unsuspected thoracic injuries.

A pneumatic antishock (MAST) garment may stabilize the patient's condition enough so that transfer to a facility providing definitive treatment is possible.

INJURIES TO THE EXTREMITIES

Diagnosis

A. Penetrating Trauma: Vascular injuries are present in 25–35% of patients with penetrating trauma to the extremities. Occasionally, vascular trauma is present without the usual physical findings, and the presence of a pulse does not rule out injury to the vessel. Arteriography is required whenever the weapon's trajectory has passed close to major blood vessels (Figs 32–8 and 32–9).

B. Blunt Trauma: Vascular injury may also occur after blunt trauma, especially if fractures and joint dislocations are present. Even if the pulse is restored with splinting and traction, an arteriogram is still necessary to rule out significant injury to the intima.

C. Posterior Dislocation of the Knee: Posterior dislocation of the knee is associated with popliteal artery injury in half of cases, and arteriography is therefore mandatory (Fig 32–1).

Treatment

Stabilize the patient, and stop hemorrhage as out-

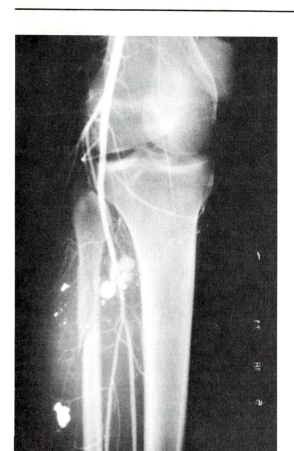

Figure 32–8. Physical examination after a gunshot wound of the leg showed a normal posterior tibial pulse and absent dorsalis pedis pulse. The arteriogram shows disruption of the anterior tibial artery near its origin, with formation of a false aneurysm.

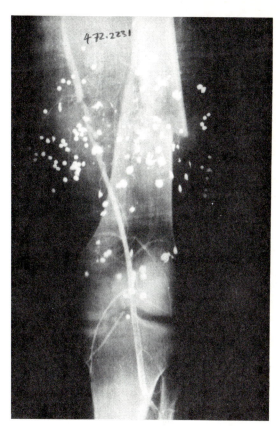

Figure 32–9. Initial examination after a short-range shotgun blast to the leg showed normal pulses. After transfer of the patient, the peripheral pulses in the leg disappeared. The arteriogram shows extensive damage to the superficial femoral artery and a distal clot in the popliteal artery.

lined above. Splint fractures. Do not clamp vessels or use a tourniquet unless injury is exsanguinating the patient and compression fails to control the hemorrhage.

Disposition

All patients with suspected vascular injury should be hospitalized for arteriography. Obtain general or vascular surgical consultation.

MAJOR VENOUS TRAUMA

Trauma to peripheral veins without associated arterial injury normally does not require operative correction; however, disruption of the central large veins (vena cava or its immediate branches: subclavian veins, iliac veins)—especially where they are not enclosed by dense fascia or muscles—requires prompt operation.

Diagnosis

Venous injury is usually manifested by hemorrhage, not ischemia.

Bleeding from the central veins presents as progressive hemorrhagic shock (Chapter 3). Superior vena cava and subclavian vein hemorrhage is usually associated with hemothorax visible on chest x-ray.

In contrast, hemorrhage from the inferior vena cava and iliac vein is more difficult to detect. The only common finding is progressive hemorrhagic shock, and many of these injuries are not suspected before they are discovered on celiotomy.

Diagnosis depends on venography (occasionally, the lesion may be visible on the venous phase of an arteriogram) and on discovery at surgery, since the condition of most patients is usually too unstable to allow detailed radiologic evaluation.

Treatment & Disposition

Surgical correction in the operating room is indicated.

II. VASCULAR EMERGENCIES NOT DUE TO TRAUMA

ACUTE ISCHEMIA

ACUTE PERIPHERAL ISCHEMIA DUE TO MAJOR ARTERIAL OCCLUSION

General Considerations

A. Mechanisms of Occlusion: Acute arterial occlusion may be caused by an embolus, thrombosis, or trauma. Embolic occlusion may be caused by the dislodgment of intravascular thrombus or tumor. Thrombi generally originate in the heart but may originate anywhere in the vascular system.

1. Cardiac emboli–Cardiac emboli generally originate in the left atrium in patients with atrial fibrillation or mitral valve disease and in the left ventricle in patients with recent myocardial infarction or ventricular aneurysm.

2. Vascular emboli–Vascular emboli originate on irregular luminal surfaces of atherosclerotic vessels (eg, ulcerative plaques or aneurysms). These emboli may contain cholesterol in the clot.

3. Tumor emboli–Tumor emboli are rare, the most common source being atrial myxomas.

4. Thrombosis–Thrombosis of an atherosclerotic artery resulting in acute ischemia is uncommon but may occur secondary to dissection of blood beneath an atherosclerotic plaque or terminal occlusion of a diseased artery or bypass graft when collateral circulation is grossly inadequate.

B. Consequences of Occlusion:

1. Ischemia–Acute occlusion of a previously patent major artery results in ischemia of the nerves, muscles, and skin distal to the artery. The severity of ischemia is inversely proportionate to the adequacy of blood flow in collateral vascular channels.

2. Reversal of ischemia–

a. Surgery–Before the development of tissue necrosis, acute ischemia can be reversed by an operation that restores patency to the occluded vessel.

b. Heparin–Administration of heparin (see Treatment, below) reduces arteriospasm and prevents propagation of thrombus distal to the site of injury, while ischemia improves as collateral vessels start to carry the circulatory flow.

c. Thrombolytics–Thrombolytic agents (eg, streptokinase, urokinase) may lyse a newly formed thrombus and reestablish perfusion.

d. Collateral blood flow–Ischemia is also reversed by spontaneous increase in collateral blood flow.

3. Irreversible effects–Within a few hours after persistent and severe occlusion, irreversible anesthesia, paralysis, and cutaneous infarction occur; the latter is manifested by a line of demarcation. During this time, developing thrombus progressively occludes the distal vessels, thereby preventing successful restoration of blood flow to the distal part.

4. Limb salvage–Salvage of the affected limb after an episode of acute ischemia depends on early recognition that ischemia has occurred and initiation of appropriate therapy before irreversible tissue damage occurs.

Diagnosis

A. Initial Findings: Coldness and numbness (and occasionally pain in the extremity) are followed by loss of motor function. Initial pallor is followed by mottled cyanosis. Severe pain is invariable after 12–18 hours.

B. Late Findings: Pain, tense swelling, and acute tenderness of a muscle belly are late findings. If these findings persist longer than 18–24 hours, irreversible ischemia with gangrene is inevitable. Pulses are absent, and there is no capillary perfusion in the affected part.

C. Collateral Flow: Tissues immediately beyond an occlusion are supplied by collateral vessels. Table 32–3 shows the level of cutaneous demarcation for common arterial occlusions. If collateral flow increases, warmth and capillary filling are restored, sensory deficit lessens, and the symptoms become those of chronic occlusion of the involved artery, eg, claudication with exercise.

D. Laboratory Studies: The results of Doppler ultrasound studies further reinforce the diagnosis of major arterial occlusion; arteriography confirms it and also serves to localize the site of the lesion.

Treatment

A. Notify a general or vascular surgeon immediately.

B. Insert a large-bore (≥ 16-gauge) intravenous catheter.

C. Obtain baseline CBC, platelet count, prothrombin time, partial thromboplastin time, and blood chemistry studies (eg, SMA-12), and send a tube of clotted blood for typing and cross-matching.

Table 32–3. Level of cutaneous demarcation for common sites of arterial occlusion.

Site of Occlusion	Level of Demarcation
Infrarenal aorta	Mid abdomen
Aortic bifurcation and common iliac arteries	Groin
External iliac artery	Upper one-third of thigh
Common femoral artery	Lower one-third of thigh
Superficial femoral artery	Upper one-third of calf
Popliteal artery	Lower one-third of calf

D. Begin a full intravenous systemic anticoagulation with heparin. Give 100 units/kg intravenously initially, with subsequent doses determined by the results of coagulation tests (eg, maintain the partial thromboplastin time between 1½ and 2½ times longer than the control time). Most adult patients require 1000–2000 units/h (given by continuous intravenous infusion). Alternatively, thrombolytic agents (eg, streptokinase, or urokinase via intra-arterial infusion) are increasingly being used to promote clot lysis.

E. In general, surgery is required to remove emboli from major arteries. In advanced ischemia, operation can usually save the extremity if it is performed within the first 12–18 hours after occlusion. When collateral circulation is adequate to permit survival of the limb, the need for and timing of operation are based on the level of chronic disability anticipated from the degree of vascular occlusion present.

Disposition

All patients with acute arterial insufficiency should be hospitalized for management.

ACUTE PERIPHERAL ISCHEMIA DUE TO SMALL-VESSEL OCCLUSION ("Blue Toe Syndrome")

Acute occlusion of a digital artery results in profound ischemia of the involved digit. The source of the emboli causing occlusion may be clots on prosthetic heart valves, mural thrombi lining the walls of peripheral aneurysms (most commonly popliteal or subclavian), ulcerative atheromatous plaques in arteries proximal to the digit (eg, iliac arteries), or septic emboli from infected heart valves.

Diagnosis
The diagnosis is made on clinical grounds. There is sudden onset of pain, cyanosis, and coldness and numbness in the affected digit. These changes generally improve spontaneously after several days. Recurrence in the same or in a different digit is the rule.

Treatment
A. Consult a vascular surgeon. Sympathectomy may be required. Proximal intra-arterial occlusive lesions may require correction to improve inflow.

B. The source of embolization must be promptly identified and corrected definitely; otherwise, recurrence is likely.

C. Long-term anticoagulation may be necessary, particularly if the heart is the source of emboli.

Disposition
Hospitalize the patient for evaluation and possible surgery.

ACUTE PERIPHERAL ISCHEMIA DUE TO VENOUS OCCLUSION

Phlegmasia cerulea dolens (venous gangrene) is a severe form of iliofemoral thrombosis characterized by massive venous occlusion. Rapidly progressive venous hypertension results in diffuse limb swelling and systemic hypovolemia. Distal ischemia occurs secondary to increased venous and tissue pressure. Cyanosis develops, and gangrene can occur.

Diagnosis
Massive acute swelling of the entire leg and cutaneous cyanosis occur early. Distal pulses are diminished or absent. Gangrene is a late finding. The diagnosis is confirmed by noninvasive means (eg, Doppler ultrasonic flow probe) or venography.

Treatment
Start intravenous heparin anticoagulation (p 566). Immediate thrombectomy or thrombolytic therapy may be necessary.

Disposition
Hospitalize all patients, and consult a general or vascular surgeon.

ACUTE VISCERAL (INTESTINAL) ISCHEMIA

Significant arterial insufficiency can cause ischemia that results in necrosis of the bowel mucosa. This may progress to full-thickness involvement in 6–48 hours. The extent of necrosis depends on the vessel involved, the adequacy of collateral perfusion, and the degree of hypoperfusion. Untreated severe intestinal ischemia results in intestinal gangrene, diffuse peritonitis, cardiovascular collapse, and death.

Etiology
A. Acute Mesenteric Vascular Occlusion: This is the cause of acute visceral ischemia in two-thirds of patients. Occlusion may be due to an embolus from a cardiac mural thrombus or to arterial thrombosis that is the end result of atherosclerotic stenosis of the involved vessel. Some patients give a history of intestinal angina. Rarely, arterial thrombosis is due to a dissecting aneurysm, connective tissue disease (eg, polyarteritis), or other condition.

Venous thrombosis occurs occasionally and is associated with portal hypertension, abdominal sepsis, hypercoagulable state, trauma, or use of oral contraceptives.

B. Nonocclusive Arteriolar Intestinal Ischemia: This is the cause of acute visceral ischemia in one-third of patients and can occur with cardiac arrhythmia, sepsis, or any prolonged hypotensive state.

Splanchnic vasoconstriction causes ischemia secondary to a low-flow state.

Diagnosis

Obscure abdominal pain and intestinal bleeding in elderly patients should suggest the diagnosis of intestinal ischemia.

A. Symptoms and Signs: Severe, poorly localized, diffuse abdominal pain is invariable in intestinal ischemia. See Chapter 7 for differential diagnosis of disorders causing acute abdominal pain. With major acute occlusion, the onset of pain is sudden. With nonocclusive ischemia, pain may develop more insidiously.

There are usually few abdominal findings early in the disease; later, abdominal distention and tenderness generally occur. Gross or occult intestinal bleeding may be present. Systemic toxicity may precede abdominal findings. Shock and generalized peritonitis occur late.

B. Laboratory Tests and Special Studies:

1. Laboratory tests–Laboratory tests show leukocytosis, metabolic acidosis, and elevated serum amylase.

2. X-ray findings–Upright plain films show ileus, absence of intestinal gas, or diffuse distention with an air-fluid level. Ischemia and intestinal necrosis are late findings. Abdominal plain films are abnormal in only 20% of cases. A barium enema (not recommended if vascular disease is strongly suspected) may show "thumbprinting" of the colonic mucosa (Fig 32–10).

3. Mesenteric arteriography–When performed early in the course of the disease, mesenteric arteriography is the definitive diagnostic procedure, since it demonstrates major vascular occlusion, if present. If it is done later, it merely delays necessary surgery and permits development of more extensive bowel necrosis and peritonitis. The catheter inserted in the superior mesenteric artery may be used to infuse

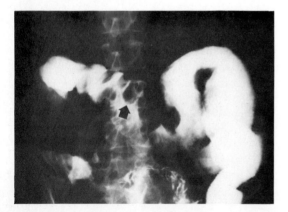

Figure 32–10. A 65-year-old woman with congestive heart failure presented with abdominal pain and bloody diarrhea. A barium enema showed "thumbprinting" (arrow) of the colonic mucosa, indicating ischemic colitis.

vasodilating agents when the cause of disease is nonocclusive arteriolar intestinal ischemia and after the primary occlusive lesion is corrected.

Treatment

A. Treat hypotension and shock with infusion of intravenous crystalloid solutions and blood, if bleeding is present.

B. Notify a vascular or general surgeon immediately to prepare for surgery.

C. Prompt operation is required to resect necrotic bowel. In some cases, the embolus can be removed or the arterial obstruction bypassed.

D. Vasodilator drugs may be used as an adjunct to management of the vascular disease in selected cases of nonocclusive ischemia; however, operation is usually required to resect necrotic bowel.

E. Begin parenteral administration of broad-spectrum antimicrobials (see Table 19–1).

Disposition

All patients with suspected or proved acute visceral ischemia should be hospitalized.

ACUTE CEREBRAL ISCHEMIA DUE TO EMBOLI

Cerebrovascular accident (stroke) due to infarction is in many cases the result of embolization of thrombotic or atheromatous debris from an extracranial vascular source. Many strokes of this type are preceded by embolic events of lesser magnitude, which result in episodes of transient hemispheric or monocular ischemia.

Diagnosis

A. Symptoms and Signs: Ischemic episodes may be defined as follows:

1. Completed stroke (CVA)–A stroke has occurred when a neurologic deficit lasts for more than 24 hours. Cerebrovascular accident represents permanent cerebral damage, although the functional defect may improve considerably over time.

2. Transient ischemic attacks (TIAs)–Episodes last for less than 24 hours and represent reversible ischemia. Transient loss of cortical function in the area of distribution of the middle cerebral artery is common, eg, aphasia with right-sided hemiparesis.

3. Amaurosis fugax–Segmental vision or transient loss of all vision in one eye due to occlusion of the retinal artery.

B. Special Examinations: Noninvasive or minimally invasive cerebrovascular testing (B mode ultrasound imaging, Doppler frequency analysis) may show an atherosclerotic lesion at the carotid bifurcation. The patient may have an associated carotid bruit, Hollenhorst plaques on funduscopic examination, or other signs of atherosclerosis.

CT scan may be needed to rule out other causes of transient ischemic attack (tumor, arteriovenous malformation).

Carotid angiography is the definitive diagnostic procedure, since it demonstrates most sclerotic and ulcerative lesions if present.

Treatment
A. Acute Cerebrovascular Accident:
1. Start an intravenous line with normal saline at the lowest rate needed to keep the vein open.

2. Obtain an emergency CT scan to rule out hemorrhage.

3. Obtain neurologic consultation (or neurosurgical consultation for intracranial hemorrhage amenable to surgery).

4. If necessary, perform emergency airway management and assist ventilation. Massive cerebrovascular accidents may be accompanied by seizures, elevated intracranial pressure, and respiratory arrest. Cerebral edema and impending transtentorial herniation may be forestalled temporarily by hyperventilation and mannitol (1 mg/kg intravenously) or furosemide (20 mg intravenously).

B. Transient Ischemic Attacks:
1. Consult a neurologist or vascular surgeon about formal evaluation and definitive treatment.

2. Anti–platelet-aggregating agents (aspirin, 325 mg orally 2 times a day) may reduce the likelihood of stroke in men.

Disposition
All patients with progressive neurologic abnormalities or attacks that increase in frequency, duration, or severity must be hospitalized. Other patients can be treated on an inpatient or outpatient basis, depending on the decision of the neurologist or vascular surgeon.

ARTERIAL ANEURYSMS

RUPTURED ABDOMINAL AORTIC ANEURYSM

True abdominal aortic aneurysms generally are atherosclerotic in origin and most commonly involve the infrarenal abdominal aorta. Rupture usually occurs spontaneously without a precipitating event. Leaking of the aneurysm into the retroperitoneum (contained rupture) often precedes free rupture into the peritoneal space and is associated with premonitory signs and symptoms that permit diagnosis and initiation of effective treatment. False aneurysms can occur at the site of a prior bypass graft anastomosis, in which case concurrent graft infection is common,

and erosion into contiguous viscera often precedes free rupture into the peritoneal space.

Diagnosis
The principal manifestations are back or abdominal pain, abdominal aortic aneurysm (confirmed by palpation, sonography, or other methods), and hypovolemia, often with shock. Ruptured abdominal aortic aneurysm is a relatively common condition in patients with shock of uncertain cause or hypovolemic shock that has no obvious source of blood loss. Ruptured abdominal aortic aneurysm should be suspected in all patients thought to have myocardial ischemia or infarction. The diagnosis should also be considered in patients with gastrointestinal tract bleeding, particularly if they have undergone previous aortic bypass grafting.

Ruptured abdominal aortic aneurysms present in 4 distinct ways:

A. Free Rupture: Free rupture into the peritoneum results in rapid exsanguination. These patients rarely reach the hospital alive. Symptoms include abrupt onset of abdominal pain, rapidly progressive hypovolemic shock, and progressive abdominal distention.

B. Contained Rupture: Sudden onset of severe abdominal or back pain in a patient with or without hypotension should suggest contained rupture of an abdominal aortic aneurysm. The patient often has a history of hypertension. A pulsatile abdominal mass is palpable in 85% of patients. The hematocrit may be normal or low. The ECG often shows myocardial ischemia.

Abdominal x-ray (particularly a cross-table lateral view) confirms the presence of an abdominal aortic aneurysm in cases associated with calcification of the vessel wall (70% of aneurysms).

A CT scan of the abdomen also confirms the presence of an aneurysm in 95% of cases. The major usefulness of this test is to establish the diagnosis in the 15% of hemodynamically stable patients in whom the diagnosis cannot be made on clinical grounds alone.

C. Rupture Into the Inferior Vena Cava: Rarely, an abdominal aortic aneurysm ruptures directly into the inferior vena cava. The patient may present with circulatory decompensation or collapse secondary to high-output heart failure. The rupture is not necessarily preceded by abdominal or back pain. A palpable pulsatile supraumbilical mass is common.

D. Rupture Into Contiguous Viscera: Rupture of an aneurysm may be manifested by bleeding into contiguous viscera, usually the duodenum or colon. This occurs almost exclusively in patients with prosthetic aortoiliac grafts and is associated with formation of a false aneurysm at the suture line. This diagnosis should be considered in *all* patients who present with gastrointestinal tract bleeding and have a history of bypass surgery for either aneurysmal or occlusive disease.

The patient may present with upper or lower gastrointestinal tract bleeding, which initially may be minor or severe. Rupture of this kind is not necessarily preceded by abdominal or back pain, and a palpable abdominal mass is uncommon.

Treatment

A. *Act quickly.* Even if the patient appears hemodynamically stable at the time of initial evaluation, the contained rupture may progress rapidly to exsanguinating hemorrhage at any time.

B. Treat hypotension and shock (Chapter 3). To reiterate briefly—

1. Begin oxygen, 4 L/min, by nasal prongs or mask.

2. Insert 2 large-bore (≥ 16-gauge) intravenous catheters by venous cutdown.

3. Obtain blood for CBC, electrolyte determinations, and renal function tests, and type and cross-match for 10 units of packed red blood cells or whole blood. Measure the hematocrit immediately and at frequent intervals thereafter. Remember the delay in equilibration of blood volume that may keep the hematocrit reading falsely elevated for 12–18 hours.

4. Give 1–3 L of crystalloid solution intravenously to restore adequate blood pressure, and follow with cross-matched blood. If the initial hematocrit is below 20%, either "universal donor" blood or type-specific blood may be necessary.

5. Insert a urinary catheter, send urine for analysis, and monitor urine output.

C. Request urgent consultation with a general or vascular surgeon, since immediate surgery is the only definitive treatment.

D. Confirm the diagnosis by one of the following:

1. **Palpation–**If an abdominal aortic aneurysm can be palpated on examination, further diagnostic tests are not needed in a patient with otherwise unexplained hypotension.

2. **X-ray–**In the stable patient or in one with an uncertain diagnosis, a routine cross-table lateral abdominal x-ray confirms the presence of an aneurysm if calcification is present in the vessel wall.

3. **Ultrasound or CT scan–**Even if an aneurysm cannot be seen on x-ray, abdominal ultrasound or CT scan generally confirms its presence. A CT scan after injection of intravenous contrast media will demonstrate the leak.

Disposition

Hospitalize all patients with suspected or documented ruptured abdominal aortic aneurysm.

VISCERAL & HYPOGASTRIC ARTERY ANEURYSM

Congenital aneurysm occurs in younger patients, whereas atherosclerotic aneurysm occurs more commonly in older patients. The splenic artery is the most commonly involved vessel. Bleeding may be con-

fined to the lesser sac of the peritoneal cavity for the first 24–48 hours. However, free rupture into the general peritoneal cavity invariably causes exsanguination. Rupture is most common during pregnancy. Hypogastric artery aneurysms may rupture into the retroperitoneum or erode into contiguous organs, in which case gastrointestinal tract bleeding or hematuria occurs.

Diagnosis

There is abrupt onset of diffuse abdominal pain. Hypotension occurs secondary to blood loss. The hematocrit is low if the bleeding is more than a few hours old. Abdominal paracentesis or peritoneal lavage may reveal gross blood. A plain film of the abdomen may show an aneurysm if it has calcified.

The only definitive diagnostic procedure is selective visceral angiography, which should be performed in the hemodynamically stable patient in whom an aneurysm is not present on a plain film.

Treatment

Start resuscitative measures, including insertion of a large-bore (≥ 16-gauge) intravenous catheter, nasogastric tube, Foley catheter, etc (see Treatment section for ruptured abdominal aortic aneurysm, above, and Chapter 3). Draw blood for CBC, and type and cross-match for 8 units of packed red blood cells or whole blood.

Notify a vascular surgeon at once, since early operation is imperative.

Disposition

Immediately hospitalize all patients with suspected or documented visceral and hypogastric artery aneurysm.

THORACIC AORTIC ANEURYSM ("Dissecting Aneurysm")

Aortic dissections result when blood under arterial pressure ruptures into and dissects the wall of the aorta. The cause is hypertension and weakening of the vessel wall due to cystic medial necrosis or other factors. Aortic dissection usually occurs just distal to the aortic valve or distal to the origin of the left subclavian artery. In the classification scheme of DeBakey, type I and type II dissections begin just distal to the aortic valves, type I extending a variable distance beyond the ascending aorta and type II being confined to the ascending aorta. Type III dissections begin in the descending aorta, usually just beyond the left subclavian artery, and progress distally or (rarely) proximally. In 20% of cases, the tear occurs in the descending thoracic aorta or abdominal aorta (DeBakey type III).

Diagnosis

A. Signs of Dissection: Signs of dissection depend on which branches of the aorta are compromised, whether the aortic valve is affected, and whether there is rupture into a contiguous space, eg, pericardium. The carotid, coronary, subclavian, or femoral pulses can be compromised and then reappear, depending on the degree of involvement with further dissection or redistribution of hematoma in the wall of the aorta. Visceral and renal blood flow may likewise be interrupted and then resume.

1. Depending on which vessels have been compromised, there may be signs of cerebrovascular accident, acute myocardial infarction, clinical findings associated with arterial occlusion of an extremity (ischemia, absent pulses), abdominal or back pain with or without hematuria or ileus, or wide difference in blood pressure measurements in the 2 arms or in an arm and a leg on the same side.

2. If the base of the aortic valve is involved, varying degrees of aortic insufficiency occur.

3. The dissection may leak into the pleura or pericardium, causing a pericardial or pleural friction rub with effusion.

4. When rupture starts, shock of sudden and catastrophic onset may occur as a result of cardiac tamponade, massive hemothorax, or bleeding into tissues surrounding the aorta.

B. Other Symptoms and Signs:
1. There may be signs of underlying disease, eg, hypertension, Marfan's syndrome.

2. "Tearing" chest pain extending to the back or extremities may occur—especially severe pain that shifts from one place to another.

C. Laboratory Findings: Hematuria may be present; the hematocrit may be normal or low.

D. Imaging: Chest x-ray may show a widened mediastinum or pleural fluid. The heart size is usually normal in acute tamponade. Retrograde aortography is the definitive diagnostic procedure, but multiple injections may be needed to demonstrate true and false lumens and the patency of arterial branches.

CT scan after injection of intravenous contrast media is less invasive than retrograde aortography and is a sensitive and specific diagnostic test. Its limitation is that the precise extent of the lesion is not defined, so that angiography may still be required if surgery is contemplated.

Digital subtraction angiography after intravenous or intra-arterial injection of contrast medium may also be helpful.

Goals of Treatment
There are 2 main goals of treatment:
A. Reduce Hypertension: Hypertension must be controlled. The forces contributing to the development of dissection are a function of increased systolic blood pressure and the force generated with each systolic contraction of the left ventricle. Accordingly, once dissection is suspected, the essential first step is to reduce systolic pressure and the rate of rise of the

left ventricular pressure wave (dp/dt) if the patient is *not* hypotensive. If the patient *is* hypotensive, treat for hypovolemic shock (Chapter 3).

B. Correct the Structural Abnormality: Surgical closure of the entrance of the dissection into the true lumen and obliteration of the false lumen complete the treatment.

Treatment
A. All Patients:
1. Insert 2 or more large-bore ($\geq$ 16-gauge) intravenous catheters or perform venous cutdowns.

2. Draw blood for CBC, electrolyte measurements, tests of renal function, and typing and crossmatching (reserve 10 units of packed red blood cells or whole blood).

3. Insert a Foley catheter; send urine for urinalysis, and monitor urine output on an hourly basis.

4. Give oxygen, 5 L/min, by mask or nasal prongs.

5. Obtain immediate vascular or thoracic surgical consultation.

B. Patients With Normotension, Hypotension, or Shock:
1. Assume that free rupture or cardiac tamponade has occurred.

2. Begin intravenous infusion of crystalloid solutions to support blood pressure; give packed red blood cells or whole blood as soon as available.

3. Obtain chest x-ray (if possible) to confirm the diagnosis.

4. Consult with the surgeon, who will decide whether immediate operation or confirmation of the diagnosis by angiography is necessary.

5. Perform immediate surgery if cardiac tamponade or gross aortic insufficiency is present.

C. Patients With Hypertension: Reduce blood pressure as much as possible consistent with adequate central nervous system function and urine output. Provide preload and afterload reduction as follows:
1. Give propranolol, 1 mg, by intravenous bolus injection. Continue administration at a rate of 1 mg every 5 minutes until beta blockade is achieved or a maximum of 0.15 mg/kg is reached.

2. Begin afterload reduction by infusion of sodium nitroprusside (25–50 µg/min, titrating to desired effect) or trimethaphan camsylate with propranolol.

3. Until nitroprusside can be started, apply nitroglycerin ointment, 1.25–5 cm (½–2 in), to the skin under an occlusive dressing.

4. If intensive blood pressure monitoring is not available, labetalol HCl, an alpha- and beta-adrenergic receptor-blocking agent, may be used effectively by itself to reduce blood pressure and left ventricular dp/dt. Give 20 mg over 2 minutes by intravenous injection. Additional doses of 40–80 mg can be given every 10 minutes (maximum dose 300 mg) until the desired blood pressure has been reached. (Alternatively, 2 mg/min may be given by intravenous infusion, titrated to desired effect.)

Disposition
Hospitalize all patients without delay. Obtain urgent cardiothoracic surgical consultation for all patients, even those already receiving medical treatment.

POPLITEAL & FEMORAL PERIPHERAL ANEURYSM

Occlusion or distal embolization of the friable lining of peripheral aneurysms results in symptoms of distal ischemia. Unlike abdominal aortic aneurysm or visceral aneurysm, rupture is rare. The most common locations of peripheral aneurysms are the popliteal artery and, secondarily, the femoral artery. Popliteal aneurysms are often bilateral and are often associated with abdominal aortic aneurysms.

Acute occlusion can result in severe distal ischemia. Distal embolization can also result in severe distal ischemia; however, it is often associated with episodes of moderate ischemia that decrease as collateral circulation improves.

Diagnosis
A. Symptoms and Signs: Symptoms are due to thrombosis, embolization, pressure from an expanding aneurysm, or (rarely) rupture. There may be an arterial mass in the popliteal fossa or the groin. The aneurysm is pulsatile unless it is thrombosed. Signs of acute arterial occlusion often coexist.

Popliteal aneurysms can cause symptoms (eg, signs of venous obstruction, weakness, sensory defects) when they compress the popliteal vein or tibial nerve. Rupture of the aneurysm is rare.

B. Imaging:
1. Plain film–A rim of calcification may be apparent in the wall of the aneurysm.
2. Arteriogram–Arteriography may not demonstrate the aneurysm if it is thrombosed, but this procedure is generally advised to define the status of the arterial circulation distal to the aneurysm.
3. Ultrasonogram–Ultrasonography is helpful in identifying the presence of an aneurysm.

Treatment
A. Notify a vascular surgeon, since immediate operation is required when severe distal ischemia has occurred secondary either to acute thrombosis or to distal embolization.

B. Elective operation is recommended for any aneurysm producing compression of adjacent structures as well as for most documented popliteal aneurysms, since the rate of complications is high if these are left untreated.

Disposition
All symptomatic patients should be hospitalized immediately.

VENOUS DISEASE

DEEP VEIN THROMBOSIS

Venous thrombosis may be due to stasis, hypercoagulability, or changes in the vessel wall. Thrombophlebitis and pulmonary embolism are common, occasionally fatal complications of venous thrombosis.

Diagnosis
A. Symptoms and Signs: Symptoms and signs vary, often depending on the location of the thrombosed segment. About one-third of patients have no clinical findings at all, whereas others may have classic manifestations.
1. Aching calf or thigh pain is common and is usually aggravated by exercise or when the limb is dependent.
2. Swelling may be mild or massive. A difference between the circumference of the affected extremity and that of the opposite side may also be present.
3. Tenderness to palpation may be present along the course of the involved veins or may be elicited in the calf with compression of the gastrocnemius muscles against the tibia.
4. Other findings include erythema, warmth, discomfort, or positive Homans' sign.
5. Clinical examination alone provides accurate diagnosis in only 50% of patients. *Note:* The diagnosis of suspected deep vein thrombosis must therefore always be confirmed by using one or more of the special tests described below, since anticoagulation therapy is not without complications.
B. Special Diagnostic Tests:
1. Venography–Contrast venography remains the standard test for deep venous thrombosis in the lower extremity. When properly performed and interpreted, it is nearly 100% sensitive and specific. However, the study cannot be performed in all patients, either because of lack of a suitable vein for cannulation or because of previous reactions to contrast media. Additionally, the procedure is invasive and may occasionally cause thrombophlebitis (2–3%) or allergic reactions. In patients with a history of previous deep vein thrombosis, the study may be difficult to interpret without old films for comparison.
2. Duplex ultrasound–Duplex ultrasound combines Doppler and ultrasound technology (B mode

and spectral) with sensitivity and specificity for thrombi in iliofemoral veins that is comparable to venography. It may be emerging as the initial imaging study of choice for proximal deep venous thrombosis. However, its accuracy is highly dependent on the skill of the operator. It is less effective for popliteal vein thrombosis and much less so for the calf.

3. Impedance plethysmography–Impedance plethysmography (IPG) noninvasively measures the electrical impedance across the calf during and after occlusion of thigh veins with a pneumatic cuff placed above the knee. The test detects most acute proximal vein thrombi but may miss those high in the iliac veins and is less sensitive to calf thromboses. IPG may be useful as a screening tool; however, its accuracy is also dependent on the technical proficiency of the operator.

4. Fibrinogen scanning–Fibrinogen scanning involves injection of radiolabeled fibrinogen into a peripheral vein and scanning the leg with a gamma camera to detect uptake by a newly formed thrombus that has incorporated the isotope. It is very sensitive to thrombi in the calf but is usually not available as a bedside test.

Treatment

For deep venous thrombosis of proximal veins of the thigh, put the patient on bed rest and elevate the limb. Thrombolytic therapy with streptokinase or urokinase is effective in treating acute deep venous thrombosis less than 7 days old and may prevent postphlebitic complications. Give 250,000 IU intravenously over 30 minutes, then 100,000 IU/h for the next 72 hours. Alternatively, start anticoagulation with intravenous heparin (p 566). Obtain consultation with a vascular surgeon in cases of massive iliofemoral thrombosis. Surgery may be required for certain patients but is controversial.

Management of calf deep venous thrombosis and the need for hospitalization are controversial. Isolated calf thrombi do not commonly produce pulmonary emboli, although they may propagate into proximal vessels. Traditional treatment has been low-dose heparin (eg, 5000 units subcutaneously twice a day), although some authors advocate serial noninvasive studies (eg, IPG or ultrasound) and treatment only if propagation occurs.

Disposition

All patients with deep venous thrombosis should be hospitalized.

SUPERFICIAL THROMBOPHLEBITIS

Superficial venous thrombosis of the upper extremity is usually iatrogenic, occurring secondary to intravenous catheterization. Lower extremity superficial venous thromboses may be associated with varicose veins, bacterial infection of surrounding tissues, trauma, or thromboangiitis obliterans. Trauma may play a part in the initial development of thrombi or may cause recurrences.

Diagnosis

Pain, tenderness, induration, and erythema are noted along the course of the involved vein, which may feel like a cord. The extremity shows only slight or no swelling, and there are no other signs of impaired venous return.

Septic thrombophlebitis usually occurs following intravenous injections (especially among intravenous drug abusers) and at venous catheter sites. It should be suspected in the presence of the above symptoms or fluctuance along a superficial vein. There may be fever and rigors. The diagnosis is confirmed if pus can be aspirated from the vein.

Treatment

A. Cases With No Complications: For uncomplicated superficial venous thrombosis, only symptomatic treatment is required. Neither bed rest nor anticoagulation is indicated. An elastic bandage at and above the level of thrombosis helps to speed remission. Elevation of the leg when the patient is sitting and nonsteroidal anti-inflammatory drugs (eg, indomethacin, 25–50 mg orally 3 times a day) are also helpful.

B. Cases With Complications: Obtain general or vascular surgical consultation for all complications. If clinical examination suggests that the thrombosis is approaching the saphenofemoral junction, ligation and division of the saphenous vein are indicated, since pulmonary embolization can result from deep venous involvement.

If septic thrombophlebitis occurs, parenteral antimicrobials are required, and the involved segment of vein must be excised or ligated and drained to prevent persistent bacteremia.

Disposition

Patients with mild, localized superficial thrombosis may be discharged. Patients with more serious disease, including suspected or documented septic thrombophlebitis, should be hospitalized.

AXILLARY-SUBCLAVIAN VEIN THROMBOSIS ("Effort Thrombosis")

Thrombosis of the subclavian and axillary veins is much less common than thrombosis of lower extremity veins. Effort thrombosis is thought to be caused by compression of the vein in the costoclavicular space. Axillary-subclavian vein thrombosis may also occur in association with heart failure, metastatic tumor in the axilla or mediastinum, indwelling venous catheters, or trauma.

Diagnosis

Symptoms are commonly preceded by muscular activity of the upper extremity. The diagnosis is generally made on clinical grounds and should be confirmed by phlebography. Pain and swelling develop within 24 hours of the inciting event and worsen with exercise. The extremity may be cyanotic. Fewer than half of patients have a palpable axillary cord. A prominent collateral venous pattern over the wall of the anterior chest and shoulder is common. Pulmonary embolism is rare. The diagnosis is confirmed by renogram. Duplex scan has a high rate of accuracy (> 90%).

Treatment

Acute symptoms respond to elevation of the arm and rest. Systemic anticoagulation with heparin is helpful to prevent progression of thrombosis and pulmonary embolization. Obtain consultation with a general surgeon or vascular surgeon as required, since elective surgery to enlarge the costoclavicular space should be considered in certain patients to relieve the cause of venous compression and prevent its recurrence.

Disposition

Hospitalization is preferred in most cases, and all patients who require systemic anticoagulation must be hospitalized.

RUPTURED VENOUS VARICOSITIES (Varicose Veins)

Rupture is an uncommon complication of varicose veins. The skin overlying varices can become thin, and erosion can occur spontaneously or with minor trauma.

Diagnosis

Bleeding from varicose veins is present and may be brisk.

Treatment

Gentle digital pressure over the bleeding site and elevation of the leg control the initial bleeding. Suture ligature of the ruptured vein may be necessary to definitively stop the bleeding. When the initial bleeding has been controlled, the leg should be wrapped in an elastic bandage or Unna's paste boot. Consult a vascular or general surgeon about elective stripping of varicose veins.

Disposition

Brief hospitalization may be advisable.

PULMONARY EMBOLISM

Pulmonary embolism is an occasional complication of venous thrombosis. It is discussed in Chapter 27.

ARTERIOVENOUS FISTULA

Arteriovenous fistulas are abnormal connections between arteries and veins. They may be congenital or acquired. Congenital lesions tend to have more diffuse connections and may involve an extremity. Acquired arteriovenous fistulas—other than those constructed to gain access for dialysis—generally occur secondary to trauma and result from erosion of the artery into a contiguous vein. The physiologic effect depends on the size of the communication.

Diagnosis

A. Symptoms and Signs: A machinery murmur is heard, and a thrill is palpable over most arteriovenous fistulas. Cardiac output may be high. Patients with congenital arteriovenous fistulas may show increased muscle mass, increased bone length, clubbing, and cyanosis of the involved limb. Polycythemia may also be present.

B. Complications: Complications include cosmetic deformity due to limb disproportion, congestive heart failure, severe arterial insufficiency, expanding false aneurysm, and hemorrhage. Arteriography delineates the precise outlines of the lesion and may be used for therapeutic embolization.

Treatment & Disposition

Patients with pain, expanding mass, heart failure, or obvious high cardiac output require hospitalization. Others may be discharged from the emergency department and referred to a vascular surgeon or general surgeon.

OTHER VASCULAR SYNDROMES

THORACIC OUTLET SYNDROME

Thoracic outlet syndrome comprises a variety of disorders caused by abnormal compression of the neural, arterial, or venous structures at the base of the neck; the most common is compression of nerve structures against the first rib. Symptoms of dysfunction of branches of the brachial plexus are far more common than symptoms secondary to compression of the axillary-subclavian artery or vein. Thoracic outlet syndrome is rarely an emergency.

Diagnosis

The diagnosis is generally made on clinical grounds.

A. Symptoms:

1. Positional paresthesias occur in the distribution of one or more trunks of the brachial plexus, most commonly in the ulnar nerve distribution.

2. Numbness of the hand may occur with occupational hyperabduction of the arm (eg, painting the ceiling), downward traction of the shoulder girdle, or abnormal sleeping position.

3. Rapid fatigue of the hand may occur in many patients when the hand is exercised with the arm elevated in an abducted position.

B. Signs:

1. A subclavian bruit can be heard in many patients when the arm is in the abducted position.

2. If venous thrombosis has occurred, dilatation of the superficial veins of the arm and anterior chest may cause the arm to swell.

3. The radial pulse may be obliterated when the arm is abducted and the patient's head turned to the opposite side. (This finding may occur in many normal people as well.)

C. Imaging: Cervical films are important in identifying a cervical rib, if present. Angiography is not useful, since any malformations observed may be similar to those seen in asymptomatic individuals.

Treatment & Disposition

Postural correction is helpful. A cervical collar may be useful. Refer the patient to a general, vascular, or thoracic surgeon for evaluation. If cervical x-ray shows acute axillary venous thrombosis, the patient should be hospitalized for treatment with anticoagulants; otherwise, hospitalization is not required.

COMPLICATIONS OF PERCUTANEOUS TRANSLUMINAL ANGIOPLASTY & RETROGRADE ANGIOGRAPHY

An increasing number of patients are undergoing percutaneous transluminal angioplasty (balloon dilatation of the arteries) and angiography via the femoral artery. These patients are observed for the development of immediate complications but are usually discharged from the hospital within 24–48 hours and may subsequently present to the emergency department with complications (Table 32–4).

Hospitalize the patient, and obtain prompt vascular or cardiothoracic surgical consultation, since many of these problems require surgical treatment.

Table 32–4. Complications of percutaneous transluminal angioplasty.

Puncture site complications
Bleeding: massive, expanding, or pulsatile hematoma
False aneurysm: pulsatile mass at puncture site
Femoral artery occlusion: loss of pulse at or proximal to puncture site, due to thrombosis at catheter site or arterial injury (eg, luminal flap)
Infection: superficial or deep, with or without arterial involvement
Dilatation site complications
Thrombosis of dilated vessel (most commonly coronary, iliac, femoral, or renal artery)
Complications distal to insertion site
Embolization (usually occurs before patient leaves the hospital)

ERGOTISM

Ergotism is caused by ergotamine tartrate or other ergot derivatives or by consumption of rye contaminated by ergot fungus. The disease is characterized by profound vasoconstriction that is almost always limited to the lower extremities.

Diagnosis

There is mottled cyanosis of the thighs and lower legs, with intense cyanosis of the feet. Prolonged vasospasm may result in distal thrombosis. Secondary tissue loss may occur. Other findings include vomiting, diarrhea, cramps, and various central nervous system symptoms.

Treatment & Disposition

Hospitalize the patient, and maintain adequate blood pressure and intravascular volume. Withdraw ergotamine medication. Vasodilators and heparin anticoagulation may be indicated. Hyperbaric oxygen therapy may be tried, although there is no evidence of benefit. Consult a general surgeon or vascular surgeon. Lumbar sympathectomy may be required.

INTRA-ARTERIAL INJECTION OF DRUGS

Inadvertent or intentional intra-arterial injection of drugs can cause intense vasospasm followed by arterial occlusion, with distal gangrene as a possible result. This is commonly known as a "hand trip" by intravenous drug abusers. Vasospasm may occur while the drug is being given, or the reaction may be delayed. Unfortunately, many patients with delayed reactions fail to seek medical attention until ischemia is advanced.

Diagnosis

There is a history of therapeutic or illicit drug injection by the parenteral route. Severe burning pain in distal arterial distribution is followed by intense vasospasm. If the vasospasm has been prolonged, gangrene of the fingers or entire hand may occur even though the arterial vasoconstriction subsequently resolves.

Treatment & Disposition

Hospitalize the patient, and obtain vascular surgical consultation. If the needle is still in place, irrigate distally with heparinized saline. Start systemic anticoagulation with heparin (p 000). Systemic vasodilating agents may be necessary to treat the intense vasospasm. Intra-arterial injection of vasodilators (eg, reserpine) is not usually beneficial. If sympathetic nerve block is indicated because of persistent severe peripheral ischemia, consult an anesthesiologist or vascular surgeon.

FROSTBITE

Arterial injury is a major pathogenetic factor in frostbite injury. See Chapter 38 for details of diagnosis and treatment.

REFERENCES

Abrams HL (editor): *Abrams Angiography: Vascular and Interventional Radiology,* 3rd ed. Little, Brown, 1983.

Betelsen S, Anker W: Phlegmasia coerulea dolens: Pathophysiology, clinical features, treatment, and prognosis. Acta Chir Scand 1968;134:107.

Borman KR, Aurbakker CM, Weigelt JA: Treatment priorities in combined blunt abdominal and aortic trauma. Am J Surg 1982;144:728.

Crawford ES: The diagnosis and management of aortic dissection. JAMA 1990;264:2537.

Daskalakis E, Bouhoutsos J: Subclavian and axillary vein compression of musculoskeletal origin. Br J Surg 1980;67:573.

Eckborn GA et al: Intra-abdominal vascular trauma: A need for prompt operation. J Trauma 1981;21:1040.

Fields WS: Selection of patients with ischemic cerebrovascular disease for arterial surgery. World J Surg 1979;3:147.

Fogarty TJ: Management of arterial emboli. Surg Clin North Am 1979;59:749.

Fry RE, Fry WJ: Extracranial carotid artery injuries. Surgery 1980;88:581.

Gaspar M: Arterial trauma. In: *Peripheral Arterial Disease.* Gaspar M, Barker WF (editors). Saunders, 1981.

Gay W: Blunt trauma to the heart and great vessels. Surgery 1982;91:507.

Gundry SR et al: Indications for aortography in blunt thoracic trauma: A reassessment. J Trauma 1982;22:664.

Killewich LA et al: Diagnosis of deep venous thrombosis: A prospective study comparing duplex scanning to contrast venography. Circulation 1989;79:810.

Kollmeyer KR: Acute and chronic arteriovenous fistulae in civilians: Epidemiology and treatment. Arch Surg 1981;116:697.

Lawrie GM et al: Improved results of operation for ruptured abdominal aortic aneurysms. Surgery 1979;85:483.

Lewis FR: Thoracic trauma. Surg Clin North Am 1982; 62:97.

Matto KL: Abdominal venous injuries. Surgery 1982;91: 497.

Ottinger LW: Mesenteric ischemia. N Engl J Med 1982; 307:535.

Perdue GD et al: Aneurysms of the internal iliac artery. Surgery 1983;93:243.

Perry MO, Snyder WH, Thal ER: Carotid artery injuries by blunt trauma. Ann Surg 1980;192:74.

Philbrick JT, Becker DM: Calf venous thrombosis: A wolf in sheep's clothing? Arch Intern Med 1988;148:2131.

Rich NM, Spencer FC: *Vascular Trauma.* Saunders, 1978.

Rogers DM et al: Mesenteric vascular problems: A 26-year experience. Ann Surg 1982;195:554.

Smelt PL et al: Emergency arteriography in extremity trauma: Assessment of indications. AJR 1981;137:807.

Snyder WH III: Vascular injuries near the knee: An updated series and overview of the problem. Surgery 1982; 91:502.

Szilagyi DE, Schwartz RL, Reddy DJ: Popliteal artery aneurysms: Their natural history and management. Arch Surg 1981;116:724.

Vogel P et al: Deep venous thrombosis of the lower extremity: US evaluation. Radiology 1987;163:747.

Hematologic Emergencies

33

Stephen H. Embury, MD, & Charles A. Linker, MD

Symptoms of bleeding or infection are common complaints in patients presenting to the emergency department. In patients with underlying hematologic disease, however, these conditions may be due to—or significantly affected by—the specific pathophysiology of the primary hematologic disorder, and a successful outcome often requires specialized diagnostic and therapeutic measures. The physician should therefore obtain the history and perform physical examination and laboratory evaluation with an emphasis on specific clues to hematologic diseases.

EVALUATION OF THE PATIENT WITH SUSPECTED BLEEDING DISORDER

Most patients with nasal, gastrointestinal, urinary, vaginal, or posttraumatic bleeding do *not* have a bleeding disorder. When bleeding is due to abnormal hemostasis, however, successful therapy depends on accurate diagnosis.

Clues to the presence of disordered hemostasis may be obtained from the medical history (Table 33–1). Perform a careful physical examination, and look specifically for evidence of a bleeding diathesis (Table 33–2). Look for an identifying necklace, bracelet, or card (eg, Medic-Alert tag) that may list a known bleeding disorder. Laboratory tests (Table 33–3) may provide the first evidence of disordered hemostasis.

Table 33–1. Medical history clues to disordered hemostasis.

Easy bruising
Petechiae
Hemorrhage during surgery or obstetric delivery
Transfusion required during surgery or obstetric delivery
Excessive bleeding after dental extraction
Bleeding into joints or deep muscles
Recurrent epistaxis
Menorrhagia
Spontaneous bleeding without obvious cause or history of trauma
Hemorrhage following anticoagulant therapy or ingestion of anti-inflammatory agents (eg, aspirin)

Table 33–2. Signs of bleeding diathesis.

Petechiae
Ecchymoses
Bleeding from multiple sites
Spontaneous bleeding without detectable cause
Evidence of prior bleeding (eg, joint deformity from hemarthroses)
Excessive bleeding at venipuncture sites

EMERGENCY MANAGEMENT OF SPECIFIC DISORDERS OF HEMOSTASIS

DISORDERED PLATELET HEMOSTASIS

There are 2 major categories of disordered platelet hemostasis: decreased number of platelets (thrombocytopenia) and abnormal platelet function. Thrombocytopenia may be due to decreased production of platelets, increased destruction, or some combination of these.

The classic sign of thrombocytopenia is petechiae, which usually occur on the lower extremities or under tight clothing (eg, waistbands). Purpura and ecchymoses may also be present. Petechiae found on other areas of the body suggest nonthrombocytopenic purpura, such as senile purpura or purpura due to amyloidosis. Only rarely does platelet *dysfunction* result in petechiae.

Patients with abnormal platelet hemostasis frequently bleed from mucosal surfaces, whereas patients with bleeding disorders due to abnormal coagulation factors are more prone to intra-articular, retroperitoneal, or deep muscle bleeding.

Emergency evaluation of platelet hemostasis should include the following:

(1) Detailed medical history, in which the patient should be asked specifically about the use of drugs known to alter platelet number or function (Table 33–4).

(2) Platelet count to detect abnormally low or high numbers of platelets.

(3) CBC to determine if platelet abnormalities are an isolated finding or part of a widespread hematologic disorder.

(4) Review of the peripheral blood smear for evi-

Table 33–3. Laboratory tests for disordered hemostasis.

CBC and peripheral blood smear
Prothrombin time
Activated partial thromboplastin time
Platelet count
Bleeding time
Adjunctive tests (eg, fibrinogen levels, factor VIII levels)

Table 33–4. Some drugs that may decrease platelet number or function.

Drugs causing thrombocytopenia
  Cytotoxic agents
  Antibiotics (eg, penicillins, cephalosporins, sulfonamides, rifampin)
  Phenylbutazone
  Thiazides
  H_2 blockers (eg, cimetidine, ranitidine)
  Gold
  Quinidine, quinine
  Heparin
  Heroin
  Alcohol
  Aspirin
  Phenytoin
Drugs causing decreased platelet function
  Aspirin
  Nonsteroidal anti-inflammatory agents (eg, indomethacin)
  Sulfinpyrazone
  Dipyridamole
  Clofibrate
  Dextran
  Semisynthetic penicillins
  Cephalosporins

dence of thrombocytopenia, thrombocytosis, or large young platelets that suggest increased platelet production.

(5) Bleeding time to assess platelet function (useful if the platelet count is normal but deranged function is suspected).

(6) Blood urea nitrogen and creatinine levels (uremia is the most common cause of acquired platelet dysfunction not due to drugs).

Treatment of significant bleeding due to platelet abnormalities depends on the diagnosis and is discussed in detail below. In general, bleeding due to decreased platelet production or intrinsic (usually inherited) qualitative platelet dysfunction is treated with platelet transfusions. Treatment intended to reverse the underlying pathologic process is used for thrombocytopenia due to peripheral platelet destruction or extrinsic qualitative platelet defects (eg, uremia).

1. IMMUNE THROMBOCYTOPENIA

Immune destruction of platelets occurs in disorders characterized by the production of platelet autoantibodies, such as idiopathic thrombocytopenic purpura, systemic lupus erythematosus, or diffuse lymphomas. Such destruction also occurs secondary to drug-induced antibody production (quinine, quinidine, sulfonamides, heroin, heparin, penicillin, cephalosporins, cimetidine, ranitidine, gold); in some infections (infectious mononucleosis and other viral infections); after transfusions; and as part of the clinical spectrum of AIDS (acquired immunodeficiency syndrome).

Diagnosis

Patients with immune thrombocytopenia (ITP), particularly patients with the idiopathic variety, are systemically well and have no clinical findings except mucosal bleeding or petechiae. The CBC reveals isolated thrombocytopenia with a normal red and white blood cell count unless there has been blood loss sufficient to cause anemia. The peripheral blood smear reveals normal red and white blood cell morphology and may demonstrate large platelets. The prothrombin and partial thromboplastin times are normal. Bone marrow aspirate or biopsy shows normal or increased numbers of megakaryocytes. Immune thrombocytopenic purpura in children is usually acute and follows a viral infection; in adults, it is often chronic. The major threats to life in immune thrombocytopenic purpura are intracranial bleeding or exsanguination due to internal bleeding.

Differential Diagnosis

Ask the patient about use of drugs (Table 33–4), and search for signs and symptoms of infection, collagen vascular disease, or cancer that may reveal the underlying cause of immune thrombocytopenia.

Splenomegaly suggests splenic sequestration as a mechanism for thrombocytopenia. Evidence of alcohol abuse should suggest drug-induced suppression of platelet production. Perform coagulation tests in all acutely ill patients with thrombocytopenia in order to distinguish immune thrombocytopenic purpura, in which results on these tests are normal, from disseminated intravascular coagulation and other complex coagulopathies. Review the peripheral blood smear for evidence of red cell fragmentation indicative of thrombotic thrombocytopenic purpura, hemolytic-uremic syndrome, disseminated intravascular coagulation, or other complex coagulopathies.

Treatment

The initial treatment of immune thrombocytopenic purpura is prednisone, 1 mg/kg/d orally, or the equivalent for parenteral administration. Platelet transfusion is usually not indicated, because transfused platelets will not survive any longer than the patient's own platelets. However, in life-threatening hemorrhage, platelet transfusion may provide transient improvement in hemostasis.

Infusion of gamma globulin may be helpful in life-threatening situations or as treatment of disease that flares in patients with chronic ITP. Give gamma globulin, 0.7 g/kg by intravenous infusion over 4–6 hours daily for 3 days. Benefit is seen in 2–5 days.

Disposition

Hospitalize patients who are actively bleeding or who have platelet counts of less than 20,000/μL, and obtain hematologic consultation. Patients without bleeding or with less severe thrombocytopenia need not be hospitalized but should be seen by a hematologist within a day.

2. THROMBOTIC THROMBOCYTOPENIC PURPURA

Thrombotic thrombocytopenic purpura is an uncommon disorder characterized by microangiopathic hemolytic anemia, thrombocytopenia, fever, fluctuating neurologic deficits, and renal complications. Patients usually present because of thrombocytopenic bleeding or neurologic abnormalities. The most common neurologic manifestations are headache, aphasia, confusion, and focal weakness, which typically wax and wane even over a matter of minutes. The pathogenesis of thrombotic thrombocytopenic purpura is not completely understood. An interaction between vascular endothelium and platelets results in abnormal platelet aggregation, which causes organ damage as a result of occlusion of small vessels by the aggregates.

Diagnosis

Thrombotic thrombocytopenic purpura should be suspected in any patient with severe thrombocytopenia. Coexisting severe hemolytic anemia, fever, evanescent neurologic findings, renal insufficiency, hematuria, or an active urinary sediment (leukocytes and casts) supports the diagnosis but is not necessarily seen at initial presentation. Examination of the peripheral blood smear is critical in confirming the diagnosis, since red blood cell fragmentation is always present and is usually dramatic. Other laboratory findings include reticulocytosis, increased serum LDH and bilirubin levels, normal coagulation tests (prothrombin, partial thromboplastin, and thrombin times; fibrinogen levels); and a negative Coombs test. Even those patients who present with thrombocytopenia as the initial manifestation of thrombotic thrombocytopenic purpura usually still demonstrate red blood cell fragmentation on the peripheral blood smear.

Differential Diagnosis

Red blood cell fragmentation does not occur in immune thrombocytopenia, which is the most common cause of isolated severe thrombocytopenia (see above). Thrombotic thrombocytopenic purpura can be distinguished from disseminated intravascular coagulation by measuring the prothrombin, partial thromboplastin, and thrombin times and fibrinogen levels; results are normal in thrombotic thrombocytopenic purpura and are usually abnormal in disseminated intravascular coagulation (see below). A negative Coombs test differentiates thrombotic thrombocytopenic purpura from Evans syndrome (immune thrombocytopenia and hemolytic anemia).

Treatment & Disposition

Thrombotic thrombocytopenic purpura is a medical emergency. Even in the absence of neurologic abnormalities, patients suspected of having this syndrome should be hospitalized for urgent hematologic consultation, since the disease may progress fulminantly. Large-volume plasmapheresis is the treatment of choice, continuing until the patient has returned to normal neurologic and hematologic status. The replacement fluid is fresh-frozen plasma (6–8% of body weight). When plasmapheresis is not immediately available, temporizing therapy is plasma infusion alone, with 40 mL/kg body weight (1000–1500 mL fresh-frozen plasma daily). Symptomatic hypervolemia should be treated with diuretics (eg, furosemide, 40–80 mg intravenously). The patient should be transferred as soon as possible to an institution that can provide plasmapheresis. Although platelet transfusions are not usually helpful because of rapid platelet consumption, patients with life-threatening bleeding and platelet counts under $10,000/\mu L$ should receive platelet transfusions, 10 units at a time; this may raise the platelet count, depending on the rate of platelet destruction. Some patients may require red blood cell transfusions to correct severe anemia. If plasmapheresis cannot be performed immediately, adjunctive therapy with platelet-inhibiting drugs or vincristine is sometimes used at the discretion of the hematologist.

3. DISSEMINATED INTRAVASCULAR COAGULATION

Disseminated intravascular coagulation is a complex coagulopathy characterized by systemic activation of coagulation processes that overwhelms the inhibitory mechanisms that normally localize coagulation. In normal hemostasis, free thrombin is restricted to the site of coagulation by a combination of protein inhibitors, rapid blood flow, and absorption onto the fibrin clot. In disseminated intravascular coagulation, circulating thrombin cleaves fibrinogen to form fibrin clots throughout the circulation. Occasionally, this results in widespread thrombosis, with end-organ ischemia and dysfunction as prominent symptoms. In most cases, thrombosis is overshadowed by generalized bleeding. Hemorrhage is caused by the combination of reduced fibrinogen level, consumption of coagulation factors, thrombocytopenia, circulating fibrin degradation products that act as anticoagulants, and excessive secondary fibrinolysis that is activated in response to widespread formation of thrombi.

The most common disorders that may result in disseminated intravascular coagulation are sepsis, hypotension, obstetric complications (eg, retained abortus), severe tissue injury (eg, crush injury or burns), brain injury, cancer (especially promyelocytic leukemia), and major hemolytic transfusion reactions.

Diagnosis

Suspect disseminated intravascular coagulation in a patient with predisposing illness who presents with signs of diffuse hemorrhage: oozing around intravenous catheters or wound sites, or frank bleeding from mucosal sites. The diagnosis is supported by a low platelet count, low levels of fibrinogen, presence of fibrin degradation products, and prolonged prothrombin time. Fibrin monomer may be present, and red blood cell fragmentation may be seen on the peripheral blood smear. The diagnosis is confirmed by sequential measurements, which document consumption of fibrinogen and platelet levels and rising levels of fibrin degradation products. *Note:* A single measurement of fibrinogen or platelet levels may be misleading because elevated levels of these components are associated with inflammatory disease.

Differential Diagnosis

Thrombocytopenia due to disseminated intravascular coagulation can be differentiated from other causes of thrombocytopenia by the additional findings of abnormal results on coagulation tests (prothrombin and partial thromboplastin times and fibrinogen level). Immune thrombocytopenia is characterized by isolated thrombocytopenia, whereas patients with thrombotic thrombocytopenic purpura have microangiopathic hemolytic anemia and thrombocytopenia but normal prothrombin and partial thromboplastin times. The coagulopathy associated with liver disease may be difficult to distinguish from disseminated intravascular coagulation, since decreased platelet counts and prolongation of prothrombin and partial thromboplastin times may be present in both disorders. However, levels of fibrinogen are usually normal and never rapidly declining in liver disease, and fibrin monomer is not present.

Treatment

The first step in treatment of disseminated intravascular coagulation is to treat the underlying cause, if possible. Obtain appropriate cultures in patients with suspected sepsis, and begin the proper antibiotic therapy as quickly as possible (Chapter 34). In patients with disseminated intravascular coagulation due to an obstetric complication (missed abortion, abruptio placentae, septic abortion, puerperal sepsis), immediate complete evacuation of the uterus is mandatory, and antibiotic therapy should be started as soon as possible (Chapter 30). Treat hypotension and shock as outlined in Chapter 3. In some patients, eg, those with advanced or untreatable cancer, disseminated intravascular coagulation may signal impending death, and no therapy is indicated.

Treatment directed specifically toward reversing disseminated intravascular coagulation is indicated when illness is not terminal and when disseminated intravascular coagulation is causing significant clinical manifestations (eg, life-threatening hemorrhage or thrombosis). When the underlying cause of disseminated intravascular coagulation is rapidly reversible (eg, treatable infection, retained abortus), the patient may be treated with replacement therapy alone. Fibrinogen levels should be raised to 150 mg/dL by the administration of cryoprecipitate (15 bags of cryoprecipitate will raise the fibrinogen level of a 70-kg [154-lb] man by about 100 mg/dL). The administration of 4 units of fresh-frozen plasma will raise the levels of all coagulation factors and antithrombin III by about 25%. The platelet count should be raised to 50,000/μL or higher; this can usually be accomplished by administering 10 units of platelets.

Patients in whom the underlying cause of disseminated intravascular coagulation is not rapidly reversible and who are threatened by bleeding or thrombosis should receive replacement therapy combined with systemic heparinization. Heparin neutralizes the effect of circulating thrombin by potentiating the activity of antithrombin III, a normally circulating anticoagulant. Since levels of antithrombin III may be reduced in disseminated intravascular coagulation, replacement therapy with fresh-frozen plasma is essential to maximize the effect of heparin. Give heparin starting with 50–100 units/kg by bolus intravenous injection, followed by 500 units/h by continuous infusion. The end point of therapy is stable or rising fibrinogen levels. The treatment of disseminated intravascular coagulation is complicated and should be undertaken in consultation with a hematologist.

Disposition

Patients with acute disseminated intravascular coagulation should be hospitalized, preferably in an intensive care unit, and should be managed on an emergency basis in consultation with a hematologist.

4. THROMBOCYTOPENIA DUE TO HEMATOLOGIC MALIGNANCY

Bleeding due to thrombocytopenia is a common presenting sign of all hematologic malignancies. In these circumstances, thrombocytopenia is usually due to diminished platelet production as megakaryocytes in bone marrow are replaced by tumor. Less commonly, thrombocytopenia is due to disseminated intravascular coagulation induced by the cancer or is due to immune thrombocytopenia complicating lymphoproliferative disease (eg, chronic lymphocytic leukemia, diffuse lymphomas).

Diagnosis

Suspect hematologic malignancy in any patient with thrombocytopenia who also has abnormalities of other cell lines. There may be a history of fevers, night sweats, or easy bruising. Physical examination may reveal lymphadenopathy, organomegaly (eg, splenomegaly), and bone tenderness, especially over the sternum. The diagnosis is confirmed by the presence of abnormal cell forms, such as immature blood cells on the peripheral smear, and by findings typical of hematologic malignancy on bone marrow examination.

Differential Diagnosis

Thrombocytopenia due to aplastic anemia is associated with anemia and neutropenia; bone marrow biopsy shows hypocellularity and no tumor cells. The presence of abnormal red blood cells (teardrop-shaped cells, nucleated red blood cells) suggests that thrombocytopenia is due to a myeloproliferative disorder such as myelofibrosis. Thrombocytopenia and evidence of microangiopathic hemolytic anemia (fragmented red blood cells on the peripheral blood smear) suggest thrombotic thrombocytopenic purpura or disseminated intravascular coagulation (see above).

Treatment

Since thrombocytopenia that is a complication of hematologic malignancy is almost always due to decreased platelet production, patients with bleeding or profound thrombocytopenia (< 10,000/μL) should receive platelet transfusions. Transfusion of 5 units of platelets will usually raise the platelet count by 30,000–50,000/μL, which should be sufficient to stop bleeding due to thrombocytopenia. Severely symptomatic anemia should be treated with transfusion of red blood cells. Treatment of the underlying hematologic condition depends on the specific diagnosis.

Disposition

Patients with known hematologic malignancy who present with mild to moderate thrombocytopenic bleeding and whose condition is otherwise stable may be treated with platelet transfusion and discharged with an appointment to see a hematologist the next day. Patients with newly diagnosed hematologic malignancy and those with serious hemorrhage should be hospitalized for evaluation and management by a hematologist.

5. THROMBOCYTOPENIA DUE TO APLASTIC ANEMIA

Aplastic anemia is characterized by reduction in bone marrow progenitor cells that results in decreased production of all hematopoietic cells. Patients may present with fatigue related to anemia, bleeding from thrombocytopenia, or infection due to neutropenia. Aplastic anemia may be caused by drugs or chemicals (eg, insecticides, chloramphenicol, phenylbutazone, sulfonamides, gold salts) or may follow viral infections. In many cases, no specific cause is identified.

The pathogenesis of aplastic anemia involves several heterogeneous factors. In some cases, bone marrow hematopoietic cells are depleted because of bone marrow injury. In other patients, however, there is an autoimmune basis for the disease. In these patients, immunosuppression is usually mediated by cytotoxic T cells; in rare patients, especially those with systemic lupus erythematosus, the responsible agent may be an IgG autoantibody.

Diagnosis

Suspect aplastic anemia in any patient with pancytopenia. There is usually no organomegaly, lymphadenopathy, or bone tenderness; the peripheral blood smear shows no abnormal cells. The diagnosis is made by bone marrow aspirate and biopsy, which show hypocellularity, reduced numbers of bone marrow progenitor cells, and absence of abnormal cellular infiltrates. The patient should be questioned about possible exposure to medications or toxic chemicals.

Differential Diagnosis

In cancer, the history and physical findings suggest that thrombocytopenia may be due to infiltration of bone marrow. The presence of abnormal cells on the peripheral blood smear suggests hematologic malignancy (blast cells) or myelofibrosis (teardrop-shaped or nucleated red blood cells). Differentiation between these disorders and aplastic anemia is based on the findings on bone marrow examination.

Treatment

Thrombocytopenic bleeding may be treated with platelet transfusion; 5 units of platelets should raise the platelet count by 30,000–50,000/μL, which is usually sufficient to stop bleeding due to thrombocytopenia.

Severe anemia should be treated with red blood cell transfusion. *Note:* Transfusions should not be given casually to patients who have never previously received a transfusion, because sensitization to blood products may compromise potential therapy with allogenic bone marrow transplantation.

Disposition

Patients with newly diagnosed pancytopenia should be hospitalized for bone marrow examination to establish the diagnosis and for initial treatment. Patients thought to have aplastic anemia may be candidates for allogenic bone marrow transplantation, which is especially successful if previous transfusion has not been performed and the patient is less than 30 years old. Alternative therapy is antithymocyte globulin. Patients with known aplastic anemia need not be hospitalized unless they have serious bleeding or infection. Patients with mild to moderate bleeding who have responded to platelet transfusion may be discharged from the emergency department with an appointment to see a hematologist within 24 hours.

6. THROMBOCYTOPENIA DUE TO ALCOHOL-INDUCED SUPPRESSION OF THROMBOPOIESIS

Alcohol is a bone marrow depressant that most commonly causes isolated modest thrombocytopenia due to ineffective thrombocytopoiesis. Platelet counts under 20,000/μL are usually caused by other disorders but may occasionally be due to excessive alcohol ingestion alone.

Diagnosis

The diagnosis of alcohol-induced suppression of thrombopoiesis is suggested by a history of excessive alcohol intake. Physical examination may reveal stigmas of alcoholic liver disease, eg, spider angiomas. The CBC may show macrocytic anemia (due to alcoholic liver disease or dietary folate deficiency) in addition to modest thrombocytopenia; the peripheral blood smear often shows target cells. Prolongation of prothrombin time due to advanced liver disease or dietary deficiency of vitamin K is not infrequent. However, thrombocytopenia may be present in the absence of these other findings. The diagnosis of alcohol-induced thrombocytopenia is often made retrospectively when the thrombocytopenia spontaneously resolves after 3–7 days of abstinence from alcohol. Bone marrow examination is usually not diagnostic, since megakaryocytes are present in normal numbers.

Differential Diagnosis

Spontaneously resolving thrombocytopenia in an alcoholic patient is not usually confused with other disorders. Persistent (> 10–12 days) severe thrombocytopenia (< 20,000 platelets per microliter) suggests that thrombocytopenia is not due to alcohol alone, and further evaluation is required.

Treatment

As noted above, thrombocytopenia related to alcohol ingestion is usually modest, and no specific treatment is required. When bleeding occurs or thrombocytopenia is severe, platelet transfusions should be performed. Infusion of 5 units of platelets will raise the platelet count by 30,000–50,000/μL and stop the bleeding.

Disposition

Patients with severe thrombocytopenia or bleeding should be hospitalized for platelet transfusion.

7. QUALITATIVE PLATELET DISORDERS

Patients with qualitative platelet abnormalities present with bleeding similar to that seen with thrombocytopenia except that the platelet count is normal and petechiae are rare. Congenital intrinsic abnormalities of platelet function are not uncommon, but associated symptoms are usually mild. Patients with von Willebrand's disease frequently present with bleeding related to extrinsic platelet dysfunction (ie, platelets are functionally abnormal because of the deficiency of factor VIII/vWF, which mediates platelet adhesion). Acquired platelet dysfunction is seen in myeloproliferative disorders and uremia and also in patients using aspirin, other nonsteroidal anti-inflammatory drugs, and semisynthetic penicillins or cephalosporins. Although aspirin exerts a marked effect on platelet function in vitro, the clinical manifestations of platelet dysfunction related to aspirin ingestion in vivo are minimal unless the patient has an underlying hemostatic defect. Patients in whom bleeding appears to be precipitated by aspirin ingestion should be evaluated for the presence of von Willebrand's disease, congenital qualitative platelet abnormalities, or other hemostatic disorders.

Diagnosis

Prolonged bleeding time in the face of a normal platelet count indicates defective platelet function. Patients with prolonged bleeding time should be asked about recent use of aspirin or other suspect drugs. Consider the possibility of uremia, and obtain blood urea nitrogen and creatinine levels. The CBC and peripheral blood smear should be examined for evidence of myeloproliferative disorders.

Patients in whom acquired platelet dysfunction (eg, uremia, medications, myeloproliferative disorder) has been ruled out probably have a congenital platelet defect or von Willebrand's disease. Assessment of bleeding time after aspirin ingestion is a useful screening test for these disorders, but definitive diagnosis requires sophisticated laboratory tests that are not available on an emergency basis. Von Willebrand's disease is best diagnosed by finding reduced levels of factor VIII antigen (VIIIR:Ag) or ristocetin cofactor (VIIIR:RCo). Intrinsic platelet abnormalities are best documented by results of in vitro platelet aggregation tests.

Differential Diagnosis

Qualitative platelet function defects may occur in some myeloproliferative disorders, such as acute leukemia, chronic myeloid leukemia, or polycythemia vera. Patients with these disorders may have very high platelet counts, mucosal hemorrhage, and prolonged bleeding time. Obtain a CBC, and look for abnormalities on the peripheral blood smear (blast cells, giant degranulated platelets). These studies should be obtained for all patients who present with a previously undiagnosed platelet function abnormality. Bone marrow examination may be necessary to confirm the diagnosis.

Treatment

Patients with intrinsic qualitative platelet dysfunction respond to platelet transfusions; 5 units of platelets should provide 30,000–50,000 of normal platelets per microliter of blood and be sufficient to stop the bleeding. Patients who have received repeated platelet transfusions often become alloimmunized and may no longer respond to treatment, in which case no effective therapy is available. Extrinsic qualitative platelet dysfunction (eg, uremia, von Willebrand's disease, the presence of platelet-inhibiting drugs in the circulation) quickly makes transfused platelets dysfunctional, and platelet transfusions are not indicated unless life-threatening hemorrhage is present. Platelet dysfunction due to aspirin ingestion should regress within 4–5 days after ingestion of the drug. Von Willebrand's disease (see below) is treated with infusion of cryoprecipitate, which provides the missing cofactor necessary for platelet function. Bleeding due to uremia is best treated with vigorous dialysis to eliminate the toxin causing the qualitative platelet abnormality. When dialysis is not possible, other forms of therapy include the infusion of cryoprecipitate (10 bags daily); desmopressin acetate (DDAVP), 0.3–0.4 µg/kg (about 25 µg for a 70-kg [154-lb] man) intravenously over 30–40 minutes; and conjugated estrogens (0.6 mg/kg/d for 5 days).

Disposition

Patients with subclinical platelet dysfunction or mild bleeding do not require hospitalization and can be referred to their primary-care physician. Patients with significant bleeding should be treated as described above and hospitalized under the care of their primary-care physician or hematologist.

8. THROMBOCYTOSIS

Thrombocytosis is defined as a platelet count exceeding 450,000/µL. Modest thrombocytosis (< 700,000/µL) frequently occurs in reaction to infection, inflammatory disorders (eg, rheumatoid arthritis or ulcerative colitis), bleeding, iron deficiency, or cancer. In reactive thrombocytosis, platelets are functionally normal and there is no associated bleeding or clotting. However, thrombocytosis may also be due to a myeloproliferative disorder such as polycythemia vera, myelofibrosis, chronic myeloid leukemia, or essential thrombocytosis. In these conditions, platelets are qualitatively abnormal and may cause bleeding or thrombosis. Patients with thrombocytosis due to myeloproliferative disorders may present with life-threatening gastrointestinal tract bleeding, since they also often have duodenal ulcers. They may also have signs of thrombotic disease (with predisposition to thrombosis of veins in the abdominal cavity, eg, hepatic, portal, or mesenteric veins).

Differential Diagnosis

Reactive thrombocytosis is diagnosed by identifi-cation of the underlying disorder and exclusion of myeloproliferative disease. The platelet count is usually under 700,000/µL and rarely exceeds 1 million/mL. Infection, iron deficiency, bleeding, trauma, cancer, and inflammatory conditions are common causes. Platelet morphology is normal, but excessive numbers of platelets are seen on the peripheral blood smear. The bleeding time is normal.

Clues to the presence of a myeloproliferative disorder include splenomegaly, abnormalities of other cells, and abnormalities of platelet morphology on the peripheral blood smear. The presence of giant, partially degranulated platelets strongly suggests a myeloproliferative disorder. Polycythemia vera is suggested by erythrocytosis and splenomegaly. Chronic myeloid leukemia is suggested by splenomegaly and a high white blood cell count with a shift to the left (see Chronic Leukemias, below). Myelofibrosis is suggested by abnormal red blood cells (teardrop-shaped and nucleated red blood cells). Essential thrombocytosis is diagnosed by persistent, unexplained elevation of the platelet count; splenomegaly and abnormal platelet morphology may also be seen. Bleeding time is frequently prolonged.

Treatment

Reactive thrombocytosis requires no treatment other than that for the underlying disorder. Patients are not at risk for development of complications associated with thrombocytosis.

Patients whose thrombocytosis is due to myeloproliferative disorders and who are not bleeding are still at risk for hemorrhagic and thrombotic complications. They should be referred to a hematologist for treatment that consists mainly of control of the platelet count through chemotherapeutic agents or radioactive phosphorus therapy.

Patients with qualitative platelet dysfunction due to thrombocytosis who present with life-threatening bleeding usually fail to respond to conventional management and will require plateletpheresis using a cell separator; give hydroxyurea, 5 g orally, if plateletpheresis is unavailable.

Disposition

Patients with thrombocytosis who are not bleeding need not be hospitalized but should be referred to a hematologist for long-term management. Patients who are bleeding should be hospitalized and hematologic consultation obtained.

ABNORMAL COAGULANT FUNCTION

The clinical pattern of bleeding seen in patients with abnormal coagulant function differs from that seen in patients with abnormal platelet hemostasis. Coagulant abnormalities generally result in bleeding from larger vessels into joint spaces and deep muscles as opposed to the small-vessel bleeding with mucosal hemorrhage and petechiae seen in patients with platelet abnormalities. Although petechiae definitively demonstrate a platelet defect, such an abnormality may coexist with one of coagulant function. Bleeding from the nose, vagina, and urinary or gastrointestinal tracts may be due to either platelet or coagulant abnormalities. Bleeding due to abnormal coagulant function is less responsive to superficial pressure than is platelet bleeding.

The physician must remember that the platelet and coagulant components of hemostasis are interdependent, as shown by the dependence of platelet aggregation on normal fibrinogen function, the combined defect of both platelet adherence and coagulation function in von Willebrand's disease, and the deficient levels and functioning of both platelets and coagulation factors seen in disseminated intravascular coagulation.

Emergency evaluation of coagulant-specific hemostasis includes (1) prothrombin time to assess both the extrinsic coagulation pathway (tissue factor and factor VII) and the common pathway (factors V and X, prothrombin, and fibrinogen) and (2) the partial thromboplastin time to assess both the intrinsic pathway (contact factors and factors VIII, IX, XI, and XII) and the factors of the common pathway (Fig 33–1). Isolated prolongation of the prothrombin time suggests abnormal levels of factor VII; isolated prolongation of the partial thromboplastin time requires consideration of abnormal levels of factors VIII, IX, XI, or XII. Combined prolongation of the prothrombin time and the partial thromboplastin time suggests an abnormality in the common pathway or a complex coagulopathy involving multiple factors.

Treatment of the patient with bleeding due to abnormal coagulant function depends on the specific diagnosis. The mainstay of therapy for these disorders is infusion of fresh-frozen plasma, but many exceptions exist. The preferred treatment for hemophilia A is infusion of cryoprecipitate or commercial factor VIII:C concentrates; for von Willebrand's disease, infusion of cryoprecipitate is the treatment of choice. Vitamin K should be replaced if the patient demonstrates deficiency. Although fresh-frozen plasma is often used to replace clotting factors in disseminated intravascular coagulation, successful treatment sometimes requires interruption of the pathophysiologic sequence of events with heparin (see above).

1. HEMOPHILIA A

Hemophilia A, the most common inherited disorder of hemostasis (1–2 persons in every 10,000 in the USA), is caused by abnormally low levels of factor VIII coagulant (VIII:C), also called antihemophilic factor. Hemophilia A occurs almost exclusively in

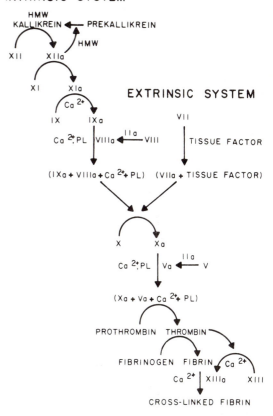

INTRINSIC SYSTEM

EXTRINSIC SYSTEM

Figure 33–1. Cascade mechanism of blood coagulation. PL, phospholipid; Ca^{2+}, calcium ion; HMW, high-molecular-weight kininogen; soluble coagulation factors are indicated by Roman numerals. (Adapted from Davie and Ratnoff. Reproduced, with permission, from Baugh RF, Hougie C: The chemistry of blood coagulation. Clin Haematol 1979;8:3).

males, since the gene encoding VIII:C is found on the X chromosome.

The severity of symptoms in hemophilia A correlates closely with the circulating level of factor VIII:C, as shown in Table 33–5. In between bleeding episodes, patients with hemophilia are usually asymptomatic and demonstrate no defect of platelet function, white cells, or red cells unless anemia has occurred as a result of extensive blood loss.

Patients commonly seek emergency medical attention for hemarthroses, hematuria, and epistaxis. Bleeding into deep tissues may result in serious complications owing to pressure on vital organs, blood vessels, or peripheral nerves. Intracranial bleeding is a life-threatening complication. Hemophiliac patients who have received multiple transfusions often develop abnormal liver function. AIDS has also developed in hemophiliac patients treated with multiple transfusions.

Table 33–5. Correlation of seveity of hemophilia A with circulating levels of factor VIII:C.

Circulating Level of Factor VIII:C	Severity	Manifestations
<1%	Severe	"Spontaneous" bleeding Postcircumcision bleeding Recurrent hemarthroses Joint deformities
1–5%	Moderate	Occasional hemarthroses Joint deformities (rare)
5–25%	Mild	Bleeding (rare) often diagnosed after dental work, trauma, or surgery

Diagnosis

Hemophilia A occurs almost exclusively in males, and the patient may report a family history of bleeding diatheses found only in males. The partial thromboplastin time but not the prothrombin time is prolonged, because factor VIII:C is the cofactor of factor IXa in the intrinsic coagulation pathway. The partial thromboplastin time is prolonged when levels of factor VIII:C are less than 30% of normal, so almost all hemophiliacs demonstrate this laboratory abnormality. When the partial thromboplastin time is prolonged, a bleeding time should be performed to exclude platelet dysfunction characterizing von Willebrand's disease. When the bleeding time is normal, a quantitative assay for levels of factor VIII:C should be performed to confirm the diagnosis of hemophilia A. Normal levels of factor VIII antigen (VIIIR:Ag) definitively distinguish hemophilia A from von Willebrand's disease, in which levels are reduced.

Treatment

The choice of treatment for bleeding in patients with hemophilia A depends on the severity of bleeding and on whether the patient has developed inhibitors to factor VIII:C.

Because of the multiple and potentially life-threatening risks associated with the infusion of blood products, transfusion therapy should be used only when necessary. For superficial cuts and abrasions and mild epistaxis, direct pressure alone or in conjunction with topical thrombin (Thrombinar, Thrombostat, others) may arrest bleeding.

In patients with mild or moderate hemophilia, intravenous infusion of desmopressin acetate (DDAVP) results in a 3- to 6-fold rise in levels of factor VIII:C, an increment often sufficient to achieve hemostatic levels (25%) of factor VIII:C. Give desmopressin acetate, 0.3–0.4 µg/kg by intravenous infusion over 30–40 minutes (about 25 µg for a 70-kg [154-lb] man).

In patients having more severe defects of factor VIII:C and uncontrolled active bleeding, replacement therapy with factor VIII:C is required; the timing and dose depend on the clinical circumstances. For in-

stance, infusion before arthrocentesis performed for hemarthrosis may result in intra-articular clotting and subsequent inability to evacuate the joint space; therefore, replacement therapy should be performed immediately after arthrocentesis. On the other hand, replacement should precede suturing of lacerations in order to prevent continued bleeding and formation of wound hematomas beneath sutures.

Replacement therapy for mild to moderately severe bleeding (mild hemarthroses or epistaxis) should raise levels of factor VIII:C to 25%; the infusion may be repeated in 24 hours. Bleeding joints should be immobilized. For major spontaneous hemorrhage or when surgery is required in a hemophiliac patient, levels of factor VIII:C should be raised to 50% of normal and should be maintained above 30% until the clot is well organized. Life-threatening hemorrhage (eg, intracranial) should be treated by maintaining levels of factor VIII:C above 50%.

The dose of factor VIII:C is based on the therapeutic level desired. By definition, normal plasma contains 1 unit/mL of all coagulants, including factor VIII:C, and plasma volume equals 40 mL/kg. An example of the required calculations is as follows: A 70-kg man has hemarthrosis and a factor VIII:C level of 1%; the desired therapeutic level of factor VIII:C is 25%. Based on the information given above, the patient's plasma volume is 2800 mL (40 mL/kg × 70 kg), and the patient's existing level of factor VIII:C is 1%. An increase of 24% is required to achieve the required level of 25%. The volume of distribution of factor VIII:C is 1.5 times the plasma volume (2800 mL × 1.5). The number of units of factor VIII:C required to achieve the desired increase of 24% is 2800 × 1.5 × 0.24 = 1008 units (about 15 units/kg).

Factor VIII:C may be obtained from blood banks either as commercial factor VIII concentrates, which are now treated to kill viruses, or as cryoprecipitate. Cryoprecipitate requires larger-volume infusions. Cryoprecipitate contains about 80–100 units of factor VIII:C per bag; the unit content of commercial concentrate is marked on the bottle.

Obtain hematologic consultation for the 10% of hemophiliac patients with circulating inhibitors to factor VIII:C and for hemophiliac patients who fail to respond to replacement therapy with decreased bleeding or normalization of the partial thromboplastin time. Such patients may require complicated therapy with factor VII–IX concentrates, high-dose factor VIII:C infusion, or animal factor VIII:C.

Intravenous analgesia is usually required in acute cases for relief of pain due to deep bleeding. Analgesic agents that inhibit platelet function (eg, aspirin, nonsteroidal anti-inflammatory agents) are contraindicated, as are intramuscular injections.

Disposition

Treat minor epistaxis, lacerations, and mild hemarthroses as described above, and refer the patient to a hematologist or primary-care physician to be seen within 24 hours. Treat major, life-threatening bleeding as described above, hospitalize the patient, and obtain hematologic consultation.

2. HEMOPHILIA B

Hemophilia B, also called Christmas disease, is similar to hemophilia A in that it is X-linked (affecting males almost exclusively) and is associated with an isolated prolongation of the partial thromboplastin time due to deficient levels of factor IX, a coagulant in the intrinsic pathway (Fig 33–1). The partial thromboplastin time may not be prolonged if there is only a mild deficiency of factor IX. In the USA, hemophilia B is seen in only one per 100,000 individuals. The type of bleeding is the same as that in hemophilia A.

Diagnosis

The diagnosis is made by the finding of low levels of factor IX in a male patient with a prolonged partial thromboplastin time. A family history of bleeding diatheses found only in males supports the diagnosis.

Treatment

As in hemophilia A, treatment is tailored to the severity of the bleeding. Hemostatic levels of factor IX are also 25%, but unlike factor VIII:C, about one-half of the infused amount of factor IX is rapidly lost from the circulation. Calculation of the required dose of factor IX is the same as for factor VIII:C except that the plasma volume is multiplied by 2 instead of 1.5. A dose of 20 units/kg will raise factor IX levels by 25%. As in hemophilia A, severe bleeding and major surgery will require higher initial levels. Sources of factor IX include fresh-frozen plasma and commercial factor IX complex (Konyne-HT, Profilnine, Proplex).

Analgesia is frequently required for relief of pain due to deep bleeding. Aspirin, nonsteroidal anti-inflammatory agents, and other drugs that inhibit platelet function are contraindicated, as are intramuscular injections.

Disposition

Patients with mild bleeding should be treated and referred to a hematologist or primary-care physician to be seen within 24 hours. Patients with more severe hemorrhage should be hospitalized under the care of a hematologist or primary-care physician with hematologic consultation.

3. VON WILLEBRAND'S DISEASE

Disordered hemostasis in von Willebrand's disease is due to a combination of 2 defects: an extrinsic platelet dysfunction and an impairment of the intrinsic coagulation pathway. Because the mechanism of inheritance is autosomal dominant, both sexes may be affected. Patients are well except for the bleeding, which follows either the pattern of bleeding due to platelet dysfunction or the pattern due to coagulant dysfunction. Abnormal platelet function is due to insufficient levels or inadequate functioning of the factor VIII:vWF, a molecule distinct from factor VIII:C. Factor VIII:vWF is produced in endothelial cells and is necessary for normal platelet adhesion. Normally, factors VIII:vWF and VIII:C are found as a stable complex in the circulation, and abnormally low levels of VIII:vWF result in a commensurate decrease in VIII:C levels because VIII:C becomes more susceptible to degradation. Defective platelet adherence is due to a primary decrease in levels of factor VIII:vWF, and abnormal coagulant activity is due to a secondary decrease in levels of factor VIII:C.

Diagnosis

Epistaxis, easy bruising, menorrhagia, prolonged bleeding after minor dental or surgical procedures, and gastrointestinal tract bleeding are common manifestations of von Willebrand's disease. Petechiae, hemarthroses, and fatal bleeding are uncommon.

Severe varieties of von Willebrand's disease may be diagnosed on the basis of a constellation of prolonged partial thromboplastin time, normal platelet count and prothrombin time, prolonged bleeding time, and decreased levels of factor VIII:C. It often is necessary to measure levels of factor VIII:vWF, ristocetin cofactor, and vWF multimers to make the diagnosis. Diagnostic difficulties occur in milder cases and when levels of factor VIII:vWF rise in reaction to certain conditions of stress (pregnancy, infection, etc). Obtain hematologic consultation to confirm the diagnosis or to clarify the diagnosis of more obscure variants of the disease. A family history of bleeding diatheses in both sexes supports the diagnosis.

Treatment

Bleeding in von Willebrand's disease is usually self-limited (though prolonged) and seldom requires specific therapy. Excessive bleeding from accessible sites may be controlled by local pressure with thrombin-soaked Gelfoam.

A. Desmopressin: Desmopressin (DDAVP) is the initial treatment of choice in patients with mild or moderate bleeding or patients known to be responsive to desmopressin. The need for blood products can be reduced along with the associated risk of transfusion-acquired diseases. Give desmopressin, 0.3 μg/kg by intravenous infusion over 20–30 minutes. Factor VIII activity and von Willebrand antigen will usually increase 3- to 5-fold. Patients can also self-administer desmopressin subcutaneously; nasal spray desmopressin for von Willebrand's disease is being investigated.

B. Cryoprecipitate and Fresh-Frozen Plasma:
Cryoprecipitate and fresh-frozen plasma are excellent sources of factor VIII:vWF. *Commercial factor VIII:C preparations do not contain sufficient amounts of factor VIII:vWF for therapy and should not be used.* Cryoprecipitate contains about 100 units of factor VIII:vWF per bag. Since the hemostatic level of factor VIII:vWF for all patients but those with severe bleeding is 25%, a dose of 10 units of factor VIII:vWF per kilogram or 0.1 bag of cryoprecipitate per kilogram is sufficient to correct the bleeding tendency. In patients with severe bleeding, hemostatic levels of factor VIII:vWF of 50% are required. Maintenance infusions are generally given every 24 hours but may need to be given more frequently.

Disposition

Patients with minor bleeding should be treated and referred to a hematologist or primary-care physician to be seen within 24 hours. Those with severe bleeding should be treated and hospitalized; obtain hematologic consultation.

4. INFREQUENT INHERITED COAGULANT DEFICIENCIES

Less common hemorrhagic disorders result from deficiencies of factors V, X, XI, prothrombin, or fibrinogen. These disorders are generally less severe than the hemophilias or von Willebrand's disease, but exceptions exist. Deficiencies of factor XII, prekallikrein, and high-molecular-weight kininogen result in remarkable prolongation of the partial thromboplastin time but no bleeding diathesis.

Diagnosis

Most patients with previously diagnosed bleeding disorders know the factor in which they are deficient. Consult a hematologist to make the diagnosis in patients with a previously undiagnosed disorder. In general, diagnosis of specific factor deficiencies is achieved by mixing the patient's plasma with various factor-deficient plasmas. Exceptions are factor XIII deficiency, which is diagnosed by the urea clot solubility test; afibrinogenemia, which is diagnosed by measuring fibrinogen levels; and dysfibrinogenemia, which is diagnosed by a discrepancy between the amount of measurable fibrinogen and the amount of functional fibrinogen.

Treatment

With the exception of fibrinogen (factor I) deficiency, treat clinically significant bleeding with fresh-frozen plasma, 5–20 mL/kg by intravenous infusion (350–1400 mL [1.1–7.7 bags] for a 70-kg [154-lb] man). Treat fibrinogen deficiency with cryoprecipitate, 0.2 bag/kg (10–20 bags for adults) by in-

travenous infusion. Factor XIII is easily replenished with 4 bags of cryoprecipitate.

Disposition

Patients with mild bleeding that has responded to therapy need not be hospitalized but should be referred for hematologic or primary-care follow-up within 24 hours. Patients with serious hemorrhage should receive initial infusion therapy as outlined above and should be hospitalized; obtain hematologic consultation.

5. HEPATIC COAGULOPATHY

Patients with severely disordered hepatic function are at risk for hemorrhage for several reasons, the most important of which is decreased hepatic production of coagulant factors. Patients with severe liver disease are susceptible to this defect because all the coagulant factors except factor VIII are synthesized by hepatocytes. When hepatic coagulopathy occurs, the liver disorder is usually so severe that other signs of liver disease are also present (eg, portal hypertension, ascites, hypersplenism, hepatic encephalopathy, or hepatorenal syndrome). The coagulopathy usually occurs in patients with decompensated hepatic cirrhosis but may also be associated with other acute or chronic liver diseases.

In addition to the low levels of coagulants, there is increased fibrinolysis due to diminished circulatory clearance of plasmin, poor clot formation due to abnormal fibrinogen production by diseased hepatocytes, abnormal coagulant function due to vitamin K deficiency (see Vitamin K Deficiency, below), and the abnormal coagulant and platelet functions that result when fibrin degradation products are not adequately cleared from the circulation. Other factors that may contribute to bleeding are thrombocytopenia due to hypersplenism, bacteremia, or alcoholic marrow suppression, and platelet dysfunction due to recent heavy alcohol consumption.

Diagnosis

Hepatic coagulopathy is the most likely diagnosis in a bleeding patient with decompensated liver disease. Usually, both the prothrombin and the partial thromboplastin times are prolonged owing to the widespread decreased levels of factors affecting the extrinsic, intrinsic, and common clotting pathways. Because of the short (6-hour) half-life of factor VII, the prothrombin time is the most sensitive index of impaired hepatic synthetic function; isolated prolongation of the prothrombin time may occur. The fibrin degradation product titer is elevated, and the thrombin time is often prolonged owing to the inhibitory effect of fibrin degradation products on fibrinogen function and the presence of abnormal fibrinogen. The platelet count is often moderately decreased.

Disseminated intravascular coagulation is the disorder most likely to be confused with hepatic coagulopathy, since the laboratory findings are similar. Both disorders also often occur in the same clinical setting, and differentiation is crucial, because their therapy may be entirely different.

In distinguishing hepatic coagulopathy from disseminated intravascular coagulation, it is useful to remember that in hepatic coagulopathy, fibrin monomer is not present and levels of factor VIII:C and fibrinogen are usually normal. However, in advanced liver disease, fibrinogen levels may be reduced. A useful clinical test is to look for the rapid fibrinogen consumption seen in disseminated intravascular coagulation but not in hepatic coagulopathy by obtaining serial (ie, every 12 hours) fibrinogen levels.

Treatment

In the absence of clinical bleeding, no replacement therapy for hepatic coagulopathy is indicated. Vitamin K, 10 mg/d orally or subcutaneously for 3 days, may partially correct coagulation abnormalities and should be given.

When clinical bleeding is present, give fresh-frozen plasma, 15–20 mL/kg intravenously (4–6 bags for a 70-kg [154-lb] man). Other treatment specific for the type of clinical bleeding present should also be administered (eg, antacids for gastrointestinal tract bleeding; nasal packing for epistaxis). Also give vitamin K, 10 mg subcutaneously, since it may result in partial resolution of the abnormality. Consider platelet transfusions if there is concurrent thrombocytopenia.

Disposition

Patients with subclinical hepatic coagulopathy should be discharged with a prescription for vitamin K, 10 mg orally daily for 3–5 days, and should be observed on an outpatient basis. Patients with clinically apparent bleeding should be hospitalized for continued monitoring and factor replacement.

6. VITAMIN K DEFICIENCY

Certain instances of coagulant-deficient types of bleeding may be due to vitamin K deficiency. Factors II, VII, IX, and X require a vitamin K–dependent γ-carboxylation of their glutamate residues for normal function; the absence of vitamin K results in the production of inert vitamin K–dependent factors. Because factor VII is in the extrinsic pathway, factor IX is in the intrinsic pathway, and factors II and X are in the common pathway, usually both prothrombin and partial thromboplastin times are prolonged in patients with abnormal hemostasis due to vitamin K deficiency. However, because the 6-hour half-life of factor VII is the shortest of any coagulant, the prothrombin time is more sensitive than the partial thromboplastin time to vitamin K deficiency, and isolated prolongation of the prothrombin time occasionally occurs.

The 2 main sources of vitamin K are diet and intestinal bacteria; deficiency occurs in 2–4 weeks if both sources are lacking. Bleeding due to vitamin K deficiency typically occurs in postoperative patients with infection who have been treated with antibiotics for long periods and who have been unable to accept oral intake. Bleeding also occurs in patients with intestinal malabsorption or severe liver disease. In the latter, decreased intestinal absorption, anorexia, and dietary neglect may cause vitamin K deficiency that contributes to the underlying hepatic coagulopathy. Bleeding due to deficiency of vitamin K may also result after treatment with warfarin. Prophylactic administration of vitamin K at birth has almost entirely eliminated the incidence of hemorrhagic disease of the newborn in the USA.

Diagnosis

The diagnosis of bleeding due to vitamin K deficiency is confirmed in patients with or without bleeding in whom a prolonged prothrombin time is restored to normal after administration of vitamin K.

Treatment

Treatment depends on clinical findings. Patients with prolonged prothrombin times without clinically evident bleeding may be treated with vitamin K replacement. The intramuscular route should be avoided because of the risk of hematoma; the intravenous route has been associated with life-threatening reactions. Vitamin K, 10 mg orally for 3–5 days, may be used in nonemergency situations, although the oral route is associated with unreliable absorption. In more urgent situations, give vitamin K subcutaneously (10–15 mg). Restoration of prothrombin time to normal occurs in 6–12 hours. In life-threatening hemorrhage, the coagulation defect can be reversed immediately by the infusion of fresh-frozen plasma, 15–20 mL/kg (4–6 bags for a 70-kg [154-lb] man) intravenously. These guidelines may not apply in patients with hemorrhage due to warfarin therapy. For instance, giving vitamin K to patients with prosthetic heart valves who require continued warfarin therapy will reverse the therapeutic effect of warfarin and require subsequent reinduction of anticoagulation. An alternative approach in these patients is to continue therapeutic doses of warfarin while treating the hemorrhage with fresh-frozen plasma. The vitamin K–dependent factors in fresh-frozen plasma are unaffected by warfarin, and therapeutic anticoagulation levels will remain after fresh-frozen plasma therapy is discontinued.

Disposition

Patients with subclinical prolongation of clotting times should be treated with oral vitamin K and referred for outpatient follow-up. Patients with significant bleeding should be treated and hospitalized for hematologic consultation and further therapy.

7. DISSEMINATED INTRAVASCULAR COAGULATION (DIC)

See p 580.

EMERGENCY EVALUATION OF THE PATIENT WITH ANEMIA

It is not unusual to learn that a patient is anemic (hematocrit < 37% in women or < 40% in men) as an incidental finding on a CBC obtained for other reasons. Asymptomatic anemias are usually mild (hematocrit ≥ 30%). Patients with more severe anemia, especially of acute onset, may present to the emergency department complaining of headache, weakness, dyspnea on exertion, dizziness, palpitations, or angina. Such patients may appear pale, with pale mucous membranes and nail beds, or may exhibit resting tachycardia or orthostatic vital signs. Obtain a hematocrit determination in patients with obvious blood loss (eg, those with blood in the stool, abnormal vaginal bleeding, or severe epistaxis), and keep in mind that early in acute bleeding the hematocrit may be normal and may not reflect the amount of blood lost.

Emergency evaluation of the patient with anemia should consider whether active or ongoing blood loss is life-threatening; whether transfusion is urgently required; and whether anemia is acute or chronic. Definitive diagnosis of the cause of anemia may not be possible in the emergency department, but initial laboratory studies should be started and appropriate follow-up arrangement made.

Is There Ongoing Blood Loss?

Hypotension, unexplained tachycardia, or orthostatic vital signs (Chapter 3) suggest that anemia is of recent onset. In addition to any obvious external blood loss, consider the possibility of active internal bleeding in victims of blunt trauma (Chapter 4), in elderly patients, in patients with a history of hypertension (eg, leaking abdominal aortic aneurysm), or in patients with known or suspected bleeding dyscrasias. Women of childbearing age should be asked about prolonged, heavy, or irregular menstrual bleeding; consider the possibility of ruptured ectopic pregnancy if there is acute anemia and pelvic pain (Chapter 30). Ask about a history of hematemesis or melena, and check samples of stool and gastric contents if gastrointestinal tract bleeding is suspected. Consider the possibility of hemolysis in any patient with an acute anemia in whom there is no evidence of blood loss.

Is Transfusion Urgently Required?

Indications for red blood cell transfusion are discussed in detail below. In general, patients with severe anemia, moderate anemia with significant symptoms, or active blood loss are candidates for urgent transfusion in the emergency department.

Is Anemia Acute or Chronic?

The rapid onset of anemia must be related to blood loss, either through bleeding (eg, gastrointestinal tract bleeding) or hemolysis. As noted above, patients with moderately severe anemia of sudden onset frequently have symptoms related to decreased oxygen delivery to the tissues. Anemia due to decreased production of erythrocytes is gradual in onset, because red blood cells normally survive for 120 days in the circulation. Past medical records are useful in evaluation of the onset of anemia, because a decrement of hemoglobin or hematocrit greater than 0.8% per day is incompatible with simple cessation of erythropoiesis. One clinical rule of thumb is that the greatest fall in hemoglobin levels that can be attributed to decreased production alone is 1 g/dL/wk.

FURTHER EVALUATION OF THE PATIENT WITH ANEMIA

Clues to the cause of anemia may be obtained from the medical history, physical examination, and laboratory tests.

Medical History

Patients should be asked about prior anemia or a family history of anemia. Ask about any recent hematemesis, melena, rectal bleeding, weight loss, abdominal pain, or use of aspirin or other medications (eg, nonsteroidal anti-inflammatory agents) or alcohol that might account for gastrointestinal tract blood loss. Obtain a detailed menstrual history in young women. Observe whether there are any constitutional symptoms (weight loss, fevers, sweats, or fatigue) that suggest cancer, infection, or inflammation. Does the patient have any chronic medical conditions (eg, renal disease, rheumatologic disease) that may be associated with anemia due to chronic disease? Ask about medication use, including over-the-counter preparations, which may cause gastrointestinal tract blood loss, bone marrow injury, or red blood cell destruction.

Physical Examination

In all patients thought to have anemia, obtain pulse and blood pressure readings in the supine, sitting, and standing positions. Orthostatic vital signs suggest an acute blood loss.

If the source of blood loss is not obvious and acute blood loss is suspected, insert a nasogastric tube to look for gastrointestinal tract bleeding (Chapter 8), obtain a stool sample for occult blood testing, and consider posttraumatic intraperitoneal bleeding.

Other physical findings that may be useful in determining the cause of anemia include evidence of cancer (cachexia, organomegaly, lymphadenopathy, masses), chronic liver disease (hepatomegaly, spider angiomas), and infection.

Laboratory Tests

Essential laboratory tests in the emergency department evaluation of anemia include a CBC, including determination of red blood cell indices (Table 33–6);

differential; and platelet count. If there is any concern about continued active bleeding, serial hematocrits and orthostatic vital signs should also be obtained to document the rapidity of blood loss. The peripheral blood smear may provide essential clues to the cause of anemia (hypochromic, microcytic cells suggest iron deficiency anemia; hypersegmented PMNs are seen in megaloblastic anemias; fragmented red blood cells are seen in microangiopathic hemolytic anemias; abnormal white blood cell forms suggest hematologic malignancy). A reticulocyte count is useful in assessing the ability of the patient's bone marrow to respond to anemia: a high count suggests a hemolytic process or other ongoing cause of blood loss, whereas a low count suggests depressed bone marrow production of erythrocytes. The reticulocyte count is normally expressed as a *percentage* of the total red blood cell count. In order to be useful in assessing the bone marrow response to blood loss, the count must be corrected for the degree of anemia. (A reticulocyte count

Table 33–6. Diagnosis of common anemias based on red blood cell indices.

Type of Anemia	Typical Values for Red Cell Indices		Common Causes	Helpful Diagnostic Clues	
	Mean Corpuscular Volume (fL)	Mean Corpuscular Hemoglobin Concentration (g/dL)		Other Clinical Findings	Common Laboratory Abnormalities
Microcytic, hypochromic	< 80	< 32	Iron deficiency	Mucositis; blood loss.	Low reticulocyte count; low serum and bone marrow iron; high serum iron-binding capacity.
			Thalassemias	Asian, black, or Mediterranean descent; family history.	High reticulocyte count; abnormal red cell morphology; normal serum iron levels.
			Chronic lead poisoning	Peripheral neuropathy; history of exposure to lead.	Basophilic stippling of red cells; elevated lead levels.
			Sideroblastic anemia (usually normocytic)	Population of hypochromic red blood cells on smear.	High serum iron; ring sideroblasts in bone marrow.
Normocytic, normochromic	81–100	32–36	Acute blood loss	Recent blood loss.	Blood in stool or nasogastric aspirate.
			Hemolysis	Hemoglobinuria; splenomegaly.	Haptoglobin low or absent; reticulocytosis; hyperbilirubinemia. LDH elevated.
			Chronic disease	Depends on cause.	Low serum iron; iron-binding capacity low or low normal.
Macrocytic, normochromic	> 101	> 36	Vitamin B_{12} deficiency	Peripheral neuropathy; glossitis.	Hypersegmented PMNs; low serum vitamin B_{12} levels; achlorhydria; macroelliptocytes.
			Folate deficiency	Alcoholism; malnutrition; glossitis.	Hypersegmented PMNs; low serum folate levels; macroelliptocytes.
			Liver disease	Signs of liver disease.	Mean corpuscular volume usually <120 fL; normal serum vitamin B_{12} and folate levels.
			Marked reticulocytosis	Variable.	Marked (> 15%) reticulocytosis.

that is only twice normal in a patient with a hematocrit of 20% would be an inadequate bone marrow response.) The reticulocyte count can be corrected for anemia by multiplying the percentage of reticulocytes by the product of the actual hematocrit divided by the expected or normal hematocrit (eg, a reported reticulocyte count of 3% in a male patient with a hematocrit of 20% would be a corrected reticulocyte count of only 1.5% [ie, $3 \times 20 \div 40 = 1.5$]). In the absence of anemia, the normal reticulocyte count is between 0.5 and 1.5% of the total red blood cell count.

Tests that may be useful in the emergency department evaluation of hemolytic anemias are listed in Table 33–7. Further laboratory evaluation of anemia should be guided by information obtained from the history, physical examination, and initial laboratory studies. Specific adjunctive tests that may be required are listed in Table 33–8. These tests are usually not available on an emergency basis.

EMERGENCY MANAGEMENT OF SPECIFIC ANEMIAS

IRON DEFICIENCY ANEMIA

In adults, iron deficiency anemia is usually the result of chronic gastrointestinal tract blood loss or, in women, losses from menstrual flow. Iron deficiency anemia due to dietary deficiency alone is uncommon in developed countries, except in infants who are breast- or bottle-fed for prolonged periods without iron supplementation or in adolescents during the adolescent growth spurt. Occult gastrointestinal blood loss is a common cause of iron deficiency anemia in older patients, and radiologic or endoscopic investigation of the gastrointestinal tract is indicated if there is documented blood in the stool.

Diagnosis

The diagnosis of iron deficiency anemia is made by the finding of decreased serum iron levels associated with an elevated total iron-binding capacity, a low serum ferritin level, or decreased bone marrow iron stores. A presumptive diagnosis can be made in the emergency department in patients with a history

Table 33–7. Tests for evaluation of hemolytic anemia.

Peripheral blood smear
Reticulocyte count (corrected)
Serum bilirubin and lactic dehydrogenase (LDH) levels
Coombs' test (direct and indirect)
Haptoglobin level

Table 33–8. Adjunctive laboratory tests for evaluation of anemia.

Serum iron and total iron-binding capacity
Ferritin level
Coombs' test
Hemoglobin electrophoresis
Glucose-6-phosphate dehydrogenase assay
Red blood cell folate levels
Serum vitamin B_{12} levels
Schilling test
Bone marrow aspirate or biopsy

or clinical evidence of blood loss, decreased hemoglobin and hematocrit levels, mean corpuscular volume under 80 fL, and mean corpuscular hemoglobin concentration under 30 g/dL. However, early in its course iron deficiency anemia may be normocytic.

Differential Diagnosis

Other causes of microcytic, hypochromic anemia are listed in Table 33–6. A family history of anemia suggests the possibility of thalassemia. The diagnosis may be confirmed by hemoglobin electrophoresis. Basophilic stippling of red blood cells in children with behavioral changes or a history of pica should suggest the possibility of lead poisoning (Chapter 39). Sideroblastic anemia is commonly a primary bone marrow disorder but may be an acquired disorder due to alcohol, chloramphenicol, or lead; the diagnosis is confirmed by the finding of "ringed" sideroblasts on bone marrow biopsy.

Treatment

In order to avoid the risk of subjecting a patient with thalassemia to iron overload, it is generally better to delay treatment of mild microcytic anemia until a definitive diagnosis has been established. Patients with severe anemia may require red blood cell transfusion.

After blood samples have been drawn for serum ferritin or serum iron and iron-binding capacity studies, stable patients in whom there is little doubt about the diagnosis (eg, young women with a history of menometrorrhagia) may be discharged from the emergency department with a prescription for iron sulfate, 325 mg orally 3 times a day; patients should be warned about side effects (black stools, possible constipation or gastrointestinal tract upset).

Disposition

Patients with mild or asymptomatic iron deficiency anemia may be discharged and advised to seek follow-up consultation with their primary-care physician in order to determine the exact cause of anemia. Symptomatic patients or those with severe anemia but no evidence of active blood loss may be discharged after receiving red blood cell transfusion in the emergency department. Be sure to obtain blood samples for all of the indicated laboratory tests for evaluation of anemia before transfusion is performed. These patients should also be advised to seek consultation with their primary-care physician. Unstable patients with continuing blood loss should be hospitalized.

ACUTE HEMOLYTIC ANEMIA

Patients who present with acute anemia without any obvious source of blood loss may have hemolytic anemia. Causes of acute hemolysis are either extracorpuscular or intracorpuscular. The intracorpuscular hemolytic anemias can be divided into abnormalities of erythrocyte membranes, hemoglobin, or metabolism.

One of the main causes of extracorpuscular hemolysis is autoimmune hemolytic anemia caused by anti–red cell antibodies. Extrinsic causes of hemolysis may also occur in association with disseminated intravascular coagulation, thrombotic thrombocytopenic purpura, physical damage to erythrocytes, and infection (eg, malaria, sepsis due to *Clostridium*).

The 2 most common causes of acute hemolysis in a previously well adult patient are autoimmune hemolytic anemia and glucose-6-phosphate dehydrogenase (G6PD) deficiency. Acute autoimmune hemolytic anemia typically results from an IgG antibody interaction with a red cell antigen, but other immunoglobulin classes (eg, IgM) may also be the cause. Because most IgG anti–red cell antibodies react optimally at body temperature, hemolytic anemia due to IgG is known as "warm-reacting" hemolytic anemia; it occurs secondary to other conditions (eg, collagen vascular diseases, lymphoproliferative disease) or use of certain medications (Table 33–9) in as many as half of patients.

IgM anti–red blood cell antibodies, on the other hand, usually react optimally at cold temperatures; patients with this type of hemolytic anemia therefore complain of onset of symptoms when they are exposed to a cold environment. Hemolysis caused by IgM antibodies is called the **cold agglutinin syndrome.** This syndrome is often idiopathic, but other causes are prior infection with *Mycoplasma pneumoniae,* infectious mononucleosis, and diffuse histiocytic lymphoma.

In the USA, hemolysis due to glucose-6-phosphate dehydrogenase deficiency occurs most commonly in blacks who have a hypofunctional mutant form of the A isoenzyme of glucose-6-phosphate dehydrogenase. This deficiency affects about 1 out of every 10 black men who are hemizygous for the deficiency and 1 in 100 black women who are homozygous. These patients experience episodes of acute hemolysis when their red cells are subject to oxidative stress, as occurs in bacterial infection; ingestion of certain drugs and chemicals (Table 33–10); or consumption of foods such as fava beans. Hemolysis is limited because only the oldest population of erythrocytes with low levels of glucose-6-phosphate dehydrogenase undergoes lysis. Hemolysis typically proceeds to a certain level, after which only younger erythrocytes that are relatively resistant to oxidative stress remain. The Mediterranean variant of this disorder (deficient B isoenzyme) is much more severe. Chronic hemolysis is common, and the acute hemolytic response to oxidative stress may be catastrophic.

Diagnosis

Any patient with acute onset of anemia without evidence of blood loss should be evaluated for evidence

Table 33–9. Medications that may induce autoimmune hemolytic anemia.

Innocent-bystander mechanism
  Stibophen
  Quinidine
  Quinine
  Sulfonamides
  Thiazides
  Isoniazid (isonicotinoylhydrazine; INH)
  Chlorpromazine
  p-Aminosalicylic acid
  Phenacetin
Hapten-mediated mechanism
  Penicillins
  Cephalosporins
  Streptomycin
Alpha-methyldopa type mechanism
  Alpha-methyldopa
  Levodopa
  Mefenamic acid
Unknown mechanism
  Ibuprofen

Table 33–10. Medications and compounds associated with glucose-6-phosphate dehydrogenase deficiency hemolysis.

Antimalarials
  Primaquine
  Quinacrine (Atabrine)
Sulfonamides
  Sulfasalazine (Azulfidine, others)
  Sodium sulfacetamide (many preparations)
  Sulfamethoxazole (Gantanol; Septra and Bactrim)
  Sulfanilamide (AVC, Vagitrol)
  Sulfapyridine
  Sulfisoxazole (Gantrisin, others)
Sulfones
  Dapsone
  Thiazolsulfone
Analgesics
  Acetanalid
Miscellaneous
  Dimercaprol (BAL)
  Methylene blue
  Nalidixic acid (NegGram)
  Naphthalene (moth balls)
  Niridazole (Ambihar)
  Nitrofurantoin (many preparations)
  Phenylhydrazine
  Toluidine blue

of hemolysis. The diagnosis of acute hemolytic anemia is suggested by a low or falling hematocrit with an elevated corrected reticulocyte count in a patient who is not bleeding. Patients with active hemolysis may have elevated serum bilirubin levels, low or absent haptoglobin, and if hemolysis is severe, free plasma hemoglobin and hemoglobinuria. The peripheral blood smear shows evidence of reticulocytosis with large bluish polychromatic cells or cells with basophilic stippling; if anemia is severe, there may be nucleated red blood cells. The definitive diagnosis often depends on demonstration of the pathophysiologic abnormality unique to the specific type of hemolytic anemia (see below).

Differential Diagnosis

The peripheral blood smear can provide valuable clues to the cause of hemolytic anemia. In acute hemolytic anemia due to warm-reacting antibodies, the smear will show microspherocytes, whereas in cold agglutinin disease the smear may show clumped red cells. The hallmark of microangiopathic hemolytic anemias (eg, disseminated intravascular coagulation, thrombotic thrombocytopenic purpura) is fragmented red blood cells. The diagnosis of acute hemolytic anemia due to a warm-reacting antibody is confirmed by a direct Coombs test demonstrating the presence of IgG on red blood cells. Cold agglutinin hemolytic anemia is diagnosed by the finding of high titers of cold agglutinins (> 1:1000) in serum and by the demonstration of a positive direct Coombs test when anticomplement reagents are used but not when antiglobulin reagents are used. Glucose-6-phosphate dehydrogenase deficiency is confirmed by finding decreased activity of this enzyme on the glucose-6-phosphate dehydrogenase assay. After an episode of hemolysis due to glucose-6-phosphate dehydrogenase deficiency, those cells with low levels of the enzyme will not be present, and measurable enzyme activity may appear to be normal. The diagnosis may therefore be confirmed only after the patient has recovered from the acute event. The diagnosis of microangiopathic hemolytic anemia (disseminated intravascular coagulation and thrombotic thrombocytopenic purpura) is discussed earlier in this chapter.

Treatment

Discontinue any medications that may be contributing to hemolysis. Initial therapy of acute hemolytic anemia is with glucocorticoids (eg, prednisone, 1 mg/kg/d orally). In acute hemolytic anemia due to cold agglutinins, corticosteroid therapy is seldom curative, and therapy with alkylating agents must often be used. In severe acute hemolytic anemia, red blood cell transfusion may be necessary, but cross-matching may be difficult. The self-limited hemolysis associated with glucose-6-phosphate dehydrogenase deficiency usually makes transfusion therapy unnecessary; the mainstay of treatment is discontinuation of any medication that may have precipitated the acute episode.

Disposition

Patients with mild to moderate acute hemolytic anemia need not be hospitalized but may be referred to a hematologist after offending medications have been discontinued and treatment has been started in the emergency department. Patients with severe anemia should be hospitalized for observation, continued therapy, and transfusion, if indicated. Obtain hematologic consultation.

SICKLE CELL ANEMIA

Sickle cell anemia is an inherited chronic hemolytic anemia caused by the substitution of valine for glutamic acid at the sixth amino acid position of the β subunit of the hemoglobin tetramer. This mutant β^s globin chain results in hemoglobin S, which is insoluble when deoxygenated. Intracellular gelation of deoxygenated hemoglobin occurs and results in morphologic sickling of red cells. This pathologic process explains the clinical manifestations of sickle cell disease, which include moderately severe chronic hemolytic anemia, recurrent acute painful episodes due to vascular occlusion, chronic and acute organ damage, intermittent episodes of more severe anemia, and shortened life expectancy. Emergency medical problems vary with the age of the patient. Acute painful episodes, aplastic or aregenerative episodes, and an acute chest syndrome occur in all age groups. Splenic sequestration and overwhelming infection occur more commonly in children.

Recurrent acute painful episodes are the most common reason for emergency department visits, but they are not life-threatening. Splenic sequestration, acute chest syndrome, overwhelming infection, and (less frequently) aregenerative episodes are potentially life-threatening. Such manifestations may occur in patients with any of the 3 major genotypic varieties of sickle cell disease: homozygous hemoglobin SS, sickle–β thalassemia, or hemoglobin SC disease.

Diagnosis

The definitive diagnosis of sickle cell disease is made by hemoglobin electrophoresis and hemoglobin solubility testing, which may not be available on an emergency basis, in which case the presence of sickled red cells on the peripheral blood smear establishes the diagnosis. Sickled red cells occur in all 3 major genotypes of sickle cell disease (above) but are not seen on the peripheral blood smear of patients with sickle cell trait (hemoglobin AS).

The diagnosis of **splenic sequestration** is made when a child presents with pain; a tender, enlarging spleen; and increased severity of anemia. Enough blood may be sequestered in the spleen to cause hypovolemic shock.

The **acute chest syndrome** often seen in patients with sickle cell anemia is characterized by chest pain, dyspnea, pulmonary infiltrates on chest x-ray, and, usually, fever and leukocytosis. In children, the upper lobes of the lungs are typically affected by infection, whereas in adults, the lower lobes are affected, usually by vaso-occlusion. In both children and adults, the major risks to life are the resulting hypoxemia and widespread sickling.

Aregenerative crises usually occur during a viral or bacterial infection, when cessation or erythropoiesis associated with extremely short lived red cells results in reticulocytopenia and rapidly falling hemoglobin levels.

Acute painful episodes are not associated with objective diagnostic signs or laboratory test abnormalities and are a diagnosis of exclusion when patients with sickle cell disease complain of severe pain with no other identifiable cause.

Overwhelming infection should be suspected in any child with sickle cell disease who is febrile and acutely ill. After appropriate diagnostic measures, including blood cultures and lumbar puncture, have been performed, start broad-spectrum antibiotics (Chapter 34).

Treatment

A. Administer oxygen, 5–10 L/min by mask or nasal prongs, to maintain oxygen saturation above 90%. Supraphysiologic levels of PO_2 should be avoided to obviate suppressed erythropoiesis and rebound vaso-occlusion.

B. Hydrate with normal saline or balanced salt solution intravenously if peripheral access can be obtained; oral hydration with water or juice can be attempted if venous access is difficult and the patient is not seriously ill.

C. Give analgesics (meperidine, hydromorphone, many others) intravenously or intramuscularly with promethazine or hydroxyzine every 45–60 minutes to relieve pain. Hydromorphone can also be given subcutaneously. Use caution when large doses of meperidine are needed, since accumulation of metabolites can cause seizures.

D. Obtain blood for CBC and, if needed, reticulocyte count. The white blood cell count is usually elevated in patients with sickle cell anemia; comparison with previous levels is often useful.

E. Search for evidence of infection. Most adults with homozygous hemoglobin S disease are functionally asplenic owing to chronic splenic infarcts and are especially susceptible to infections caused by encapsulated organisms, particularly *Salmonella*.

F. Patients with splenic sequestration or aregenerative (aplastic) crises require red blood cell transfusions to maintain their usual hemoglobin level.

G. Perform partial exchange transfusion to replace sickled red cells with normal red blood cells in patients with intractable pain or severe hypoxemia. In a 70-kg (154-lb) adult patient, remove 2 units (1000 mL) of whole blood while maintaining blood volume with normal (0.9%) saline, and then infuse 4–5 units of packed red blood cells (1000–1250 mL).

Disposition

Management of acute painful episodes can be attempted in the emergency department, but if pain does not diminish satisfactorily within 4–6 hours or with 3–4 doses of parenteral analgesic medication, the patient may require hospitalization for continued analgesia, intravenous hydration, oxygen inhalation therapy, and possibly partial exchange transfusion.

Splenic sequestration, acute chest syndrome, serious infection, and aregenerative crises are medical emergencies, and patients with these complications must be hospitalized.

Patients with sickle cell disease usually make frequent and recurrent visits to the emergency department. Drug addiction is common, and drug-seeking behavior can make management difficult. This problem can be mitigated if individual protocols setting guidelines and limits are established between the patient and the primary-care provider and approved by the emergency department. Prompt treatment should be instituted whenever patients with protocols arrive in the emergency department, but increased frequency of emergency visits and evidence of abuse necessitate review of overall patient management by the primary-care provider.

EMERGENCY MANAGEMENT OF THE PATIENT WITH POLYCYTHEMIA

In polycythemia, elevated hematocrit levels (> 55% for men and > 46% for women) are due to increased total red blood cell mass. Primary polycythemia (**polycythemia vera**) is a myeloproliferative disorder in which increased red blood cell mass is due to proliferation of an abnormal clone of hematopoietic progenitor cells; increased numbers of leukocytes and platelets may be noted as well. Most of the emergencies associated with polycythemia are related either to thrombotic events (eg, cerebral thrombosis, myocardial infarction, deep venous thrombosis, mesenteric vascular thrombosis) or to bleeding due to dysfunctional platelets (see Qualitative Platelet Disorders, above). **Secondary polycythemia** may result either from hypoxemia or from increased erythropoietin production (Table 33–11). Conditions causing secondary polycythemia produce isolated eleva-

Table 33–11. Common causes of secondary polycythemia.

Cyanotic congenital heart disease
Chronic pulmonary disease
Heavy cigarette smoking
Hypoventilation syndromes (eg, Pickwickian syndrome, Ondine's curse)
Abnormal hemoglobins with increased oxygen affinity
Cystic kidney disease, hydronephrosis, bilateral renal arterial stenosis
Tumors (especially of kidney, liver, uterus, or cerebellum)
Residence at high altitude
Adrenal abnormalities

tion of the red cell count, with normal leukocyte and platelet counts. Clinical consequences of secondary polycythemia are similar to those of polycythemia vera except that the disease does not progress to myelofibrosis or leukemia.

Another condition characterized by high hematocrit levels is **spurious polycythemia,** in which the hematocrit is elevated because of decreased plasma volume. Patients with spurious polycythemia are typically hypertensive, under stress, or obese, and they may be taking diuretics.

Diagnosis

The diagnosis of polycythemia vera is based on the finding of normal hemoglobin-oxygen saturation values (> 92%) in the presence of increased total red cell mass and normal plasma volume. Other useful diagnostic clues include splenomegaly, leukocytosis, thrombocytosis, increased leukocyte alkaline phosphatase values, and elevated serum levels of vitamin B_{12}. Symptoms include headache, dizziness, pruritus, and gastrointestinal disturbances related to peptic ulcer disease.

Diagnostic tests *must* include radioisotopic studies of red cell mass and plasma volume in order to differentiate patients with spurious polycythemia (decreased plasma volume) from those with polycythemia vera or secondary polycythemia (increased red cell mass). Erythropoietin assay is also useful (levels close to 0 are found in patients with polycythemia vera, whereas elevated levels are noted in patients with secondary polycythemia). Arterial blood gas and carboxyhemoglobin determinations, excretory urography, sonography, CT scan, serum electrolyte determinations, renal and hepatic function tests, and hemoglobin-oxygen affinity testing may be required to detect causes of secondary polycythemia.

Treatment

Patients who need treatment for polycythemia (reduction of hematocrit and blood viscosity) usually have polycythemia vera; occasional patients with secondary or spurious polycythemia also need treatment. Long-term management of polycythemia vera is directed toward reduction of total red cell mass by phlebotomy or chemotherapy. Systemic symptoms and complications due to abnormal platelet function require therapy with either radioactive phosphorus or chemotherapeutic agents.

Emergencies due to thrombosis are managed in the standard manner (Chapter 32) but may also require reduction of blood viscosity by phlebotomy.

Patients with polycythemia vera who require surgery (eg, for mesenteric vascular occlusion) must undergo vigorous preoperative phlebotomy in order to avoid postoperative thrombotic complications.

When hemorrhage due to the qualitative platelet defect associated with polycythemia vera occurs, hemostasis is restored by reducing the platelet count to normal with plateletpheresis or cytotoxic chemotherapy (hydroxyurea, 5 g orally). These procedures should not be started without hematologic consultation.

Disposition

Patients without symptoms should be referred to a hematologist. Those with thrombotic complications or significant bleeding should be hospitalized, and hematologic consultation obtained.

EMERGENCY EVALUATION OF THE PATIENT WITH WHITE BLOOD CELL DISORDERS

Emergencies that stem from abnormalities of the white blood cells typically result from too few leukocytes, too many leukocytes, or the metabolic or anatomic consequences of abnormal white blood cell production. Abnormalities in white blood cells may be a manifestation of a primary hematologic disorder (eg, leukemia) or the consequence of a nonhematologic condition (eg, myelotoxic drugs).

NEUTROPENIA

The neutrophil (granulocyte, PMN) is the main blood component protecting the body against bacterial or fungal infection. Neutropenia—a reduction in the absolute number of circulating neutrophils—therefore predisposes to bacterial and fungal infections and to breakdown in mucosal surfaces, with resulting stomatitis. Neutropenia is not associated with an increased incidence or severity of viral or protozoan infections.

The normal neutrophil count is between 1800 and $8000/\mu L$; however, the risk of infection does not rise appreciably until the count is under $1000/\mu L$, and the incidence of infection rises sharply when the count drops below 500/μL. Patients with severe neutropenia (< 100/μL) almost invariably develop infection within a matter of days.

Differential Diagnosis of Neutropenia

Neutropenia may result from decreased bone marrow production or increased peripheral destruction of neutrophils. Bone marrow disorders that commonly cause neutropenia include aplastic anemia, leukemia, myeloproliferative diseases, lymphomas, other infiltrating diseases of bone marrow, and megaloblastic anemia. Chemotherapeutic agents and therapeutic irradiation commonly cause neutropenia as a consequence of their injurious effects on bone marrow precursors. Medications known to cause decreased bone marrow production of neutrophils include chloramphenicol, phenylbutazone, procainamide, phenothiazines, sulfonamides, antithyroid medications, and chlorpropamide.

Patients with normal bone marrow may develop neutropenia because of increased *peripheral* consumption of neutrophils. Patients with septicemia or infection of any cause (bacterial, mycobacterial, fungal, viral) may develop neutropenia during the illness. Immune neutropenia analogous to immune thrombocytopenic purpura may arise as an isolated occurrence or as part of a generalized immunologic disorder such as systemic lupus erythematosus or rheumatoid arthritis. Medications (eg, penicillins, cephalosporins) may cause neutropenia by inducing autoantibody formation or, occasionally, by causing the abrupt complete disappearance of granulocytes from the circulation (agranulocytosis).

Obtain a meticulous medication history when evaluating the patient with neutropenia. Carefully examine the patient for stomatitis, organomegaly, lymphadenopathy, and bony tenderness. Obtain a platelet count and hematocrit determination, and examine the peripheral blood smear for leukemic cells. The white blood cell differential is useful in evaluating neutropenia, since patients in whom neutrophils constitute the majority of circulating white blood cells typically have less severe hematologic conditions than patients in whom neutrophils represent only a small portion of the total white blood cell count.

Treatment

Discontinue any medications that may be causing neutropenia. Febrile neutropenic patients or those with severe neutropenia (< 500/μL) should be hospitalized. In febrile neutropenic patients, obtain cultures (blood, sputum, urine, ascites fluid) as soon as possible, and follow with empiric broad-spectrum antibiotics (Chapter 34), since bacterial infection may be rapidly fatal in the face of inadequate host defenses. One appropriate regimen for adults is tobramycin, 1.7 mg/kg intravenously every 8 hours (adjusted to renal function); plus ticarcillin, 3 g intravenously every 4 hours. *Note: The usual symptoms and signs of infection may be absent owing to a deficient host inflammatory response.*

Definitive treatment of neutropenia apart from the complicating infection depends on the precise diagnosis.

Disposition

Patients who are afebrile, with mild neutropenia (> 1000/μL), should be evaluated by a hematologist as soon as possible. Hospitalize patients with significant infections and those with severe neutropenia (< 500/μL), and obtain immediate hematologic consultation.

LEUKOCYTOSIS

Elevated white blood cell counts may represent an appropriate response to infection or may constitute an autonomous proliferation of cells due to a primary hematologic disorder. Elevation of the white blood cell count is not in itself a problem except in the unusual case of acute leukemia complicated by hyperleukocytosis (circulating blast cell counts > 100,000/μL), when the increased whole blood viscosity due to increased numbers of white blood cells having reduced deformability results in leukostasis and circulatory compromise.

Leukocytosis may be defined as a total white blood cell count in excess of 12,000/μL. Lymphocytosis is a lymphocyte count above 4000/μL, and granulocytosis is a granulocyte count above 8000/μL.

1. CHRONIC LEUKEMIAS

Chronic myelogenous leukemia is a clonal disorder of the hematopoietic stem cell that results in increased production of all blood cell lines, especially granulocytes. In chronic leukemias (unlike in acute forms), production of red cells and platelets is not diminished and may even be increased. Patients most commonly present with systemic symptoms, eg, fatigue, malaise, low-grade fever. Less common manifestations include bony tenderness, acute gout, and discomfort in the region of the spleen. Occasionally, patients are asymptomatic, and an elevated white blood cell count or splenic enlargement is noted only by chance. The white blood cell count is usually between 50,000 and 200,000/μL. Moderate anemia occurs occasionally. The platelet count is usually elevated, though it may be normal or even modestly reduced. The peripheral blood smear characteristically shows neutrophils as the dominant cells with lesser numbers of band cells, metamyelocytes, and myelocytes. Blast cells and promyelocytes usually constitute less than 5% of the total white count.

Chronic lymphocytic leukemia is an indolent disease characterized by gradual accumulation of immunoincompetent B lymphocytes. In the early stages, these cells accumulate in the bone marrow and the peripheral blood; later they cause lymphadenopathy and organomegaly, and bone marrow failure and tissue infiltration occur. Many patients are asymptomatic, and the disease is discovered accidentally on routine blood counts. Other patients present with fatigue or lymphadenopathy.

Differential Diagnosis of Chronic Leukemia

Chronic myelogenous leukemia must be distinguished from the reactive leukocytosis that characterizes the response to infection. Reactive leukocytosis rarely produces white blood cell counts above 50,000/μL and does not usually cause thrombocytosis or splenomegaly. Chronic myelogenous leukemia can be diagnosed on the basis of a lack of underlying infection, extremely high white blood cell count, characteristic findings on the differential (see above), and the presence of splenomegaly. A low or absent leukocyte alkaline phosphatase level confirms the diagnosis, as does the presence of the Philadelphia chromosome. Differentiating chronic myelogenous leukemia from acute leukemia occasionally may require bone marrow examination.

Chronic lymphocytic leukemia must also be distinguished from the reactive lymphocytosis signifying response to a viral infection. Lack of evidence of underlying infection and lymphocytosis persisting for more than 1 month in the absence of signs of infection virtually confirm the diagnosis of chronic lymphocytic leukemia. The peripheral blood smear shows more than 15,000 lymphocytes per microliter; their morphology is indistinguishable from that of the small lymphocytes usually seen in peripheral blood. Morphology of cells on the peripheral blood smear distinguishes chronic lymphocytic leukemia from reactive lymphocytosis, in which lymphocytes are usually larger and more varied, with more abundant cytoplasm. Morphologic differences also distinguish chronic lymphocytic leukemia from acute lymphoblastic leukemia, in which cells are larger and less mature.

Treatment & Disposition

Treatment of chronic myelogenous leukemia is usually not urgently required. However, patients with white blood cell counts higher than 300,000/μL should receive urgent hematologic consultation, and patients with symptoms of leukostasis, eg, respiratory insufficiency, abnormal mental status, or priapism, should be hospitalized for hematologic consultation and emergency treatment. Initial treatment measures include hydration, alkalization of the urine, and allopurinol, 300 mg orally. When hematologic consultation is not immediately available, give hydroxyurea, 5 g orally once.

Treatment of chronic lymphocytic leukemia is rarely required on an emergency basis; even very high white blood cell counts (> 500,000/μL) are usually well tolerated.

2. ACUTE LEUKEMIA

Acute leukemia is malignancy of hematopoietic progenitor cells in which a leukemic cell population replaces and suppresses normal bone marrow cells, resulting in bone marrow failure with anemia, neutropenia, and thrombocytopenia. The usual causes of illness and death are infection and bleeding related to neutropenia and thrombocytopenia, respectively. Less commonly, complications and death result from direct organ infiltration.

These rapidly progressive malignant disorders are uniformly fatal without treatment.

Effective treatment is now available for most patients with acute leukemia, and young patients are treated with intent to cure and not simply to palliate symptoms.

Diagnosis

Suspect acute leukemia in any patient with leukocytosis or lymphocytosis who also has abnormal white blood cells on the peripheral blood smear (eg, blast cells). Such patients characteristically have moderate or severe anemia and thrombocytopenia, although the hematocrit and platelet count may be normal. Some patients with acute leukemia may present with neutropenia; blast cells may be absent in about 10% of cases (aleukemic leukemia).

Definitive diagnosis of acute leukemia is based on bone marrow examination showing more than 30% blast cells in bone marrow. Differentiation between acute myelogenous leukemia and acute lymphoblastic leukemia is made on the basis of morphologic, histochemical, and immunologic examination of cells.

Differential Diagnosis of Acute Leukemia

Acute myelogenous leukemia is distinguished from chronic myelogenous leukemia by the increased proportion of blast cells on the peripheral blood smear. When the white blood cell count is low, acute leukemia can be distinguished from other causes of pancytopenia (eg, aplastic anemia) only by bone marrow examination. Acute lymphoblastic leukemia is distinguished from virus-induced lymphocytosis and from chronic lymphocytic leukemia by the presence of more immature lymphoblastic cells.

Treatment

Patients with documented or suspected acute leukemia should be hospitalized. Fever should be presumed to be due to infection. Obtain appropriate material for culture, and begin emergency treatment with empiric broad-spectrum antibiotics such as an aminoglycoside plus a semisynthetic penicillin (Chapter 34). Bleeding may be due to isolated thrombocytopenia or to disseminated intravascular coagulation, which may be caused by sepsis or the leukemia itself.

Patients with hyperleukocytosis (blast cell counts > 100,000/μL) should be treated on an emergency basis, with immediate hematologic consultation. Initial treatment measures include hydration, alkalization of urine, and allopurinol, 300 mg orally. Red blood cell transfusion should be avoided, if possible, since it may increase the viscosity of whole blood to the point that circulatory compromise occurs. When hematologic consultation is not immediately available, give hydroxyurea, 5 g orally, to reduce the white blood cell count. Allopurinol should be given simultaneously.

Disposition

Patients with acute leukemia should be hospitalized immediately for urgent hematologic consultation.

INFECTIOUS MONONUCLEOSIS

Infectious mononucleosis is caused by systemic infection with Epstein-Barr virus, a DNA virus that preferentially infects epithelial cells and B lymphocytes.

Diagnosis

The diagnosis of infectious mononucleosis is suggested by the combination of fever, pharyngitis (which may be exudative), and cervical lymphadenopathy, especially of the posterior cervical chain. Splenomegaly, palatal petechiae, periorbital edema, and maculopapular skin rashes are also common. Life-threatening complications include encephalitis and upper airway obstruction from lymphoid hypertrophy. Clinical hepatitis occurs frequently. The white blood cell count is elevated, and the peripheral blood smear shows lymphocytosis in which at least 10% of lymphocytes are "atypical"—large, varied, and with abundant basophilic cytoplasm. The diagnosis is confirmed by demonstration of heterophil antibody, which is present within the first 2 weeks of illness. Patients with initially negative results on a heterophil agglutination test (eg, Monospot) should be retested in 1–4 weeks. Specific tests for Epstein-Barr virus antibody are also available; these are especially useful in children, in whom false-negative results on heterophil antibody tests occur frequently. Patients with a clinical syndrome suggestive of infectious mononucleosis but with negative results on heterophil testing may have cytomegalovirus infection or other viral infections.

Differential Diagnosis

Infectious mononucleosis can be distinguished from acute lymphoblastic leukemia by the morphology of individual lymphocytes. The atypical lymphocytes of infectious mononucleosis have a more mature nuclear chromatin pattern and more abundant cytoplasm. Patients with infectious mononucleosis characteristically do not have other cytopenias, though hemolytic anemia and immune thrombocytopenia are occasional complications. Patients with mononucleosis due to cytomegalovirus usually do not have pharyngitis; culture and serologic tests for cytomegalovirus are positive.

Treatment & Disposition

Patients with infectious mononucleosis usually do not have to be hospitalized unless they have debilitating systemic symptoms, hepatitis, or life-threatening complications, such as idiopathic thrombocytopenic purpura, airway obstruction, or cerebritis, which require corticosteroid therapy and hospitalization. Patients with severe pharyngitis or periorbital edema may benefit from a short course of high-dose corticosteroids, eg, prednisone, 40–60 mg orally daily tapering over 10–14 days. Activity should be restricted to minimize risk of splenic injury, since associated splenic hypertrophy is common. Patients should receive follow-up care from their primary-care physician.

MULTIPLE MYELOMA

Multiple myeloma, a neoplasm of a single clone of plasma cells, affects middle-aged to elderly patients. Infiltration of bone marrow by malignant plasma cells may result in diffuse osteoporosis or lytic bone disease with impending or actual fracture. Bone marrow failure with anemia, thrombocytopenia, or neutropenia may occur. The malignant plasma cells may form extramedullary tumors, most commonly in the skin, paranasal sinuses, or lymph nodes. On occasion, the cells may infiltrate other organs and cause meningitis or plasma cell leukemia.

Almost all malignant plasma cells secrete either a complete immunoglobulin or an immunoglobulin light chain. Levels of the secreted paraprotein occasionally become so high that blood viscosity rises, resulting in sludging in the microcirculation (hyperviscosity syndrome). Such patients often present with headache, nausea and vomiting, vertigo, mucosal bleeding, or congestive heart failure. Heart failure is due to the expanded plasma volume associated with the high intravascular concentration of paraprotein. If untreated, hyperviscosity syndrome progresses to mental status abnormalities, coma, and death.

Hypercalcemia is a frequent complication resulting either from direct bone lysis or from the indirect effect of a humoral factor secreted by plasma cells (osteoclast-activating factor). Hypercalcemia predisposes to renal failure, especially if patients have light-chain disease. Most patients with multiple myeloma demonstrate markedly diminished levels of normal immunoglobulin and severely impaired ability to generate specific antibodies, with resulting increased incidence of infection, especially that caused by *Streptococcus pneumoniae* and *Haemophilus influenzae*.

Diagnosis

Multiple myeloma should be suspected in an older patient presenting with anemia, proteinuria, hypercalcemia, acute renal failure, elevated sedimentation rate, diffuse osteoporosis, or lytic bone disease. Patients with multiple myeloma commonly present because of fatigue, bone pain, hypercalcemia, or infection.

Physical examination often fails to reveal any significant findings. Patients with hyperviscosity syndrome may have engorged retinal veins, congestive heart failure, and mucosal bleeding. The peripheral blood smear may show marked erythrocyte rouleau formation, an early clue to the diagnosis. Circulating plasma cells are rare.

Definitive diagnosis is based on the finding of a monoclonal paraprotein on serum or urine protein electrophoresis, the presence of lytic bone disease, plasma cell infiltration of bone marrow, or plasmacytoma.

Treatment

Chemotherapy—usually a combination of melphalan and prednisone—is the mainstay of treatment; occasionally, more aggressive chemotherapeutic regimens are required.

Treat hyperviscosity syndrome with plasmapheresis, which is most conveniently performed with a cell separator machine. Patients may benefit significantly from manually performed low-volume plasmapheresis, however. Removal of as little as 2 units (500 mL each) of blood from the patient by phlebotomy may reduce serum viscosity enough to avoid severe symptoms. Depending on the severity of anemia and the facilities available, the volume removed should be replaced either with saline or with a combination of saline and red blood cells.

Treat hypercalcemia as outlined in Chapter 36; prednisone is especially helpful in hypercalcemia due to multiple myeloma.

Treat pathologic fractures in consultation with an orthopedist and a hematologist. Impending fractures in critical areas such as vertebrae or weight-bearing bones should be identified so that prophylactic therapy can be started.

Treat pneumonia with a regimen appropriate for pneumococcal disease. Recurrent infections may be prevented by prophylactic infusion of intravenous immunoglobulin (0.7 g/kg) every 3–4 weeks.

Disposition

Patients with multiple myeloma should be referred to a hematologist within several days for definitive therapy. Patients may require hospitalization with hematologic consultation for treatment of hypercalcemia, fractures or impending fractures, hyperviscosity syndrome, or other severe complications.

WALDENSTRÖM'S MACROGLOBULINEMIA

Waldenström's macroglobulinemia is a neoplastic disease of plasma cells which differs from multiple myeloma in that the malignant cells are more lymphocytic in morphology and secrete an IgM paraprotein (rather than other immunoglobulins). Organomegaly and lymphadenopathy are more common in patients with macroglobulinemia than in those with multiple myeloma. Destructive bony disease is rare. Because IgM is distributed mainly in the intravascular compartment of blood (75% of total body IgM is found in the intravascular circulation as opposed to 50% of total body IgG) and because IgM increases blood viscosity to a higher level than does IgG, patients with macroglobulinemia experience more severe symptoms of hyperviscosity syndrome than do patients with multiple myeloma.

Diagnosis

The diagnosis is confirmed by demonstration of malignant plasma cells in bone marrow and a monoclonal IgM paraprotein spike on serum electrophoresis. Clinical features suggestive of the diagnosis are organomegaly, lymphadenopathy, and hyperviscosity syndrome (mental status abnormalities, nausea and vomiting, vertigo, mucosal bleeding, and congestive heart failure).

Treatment

Treat hyperviscosity syndrome with emergency plasmapheresis as described above. When cell separator facilities are unavailable, perform phlebotomy, and replace fluids with intravenous crystalloid solutions to achieve the same results. Definitive treatment of macroglobulinemia includes chemotherapy and is usually not required on an emergency basis.

Disposition

Patients with macroglobulinemia should be referred to a hematologist within 1 week unless there are complications such as hyperviscosity syndrome that require emergency hospitalization.

PRINCIPLES OF TRANSFUSION THERAPY

Many patients presenting to the emergency department require urgent replacement of one or more components of blood or blood products. Safe and effective use of blood products requires an understanding of typing, screening, and cross-matching procedures as well as knowledge of available products.

Blood Typing & Screening

The 2 red cell antigen groups that are of primary clinical importance are the ABO and the Rh antigen systems. There are 2 antigens, A and B, in the ABO system. An individual may have only A antigens (type A blood), only B antigens (type B blood), a mixture of A and B antigens (type AB blood), or neither antigen (type O blood). The serum of a given individual contains antibodies to whichever of the AB antigens is not present on that person's own red blood cells. Thus, a person with type A blood has circulating antibodies to B antigen, and a person with type B blood has antibodies to A antigen. Individuals with type O blood have both anti-A and anti-B antibodies, and patients with type AB blood have neither anti-A nor anti-B antibodies. The titer of these naturally occurring antibodies varies greatly among individuals. The Rh system is based on the presence or absence of C, D, or E antigens on red blood cells. Rh-positive individuals have one of these antigens on their cells, whereas Rh-negative patients do not. In contrast to the ABO blood group antigens, circulating antibodies to C, D, or E antigens are not found in Rh-negative patients unless they have been exposed to Rh-positive blood (eg, through transfusion or transplacental passage of Rh-positive red blood cells from fetus to mother during delivery). There are many other erythrocyte antigens (Lewis, Kell, I, etc) that are less commonly of clinical significance.

Blood typing is performed by suspending red blood cells obtained from a tube of clotted blood in saline and then adding commercially available specific antisera to the suspension and watching for agglutination. For example, the addition of anti-A antiserum to a suspension of red blood cells carrying A antigen causes an easily detectable agglutination reaction. Red blood cells are tested against anti-A, anti-B, and anti-D serum, so that the patient's blood may be classified as one of the 4 ABO types and as either Rh-positive or Rh-negative.

The patient's **serum** is also tested against a panel of commercially available red blood cells (which includes all of the common, clinically important red blood cell antigens) in order to determine which circulating antibodies are present. This procedure serves as a confirmation of red blood cell typing (ie, an individual with type A blood should have anti-B but not anti-A antibody in the serum). Serum testing detects clinically significant titers of antibodies to antigens other than those of the ABO and Rh systems. Once a patient's blood is typed and screened, compatible donor units can usually be cross-matched within 30 minutes.

Cross-Matching

The **major cross-match** is performed by incubating donor cells of the appropriate ABO and Rh group with the recipient's serum. The cells are then washed and antiglobulin serum added (indirect Coombs test); if antibodies from the recipient's serum have become bound to donor red blood cell antigens, then addition of antiglobulin causes an easily detectable agglutination reaction which indicates that the donor cells are incompatible with the recipient's serum. If there is no agglutination, the donor cells are acceptable for transfusion. It is unusual to detect clinically significant antibodies during cross-matching that have not already been detected by the serum screening procedure described above. All donor serum is prescreened for antibodies to common and clinically significant red blood cell antigens, and donor serum with common antibodies is not used for transfusions. Because of this prescreening, the **minor cross-match** (incubation of donor serum with the recipient's red blood cells) is no longer necessary.

Once compatible donor cells have been identified, they are set aside for the individual for whom they were cross-matched and are therefore not available for use by other patients. Because of this and because cross-matching is more time-consuming and expensive than typing and screening alone, *only* typing and screening should be performed when the need for blood is not definitely established (eg, for surgical procedures in which blood loss is usually minimal or for stable patients with blood in the stool but whose hematocrit is not yet known). Once the need for transfusion has been established, cross-matching can be performed, and blood is then usually ready for transfusion within 30–60 minutes.

Blood & Blood Products

Table 33–12 lists the commonly available blood products as well as the approximate volumes in each unit. A clotted specimen of the patient's blood should be sent for typing and screening whenever blood components containing red blood cells are to be transfused.

Indications for Specific Types of Red Blood Cell Transfusions

A. Universal Donor Blood: Universal donor blood is O-negative whole blood known to have low titers of anti-A and anti-B antibodies. It is given only in dire emergencies, when blood must be adminis-

Table 33–12. Blood products commonly used in emergencies.

Product	Volume	Indications	Contraindications	Comments
Whole blood	1 unit = 500 mL (hematocrit 35–40%).	Hypovolemic shock due to blood loss.	None.	Not a source of viable platelets or labile procoagulants.
Packed red blood cells	1 unit = 300 mL (hematocrit 65–80%).	Symptomatic anemia without shock.	Do not use if anemia can be corrected by medication (eg, iron).	Platelets or white blood cells may be removed during processing.
Leukocyte-poor red blood cells	1 unit = 300 mL (hematocrit 65–80%).	Patients with frequent febrile transfusion reactions.	Same as for packed red blood cells.	At least 70% of leukocytes have been removed by centrifugation, filtration, or sedimentation.
Washed red blood cells	1 unit = 300 mL (hematocrit 65–80%).	Patients with prior allergic reactions to plasma proteins in donor blood.	Do not use if anemia can be corrected by medication.	85% of leukocytes and about 99% of original plasma have been removed. More expensive than leukocyte-poor red blood cells.
Frozen red blood cells	1 unit = 250 mL (hematocrit 65–80%).	Storage form for rare blood types or for autologous transfusion of patients whose blood is difficult to cross-match.	Same as for packed red blood cells.	Can be stored for up to 3 years. Must be thawed and washed before administration. More expensive.
Platelets	1 unit (platelet pack) = 40–70 mL; each unit has at least 5.5×10^{10} platelets.	Patients with thrombocytopenic bleeding due to decreased platelet production; patients with bleeding due to abnormal platelet function.	Generally not useful in patients with rapid platelet destruction (eg, immune thrombocytopenic purpura).	Trace amounts of red blood cells account for pink color in some units.
Fresh-frozen plasma or plasma frozen within 24 hours after donation	1 unit = 180–300 mL; each unit contains about 200 units of factor VIII and 200–400 mg of fibrinogen.	Patients with multiple clotting factor deficiencies or deficiencies for which more specific therapy is not available.	Do not use when coagulopathy can be corrected with more specific therapy (eg, vitamin K, factor VIII concentrates).	Use fresh-frozen plasma no later than 6 hours after thawing. Associated with high risk of infectious complications.
Cryoprecipitate (antihemophilic factor; AHF)	1 unit (bag) contains ≥80 units of factor VIII:C and at least 150 mg of fibrinogen in <15 mL of plasma.	Hemophilia A, von Willebrand's disease; replacement of fibrinogen or factor XIII.	Use only for specified indications.	Associated with increased risk of infectious complications, since this is pooled multiple-donor product.

tered without the benefit of typing, eg, a trauma victim with active bleeding refractory to treatment and persistent shock despite the infusion of 3 L or more of crystalloid solutions. Significant transfusion reactions, including hemolytic reactions, may occur as a result of the interaction of the recipient's red blood cells with anti-A and anti-B antibodies present in donor serum.

B. Type-Specific Whole Blood: Type-specific whole blood can be administered in critical situations when there is need for rapid administration of blood but still enough time for typing of the recipient's blood. Transfusions of this sort may cause significant transfusion reactions (including hemolytic reactions) owing to the presence of antibodies to red blood cell antigens other than those of the ABO system.

C. Cross-Matched Whole Blood: Cross-matched whole blood should be reserved for patients who have *significant* hypovolemia with *acute* blood loss. There

are a number of reasons for this precaution: Transfusion of unnecessary antigens and antibodies is avoided, equal oxygen-carrying capacity can be delivered in a smaller volume with packed red blood cells, and more efficient use of donated blood is achieved when it is separated into specific components for specific indications.

D. Packed Red Blood Cells: Transfusion of packed red blood cells is indicated whenever a patient has severely symptomatic anemia. Transfusion should not be used for mild or moderate anemia in asymptomatic younger patients. Packed red blood cells are also the treatment of choice for patients with active blood loss due to trauma or for patients with bleeding from gastrointestinal tract, vaginal, or other sources whose condition can be stabilized with administration of crystalloid solutions.

E. Leukocyte-Poor Red Blood Cells: Patients with a history of frequent febrile transfusion reactions attributed to the presence in their serum of antibodies to white blood cells or platelets (see below) may require leukocyte-poor units.

F. Washed Red Blood Cells: Patients who have had allergic reactions attributed to the presence of antibodies to plasma proteins in donor units (see below) may require the transfusion of red cells that have been washed to remove most of the plasma proteins.

G. Frozen Red Blood Cells: Frozen red blood cells have a shelf life which is considerably longer than that of red blood cells stored by conventional means. However, the costs of maintaining frozen red blood cells currently limit their use to maintenance stores of rare donor blood types or storage of blood for autotransfusion for patients with rare blood types or with blood that is difficult to cross-match.

Preparation for Red Blood Cell Transfusion

Insert an intravenous catheter ($\geq$ 18-gauge) securely in a peripheral vein. Keep the line open with infusion of normal saline, since glucose-containing solutions and hypo-osmolar solutions may damage transfused red blood cells.

EMERGENCY DIAGNOSIS & TREATMENT OF TRANSFUSION REACTIONS

Several types of transfusion reactions may occur in the emergency department. Signs and symptoms may develop within minutes to hours of the onset of the transfusion. *Note:* Because the signs and symptoms of minor allergic reactions may mimic those of major life-threatening reactions, *transfusion must be stopped immediately in a patient who manifests any untoward sign or symptom.*

Hemolytic Reaction

The most important transfusion reaction is the **hemolytic reaction,** in which a major incompatibility results in intravascular hemolysis (usually because transfused blood has been mislabeled or blood has been given to the wrong patient). The patient may complain of chills, dyspnea, back or chest pain, nausea and vomiting, and pruritus. Fever, tachycardia, tachypnea, wheezing, urticaria, red urine (from free hemoglobin), hypotension, or frank anaphylactic shock may develop rapidly. Renal failure may follow hemolytic transfusion reactions either as a result of the toxic effects of lysed red cells or because of acute tubular necrosis due to hypotension. Disseminated intravascular coagulation develops in about half of patients with major hemolytic reactions. *A hemolytic transfusion reaction is life-threatening; transfusion must be stopped immediately.* Patients in shock should be treated as described in Chapter 3 with intra-venous infusion of normal saline or a balanced salt solution (eg, lactated Ringer's injection) to maintain adequate tissue perfusion. If intravenous fluid replacement alone fails to maintain adequate urine output (0.5–0.7 mL/kg/h) or if the patient shows signs of volume overload (eg, congestive heart failure), give furosemide, 20 mg intravenously. If the patient's volume status permits, osmotic diuresis with mannitol, 12.5 g intravenously over 3–5 minutes, may prevent development of renal failure following a hemolytic transfusion reaction.

Once urgent treatment has been started, the diagnosis of a hemolytic reaction should be confirmed by checking the identification of the transfused blood and the patient's identification tag. A clotted sample of the patient's blood and the donor bag with any remaining blood should be sent to the blood bank for retyping and cross-matching. Gross hemolysis can be detected by obtaining an anticoagulated sample of the patient's blood and spinning it in a hematocrit tube; a red supernatant denotes more than 20–25 mg/dL of free hemoglobin in the plasma. Specimens should also be sent for plasma hemoglobin and haptoglobin and urine hemoglobin measurements. In addition, coagulation studies (platelet count, prothrombin and partial thromboplastin times, and fibrinogen level) should be obtained for detection of disseminated intravascular coagulation, a possible complication of hemolytic transfusion reaction.

All patients with suspected hemolytic transfusion reactions should be hospitalized.

Allergic Reactions

Allergic reactions are usually minor and complicate about 1% of transfusions. They typically represent a reaction to transfused plasma proteins. Patients complain of pruritus and may develop urticaria and fever; occasionally, a more severe anaphylactic reaction occurs, with bronchospasm, airway edema, or shock. *The transfusion must be stopped.* Minor reactions may be treated with an antihistamine (eg, diphenhydramine, 50 mg intravenously). More severe reactions should be treated as described in Chapter 3 with epinephrine, 0.3–0.5 mL of 1:1000 solution subcutaneously or intramuscularly. For severe anaphylactic reactions, give epinephrine, 1–5 mL of 1:10,000 solution intravenously or via an endotracheal tube, repeating every 10 minutes as needed. (For children, give 0.01 mg/kg of 1:1000 solution subcutaneously or intramuscularly [maximum 0.3 mL], or 0.1 mL/kg of 1:10,000 solution intravenously or via an endotracheal tube.) Patients with a history of minor transfusion reactions may be pretreated with diphenhydramine, 50 mg orally, and acetaminophen, 650 mg orally.

Allergic reactions can be avoided by using washed red blood cells, in which the washing removes most of the donor's plasma proteins. In patients with major allergic reactions, samples of the patient's and the donor's blood should be sent to the blood bank to rule out the possibility of a hemolytic reaction.

Patients with minor allergic transfusion reactions may be discharged from the emergency department; patients with more significant transfusion reactions (eg, anaphylactic reaction) should be hospitalized after they are stabilized.

Febrile Reactions

Fever may occur in many types of transfusion reactions, including hemolytic reactions, in response to transfusion of bacterial pyrogens in contaminated units (rare) or as a result of the reaction of recipient antibodies to antigens on transfused white blood cells or platelets. If fever is the only sign or symptom, antipyretics should be given and the transfusion continued. However, differentiation of a minor febrile reaction from the early manifestations of a more serious reaction may be difficult, and the transfusion should be discontinued if there is any doubt at all about the type of reaction involved. Leukocyte-poor red blood cells may be useful in patients with a history of febrile transfusion reactions.

Complications of Massive Transfusions

The transfusion of large amounts of stored blood (> 10 units) in a short period of time (hours) may lead to several complications. **Hypothermia** from the transfusion of large amounts of refrigerated blood can be avoided by the use of a blood warmer (if this is not available, running the infusion tubing through a pan of warm water can serve the same purpose).

Platelet depletion may occur because of poor platelet survival in stored blood. In addition, **dilution of coagulation factors** may occur because of low levels of certain factors (V and VIII) in stored blood. Both complications can be avoided by transfusing 1 unit of *fresh* blood for every 4 or 5 units of stored blood transfused in a 10- to 12-hour period. An alternative method is to transfuse 4 units of platelets and 1 unit of fresh-frozen plasma with every 5 units of stored blood transfused. **Hypocalcemia** from citrate-mediated chelation of calcium is rare, especially if packed red blood cells have been transfused. If large amounts of stored whole blood are given over a short period of time (> 2000 mL of citrated whole blood or plasma over 15–20 minutes), give calcium gluconate, 10 mL of a 10% solution intravenously over 5 minutes. Hypocalcemia is discussed in Chapter 36.

Other Complications of Transfusion

Transfusion of blood and blood products is associated with the transmission of infectious agents. Although screening of donors for evidence of hepatitis B has markedly decreased the incidence of transfusion-associated hepatitis B, the transmission of non-A, non-B hepatitis, cytomegalovirus, and AIDS virus is an important complication of transfusion. Currently, the only ways of decreasing the chance of transmitting these agents are to avoid unnecessary transfusions and to use blood from volunteer donors. A serologic test to screen donors for evidence of exposure to the human immunodeficiency virus (HIV) is currently employed in the USA.

REFERENCES

Ballas SK: Treatment of pain in adults with sickle cell disease. Am J Hematol 1990;34:49.

Barlogie B et al: Plasma cell myeloma: New biological insights and advances in therapy. Blood 1989;73:865.

Berchtold P, McMillan R: Therapy of chronic idiopathic thrombocytopenic purpura in adults. Blood 1989;74:2309.

Berlin NI (editor): Polycythemia vera: An update. (2 parts.) Semin Hematol 1986;23:131,167. [Entire issue.]

Champlin R et al: Postremission chemotherapy for adults with acute myelogenous leukemia: Improved survival with high-dose cytarabine and daunorubicin consolidation treatment. J Clin Oncol 1990;8:1199.

Cook JD: Clinical evaluation of iron deficiency. Semin Hematol 1982;19:6.

Embury SH, Mentzer WC: Sickle cell anemia. Pages 690–695 in: *Current Therapy in Emergency Medicine.* Callaham ML (editor). Decker, 1987.

Feinstein DI: Treatment of intravascular coagulation. Semin Thromb Hemost 1988;14:351.

Foon KA, Rai KR, Gale RP: Chronic lymphocytic leukemia: New insights into biology and therapy. Ann Intern Med 1990;113:525.

Frank MM et al: Pathophysiology of immune hemolytic anemia. Ann Intern Med 1977;87:210.

de la Fuente B et al: Response of patients with mild and moderate hemophilia A and von Willebrand disease to treatment with desmopressin. Ann Intern Med 1985;103:6.

Kasper CK (editor): *Recent Advances in Hemophilia Care.* Liss, 1990.

Loughran TP Jr, Storb R: Treatment of aplastic anemia. Hematol Oncol Clin North Am 1990;4:559.

Mollison PL, Engelfriet CP, Contreras M: *Blood Transfusion in Clinical Medicine,* 8th ed. Blackwell, 1987.

Moroose R, Hoyer LW: von Willebrand factor and platelet function. Annu Rev Med 1986;37:157.

Petz LD: Red cell transfusion problems in immunohematologic disease. Annu Rev Med 1982;33:355.

Rose EH, Aledort LM: Nasal spray desmopressin (DDAVP) for mild hemophilia A and von Willebrand disease. Ann Intern Med 1991;114:563.

Silver RT: Chronic myeloid leukemia. Hematol Oncol Clin North Am 1990;4:319.

Infectious Disease Emergencies

34

Pamela H. Nagami, MD, & Phyllis A. Guze, MD

IMMEDIATE MANAGEMENT OF LIFE-THREATENING PROBLEMS

SEPTIC SHOCK

Infection must be suspected and actively sought in any acutely ill patient who presents with no other obvious cause of illness. Patients who are especially susceptible to infections include immunocompromised individuals and those whose natural mechanical barriers of defense have been breached or manipulated through injury or surgery. Examples of the latter group include patients who have undergone surgical or other manipulation of the urinary, biliary, or gynecologic tracts; those who have temporary or indwelling intravenous catheters (eg, Hickman); those who have experienced trauma, tracheostomy, or other operation (especially abdominal procedures); and those with burns or respiratory infections. The incidence of bacteremia and sepsis is increased in elderly patients; those with diabetes mellitus, leukemia, severe granulocytopenia, genitourinary tract diseases, or cirrhosis; and those receiving corticosteroids, immunosuppressive agents, cancer chemotherapy, or radiation treatment.

The classic clinical pattern of abrupt onset of chills followed by fever and hypotension is present in only 30–40% of patients in septic shock. Other presenting symptoms include hypothermia, oliguria, aberration of mental function, unexplained hypotension, or metabolic acidosis.

Immediate Measures

A. Maintain Airway and Ventilation: Give oxygen, 4 L/min, by nasal prongs or mask. Listen for stridor and other evidence of upper airway obstruction, especially in children, and make sure that intubation or cricothyrotomy equipment is readily at hand.

B. Obtain Complete Vital Signs:

1. Signs of septic shock–Hypotension in septic shock results from (1) hypovolemia caused by pooling of blood in the microcirculation and (2) loss of fluid from the vascular space due to a generalized increase in capillary permeability. Opening of arteriovenous shunts decreases peripheral resistance, which further decreases arterial blood pressure. Early in septic shock, therefore, the extremities may be warm and dry, but as shock progresses, they become cold and clammy. Hypotension, tachycardia, hyperventilation, altered sensorium, and oliguria may be present as well.

2. Fever or hypothermia–Rectal or tympanic membrane temperature measurements are preferred to oral or axillary readings in seriously ill patients. If a clinical thermometer fails to provide a temperature reading, use a laboratory thermometer capable of recording temperatures as low as 20 °C (68 °F) (room temperature).

C. Treat Shock:

1. Insert a large-bore (≥ 18-gauge in adults) intravenous catheter, and obtain a venous blood sample for CBC with differential, platelet count, prothrombin time, partial thromboplastin time, electrolyte studies, and renal and liver function tests. A Swan-Ganz catheter may be necessary for hemodynamic monitoring.

2. Obtain arterial blood gas and pH measurements. Respiratory alkalosis may be present early in septic shock but usually progresses to metabolic acidosis.

3. Monitor cardiac rhythm. Obtain a 12-lead ECG, and begin continuous cardiac monitoring. The stress of sepsis or shock can precipitate or worsen myocardial ischemia in patients with coronary artery disease. Also, shock of any cause may predispose to cardiac arrhythmias due to electrolyte and acid-base abnormalities.

4. Begin volume replacement. Initial fluid replacement should be with crystalloid solutions such as balanced salt solutions, since capillary endothelial integrity is damaged and administration of colloid solutions may result in extravasation of protein into the interstitium, thus aggravating interstitial edema (Chapter 3). In general, 1–2 L of crystalloid solution given over 30–60 minutes (adult dose) will improve blood pressure and urine output. Administer additional amounts based on the results of central venous or pulmonary arterial wedge pressure measurements.

5. Correct acidosis. Use of a sodium bicarbonate infusion, 0.5–1 meq/kg, to maintain arterial blood pH above 7.1 may be considered.

6. Give inotropic agents. Dopamine should be used if shock cannot be relieved by fluid replacement therapy alone. Follow the dosage guidelines given in the table on the inside front cover.

7. Give other special drugs as necessary.

a. Corticosteroids–Two large clinical trials have shown that glucocorticoid therapy provides no benefit for patients with septic shock and may even be harmful. Therefore, glucocorticoids should not be administered to patients with sepsis or septic shock, unless adrenal insufficiency is suspected (eg, meningococcemia with adrenal hemorrhage). If adrenal insufficiency is suspected, replacement doses of hydrocortisone, 100-mg bolus intravenously, then 50–100 mg intravenously every 6 hours, should be administered.

b. Heparin–Disseminated intravascular coagulation may occur in septic shock. If the treatment of septic shock is successful, consumption of coagulation factors usually ceases and rapid regeneration occurs. The use of heparin in disseminated intravascular coagulation is a measure of last resort. Give 50–100 units/kg intravenously initially, followed by 500–

1000 units every hour by continuous intravenous drip (infusion pump preferred). Response to heparin is indicated by slowing of bleeding and a rise within 12 hours of the levels of factors V and VIII and of fibrinogen. Platelet counts may rise at a slower rate. Discontinue heparin therapy when the cause of disseminated intravascular coagulation has been corrected and coagulation factors have been restored to homeostatic levels. (See also Chapter 33.)

c. Naloxone–Some animal and clinical trials have shown that naloxone (Narcan, others) may reverse the hypotension associated with septic shock. Administration of 0.1 mg/kg as an intravenous bolus, followed by 0.7 mg/kg/h by continuous intravenous infusion, has been suggested. Use of naloxone has fallen into disfavor.

8. Insert an indwelling urinary catheter to monitor urine output. Remove the catheter once the patient's condition stabilizes, usually in 12–24 hours.

D. Search for Source of Infection: Thoroughly but rapidly examine the patient for an obvious source of infection. Pay special attention to the following sites:

1. Skin and nails–Look carefully for a rash, petechiae, purpura, abscesses, ulcers, an infected intravenous catheter insertion site, needle marks (intravenous drug use), and splinter hemorrhages. Be sure to examine the patient's scalp, back, perineum, mucosal surfaces (conjunctivas, oral cavity), and palms and soles (including web spaces).

2. Check for signs of meningeal irritation (nuchal rigidity, etc) (Chapter 13).

3. Listen for heart murmurs or abnormal lung sounds.

4. Examine the abdomen, and perform a rectal examination, since rectal abscesses are frequently overlooked on physical examination.

5. Percuss and palpate all joints and vertebrae.

6. Perform a bimanual pelvic examination in all female patients.

E. Perform Diagnostic Laboratory Tests:

1. Blood cultures–Obtain 2 sets of blood cultures (aerobic and anaerobic) from separate sites in all seriously ill patients.

2. Gram staining and culture–Obtain Gram-stained smears and culture of all accessible body fluids, purulent material, and other potentially infected tissue. Typical sources of infection include urine, pulmonary secretions, cerebrospinal fluid, surgical wounds and drains, intravenous catheter sites, ascitic fluid, and decubitus ulcers. Microscopic examination of the buffy coat of a centrifuged blood sample may sometimes identify the causative organism, particularly in meningococcemia.

3. Radiologic studies–Chest x-ray, sinus films, abdominal x-ray series, bone and soft tissue films, and other studies should be obtained as needed.

F. Start Antibiotic Treatment: Antibiotic treatment should be specific for the infecting organism; however, the causative agent is frequently not known when the patient presents for treatment. Empiric antibiotic therapy chosen on the basis of an educated "best guess" about the possible causative organisms may be used until the infectious agent is positively identified. Follow the recommendations set forth in Table 34–1.

Note: Antibiotic treatment for acute bacterial meningitis and meningococcemia should be started in the emergency department immediately after samples for culture have been obtained.

The most common route of entry for infective organisms is the genitourinary tract, followed in order of decreasing incidence by the respiratory tract, wounds (including decubitus ulcers), and the gastrointestinal tract. Numerically, aerobic gram-negative bacilli are the most common organisms *(Escherichia coli, Klebsiella, Proteus, Enterobacter,* and *Pseudomonas).* Common gram-positive pathogens include *Staphylococcus aureus,* the pneumococcus, enterococci, and viridans streptococci. Anaerobic bacteria (notably *Bacteroides fragilis*) are becoming increasingly important causative organisms.

G. Provide Surgical Treatment as Needed: Antibiotics and volume replacement are fruitless if the emergency physician fails to incise and drain abscesses or debride infected necrotic tissue. Possible sources of sepsis (eg, intra-abdominal abscess, biliary obstruction with cholangitis, perirectal abscess, septic abortion, or any other disorder requiring surgery) must be identified as soon as possible.

Disposition

Hospitalization in an intensive care unit is required for all patients in septic shock or those seriously ill with an infection.

EVALUATION OF THE IMMUNOCOMPROMISED PATIENT WITH SUSPECTED INFECTION

Diagnosis

A. Classification of Immune Dysfunction: Identification of the type of immune dysfunction will often enable the physician to predict the agent causing infection, so that differential diagnosis and, in some cases, treatment may be started in the emergency department. Types of immune dysfunction include the following:

1. Granulocytopenia–Patients with circulating granulocyte counts below 500/μL are especially susceptible to infections caused by gram-negative bacilli (including *Pseudomonas aeruginosa*) and staphylococci. Profound granulocytopenia is usually due to myelosuppressive therapy or irradiation, which in addition to causing toxic effects on the bone marrow, damages the mucosa in the alimentary canal. Bowel flora may thereby enter the bloodstream and cause septicemia and secondary pneumonia. Perirectal and perineal infections are also common.

Table 34–1. Suggested empiric antibiotics in septic shock.

Suspected Site of Infection or Predisposing Factor	Common Pathogens	Antibiotics[1]
Genitourinary tract	Aerobic gram-negative bacilli (*Escherichia coli, Klebsiella, Proteus, Pseudomonas*); group D streptococci.	Ampicillin plus aminoglycoside. (Third-generation cephalosporin may be substituted for aminoglycoside.)
Respiratory tract[2]	*Streptococcus pneumoniae; Staphylococcus aureus;* aerobic gram-negative bacilli; anaerobes, *Haemophilus influenzae.*	Ampicillin or cefotaxime, plus aminoglycoside. (Metronidazole or PRSP[3] may be added.)
Below the diaphragm: Intra-abdominal abscess; decubitus ulcers; pelvic or perirectal abscess	Aerobic gram-negative bacilli; anaerobes (including *Bacteroides fragilis*); viridans and group D streptococci.	Ampicillin plus metronidazole plus aminoglycoside. (Clindamycin may be substituted for metronidazole and a third-generation cephalosporin, or aztreonam may be substituted for aminoglycoside.)
Biliary tree	Aerobic gram-negative bacilli; group D streptococci, anaerobes.	Ampicillin plus aminoglycoside. (Clindamycin or metronidazole may be added.)
Skin, bone, or joint	*S aureus;* streptococci; aerobic gram-negative bacilli, *Clostridium* or other anaerobes; *H influenzae* in children less than 5 years.	PRSP[3] plus aminoglycoside or cefotaxime. (Metronidazole may be added.)
Immunocompromised host (immunosuppressive drugs; corticosteroids; cancer)	Usual pathogens, as well as higher incidence of aerobic gram-negative bacilli (including *Pseudomonas*); staphylococci; yeasts (especially *Candida albicans*).	APP[4] plus aminoglycoside, or ceftazidime + APP[4]. (Vancomycin may be added.)
Unknown	*S pneumoniae; S aureus; Neisseria meningitidis;* aerobic gram-negative rods; *H influenzae* in children less than 5 years.	Ampicillin plus aminoglycoside. (PRSP[3] may be added; in children less than 5 years, substitute cefotaxime for aminoglycoside.)

[1]For doses of antibiotics, see Table 34–13. Use high initial doses of antibiotics in septic shock.
[2]When possible, choice of antibiotics should be guided by sputum Gram's stain.
[3]PRSP = Penicillinase-resistant synthetic penicillins (methicillin, oxacillin, nafcillin).
[4]APP = Antipseudomonal beta-lactamase–susceptible penicillins (carbenicillin, ticarcillin, mezlocillin, azlocillin, piperacillin).

2. Cellular immune dysfunction—Defects in cell-mediated immunity may be due to underlying disease (eg, congenital defects in cell-mediated immunity, Hodgkin's disease, acquired immunodeficiency syndrome [AIDS]) or may occur as a result of antineoplastic or immunosuppressive treatment (eg, treatment of lymphoma or transplant rejection). Patients with this type of immune dysfunction are especially susceptible to infection caused by intracellular pathogens such as *Listeria monocytogenes, Mycobacterium* species, *Cryptococcus neoformans* and other fungi, and herpes viruses (herpes simplex, cytomegalovirus), as well as *Pneumocystis carinii.*

3. Humoral immune dysfunction—Defects in opsonizing antibody production occur in untreated patients with multiple myeloma and in patients who have undergone splenectomy. These patients are susceptible to infections caused by encapsulated organisms, particularly *Streptococcus pneumoniae* and *Haemophilus influenzae.* Patients with multiple myeloma usually develop pneumonia; splenectomized patients may develop overwhelming sepsis.

B. Symptoms and Signs: Fever is the most reliable sign of infection in immunocompromised patients and must never be ascribed to an underlying disease until infection has been ruled out. Localized collections of pus (abscesses or fluctuant areas) are generally absent in neutropenic patients, and the only

sign of serious infection may be an area of localized tenderness or redness in a febrile patient. In patients thought to have AIDS, helpful diagnostic clues are inclusion in a recognized high-risk group (eg, homosexual men or intravenous drug abusers [Table 34–11]) and history of a prodrome of low-grade fever, lymphadenopathy, weight loss, and oropharyngeal candidiasis. In all immunocompromised patients, careful examination of the lungs, skin, and mucous membranes for signs of infection is important. The lungs may show signs of pneumonia, and signs of disseminated infection may be found in skin and mucous membranes (eg, the ulcerated pustules characteristic of ecthyma gangrenosum in patients with sepsis caused by *Pseudomonas,* and perirectal cellulitis in patients with neutropenia).

C. Laboratory and X-Ray Findings: Determination of the absolute number of circulating granulocytes is mandatory in the evaluation of immunocompromised patients. For example, if the patient's white cell count is 1500 with a total of 10% mature and immature PMNs, then the granulocyte count is 150/μL. In patients with AIDS, the total lymphocyte count is frequently less than 1000/μL. The presence of anemia or thrombocytopenia should also be assessed. Samples of blood, urine, and (when obtainable) sputum should be sent for Gram staining and culture in all immunocompromised patients. A chest x-ray will often show signs of pneumonia, even in patients with very low white blood cell counts. Bilateral interstitial and alveolar infiltrates radiating from the hilum characterize *P carinii* pneumonia, which is common in patients with AIDS and occasionally occurs in other immunocompromised patients. Other studies (eg, sinus films) should be obtained depending on localizing symptoms and signs. Successful diagnosis in these patients often depends on examination of tissue samples (eg, lung tissue obtained by transbronchial or open lung biopsy). For the evaluation of pneumonia in AIDS patients, see p 638.

Treatment

A. Antibiotics: In febrile patients with granulocyte counts under 1000/µL, antibiotic therapy should be started immediately after material for routine cultures has been obtained. Circumstances that strengthen the directive for urgent empiric therapy include **(1)** a rapidly falling granulocyte count, **(2)** a very low granulocyte count (< 500/µL further increases the risk of infection; < 100/µL is commonly associated with fulminant infection), and **(3)** other clinical findings suggesting infection. High doses of intravenous antibiotics should be given at frequent intervals (Tables 34–1 and 34–13).

Well-tested antibiotic regimens of comparable efficacy include the following: **(1)** an aminoglycoside combined with an extended-spectrum penicillin such as ticarcillin, mezlocillin, or piperacillin (the regimen preferred by the authors); **(2)** an aminoglycoside combined with a third-generation cephalosporin; or **(3)** anti-*Pseudomonas* penicillin (eg, piperacillin, mezlocillin) and ceftazidime.

B. Isolation: Neutropenic patients should be hospitalized in private rooms, and strict hand-washing precautions should be observed. Protective isolation as usually practiced (masks and gowns) does not appear to be effective. Patients should be prescribed a diet free of fresh fruits and vegetables, which are often heavily contaminated with gram-negative bacilli.

Disposition

All immunocompromised patients with new findings of fever or other signs of infection should be hospitalized.

SERIOUS INFECTIONS PRESENTING WITH FEVER & RASH

The combination of fever and an exanthem with or without an enanthem (mucosal eruption) is considered separately here, because early recognition of a few classic infectious diseases and prompt institution of appropriate empiric antimicrobial therapy will reduce the incidence of severe illness and death.

1. ACUTE MENINGOCOCCEMIA

Diagnosis

A. Symptoms and Signs: Meningococcemia often follows a mild upper respiratory tract infection. Onset may be acute or subacute, with fever and malaise, with or without symptoms and signs of meningitis and septic shock. A petechial rash appears early in the course of illness, usually on the trunk and lower portion of the body and over pressure points, eg, under elastic underwear or stockings. The petechiae are small (1–2 mm), irregular, gunmetal gray, and often palpable. Petechiae may become confluent (purpura) or may progress to form vasculitic ulcers. Mucosal petechiae (eg, on the palpebral conjunctiva) also occur. Early in the disease, the number of petechiae correlates with the degree of thrombocytopenia and with the probability of disseminated intravascular coagulation.

B. Laboratory Findings: Results of routine laboratory studies are consistent with findings of bacteremia with or without sepsis. All patients should be evaluated for disseminated intravascular coagulation (prothrombin time, partial thromboplastin time, and levels of fibrinogen and fibrin degradation products). Blood cultures should always be obtained. Because subclinical meningitis is common in meningococcemia, most patients thought to have meningococcemia should undergo lumbar puncture. Special laboratory studies that confirm the diagnosis include the following:

1. Bacteria on stained smear–Meningococci (gram-negative kidney bean–shaped diplococci) may be found in stained smears of the buffy coat of a centrifuged blood sample or in material taken from petechial skin lesions. If meningitis has developed, meningococci and PMNs may often be seen on careful examination of Gram-stained smears of cerebrospinal fluid.

2. Meningococcal polysaccharide antigen–Special tests for meningococcal polysaccharide antigen in cerebrospinal fluid and urine may confirm the diagnosis in patients who have been treated with antimicrobials before hospitalization or in whom routine cultures have yielded negative results.

Differential Diagnosis

Rickettsial infections, septicemia caused by organisms other than meningococci (*H influenzae, S pneumoniae, S aureus*, etc), and atypical measles may resemble meningococcemia. Bleeding diatheses (eg, idiopathic thrombocytopenic purpura) and cutaneous vasculitides (eg, Henoch-Schönlein purpura) may also be confused with meningococcemia.

Complications

Complications of meningococcemia include the following:

A. Septic Shock: Septic shock is a common complication of meningococcemia. Myocarditis is often found at autopsy and may contribute to vascular collapse.

B. Disseminated Intravascular Coagulation: Disseminated intravascular coagulation is frequently diagnosed in meningococcemia, particularly if sensitive tests are used (eg, presence of fibrin degradation products). Therapy is directed mainly at treating the underlying sepsis while giving supportive care. Heparin therapy is controversial and is rarely used.

C. Adrenal Hemorrhage: Waterhouse-Friderichsen syndrome is characterized by shock and vascular collapse caused by endotoxemia and glucocorticoid deficiency due to adrenal hemorrhage.

D. Metastatic Infection: Meningitis, arthritis, and pericarditis are common complications.

Treatment

A. Begin supportive therapy for shock, if present.

B. Give intravenous antibiotics.

1. Prior to confirmation by culture or in the absence of a positive meningococcal polysaccharide antigen test, empiric treatment with ceftriaxone, 50–100 mg/kg/d (maximum 4 g/d in 2 divided doses), or cefotaxime, 100–200 mg/kg/d (maximum 12 g/d in 4–6 divided doses), is appropriate. When meningococcal disease is confirmed, the treatment of choice is aqueous penicillin G, 300,000 units/kg/d (up to 24 million units/d) in 6 divided doses.

2. Chloramphenicol, 100 mg/kg/d (up to 4 g/d) in 4 divided doses, should be used when there is a history of serious allergy to penicillin (eg, anaphylaxis, hives) and may also be used if rickettsial infection (eg, Rocky Mountain spotted fever) enters the differential diagnosis in endemic areas. Alternatively, doxycycline, 100 mg by vein (adult dose) every 12 hours, may be added to one of the above-cited beta-lactams to treat possible Rocky Mountain spotted fever.

C. Consider corticosteroid therapy.

1. If shock is present (presumptive Waterhouse-Friderichsen syndrome), treat adrenal insufficiency by giving replacement doses of cortisol, eg, hydrocortisone sodium phosphate or succinate, 100 mg intravenously every 6 hours (Chapter 35).

2. Pharmacologic doses of corticosteroids have been given, although they have been shown to be ineffective (see Septic Shock, p 606).

Disposition

Patients with meningococcemia should be hospitalized in an intensive care unit.

Prophylaxis of Exposed Contacts

A. Indications:

1. Residential groups–The value of antimicrobial prophylaxis in military barracks, dormitories, camps, residential schools, and day-care institutions is well established.

2. Households–For household members, the risk of secondary infection is about 1–2% (400 times that of unexposed individuals); the risk is greater in very young individuals and in those who live in crowded conditions.

3. Health care and hospital personnel–Health care professionals and other hospital personnel are at minimal risk of infection. Prophylaxis is not recommended unless close contact with secretions (mouth-to-mouth) has occurred.

B. Antimicrobial Prophylaxis: The most acceptable drug for antimicrobial prophylaxis is rifampin, 600 mg orally twice daily for 2 days in adults. For children 1–12 years of age, give 10 mg/kg twice daily; reduce this amount to 5 mg/kg twice daily for children 3–12 months of age.

C. Vaccination: Immunization with meningococcal polysaccharide vaccine should be considered as an adjunct to antibiotic chemoprophylaxis for household and intimate contacts of patients with meningococcal disease if the infection was caused by a vaccine serotype (A, C, Y, or W135).

2. ROCKY MOUNTAIN SPOTTED FEVER

Rocky Mountain spotted fever is an acute febrile tick-borne illness caused by *Rickettsia rickettsii*. Although it has been reported in almost all states in the USA, it is most common in the South Atlantic and South Central states and in Oklahoma. Most cases occur in the warm months, when ticks are most active. Eighty percent of patients have a history of tick bite.

Diagnosis

A. Symptoms and Signs: Following an incubation period of about 1 week, there is sudden onset of fever, chills, malaise, myalgias, and severe frontal headache. On the second to fifth day of illness, a pink, macular rash 1–4 mm in diameter appears on the palms, soles, hands, feet, wrists, and ankles. Over the next 24–48 hours, the rash becomes petechial, purpuric, and even gangrenous and spreads centripetally to involve the rest of the body. (At this stage, the rash may mimic the lesions of fulminant meningococcemia, although in meningococcemia, the skin eruption appears earlier in the disease.) There may be diffuse edema due to capillary leakage, and hypotension, splenomegaly, and delirium may be seen.

B. Laboratory Findings: Results on ordinary laboratory tests are not exceptional. The white cell count is usually not elevated. Hyponatremia, hypochloremia, and hypoalbuminemia may be present. Thrombocytopenia may occur as an isolated finding or in association with disseminated intravascular coagulation, which is common in Rocky Mountain spotted fever. The cerebrospinal fluid is usually normal, but protein levels may be elevated and there may be a few mononuclear cells. There is no specific laboratory test generally available for the diagnosis of Rocky Mountain spotted fever during the acute stage. The diagnosis must be made on clinical grounds.

Treatment

A. To be most effective, antimicrobial therapy must be started early. Give tetracycline, 500 mg orally 4 times daily, or doxycycline, 100 mg orally 2 times daily. For children less than 8 years of age, give chloramphenicol, 50–100 mg/kg/d orally or intravenously in 4 divided doses. Severely ill patients may be treated with doxycycline or chloramphenicol intravenously.

B. Give appropriate supportive therapy for shock, if present.

Disposition

Hospitalization is required for all patients except those with the mildest symptoms, and patients severely ill with Rocky Mountain spotted fever should be managed in an intensive care unit.

3. INFECTIVE ENDOCARDITIS

Infective endocarditis denotes infection of the endothelial surface of the heart, most often of the cardiac valves. The disease may be either acute or subacute and may affect normal valves, previously damaged cardiac valves, or prosthetic cardiac valves. It is usually caused by bacteria, but fungi are also important pathogens, especially in intravenous drug abusers with acute endocarditis. Seeding of bacterial emboli or deposition of immune complexes in the skin may cause characteristic skin lesions that can alert the physician to the correct diagnosis before progressive damage to the heart leads to circulatory collapse.

Diagnosis

A. Symptoms and Signs: Patients usually present with fever and malaise. In subacute endocarditis, there may be a history of anorexia, night sweats, and weight loss. Patients may also present in cardiac failure, with a stroke due to cerebral embolism, or with a cold extremity due to arterial emboli. In infective endocarditis of the tricuspid valve (usually seen in intravenous drug abusers), acute, often bilateral, embolic pneumonia is a common initial manifestation. Examination of the heart often reveals a murmur, although heart murmurs are often absent in right-sided endocarditis. Characteristic (but not specific) cutaneous and mucosal lesions in bacterial endocarditis include conjunctival and palatal petechiae, subungual (splinter) hemorrhages, Osler nodes, and Janeway lesions. Osler nodes are tender erythematous nodules with opaque centers that appear on the pulp of the fingertips and toes. Janeway lesions are nontender red or maroon macules or nodules that de-

velop on the palms and soles. Careful ophthalmoscopic examination may also reveal Roth spots (pale oval areas surrounded by hemorrhage) near the optic disk.

B. Laboratory Findings: Laboratory findings are variable and nonspecific in infective endocarditis. There may be a normochromic, normocytic anemia, especially in patients with subacute disease. The white cell count may be elevated, especially in acute disease. The erythrocyte sedimentation rate is usually elevated. Microscopic hematuria is present in 30–50% of patients. Immune-complex glomerulonephritis with renal failure may occur. Echocardiography (both M-mode and 2-dimensional) may be useful in demonstrating valvular vegetations or other signs of valvular damage. Esophageal echocardiography may demonstrate vegetations not detectable by conventional echocardiography. Definitive diagnosis depends on isolating the causative microorganism in blood cultures. Gram-stained smears of aspirates from skin lesions (usually Janeway lesions) may occasionally permit rapid diagnosis. In patients with embolic pneumonia, Gram-stained smears of sputum may demonstrate the causative agent (usually *S aureus*); however, in intravenous drug abusers, possible concurrent infection with other organisms (streptococci, gram-negative bacilli) must be treated pending results of blood cultures.

Treatment

In patients who are not acutely ill and in whom symptoms and signs of cardiac failure or major emboli are absent, antibiotic therapy may be withheld pending results of blood cultures. In all other patients, empiric antimicrobial therapy should be started after samples of blood, urine, and (when present) sputum and aspirates from skin lesions have been obtained for culture.

A. Abnormal Cardiac Valve or Congenital Heart Disease: The usual pathogens in patients with abnormal cardiac valves or congenital heart disease are viridans and group D streptococci. Aqueous penicillin G, 150,000–300,000 units/kg/d intravenously in 6 divided doses, plus gentamicin, loading dose of 1.5 mg/kg, followed by 1 mg/kg every 8 hours with adjustment for blood levels, is an acceptable empiric regimen. Vancomycin, 15 mg/kg (maximum 1 g) intravenously every 12 hours, may be substituted for penicillin.

B. Prosthetic Cardiac Valves: Many pathogens cause prosthetic valve endocarditis. Infection occurring less than 6 months postoperatively may be caused by *S aureus, Staphylococcus epidermidis,* gram-negative aerobic bacilli, diphtheroids, and fungi. Infection occurring more than 6 months after prosthetic valve insertion is usually caused by viridans streptococci, aerobic gram-negative bacilli, enterococci, and staphylococci. Because growth of some of these organisms requires multiple blood cultures using special techniques, it is best to avoid early empiric therapy whenever possible. In a patient who requires immediate surgery because of hemodynamic decompensation, empiric therapy may be started with vancomycin and gentamicin, in the doses given in ¶ A.

C. Parenteral Drug Abuse: The usual pathogens in infective endocarditis in intravenous drug abusers are *S aureus, Pseudomonas* species, and streptococci, including group D streptococci. Empiric therapy should include the following antibiotics given intravenously: vancomycin, 1 g every 12 hours; and gentamicin, 1.5 mg/kg loading dose, followed by 1 mg/kg every 8 hours with adjustment for blood levels. Penicillin, 12 million units/d in 6 divided doses; and nafcillin, oxacillin, or methicillin, 12 g/d in 4 divided doses; may be substituted for vancomycin in patients with compromised renal function.

Disposition

Patients with suspected infective endocarditis should be hospitalized. Obtain cardiothoracic surgical consultation for patients with infected prosthetic heart valves, new onset of cardiac failure, or emboli in major vessels, because emergency valve replacement is frequently necessary.

4. DISSEMINATED GONOCOCCEMIA

Gonococcal bacteremia occurs in about 1–3% of patients with infections and is the leading cause of acute septic arthritis in adults (see Septic Arthritis, p 620). A presumptive diagnosis based on the characteristic clinical picture is usually possible in a sexually active patient.

Diagnosis

A. Symptoms and Signs: Disseminated gonococcemia begins as a subacute febrile illness with migratory polyarthralgia. Typically, in the first week of illness, 5–40 discrete lesions develop on the extremities; the face and trunk are spared. Lesions vary and range from petechiae and erythematous, palpable purpura to vesiculopustules with an erythematous halo, and they often have necrotic centers. About one-fourth of patients have tenosynovitis, usually affecting the wrist or ankle. Acute septic arthritis, affecting one or more large joints, may follow disseminated gonococcemia or occur in its absence.

B. Laboratory Findings: The white cell count may be elevated. Blood cultures (especially with the more sensitive sodium polyanetholesulfonate–free media) are often positive in disseminated gonococcemia, although Gram staining and cultures of skin lesions are generally negative. Cultures from all sites are negative in as many as 50% of patients, and a presumptive diagnosis is based instead on the patient's prompt response to ceftriaxone therapy.

Treatment

A. Antimicrobial Therapy: Give ceftriaxone, 1 g intramuscularly or intravenously every 24 hours, or alternative regimen.

B. Arthrocentesis: Arthrocentesis should be performed as often as necessary to prevent reaccumulation of fluid in an infected joint. Open drainage is usually not necessary in gonococcal arthritis.

Disposition

Most patients with septic arthritis should be hospitalized, but outpatient treatment with daily visits for joint aspiration is an acceptable alternative in reliable patients. Many patients with only dermatitis or tenosynovitis may be managed as outpatients with close follow-up.

5. TOXIC SHOCK SYNDROME

Toxic shock syndrome results from absorption of toxin from localized *S aureus* colonization or infection. In the past, most cases have occurred in young women who have vaginal colonization with *S aureus* that produces exotoxin C; however, increasing numbers of cases unrelated to vaginal colonization are being seen, eg, following wound and sinus infection.

Diagnosis

Toxic shock syndrome usually starts abruptly during menses. It occurs most commonly in women using tampons or contraceptive sponges, but some cases have resulted (in men, women, and children) from localized staphylococcal infections such as abscesses. Rarely, *Streptococcus pyogenes* can produce a similar syndrome with or without antecedent pharyngitis.

A. Symptoms and Signs: There is a short prodrome consisting of various combinations of the following: feverishness, myalgia, vomiting, diarrhea, and pharyngitis. Patients then develop shock (systolic blood pressure < 80 mm Hg) with fever (> 39 °C [102.2 °F]) and signs of multiple organ dysfunction. At the time of presentation to the emergency department or within 24 hours of admission to the hospital, a diffuse, blanching, macular erythema appears, accompanied by signs of mucous membrane inflammation (pharyngitis, conjunctivitis, vaginitis, and strawberry tongue). The rash fades in about 3 days, but desquamation of the hands and feet occurs in all patients 5–12 days after the rash disappears. Patients typically prefer to remain motionless in bed because of intense myalgias. Confusion and agitation occur in half of patients. Pedal edema is common.

B. Laboratory Findings: Laboratory findings reflect dysfunction of several organ systems. There may be leukocytosis and thrombocytopenia, elevated blood urea nitrogen and creatinine levels, hyperbilirubinemia, elevated hepatic enzymes, and sterile pyuria. The prothrombin and partial thromboplastin times may be elevated, with or without thrombocytopenia. Other laboratory abnormalities include acidosis, elevated CK levels (indicating rhabdomyolysis), hypocalcemia, decreased serum albumin and total protein due to capillary leakage, and elevated liver enzyme levels. Cultures of material from the vagina or cervix are usually positive for *S aureus*. Blood cultures are generally negative.

Treatment & Disposition

Remove the vaginal tampon if present. Begin volume replacement with saline or colloid solutions and with vasopressors, if necessary. Admit the patient to an intensive care unit, and monitor hemodynamic status. Start treatment with a first-generation cephalosporin, penicillinase-resistant synthetic penicillin, or vancomycin intravenously.

6. GROUP A STREPTOCOCCAL INFECTIONS ASSOCIATED WITH A TOXIC SHOCK–LIKE SYNDROME

An infection with group A streptococci that is remarkable for severity of local tissue destruction, life-threatening systemic toxicity, and a toxic shock–like syndrome has recently been described in adults. Clinical isolates frequently produce pyrogenic exotoxin A. The portal of entry may be the skin or mucous membranes or it may occur subsequent to a surgical procedure, but many patients do not have obvious evidence of a portal of entry.

Diagnosis

A. Symptoms and Signs: Pain is the most common initial symptom and is frequently severe and abrupt in onset. The pain usually involves the extremity but may be intra-abdominal. Before onset, some patients complain of an influenzalike syndrome characterized by fever, chills, myalgia, vomiting, and diarrhea. Patients often have oral temperatures above 37 °C (98.6 °F), may have confusion that rapidly deteriorates to coma, or may be combative. Shock is apparent at the time of presentation or within hours with evidence of hypotension, renal dysfunction, and respiratory failure. Most patients present with soft tissue infection, such as cellulitis or necrotizing fasciitis. Deeper infections may be present, including osteomyelitis, myometritis, peritonitis, suppurative phlebitis, and endophthalmitis. A major difference between these patients and patients with staphylococcal toxic shock syndrome is that these patients have extensive soft tissue infection and bacteremia. Mortality is approximately 30%.

B. Laboratory Findings: Laboratory findings reflect dysfunction of several organ systems. There may be leukocytosis and thrombocytopenia. The hematocrit is initially normal but may drop within 48–

72 hours. Serum creatinine and creatine kinase levels are elevated, but calcium and albumin levels are low. Microscopic hematuria is often present and correlates with the presence of renal impairment. Group A streptococci are cultured from the blood, body fluid, or tissues of all patients who have not received prior antibiotic therapy.

Treatment & Disposition

Intensive fluid replacement, central venous or pulmonary capillary wedge pressure monitoring, and timely surgical debridement are essential. Start antibiotic therapy with intravenous penicillin or a cephalosporin. Patients should be admitted to the intensive care unit.

7. LYME BORRELIOSIS

Lyme borreliosis (Lyme disease, Lyme arthritis) is a chronic disease caused by the spirochete *Borrelia burgdorferi*. Transmission is by several species of ticks *(Ixodes, Amblyomma, Rhipicephalus)* and occurs throughout the USA, with highest prevalence in the Northeast and Midwest. It has been recognized in Europe, Asia, and Australia. In stage 1, a rash is present, sometimes accompanied by fever. Timely treatment at this stage may prevent disease progression.

Diagnosis

A. Symptoms and Signs: Between 3 and 32 days following the tick bite, which may go unnoticed by the patient, a gradually expanding area of redness with clearing (erythema migrans) occurs at the bite site. The involved skin is warm but not particularly tender to touch. About half of affected patients will develop smaller lesions of similar morphology at areas remote from the bite site over ensuing days to weeks. In stage 1 disease (erythema migrans), often there is fever, chills, malaise, and regional lymphadenopathy. In stage 2 (days to weeks after infection), symptoms related to the multisystemic nature of Lyme borreliosis often appear, such as meningitis, hepatitis, sore throat, dry cough, heart block and other cardiac abnormalities, musculoskeletal pain, and neuropathy. Fatigue and lethargy are prominent and may persist for months after the skin lesions have disappeared. A persistent illness (stage 3) may linger for months to years and usually involves the musculoskeletal system (chronic arthritis), neurologic system (both central and peripheral), and skin (acrodermatitis chronica atrophicans). Patients in stage 3 illness respond slower to treatment and have higher failure rates than patients in stages 1 and 2.

B. Laboratory Findings: Laboratory testing is currently not reliable or standardized. Diagnosis depends on recognition of the pathognomonic rash. Serodiagnosis by either indirect immunofluorescence or ELISA may be negative in early infection. Nonspecific laboratory abnormalities include an elevated erythrocyte sedimentation rate, mild anemia, and transient elevations in SGOT (AST), SGPT (ALT), and LDH enzyme levels.

Treatment & Disposition

The treatment of choice for early Lyme borreliosis is tetracycline, 250 mg or 500 mg orally 4 times daily for at least 10 days, or for 20 or 30 days if symptoms persist or recur. For children under the age of 12 years, give amoxicillin or penicillin V, 50 mg/kg (not less than 1 g/d and not more than 2 g/d) in 3 divided doses for the same duration as for adults. For pediatric patients with penicillin allergy, give erythromycin, 30 mg/kg/d in 4 divided doses for 15–30 days. For more serious disease (eg, Lyme carditis or meningitis), intravenous therapy with ceftriaxone, 2 g/d, or penicillin G, 20 million units/d in divided doses, for 14–21 days is recommended.

8. EXANTHEMATOUS DISEASES OF CHILDHOOD

A detailed discussion of the many childhood exanthems is beyond the scope of this chapter. Table 42–24 summarizes the clinical features and differential diagnosis of common exanthematous diseases of childhood.

EMERGENCY MANAGEMENT OF SPECIFIC DISORDERS

MENINGITIS & MENINGOENCEPHALITIS

Acute bacterial meningitis is a life-threatening medical emergency. The current mortality rate is 10–30%, and survival depends on prompt recognition and early treatment.

Diagnosis

A. Symptoms and Signs: Patients with meningitis present with fever, headache, nuchal rigidity, and mental dysfunction. Seizures and cranial nerve deficits are also common. Infants with meningitis may show only vomiting, lethargy, irritability, and poor feeding. Elderly patients may present only with low-grade fever and delirium. The headache of meningitis is continuous and throbbing and, though generalized, is usually most prominent over the occiput. The pain is increased by head shaking, jugular vein compression, or any other maneuver that increases intracranial pressure (eg, coughing, sneezing, straining at stool). Neck stiffness and other signs of menin-

geal irritation (Chapter 13) must be sought with care, since they may not be obvious early and may disappear during coma. **Note: Do not** perform lumbar puncture in patients with signs of intracranial infection who also have papilledema or focal neurologic findings (other than cranial nerve deficits); these patients may have intracranial mass lesions, and herniation of the brain may occur if lumbar puncture is performed.

Patients with meningitis may be divided into 2 groups on the basis of the presentation of the disorder.

1. Acute presentation–Symptoms and signs have been present for less than 24 hours and are rapidly progressive. The causative organisms in these patients are usually pyogenic bacteria, and the mortality rate is about 50%.

2. Subacute presentation–Symptoms and signs have been present for 1–7 days. Meningitis in this group of patients is due to bacteria, viruses, or fungi, and the death rate in cases due to bacterial infection is much lower than in patients with acute presentation of disease.

B. Laboratory Findings: Perform lumbar puncture immediately in the absence of papilledema and focal neurologic findings (except cranial nerve deficits). Draw blood for serum glucose measurement and for culture. Gram staining of cerebrospinal fluid will often enable the physician to make a presumptive identification of the causative agent. Even if no organisms are seen on Gram-stained smears of cerebrospinal fluid, bacterial meningitis is a likely diagnosis and warrants empiric antimicrobial therapy if total cerebrospinal fluid leukocytes number more than 1000/μL, if PMNs make up at least 85% of the white cells in cerebrospinal fluid, or if the cerebrospinal fluid glucose is less than 50% of the serum glucose level in a simultaneously drawn blood sample. The differential diagnosis in patients in whom PMNs are less than 85% of the cerebrospinal fluid white cell count must consider a number of disorders (Table 34–2). **Note:** Prior therapy with a few doses of oral or parenteral antimicrobials will often result in sterile cerebrospinal fluid cultures and may lead to a misleading white cell count or Gram-stained smear of cerebrospinal fluid. Counterimmunoelectrophoresis of cerebrospinal fluid may be helpful. Other laboratory findings in bacterial meningitis are variable.

Treatment

A. Antimicrobial Therapy:

1. Acute presentation–When bacterial meningitis is suspected, begin administration of appropriate antibiotics immediately (Table 34–3). Give the first dose as soon as samples of cerebrospinal fluid and blood have been collected for tests; the goal is to begin intravenous administration of antimicrobials within 30 minutes after a patient with acute presentation of meningitis has sought treatment. If lumbar puncture must be delayed for anatomic studies (CT

Table 34–2. Some causes of acute lymphocytic meningitis.[1]

Early or partially treated bacterial meningitis
Viral meningitis and meningoencephalitis (including HIV)
Tuberculous or fungal meningitis
Syphilis
Parameningeal infection (eg, brain abscess)
Central nervous system collagen vascular disease
Central nervous system tumor, leukemia, lymphoma, or
 carcinomatosis
Intracranial injury (eg, subdural hematoma)
Subarachnoid hemorrhage

[1]PMNs in cerebrospinal fluid are less than 85% of the total white cell count.

scan or angiogram), obtain 2 blood samples for culture, and begin appropriate antimicrobials; perform lumbar puncture if mass lesion has been excluded, and obtain cerebrospinal fluid for microscopic examination and culture as soon as possible.

2. Subacute presentation–Treatment is based on results of Gram staining of cerebrospinal fluid and other tests. If meningitis is likely but Gram staining is negative, begin empiric therapy based on the patient's clinical characteristics (Table 34–3) pending results of cerebrospinal fluid cultures.

3. Suspected brain abscess–In patients thought to have brain abscess, begin intravenous therapy with a combination of penicillin (200,000 units/kg/d intravenously in 4–6 divided doses) and metronidazole (30 mg/kg/d intravenously in 4 divided doses), or a third-generation cephalosporin (cefotaxime, ceftazidime [maximum dose]) and metronidazole. Obtain an emergency CT scan.

B. Supportive Care: General supportive care measures should be started in the emergency department. Protect the patient's airway, and provide padded bed rails or restraints for agitated or delirious patients. If seizures occur, begin anticonvulsant therapy (Chapter 11). Avoid overhydration, which may worsen cerebral edema. In children older than 2 months of age with bacterial meningitis, dexamethasone, 0.6 mg/kg/d in 4 divided doses for 4 days, has been shown to reduce neurologic sequelae and hearing loss.

Disposition

Immediate hospitalization is warranted for all patients except for those with aseptic (viral) meningitis who appear well and can be observed at home by a third party.

PNEUMONIA & BRONCHIOLITIS

Pneumonia and bronchiolitis are common emergency department problems that demand prompt diagnosis and treatment. Although virtually any microorganism can cause pneumonia, only a few agents actually cause the disease in most cases. The common pathogens differ with the age and immune status of the patient (Table 34–4).

Table 34–3. Empiric antibiotic therapy of bacterial meningitis by type of patient.

Type of Patient	Pathogen[1]	Antibiotics of Choice Pending Results of Cultures and Susceptibility Tests (Give Intravenously)
All adult patients	*Streptococcus pneumoniae, Neisseria meningitidis, Haemophilus influenzae,* or unknown pathogen	Penicillin G, 20–24 million units in 6 divided doses; or cefotaxime, 150–200 mg/kg (maximum 12 g) in 4 divided doses; or ceftriaxone, 4 g in 2 divided doses. (Chloramphenicol, 75 mg/kg/d, maximum 4 g, in 4 divided doses, may be used.)[2]
Partially treated (patient has already received antibiotics)	Unknown pathogen	Same as above.
Newborn (< 2 months of age)	*Eschericia coli,* group B streptococci, *Listeria monocytogenes,* or unknown pathogen	Ampicillin, 200 mg/kg/d[3] in 6 divided doses; plus cefotaxime, 200 mg/kg/d in 4 divided doses; or gentamicin, 7.5 mg/kg/d in 3 divided doses.
Infant (> 2 months of age)	*H influenzae, N meningitidis, S pneumoniae,* or unknown pathogen	Ampicillin, 200 mg/kg/d in 6 divided doses; plus cefotaxime, 200 mg/kg/d in 4 divided doses; or ceftriaxone, 100 mg/kg/d in 2 divided doses.
Immunosuppressed adult patient with hospital-acquired infection; patient with open cranial wound	Unknown pathogen, *Staphylococcus* species, gram-negative bacilli, including pseudomonas	Ceftazidime, 6 g in 3 divided doses; plus vancomycin, 2 g in 2 divided doses. (Ampicillin, 200 mg/kg/d in 6 divided doses may be added if *Listeria* infection is suspected.)

[1]Cerebrospinal fluid Gram staining may be used to guide therapy if it can be obtained without delay.
[2]If cerebrospinal fluid Gram staining is clearly indicative of *Streptococcus pneumoniae* or *Neisseria meningitidis,* penicillin G, 20–40 million units in 6 divided doses, may be given initially.
[3]Doses are for newborn more than 7 days old.

Table 34–4. Causative agents of pneumonia according to type of patient.

Type of Patient	Common Pathogens	Less Common Pathogens of High Virulence
Neonate (< 2 months of age)	Escherichia coli Group B streptococci Viruses[1]	Listeria monocytogenes Staphylococcus aureus
Infant or young child (2 months to 5 years of age)	Viruses[2] Chlamydia trachomatis Mycoplasma pneumoniae	S aureus Haemophilus influenzae Streptococcus pneumoniae
Child (5–14 years of age)	M pneumoniae S pneumoniae Viruses (influenza, adenoviruses) C pneumoniae	S aureus (especially after influenza) H influenzae Mycobacterium tuberculosis Group A streptococci Mixed aerobic-anaerobic infection[3] S aureus
Adult	Mixed aerobic-anaerobic infection[3] M pneumoniae S pneumoniae H influenzae C pneumoniae	Klebsiella pneumoniae and other aerobic gram-negative bacilli Legionella pneumophila M tuberculosis
Immunocompromised patient	Aerobic gram-negative bacilli S pneumoniae H influenzae S aureus Pneumocystis carinii	M tuberculosis Nocardia Fungi Cytomegalovirus

[1]Prinicipally cytomegalovirus, herpes simplex virus, and rubella.
[2]Principally respiratory syncytial virus and parainfluenzae viruses.
[3]Mixed infection with oropharyngeal flora (aerobic and anaerobic streptococci, Bacteroides and Fusobacterium species) following aspiration of oropharyngeal secretions.

1. PNEUMONIA IN NEONATES (Age < 2 Months)

Diagnosis

A. Symptoms and Signs: Neonates with pneumonia often have widely disseminated infection caused by group B streptococci, gram-negative bacilli, viruses, and other pathogens. Patients present with fever or labile temperature, poor feeding, irritability, jaundice, and apneic spells. Concurrent meningitis is frequent in bacterial infections.

B. Laboratory and X-Ray Findings: Draw samples of blood, urine, and cerebrospinal fluid for culture for bacteria and viruses. Order routine blood tests and chest x-ray.

Treatment

Begin any necessary resuscitative measures, and pending identification of the causative organism, begin intravenous antibiotic therapy with ampicillin, 200 mg/kg/d in 6 doses, plus gentamicin or tobramycin, 7.5 mg/kg/d in 3 divided doses. A third-generation cephalosporin (eg, ceftriaxone, cefotaxime) may be substituted for the aminoglycoside.

Disposition

Neonates with pneumonia should be hospitalized in a neonatal intensive care unit.

2. PNEUMONIA IN INFANTS & CHILDREN (Age 2 Months to 5 Years)

Pulmonary infections in infants and young children include the following:

A. Chlamydia trachomatis Pneumonia: *Chlamydia trachomatis* pneumonia is an afebrile, interstitial disease in infants 4–12 weeks of age and is characterized by staccato cough, hyperaeration of the lungs, and eosinophilia in peripheral blood.

B. Bronchiolitis: The most common manifestations of lower respiratory tract infection in infants 2–8 months old are wheezing and hyperinflated lungs without signs of consolidation or pulmonary infiltrates. Respiratory syncytial virus and parainfluenza virus are the organisms most frequently isolated in cultures from infants with bronchiolitis. Respiratory failure requiring endotracheal intubation may occur.

C. Bacterial Pneumonia: In infants and young children, bacterial pneumonia is usually caused by *S pneumoniae, H influenzae,* and *S aureus.* Concurrent meningitis, epiglottitis, or otitis media occurs in up to 43% of children with pneumonia due to *H influenzae.* Sixty percent of these infections occur within the first year of life, and the illness can be catastrophic.

Diagnosis

A. Symptoms and Signs: In infants, tachypnea

out of proportion to fever is the most common sign of lower respiratory tract infection. Thus, it is important to measure the rate of respiration *before* the infant is disturbed by attempts at auscultation. Grunting respirations secondary to air trapping and expiratory obstruction suggest pneumonia. Localized findings (rales, decreased breath sounds) are more common in children over 1 year of age.

B. Laboratory and X-Ray Findings: A peripheral leukocyte count over 15,000/µL suggests bacterial pneumonia, although lower counts do not exclude the diagnosis. Arterial blood gas measurements should be obtained to assess the adequacy of ventilation. Electrolyte measurements and blood urea nitrogen levels are useful in assessing the degree of dehydration, the most frequent complication of pneumonia in infants and children. Gram-stained smears of sputum, when obtainable, can be diagnostic. Chest x-rays in children under 1 year of age with bronchiolitis usually show only hyperaeration with or without atelectasis. Lobar consolidation, pneumatoceles (caused by *S aureus*) and pleural effusions (due to *H influenzae* and *S aureus*) suggest bacterial pneumonia. Blood cultures are frequently positive in pneumonia due to *H influenzae*. In infants who are immunosuppressed or seriously ill with pneumonia, diagnostic pneumocentesis may be indicated and is usually well tolerated when performed by a physician expert in the procedure. Pleural fluid, when present, will also often yield the causative agent.

Treatment

Antibiotic therapy is indicated in any infant or young child with lobar consolidation, pneumatocele, or pleural effusion. Antibiotics are also indicated if Gram-stained smears of sputum show many neutrophils and a predominant microorganism, or if bacteria are seen on Gram-stained smears of pleural fluid or lung aspirate. The choice of antibiotics depends, in part, on x-ray findings: lobar infiltrates *(S pneumoniae, H influenzae)*, pneumatoceles *(S aureus)* pleural effusions *(S aureus, H influenzae)*. It also depends on the morphology of any organisms seen on Gram-stained smears. Empiric antibiotic therapy includes the following choices, alone or in combination:

A. Cefuroxime, 50–100 mg/kg/d intravenously in 3 divided doses, or cefotaxime, 100–200 mg/kg/d intravenously in 3–6 divided doses, is a good empiric choice for *H influenzae.*

B. Oxacillin, methicillin, or nafcillin, 200 mg/kg/d intravenously in 4–6 doses, may be added if *S aureus* is strongly suspected (eg, pneumatoceles, immunocompromised child, child with sickle cell disease).

Antibiotic therapy may be withheld in clinically stable patients who show only hyperaeration or atelectasis on chest x-ray.

Aerosolized ribavirin is generally recommended for the treatment of severe lower respiratory infection due to respiratory syncytial virus. A solution of 20 mg/mL is administered via a specific small-particle aerosol generator (available on loan from Viratek, Inc.) through an oxygen mask. It is given 12–18 hours per day for at least 3 and no more than 7 days. Treatment may be begun empirically, but the diagnosis of respiratory syncytial virus infection should be confirmed by viral culture or direct immunofluorescence.

Pneumonia thought to be due to *Chlamydia trachomatis* should be treated with erythromycin, 50 mg/kg/d in 4 divided doses (orally or intravenously), depending on the patient's condition.

Disposition

A. Severely ill infants (respiratory distress, severe hyperthermia, arterial $PO_2 < 70$ mm Hg on room air) should be hospitalized.

B. Hospitalized infants who are less seriously ill may be observed closely and diagnostic measures deferred unless their clinical status worsens. Antibiotics should be withheld until adequate samples have been obtained for culture.

C. Infants with mild pneumonia thought to be viral in origin may be observed on an outpatient basis without specific diagnostic measures or antibiotic therapy. Follow-up at 24-hour intervals is mandatory until it is established that recovery is well under way.

3. PNEUMONIA IN OLDER CHILDREN (Age 5–14 Years)

In children 5–14 years of age, *Mycoplasma pneumoniae* is the commonest cause of pneumonia. Viruses (adenoviruses) and bacteria (*S pneumoniae, S aureus,* and others) also cause pneumonia.

Diagnosis

A. Symptoms and Signs: Infection due to *M pneumoniae* usually develops insidiously with fever and malaise followed in 3–5 days by nonproductive cough, hoarseness, and sore throat, with or without chest pain. Physical examination may disclose pharyngeal erythema and areas of fine rales, wheezes, or dullness, especially over the lower lobes. Myringitis occurs in about 15% of cases, occasionally with the development of tympanic bullae. Maculopapular rashes are common. Pneumonia due to *S pneumoniae, H influenzae,* or *S aureus* often follows a viral upper respiratory tract infection and is characterized by the abrupt onset of fever, chills, tachypnea, and cough accompanied by signs of lobar consolidation or bronchopneumonia.

B. Laboratory and X-Ray Findings: In pneumonia due to *M pneumoniae,* the white cell count is usually normal or slightly elevated, and chest x-ray reveals scattered segmental infiltrates, atelectasis, interstitial disease, or (less frequently) lobar consolidation.

Positive results on a rapid cold agglutination test correlate strongly with a diagnosis of mycoplasmal pneumonia. To perform this test, add 3 drops of blood to the liquid anticoagulant contained in the small blue-topped tubes used for coagulation studies. Immerse the tube for 15 seconds in crushed ice, and then rotate it slowly in a horizontal position, and examine the contents for hemagglutination that disappears as the tube rewarms. The rapid test should be confirmed by cold agglutinin titers (> 1:32).

In pneumonia due to bacteria other than *M pneumoniae*, the white cell count usually exceeds 15,000/μL. Chest x-ray abnormalities include patchy infiltrates, increased bronchovascular markings, lobar consolidation, cavitary infiltrates, and pleural effusions or empyema. Gram-stained smears of sputum may enable the physician to make a presumptive diagnosis if there are numerous PMNs, few epithelial cells, and a predominant microorganism. Pleural fluid should be examined if present. Blood cultures should always be obtained.

Treatment & Disposition

A. Mildly ill patients who cannot produce sputum should be started on erythromycin (base or estolate, 50 mg/kg/d orally), which is active against *M pneumoniae* and *S pneumoniae*. A tetracycline may be substituted in children 8 years of age or older but is not recommended when pneumococcal infection is strongly suspected. If a good sputum specimen can be obtained, therapy may be guided by the results of Gram-stained smears. Close follow-up is essential until it is established that recovery is well under way.

B. More severely ill children who require hospitalization should be evaluated by means of blood cultures and by nasotracheal aspiration, transtracheal aspiration, or pneumocentesis for bacteriologic diagnosis.

C. Empiric antibiotic therapy (before culture results are received) is warranted in seriously ill patients. For possible regimens, see Treatment in the preceding section.

4. PNEUMONIA IN TEENAGERS & ADULTS (Age 15 Years & Older)

In teenagers and young adults, *M pneumoniae* and *S pneumoniae* are the microorganisms most commonly causing pneumonia. In older adults, *S pneumoniae* is the most common, although many other pathogens also cause the disease. Aspiration pneumonia due to mixed anaerobic and aerobic flora is common in patients with depressed consciousness. Alcoholics are predisposed to severe pneumonia due to

Klebsiella pneumoniae and other gram-negative bacilli. Patients with chronic lung disease may develop pneumonia due to *H influenzae*. *Legionella* species are an uncommon but important cause of community-acquired pneumonia in middle-aged adults; special diagnostic tests (sputum for direct fluorescent antibody) and treatment with erythromycin is required for successful management of disease caused by this pathogen.

Diagnosis

A. Symptoms and Signs: The clinical signs of pneumonia due to *M pneumoniae* are similar to those in younger patients. In pneumonia due to other bacteria, there is often abrupt onset of malaise, fever with or without rigors, productive cough, and pleuritic chest pain. Rales and signs of consolidation are noted on physical examination. Elderly or debilitated patients may manifest only fever and obtundation. In Legionnaires' disease, high, spiking fevers, diarrhea, and delirium are especially common. Foul-smelling sputum and involvement of dependent parts of the lung suggest aspiration pneumonia due to mixed anaerobic and aerobic flora.

B. Laboratory and X-Ray Findings: Chest x-ray findings are similar to those described for mycoplasmal and other bacterial pneumonias in older children, except that pneumatoceles do not occur in adults. Bilateral pneumonia indicates severe or atypical disease (eg, septic emboli due to endocarditis; viral pneumonia). In pneumonia due to *M pneumoniae*, the white cell count is usually normal or only slightly elevated. In pneumonia due to other bacteria, leukocytosis commonly exceeds 15,000/μL. In elderly or critically ill patients, however, leukopenia with a shift to the left is not uncommon and is a poor prognostic sign. Gram-stained smear of a good sputum sample (many PMNs, few buccal epithelial cells) is the most important diagnostic test in acute pneumonia. Characteristic findings on Gram-stained smears are described in Table 34–5. Positive results on a cold agglutination test are valuable findings favoring a diagnosis of mycoplasmal pneumonia. In general, all but the smallest pleural effusions should be aspirated to rule out empyema. Fluid should be sent to the laboratory for Gram staining and culture and for measurement of protein, LDH, glucose, and pH. Blood cultures and arterial blood gas measurements should be obtained in all patients severely ill with pneumonia. Results on other laboratory tests are less specific: Prerenal azotemia is common in elderly patients; in Legionnaires' disease, hyponatremia, hypophosphatemia, and elevated liver enzyme levels are sufficiently common to be important diagnostic clues.

Treatment

Treatment should be based on the findings on

Table 34–5. Treatment of pneumonia in adults.

Microorganism	Findings on Gram-Stained Smears of Sputum	Antibiotics of First Choice	Alternative Regimens
Streptococcus pneumoniae	Gram-positive diplo-cocci or short chains	**Outpatients**	
		Procaine penicillin G, 600,000 units intra-muscularly, followed by amoxicillin, 500 mg orally 4 times daily for 10 days.	Erythromycin, 250–500 mg orally 4 times daily. Cephalexin, 500 mg orally 4 times daily for 10 days.
		Inpatients (Uncomplicated illness)	
		Penicillin G, 0.5–1 million units intrave-nously 4–6 times daily. Procaine penicillin G, 600,000 units intra-muscularly every 12 hours.	Cefazolin, 1–2 g intravenously 3 times daily. Erythromycin 250–500 mg intravenously 4 times daily.
Haemophilus in-fluenzae	Small gram-negative coccobacillary or pleo-morphic forms	**Outpatients**	
		Trimethoprim-sulfamethoxazole, 2 single-strength (trimethoprim, 80 mg; sulfame-thoxazole, 400 mg) or 1 double-strength tablet orally 2 times daily for 10 days.	Amoxicillin-clavulanic acid, 500 mg orally 3 times daily for 10 days, or cefaclor, 500 mg orally 3 times daily for 10 days.
		Inpatients	
		Cefuroxime, 750 mg–1.5 g intravenously every 8 hours.	Trimethoprim, 10 mg/kg/d, and sulfame-thoxazole, 50 mg/kg/d intravenously in 2 di-vided doses.
Staphylococcus aureus	Gram-positive cocci in clusters	Nafcillin, oxacillin, or methicillin, 2 g intrave-nously 4–6 times daily.	Cefazolin, 2 g intravenously every 8 hours. Vancomycin, 750 mg–1.0 g intravenously every 12 hours.
Mixed aerobic and anaerobic organisms	Abundant, often foul-smelling sputum with many leukocytes and mixed bacterial flora	**Community-acquired illness (Non–nursing home patients)**	
		Penicillin G, 2 million units intravenously, 4–6 times daily.[1]	Clindamycin, 600–900 mg intravenously every 8 hours.
		Nursing home or recently hospitalized patients	
		Penicillin G, 2 million units intravenously, 4–6 times daily; plus gentamicin or tobramy-cin, 5 mg/kg/d intramuscularly or intrave-nously in 3 divided doses.[1]	Clindamycin, 600–900 mg intravenously every 8 hours; plus gentamicin or tobramycin, 5 mg/kg/d intramuscularly or in-travenously in 3 divided doses.
Legionella species	Leukocytes with scant or no bacteria	Erythromycin, 1 g intravenously 4 times daily.[2]	Doxycycline[3], 100 mg intravenously or orally every 12 hours. Trimethoprim (160 mg) and sulfamethoxa-zole[3] (800 mg), intravenously every 8 hours or orally every 12 hours. Ciprofloxacin[3], 750 mg orally every 12 hours.
Mycoplasma pneumonia E Chlamydia pneu-monia	Leukocytes with scant or no bacteria	**Uncomplicated illness**	
		Erythromycin, 500 mg orally 4 times daily for 10 days.	Tetracycline, 500 mg orally 4 times daily for 10 days. Doxycycline, 100 mg intravenously or orally every 12 hours, is also effective.

[1]May add metromidazole, 15 mg/kg loading dose followed by 30 mg/kg/d intravenously in 4 divided doses (usually 500 mg intrave-nously every 6 hours).

[2]May add rifampin, 600 mg orally twice daily, in severely ill patients.

[3]Efficacy not confirmed by controlled evaluations.

Gram-stained smears of respiratory secretions or pleural fluid and on the clinical setting (Table 34–5).

A. Severely Ill Patients: In seriously ill patients with equivocal results on Gram-stained smear of sputum, empiric broad-spectrum antibiotic therapy is warranted pending results of culture. The high prevalence of *H influenzae* resistant to ampicillin (up to 30% in some communities) has made the drug less useful in empiric therapy. In such patients, a second- or third-generation cephalosporin given intravenously (eg, cefuroxime, 1.5 g every 8 hours, or ceftriaxone, 2 g every 8 hours) is satisfactory therapy for the nonimmunocompromised patient with community-acquired pneumonia. Alternatively, one may give an intravenous combination of penicillin G, 6 million units/d in 6 divided doses; methicillin, oxacillin, or nafcillin, 9–12 g/d in 4 divided doses; and gentamicin or tobramycin, 5 mg/kg/d in 3 divided doses.

B. Moderately Ill Patients: Moderately ill patients should be hospitalized and treated with parenteral antibiotics. The choice of antibiotic should be based on findings on Gram-stained smears and clinical symptoms and signs.

C. Mildly Ill Patients: Mildly ill patients may be treated on an outpatient basis with trimethoprim-sulfamethoxazole, 2 single-strength tablets orally every 12 hours, or amoxicillin-clavulanate, 250 or 500 g orally every 8 hours for 10 days. In areas where *H influenzae* resistant to ampicillin is not prevalent, ampicillin or amoxicillin may be substituted. If Gram-stained smears of sputum and the clinical presentation suggest mycoplasmal or chlamydial pneumonia, patients may be treated with erythromycin, tetracycline, or doxycycline.

Disposition

Hospitalization is indicated for most older patients with pneumonia, especially if there is preexisting pulmonary disease, and is *required* for all patients with bilateral bacterial pneumonia, regardless of age. Patients who appear well enough to be treated on an outpatient basis should be seen or telephoned daily until recovery is well under way.

SEPTIC ARTHRITIS
(See also Chapter 15.)

Septic arthritis is a medical emergency. When it is left untreated, bacterial infection rapidly destroys articular cartilage, causing permanent damage to the joint. Certain clinical settings may point to a specific pathogenic organism (Table 34–6). Septic arthritis typically affects only one or a few asymmetrically distributed joints. Joint infection superimposed on rheumatoid arthritis is not uncommon, so that in patients with rheumatoid arthritis, any joint that develops inflammation out of proportion to that in other affected joints should be aspirated to rule out the possibility of infection. Rarely, acute arthritis is caused by fungi, mumps, or hepatitis B virus, or, in women, may be due to wild or vaccine strains of rubella virus. Aspiration of the affected joint in the emergency department is often necessary to differentiate septic arthritis from other causes of synovitis, such as gout or pseudogout.

Diagnosis

A. Symptoms and Signs: Patients with septic arthritis usually have acute or subacute onset of pain, erythema, swelling, and limitation of motion in the affected joints. The arthritis more commonly affects the large joints, especially the knee. Systemic symptoms and signs of infection (malaise, fever, and leukocytosis) are common but not always present.

B. Laboratory Findings: Definitive diagnosis is established by demonstration of the infecting organism in synovial tissue or joint fluid. Blood cultures may be positive when cultures of joint fluid are negative and should be obtained in all patients thought to have septic arthritis.

1. Joint fluid analysis–(See Table 15–2.) Joint fluid shows high leukocyte counts, usually over $40,000/\mu L$, although the count may not be strikingly elevated early in the disease. The higher the white cell count in joint fluid, the greater the likelihood of bacterial or fungal arthritis. The glucose content of synovial fluid is usually lower than normal but may occasionally be normal. If no antimicrobial therapy has been given, smears and cultures of joint fluid often reveal the causative organism. Results of other laboratory tests are variable, and plain films of affected joints are usually negative early in the disease.

2. Gonococcal arthritis–In gonococcal arthritis, Gram-stained smears and cultures of joint fluid are negative in 50–75% of cases, although in most patients, cultures of exudate from the cervix, urethra, pharynx, or rectum demonstrate gonococci. Because the gonococcus is a fastidious organism, demonstration of its growth in cultures depends upon prompt processing of specimens by the laboratory. Since special handling is also required, all specimens submitted should bear the instruction "Rule out gonorrhea." Prompt response to antimicrobial therapy helps to confirm the diagnosis in gonococcal arthritis.

Treatment

A. Aspirate affected joints, and repeat as often as necessary to evacuate reaccumulating joint fluid. Aspiration is necessary to minimize enzymatic and toxic damage to articular cartilage. Open drainage is usually not necessary except for infections in inaccessible joints, such as the hip. Open drainage is almost never required in gonococcal arthritis.

B. High doses of intravenous antibiotics should be given. Intra-articular instillation of antibiotics is unnecessary, since high antibiotic levels are attained in synovial fluid when drugs are given intravenously.

Table 34–6. Septic arthritis.

Patient Group	Microorganisms	Joints Typically Affected	Common Associated Findings	Antibiotics of Choice[1]
Children Age 2 months to 5 years	*Haemophilus influenzae, Staphylococcus areus,* streptococci	Knee, hip, ankle	Sometimes none; bacteremia, contiguous osteomyelitis, cellulitis	PRSP[2] plus cefotaxime, or cefotaxime alone
Age over 3 years	*S aureus,* streptococci	Hip, knee, ankle	Often none	Nafcillin, oxacillin, or methicillin
Sexually active patients	*Neisseria gonorrhoeae*	One or more large joints	Urethritis, tenosynovitis, skin lesions	Ceftriaxone
Patients with sickle cell anemia	*Streptococcus pneumoniae, S aureus, Salmonella* species	Usually large joints	Sickle cell crisis	Ampicillin and chloramphenicol or cefotaxime
Patients with rheumatoid arthritis	*S aureus*	One or more joints	Advanced rheumatoid arthritis, decubitus or vasculitic ulcers, corticosteroid therapy, prior arthrocentesis	Nafcillin, oxacillin, methicillin, or vancomycin
Intravenous drug abusers	*S aureus*	Any joint	Staphylococcal endocarditis	Nafcillin, oxacillin, methicillin, or vancomycin
	Gram-negative bacilli especially *Serratia marcescens* and *Pseudomonas aeruginosa*	Sternoclavicular, sternochondral, or sacroiliac joint	Contiguous osteomyelitis or abscess	Aminoglycoside with APP[3]
Debilitated, immunosuppressed, or elderly patients	Aerobic gram-negative bacilli	Usually large joints	Concurrent or recent extraarticular infection with or without bacteremia	Aminoglycosides with ticarcillin or a third-generation cephalosporin
	S aureus			Nafcillin, oxacillin, methicillin, or vancomycin

[1]Give antibiotics intravenously and in high doses (Table 34–13).
[2]PRSP = Penicillinase-resistant antistaphylococcal penicillin (nafcillin, oxacillin, methicillin).
[3]APP = Antipseudomonal penicillin (carbenicillin, ticarcillin, mezlocillin, azlocillin, piperacillin).

If no organisms are seen on Gram-stained smears of synovial fluid but other findings suggest septic arthritis, empiric antibiotic therapy based on the type of patient and clinical findings (Table 34–6) should be started pending results of culture and sensitivity testing.

Disposition

Hospitalize all patients with suspected or documented septic arthritis.

OSTEOMYELITIS

Osteomyelitis is an infection of bone that affects all age groups. The infecting organisms are bacteria (most often), mycobacteria, or fungi. For purposes of discussion, osteomyelitis can be classified into different groups on the basis of the pathogenic mechanism: (1) hematogenous osteomyelitis, (2) osteomyelitis secondary to a contiguous focus of infection; and (3) osteomyelitis associated with peripheral vascular disease. Hematogenous osteomyelitis is common in children, although its incidence is increasing in older age groups. Hematogenous osteomyelitis in adults usually involves the vertebral bodies. Spread of disease from a contiguous focus of infection is the most common pathogenic mechanism in adults. Osteomyelitis associated with vascular insufficiency is seen almost exclusively in adults with diabetes mellitus or severe peripheral vascular disease.

In both children and adults, the most commonly involved bones are the long bones, especially those of the lower extremities; this is particularly true in children. Orthopedic procedures or traumatic wounds predispose to osteomyelitis of the extremities.

Diagnosis

A. Symptoms and Signs:

1. **Hematogenous osteomyelitis–**In children, abrupt onset of high fever, systemic toxicity, and physical findings of local suppuration surrounding the involved bone (local pain, swelling, and tenderness) are typical. The child is often unwilling to move the affected extremity.

In adults, the disease may be more indolent, particularly in patients with vertebral osteomyelitis. About half of patients may have pain, swelling, chills, and fever. Patients with vertebral osteomyelitis may have low-grade or intermittent fever or back pain which may be either severe or only "nagging" and which may not cause extreme discomfort or immobility until late in the disease. Focal tenderness over the dorsal spines of the involved vertebral bodies may be the only physical finding.

2. Osteomyelitis secondary to contiguous infection–The most common predisposing factor is postoperative infection, such as that following open reduction of fractures. Extension of soft tissue infection to bone from infected fingers and toes, infected teeth, or infected sinuses also occurs. Most patients are over 50 years of age and may present with fever, swelling, and erythema in the initial episode. During recurrences, sinus formation and drainage are the major presenting signs.

3. Osteomyelitis associated with vascular insufficiency–Patients with osteomyelitis associated with vascular insufficiency invariably have diabetes mellitus or severe peripheral vascular disease. The toes and small bones of the feet are usually affected. Local signs and symptoms such as pain, swelling, redness, or frank cellulitis with deep ulcers in the soft tissue are prominent. Pain is often absent because of diabetic neuropathy.

B. Laboratory Studies: Routine laboratory tests are of limited value in the diagnosis of osteomyelitis. The leukocyte count is often elevated in acute disease but may be normal in more chronic infection. The erythrocyte sedimentation rate is elevated in most patients.

Radiographic procedures are the primary diagnostic tool, although plain films may not show signs of disease for 10–14 days after onset of symptoms. The earliest visible x-ray changes are adjacent soft tissue swelling and periosteal reaction. Lytic lesions and areas of sclerosis may then develop. If osteomyelitis is suspected and plain films fail to show any signs of disease, CT scan or technetium bone scan should be performed. The diagnosis is confirmed by culture and histologic examination of bone. Bacteriologic findings vary, and cultures should be obtained from bone (needle aspiration, surgical biopsy) or blood (results are positive in 50% of cases in patients with acute hematogenous osteomyelitis).

Treatment

The most important therapeutic measures are systemic antibiotics and surgery to drain abscesses or debride necrotic tissue. The selection of an antibiotic depends on identification of the causative organism. If the disease is uncomplicated (ie, involves a long bone in a patient without underlying medical problems), if the patient is a child, or if the patient is critically ill, then antistaphylococcal therapy should be initiated, since *S aureus* is the most common infecting organism. See Table 34–7 for the pathogens most often associated with osteomyelitis in different patient groups and the suggested antibiotic regimens for each.

Surgery in acute osteomyelitis should be limited to biopsy for diagnosis, drainage of suppurative areas, and debridement of necrotic bone. Surgical drainage is also indicated if neurologic abnormalities are present or develop in vertebral or cranial osteomyelitis or if infection spreads to the hip joint in a child.

Disposition

Patients with acute osteomyelitis should be hospitalized for intravenous antimicrobial therapy.

PHARYNGITIS

Acute pharyngitis is inflammation of the pharynx often caused by viral and bacterial infections. The physician's most important task in the evaluation of pharyngitis is to identify and treat group A streptococcal infection and to recognize less common causes of pharyngitis associated with more serious systemic illness. Viral infections are responsible for many cases of sore throat.

Diagnosis

A. Symptoms and Signs:

1. Group A streptococcal infection–The signs and symptoms of pharyngitis caused by group A streptococci vary and include fever, sore throat, anterior cervical adenopathy, headache, beefy red pharynx, tonsillar exudate, lymphatic hyperplasia, and scarlatiniform rash. The so-called classic findings of high fever, pharyngeal exudate, and anterior cervical adenopathy only suggest streptococcal pharyngitis and do not confirm the diagnosis. The 3 clinical features that are most helpful in differentiating streptococcal from viral pharyngitis are fever of 38.9 °C (102 °F) or higher, painful cervical adenitis, and absence of flulike symptoms such as cough and coryza.

2. Infectious mononucleosis–Acute infection by Epstein-Barr virus (the etiologic agent of infectious mononucleosis), by adenovirus, or by the human immunodeficiency virus (HIV) may produce an exudative pharyngitis with fever, posterior cervical adenopathy, malaise, and enlarged spleen. Patients with acute cytomegalovirus infection may have pharyngeal soreness, but examination shows a few findings of note.

3. Diphtheria–Diphtheria should be considered in patients with exudative or membranous pharyngitis in whom the status of immunization for diphtheria is either incomplete or in question. The characteristic tonsillar or pharyngeal membrane varies from light to dark gray and is firmly attached to the tonsillar and pharyngeal mucosa. Toxemia and tachycardia out of proportion to the degree of fever are other clues.

4. Vincent's angina–Vincent's angina is a membranous pharyngitis caused by a mixture of anaerobic and microaerophilic bacteria and spirochetes. It is generally encountered in children and young adults and characterized by foul breath, cervical lymphadenitis, and low-grade fever in association

Table 34–7. Acute osteomyelitis.

Patient Group	Organisms	Clinical Findings	Antibiotics[1] (Alone or Combination)
Newborns	Staphylococcus aureus, Escherichia coli	High incidence of multiple bone involvement; rapidly lytic lesions; infants exposed to complications during pregnancy or delivery.	PRSP,[2] or vancomycin plus aminoglycoside or cefotaxime.
	Group B streptococcus	Healthy neonate; single bone, often in the upper limb.	Ampicillin or penicillin. Consider adding aminoglycoside.
Children (≤ 15 years of age)	S aureus, streptococci, Haemophilus influenzae	Hematogenous spread; long bones.	PRSP.[2] Consider adding cefotaxime.
Adults	S aureus, streptococci, Enterobacteriaceae	Vertebral osteomyelitis.	PRSP,[2] aminoglycoside, penicillin G, third-generation cephalosporin.
Intravenous drug abusers	S aureus, Pseudomonas, Seratia, Candida	Involvement of vertebrae, ribs, sternoclavicular joint, pelvis.	PRSP,[2] aminoglycoside. Treat Candida infection only after organism has been identified in culture.
Patients with hemoglobinopathy (SS, SC)	Streptococci, S aureus, Salmonella	Vertebrae or long bones.	Penicillin G, PRSP,[2] ampicillin, chloramphenicol, trimethoprim-sulfamethoxazole cefotaxime.
Diabetics Patients with peripheral vascular disease	Mixed infections common (S aureus, streptococci, aerobic gram-negative bacilli, anaerobes [including Bacteroides fragilis])	Toes and small bones of feet.	First- or third-generation cephalosporin, aminoglycoside PRSP,[2] metronidazole.
Immunocompromised patients	Fungi (Candida, Aspergillus, Rhizopus), aerobic gram-negative bacilli, gram-positive cocci	Vertebral disease most common; associated with prolonged intravenous therapy and parenteral nutrition.	Diagnosis confirmed by biopsy. Culture must be obtained before therapy is started.

[1]See Table 34–13 for parenteral dosage.
[2]PRSP = Penicillinase-resistant antistaphylococcal penicillin (nafcillin, oxacillin, methicillin).

with membranous pharyngitis. Removal of the necrotic gray pseudomembrane usually results in bleeding.

Other causes of pharyngitis include *M pneumoniae, N gonorrhoeae, Chlamydia trachomatis,* and secondary syphilis. See Chapter 26 for discussion of peritonsillar abscess, Ludwig's angina, epiglottitis, and parapharyngeal and retropharyngeal abscesses.

B. Laboratory Findings: Definitive diagnosis of group A streptococcal pharyngitis can be made by results on culture of exudate from the throat and demonstration of a rise in titers to ASO or other streptococcal products, since many people are asymptomatic carriers of group A streptococci.

The American Heart Association has revised its recommendations for throat cultures before antibiotic therapy. Throat cultures are considered "valuable" for children and adolescents and "not as essential" for adults. They are indicated primarily to avoid the unnecessary use of antibiotics for the 70–80% of adult patients with pharyngitis due to viruses. In the patient with culture-proved streptococcal pharyngitis, follow-up test-of-cure throat cultures are not indicated unless the patient remains symptomatic. Cultures of

asymptomatic family members and contacts should be reserved for special circumstances, eg, if the patient has a history of rheumatic fever or if there is an epidemic of group A streptococcal pharyngitis. An elevated white cell count (≥ 12,000/μL) suggests bacterial pharyngitis. Obtain a heterophil agglutination test or mononucleosis spot test in patients thought to have infectious mononucleosis.

Treatment

Begin empiric treatment in children and young adults if they have the classic signs and symptoms of streptococcal pharyngitis, scarlatiniform rash, or a history of rheumatic fever or valvular heart disease, or if illness occurs during an epidemic of group A streptococcal infection. A throat culture is not necessary in most cases because its results would not influence the management strategy. Effective antibiotic regimens are penicillin V, 250 mg orally 4 times a day for 10 days, or benzathine penicillin G, 1.2 million units intramuscularly (children < 10 years of age, 600,000 units; children 10–15 years of age, 900,000 units). For a patient with penicillin allergy, erythromycin, 250 mg orally 4 times a day for 10 days, is suggested. For both penicillin V and erythromycin, a full 10 days of therapy is necessary to eradicate infection and prevent rheumatic fever.

Patients with a sore throat but no other features of streptococcal pharyngitis should receive symptomatic therapy (throat lozenges, saline gargles). A throat culture is not necessary. Patients with sore throat and one or 2 features (fever, exudate, or adenopathy) have an intermediate chance of having streptococcal pharyngitis. A throat culture may be useful to avoid unnecessary use of antibiotics and to provide reassurance to the patient. Antibiotic treatment should be withheld until the results of the culture are known.

Disposition

Patients with pharyngitis without complications may be treated on an outpatient basis. Patients thought to have diphtheria, Vincent's angina, epiglottitis, or possible localized abscess should be hospitalized.

URINARY TRACT INFECTION

1. ACUTE LOWER URINARY TRACT INFECTION (Uncomplicated Cystitis)

Uncomplicated bacterial cystitis is defined as urinary tract infection confined to the bladder. It affects women more commonly than men and tends to recur even in the absence of anatomic abnormalities. Many patients with apparent lower urinary tract infection also have asymptomatic involvement of the upper urinary tract (absence of fever, chills, flank pain).

Most cystitis is caused by bacterial infection, usually *E coli* and other enteric gram-negative bacilli, *Staphylococcus saprophyticus,* and enterococcus *(Streptococcus faecalis).* However, adenovirus infection is a common cause of acute hemorrhagic cystitis in children and, occasionally, young adults.

Diagnosis

A. Symptoms and Signs:

1. A history of urinary tract infections is frequently elicited.

2. Dysuria and urinary frequency and urgency are the most common symptoms in adults, although they may be absent in children. The patient may report that the urine is cloudy, smelly, or dark.

3. Suprapubic discomfort and tenderness are common.

4. The patient is usually afebrile or has a low-grade fever. The presence of high fever (> 38.3 °C [101 °F]) or rigors is inconsistent with a diagnosis of uncomplicated cystitis and suggests pyelonephritis.

5. Nausea and vomiting, though uncommon in adults, are not unusual in children with uncomplicated cystitis.

B. Laboratory Findings:

1. Urinalysis–Accurate diagnosis of urinary tract infection depends on obtaining a urine specimen uncontaminated by perineal secretions. The presence of squamous epithelial cells or of mixed flora on Gram-stained smears suggests contamination, and the specimen should be discarded and a better one obtained (see Dysuria in Chapter 31). Urine should be examined while it is fresh (within 1 hour) or should be refrigerated if delay is expected.

a. Chemistry–Mild degrees of proteinuria and hematuria are common on dipstick tests of urine. If the infection is caused by a urea-splitting bacterium (eg, *Proteus mirabilis*), urinary pH may be abnormally high (pH 6–8). The leukocyte esterase dipstick test is a reliable indicator of infection. Chemical tests for the presence of bacteria in urine (eg, nitrate reduction) are not sensitive and specific enough to be generally recommended.

b. Sediment–Many leukocytes and often some erythrocytes are present. Clumps of leukocytes must be differentiated from white blood cell casts, which signify upper urinary tract involvement. In most cases, numerous bacteria are visible.

c. Gram-stained smears–Microscopic examination of Gram-stained specimens of urinary sediment from centrifuged urine usually shows bacteria of a single morphologic type. If uncentrifuged urine is examined and if there is an average of one bacterium per oil-immersion field, there is about an 80% probability that there are 10^5 organisms per milliliter of urine (strongly indicative of infection).

2. Urine culture–In women of childbearing age with a history of recurrent cystitis (2–3 times per year) who are otherwise healthy, treatment may be started on the basis of the results of urinalysis alone, and urine culture may be postponed until 1 week after treatment (test-of-cure culture) or may be omitted in patients who do well. In all other patients, quantitative urine cultures should be obtained. Growth of at least 100,000 (10^5) organisms of a single species per milliliter of urine indicates a high probability of active urinary tract infection. However, in symptomatic but otherwise healthy young women with pyuria, smaller numbers (10^2–10^4/mL) of bacteria (especially a single species) are significant and indicate the need for therapy (see Dysuria-Frequency Syndrome, below).

Treatment

A. Antimicrobials:

1. Nonpregnant women of childbearing age who have a history of recurrent cystitis and findings compatible with uncomplicated cystitis may be treated with a short course (3 days) of therapy. Single-dose therapy has fallen into disfavor because of the frequency of relapse and because it requires that the patient be seen at a follow-up appointment 2–4 days later for a test-of-cure urine culture. All other patients should receive multidose therapy for at least 7–10 days. Because men often harbor occult infection in the prostate or kidney, some authorities recommend that treatment be extended for at least 3 weeks in an effort to prevent relapse of infection.

2. Select an antimicrobial from those set forth in Table 34–8. Trimethoprim-sulfamethoxazole and ciprofloxacin, because of their good penetration into the prostate and high level of activity against uropathogens, are recommended for men with urinary tract infection who have normal serum creatinine levels.

B. Adjunctive Measures: Phenazopyridine (Pyridium, many others), 200 mg orally 3 times a day, may help relieve severe dysuria (warn the patient that urine will turn orange). Give the drug only for 2–3 days.

C. Follow-Up: In uncomplicated cystitis, follow-up urine cultures are optional in patients who respond to therapy. Patients treated with single-dose or 3-day therapy whose symptoms recur should have a urine culture and be treated with a 10-day course of therapy.

Disposition

Infants, children, and men with diagnosed urinary tract infection should be treated and referred to a urologist. Urologic referral is also recommended for women with frequent recurrences of cystitis (monthly) and probably also for those who have had 3 or more infections in 1 year, although the latter recommendation is controversial. Hospitalization is not indicated for patients with uncomplicated cystitis.

2. DYSURIA-FREQUENCY SYNDROME

The dysuria-frequency syndrome (urethral syndrome) occurs by definition only in women, usually

Table 34–8. Antimicrobials for treatment of acute urinary tract infection.[1]

Multidose therapy (3 days or 7–10 days)[2]
  Trimethoprim-sulfamethoxazole, 1 double-strength
    (trimethoprim 160 mg; sulfamethoxazole, 800 mg) tablet
    twice daily
  Sulfisoxazole, 1 g orally 4 times daily (loading dose
    unnecessary)
  Nitrofurantoin, 100 mg orally 4 times daily
  Ciprofloxacin, 500 mg orally twice daily
Single-dose therapy[3]
  Trimethroprim-sulfamethoxazole, 2 double-strength tablets
    orally

[1]This is not a complete list. The drugs shown are selected because they are effective and nontoxic.
[2]Dosages shown are for adults.
[3]Single-dose therapy is no longer recommended but may be used for uncomplicated cystitis with close patient follow-up (see text).

young women. These patients have symptoms of lower urinary tract infection but have urine cultures that are sterile or contain fewer than 105 organisms per milliliter of urine. Patients with dysuria-frequency syndrome may be divided into 2 groups: those with accompanying pyuria (> 10 leukocytes per × 100 field) and those without. In women with pyuria, symptoms are usually due either to a low-grade bacterial cystitis (bacteriuria with < 100,000 organisms per milliliter of urine) or to chlamydial urethritis with or without accompanying chlamydial cervicitis. *N gonorrhoeae* also causes urethritis and must be ruled out. Herpes simplex virus causes urethritis during primary infection and, on occasion, during recurrent infection. In some patients with pyuria and in most patients who lack pyuria, no causative agent can be identified.

Diagnosis

A. Symptoms and Signs: The principal symptoms are those of cystitis: dysuria, urgency, and frequency. The dysuria is "internal" dysuria as opposed to the "external" dysuria which is seen in vaginitis or genital herpes simplex infection and which results from urine coming in contact with denuded skin. Findings on physical examination are normal except that there may be urethral inflammation or mucopurulent cervical discharge and cervical edema in patients whose symptoms are due to gonococcal or chlamydial infection. Pelvic examination is important to rule out vaginitis, which may also cause dysuria.

B. Laboratory Findings: The urine may be normal or contain PMNs with few or absent bacteria. Swabs of urethral discharge should be obtained for smear and culture for *N gonorrhoeae* in patients with a history of gonorrhea, in those with multiple sexual partners, and in those whose recent sexual partner has had urethritis. Urine culture shows scant growth (< 10^5 bacteria per milliliter) or no growth of organisms. A cervical swab for *Chlamydia* antigen (fluorescent or ELISA slide test) is indicated in sexually active women with cervicitis accompanying this syndrome, since this organism causes concurrent cervicitis and urethritis (p 630). Results of other laboratory tests are normal.

Treatment

Antimicrobial therapy is usually reserved for those patients with pyuria. Tetracyclines and erythromycin are the most effective drugs for suspected chlamydial infection; other bacterial pathogens may be resistant to these drugs. Optimal treatment of chlamydial infection requires 7 days of therapy. Short-course, 3-day therapy may be tried initially in patients with low-grade bacteriuria (< 10^5 organisms per milliliter). None of the single-dose regimens listed provide reliable empiric therapy for both chlamydial and bacterial infection. Multidose regimens for *Chlamydia* include (**1**) doxycycline, 100 mg orally 2 times a day for 7 days; (**2**) tetracycline, 500 mg orally 4 times a day for 7 days; or (**3**) erythromycin, 500 mg 4 times daily for 7 days.

Disposition

Because of the difficulties of empiric therapy in the urethral syndrome, a follow-up visit to a primary-care physician should be arranged. If ordinary bacterial cultures of urine are sterile in patients with pyuria, the patient's sexual partners should probably be screened for urethritis and *Chlamydia* infection.

3. PYELONEPHRITIS
(Upper Urinary Tract Infection)

Acute pyelonephritis is symptomatic inflammatory bacterial infection of the kidney. Because it most commonly results from ascending spread of infection up the ureters from the bladder, it is usually caused by the same organisms that cause cystitis *(E coli, P mirabilis)*. In elderly men, pyelonephritis may be caused by *S faecalis*. In patients who have received prior antimicrobial therapy (eg, during recent hospitalization, because of chronic indwelling Foley catheter) the infecting organisms may be resistant to commonly used antimicrobials. *Pregnant patients are especially prone to upper urinary tract infection.* Because pyelonephritis in pregnancy is associated with an increased risk of premature delivery, pregnant patients with urinary tract infection should always receive multidose antimicrobial therapy.

Diagnosis

A. Symptoms and Signs: Pyelonephritis is characterized by symptoms of cystitis (dysuria, urgency, and frequency) accompanied by flank pain and tenderness. Fever, rigors, and—in patients with complicating bacteremia or endotoxemia—systemic signs of sepsis (eg, hypotension, delirium) may be present. In pyelonephritis occurring as a complication of nephrolithiasis, severe flank pain radiating to the groin may be the most prominent symptom. In patients with sickle cell disease, diabetes, or nephropathy caused by analgesic abuse, necrosis of the renal papillae with sloughing into the ureters occurs as a complication of renal infection, and the patient may present with symptoms of ureteral obstruction that mimic nephrolithiasis. It is important to identify patients with ureteral obstruction, as they are often very ill.

B. Laboratory Findings:

1. Urine—The findings on urinalysis, microscopic examination, and culture are the same in cystitis (see above) except that leukocyte casts are seen only with pyelonephritis. Gross hematuria and pain suggest pyelonephritis complicating urolithiasis.

Send urine for culture and susceptibility testing in all patients with suspected pyelonephritis.

2. Blood—Blood cultures should be obtained in all patients with pyelonephritis who are ill enough to receive intravenous therapy.

3. Other laboratory studies—Serum electrolyte, blood urea nitrogen, and creatinine measurements should be obtained, since azotemia may be present. The white cell count is usually elevated. A normal or low white cell count with a shift to the left in a patient with suspected pyelonephritis is often a sign of sepsis, indicating the need for hospitalization.

C. X-Ray Findings and Other Examinations: Some authorities suggest that excretory urography be performed in all nonpregnant women with pyelonephritis after the infection has cleared. In patients with pyelonephritis in whom urinary obstruction is suspected, radiologic and other examinations should be performed as soon as possible (see Urolithiasis in Chapter 31). Ultrasonography is a safe and sensitive means of assessing hydronephrosis and may reveal intrarenal and perinephric abscesses. Remember that in pregnancy some degree of ureteral dilatation (usually greater in the right ureter than in the left) is normal.

Treatment

A. Antimicrobials:

1. Outpatients may be treated with trimethoprim-sulfamethoxazole, 1 double-strength tablet (trimethoprim, 160 mg; sulfamethoxazole, 800 mg) twice daily; or ciprofloxacin, 500 mg orally twice daily. Ampicillin or amoxicillin, 500 mg orally 4 times daily, should be used only if the organism is shown to be sensitive to ampicillin on susceptibility testing or if the patient is in an area where ampicillin-resistant *E coli* is uncommon. Patients should be treated for at least 14 days. Patients with anatomic abnormalities of the urinary tract or concomitant prostatitis may require up to 6 weeks of therapy.

2. Inpatients may be treated with a first- or third-generation cephalosporin equivalent to cephalothin, 4–6 g/d intravenously. Ampicillin, 4–6 g/d, may be used to treat susceptible organisms. In patients with suspected bacteremia or suspected infection due to antibiotic-resistant organisms, an aminoglycoside (Table 34–1) should be added.

B. General Measures:

1. If vomiting or dehydration is present, begin intravenous fluid replacement with crystalloid solutions.

2. Provide analgesia for flank pain as needed.

3. Give antipyretics for high fever regularly (rather than as needed) until the patient is afebrile.

Disposition

A. Patients who meet the criteria listed below or who have any of the following conditions should be hospitalized:

1. Severe unilateral costovertebral angle tenderness (possible renal carbuncle or perinephric abscess).

2. Suspected bacteremia (high fever, rigors, hypotension, or shock).

3. Complicating conditions, eg, severe vomiting unresponsive to antiemetic medication, azotemia, electrolyte abnormalities, pregnancy, or poorly controlled diabetes.

4. Suspected or known anatomic abnormalities (obstruction, papillary necrosis, etc).

5. Recent hospitalization, especially if the patient received an indwelling urinary catheter (the danger is development of a nosocomial infection resistant to treatment with the usual antimicrobials).

6. Infants, children, older men (> age 45 years), debilitated or elderly patients of either sex.

B. Patients who are not hospitalized should receive a follow-up appointment within 1–2 days to assess the response to therapy.

C. Some patients with pyelonephritis, especially young women, may not be sick enough for hospitalization but do not appear well enough to be treated at home. In these patients, a 12- to 24-hour period of intravenous antimicrobial therapy, intravenous hydration, and observation in the emergency department may be indicated. If rapid resolution of signs and symptoms occurs, the patient may be discharged with a prescription for oral antimicrobials and a follow-up appointment in 1–2 days.

DISEASES OF THE FEMALE GENITOURINARY TRACT
(See also Sexually Transmitted Diseases.)

1. PELVIC INFLAMMATORY DISEASE

Infection of the uterine tubes may be acute or chronic and unilateral or bilateral. It may lead to pyosalpinx or tubo-ovarian abscess. Pelvic peritonitis is frequently present as well. Causative agents include *C trachomatis, N gonorrhoeae,* anaerobic bacteria (which include *Bacteroides* and gram-positive cocci), facultative gram-negative bacilli (such as *E coli*), *Mycoplasma hominis,* and rarely *Actinomyces israelii.* In the individual patient it is often impossible to differentiate among these agents, and treatment regimens that are active against the broadest possible range of these pathogens should be used. Salpingitis must be distinguished from ectopic pregnancy, appendicitis, and ruptured ovarian cyst (see Table 30–2).

Diagnosis
A. Symptoms and Signs: Patients are usually young (< 30 years old) and sexually active. Symptoms include fever (sometimes with rigors), severe pelvic pain (usually bilateral) that may be either continuous or crampy, dyspareunia, menstrual disturbances, vaginal discharge, and gastrointestinal disturbances (anorexia, nausea and vomiting, constipation). Patients are usually menstruating or else have just finished their periods.

Physical examination in acute cases discloses marked tenderness on manipulation of the cervix and palpation of the adnexa. There is a unilateral tender adnexal mass if tubo-ovarian abscess or pyosalpinx is present.

B. Laboratory Tests and Special Examinations: There is usually leukocytosis or an elevated erythrocyte sedimentation rate. A serum pregnancy test should be obtained to detect pregnancy and to rule out ectopic pregnancy. Culdocentesis (see Fig 30–1) is a valuable diagnostic aid. Purulent fluid should be cultured for aerobic and anaerobic pathogens and specifically for *N gonorrhoeae* and *Chlamydia.* Ultrasonography may be helpful for detecting or assessing the size of tubo-ovarian abscess.

Treatment
A. Antibiotic Therapy: The treatment of choice is not established. No single agent is active against the entire spectrum of pathogens. Several antibiotic combinations do provide a broad spectrum of activity against the major pathogens, but none have been adequately evaluated. Treatment with penicillin, ampicillin, amoxicillin, or a cephalosporin alone is not recommended. The following regimens are recommended by the Centers for Disease Control:

1. Outpatients–

a. Cefoxitin, 2 g intramuscularly, plus probenecid, 1 g orally, or ceftriaxone, 250 mg intramuscularly, are the preferred treatments. This initial treatment should be followed by doxycycline, 100 mg orally twice daily for 10–14 days.

b. Tetracycline, 500 mg orally every 6 hours, may be substituted for doxycycline but is less well absorbed, is less active against certain anaerobes, and requires more frequent dosing than doxycycline; these are potentially important drawbacks of its use in the treatment of pelvic inflammatory disease.

2. Hospitalized patients–

a. Doxycycline, 100 mg intravenously or orally twice daily, plus cefoxitin, 2 g intravenously every 6 hours, or cefotetan, 2 g intravenously every 12 hours, should be given. Continue to administer the drugs intravenously for at least 48 hours after the patient's condition improves. Then continue doxycycline, 100 mg orally twice daily to complete 10–14 days of therapy.

b. Clindamycin, 900 mg intravenously every 8 hours, plus gentamicin, 2 mg/kg intravenously as a loading dose followed by 1.5 mg/kg every 8 hours, in patients with normal renal function. Continue to administer the drugs intravenously for at least 48 hours after patient's condition improves. Then continue clindamycin, 450 mg orally 5 times daily to complete 10–14 days of therapy.

c. Pelvic inflammatory disease in prepubertal children is rare. These patients may receive either cefuroxime, 150 mg/kg intravenously daily, or ceftriaxone, 100 mg/kg intravenously daily plus erythromycin, 40 mg/kg/d in 4 doses intravenously. Alternatively, sulfasoxazole, 100 mg/kg/d in 4 doses intravenously, or, in children older than 7 years, tetracycline, 30 mg/kg/d in 3 doses intravenously, may be given. Continue the intravenous regimen as recommended above for hospitalized adults. Thereafter, continue the erythromycin, sulfasoxazole, or tetracycline orally to complete at least 14 days of therapy. *Note:* Pelvic infection in prepubertal children should raise the suspicion of child abuse.

B. Reevaluation: Patients who are not hospitalized should be reevaluated in 2–4 days and hospitalized if their condition has not markedly improved.

C. Adjunctive Measures:

1. Relieve pain. Narcotics are frequently required.

2. If present, an IUD should be removed as soon as adequate antibiotic levels are achieved in the blood.

3. Surgery should be delayed at least 2–3 days until the effect of antibiotic therapy can be assessed, even if pyosalpinx or tubo-ovarian abscess is present. Pelvic abscesses often regress with antibiotic therapy alone or may drain externally via the vagina or rectum. Repeated ultrasound examinations help to determine the patient's progress.

Disposition

Generally accepted indications for admission are listed in Table 34–9. Many experts hospitalize all but the mildest cases of pelvic inflammatory disease because of the severity of long-term sequelae.

2. VAGINITIS

Vaginitis is a common and annoying disorder that in the absence of other symptoms or signs rarely indicates serious disease. Common pathogens include *Candida albicans, Trichomonas vaginalis, Gardnerella vaginalis* with anaerobic bacteria (bacterial

Table 34–9. Indications for hospitalization for patients with acute pelvic inflammatory disease.

Diagnosis is uncertain.
Surgical emergencies such as appendicitis and ectopic pregnancy cannot be excluded.
Pelvic or tubo-ovarian abscess is suspected.
The patient is an adolescent.
Severe illness (vomiting) precludes outpatient management.
Patient is pregnant.
Patient is unable to follow or tolerate an outpatient regimen.
Patient has failed to respond to outpatient therapy.
Clinical follow-up 48–72 hours after the start of antibiotic treatment cannot be arranged.

vaginosis), and gonococci (in prepubertal girls). Other common causes are estrogen deficiency (atrophic vaginitis) and vaginal foreign body. Systemic antibiotics (especially tetracyclines), oral contraceptives, diabetes mellitus, primary genital herpes simplex virus infection, and pregnancy predispose to development of candidiasis.

Less common causes include allergy, cervicitis, polyps, tumors, vaginal ulcer, shigellosis, irradiation for cancer, and certain bubble bath preparations.

Diagnosis

A. Symptoms and Signs: Vaginal discharge and pruritus are the chief symptoms. Vaginal discharge with varying degrees of inflammation of the vaginal wall (minimal in atrophic vaginitis) is usually found. Search for foreign bodies in the vagina, particularly in young girls, and examine for associated disorders (eg, salpingitis).

B. Laboratory Tests:

1. Examination of smears–

a. Gram's stain–Look for *Candida* and *G vaginalis* (small gram-negative rods usually closely associated with epithelial cells ["clue cells"]). Methylene blue stain also demonstrates these cells. Vaginitis due to *Candida* or *Trichomonas* is usually associated with a polymorphonuclear exudate, whereas inflammatory cells are absent in bacterial vaginosis caused by *G vaginalis.* In prepubertal girls with gonococcal vulvovaginitis, Gram's stain of smears usually shows typical gram-negative intracellular diplococci, but cultures should be performed to confirm the diagnosis.

b. Saline wet mount–Look for motile trichomonads. *Candida* and clue cells of *G vaginalis* may also be seen.

c. KOH (potassium hydroxide) wet mount–Addition of a few drops of potassium hydroxide to a sample of vaginal secretions releases a typical amine odor ("fishy") in cases of bacterial vaginosis due to *G vaginalis.* Microscopic examination reveals *Candida* in cases of *Candida* vaginitis, but Gram staining is more sensitive and specific.

2. Urinalysis–Obtain a clean-catch urine specimen for analysis and culture if dysuria is present (Chapter 31).

3. Other tests–Fasting blood glucose measurements should be obtained in cases of recurrent candidiasis to rule out diabetes mellitus.

Treatment

A. General Measures:

1. Avoid systemic antibiotic therapy, if possible.

2. Advise adequate perineal ventilation. Patients should wear loose cotton underpants with skirts and avoid pantyhose and tight pants.

3. Sitz baths may give relief.

4. Occasional douches with white vinegar (2 tablespoons per quart [30 mL/L] of warm water) may provide symptomatic relief but seldom influence recovery.

5. Advise the patient to avoid intercourse for a few days after treatment.

6. Treat both the patient and her partner, as described below.

B. Specific Measures:

1. *C albicans* **vaginitis–**

a. **Imidazole regimens–**

(1) Miconazole nitrate (vaginal suppositories, 200 mg) or clotrimazole (vaginal suppositories, 200 mg), intravaginally at bedtime for 3 days are effective; or

(2) Butoconazole (2% cream, 5 g), intravaginally at bedtime for 3 days; or

(3) Terconazole, 80-mg suppository or 0.4% cream, intravaginally at bedtime for 3 days.

b. **Reinfection–**The male partner should wear a condom, or both should abstain from intercourse for 2–3 days; if the man has balanitis or if vaginitis due to *C albicans* recurs promptly after treatment has been stopped, the man should be treated with an antifungal cream (see ¶B1, above) applied to the penis twice daily for 1 week. Balanitis due to *Candida* occurs almost exclusively in uncircumcised men. Occasionally, the patient's gastrointestinal tract is a reservoir for *Candida,* in which case oral nonabsorbable antifungal preparations (eg, nystatin) are necessary.

2. *T vaginalis* **vaginitis–**Give both the patient and her sexual partner metronidazole, 2 g orally in a single dose (eight 250-mg tablets). This regimen produces cure in about 95% of cases. Metronidazole may be weakly carcinogenic and may be teratogenic (it is contraindicated in early pregnancy and during lactation, and its safety during the rest of pregnancy has not yet been established). Gastrointestinal upset and a metallic taste in the mouth are common. Because metronidazole also exerts an effect similar to that of disulfiram (nausea and vomiting after consumption of alcohol), patients should avoid alcohol for 48 hours after taking the medication. An alternative regimen is metronidazole, 250 mg orally 3 times daily for 7 days.

Resistance of *T vaginalis* to metronidazole has been observed but is rare. In case of proved treatment failure, the patient should be treated again with the same regimen. Persistent treatment failure should be addressed in consultation with an expert.

3. **Bacterial vaginosis–** Several species of vaginal bacteria (including *G vaginalis*) interact to produce this syndrome. Metronidazole, 500 mg orally twice daily for 7 days is an effective treatment. Warn the patient about side effects (see *T vaginalis* vaginitis, above). Clindamycin, 300 mg orally 2 times a day for 7 days, may be used in pregnant patients. Recent studies suggest that bacterial vaginosis may be a factor in premature rupture of membranes and premature delivery, and so close clinical follow-up of pregnant women is essential.

Treatment of male sexual partners does not reduce the risk of recurrence of bacterial vaginosis in the index case.

4. **Atrophic vaginitis–**Prescribe estrogen suppositories or creams. Diethylstilbestrol, one 0.5-mg vaginal suppository every 3 days for 3 weeks, followed by 1 week without treatment, may be tried.

5. **Gonococcal vaginitis–**See Gonorrhea, below.

Disposition

Patients should be given a follow-up appointment in 7–10 days with a gynecologist or primary-care physician so that results of treatment can be assessed and follow-up cultures obtained.

3. GENITAL ABSCESSES

Vulvar abscesses may arise in a sebaceous gland or Bartholin's gland (Bartholin's cyst). Skene's glands, adjacent to the urethra, may also be the site of abscess formation. *N gonorrhoeae* is responsible for some vulvar abscesses; the remainder are caused by a variety of bacteria, often in mixed culture.

Diagnosis

The patient complains of tender swelling of the labia majora that is confirmed by examination. Gram's stain and culture of pus from the abscess help to identify the causative organism. Endocervical culture for *N gonorrhoeae* should be performed, if possible.

Treatment

A. Nonfluctuant Lesions: If lesions are not fluctuant, incision and drainage is not indicated. If gonorrhea is suspected, give ceftriaxone, 250 mg intramuscularly. In addition, treat all cases with a broad-spectrum oral antibiotic such as amoxicillin-clavulanate, 500 mg 3 times daily. Apply warm (43 °C [about 110 °F]) compresses, and prescribe sitz baths (38 °C [about 100 °F]). Ask the patient to return in 1–2 days for reevaluation of the need for incision and drainage.

B. Fluctuant Lesions: When drainage is performed, pack the abscess. Administer antimicrobials as described above. Have the patient return in 2–3 days.

Disposition

Gynecologic follow-up is mandatory, since surgery (marsupialization) may be necessary. Occasionally, marsupialization may be performed at the time of diagnosis of acute bartholinitis.

4. MUCOPURULENT CERVICITIS

The presence of mucopurulent endocervical exudate strongly suggests cervicitis due to chlamydial or gonococcal infection.

Diagnosis

A. Symptoms and Signs: Vaginal discharge and pruritus may be present. Mucopurulent endocervical exudate may be observed.

B. Laboratory Tests:

1. Swab test–Mucopurulent secretion from the endocervix may appear yellow or green when viewed on a white cotton-tipped swab. Cervicitis is present if there is bleeding when the first swab culture for gonococci is taken or if there is erythema or edema within a zone of cervical ectopy.

2. Gram's stain–Gram-stained smear of endocervical secretions shows greater than 10 PMNs per microscopic oil-immersion field. The presence of gram-negative diplococci suggests infection with *N gonorrhoeae* but is not diagnostic. Culture is necessary to confirm infection with *N gonorrhoeae*.

3. Slide test–Fluorescent antibody or ELISA slide test should be used to diagnose *Chlamydia*.

Treatment

A. If *N gonorrhoeae* is suspected or found on Gram's stain of endocervical or urethral discharge, treatment should be given as recommended for uncomplicated gonorrhea in adults (p 632).

B. If *N gonorrhoeae* is not suspected, treatment should be as recommended for chlamydial infection in adults (p 632).

DISEASES OF THE MALE GENITOURINARY TRACT
(See also Sexually Transmitted Diseases.)

1. ACUTE BACTERIAL PROSTATITIS

Diagnosis

A. Symptoms and Signs: Patients with acute bacterial prostatitis often have chills, fever, low back and perineal pain or pressure, malaise, dysuria, urgency, and difficulty voiding or decreased urinary stream. Recurring attacks of acute prostatitis are common. Urethral discharge may be present if prostatitis is secondary to urethritis (uncommon). The prostate is tender and enlarged. Prostatic abscess should be suspected when there is localized prostatic tenderness, swelling, or fluctuance. *Prostatic massage is contraindicated in severe, acute prostatitis because it may induce bacteremia.* A simple rectal examination may be performed, however.

B. Laboratory Findings: When acute bacterial prostatitis is suspected based on the patient's symptoms and on physical examination, presumptive diagnosis may be made based on the results of urinalysis and urine Gram's stain and culture. The bacterial pathogen found in the urine will usually be the same as that infecting the prostate. The presence of bacteria should be confirmed by culture and susceptibility testing. Leukocytosis is common. Azotemia suggests obstructive uropathy.

Blood cultures should be performed in all patients with high fever or rigors.

Treatment

A. Antimicrobials: Trimethoprim-sulfamethoxazole, 1 double-strength tablet (trimethoprim, 160 mg; sulfamethoxazole, 800 mg) twice daily for 14 days is the outpatient treatment of choice for acute bacterial prostatitis of moderate severity due to gram-negative bacilli. Ciprofloxacin, 500–750 mg orally twice daily, is also effective. Enterococcal prostatitis may require inpatient treatment with intravenous ampicillin and gentamicin. Other inpatient regimens include trimethoprim-sulfamethoxazole (trimethoprim component, 10 mg/kg/d) intravenously in 2 divided doses, or an aminoglycoside. Gonococcal prostatitis is uncommon and should be managed in consultation with a urologist.

B. Adjunctive Measures:

1. Analgesics (often including a narcotic) should be provided.

2. Hot sitz baths may provide relief.

3. Bed rest is usually helpful.

Disposition

Patients with acute bacterial prostatitis causing systemic symptoms (high fever, rigors) or with suspected prostatic abscess should be hospitalized for treatment with parenteral antibiotics and consultation with a urologist.

Patients who are not hospitalized should return for follow-up in 3–4 days to make sure that recovery is progressing and again 7–10 days after stopping antimicrobial therapy for a test-of-cure culture of expressed prostatic secretions or of urine. Refer the patient to a urologist or source of regular medical care.

2. ACUTE EPIDIDYMITIS

Epididymitis usually results from retrograde spread of urethral or urinary tract infection into the epididymis. Epididymitis is therefore usually caused by the same pathogens causing urethritis (eg, gonococci, *Chlamydia*) or urinary tract infection (eg, *E coli*). The former pathogens are found more commonly in men less than 35 years of age, whereas *E coli* is seen more often in men over 35 years of age.

Diagnosis

There is pain and tenderness of the epididymis on

one or both sides. Epididymitis must be differentiated from testicular torsion and from torsion of the testicular appendage. The principal differentiating features are discussed in Chapter 31. In orchitis the involved testicle is diffusely and tensely swollen, warm, firm, and tender.

Urethritis or urinary tract infection usually coexists with epididymitis, and evidence of these conditions must be sought with appropriate laboratory tests. At a minimum, Gram's or methylene blue stain of urethral exudate (or swab of material in the anterior urethra if no exudate can be obtained) and a clean-voided midstream urine specimen should be obtained for analysis.

Treatment
A. Antimicrobials:
1. Epididymitis with urinary tract infection– Give trimethoprim-sulfamethoxazole, 1 double-strength tablet (trimethoprim, 160 mg; sulfamethoxazole, 800 mg) twice daily for 10 days. See the sections on urinary tract infections for further details.

2. Epididymitis in sexually active heterosexual men less than 35 years of age–Regardless of whether *N gonorrhoeae* is demonstrated, the Centers for Disease Control recommends treatment for gonorrhea and *Chlamydia*. Administer ceftriaxone, 250 mg intramuscularly, followed by doxycycline, 100 mg orally 2 times daily, or tetracycline, 500 mg orally 4 times daily, for 10 days.

B. Adjunctive Measures:
1. Prescribe analgesics as needed.
2. Hot sitz baths may be helpful.
3. Bed rest and scrotal elevation for 1–2 days will provide symptomatic relief; if the patient must be ambulatory, an athletic supporter may be helpful.

Disposition
Refer the patient to a urologist or primary-care physician within a few days. Hospitalization is indicated for orchitis that does not respond within 48 hours to oral therapy and adjunctive measures.

SEXUALLY TRANSMITTED DISEASES

The management of all sexually transmitted diseases should include counseling regarding safe sexual practices and the performance of an HIV antibody test in consenting patients.

1. GONORRHEA

N gonorrhoeae causes primary genitourinary tract infections, localized infections, and the disseminated arthritis-dermatitis syndrome. The disseminated arthritis-dermatitis syndrome is discussed on p 612.

Diagnosis
A. Symptoms and Signs: In men, gonococcal urethritis is characterized by acute onset of dysuria, sometimes with hematuria, and a copious creamy urethral discharge. Less profuse urethral discharge requiring milking of the penile urethra may also occur. Local extension of infection may produce inflammation of preputial glands, epididymitis, seminal vasculitis, and prostatitis. In women, gonococcal cervicitis may be asymptomatic or present with vaginal discharge or symptoms of accompanying urethritis (eg, dysuria, frequency). Occasionally, a Bartholin gland abscess may be the initial complaint. Patients with gonococcal salpingitis complain of lower abdominal pain (unilateral and bilateral), vaginal discharge, and metromenorrhagia. Pain on cervical motion and adnexal tenderness is usual; nausea and vomiting and marked abdominal tenderness or rebound suggest pelvic peritonitis. Criteria for hospitalization of patients with salpingitis are given in Table 34–9.

Rectal infection with *N gonorrhoeae* is usually asymptomatic, although patients occasionally present with proctitis (rectal pain, discharge, tenesmus, and constipation). Pharyngeal infection is almost always asymptomatic.

Patients with gonococcal conjunctivitis present with marked conjunctival erythema and purulent discharge, often unilateral. In adults, it usually follows contact between contaminated fingers and the eye.

B. Laboratory Findings: In men, obtain a Gram-stained smear of urethral discharge, examine it microscopically, and obtain culture and antimicrobial susceptibility testing. The presence of leukocytes (usually PMNs) and intracellular gram-negative diplococci on the smear is more than 99% specific for gonorrhea. A smear showing only PMNs with no gram-negative diplococci is a predictor of a negative gonococcal culture in over 90% of patients, although culture for gonococci is generally recommended. These patients should be treated for nongonococcal urethritis. Culture of the pharynx and rectum is necessary if there is a history of oral or receptive rectal intercourse, since negative results on Gram-stained smears from these areas do not rule out gonorrhea.

In women, findings on Gram-stained smears of cervical secretions may suggest gonorrhea (PMNs with intracellular gram-negative diplococci), but culture should be performed to confirm the diagnosis in all patients. Culture of rectal secretions is recommended in all women, because it is sometimes the only site yielding positive cultures. Culture of pharyngeal secretions is necessary in patients with a history of oral sexual intercourse (fellatio).

Express the exudate in purulent conjunctivitis, and examine a Gram-stained smear. Gram-negative diplococci confirm a diagnosis of gonococcal conjunctivitis. Send a sample of the exudate for culture.

A serologic test for syphilis (eg, VDRL) should be performed in all patients.

Treatment

A. Because there has been worldwide spread of strains of *N gonorrhoeae* that are resistant to penicillin, amoxicillin, and tetracycline, these agents are no longer recommended for empiric treatment of gonococcal infections. Owing to the high frequency of coexisting chlamydial infection (up to 45%), a tetracycline or doxycycline regimen should follow treatment of gonococcal infections. The recommended regimen is ceftriaxone, 250 mg intramuscularly, followed by doxycycline, 100 mg orally twice daily, or tetracycline, 500 mg orally 4 times daily, for 7 days.

B. Patients with gonococcal conjunctivitis must be hospitalized and should receive ophthalmologic consultation. Therapy consists of ceftriaxone, 1 g intramuscularly or intravenously once a day for at least 5 days, combined with immediate and at least hourly irrigation of the eye with saline or buffered ophthalmic solutions. Simultaneous ophthalmic infection with *C trachomatis* can also occur. Careful ophthalmic follow-up is necessary to prevent ocular complications.

Disposition

A. Hospitalization is not indicated for patients with localized gonococcal infection, except for gonococcal conjunctivitis.

B. Table 34–9 provides guidelines for hospitalization in women with acute salpingitis. Many experts recommend hospitalization for all patients with pelvic inflammatory disease.

C. Sexual partners of patients with gonorrhea must be notified and treated.

D. Cases of gonorrhea must be reported to the Public Health Department.

2. NONGONOCOCCAL URETHRITIS (Nonspecific Urethritis)

Nongonococcal urethritis, or nonspecific urethritis, is due to infection with *C trachomatis* in over half of cases. Genital mycoplasmas *(Ureaplasma),* herpes simplex virus, and *Trichomonas* are occasional causes.

Diagnosis

A. Symptoms and Signs: Most male patients have urethral discharge and dysuria. Symptoms are often insidious in onset, with urethral discharge that is scanty, mucoid, watery, and most prominent in the morning.

Women may be asymptomatic or may complain of dysuria or frequency. Infection may involve the cervix as well and extend to the oviducts (cervicitis, salpingitis), producing low-grade symptoms.

B. Laboratory Findings: Urethral discharge should be stained with Gram's stain and examined microscopically. The presence of more than 4 leukocytes per high-power field confirms the diagnosis of urethritis. If no organisms morphologically consistent with gonococci are found, then a presumptive diagnosis of nongonococcal urethritis can be made. A Gram-stained smear with findings diagnostic of gonorrhea does not rule out nongonococcal urethritis, since dual infection with *Chlamydia* and the gonococcus is common, particularly in a heterosexual population. The specimen should be sent for culture to definitely rule out gonorrhea. A variety of slide tests for *Chlamydia* are now available; follow the manufacturer's instructions.

A serologic test for syphilis should also be performed.

Treatment

If nongonococcal urethritis is suspected (negative or equivocal findings on Gram-stained smear with culture results pending) or documented (culture negative for *N gonorrhoeae*), treat for nongonococcal urethritis (p 632). Sexual partners should also be treated.

Disposition

Patients with nongonococcal urethritis can be treated on an outpatient basis. Women with salpingitis or pelvic inflammatory disease often require hospitalization (Table 34–9).

3. GENITAL HERPES SIMPLEX VIRUS INFECTION

Herpes simplex virus is a major cause of recurrent genital lesions. The initial (primary) infection is the most severe, although it may occasionally be asymptomatic. After the primary lesion has healed, the virus remains latent in the paraspinous ganglia, where it periodically causes reactivation of infection owing to a variety of stimuli.

Genital infection is usually caused by herpes simplex virus type 2, and about 99% of patients with recurrent disease will be infected by type 2 virus. Spread of infection is almost exclusively by sexual intercourse.

Diagnosis

Obtain a serologic test for syphilis (eg, VDRL) to rule out coexisting syphilis.

A. First Clinical Episode of Genital Herpes Simplex: The first clinical attack of herpes simplex is usually the most severe. Patients may present with fever, malaise, myalgias, and arthralgias. Aseptic meningitis occurs in 10–20% of cases, particularly in women. Associated symptoms may include dysuria, dyspareunia, and urinary retention. Successive crops of grouped vesicles on an erythematous base denude, form ulcers, and heal by secondary intention, usually in 2–3 weeks but sometimes not until after 6 weeks. Genital edema is common. Local pain and regional adenopathy are usually marked. In men, the glans and penile shaft are involved. In women, the vulva, vagina, and cervix are the usual sites of involvement. Herpetic proctitis (in men or women) presents with fever, tenesmus, obstipation, and rectal pain.

B. Recurrent Herpes Simplex Episodes: Recurrent infection is common and may be triggered by a variety of stimuli (eg, friction, menstruation, sexual intercourse, pregnancy, or stress). Recurrent attacks are frequently heralded by a prodrome consisting of local itching, pain, or aching in the buttocks or leg. Initially, a papule develops that rapidly vesiculates, breaks down into an ulcer, and then heals, usually within 7–10 days. The virus may be recovered as long as lesions are moist. Patients should avoid direct skin-to-skin contact until the area is completely dried and healed.

The presence of herpes simplex virus may be confirmed by the Tzanck test (about 60% sensitivity and 80% specificity), direct tests (eg, immunofluorescence) for herpes simplex antigens (about 70% sensitivity and 95% specificity), or virus culture (see Table 40–8). Virus culture is recommended in most cases.

Treatment

A. Antipyretics and analgesics may help to relieve systemic symptoms.

B. The acyclovir regimens listed accelerate resolution of the signs and symptoms of herpetic eruptions but do not affect the subsequent risk, frequency, or severity of recurrences after the drug is discontinued.

1. First clinical episode–All patients with a first clinical episode of genital herpes should be treated with acyclovir, 200 mg orally 5 times daily for 7–10 days or until clinical resolution occurs. For patients with severe disease or complications necessitating hospitalization, give intravenous acyclovir, 5 mg/kg every 8 hours for 5–7 days or until clinical resolution occurs. These treatments shorten the median course of first episodes by about 50% (approximately 7 days).

2. First clinical episode of herpes proctitis– Give acyclovir, 400 mg orally 5 times daily for 10 days or until clinical resolution occurs.

3. Recurrent episodes–Since benefit to the patient may be minimal, treatment for recurrent episodes should be limited to those patients who typically have severe symptoms and are able to begin therapy at the beginning of the prodrome or within 2 days of onset of lesions. Acyclovir, 200 mg orally 5 times daily for 5 days, may be used.

Immunocompromised patients, especially AIDS patients, with extensive, ulcerative, or progressive mucocutaneous herpes should be treated with oral acyclovir, 200 mg 5 times daily or 400 mg 2–3 times daily until the lesion has healed. Continuous therapy (with 200–400 mg twice daily) may be necessary in some patients. Hospitalization for intravenous acyclovir (5 mg/kg every 8 hours) may be warranted if the patient is unable to take medications orally or if the lesions are extensive.

4. Suppressive therapy–In patients having more than 6 episodes of recurrence yearly, suppressive daily therapy can often reduce the frequency of recurrence. Give 200 mg orally 2–5 times daily or 400 mg twice a day. Discontinue after 1 year to reassess recurrence rate.

C. Antibiotics are not necessary unless Gram-stained smears suggest bacterial superinfection. Women with primary genital herpes frequently have associated *Candida* vaginitis; treat as described above.

D. Bathe the exposed affected areas with warm tap water, or apply warm compresses every 4 hours.

E. Since lesions shed infectious virus, patients should avoid manipulating lesions with their bare hands and should wash their hands after exposure (autoinoculation of the eye or other sites may occur). Any other contact with the lesions (eg, sexual) should be avoided until they have healed.

Disposition

A. Hospitalization is occasionally indicated for patients with primary herpes simplex infection because of severe pain, systemic symptoms, and other complications (urinary retention, obstipation, aseptic meningitis, dehydration). Hospitalization is also required for patients with extensive, large, or rapidly progressive lesions.

B. Patients with genital herpes simplex infection are often frightened and confused about the nature and transmission of the disease and may suffer both physically and psychologically. Counseling should be initiated and provided in the emergency department, if possible, and patients should be referred to a gynecologist or primary-care provider who is experienced in treating herpes simplex infection and who can explain the disease, answer any questions, and provide information on various methods of treatment, so that the patient can make an informed evaluation of the associated efficacy, risks, and side effects.

C. Obtain obstetric consultation in pregnant patients with herpes simplex infection.

4. SYPHILIS

Disease following infection due to *Treponema pallidum* may be divided into the primary, secondary, latent, and tertiary stages. Primary and secondary disease, the infectious stages, are discussed below. Infection with *T pallidum* has been identified as an important risk factor for HIV infection. All consenting patients with early syphilis should have an HIV antibody test.

Diagnosis

A. Symptoms and Signs:

1. Primary disease–A chancre develops at the site of entry of the spirochete between 10 days and 6 weeks after exposure. The ulcer, located on the genitals or occasionally on extragenital sites (finger, mouth) is nontender with a depressed center and rolled, pearly edges. Associated inguinal adenopathy, if present, is usually firm, hard, and nontender.

2. Secondary disease–Secondary disease develops about 4 weeks after the appearance of the chancre. Clinical manifestations reflect the presence of spirochetes in the bloodstream. Most common is a rash that ranges from macular to maculopapular to plaques (condylomata lata). The rash is generally distributed over the thorax, abdomen, and extremities; may involve the palms and soles; and is nonpruritic. Associated findings may include low-grade fever, generalized lymphadenopathy, hepatitis, meningitis, alopecia, and weight loss.

B. Laboratory Findings:
The diagnosis of infectious syphilis is confirmed by serologic testing or by positive results on microscopic darkfield examination of scrapings from the chancre or lesions of secondary disease. Obtain blood for serologic (VDRL or RPR) testing; if results are positive, perform a treponemal antibody test (eg, FTA-ABS or MHA-TP).

Treatment

A. Infectious Syphilis:

1. Benzathine penicillin G, 2.4 million units intramuscularly, is the treatment of choice. Patients who claim to be allergic to penicillin should, optimally, have skin testing and, if necessary, desensitization.

2. Doxycycline, 100 mg orally twice daily, or tetracycline, 500 mg 4 times a day, for 14 days is a alternative regimen for nonpregnant penicillin-allergic patients.

3. Erythromycin, 500 mg orally 4 times daily for 14 days, can be used in patients who cannot take penicillin, doxycycline, or tetracycline and who are reliable and can be followed closely.

B. Jarisch-Herxheimer Reaction:
Aspirin or acetaminophen may be prescribed for the Jarisch-Herxheimer reaction that commonly occurs within a few hours after treatment for secondary syphilis has been started. The reaction is characterized by malaise, headache, fever, faintness, and intensification of the rash. Patients with secondary syphilis who are released from the emergency department following penicillin therapy should be warned about the symptoms of the reaction and should be told that it is *not* due to penicillin allergy.

C. Syphilis in HIV-Infected Patients:
A lumbar puncture should be performed in HIV-infected patients with early syphilis because of the increased risk of treatment failure and central nervous system relapse. If the cerebrospinal fluid cell count is normal and the VDRL test nonreactive, give benzathine penicillin G therapy, 1–3 doses. Serum VDRL tests must be repeated at monthly intervals for at least 3 months. Tetracyclines are probably inadequate therapy for HIV-infected patients with syphilis. Ceftriaxone, 250 mg intramuscularly once a day for 10 days, can be tried.

Disposition

Patients may be treated on an outpatient basis. Cases of syphilis must be reported to the Public Health Department. Sexual partners of patients should be notified and treated. Arrangements must be made for follow-up serologic testing.

5. MINOR SEXUALLY TRANSMITTED DISEASES

Chancroid, lymphogranuloma venereum, and granuloma inguinale are less commonly encountered sexually transmitted diseases. Table 34–10 compares these infections.

SKIN & SOFT TISSUE INFECTIONS

1. SUPERFICIAL SOFT TISSUE INFECTIONS

Superficial soft tissue infections (impetigo, erysipelas, cellulitis) are rarely emergencies. However, these infections may be potentially life- or limb-threatening in 3 situations: (**1**) infection around the face and hand; (**2**) cellulitis in the presence of diabetes, peripheral vascular disease, or venous or lymphatic insufficiency; and (**3**) local infection in the presence of immunodeficiency, particularly leukopenia, leukemia, or AIDS.

Diagnosis

A. Symptoms and Signs:

1. Impetigo–Impetigo is a superficial skin infection seen mainly in children and is usually due to group A streptococci. Less commonly, staphylococci alone or in conjunction with streptococci may cause the disease. Impetigo begins as small vesicles that rapidly pustulate and rupture easily. The purulent discharge dries, forming the characteristic thick, golden-yellow, "stuck-on" crusts. Exposed areas are the most common sites of lesions. Mild regional lymphadenopathy is common. The lesions are painless and often pruritic; systemic symptoms are minimal.

Table 34–10. Minor sexually transmitted diseases.

	Chancroid	Lymphogranuloma Venereum	Granuloma Inguinale
Etiologic agent	*Haemophilus ducreyi*	*Chlamydia trachomatis*	*Calymmatobacterium granulomatis*
Clinical findings	Shallow, painful, soft ulcer appears 2–5 days after infection. Multiple lesions are common. Regional lymphadenitis, unilateral bubo.	Evanescent, painless vesicle or papule followed in 10–30 days by painful buboes. Proctitis, rectal strictures and fissures, lymphatic obstruction with secondary elephantiasic changes.	Insidious onset, usually painless. Papule or nodule erodes to leave irregular ulcer with red granular base. Pseudobuboes may be present. No true lymphadenitis in absence of secondary infection.
Confirmation of diagnosis	Clinical appearance; negative darkfield and serologic tests for syphilis; culture; Gram's stain.	Clinical appearance; complement fixation or immunofluorescent antibody tests; culture.	History and clinical appearance; Donovan bodies in scraping; negative darkfield and serologic tests for syphilis.
Treatment	Erythromycin, 500 mg orally 4 times a day for 7 days; or ceftriaxone, 250 mg intramuscularly in a single dose; or trimethoprim-sulfamethoxazole, 1 double-strength (trimethoprim, 160 mg; sulfamethoxazole, 800mg) tablet orally twice a day for 7 days.	Tetracycline, 500 mg 4 times a day; or doxycycline, 100 mg twice a day; or erythromycin, 500 mg 4 times a day; or sulfamethoxazole, 1 g twice a day; all given orally for at least 2 weeks.	Tetracycline, 500 mg orally 4 times a day for at least 2 weeks. Not yet fully evaluated are doxycycline, 100 mg orally twice a day; or erythromycin, 500 mg orally 4 times a day; or sulfamethoxazole, 1 g orally twice a day for at least 2 weeks.
Management of lesions	Aspirate fluctuant lymph nodes through healthy adjacent skin. Incision and drainage is contraindicated. Remove necrotic material.	Aspirate fluctuant lymph nodes through healthy adjacent skin. Incision and drainage is contraindicated. Late sequelae such as stricture as fissure may require surgical treatment.	Apply local compresses, and start symptomatic treatment.

Ecthyma is a deeper form of impetigo that is associated with ulceration and scarring. It occurs frequently on the legs, often as a complication of debility or infestation with ectoparasites.

Bullous impetigo, due to *S aureus,* occurs mostly in newborns and younger children. The lesions begin as vesicles and then progress to flaccid bullae containing clear yellow fluid. The bullae quickly rupture and form thin, light brown crusts. Bullous impetigo, like staphylococcal scalded skin syndrome, is a response to a staphylococcal exfoliative toxin.

Staphylococcal scalded skin syndrome, the most severe manifestation of skin disease caused by an exfoliative toxin, is characterized by widespread bullae and exfoliation. It usually occurs in younger children but may rarely develop in adults. It begins abruptly with fever, skin tenderness, and a scarlatiniform rash. Large, flaccid, clear bullae form and promptly rupture, resulting in separation of sheets of skin.

2. Erysipelas–Erysipelas is a distinctive superficial cellulitis characterized by prominent lymphatic involvement. It is almost always due to group A streptococci (rarely *S aureus*) and is more common in infants, young children, and older adults. The face is most often involved. The lesion is painful and has a bright red edematous, indurated ("peau d'orange") appearance and an advancing raised border that is sharply demarcated from adjacent normal skin. A common form of the disease affects the bridge of the nose and the cheeks. Fever is common. Erysipelas is usually limited to the dermis and lymphatics but can occasionally extend more deeply to produce cellulitis and bacteremia.

3. Cellulitis–Cellulitis is an acute spreading infection of the skin that extends deeper than erysipelas. Group A streptococci and *S aureus* are the most common causative agents. Previous trauma or underlying skin lesions (furuncle, ulcer) predispose to the development of cellulitis. Local tenderness, pain, and erythema develop within several days and rapidly intensify. The lesion has poorly demarcated borders, and the skin is red, hot, and edematous. Malaise, fever, and chills may develop. Regional lymphadenopathy is common, and bacteremia may occur. Local abscesses and superinfection with gram-negative bacilli may develop. In older patients, cellulitis in the lower extremity may be complicated by thrombophlebitis. In patients with diabetes or peripheral vascular disease, cellulitis in the lower extremity may be caused by gram-negative bacilli and anaerobes, in addition to streptococci and staphylococci.

B. Laboratory Studies: Leukocytosis with a shift to the left may be present. Obtain Gram-stained smear and culture of material from vesicles, bullae, or exudate. Examination of material aspirated at the leading edge of cellulitis may reveal the causative organism. Obtain blood cultures in patients with high fever, chills, or rapid progression of infection.

Treatment

A. Impetigo and Ecthyma: Penicillin is the drug of choice and is administered either as a single intramuscular injection of benzathine penicillin G (300,000–600,000 units for children; 1,200,000 units for adults) or as oral penicillin (125–500 mg every 6 hours for 10 days). Erythromycin (30–50 mg/kg/d orally in divided doses every 6 hours for 10 days for children; 250–500 mg orally every 6 hours for adults) is an alternative for patients allergic to penicillin. It is helpful to remove crusts by soaking them with soap and water.

Bullous impetigo responds to treatment with a penicillinase-resistant penicillin (eg, dicloxacillin); erythromycin may be substituted in patients allergic to penicillin.

Staphylococcal scalded skin syndrome is treated with a penicillinase-resistant penicillin (eg, nafcillin, 50–100 mg/kg/d intravenously in newborns; 100–200 mg/kg/d intravenously in older children). Topical treatment consists of application of cool saline compresses. Corticosteroids should not be used.

B. Erysipelas: Mild cases in adults may be treated with procaine penicillin G (600,000 units intramuscularly once or twice daily) or with oral penicillin (250–500 mg every 6 hours) for 2 weeks. Erythromycin (250–500 mg orally every 6 hours) is a suitable alternative. For more extensive erysipelas, hospitalization for treatment with parenterally administered aqueous penicillin G (600,000–2,000,000 units intravenously every 6 hours) is required.

C. Cellulitis: Mild, early cellulitis may be treated with oral antibiotics. Because S aureus may be involved, empiric therapy is with a penicillinase-resistant penicillin (eg, dicloxacillin) or a first-generation cephalosporin. For more severe infections thought to be caused by streptococci and staphylococci, give penicillinase-resistant penicillin intravenously (eg, nafcillin, oxacillin, or methicillin, 1–2 g every 4 hours) with or without penicillin G. A first-generation cephalosporin equivalent to cefazolin, 1–2 g every 8 hours, is an acceptable alternative in patients who are not critically ill. Vancomycin (1–2 g/d intravenously) is an alternative in patients allergic to penicillin. If superinfection with gram-negative bacteria is present or suspected (eg, in an immunocompromised patient), add an aminoglycoside such as gentamicin or amikacin. Local care includes immobilization and elevation of the involved limb.

Disposition

Patients with cellulitis that has progressed rapidly over the preceding 12 hours, or with lymphangitis, can be treated with parenteral antibiotic therapy in the emergency department if they are reliable and follow-up within 12–24 hours can be arranged. Hospitalize patients who worsen despite parenteral antibiotic therapy, are unreliable, or cannot be closely followed in an outpatient setting. Cellulitis involving the face or hand usually requires hospitalization for parenteral antibiotic therapy. The presence of diabetes, venous or lymphatic insufficiency, or systemic symptoms usually requires inpatient or outpatient parenteral therapy.

2. DEEP SOFT TISSUE INFECTIONS

Deep soft tissue infections involve subcutaneous tissues and may also involve muscles and fascial planes. Classification of these infections is complicated by use of varied nomenclature. Most of these infections are due to anaerobic and aerobic gram-positive and gram-negative organisms.

Infected Vascular Gangrene & Cellulitis

Infected vascular gangrene and cellulitis is a mixed infection occurring mostly in the lower extremities in patients with peripheral vascular disease or diabetes mellitus. Anaerobic organisms, aerobic gram-negative bacilli, and staphylococci may be involved. An underlying ulcer is often the source of infection that may spread to involve not only superficial and deep soft tissue but also muscles or an entire limb. Gas formation may occur. Edema and foul-smelling pus are noticeable. Pain and tenderness may be present.

Hospitalization is required for surgical debridement and intravenous therapy with a combination of antibiotics (eg, cefoxitin alone, or clindamycin plus gentamicin). Underlying osteomyelitis is common if an ulcer is present. Amputation is sometimes necessary.

Clostridial Anaerobic Cellulitis

Clostridial anaerobic cellulitis is a necrotizing clostridial infection of devitalized subcutaneous tissue. The deep fascia is not appreciably involved and there is ordinarily no associated myositis. Gas formation is common and often extensive. Onset of infection is gradual after an incubation period of several days. Local pain, swelling, and systemic toxicity are not prominent. A thick, dark, sometimes foul-smelling drainage is characteristic. Frank crepitus is present. Gram-stained smears of drainage material show numerous blunt-ended, thick, gram-positive bacilli. Soft tissue x-rays show abundant gas. Cultures for aerobic and anaerobic organisms should be obtained.

Hospitalize the patient for treatment with high doses of intravenous penicillin (chloramphenicol in patients allergic to penicillin) and surgery.

Nonclostridial Anaerobic Cellulitis

A clinical picture similar to clostridial cellulitis can be produced by nonclostridial anaerobic bacteria alone or in mixed infection with aerobic gram-negative and gram-positive organisms.

Antimicrobial therapy is based on the findings on Gram-stained smears of drainage material. Since these are frequently mixed infections, several antibiotics may be needed (eg, cefoxitin, or clindamycin, or penicillin, plus an aminoglycoside). Surgical incision and drainage is necessary.

Synergistic Necrotizing Cellulitis

Synergistic necrotizing cellulitis is a rapidly progressive infection with high fever and systemic manifestations caused by infection with anaerobes and aerobic gram-negative bacilli. It occurs most commonly on the perineum and lower extremities and has a high mortality rate. The disease is first manifested as skin ulcers from which drains foul-smelling, reddish-brown ("dishwater") pus. Circumscribed areas of blue-gray gangrene surround these drainage sites, but intervening skin appears normal. Local pain and tenderness are marked. Tissue gas is noted in about one-fourth of patients.

Hospitalization for prompt surgical incision and drainage of necrotic tissue must be combined with antimicrobial therapy (eg, clindamycin plus gentamicin).

Necrotizing Fasciitis

Necrotizing fasciitis is a mixed anaerobic and aerobic infection that rapidly dissects deep fascial planes and produces severe toxicity associated with a high mortality rate. It most commonly occurs on the extremities but may occur on the abdomen in patients with diabetes mellitus, especially after abdominal surgery, or on the perineum or scrotum (Fournier's gangrene) in patients with diabetes mellitus, especially after urinary tract manipulation. The affected area is initially erythematous, swollen, and painful. Bullae containing serosanguineous material appear, and subcutaneous gas is common. Systemic toxicity with high fever is prominent. When a lesion is probed with a hemostat through a limited incision, the instrument passes easily along a plane just superficial to the deep fascia, a distinguishing feature that does not occur with ordinary cellulitis. Leukocytosis is present. About half the cases are due to group A streptococci alone; the remainder are due to mixtures of gram-positive and gram-negative bacteria, both aerobic and anaerobic.

Hospitalization for prompt surgical therapy with extensive incision and excision of necrotic tissue is of paramount importance. The initial empiric antimicrobial therapy (eg, cefoxitin alone, or clindamycin plus gentamicin) should be altered based on results of Gram-stained smears and cultures of tissue biopsies.

Clostridial Myonecrosis

Clostridial myonecrosis (gas gangrene) is a necrotizing infection of fascia and muscle. Infection most commonly occurs following surgical procedures or as a result of contaminated wounds. Patients with peripheral vascular disease, diabetes mellitus, and neoplastic diseases are especially at risk for this infection. The incubation period is usually less than 3 days. Severe pain is the earliest symptom, followed by intense swelling and edema. A thin, hemorrhagic exudate may be seen. The skin is exquisitely tender to the touch and has a bronze to dusky discoloration that

darkens with time. Bullae may appear and are filled with serosanguineous fluid. Crepitus is uncommon early in the disease. There may be a watery brown discharge with a peculiar sweet smell. Systemic symptoms of tachycardia and low-grade fever are usually present. Gram-stained smears may demonstrate *Clostridium perfringens,* but surgical exploration is necessary for confirmation of the diagnosis.

Hospitalization for prompt, complete excision of necrotic muscle is mandatory. Penicillin G (300,000 units/kg/d intravenously) or chloramphenicol (50–100 mg/kg/d) in the patient allergic to penicillin is recommended. Since some species of *Clostridium* are resistant to clindamycin and cefoxitin, these agents should not be used as initial empiric drugs in suspected cases of clostridial myonecrosis. General supportive measures include administration of oxygen and adequate volume replacement to counteract shock. Hyperbaric oxygen, though useful, is not a substitute for immediate surgery.

AIDS
(Acquired Immunodeficiency Syndrome)

AIDS is the end stage of chronic infection by a lymphotropic retrovirus named human immunodeficiency virus (HIV). Transmission occurs by sexual contact, perinatally, and by contact with infected blood (transfusion, needle sharing, occupational exposure). The virus causes slow destruction of the helper T cell subset and, in most infected individuals, eventually leads to fatal immunodepression. Opportunistic infections (eg, *Pneumocystis carinii* pneumonitis), malignancies (eg, Kaposi's sarcoma), and a primary HIV-induced dementia and wasting syndrome account for most deaths.

The most common emergencies in AIDS are pneumonia (usually due to *P carinii*) and central nervous system infection (cryptococcosis, toxoplasmosis) or tumor. Overwhelming infection due to encapsulated microorganisms *(S pneumoniae, H influenzae)* also cause pneumonia and meningitis with sepsis.

Patients may also present to the emergency department with oropharyngeal and esophageal thrush *(C albicans)* or with dehydration due to diarrhea.

Diagnosis

Table 34–11 sets forth common emergencies seen in patients with AIDS or AIDS-related conditions; these are classified by presenting clinical findings.

Note: Some of the conditions causing emergencies in patients with AIDS may be the first clinical manifestation of AIDS in a patient not previously known to have the disease. An HIV antibody test should be performed on consenting patients who present with syndromes suggestive of HIV infection or with sexually transmitted diseases if the antibody status is un-

Table 34–11. Common emergencies in AIDS, AIDS-related conditions, and AIDS risk group patients.

Presenting Findings[1]	Common Causes	Helpful Diagnostic Tests
Pulmonary Cough, dyspnea; pulmonary infiltrates (often with fever)	*Pneumocystis carinii* *Mycobacterium tuberculosis* Pneumococci *Haemophilus influenzae*	Arterial blood gas measurements Chest x-ray Giemsa, acid-fast, and Gram staining of sputum; culture Bronchoscopy with lavage and biopsy
Neurologic Seizures; focal neurologic deficit; encephalopathy; hydrocephalus	*Toxoplasma gondii* Cryptococcal or tuberculous meningitis Cerebral lymphoma Encephalitis (HIV, herpesvirus)	CT scan, MRI Lumbar puncture (after CT scan) Brain biopsy
Systemic Fever; rigors; night sweats	Neutropenia with sepsis Cryptococcal infection Disseminated mycobacterial infection (several species) Sinusitis *Pneumocystis carinii* Cytomegalovirus *Salmonella*	CBC Blood cultures (viruses, bacteria, fungi, mycobacteria) Lumbar puncture and cerebrospinal fluid examination Chest x-ray
Gastrointestinal Diarrhea; dehydration	*Cryptosporidium* *Shigella* *Salmonella* *Campylobacter jejuni* *Entamoeba histolytica*	Culture of stool, and microscopic examination for parasites
Hematologic Bleeding; purpura	Thrombocytopenia Intestinal or pulmonary Kaposi's sarcoma (rare)	CBC and platelet count Endoscopy

[1]Findings are given in approximate order of frequency.

known, regardless of whether the patient appears to be at epidemiologic risk for AIDS.

Treatment & Disposition

A. Pulmonary Presentation:

1. Obtain arterial blood gas measurements to evaluate the degree of pulmonary dysfunction. Dyspnea and hypoxemia even without chest x-ray findings may be evidence of *P carinii* infection.

2. Begin oxygen, 5–10 L/min, by nasal prongs or mask. Repeat arterial blood gas determinations if initial PO_2 is under 60 mm Hg or if PCO_2 is over 40 mm Hg.

3. Obtain posteroanterior and lateral chest x-rays.

4. Obtain expectorated or induced sputum for Gram, acid-fast, and methenamine silver staining for pathogenic bacteria, mycobacterium species, and *Pneumocystis,* respectively. Begin empiric antimicrobial therapy if bacterial pneumonia is suspected (rigors, pleurisy, total white blood cell count > 15,000/µL or neutrophil count < 500/µL, lobar infiltrates on chest x-ray). See Pneumonia & Bronchiolitis, above, for details; otherwise, begin empiric treatment for *P carinii* pneumonia, pending diagnostic studies, as follows: give trimethoprim-sul-

famethoxazole (15–20 mg/kg of trimethoprim component) orally or intravenously in 4 divided doses. In patients allergic to sulfonamides, give pentamidine, 3–4 mg/kg by intravenous infusion over 1 hour. Preliminary evidence suggests that corticosteroids are beneficial when administered early to patients hospitalized with severe pneumocystic pneumonia (PaO_2 < 70 mm Hg on room air). Give prednisone, 60 mg orally every 24 hours, or methylprednisolone, 40 mg intravenously every 8 hours.

5. Hospitalize the patient if new pulmonary infiltrates are present, if arterial PO_2 is under 80 mm Hg or PCO_2 is over 40 mm Hg, or if dyspnea is severe or rapidly progressive. Patients not requiring hospitalization may be referred for further evaluation to a pulmonary physician, infectious disease specialist, or physician experienced in the treatment of patients with AIDS.

B. Neurologic Presentation:

1. Control the airway by positioning the patient on one side and applying suction frequently; insert an endotracheal tube if the gag reflex is markedly depressed or if the patient is obtunded.

2. Treat seizures with intravenous anticonvulsants (Chapter 11).

3. Obtain an emergency CT or MRI scan (arteriography or radionuclide brain scan may be used instead, but both are less satisfactory).

4. If the CT or MRI scan shows focal lesions or increased intracranial pressure, seek urgent neurosurgical consultation. Otherwise, perform lumbar puncture to obtain cerebrospinal fluid for cell count, protein and glucose determinations, cryptococcal antigen titer, Gram and acid-fast staining, and cultures for viruses, bacteria, mycobacteria, and fungi.

5. Hospitalize all patients for further evaluation and treatment.

C. Systemic Presentation (Fever):

1. Obtain CBC with differential and platelet count.

2. Culture blood for bacteria, mycobacteria, and

fungi. Consider lumbar puncture to obtain cerebrospinal fluid if the patient has a headache or meningeal signs. Obtain chest x-ray and room air arterial blood gas measurement for all suspected HIV-positive patients with new-onset fever. Consider sinus x-rays, since occult bacterial sinusitis is common in these patients.

3. If the absolute neutrophil count is under 500/mL, begin empiric antimicrobial therapy for possible bacteremia. Follow the recommendations for the immunocompromised host given in Table 34–1.

4. Severely ill patients will require hospitalization. Others may be managed as outpatients with close follow-up.

D. Gastrointestinal Presentation:

1. Treat hypovolemic shock, if present, with

Table 34–12. Commonly used oral antimicrobial agents.

Antimicrobial	Common Clinical Indications	Dosage Adults	Dosage Children
Penicillin V	Pharyngitis, mild pneumonia, animal and human bites, streptococcal skin infections	250–500 mg every 6 hours	25–50 mg/kg/d in 4 divided doses
Ampicillin	Acute bronchitis, urinary tract infection, otitis media, sinusitis	250–500 mg every 6 hours	50–100 mg/kg/d in 3–4 divided doses
Amoxicillin	Same as for ampicillin	250–500 mg every 8 hours	40 mg/kg/d in 3 divided doses
Amoxicillin/clavulanic acid	Cellulitis, human and animal bites, sinusitis, mild pneumonia or bronchitis	250–500 mg every 8 hours	40 mg/kg/d based on amoxicillin in 3 divided doses
Dicloxacillin	Skin infections, chronic osteomyelitis	500 mg every 6 hours	12.5–25 mg/kg/d in 4 divided doses
Cephalexin or cephradine	Skin infections, bronchitis or mild pneumonia (**not** due to *H influenzae*)	250–500 mg every 6 hours	25–50 mg/kg/d in 4 divided doses
Cefaclor	Skin infections, mild pneumonia or bronchitis (due to *H influenzae*), otitis media, sinusitis	250–500 mg every 8 hours	20–40 mg/kg/d in 3 divided doses
Clindamycin	Chronic sinusitis, pneumonia (occasionally)	150–450 mg every 6–8 hours	8–25 mg/kg/d in 3–4 divided doses
Erythromycin	Pharyngitis, streptococcal skin infections, mild pneumonia, bronchitis, sinusitis	250–500 mg every 6 hours	30–50 mg/kg/d in 4 divided doses
Tetracycline[1]	Acute bronchitis, gonorrhea, nongonococcal urethritis or cervicitis, urethral syndrome, pneumonia, including *Mycoplasma* infections	250–500 mg every 6 hours	20–40 mg/kg/d in 4 divided doses[1]
Doxycycline[1]	Same as for tetracycline	100 mg every 12 hours	2–4 mg/kg/d in 2 divided doses[1]
Sulfonamides	Urinary tract infection	0.5–1 g every 6 hours	150 mg/kg/d in 4 divided doses
Trimethoprim-sulfamethoxazole	Urinary tract infection, prostatitis, epididymoorchitis, acute bronchitis, otitis media, acute sinusitis, shigellosis	1 double-strength (trimethoprim, 160 mg; sulfamethoxazole, 800 mg) tablet twice daily	8–10 mg/kg/d of the trimethoprim component in 2 divided doses
Ciprofloxacin[2]	Bronchitis, urinary tract infection, infectious diarrhea,[3] cellulitis, sinusitis, bronchitis	250–750 mg every 12 hours	. . .
Norfloxacin[2]	Urinary tract infection, prostatitis, infectious diarrhea	400 mg every 12 hours	. . .
Nitrofurantoin	Urinary tract infection	50–100 mg every 6 hours	5–7 mg/kg/d in 4 divided doses

[1]Should not be used in children under 8 years of age.

[2]Contraindicated in children; often not active against *Streptococcus pneumoniae*.

[3]Because of its expense, ciprofloxacin is not routinely the first drug of choice for this indication, but it may be required in areas where enteric pathogens are resistant to trimethoprim-sulfamethoxazole.

infusion of intravenous crystalloid solution (Chapter 3).

2. Obtain stool samples for culture for enteric pathogens and *Mycobacterium avium-intracellulare* and for intestinal parasite studies (in most laboratories, examinations for *Cryptosporidium* are not routine procedures and must be specially requested). Obtain blood cultures if the patient is febrile.

3. Patients should be hospitalized if they are in shock or dehydrated (or if vomiting precludes maintenance of adequate oral hydration) or if they have evidence of dysentery (blood or neutrophils in stool) or sepsis (high fever, rigors). Patients without these signs may be referred to a gastroenterologist, infectious disease specialist, or AIDS expert for further evaluation.

E. Hematologic Presentation:

1. Treat hypotension or shock, if present, with intravenous infusion of crystalloid solutions (Chapter 3).

2. Document thrombocytopenia with a platelet count; obtain a CBC and differential to search for other cytopenias. Determine prothrombin and partial thromboplastin times.

3. Type and cross-match for 10 units of platelets; request cross-matched packed red cells in addition if the hematocrit is below 30%.

Table 34–13. Commonly used parenteral antimicrobial agents.

Antimicrobial	Daily Dosage in Patients With Normal Renal Function (Intravenous Unless Otherwise Specified)		Usual Dosage Interval
	Adults	**Children**	
Aminoglycosides			
Amikacin	15 mg/kg intramuscularly or intravenously	15–30 mg/kg	Every 8–12 hours
Gentamicin or tobramycin	3–5 mg/kg intramuscularly or intravenously	3–7.5 mg/kg	Every 8 hours
Cephalosporins			
Cephalothin	4–12 g	60–100 mg/kg	Every 4–6 hours
Cefazolin	1.5–6 g	50–100 mg/kg	Every 8 hours
Cefoxitin	4–12 g	80–160 mg/kg/d	Every 4–6 hours
Ceftriaxone	1–4 g	50–100 mg/kg	Every 12–24 hours
Cefuroxime	1.5–9 g	100–200 mg/kg	Every 8 hours
Cefotaxime[1]	4–12 g	100–200 mg/kg	Every 6–8 hours
Macrolides; lincomycins			
Clindamycin	1–3 g	10–40 mg/kg	Every 8 hours
Erythromycin	1–4 g	30–50 mg/kg	Every 6 hours
Penicillins			
Aqueous penicillin G	2.4–24 million units	150,000–250,000 units/kg	Every 4–6 hours
Procaine penicillin G	1.2–4.8 million units intramuscularly	25,000–50,000 units/kg intramuscularly	Every 12–24 hours
Benzathine penicillin G	600,000–1.2 million units intramuscularly	50,000 units/kg intramuscularly	Every 15–30 days
Ampicillin	4–12 g	100–300 mg/kg	Every 4–6 hours
Nafcillin, methicillin, or oxacillin	4–12 g	100–200 mg/kg	Every 4–6 hours
Piperacillin; mezlocillin	12–24 g	200–300 mg/kg	Every 4–6 hours
Ticarcillin	12–30 g	150–300 mg/kg	Every 4–6 hours
Miscellaneous			
Ampicillin/sulbactam	4–8 g ampicillin/2–4 g sulbactam	100–200 mg/kg ampicillin/50 mg/kg sulbactam	Every 6 hours
Aztreonam	6–8 g	30 mg/kg	Every 6–8 hours
Chloramphenicol	4 g	50–100 mg/kg	Every 6 hours
Metronidazole	15 mg/kg loading dose, then 30 mg/kg/d	30 mg/kg	Every 6 hours
Trimethoprim-sulfamethoxazole	8–20 mg/kg of the trimethoprim component	8–20 mg/kg of the trimethoprim component	Every 6–12 hours
Vancomycin	2 g	30–60 mg/kg	Every 8–12 hours

[1]Ceftizoxome may be substituted.

AIDS & HIV INFECTION IN THE GENERAL STD SETTING*

The acquired immunodeficiency syndrome (AIDS) is a late manifestation of infection with human immunodeficiency virus (HIV). Most people infected with HIV remain asymptomatic for long periods. HIV infection is most often diagnosed by using HIV antibody tests. Detectable antibody usually develops within 3 months after infection. A confirmed positive antibody test means that a person is infected with HIV and is capable of transmitting the virus to others. Although a negative antibody test usually means a person is not infected, antibody tests cannot rule out infection from a recent exposure. If antibody testing is related to a specific exposure, the test should be repeated 3 and 6 months after the exposure.

Antibody testing for HIV begins with a screening test, usually an enzyme-linked immunosorbent assay (ELISA). If the screening test is positive, it is followed by a more specific confirmatory test, most commonly the Western blot assay. The P24 antigen test may be positive in newly infected patients who have not seroconverted to a positive HIV antibody test. However, a negative P24 antigen test does not rule out HIV infection.

The time between infection with HIV and development of AIDS ranges from a few months to ≥ 10 years. Most people who are infected with HIV will eventually have some symptoms related to that infection. In one cohort study, AIDS developed in 48% of a group of gay men $\leq$10 years after infection; but additional AIDS cases are expected among those who have remained AIDS-free for > 10 years.

Therapy with zidovudine (ZDV—previously known as azidothymidine) has been shown to benefit HIV-infected patients with a CD4 [T4] lymphocyte count less than 500/mm^3. At doses of 100 mg orally every 4 hours while awake (500 or 600 mg/d), serious side effects, usually anemias and cytopenias, have been uncommon during therapy with ZDV until late stages of infection.

PREVENTING THE SEXUAL TRANSMISSION OF HIV

The only way to prevent AIDS is to prevent the initial infection with HIV. Prevention of sexual transmission of HIV can be ensured in only 2 situations: (1) sexual abstinence or (2) choosing only sex partners who are not infected with HIV.

Many HIV-infected persons are asymptomatic and are unaware that they are infected. Therefore, without an antibody test, infected persons are difficult to identify. AIDS case surveillance and HIV seroprevalence studies allow estimation of risk for persons in different areas; however, these population estimates may have a limited impact on an individual's sexual decisions. Although knowledge of antibody status is desirable before a sexual relationship is initiated, this information may not be available. Therefore, individuals should be counseled that when they initiate a sexual relationship they should use sexual practices that reduce the risk of HIV transmission.

Sexual practices may influence the likelihood of HIV transmission during sexual contact with an infected partner. Women who practice anal intercourse with an infected partner are more likely to acquire infection than women who have only vaginal intercourse. The relative risk of transmission by oral-genital contact is probably somewhat lower than the risk of transmission by vaginal intercourse. Other STD or local trauma that breaks down the mucosal barrier to infection would be expected to increase the risk of HIV transmission. Condoms supplement natural barriers to infection and therefore reduce the risk of HIV transmission.

WHEN TO TEST FOR HIV

Voluntary, confidential, HIV antibody testing should be done routinely when the results may contribute either to the medical management of the person being tested or to the prevention of further transmission.

*Modified and reproduced, with permission, from Centers for Disease Control: Sexually transmitted diseases: Treatment guidelines. MMWR (Sept 1) 1989;38(No. S-8):5. STD = Sexually transmitted disease.

(*Continued on next page*)

Testing is important for persons with symptoms of HIV-related illnesses or with diseases such as syphilis, chancroid, herpes, or tuberculosis, for which a positive test result might affect the recommended diagnostic evaluation, treatment, or follow-up. HIV counseling and testing for persons with STD is a particularly important part of an HIV prevention program, because patients who have acquired an STD have demonstrated their potential risk for acquiring HIV.

Because no vaccine or cure is available, HIV prevention requires changes in behavior by people at risk for transmitting or acquiring infection. Therefore, patient counseling must be an integral part of any HIV testing program in an STD clinic. Counseling should be done both before and after HIV testing.

PRETEST COUNSELING

Pretest counseling should include assessment of the patient's risk for HIV infection and measures to reduce that risk.

Users of illicit intravenous (IV) drugs should be advised to stop using drugs. If they do not stop, they should not share needles. If needle-sharing continues, injection equipment should be cleaned with bleach between uses. Sexually active persons who have multiple partners should be advised to consider sexual abstinence or to enter a mutually monogamous relationship with a partner who has also been tested for HIV. Condoms should be used consistently if either or both partners are infected or have other partners. Similarly, heterosexuals with STD other than HIV should be encouraged to bring their partners in for HIV testing and to use condoms if they are not in a mutually monogamous relationship with an uninfected partner.

POSTTEST COUNSELING & EVALUATION

Persons who have negative HIV antibody tests should be told their test result by a person who understands the need to reduce unsafe sexual behaviors and can explain ways to modify sexual practices to reduce risks.

Antibody tests cannot detect infections that occurred in the several weeks before the test (see above). Persons who have negative tests should understand that the negative test result does not signify protection from acquiring infection. They should be advised about the ways the virus is transmitted and how to avoid infection. Their partners' risks for HIV infection should be discussed, and partners at risk should be encouraged to be tested for HIV.

Persons who test positive for HIV antibody should be told their test result by a person who is able to discuss the medical, psychological, and social implications of HIV infection. Routes of HIV transmission and methods to prevent further transmission should be emphasized.

Risks to past sexual and needle-sharing partners of HIV antibody–positive patients should be discussed, and they should be instructed in how to notify their partners and to refer them for counseling and testing. If they are unable to notify their partners or they are not sure that their partners will seek counseling, physicians or health department personnel should assist, using confidential procedures, to ensure that the partners are notified. Infected women should be advised of the risk of perinatal transmission (see below), and methods of contraception should be discussed and provided. Additional follow-up, counseling, and support systems should be available to facilitate psychosocial adjustment and changes in behavior among HIV antibody–positive persons.

PERINATAL INFECTIONS

Infants born to women with HIV infection may also be infected with HIV; this risk is estimated to be 30–40%. The mother in such a case may be asymptomatic and her HIV infection not recognized at delivery. Infected neonates are usually asymptomatic, and currently HIV infection cannot be readily or easily diagnosed at birth. (A positive antibody test may reflect passively transferred maternal antibodies, and the infant

(*Continued on next page*)

must be observed over time to determine if neonatal infection is present.) Infection may not become evident until the child is 12–18 months of age. All pregnant women with a history of STD should be offered HIV counseling and testing. Recognition of HIV infection in pregnancy permits health-care workers to inform patients about the risks of transmission to the infant and the risks of continuing pregnancy.

ASYMPTOMATIC HIV INFECTIONS

As more HIV-infected persons are identified, primary health-care providers will need to assume increased responsibility for these patients. Most internists, pediatricians, family practitioners, and gynecologists should be qualified to provide initial evaluation of HIV-infected individuals and follow-up of those with uncomplicated HIV infection. These services should be available in all public health clinics.

Health-care professionals who identify HIV-positive patients should provide posttest counseling and medical evaluation (either on site or by referral)—including a physical examination, complete blood count, lymphocyte subset analysis, syphilis serology, and a purified protein derivative (PPD) skin test for tuberculosis. Psychosocial counseling resources should also be available.

All clinics and providers should establish and maintain contacts with resources in their regions for persons concerned about HIV infection, and they should refer patients when necessary. Possible resources for referral include counseling services, support groups, social workers, physicians, and clinics.

4. Hospitalize the patient for further evaluation and treatment. Obtain urgent hematologic consultation.

Other Conditions Seen in AIDS or AIDS-Related Conditions

A. Thrush: Oropharyngeal candidiasis (thrush) is common in patients with AIDS or AIDS-related conditions, even if they have not received previous antimicrobial therapy. Although thrush does not in itself denote AIDS, HIV-infected patients with thrush are at high risk for subsequent development of AIDS.

Patients may complain of a dry or sore mouth or may be asymptomatic. Raised white plaques are present on the buccal mucosa or elsewhere in the oral cavity; Gram staining shows *Candida*. Culture is unnecessary. Ask about symptoms of esophagitis (pain on swallowing) that might be due to *Candida;* the presence of endoscopically verified *Candida* esophagitis confirms the diagnosis of AIDS. Also ask about symptoms in other organ systems (eg, lung) that might be early manifestations of AIDS.

Prescribe clotrimazole troches to be dissolved in the mouth 4–5 times a day. Nystatin suspension or suppositories are also effective but much less palatable. Patients with thrush that is refractory to topical therapy may respond to ketoconazole, 200–400 mg orally once a day, but this drug should not be used for initial therapy.

Refer the patient to a physician or clinic experienced in the management of patients with AIDS.

B. Folliculitis: Folliculitis is common with HIV infection. *S aureus* is the usual pathogen.

Red papules are found at the base of hair shafts; pustulation is common, and regional adenopathy may occur. Fever and leukocytosis are absent. Gram-stained smears of pus will reveal the causative agent; culture is necessary only for cases that are refractory to antimicrobial therapy.

Begin dicloxacillin, 500 mg orally 4 times a day for 7–10 days. Erythromycin (same dose) or clindamycin (300 mg orally 3 times a day) may be used in patients allergic to penicillin. Regular bathing with a hexachlorophene-containing soap (eg, pHiso-Hex) may be helpful. Refer the patient to a physician or clinic experienced in treating patients with AIDS.

Universal Precautions

The Centers for Disease Control advocates the concept of "universal precautions," ie, that all patients should be considered potentially infectious for HIV and other blood-borne pathogens and appropriate precautions should be taken at all times to prevent transmission. Barrier precaution, glove use in particular, should be followed whenever contact with bodily fluids is a possibility. Proper handling of needles and other sharp objects (eg, not recapping) both during and after patient care should be taught to all workers who have potential contact with possible HIV-infected materials. Needlestick and other sharp object exposures account for up to 90% of documented nosocomial transmissions. Emergency department and hospital-wide guidelines modeled after the Centers for Disease Control recommendations should be instituted.

HIV transmission occurs by the same routes as hepatitis B but with less efficiency. Exposures as the result of needlestick injuries carry a 1:200 risk of HIV infection (versus 1:20 for hepatitis B). Mucous membrane exposure to blood and exposure of broken skin to HIV-infected blood has also resulted in infection. Other body fluids (tears, cerebrospinal fluid, saliva) may also contain virus but in lower titers than those found in blood. Transmission by these fluids has not been definitely documented but is theoretically possible. AIDS is not transmitted by casual contact.

At least 2 occupational HIV infections to health care workers have occurred during needlestick injuries sustained during cardiopulmonary resuscitative procedures commonly done in the emergency department. The crowding of personnel about the patient's bedside and the urgency of these procedures put health care workers at higher risk of injury at such times. Inadequate precaution becomes most frequent during management of seriously ill or injured patients.

Recent studies show unexpectedly high seroprevalence rates for HIV infection in patients presenting to the emergency department for conditions *not* suggestive of HIV infection (18–22% for men 25–44 years old in sentinel hospitals in New York City). Therefore, universal precautions to HIV exposure are mandatory at all times with all patients.

ANTIMICROBIAL USE IN THE EMERGENCY DEPARTMENT

Many patients present in the emergency department with illnesses requiring treatment with antimicrobial agents. Tables 34–12 and 34–13 list some of the commonly used oral and parenteral antimicrobial agents, the indications for their administration, and dosages.

REFERENCES

General

The choice of antimicrobial drugs. Med Lett Drugs Ther 1990;32:41.

Dershewitz RA (editor): *Ambulatory Pediatric Care.* Lippincott, 1988.

Hathaway WE et al (editors): *Current Pediatric Diagnosis & Treatment,* 10th ed. Appleton & Lange, 1990.

Mandell GL, Douglas RG, Bennett J (editors): *Principles and Practice of Infectious Diseases,* 3rd ed. Churchill Livingstone, 1990.

Rubin RH, Young LS (editors): *Clinical Approach to Infection in the Compromised Host,* 2nd ed. Plenum, 1988.

Safety of antimicrobial drugs in pregnancy. Med Lett Drugs Ther 1987;29:61.

Septic Shock

Harris RL et al: Manifestations of sepsis. Arch Intern Med 1987;147:1895.

Jacobson MA, Young LS: New developments in the treatment of gram-negative bacteremia. West J Med 1986;144:185.

Nicholson DP: Review of corticosteroid treatment in sepsis and septic shock: Pro or con. Crit Care Clin 1989;5:151.

Parker MM, Pacillo SE: Septic shock. JAMA 1983;250:3324.

Evaluation of the Immunocompromised Patient With Suspected Infection

Brown AE, Armstrong D (editors): Symposium on infectious complications of neoplastic disease. (Part 1.) Am J Med 1984;76:413.

Hughes WT et al: Guidelines for the use of antimicrobial agents in neutropenic patients with unexplained fever. J Infect Dis 1990;161:381.

Rubin RH, Young LS (editors): *Clinical Approach to Infection in the Compromised Host.* Plenum, 1988.

Serious Infections Presenting With Fever & Rash

Helmick CG, Bernard KW, D'Angelo LJ: Rocky Mountain spotted fever: Clinical, laboratory, and epidemiological features of 262 cases. J Infect Dis 1984;150:480.

Hermans PE: The clinical manifestations of infective endocarditis. Mayo Clin Proc 1982;57:15.

Kline PP: Fever and rash. Emergency Decisions (April) 1988;27.

Peltola H: Meningococcal disease: Still with us. Rev Infect Dis 1983;5:71.

Rahn DW, Malawista SE: Lyme disease: Recommendations for diagnosis and treatment. Ann Intern Med 1991;114:472.

Steere AC: Lyme disease. N Engl J Med 1989;321:586.

Stevens DL et al: Severe group A streptococcal infections associated with a toxic shock–like syndrome and scarlet fever toxin A. N Engl J Med 1989;321:1.

The toxic shock syndrome. Ann Intern Med 1982;96 (Suppl):831.

Meningitis & Meningoencephalitis

Ho DD, Hirsch MD: Acute viral encephalitis. Med Clin North Am 1985;69:415.

Tunkel AR, Wispelwey B, Scheld WM: Bacterial meningitis: Recent advances in pathophysiology and treatment. Ann Intern Med 1990;112:610.

Pneumonia

Chase RA, Trenholme GM: Overwhelming pneumonia. Med Clin North Am 1986;70:945.

Grayston JT et al: A new respiratory tract pathogen: *Chlamydia pneumoniae* strain TWAR. J Infect Dis 1990;161:618.

Levy M et al: Community-acquired pneumonia: Importance of initial noninvasive bacteriologic and radiographic investigations. Chest 1988;92:43.

Siegel D: Management of community-acquired pneumonia in outpatients. West J Med 1985;142:45.

Verghese A, Berk SL: Bacterial pneumonia in the elderly. Medicine 1983;62:271.

Wilson WR, Cockerill FR, Rosenow EC III: Pulmonary disease in the immunocompromised host. Mayo Clin Proc 1985;60:1610.

Septic Arthritis

Chandrasekar PH, Narula AP: Bone and joint infections in intravenous drug abusers. Rev Infect Dis 1986;8:904.

Dan M: Septic arthritis in young infants: Clinical and microbiologic correlations and therapeutic implications. Rev Infect Dis 1984;6:147.

Gainor BJ: Septic arthritis: Common pitfalls. Orthop Rev 1989;18:555.

Jackson MA, Nelson JD: Etiology and medical management of acute suppurative bone and joint infections in pediatric patients. J Pediatr Orthop 1982;2:313.

Koss PG: Disseminated gonococcal infections. Cleve Clin Q 1985;52:161.

Osteomyelitis

Gentry LO: Osteomyelitis: Options for diagnosis and management. Antimicrob Agents Chemother 1988;21 (Suppl C):115.

Waldvogel FA, Vasey H: Osteomyelitis: The past decade. N Engl J Med 1980;303:360.

Pharyngitis (Sore Throat)

Hayden GF, Hendley JO, Gwaltney JM Jr: Management of the ambulatory patient with a sore throat. Curr Clin Top Infect Dis 1988;9:62.

Levy ML, Ericsson CD, Pickering LK: Infections of the upper respiratory tract. Med Clin North Am 1983;67:153.

Rheumatogenic group A streptococci and the return of rheumatic fever. Adv Intern Med 1990;35:1.

Shulman ST et al: Prevention of rheumatic fever: A statement for health professionals by the Committee on Rheumatic Fever and Infective Endocarditis of the Council on Cardiovascular Disease in the Young. Circulation 1984;70:1118.

Urinary Tract Infections

Johnson JR, Stamm WE: Urinary tract infections in women: Diagnosis and treatment. Ann Intern Med 1989;111:906.

Lipsky BA: Urinary tract infections in men: Epidemiology, pathophysiology, diagnosis, and treatment. Ann Intern Med 1989;110:138.

Martens MG: Pyelonephritis. Obstet Gynecol Clin North Am 1989;16:305.

Stamm WE, Huoten TM, Johnson JR: Urinary tract infections from pathogenesis to treatment. J Infect Dis 1989;159:400.

Diseases of the Female Genitourinary Tract

Chantigian PD: Vaginitis: A common malady. Prim Care 1988;15:517.

Hemsell DL: Acute pelvic inflammatory disease: Etiologic and therapeutic considerations. J Reprod Med 1988;33:119.

Swinker ML: Salpingitis and pelvic inflammatory disease. Am Fam Physician (Jan) 1985;31:143.

Diseases of the Male Genitourinary Tract

Drotman DP: Epidemiology and treatment of epididymitis. Rev Infect Dis 1982;4(Suppl):S788.

Stewart C: Prostatitis. Emerg Med Clin North Am 1988;6:391.

Sexually Transmitted Diseases

Centers for Disease Control: Sexually transmitted diseases: Treatment guidelines. MMWR 1989;38(No. S-8):5.

Fraiz J, Jones RB: Chlamydial infections. Annu Rev Med 1988;39:357.

Holmes KK et al (editors): *Sexually Transmitted Diseases,* 2nd ed. McGraw-Hill, 1990.

Lucas LM, Smith DL: Nongonococcal urethritis: Diagnosis and management. J Gen Intern Med 1987;2:199.

Lukehart SA et al: Invasion of the central nervous system by *Treponema pallidum:* Implications for diagnosis and treatment. Ann Intern Med 1988;109:855.

McNabney WK, Barnes WG: Urethral and endocervical culturing: Gonorrhea and chlamydia. Ann Emerg Med 1986;15:333.

Thin RN: Management of genital herpes simplex infections. Am J Med 1988;85:3.

Soft Tissue Infections & Cellulitis

Ahrenholz DH: Necrotizing soft-tissue infections. Surg Clin North Am 1988;68:199.

Boulton AJ: The diabetic foot. Med Clin North Am 1988;72:1513.

Finch R: Skin and soft-tissue infections. Lancet 1988;1:164.

Reboli AC, Del Bene VE: Oral antibiotic therapy of dermatologic conditions. Dermatol Clin 1988;6:497.

Suss SJ, Middleton DB: Cellulitis and related soft tissue infections. Am Fam Physician 1987;36:3.

AIDS (Acquired Immunodeficiency Syndrome)

Baroff LJ, Talan DA, Torres M: Prevalence of HIV antibody in a non–inner city university hospital emergency department. Ann Emerg Med 1991;20:782.

Becherer P, Wilson SE: Management of early HIV-1 infection in adults. Postgrad Med 1989;86:101.

Centers for Disease Control: Guidelines for prevention of transmission of human immunodeficiency virus and hepatitis B virus to health care and public safety workers. MMWR 1989;38:S-6.

Glatt AE, Chirgwin K: *Pneumocystis carinii* pneumonia in human immunodeficiency virus–infected patients. Arch Intern Med 1990;150:271.

Kelen GD: Human immunodeficiency virus and the emergency department: Risks and risk protection for health care providers. Ann Emerg Med 1990;19:242.

Kelen GD et al: Human immunodeficiency virus infection in emergency department patients. JAMA 1989;262:516.

Kelen GD et al: Unrecognized human immunodeficiency virus infection in emergency department patients. N Engl J Med 1988;318:1645.

Montaner JSG et al: Corticosteroids prevent early deterioration in patients with moderately severe *Pneumocystis carinii* pneumonia and the acquired immunodeficiency syndrome (AIDS). Ann Intern Med 1990;113:14.

Sande MA, Volberding PA: *The Medical Management of AIDS,* 2nd ed. Saunders, 1990.

Terwilliger EF, Sodroski JG, Haseltine WA: Mechanisms of infectivity and replication of HIV-1 and implications for therapy. Ann Emerg Med 1990;19:233.

Witt DJ, Craven DE, McCabe WR: Bacterial infections in adult patients with the acquired immune deficiency syndrome (AIDS) and AIDS-related complex. Am J Med 1987;82:900.

Antimicrobial Use in the Emergency Department

Rehm SJ, McHenry MC: Oral antimicrobial drugs. Med Clin North Am 1983;67:57.

Metabolic & Endocrine Emergencies

35

J. Blake Tyrrell, MD, David C. Aron, MD, & John H. Karam, MD

I. EMERGENCY MANAGEMENT OF CARBOHYDRATE DISORDERS (See also Chapter 10.)

Coma or altered mental status in patients with diabetes mellitus may be related to the diabetes or may occur from a variety of causes not directly related to diabetes, eg, cerebrovascular accidents, encephalitis, alcohol or other drug toxicity, and head trauma (Chapter 10).

Coma due to carbohydrate disorders may be classified as follows:

A. Diabetic Ketoacidosis (Hyperglycemic Hyperosmolar Coma Associated With Ketosis): Diabetic ketoacidosis is usually insidious in onset and is characterized by increasing fatigue, nausea and vomiting, progressive stupor, dehydration, and rapid deep breathing (Kussmaul breathing). Diabetic ketoacidosis is associated with severe insulin deficiency.

B. Hyperglycemic Hyperosmolar Nonketotic Coma: Patients in deep hyperosmolar nonketotic coma are generally flaccid and have quiet breathing. Dehydration is common. Endogenous insulin production is moderately deficient but sufficient to prevent ketosis.

C. Hypoglycemic Coma: Hypoglycemic coma has a relatively rapid onset and usually results from excessive doses of insulin or oral hypoglycemic agents. Patients in hypoglycemic coma have mild hypothermia, usually associated with normal hydration. The skin may be clammy and diaphoretic. The patient may be breathing normally, or hypoventilation may be present.

D. Lactic Acidosis: Lactic acidosis is often present in diabetic patients who have suffered severe cardiovascular collapse. In patients with lactic acidosis who are dehydrated and who have Kussmaul breathing, arterial blood pH is 7.1 or less.

Diagnostic Laboratory Methods

Blood chemistry measurements confirm the diagnosis of diabetes mellitus. A glucose meter or glucose oxidase paper strips such as Chemstrip bG, used with a fresh drop of blood, provide a convenient means of rapid estimation of blood glucose concentration in the emergency department or outside a hospital setting. *Note:* Blood in fluoride anticoagulant (gray-topped specimen tube) cannot be used for paper strip testing because enzymes on the strip are inactivated by fluoride. Plasma ketones can be measured using crushed Acetest tablets. Table 35–1 outlines the laboratory differentiation of coma due to disorders of carbohydrate metabolism.

DIABETIC KETOACIDOSIS

Diabetic ketoacidosis is an acute complication of diabetes mellitus that may result from failure to take an adequate amount of insulin or may occur as the first manifestation of diabetes in a previously undiagnosed diabetic. In many instances, ketoacidosis is precipitated by conditions that increase the patient's requirements for insulin, eg, infection or trauma. Recurrent episodes of severe ketoacidosis in juvenile-onset diabetics (particularly teenagers) often indicate poor patient compliance and require family counseling and ongoing education.

When dehydration occurs secondary to osmotic diuresis, impaired renal blood flow reduces the ability of the kidney to excrete glucose, and this defect exacerbates the hyperosmolality. Severe hyperosmolality correlates closely with central nervous system depression and coma, whereas prolonged acidosis can compromise cardiac output and reduce vascular tone and thereby contribute to circulatory collapse in the dehydrated patient.

Diagnosis

A. History:

1. Determine whether there is a personal history of diabetes. If the patient is known to be an insulin-dependent diabetic, ascertain if insulin has been given on a regular basis and if the dosage has been adequate.

2. Inquire about possible predisposing factors (infection, etc).

B. Symptoms and Signs:

1. Polyuria, dry mouth, and polydipsia with marked fatigue and nausea and vomiting.

2. Kussmaul breathing due to acidosis. Fruity breath odor due to acetone.

3. Abnormal mentation, varying from slight confusion to stupor or coma.

4. Orthostatic hypotension with tachycardia and poor skin turgor, indicating dehydration and salt depletion. Some patients may present in frank shock.

5. Hypothermia may be an associated finding.

6. Signs of a possible precipitating event (infection, trauma, etc) should be sought on examination.

C. Laboratory Findings:

1. Marked (4+) glycosuria and strong ketonuria with hyperglycemia and ketonemia–Patients with moderately severe diabetic ketoacidosis generally have a plasma glucose in the range of 350–900 mg/dL and a positive acetoacetate (Acetest) response at a plasma dilution of 1:3 or higher. Unlike acetoacetate, β-hydroxybutyrate, which makes up the bulk of the keto acid content of plasma and urine, is not measured in the nitroprusside reaction of Acetest tablets or Ketostix.

2. Acidosis–Acidosis may be severe, with low arterial blood pH (6.9–7.2) and reduced blood bicarbonate (5–10 meq/L); PCO_2 is generally low (10–20 mm Hg) as a result of hyperventilation.

3. Serum potassium–Despite total body potas-

Table 35–1. Laboratory diagnosis of coma due to disorders of carbohydrate metabolism.[1]

	Urine		Plasma		
	Sugar	**Acetone**	**Glucose**	**Bicarbonate**	**Acetone**
Often related to diabetes					
Hypoglycemia	0[2]	0 or +	Low	Normal	0
Diabetic ketoacidosis	+ + + +	+ + + +	High	Low	+ + + +
Nonketotic hyperglycemia	+ + + +	0 or +	High	Normal or slightly low	0
Lactic acidosis	0 or +	0 or +	Normal, low, high	Low	0 or +
Unrelated to diabetes					
Alcohol or other durgs	+ or 0	0 or +	May be low	Normal or low[3]	0 or +
Cerebrovascular accident or head trauma	+ or 0	0	Often high	Normal	0
Uremia	0 or +	0	High or normal	Low	0 or +

[1]Modified and reproduced, with permission, from Krupp MA, Schroeder SA, Tierney LM Jr (editors). *Current Medical Diagnosis & Treatment 1987.* Appleton & Lange, 1987.
[2]Leftover urine in bladder might still contain sugar from earlier hyperglycemia.
[3]Alcohol can elevate plasma lactate as well as keto acids to reduce pH.

sium depletion resulting from protracted polyuria or vomiting, serum potassium is usually normal or slightly elevated owing to acidosis that shifts potassium from the cells into plasma. When the acidosis subsides, potassium returns to the cells and hypokalemia becomes evident. With profound potassium depletion (300–400 meq), the serum potassium concentration may be subnormal before therapy of the ketoacidosis (see Fig 36–2).

4. Serum sodium–There is mild to moderate hyponatremia (125–130 meq/L). This is due to loss of sodium in body fluids (eg, in urine, vomitus) as well as from a shift of intracellular water to the extracellular (and intravascular) compartment as a result of the osmotic effects of severe hyperglycemia. Serum sodium should be corrected for the presence of hyperglycemia by adding 1.8 meq/L of sodium for every 100 mg/dL glucose above normal.

5. Serum phosphate–Serum phosphate is elevated to 6 or 7 mg/dL as a consequence of insulin deficiency and prerenal azotemia, whereas total body phosphate is generally depleted secondary to osmotic diuresis.

6. Severe volume depletion–Severe volume depletion is associated with elevated hematocrit and azotemia.

7. Serum creatinine–Serum creatinine may be spuriously elevated out of proportion to that expected for prerenal azotemia. The high levels are caused by interference of acetoacetate in the automated assay for creatinine.

Treatment in the Emergency Department

A. Ensure Ventilation:

1. Protect the airway–Obtunded patients without a functioning gag reflex should be positioned so that aspiration will not occur. Intubation may be necessary.

2. Administer oxygen–Give 4–6 L/min, by mask or nasal prongs, until arterial blood gas measurements are known. Oxygen may be discontinued if the arterial PO_2 is 75 mm Hg or higher.

B. Give Fluids to Correct Hyperosmolality and Dehydration: Insert a large-bore intravenous catheter ($\geq$ 16-gauge), and begin administration of isotonic fluids (normal saline is satisfactory), at least 1 L in the first 1–2 hours; administer fluids more rapidly if the patient is hypotensive or in shock.

C. Give Insulin: An initial loading dose of regular insulin, 0.15–0.3 unit/kg (usual dose, 10 units) by rapid intravenous injection, should be given as soon as the diagnosis of diabetic ketoacidosis is made. This loading dose permits rapid achievement of adequate therapeutic levels of insulin and avoids delay in obtaining an effective insulin concentration at tissue receptor sites. This may be followed by a continuous infusion or periodic (hourly) intravenous or intramuscular administration of regular insulin beginning with a dose of 0.1–0.15 unit/kg/h; the dosage is modulated

depending on the therapeutic response. If hypotension is present, use only the intravenous route.

D. Treat Severe Acidosis: Some experts feel that severe acidosis (pH < 7.1) should be partially corrected with bicarbonate, which can be conveniently given by adding 44–88 meq (1–2 ampules) of sodium bicarbonate to 900 mL of *hypotonic* (0.45%) saline and infusing as described above until pH reaches 7.1 or serum bicarbonate levels reach 15 meq/L. Mild to moderate acidosis (pH $\geq$ 7.2) is well tolerated, can be quickly corrected with administration of insulin and fluids, and *should not* be treated with alkali. Other experts feel that the administration of bicarbonate for any degree of acidosis may be detrimental, leading to paradoxical cerebrospinal fluid acidosis, hyperosmolarity, and hypernatremia. Furthermore, clinical trials have failed to show an improved outcome when bicarbonate is used.

E. Provide Supportive Measures:

1. Insert a nasogastric tube–Use a nasogastric tube to drain the stomach (gastric atony and retention are common) and prevent aspiration.

2. Monitor urine output–Use an indwelling or condom catheter if urine output cannot otherwise be monitored. Use strict aseptic technique and a closed drainage system to prevent infection.

3. Treat sepsis–If infection is thought to be a precipitating cause of ketoacidosis, quickly obtain appropriate cultures (including one or 2 blood cultures), and institute empiric antimicrobial therapy (see Table 3–6).

F. Prepare Flow Sheet: Since frequent assessment of physical findings and laboratory data is essential to the proper treatment of diabetic ketoacidosis, the physician should prepare a comprehensive flow sheet that includes vital signs, serial laboratory data, and treatment given (Fig 35–1). Essential baseline blood chemistry measurements include glucose, ketones, electrolytes, arterial blood gases and pH, blood urea nitrogen, creatinine, and phosphate.

Plasma glucose and potassium levels should be recorded hourly, and electrolytes and pH should be measured at least every 2–3 hours. Fluid intake and output and therapy given should also be recorded on this sheet.

Disposition

Hospitalize the patient at once. Elderly or deeply comatose patients or those who show signs of cardiovascular collapse or cardiac arrhythmias should be admitted to an intensive care unit, where cardiac and ventilatory status can be closely monitored.

Continuing Treatment

Each case must be managed individually, and the physician should take into account the specific deficits present and the responses to initial therapy.

A. Insulin Replacement: Use only regular insulin for the management of diabetic ketoacidosis.

DIABETIC KETOACIDOSIS FLOW SHEET

Name_____

Hospital No._____

Age_____ Initial weight_____

Initial level of consciousness

_____ Alert

_____ Lethargic

_____ Semicomatose

_____ Comatose

DATE									
TIME									
BLOOD PRESSURE									
PULSE									
BLOOD									
Creatinine									
Blood urea nitrogen									
Glucose									
Acetone									
Hematocrit									
pH									
P_{O_2}									
P_{CO_2}									
Na^+									
K^+									
HCO_3^-									
Cl^-									
URINE									
Volume									
Glucose									
Acetone									
REGULAR INSULIN									
Intravenous									
Intramuscular									
Units									
INTRAVENOUS FLUIDS									
Type									
Amount									
Potassium									
OTHER									

Figure 35–1. Flow sheet for diabetic ketoacidosis.

1. Initial dose—Regular insulin, an initial loading dose of 0.3 unit/kg body weight as an intravenous bolus, should be given in the emergency room. This is then followed by 0.15 unit/kg/h, either continuously infused (with an infusion pump) or injected intramuscularly, which is sufficient to replace the insulin deficit in most patients.

2. Continuous infusion—To avoid adsorption and loss of insulin onto the container or intravenous tubing, the first 50 mL of the insulin solution that flows through the infusion tubing is discarded before the infusion is started. This practice saturates the infusion tubing with adsorbed insulin molecules, thereby preventing further loss of insulin from the infusate.

3. Repeat dose—If the plasma glucose level fails to fall at least 80–100 mg/dL in the first hour, a repeat loading dose is recommended. (Insulin therapy is greatly facilitated when the plasma glucose level can be measured or estimated using a glucose reflectance meter within a few minutes of drawing blood.)

4. Insulin resistance—In the rare patient with insulin resistance, the insulin dose must be doubled every 2–4 hours if severe hyperglycemia does not fall more than 30–40 mg/dL/h during initial therapy.

B. Fluid, Sodium, and Glucose Replacement:

1. Initial fluids—In most adult patients the fluid deficit is as high as 5–10 L. Initially, normal (0.9%) saline solution is preferred to restore plasma volume; it should be infused rapidly to provide 1000 mL/h for the first 1–2 hours to help stabilize blood pressure and reduce hyperosmolality. In addition, by improving renal blood flow, the clearance of glucose and hydrogen ion are enhanced.

2. Follow-up fluids—After the first 2 L of fluid have been replaced, saline solution, 0.45%, should be infused at a rate of 300–400 mL/h, since water deficit exceeds sodium loss in uncontrolled diabetes with osmotic diuresis. This also lessens the chances of post-treatment hyperchloremia, which is aggravated when normal (0.9%) saline is used to correct fluid losses. A benign transient hyperchloremic acidosis is commonly seen following treatment owing to a deficit of bicarbonate anion resulting from the loss of keto acids in the urine before therapy.

3. Glucose—When blood glucose falls below 300 mg/dL, glucose solutions, 5% (eg, 5% dextrose in 0.45% saline), should be infused in order to prevent hypoglycemia and reduce the likelihood of cerebral edema that can result from too rapid a decline in blood glucose.

4. Subcutaneous insulin—Continue infusion of insulin until acidosis and ketonemia have cleared. Since these insulin-deficient patients are prone to ketosis and may quickly slip back into ketoacidosis if insulin is not adequately replaced, they should receive subcutaneous insulin at regular intervals, with dosage based on frequent monitoring of blood glucose levels. Start subcutaneous insulin during the last hour of insulin infusion to prevent a period of insulin deficiency following discontinuation of intravenous insulin.

C. Correction of Acidosis: *Caution:* The use of sodium bicarbonate has been questioned by some because of the following potential consequences of rapid correction of acidosis: (**1**) hypokalemia from rapid shifts of potassium into cells; (**2**) tissue anoxia from reduced dissociation of oxygen from hemoglobin; and (**3**) cerebral acidosis resulting from a reduction of cerebrospinal fluid pH. Bicarbonate does not cross the blood-brain barrier; it generates carbonic acid in the plasma that readily diffuses as CO_2 into the cerebrospinal fluid while the bicarbonate remains in the plasma. These considerations are less important when acidosis is severe, and 1–2 ampules of sodium bicarbonate (44 meq per 50-mL ampule) added to 1 L of hypotonic (0.45%) saline solution should probably be administered whenever the blood bicarbonate level is below 9 meq/L or arterial blood pH is less than 7.1. To date, however, randomized clinical trials have not shown an improved survival rate with bicarbonate administration.

D. Correction of Potassium Deficit: Total body potassium loss from polyuria as well as from vomiting may be greater than 200 meq. However, because of potassium shift from cells due to the acidosis, serum potassium is usually normal or high until after the first few hours of treatment, when acidosis improves and serum potassium returns into cells. Potassium replacement is seldom indicated at the onset of therapy if pretreatment serum potassium levels are 5–6 meq/L or higher (see Fig 36–2). However, once a satisfactory urine output is established and serum potassium levels fall below 5 meq/L, potassium chloride in doses of 10–30 meq/h should be infused. There is generally no need for potassium replacement until after 1–2 hours of therapy, except in rare cases of severe potassium depletion when initial levels of serum potassium are below 4 meq/L despite severe acidosis. In this instance, potassium therapy should be started immediately. An ECG (see Fig 36–1) can be helpful in monitoring the patient and reflecting the state of potassium balance at the time but should not replace accurate measurement of serum electrolytes. Cardiac arrhythmias can occur in the presence of either high or low potassium levels and are a serious prognostic sign.

E. Correction of Hypophosphatemia: Certain theoretic advantages have been proposed for correcting the hypophosphatemia that occurs during insulin treatment of diabetic ketoacidosis. Replacing phosphate helps to restore the buffering capacity of the plasma, thereby facilitating renal excretion of hydrogen; it also corrects the impaired dissociation of oxygen from hemoglobin by regenerating 2,3-diphosphoglycerate and to some extent enhances insulin activity. However, prospective randomized studies have failed to confirm the benefit of adding phosphate to the therapeutic regimen in treating diabetic ketoacidosis, whereas severe tetany due to excessive amounts of phosphate has been reported from several centers. Therefore, replace phosphate when serum levels below 1.5 mg/dL occur, or if an accompanying disorder causing hypophosphatemia is present (eg, chronic malabsorption, alcohol withdrawal, or chronic malnutrition) and not as a routine measure in treating diabetic ketoacidosis.

1. Phosphate replacement–To minimize the risk of inducing tetany from excessive replacement of phosphate, an average deficit of 40–50 mmol of phosphate in adults with diabetic ketoacidosis should be replaced with intravenous infusion at a rate no faster than 3–6 mmol/h. Since the potassium deficit is typically about 2–3 times that of phosphate, attempts to combine potassium and phosphate replacement by using only intravenous potassium phosphate to correct the potassium deficit have led to serious phosphate overdose resulting in severe hypocalcemic tetany. For this reason, potassium should be replaced with the potassium chloride salt, and phosphate replacement, if needed, should be conducted separately, with allowances made for the small amounts of potassium also being replaced (4–5 meq/h, as indicated below).

2. Dose–A sterile stock solution available from Abbott Laboratories provides a mixture of 1.12 g KH_2PO_4 and 1.18 g K_2HPO_4 in a 5-mL single-dose vial representing 22 meq potassium and 15 mmol phosphate (27 meq). Five milliliters of this stock solution in 2 L of either 0.45% saline or 5% dextrose in water, infused at 400 mL/h, will replace the phosphate at the optimal rate of 3 mmol/h and will provide 4.4 meq potassium per hour. If serum phosphate remains below 2 mg/dL, the infusion may be repeated.

HYPERGLYCEMIC HYPEROSMOLAR NONKETOTIC COMA

Hyperglycemic hyperosmolar nonketotic coma or state occurs in patients with non–insulin-dependent diabetes (type II); most patients are at least middle-aged to elderly. There is accompanying dehydration due to inadequate intake of water. Underlying renal insufficiency or congestive heart failure is common, and the presence of either worsens the prognosis.

A precipitating event such as pneumonia, burns, cerebrovascular accident, or recent surgery is often present. Certain drugs such as phenytoin, diazoxide, glucocorticoids, immunosuppressives, and diuretics have been implicated in pathogenesis, as have procedures such as peritoneal dialysis when fluids containing high glucose are used.

Diagnosis

A. Symptoms and Signs: Onset is frequently insidious over a period of days or weeks. Symptoms and signs include the following:

1. Weakness, polyuria, and polydipsia.

2. Reduced fluid intake–A history of reduced intake of fluid is common and is caused by inappropriate lack of thirst, gastrointestinal upset, or inaccessibility of fluids to elderly, bedridden patients.

3. Profound dehydration–Dehydration is often more severe than in ketoacidosis, because the lack of toxic features delays recognition of the syndrome and start of therapy. Signs of dehydration include dry mucous membranes, poor skin turgor, sunken eyes, etc.

4. Lethargy and confusion–Lethargy and confusion progress to convulsions and deep coma.

5. Kussmaul breathing is not present.

B. Laboratory Findings:

1. Severe hyperglycemia is present, with blood glucose values ranging from 800 to 2400 mg/dL.

2. Early hyponatremia–When dehydration is less severe, dilutional hyponatremia as well as urinary sodium losses may reduce serum sodium to 120–125 meq/L, which protects to some extent against extreme hyperosmolality. For an estimate of the true serum sodium level, measured serum sodium should be corrected for the presence of hyperglycemia by adding 1.8 meq/L of sodium for every 100 mg/dL glucose above normal.

3. Late hypernatremia–Once dehydration progresses further, serum sodium can exceed 140 meq/L. This lack of fluid to dilute serum electrolytes results in profound hyperosmolality and coma.

4. Serum osmolality readings of 330–440 mosm/kg H_2O are found. A convenient method of estimating serum osmolality is as follows (normal values in humans are 280–295 mosm/kg H_2O):

$$\text{Serum osmolality (mosm/L)} = 2[Na^+] + \frac{\text{Glucose (mg/dL)}}{18} + \frac{\text{Blood urea nitrogen (mg/dL)}}{2.8}$$

These calculated estimates are usually 10–20 mosm/kg H_2O lower than values recorded by standard cryoscopic techniques in patients in diabetic coma. *Note:* The degree of mental status impairment directly correlates with the osmolality. If serum osmolality is *less than* 330 mosm/kg H_2O, other causes of coma (eg, poisoning or trauma) should be considered.

5. Ketosis and acidosis are usually absent or mild. Prerenal azotemia is the rule. Blood urea nitrogen elevations to 90 mg/dL resulting from dehydration are typical.

Treatment

Initial management is the same as for diabetic ketoacidosis (ie, protect airway, give oxygen, and insert an intravenous catheter).

A. Fluids:

1. Saline solution–Hypotonic (0.45%) saline is preferable to isotonic saline solution as initial therapy, especially in the presence of hypernatremia, congestive heart failure, or renal insufficiency. Rapid correction of hyperosmolality, however, may precipitate cerebral edema, particularly in children. Some authorities therefore recommend isotonic saline. As much as 4–6 L of 0.45% saline may be required in the first 10 hours. The objective is to restore urine output to 50 mL/h or more. Since these patients are often older and may have compromised cardiovascular function, the prognosis is often guarded because of the difficulties in replacing fluids without precipitating heart failure. In elderly patients or those with cardiac disease, a central venous pressure line or even a Swan-Ganz catheter is a crucial adjunct to fluid therapy. When diseased myocardium shows poor compliance, patients may develop pulmonary edema even with relatively slight fluid excesses.

2. Dextrose in water–Plasma glucose should not be allowed to fall too rapidly. Therefore, intravenous fluids should be changed to 5% dextrose in water (or hypotonic saline) once plasma glucose falls to 250 mg/dL. Rehydration alone often produces a dramatic fall in blood glucose concentration.

B. Insulin Dosage: In the absence of ketoacidosis, less total insulin is usually needed to reduce hyperglycemia. However, critically ill or profoundly ill patients should receive treatment similar to that for diabetic ketoacidosis, above (an intravenous loading dose and continuous infusion of insulin). More stable patients (eg, those with minimal dehydration or a normal level of consciousness) may be given 10–15 units of regular insulin intravenously as well as 10–15 units intramuscularly, immediately, followed by 10 units intramuscularly or subcutaneously every 2–3 hours, depending on the initial response.

C. Potassium Dosage: In the absence of acidosis, there is less likelihood of hyperkalemia initially, and potassium replacement can be started earlier than in ketoacidosis. Once it is determined that renal failure with hyperkalemia is not present, potassium chloride, 10–20 meq/h, can be given, starting with the initial bottle of fluid.

D. Phosphate Replacement: Phosphate can be given at a relatively low rate of 3 mmol/h for up to 5 hours if renal failure is not present. Phosphate replacement is given as for diabetic ketoacidosis, and with the same precautions. Hypocalcemia due to overaggressive phosphate replacement can be a particular hazard to cardiac function in elderly patients on digitalis therapy.

E. Special Examinations: Search vigorously for underlying causes of coma. Obtain blood, urine, and sputum samples for culture. Serial ECGs and myocardial enzyme measurements are necessary to rule out silent myocardial infarction.

Disposition

Hospitalization is indicated for all patients.

HYPERGLYCEMIA WITHOUT KETOACIDOSIS

Hyperglycemia without ketoacidosis is commonly seen in the emergency department. Patients usually have non–insulin-dependent diabetes mellitus (type II) and frequently are overweight. They may have known diabetes and seek treatment because of elevated glucose level found on self-monitoring, or they may have no prior history of elevated serum glucose.

Diagnosis

A. Symptoms and Signs: Patients often are asymptomatic, and hyperglycemia is found on incidental laboratory examination or self-test with glucose oxidase paper strips or glucose meter measurements. Symptoms, when present, are usually mild.

1. Characteristic symptoms–Blurred vision, polyuria, polydipsia, and less commonly polyphagia are often present.

2. Hypovolemia–Orthostatic symptoms of lightheadedness (often reported as dizziness), weakness, and near-syncope may be present. Blood pressure and pulse taken in the supine, sitting, and upright positions show mild to moderate systolic pressure drop and pulse rise; frank shock due to isolated hyperglycemia is uncommon.

3. Frequent infections–Recurrent urinary tract infections and, in women, frequent vaginal fungal infections occur as a consequence of glycosuria and defective cell-mediated immune response. Evidence of infection at other sites may also be present.

4. Skin ulcers–Skin ulcers, especially of the lower extremities, develop owing to poor wound healing and may show concomitant infection.

5. Autonomic and peripheral neuropathy– Disordered motility of the gastrointestinal tract, urinary retention due to bladder atrophy, and hypoesthesia or dysesthesia in a stocking-glove distribution may be present.

B. Laboratory Findings:

1. Random blood glucose > 200 mg/dL or fasting blood glucose > 140 mg/dL on several occasions establishes the diagnosis of diabetes mellitus. Elevated glycosylated hemoglobin is helpful but is not available in the emergency setting.

2. Acidosis is absent on serum electrolyte measurement.

3. Renal function tests should be obtained to detect renal insufficiency.

4. Urinalysis should be obtained routinely to detect urinary tract infection that may exacerbate the hyperglycemia or be a consequence of it. Tests for evidence of suspected infection at other sites should also be performed.

5. An ECG to detect myocardial ischemia or infarction should be obtained in most patients, especially if no other cause of hyperglycemia is found. Patients with diabetes mellitus have an increased incidence of asymptomatic ("silent") myocardial infarction or atypical presentation.

Treatment

A. Fluids: Replace fluid loss by intravenous infusion of non–glucose-containing solutions (eg, normal saline), 200–1000 mL/h (rate depending on severity of dehydration, patient size, and cardiac and renal status). Mild dehydration in asymptomatic patients can be treated with water or non–glucose-containing fluids orally. Fluid replacement alone can often reduce blood glucose level.

B. Insulin: Patients whose blood glucose is greater than 400–450 mg/dL should be treated with regular insulin, 5–10 units/h until glucose level is in the range of 250–300 mg/dL.

C. Oral Hypoglycemic Agents: In general, these agents are not recommended for the emergent treatment of hyperglycemia or for patients with type I diabetes mellitus. They are useful for outpatient treatment after the patient is discharged from the emergency department. Patients who discontinued their oral hypoglycemic medication should be restarted on their usual regimen. Patients already taking oral agents may need the dose adjusted if an underlying disorder causing the acute or subacute elevation in blood glucose is not found or cannot be rapidly treated. Patients with new-onset diabetes mellitus requiring treatment (eg, blood glucose > 300–350 mg/dL) can be started on glyburide, 2.5–5 mg/d, or glipizide, 5 mg/d.

D. Other Causes: Treat any underlying condition that may be causing the blood glucose elevation (eg, treat infections with the appropriate antibiotic).

Disposition

Most patients with hyperglycemia without ketoacidosis can be treated in the emergency department and discharged home for follow-up care with a primary-care physician or diabetes specialist within 1–3 days. Hospitalization is indicated for patients with underlying conditions that require hospitalization and for patients with hyperglycemia (> 400 mg/dL) that is refractory to treatment with 10–20 units of regular insulin and hydration.

HYPOGLYCEMIA

Etiology

Hypoglycemia may occur for many reasons (Table 35–2). Most commonly, hypoglycemia results from the effects of endogenous or exogenous insulin excess.

A. Exogenous Insulin: In diabetics, severe hypoglycemia associated with coma most commonly results from an excess of insulin that may be due to (1) delay in eating a meal, (2) unusual physical exertion, (3) an excessive dose of exogenous insulin, (4)

Table 35–2. Conditions associated with hypoglycemia.

Insulin-mediated hypoglycemia
  Excessive dose of exogenous insulin in diabetic patients
  Surreptitious administration of exogenous insulin or sulfonyl-urea in patients with factitious hypoglycemia
  Spontaneous release of excessive quantities of endogenous insulin from pancreatic B cell adenoma, carcinoma, or nesidioblastic islets
  Reactive (postprandial) hypoglycemia
Hypoglycemia due to non–insulin-mediated causes
  Extrapancreatic tumors
  Chemically induced hypoglycemia (ethanol, akee fruit, etc)
Hypoglycemia due to counterregulatory deficiency
  Addison's disease
  Hypopituitarism
  Myxedema
  Severe cachexia
  Hepatic failure
Hypoglycemia of severe renal failure in dialysis

unusual fluctuations in insulin absorption from varying injection sites, or (5) impaired counterregulatory mechanisms due to autonomic neuropathy.

Severe hypoglycemia may also occur in diabetics taking sulfonylurea drugs, particularly patients with reduced renal clearance. Surreptitious administration of insulin (or, rarely, sulfonylureas) to diabetics or nondiabetics has resulted in hypoglycemic coma.

B. Pancreatic B Cell Tumor: In nondiabetics, the most common insulin-mediated cause of hypoglycemic stupor or coma is excessive release of endogenous insulin by a pancreatic B cell tumor.

C. Alcohol: Severe hypoglycemia is seen in patients after excessive ethanol intake combined with limited food intake and is due to depleted hepatic glycogen and reduced gluconeogenesis.

D. Postprandial (Reactive) Hypoglycemia: Postprandial hypoglycemia is usually associated with adrenergic manifestations but is rarely severe enough to result in depressed levels of consciousness.

Diagnosis

Look first for a bracelet, necklace, or card identifying the patient as diabetic.

A. Moderate Hypoglycemia: (Blood glucose 30–50 mg/dL.)

1. Tachycardia; sweating; and clammy, wet skin may not be present but are valuable diagnostic clues. Beta-adrenergic blockade (eg, with propranolol) blocks the tachycardic manifestations of hypoglycemia.

2. Paresthesias about the face or hands occur frequently.

3. Increasing irritability may be noted.

4. The patient may complain of hunger.

B. Severe Hypoglycemia: (Blood glucose < 30–35 mg/dL.) Clinical manifestations are mainly a result of impaired function of the central nervous system and include the following:

1. Mental confusion and bizarre behavior.

2. Seizures.

3. Coma. Patients in deep *hypoglycemic* coma appear adequately hydrated, are generally flaccid, and have quiet breathing. Focal neurologic findings are rare.

4. Lack of Kussmaul breathing. Patients in *ketotic hyperglycemic* coma who are severely dehydrated and have acidosis exhibit Kussmaul breathing; breathing in hypoglycemic coma is normal or depressed (hypoventilation).

5. Mild hypothermia (32.2–35 °C [90–95 °F]) is common and is a valuable diagnostic clue.

C. Serum Glucose Determination: Draw blood by inserting an indwelling catheter or needle carefully into a large brachial or antecubital vein and withdrawing blood before any infusion is begun. Immediately measure glucose using a drop of fresh blood and glucose oxidase paper strips (eg, Chemstrip bG) or glucose meter. Send remaining blood to the laboratory for serum glucose measurement.

Treatment

A. Airway: Make sure there is an adequate airway, and prevent injury to the tongue in case seizures occur.

B. Emergency Measures:

1. Intravenous glucose–Give 50% dextrose in water, 50 mL at 10 mL/min, to any comatose patient. Patients seldom require more than 20–50 mL of 50% dextrose in water to correct hypoglycemia. More rapid infusion or an excessive amount may cause symptomatic hypokalemia, particularly if the glucose is infused into a central vein. (If chronic alcohol ingestion is suspected, give thiamine, 100 mg intramuscularly or intravenously, before giving dextrose in order to prevent Wernicke's encephalopathy.) Most patients regain consciousness rapidly (5–10 minutes). However, if hypoglycemia has been severe and prolonged, full restoration of neurologic function may not occur until later, and a residual neurologic deficit may persist. Administration of an additional 50 mL of 50% dextrose in water may be needed to maintain consciousness in some patients. Hypoglycemia caused by ingestion of long-acting oral hypoglylcemic agents (eg, chlorpropamide) or by the presence of long-acting insulin in the patient's system should be treated with continuous infusion of glucose to prevent recurrent episodes. Give 5% dextrose in water at 100–125 mL/h.

2. Oral feedings–Patients should be given oral feedings of fruit juice as soon as they regain consciousness. When patients who take longer-acting insulin (NPH or lente) or chlorpropamide develop reactions, they should be observed for the possibility of relapse over the next 12–48 hours. High-protein food such as milk should be given in addition to carbohydrates, and 5% dextrose in water, infused at a rate of 100–125 mL/h, may be useful.

3. Glucagon injection–If intravenous glucose is not available to treat hypoglycemic coma, glucagon, 1 mg intramuscularly, should be given. *Glucagon should be carried by all insulin-requiring diabetic patients.* Consciousness is usually restored after a 10- to 15-minute interval, and oral feedings can then be resumed. The families of insulin-treated patients should be taught how to administer glucagon.

Disposition

Uncomplicated hypoglycemic coma due to insulin excess in a diabetic patient rarely requires hospitalization. Other patients may warrant brief hospitalization (1–2 days) so that the cause of hypoglycemia can be investigated in order to prevent recurrences. Hospitalization is usually warranted for patients with hypoglycemia due to excessive long-acting insulin preparations or long-acting oral hypoglycemic agents. Patients should not be discharged until they have been observed for an adequate period of time while no longer receiving parenteral dextrose infusions. Patients should be discharged into the care of a responsible person who can observe for signs of recurrent hypoglycemia.

LACTIC ACIDOSIS

Overproduction of lactic acid accompanied by impaired removal of lactic acid by the liver can result in excessive lactic acid accumulation (> 7 mmol/L) and profound metabolic acidosis.

Etiology

Lactic acidosis may occur in any severely ill patient with cardiac decompensation; respiratory or hepatic failure; shock; acute septicemia; acute infarction of lung, bowel, or extremities; leukemia; or terminal metastatic cancer. Hyperlactatemia has also been produced by toxic overdoses of phenformin, alcohol, or isoniazid, particularly in patients with predisposing factors affecting lactate or phenformin excretion, eg, renal dysfunction, liver disease, alcoholism, or cardiopulmonary decompensation. Now that phenformin is no longer available for general use in the USA, cases of spontaneous lactic acidosis have virtually disappeared.

Diagnosis

A. Symptoms and Signs: The clinical presentation of lactic acidosis varies with the underlying illness. Lactic acidosis is usually secondary to tissue hypoxia or vascular collapse.

1. Characteristic symptoms–Marked hyperventilation and weakness are characteristic.

2. Lack of other symptoms–In the idiopathic (spontaneous) variety, the onset is rapid (usually over a few hours); blood pressure is initially normal; peripheral circulation is good; and cyanosis is absent.

Weakness and hyperventilation may be the only manifestations at onset.

B. Laboratory Findings:

1. Plasma bicarbonate levels and blood pH are both quite low and indicate the presence of severe metabolic acidosis.

2. Ketones are usually absent from plasma and urine or are at most minimally elevated. Nitroprusside tests for ketones, however, are generally inadequate when high levels of lactate are present.

3. The first clue to lactic acidosis may be a high anion gap (serum sodium minus the sum of chloride and bicarbonate anions [in meq/L]). An anion gap greater than 15 indicates an abnormal excess of unmeasured anions. If this cannot be clinically explained by an excess of keto acids (diabetes), inorganic acids (uremia), or anions from drug overdose (salicylates, methyl alcohol, ethylene glycol), lactic acidosis is probably the correct diagnosis.

4. In the absence of azotemia, hyperphosphatemia may be a clue to the presence of lactic acidosis. This may result from exaggerated anaerobic glycolysis.

5. The diagnosis of lactic acidosis is confirmed by demonstrating a plasma lactic acid level of 7 mmol/L or higher in a sample of blood that is promptly chilled and centrifuged. Values as high as 30 mmol/L have been reported. Normal plasma values average 1 mmol/L, with a normal lactate/pyruvate ratio of 10:1. This ratio is greatly exceeded in lactic acidosis.

In collecting samples, it is essential to chill the blood rapidly and to centrifuge it to remove red cells, whose continued glycolysis at room temperature is a common source of error in reports of high plasma lactate. Frozen plasma remains stable for subsequent assay.

Treatment

A. Emergency Measures: Supportive care to maintain satisfactory tissue perfusion with blood that is adequately oxygenated should be initiated while efforts are being made to identify and correct the underlying cause of lactic acidosis. Therapy involves correction of severe acidosis, supportive care, and specific treatment of the illness causing lactic acidosis.

1. Oxygen–Give oxygen, 10 L/min, by mask, and support ventilation as needed.

2. Fluid–Give 500–2000 mL of physiologic (0.9%) saline to restore adequate blood pressure and cardiac output.

3. Sodium bicarbonate–Alkalization with intravenous sodium bicarbonate to keep the pH above 7.2 is advocated by some authorities. Sodium bicarbonate (1–2 ampules in 1 L of 5% dextrose in water) may be used. One 50-mL ampule contains 44 meq. As much as 2000 meq in 24 hours has been used. *Caution:* The benefit of bicarbonate therapy is often outweighed by its tendency to cause hyperosmolality, paradoxical cerebrospinal fluid acidosis, and pulmonary edema when given in the high doses required. Clinical trials have not proved the benefit of bicarbonate administration.

B. Antibiotics: If overwhelming infection is suspected, empiric administration of antibiotics (see Table 3–6) is indicated after appropriate cultures have been obtained.

C. Hemodialysis: Hemodialysis may be useful when large sodium loads are poorly tolerated and is particularly useful when phenformin is the cause of lactic acidosis, since both phenformin and lactate are dialyzable.

D. Dichloroacetate: Dichloroacetate, an experimental anion that facilitates pyruvate removal by activating pyruvate dehydrogenase, reverses certain types of lactic acidosis in animals and has been used in treating some types of lactic acidosis in humans with fair results. Methylene blue is not useful.

Disposition

All patients with persistent lactic acidosis require hospitalization. The prognosis is generally guarded.

ALCOHOLIC KETOACIDOSIS

Although ketonemia is well documented in starved individuals, accumulation of keto acids sufficient to produce clinical signs of acidosis is relatively infrequent in simple starvation. However, a number of cases of ketoacidosis have been reported in alcoholics who have been unable to retain food during a severe drinking bout. Alcoholic ketoacidosis occurs almost exclusively in patients with a history of markedly reduced food intake in whom lipolysis is increased further by a sympathetic discharge provoked by alcohol.

Diagnosis

A. Symptoms and Signs: The main clinical features of alcoholic ketoacidosis are as follows:

1. Recent alcoholic binge followed by anorexia and vomiting.

2. Kussmaul breathing.

3. Dehydration.

B. Laboratory Findings:

1. Severe metabolic acidosis (pH 6.9–7.2) with low serum bicarbonate levels.

2. Plasma glucose ranging from hypoglycemic values (25–50 mg/dL), seen occasionally, to moderately elevated levels (140–260 mg/dL).

3. Ketones in plasma at several dilutions. *Note:* β-hydroxybutyric acid predominates over acetoacetic acid. Thus, ketonuria may not be indicated by reagent test strips that react only to acetoacetate.

4. Slight to moderate elevations of plasma lactate.

5. Hypophosphatemia (1–1.5 mg/dL) is common.

6. Blood alcohol levels may not be elevated at the time of hospital admission.

Treatment

Therapy is aimed at correcting dehydration and acidosis with intravenous fluids and restoring glucose homeostasis.

1. If blood glucose is low, give glucose, 1 ampule of 50 mL of 50% dextrose in water after giving thiamine 100 mg intravenously or intramuscularly, followed by a continuous infusion of 5% dextrose in water or in hypotonic (0.45%) saline.

2. Give 1000 mL/h normal (0.9%) saline solution for the first 1–2 hours, followed by continuous infusion of 5% dextrose in hypotonic (0.45%) saline to replace fluid loss.

3. If pH is below 7.1, sodium bicarbonate, 1 or 2 ampules (44 meq/ampule) in 1 L of hypotonic (0.45%) saline (with or without glucose, as needed) may be given (see Correction of Acidosis, p 651).

4. Insulin is seldom required, since acidosis often resolves with fluid replacement.

5. As described in the section on treatment of diabetic ketoacidosis, monitor electrolyte levels, and replace phosphate at a rate of 3–6 mmol/h for five 1-hour periods or until the phosphate level reaches 3–4 mg/dL.

Disposition

Patients should be hospitalized for acute care.

II. EMERGENCY MANAGEMENT OF OTHER METABOLIC & ENDOCRINE ABNORMALITIES

THYROID DISORDERS

THYROID STORM

Thyroid storm is a *life-threatening emergency* characterized by exaggerated manifestations of thyrotoxicosis plus fever, cardiac decompensation, central nervous system dysfunction, and gastrointestinal signs and symptoms. It can be prevented by prompt diagnosis and treatment of thyrotoxicosis and aggressive therapy of hyperthyroidism in patients with complicating general medical illnesses.

Etiology

The clinical syndrome is usually precipitated by intercurrent stress, most frequently infection, surgery, or trauma in a patient with poorly treated or untreated thyrotoxicosis. Thyroid storm may also occur after drug ingestion, metabolic abnormalities such as diabetic ketoacidosis, and (rarely) after radioactive iodine therapy for hyperthyroidism. Total levels of circulating thyroid hormones (T_4 and T_3) in thyroid storm do not differ significantly from those usually observed in hyperthyroidism; however, serum concentrations of free thyroxine are usually increased.

Diagnosis

A clinical diagnosis is crucial, since the death rate is high if the disease is unrecognized. A presumptive diagnosis of thyroid storm should be made in patients with a history or current manifestations of thyrotoxicosis who have fever, rapidly worsening symptoms, and cardiac or central nervous system manifestations. Physical manifestations that should suggest the diagnosis are thyromegaly, which is almost always present; a thyroid bruit; atrial arrhythmias in patients with no antecedent cardiac disease; and ophthalmologic signs of thyrotoxicosis, which include proptosis, stare, and lid retraction. The ophthalmopathy and pretibial myxedema of Graves' disease are less commonly observed.

A. Early Symptoms and Signs:

1. Most patients have symptoms of preceding thyrotoxicosis. With the onset of thyroid storm, fever, anxiety, tremulousness, tachycardia, weakness, and delirium are noted. In acutely ill patients, the history may be unobtainable.

2. Apathetic hyperthyroidism may occur in elderly patients, in which case the symptoms of hyperthyroidism may be unrecognized.

B. Late Symptoms and Signs: With fully developed thyroid storm, the following are noted:

1. Fever is characteristic and may exceed 40 °C (104 °F). It may be due either to the thyrotoxicosis per se or to an intercurrent infection. For this reason, fever should always arouse concern when it occurs in patients with thyrotoxicosis.

2. Exaggerated manifestations of thyrotoxicosis, including increasing anxiety, nervousness, tremor, sinus tachycardia, sweating, and warm skin, occur.

3. Cardiac findings, include wide pulse pressure, hyperdynamic precordium, atrial fibrillation, and congestive failure are seen.

4. Nervous system findings of generalized weakness, proximal myopathy, agitation, confusional states, or psychosis occur.

5. Gastrointestinal symptoms are usually present and may include nausea and vomiting, diarrhea, and abdominal pain. Jaundice and hepatic tenderness may be present.

6. Dehydration may be profound in patients with hyperpyrexia, vomiting, and diarrhea.

7. Death occurs either from hypovolemic shock,

coma, or congestive heart failure and tachyarrhythmias.

C. Laboratory Findings:

1. Results of thyroid function tests are generally unobtainable in the acute situation. Previous tests confirm the presence of thyrotoxicosis but cannot establish the diagnosis of thyroid storm.

2. There are no characteristic electrolyte abnormalities; hypokalemia, mild hypercalcemia, hypoglycemia or hyperglycemia, and hyponatremia or hypernatremia may be seen.

3. Lymphocytosis and abnormal liver function tests are commonly noted. Other routine laboratory studies are not helpful.

D. Electrocardiographic Findings:
The ECG is usually abnormal; common findings are sinus tachycardia, increased QRS and P wave voltage, nonspecific ST–T wave changes, and atrial arrhythmias, usually fibrillation or flutter. First-degree heart block or intraventricular conduction defects may occur.

Treatment

A. Emergency Measures:

1. Maintain the airway, and give oxygen, 5–10 L, by mask or nasal cannula, if required.

2. Insert a large-bore ($\geq$ 16-gauge) intravenous catheter.

3. Draw blood samples for T_3 and T_4 (or free T_4) radioimmunoassay, CBC, serum glucose and electrolyte measurements, tests of renal and hepatic function, and arterial blood gas determinations.

4. Begin infusion of electrolyte and glucose solutions (eg, 5% dextrose in normal saline), and alter as indicated by results of electrolyte and glucose determinations.

5. Begin electrocardiographic monitoring, and obtain 12-lead ECG.

6. Give vasopressors if hypotension is unresponsive to volume replacement (use pulmonary capillary wedge pressures as a guide) (Chapter 3).

7. Treat congestive heart failure and arrhythmias, if present (Chapters 28 and 29).

8. Glucocorticoids inhibit peripheral conversion of T_4 to T_3, and their use is generally accepted, although there is no specific evidence of efficacy in thyroid storm. Administer cortisol (hydrocortisone sodium phosphate or sodium succinate), 100–300 mg bolus intravenously, followed by 200–400 mg/24 h intravenously in divided doses every 6 hours, and then taper the dose over 3–5 days as the clinical situation warrants.

B. Specific Therapy:

1. Block hormone action–Propranolol and other beta-adrenergic antagonists block the peripheral effects of excess thyroid hormone; they also decrease conversion of T_4 to T_3 and are the agents of choice for atrial arrhythmias. In severe cases, give 1–10 mg of propranolol intravenously (1 mg/min) every 3–6 hours as required to control cardiac rate or

tachyarrhythmias. The desired end point is sinus rhythm with a rate less than 100 beats/min. When the heart rhythm and rate are controlled, oral or nasogastric administration may be substituted (160–400 mg/24 h in divided doses every 6 hours). Oral administration alone may be used in mild cases. Propranolol should be continued until definitive therapy of hyperthyroidism is undertaken. Congestive heart failure in thyroid storm or severe thyrotoxicosis is not an absolute contraindication to propranolol if heart failure is due to tachyarrhythmia or high-output failure.

2. Block hormone synthesis–Thiourea compounds block thyroid hormone synthesis and should be administered orally or by nasogastric tube in all cases of thyroid storm. Propylthiouracil is the drug of choice, since it also inhibits peripheral conversion of T_4 to T_3. Give propylthiouracil, 800–1200 mg as an initial loading dose, followed by 300 mg every 6 hours until the acute episode has resolved. The dosage may then be tapered, but propylthiouracil should be continued until definitive therapy is undertaken. Certain iodinated radiographic contrast agents (eg, ipodate sodium [Bilivist, Oragrafin]) are potent inhibitors of peripheral T_4 to T_3 conversion and may be useful adjuncts.

3. Block hormone release–Iodide compounds in high dosage decrease thyroid hormone release in thyrotoxicosis and can rapidly decrease circulating thyroid hormone levels. *These compounds should be given 2–4 hours after administration of propylthiouracil.*

a. Give sodium iodide, 1 g every 8 hours by continuous intravenous infusion, during the acute episode.

b. Alternatively, give Lugol's iodine solution (8 mg iodide/drop), 10 drops every 8 hours; or saturated solution of potassium iodide (eg, SSKI, 40 mg iodide/drop), 5–10 drops every 8 hours orally or by nasogastric tube.

c. Continue iodine therapy orally for approximately 2 weeks following resolution of the acute episode using the dosage shown in ¶b, above.

d. Give cortisol (hydrocortisone sodium phosphate or sodium succinate), 100 mg intravenously every 6 hours, to treat relative adrenal insufficiency, which may be present. Corticosteroids also inhibit release of thyroid hormone and conversion of T_4 to T_3 peripherally.

e. Removal of thyroid hormones by plasmapheresis or by peritoneal dialysis should be considered in patients not responsive to the above measures.

C. Supportive Measures:

1. Identify and treat precipitating factors, particularly infections. Take samples of blood and other appropriate material for culture. Begin empiric antimicrobial treatment if infection is suspected (see Table 3–6).

2. Administer vitamin supplements (especially B vitamins); give vitamin B_1 (thiamine), 50–100 mg intravenously daily; vitamin B_2 (riboflavin), 40–50 mg intravenously daily; and niacinamide, 100–200 mg intravenously daily. This may be conveniently given as a vitamin B complex mixture (Solu-B-Forte, many others).

3. Treat hyperthermia as needed with acetaminophen, 325–650 mg orally every 4–6 hours. A cooling blanket may also be necessary.

Disposition

Hospitalization in an intensive care unit is indicated in all cases of thyroid storm.

MYXEDEMA COMA

Myxedema coma is a rare complication of severe hypothyroidism and is due to profound thyroid hormone deficiency that results in encephalopathy. The pathophysiology involves respiratory failure with hypoxemia and hypercapnia related to respiratory center depression, respiratory muscle abnormalities, and other factors. Disordered cerebral metabolism, hypothermia, hypoglycemia, hyponatremia, and impaired drug metabolism may also contribute to the syndrome. Myxedema coma may develop insidiously, especially in the elderly, or may be precipitated abruptly by infection, drugs, anesthesia, or stress. The death rate is high (40–60%), particularly in elderly patients and in those who have concurrent chronic underlying disease. Myxedema coma may be prevented by prompt diagnosis and treatment of hypothyroidism.

Diagnosis

A presumptive diagnosis of myxedema coma should be made when clinical manifestations of hypothyroidism are accompanied by disturbances of consciousness, hypothermia, hypoventilation, or hypotension.

A. History: The history (if available) is usually that of classic hypothyroidism and may include discontinuation of thyroid medication, previous radioactive iodine treatment, thyroidectomy, or drug administration (eg, sedatives, iodides, or amiodarone).

B. Preceding Symptoms and Signs:

1. Cold intolerance, dry skin, constipation, weakness, increased sleep, lethargy, depression, slow speech, and weight gain.

2. Irregular menses.

3. Muscle cramps, paresthesias, angina, or seizures.

4. Apathy, ataxia, inappropriate humor ("myxedema wit"), or psychosis (in severely hypothyroid patients).

C. Late Symptoms and Signs: As myxedema coma develops, the following are noted:

1. Increasing lethargy, disorientation, or unresponsiveness progressing to frank coma.

2. Grand mal seizure (a frequent presenting event).

3. Hypothermia, hypoventilation, and hypotension.

4. Signs of severe hypothyroidism, eg, bradycardia, facial puffiness, especially around the eyes; coarse dry skin with pallor and a yellowish cast (due to carotenemia); hair loss; thinning of the eyebrows; enlargement of the tongue; delayed return phase of deep tendon reflexes.

5. Examination of the thyroid frequently reveals a thyroidectomy scar, goiter, or no palpable thyroid tissue.

6. There may be cardiomegaly, distant heart sounds, ileus, and urinary retention.

7. Infection, a common precipitating event, may be masked by the profound metabolic disorder.

D. Laboratory Findings:

1. On thyroid function tests, free T_4, total T_4, and free T_4 index are low, as is total T_3 (by radioimmunoassay). Blood for TSH measurement should be drawn before treatment is started. Elevated TSH levels confirm a diagnosis of primary hypothyroidism, whereas TSH is low or undetectable in secondary hypothyroidism. (Primary hypothyroidism is far more common than secondary hypothyroidism.)

2. Blood gas measurements reveal hypoxemia, hypercapnia, and respiratory or mixed acidosis.

3. Dilutional hyponatremia is common, and hypoglycemia may be present.

4. Miscellaneous abnormalities include hypercholesterolemia, elevated creatine phosphokinase, and increased cerebrospinal fluid protein.

E. X-Ray Findings: Chest x-ray frequently shows an enlarged cardiac silhouette that may be due to pericardial effusion.

F. Electrocardiographic Findings: The ECG shows bradycardia, low voltage of the QRS complex in all leads, and flattening or inversion of T waves. Conduction abnormalities may be present.

Treatment

A. General and Supportive Measures:

1. Treat respiratory failure, hypoxemia, and CO_2 retention with intubation, pulmonary toilet, oxygen, and mechanical ventilation as required (Chapter 5).

2. Begin electrocardiographic monitoring.

3. Insert a large-bore ($\geq$ 16-gauge) intravenous catheter.

4. Draw blood samples for T_3 and T_4 radioimmunoassay, resin T_3 uptake (or free T_4), TSH, cortisol, CBC, serum glucose and electrolyte determinations, renal and hepatic function tests, and arterial blood gas measurements.

5. Support blood pressure if hypotension is present. Give crystalloid solution (normal saline or lactated Ringer's injection). Do not give excess free water; avoid hypotonic solutions. *Caution:* Patients with myxedema frequently demonstrate decreased responsiveness to vasopressors, and arrhythmias may occur when vasopressors are administered along with thyroid hormone.

6. Correct hypoglycemia by administration of 50% glucose initially and then 5% glucose by infusion.

7. Treat hypothermia with passive rewarming; avoid rapid, active external rewarming, which may cause serious arrhythmias or circulatory collapse due to peripheral vasodilatation (Chapter 38).

8. Treat ileus, which may simulate a "surgical" abdomen, by insertion of a nasogastric tube (occasional patients will require cecostomy), and treat urinary retention by catheter drainage.

9. Administer cortisol (hydrocortisone sodium phosphate or sodium succinate), 100 mg/24 h intravenously in divided doses every 6 hours, or equivalent doses of synthetic corticosteroids. Patients with primary hypothyroidism may have decreased adrenal reserve, and panhypopituitarism is usual in those with secondary hypothyroidism.

10. Correct hyponatremia by restricting free water intake. Since hyponatremia usually resolves with treatment of the hypothyroidism, other interventions are not usually required.

11. Avoid administration of all unnecessary drugs, especially those with central nervous system depressant effects, since patients with hypothyroidism have decreased drug metabolism and hence increased sensitivity to many pharmacologic agents.

12. Identify and treat the precipitating cause of myxedema coma. Signs of infection may be masked by the metabolic disorder. If infection is suspected, give antibiotics empirically until results of cultures and susceptibility testing are available (see Table 3–6).

13. Note that recovery from myxedema coma is slow, since reversal of severe metabolic abnormalities is required.

B. Specific Therapy: Initial replacement of thyroid hormone is best given as levothyroxine, 300–500 μg as a single loading dose intravenously, which will replenish body stores; this is followed by 50–100 μg/d intravenously until the patient is able to take oral medication. Patients with known atherosclerotic cardiac disease present a difficult problem in management, since administration of thyroid hormone may precipitate arrhythmias, angina, or myocardial infarction. In these patients, the risk of cardiac disturbances must be weighed against the high death rate associated with myxedema coma.

Disposition

Hospitalization in an intensive care unit is indicated for patients in myxedema coma.

ADRENAL DISORDERS

ACUTE ADRENAL INSUFFICIENCY (Addisonian Crisis)

The loss of adrenal glucocorticoid or mineralocorticoid secretion has life-threatening consequences, since these hormones are required for maintenance of blood pressure, blood volume, glucose homeostasis, and a variety of other functions.

Classification

A. Primary adrenocortical insufficiency (Addison's disease) results from destruction of the adrenal cortex by a number of processes, of which the idiopathic (autoimmune) and granulomatous (due to tuberculosis or histoplasmosis) forms account for over 90% of cases. Adrenal insufficiency may also result from metastases to the adrenals and from AIDS. These processes result in deficiency of both glucocorticoids and mineralocorticoids. Medications such as aminoglutethimide and ketoconazole also may inhibit adrenal function.

B. Secondary adrenocortical insufficiency (ACTH deficiency) is most commonly caused by exogenous glucocorticoid administration and also by hypothalamic-pituitary disorders (frequently accompanied by panhypopituitarism). These disorders are characterized primarily by glucocorticoid deficiency; mineralocorticoid secretion (largely controlled by the renin-angiotensin system) is usually unimpaired.

C. Acute adrenal crisis may occur in either primary or secondary adrenal insufficiency, and there is usually a history of chronic symptoms. The acute crisis is usually precipitated by acute stress, eg, infection, hemorrhage, trauma, surgery, or abrupt cessation of glucocorticoid therapy. Acute destruction of the adrenal cortex due to hemorrhage (eg, in Waterhouse-Friderichsen syndrome) is an unusual type of acute adrenal crisis and is most frequently caused by septicemia in children and by anticoagulant therapy in adults.

Clinical Presentation

A. Preceding Manifestations:

1. Primary adrenocortical insufficiency leads to the following:

a. Hyperpigmentation of skin creases, extensor surfaces, scars, and the buccal mucosa.

b. Weakness and fatigue.

c. Anorexia and weight loss.

d. Nausea and vomiting and diarrhea.

e. Salt craving and postural hypotension.

2. Acute bilateral adrenal hemorrhage leading to

adrenal insufficiency is not accompanied by the above chronic manifestations but should be suspected in the following situations:

a. Patients with sepsis (eg, meningococcemia) who have rapid or unexplained deterioration.

b. Adults with major medical illnesses who have abdominal, flank, or chest pain; dehydration; hypotension; shock; or fever (especially if anticoagulants have been used).

3. Secondary adrenal insufficiency may present with acute adrenal insufficiency; in these patients it is preceded by one of the following:

a. History of or physical features characteristic of chronic glucocorticoid administration.

b. Symptoms of hypopituitarism (hypogonadism, hypothyroidism) and manifestations of a hypothalamic or pituitary tumor (including headache, visual field defects, or enlargement of the sella turcica) in patients with hypothalamic or pituitary disorders.

B. Symptoms and Signs of Acute Crisis:
1. Rapid worsening of preceding symptoms and severe weakness.

2. Fever.

3. Increased nausea and vomiting with nonspecific abdominal pain.

4. Rapid dehydration and hypovolemia.

5. Hypotension and shock.

6. Altered mental status ranging from lethargy to coma.

C. Laboratory Findings: The classic features of primary adrenocortical insufficiency are as follows:

1. Hyponatremia and hyperkalemia are present in 88% and 64% of patients, respectively. The finding of these 2 conditions together should suggest the diagnosis; however, their absence does not rule out acute adrenal insufficiency.

2. Azotemia.

3. Anemia of chronic disease, eosinophilia, and lymphocytosis.

4. Hypoglycemia or hypercalcemia in a few cases.

In secondary adrenocortical insufficiency, potassium, blood urea nitrogen, and serum creatinine are usually normal. There may be hyponatremia, anemia, eosinophilia, lymphocytosis, and hypoglycemia.

D. Imaging: Chest x-rays may reveal a small heart. Calcification of the adrenals may be present as a result of tuberculosis or histoplasmosis. Procedures such as computed tomographic (CT) scan or magnetic resonance imaging (MRI) may reveal adrenal masses or enlargement in patients with adrenal hemorrhage, invasive disorders, infection, or metastases. The adrenals are atrophic or absent in patients with autoimmune destruction.

E. Electrocardiographic Findings: The ECG may reveal low voltage in all leads and changes secondary to the electrolyte abnormalities.

Diagnosis

Perform a rapid ACTH stimulation test, and obtain a baseline plasma sample for ACTH measurement before initiation of glucocorticoid therapy.

A. Draw blood for baseline plasma cortisol and ACTH determination.

B. Give synthetic human $ACTH_{1-24}$ (cosyntropin [Cortrosyn, others]), 0.25 mg intravenously.

C. Draw blood for plasma cortisol measurement 30 and 60 minutes after the ACTH injection. In severely ill patients who require immediate therapy, the test may be limited to 30 minutes.

D. Normally, plasma cortisol concentration should increase by 5–8 µg/dL and reach a peak greater than 15–18 µg/dL. Normal responses vary with the cortisol assay used.

E. Basal ACTH levels are usually markedly elevated in patients with primary adrenal insufficiency but are normal or low in those with secondary forms (ACTH deficiency).

Treatment

A. Emergency Treatment: Cortisol (hydrocortisone) is the drug of choice, since both mineralocorticoid and glucocorticoid effects are necessary in acute adrenal crisis.

1. Give cortisol as hydrocortisone sodium phosphate or hydrocortisone sodium hemisuccinate; an initial dose of 100 mg intravenously is followed by 100 mg every 6 hours for 24 hours. If progress is satisfactory, the dose is reduced to 50 mg every 6 hours on the second day and then tapered to oral maintenance levels (20–30 mg/d in 2 doses: two-thirds in the morning and one-third in the late afternoon) by the fourth to fifth day.

2. *Caution:* Synthetic glucocorticoids (eg, prednisolone or dexamethasone) cause less sodium retention and should not be used in acute situations, particularly since parenteral mineralocorticoid therapy is no longer available.

3. *Caution:* Avoid *intramuscular* cortisone acetate in the treatment of acute adrenal crisis, since it is poorly absorbed, does not reach adequate blood levels, and does not have adequate biologic activity, as evidenced by failure to suppress the elevated plasma ACTH levels of primary adrenal insufficiency.

4. Added mineralocorticoid therapy is not required initially with the doses of hydrocortisone described above. However, in primary adrenocortical insufficiency, as the dose of hydrocortisone is tapered (below 40–60 mg/d), most patients also require mineralocorticoid support in the form of fludrocortisone acetate (Florinef), 0.05–0.1 mg orally daily.

B. General and Supportive Measures:
1. Insert a large-bore (≥ 16-gauge) intravenous catheter (central venous pressure monitoring may be required); draw blood samples for glucose and electrolyte determinations, renal function tests, and CBC. Perform a rapid ACTH stimulation test, and obtain plasma for ACTH measurement as described above.

2. Monitor body weight, fluid intake, and urine

output. Check serum electrolytes, glucose, and renal function every 4–6 hours initially and then once or twice daily until they are stable.

3. Replace fluid volume and electrolyte deficits, and correct hypoglycemia. Dehydration may be profound, and fluid deficits may exceed 20% of total body water.

a. Initial therapy–Give 5% dextrose in normal saline, 500 mL/h for 2–4 hours.

b. Subsequent therapy–Fluid volume and electrolyte replacement should later be determined by the blood pressure, serum electrolytes, and urine output.

c. Serum potassium–Although initial serum potassium is usually increased, there is frequently a deficit of total body potassium; replacement therapy should therefore be started when serum potassium begins to fall after hydration and cortisol administration.

4. Although most patients respond well to crystalloid solutions and glucocorticoid therapy, those with severe shock may require blood or colloids.

5. Vasopressors are frequently ineffective unless preceded and accompanied by adequate glucocorticoid and fluid therapy.

6. Avoid unnecessary procedures that may further provoke hypotension or dehydration. Avoid sedatives and narcotics.

7. Begin treatment of the underlying cause, usually an infection. Look for associated conditions such as hypothyroidism or panhypopituitarism.

Disposition

All patients with clinically suspected or documented addisonian crisis must be hospitalized. If the patient is hypotensive or in shock, hospitalization in the intensive care unit is preferred.

PHEOCHROMOCYTOMA (Catecholamine Crisis)

Excess circulating catecholamines may lead to severe or malignant hypertension or to acute hypertensive crisis (Chapter 28). Excessive amounts of circulating catecholamines are usually due to pheochromocytoma, a chromaffin cell tumor, of which 90% arise from the adrenal medulla. Catecholamine crisis may also result from increased intake of catecholamine precursors (drugs such as ephedrine or amphetamine or foods containing tyramine, such as aged cheese, Chianti wine) in patients unable to metabolize them, eg, those taking monoamine oxidase inhibitors. Abrupt cessation of therapy with clonidine may also produce a syndrome of severe hypertension with excessive catecholamines.

Diagnosis
A. History:
1. Classic manifestations during acute episodes

include attacks of headache, sweating, pallor, and heat intolerance; palpitations, nervousness, and apprehension; and nausea and vomiting.

2. Weight loss and symptoms of hyperglycemia may also occur.

3. A history of medications used usually identifies those patients with catecholamine crisis secondary to monoamine oxidase inhibitor therapy or clonidine withdrawal.

4. Patients with acute hypertensive crises, myocardial infarction, stroke, or acute anxiety and panic attacks may have elevated catecholamines without pheochromocytoma, and this must be considered in the differential diagnosis.

B. Symptoms and Signs:
1. Hypertension is usually sustained, with superimposed paroxysmal exacerbations during which the blood pressure may exceed 220/150 mm Hg. A few patients are normotensive between paroxysmal attacks. Hypertension may be accompanied by headache, visual disturbances, papilledema, retinal hemorrhages, encephalopathy, congestive heart failure and pulmonary edema, aortic dissection, or hemorrhagic stroke.

2. Postural tachycardia and hypotension are usually present and are important diagnostic clues.

3. Anxiety, apprehension, or irritability is noted.

4. Increased sweating with warm skin occurs.

5. Sinus tachycardia is common, and tachyarrhythmias may occur, especially in patients with excessive epinephrine secretion.

6. Hypertensive retinopathy may be found in those with long-standing disease.

7. Mucosal neuromas and a marfanoid appearance suggest multiple endocrine neoplasia type IIB.

8. Recklinghausen's disease is associated with pheochromocytoma, and these patients have cutaneous neurofibromatosis and café au lait spots.

C. Laboratory Examination and Special Tests:
1. Definitive diagnosis depends on the demonstration of elevated catecholamines or their metabolites in serum or urine. Potentially dangerous provocative tests are rarely necessary, since patients with sustained hypertension have elevated basal catecholamine secretion. In patients with episodic symptoms, 24-hour urine collections may show normal levels; however, catechol excess can be demonstrated in 3-hour collections during episodes.

2. Increased hematocrit due to volume depletion frequently occurs, and the white blood cell count may be elevated, with increased PMNs.

3. Hyperglycemia is often present.

4. The ECG shows sinus tachycardia and various other abnormalities, including (**a**) myocardial infarction, (**b**) ST depression in limb and anterior precordial leads due to subendocardial ischemia, (**c**) transient ST elevation simulating transmural myocardial infarction, (**d**) marked diffuse T wave inversion with prolonged QT interval similar to the pattern seen in cerebrovascular accident, and **(e)** tachyarrhythmias and ectopic beats.

5. Current procedures that effectively localize pheochromocytoma are CT scan, MRI, and isotope scanning with MIBG (^{131}I-metaiodobenzylguanidine).

Treatment

The patient presenting with hypertensive crisis should be treated immediately as detailed in Chapter 28. Prepare the patient for admission to the intensive care unit.

A. General and Supportive Measures:

1. Insert a large-bore ($\geq$ 16-gauge) intravenous catheter.

2. Begin cardiac monitoring; an arterial pressure line may be required to monitor the blood pressure.

3. Draw blood for routine studies (CBC, serum electrolytes, glucose, and hepatic and renal function) and subsequent catecholamine determination.

4. Replace volume deficits, and correct electrolyte abnormalities as required.

5. Avoid all unnecessary drugs and invasive procedures that may further provoke excess catecholamine secretion.

6. Begin 24-hour urine collection for fractionated catecholamines, metanephrine, and VMA (4-hydroxy-3-methoxymandelic acid; vanillylmandelic acid).

B. Specific Measures:

1. Sodium nitroprusside, 0.5–10 μg/kg/min by continuous intravenous infusion using an infusion pump, is very effective in the treatment of acute hypertensive crisis due to pheochromocytoma and is the drug of choice for management of intraoperative hypertension. It generally affords more stable control of hypertension than do intermittent doses of phentolamine. See Chapter 28 for further details.

2. Alpha-adrenergic blockage with phentolamine was the traditional method of acute therapy for pheochromocytoma.

a. Give phentolamine, 1–2 mg intravenously every 5 minutes initially. *Caution:* Higher initial doses may cause sudden severe hypotension. If no response is seen, increase the dose as necessary to 5 mg intravenously every 5 minutes until adequate control of blood pressure is achieved.

b. Maintain the patient on phentolamine, 1–5 mg intravenously every 2–4 hours as required.

c. As soon as oral intake is possible, give phenoxybenzamine, a long-acting alpha-adrenergic blocker that can be given twice daily. The initial dose is 10 mg twice daily, which is then increased in increments of 20 mg/d until blood pressure is well controlled, with mild orthostatic hypotension, and until other symptoms, especially sweating, are abolished. Many patients require 100–200 mg of phenoxybenzamine per day to achieve normotension and prevent hypertensive episodes.

d. Orthostatic hypotension is quite common during initial therapy and after increases in dosage; it frequently resolves or becomes less severe if phenoxybenzamine is continued (presumably as a result of volume expansion). Orthostatic hypotension can be managed by keeping the patient recumbent and correcting volume depletion; the phenoxybenzamine should not be withheld or discontinued unless severe symptomatic hypotension is present.

3. Beta-adrenergic blockade is usually administered only to patients with severe tachycardia or tachyarrhythmias. These symptoms are most prominent in patients with excessive epinephrine secretion. Beta blockade should be initiated with propranolol, 1–2 mg intravenously at a rate of 1 mg/min and repeated every 5 minutes to a total dose of 10 mg; maintenance therapy is with propranolol, 20–80 mg orally every 6 hours. *Caution:* Alpha blockade, as described above, should be done first in order to prevent unopposed alpha (vasoconstrictive) activity following beta blockade. Recently, labetalol hydrochloride, an adrenergic blocking agent with both alpha and beta effects, has been shown to be effective in the treatment of pheochromocytoma. In milder cases, it may be useful as the sole agent. Give 20 mg intravenously slowly, then 40–80 mg intravenously every 10 minutes until the desired effect is achieved or 300 mg has been given. Oral dosing can begin when the blood pressure begins to rise.

4. Preoperative management measures are as follows:

a. Give phenoxybenzamine orally in increasing doses until symptoms are abolished and blood pressure is less than 160/90 mm Hg for 3 consecutive days. In uncomplicated cases, this may require 2–6 weeks; however, in patients with myocardial ischemia or infarction, 3–6 months of treatment may be required before the patient is ready for surgery.

b. Continue phenoxybenzamine up to and including the morning of surgery. With adequate alpha blockade, postoperative hypotension is unusual, and when it does occur, it can be corrected with blood and volume replacement.

Disposition

Hospitalization in an intensive care unit is mandatory in all cases.

DISORDERS OF ANTIDIURETIC HORMONE

INAPPROPRIATE SECRETION OF ANTIDIURETIC HORMONE (SIADH)

The syndrome of inappropriate secretion of antidiuretic hormone (SIADH) results in hyponatremia and hypotonicity of plasma. Hyponatremia and decreased plasma osmolality result from decreased free water excretion; the resulting increase in the volume of extracellular fluid leads to continued urinary sodium excretion in the face of hyponatremia.

Etiology

SIADH is caused by a variety of disorders of which the most common are tumor production, central nervous system disorders, lung disease, and drugs. Myxedema may cause a clinically similar syndrome, and it is important to remember that ADH may play a role in the hyponatremia produced by numerous conditions.

Diagnosis

Classic SIADH is characterized by the following:

(1) Hyponatremia with lower than normal plasma osmolality in the absence of dehydration or volume depletion.

(2) Failure of the kidney to dilute the urine to the greatest extent possible (ie, to less than 100 mosm/kg H_2O despite reduced plasma osmolality). Urine osmolality is frequently greater than 300 mosm/kg H_2O and is usually greater than serum osmolality.

(3) Continued sodium excretion (usually > 20 meq/L) despite hyponatremia.

(4) Normal adrenal and thyroid function.

(5) Absence of hepatic, renal, or cardiac failure.

A. Symptoms and Signs: The clinical presentation of SIADH depends on the level of hyponatremia and the degree of water intoxication (Chapter 36). Manifestations of the underlying disease may include evidence of cancer, central nervous system disease, pulmonary disease, or a history of use of certain medications (eg, chlorpropamide). The differential diagnosis of hyponatremic states is discussed in Chapter 36.

1. In milder cases (serum sodium > 120 meq/L), there may be no clinical manifestations.

2. When serum sodium is moderately depressed (115–120 meq/L), neurologic manifestations predominate and include anorexia, nausea and vomiting, personality changes, depressed tendon reflexes, and muscle weakness.

3. With severe hyponatremia (serum sodium < 115 meq/L), coma, seizures, bulbar palsy, hypo-

thermia, and altered patterns of respiration may occur.

4. Edema is unusual even with severe hyponatremia and water intoxication.

B. Laboratory Findings: Hyponatremia is the classic feature of SIADH. In severe cases, serum sodium may be less than 110 meq/L. Hypo-osmolality of plasma also occurs. There is persistent urinary excretion of sodium (> 20 meq/L), and urine osmolality is inappropriately high for the degree of hyponatremia and plasma hypo-osmolality. Blood urea nitrogen and uric acid levels may be below normal.

Indices of renal, hepatic, cardiac, thyroid, and adrenal function are normal.

Treatment
(See also Chapter 36.)

A. General and Supportive Measures:

1. Insert a large-bore (≥ 16-gauge) intravenous catheter, and keep the line patent with an infusion of normal saline.

2. Draw blood for measurement of serum sodium, electrolytes, creatinine, blood urea nitrogen, osmolality, cortisol, and thyroid function determinations.

3. Send urine for urinalysis and measurement of urinary osmolality, electrolytes, and specific gravity.

4. Monitor and record intravascular volume, body weight, intake, and urine output. Measure serum and urine electrolytes and osmolality every 4–6 hours during the acute phase and then once or twice daily until the patient's condition has stabilized.

5. Assess the patient for evidence of renal, hepatic, or cardiac dysfunction. Obtain a history of drugs and medications used by the patient. Evaluate as appropriate for clinical evidence of cancer, central nervous system disease, or pulmonary disease.

B. Specific Therapy: *Caution:* Overly rapid correction of hyponatremia can cause neurologic complications such as seizures and has been implicated in the development of central pontine myelinolysis.

1. Fluid restriction is the treatment of choice.

a. Mild SIADH–(Serum sodium > 120 meq/L.) Total intake should be limited to 1000 mL/24 h and the response of serum sodium and plasma osmolality carefully monitored.

b. More severe SIADH–(Serum sodium < 120/meq/L.) Restrict fluids to 500 mL/24 h or less. Patients with significant neurologic symptoms should be treated for severe SIADH as described below.

c. Severe SIADH–(Serum sodium < 110 meq/L.) Use furosemide and isotonic or hypertonic saline to increase serum sodium concentration. Although many authorities have cautioned to limit the rate of correction to 1–2 meq of saline per hour, this caution has been called into question by a clinical trial that showed no detriment as a result of more rapid correction.

(1) Furosemide (1 mg/kg body weight intravenously) is used with isotonic saline—or, in the most severe cases, hypertonic saline (3% or 5%)—since it causes excretion of hypotonic urine, inducing negative water balance (excretion of free water). Subsequent doses are given as required to maintain the output of hypotonic urine.

(2) Monitor sodium and potassium losses *hourly,* and replace the losses. Continue until serum sodium increases to 125–130 meq/L (usually 8–10 hours). Fluid restriction should then be instituted to prevent recurrent hyponatremia.

(3) Hypertonic (3%) sodium chloride alone has also been used in severe SIADH. However, the sodium is rapidly excreted, and the effect is transient. In addition, further volume expansion may cause congestive heart failure and pulmonary edema.

2. Patients with recurrent or persistent SIADH—which is usually due to ectopic ADH production by cancer—may require chronic fluid restriction. In severe cases, give demeclocycline (demethylchlortetracycline), an inhibitor of ADH action, 600–1200 mg orally daily. The drug is not useful in acute situations, since the onset of action may require 5–8 days; azotemia is the most common adverse effect. Lithium and phenytoin appear to be less effective.

Disposition

A. Responsible patients with mild SIADH (serum sodium > 125 meq/L without neurologic symptoms) may be managed on an outpatient basis with restriction of fluid intake and close follow-up.

B. Patients with more severe SIADH and those who may not follow proposed treatment recommendations should be hospitalized. Patients treated with hypertonic saline should be admitted to an intensive care unit.

CENTRAL DIABETES INSIPIDUS

Central diabetes insipidus is due to antidiuretic hormone (ADH) deficiency and leads to an inability to concentrate the urine, with consequent polyuria, volume depletion, and hyperosmolality, which stimulate thirst and lead to polydipsia. The conscious patient with an intact thirst mechanism and access to water compensates for water loss by increased intake. However, severe dehydration and volume depletion may occur in patients with decreased fluid intake caused by decreased level of consciousness, defective thirst mechanism (usually secondary to hypothalamic mass lesions), or no access to fluids.

Etiology

Central diabetes insipidus is most frequently caused by invasive or infiltrative lesions of the hypothalamus, including craniopharyngioma, primary or metastatic hypothalamic tumors, chronic infection (tubercular, syphilitic, fungal), sarcoid, and histiocytic disorders (multifocal eosinophilic granuloma Hand-Schüller-Christian disease). Pituitary surgery is a frequent cause of transient diabetes insipidus; unusual causes include trauma, vascular accident, or hemorrhage. Familial and idiopathic types also occur.

Diagnosis

A presumptive diagnosis of central diabetes insipidus may be made if volume depletion, hypernatremia, and serum hyperosmolality are accompanied by polyuria and low specific gravity and hypo-osmolality of urine. The response to administration of ADH is also diagnostically useful, because in central diabetes insipidus, there is a rapid decrease in urine volume with increased urine specific gravity and osmolality; patients with nephrogenic diabetes insipidus fail to respond.

A. Symptoms and Signs:

1. ADH deficiency–

a. Thirst (with a particular craving for cold liquids) may be so intense as to awaken the patient from sleep.

b. Polyuria and nocturia occur.

c. Fluid intake and urine output range from 5 L to as much as 20 L per day. The specific gravity of urine is less than 1.006.

d. Weight loss, fatigue, lethargy, and somnolence are often present.

2. Hypernatremia and hyperosmolality–

a. Irritability, delirium, or confusion may be seen.

b. Fever, dizziness, muscle cramps, and headache may also occur.

c. Physical signs depend on the degree of dehydration and hyperosmolality. Patients with marked volume deficits typically have hypotension, tachypnea, tachycardia, and decreased levels of consciousness. Fever may be present. With severe dehydration, shock and coma supervene.

3. Patients with chronic hypothalamic lesions may also manifest visual field defects and anterior pituitary insufficiency.

B. Laboratory Findings: Hypernatremia and hyperosmolality are found in uncompensated patients. Serum sodium may be 160 meq/L in severe cases, and prerenal azotemia is usual in these patients. Specific gravity and osmolality of urine are low in proportion to serum osmolality.

Differential Diagnosis

Rule out primary, or "psychogenic," polydipsia, in which increased fluid intake leads to polyuria with dilute urine, and other disorders of the renal concentrating mechanisms that do not respond to ADH administration, eg, nephrogenic diabetes insipidus, chronic renal disease, hypokalemia, hypercalcemia, renal amyloidosis, multiple myeloma, and Sjögren's syndrome. Drugs such as lithium, methoxyflurane, and demeclocycline also affect the renal concentrating mechanisms and induce transient nephrogenic diabetes insipidus.

Treatment

A. General Measures:

1. Insert a large-bore (≥ 16-gauge) intravenous catheter, and draw blood samples for measurement of electrolytes, osmolality, glucose, calcium, and cortisol and for renal and thyroid function tests. Measure plasma ADH, which, if very low, may be diagnostic.

2. Obtain urine specimens for routine urinalysis and specific gravity and osmolality measurements.

3. Monitor volume status, body weight, fluid intake, and urine output and specific gravity.

B. Volume and Electrolyte Deficits: (See also Chapter 36.)

1. Give water orally if the patient is conscious.

2. If shock is present, restore intravascular volume with saline, 0.45% or 0.9%, intravenously.

3. With severe hypernatremia (serum sodium concentration > 150 meq/L) or obtundation without shock, give 5% dextrose in water intravenously, and replace half of the volume deficit during the first 12–24 hours. Do not give fluid more rapidly than this, since excessively rapid lowering of the serum sodium concentration and osmolality may result in cerebral edema with coma or seizures. See Chapter 36 for further details of treatment of severe hypernatremia.

4. When serum sodium decreases to less than 150 meq/L, sodium chloride, 0.45% or 0.9%, is substituted for 5% dextrose in water depending on the amount of sodium depletion.

C. Specific Measures: ADH therapy should begin with fluid replacement.

1. Desmopressin acetate (DDAVP), a long-acting vasopressin analog, is the current drug of choice. The parenteral dose is 1–4 µg given intravenously or subcutaneously every 12–24 hours. The next dose is administered when polyuria recurs (> 200 mL/h). In alert patients and for maintenance therapy, desmopressin acetate is given by nasal inhalation. The usual dose is 10 µg (range 5–20 µg) every 12–24 hours.

2. Aqueous vasopressin (Pitressin), 5–10 units subcutaneously every 3–6 hours; or lysine vasopressin (lypressin; Diapid), 2 sprays to each nostril every 3–6 hours, may also be used. These preparations have the disadvantage of a short duration of action.

3. Adjust the ADH dose and timing to relieve thirst and polyuria. Avoid set dosage schedules, since excessive ADH administration may cause volume overload, hyponatremia, and water intoxication.

Disposition

Hospitalize all patients for definitive diagnosis and treatment.

PITUITARY DISORDERS

PITUITARY APOPLEXY

Pituitary apoplexy occurs almost exclusively in patients with pituitary tumors and is due to hemorrhagic infarction of the pituitary tumor or the pituitary gland itself. Chronic hemorrhage into the pituitary gland or gradual infarction of it may occur without symptoms. However, *sudden* hemorrhage or infarction is a *medical emergency*.

The clinical manifestations result from (1) leakage of blood or necrotic tissue into the subarachnoid space, (2) the development of a rapidly expanding hemorrhagic intrasellar mass lesion with pressure on the optic chiasm, cavernous sinuses, cranial nerves, and adjacent structures (hypothalamus and internal carotid arteries), and (3) acute hypopituitarism.

Precipitating events include the use of anticoagulants, radiation therapy, trauma, hypertension, estrogen therapy, or respiratory infections. Sheehan's syndrome (peripartum pituitary necrosis) represents vasospastic infarction secondary to intrapartum hemorrhage and shock. Patients usually present with failure to lactate and then develop other signs and symptoms of hypopituitarism.

Diagnosis

A. Symptoms and Signs: Neurologic symptoms are most prominent, and transient neurologic symptoms frequently precede the acute event over several days. The usual symptoms and signs include the following:

1. Increasing headache, diplopia, blurred vision, visual loss, and visual field defects (especially bitemporal hemianopia).

2. Extraocular motor palsies are common.

3. Altered mental status with lethargy, confusion, and delirium that may progress to coma.

4. Nausea and vomiting.

5. Less commonly, paresthesias, ataxia, seizures, and focal hemispheric symptoms.

6. Symptoms of the preexisting pituitary adenoma, eg, previous headache, visual defects, and hypopituitarism.

7. Meningeal irritation may be prominent, and there may be mild hemispheric dysfunction.

8. Fever is common and may result from subarachnoid bleeding, acute hypoadrenalism, or hypothalamic compression.

9. Hypotension is present in those with acute adrenal insufficiency.

10. Respiratory failure may occur because of hypothalamic compression or increased intracranial pressure.

B. Laboratory Findings:

1. Hypernatremia or hyponatremia may occur as a result of diabetes insipidus or SIADH, respectively.

2. The cerebrospinal fluid is xanthochromic or grossly bloody, with elevated pressure. Analysis reveals elevated protein concentration and increased numbers of red and white cells.

C. Imaging: MRI and CT scan are the most rapid and accurate means of diagnosis; they reveal an enlarged sella turcica, suprasellar extension of the hemorrhagic pituitary adenoma, and compression of the cavernous sinuses.

Treatment

A. Insert a large-bore (≥ 16-gauge) intravenous line. Draw blood for CBC, electrolyte determination, thyroid function tests, and growth hormone, cortisol, and prolactin measurements.

B. Begin cardiac monitoring.

C. Administer a soluble cortisol preparation (hydrocortisone sodium succinate or phosphate), 100 mg intravenously, and then treat as for acute adrenocortical insufficiency (p 660).

D. Correct electrolyte abnormalities, and treat diabetes insipidus or SIADH as required.

E. Obtain an emergency CT or MRI scan.

F. Emergency neurosurgical decompression of the sella turcica may be required in patients with decreasing consciousness, deteriorating visual acuity or visual fields, or increasing extraocular motor palsies, indicating cavernous sinus compression.

Disposition

Hospitalization and neurosurgical consultation are indicated. Surgery is the definitive treatment of pituitary apoplexy, although not every patient will require operation; some patients recover without sequelae on conservative management alone.

REFERENCES

General

DeGroot LJ (editor): *Endocrinology,* 2nd ed. Saunders, 1989.

Felig P et al (editors): *Endocrinology and Metabolism,* 2nd ed. McGraw-Hill, 1987.

Wilson J, Foster DW (editors): *Williams Textbook of Endocrinology,* 8th ed. Saunders, 1992.

Hyperglycemic Emergencies

Davgirdas JT et al: Hyperosmolar coma: Cellular dehydration and serum sodium concentration. Ann Intern Med 1989;110:855.

Fisher JN, Kitabchi AE: A randomized study of phosphate therapy in the treatment of diabetic ketoacidosis. J Clin Endocrinol Metab 1983;57:177.

Foster DW, McGarry JD: The metabolic derangements and treatment of diabetic ketoacidosis. N Engl J Med 1983;309:159.

Fulop M: The treatment of severely uncontrolled diabetes mellitus. Adv Intern Med 1984;29:327.

Keller U: Diabetic ketoacidosis: Current views on pathogenesis and treatment. Diabetologia 1986;29:71.

Kitabchi AE, Rumbak M: The management of diabetic emergencies. Hosp Pract (June) 1989;24:129.

Morris LR, Murphy MB, Kitabchi AE: Bicarbonate therapy in severe diabetic ketoacidosis. Ann Intern Med 1986;105:836.

Pope DW, Dansky D: Hyperosmolar hyperglycemic nonketotic coma. Emerg Med Clin North Am 1989;7:849.

Rosenblum AL: Intracerebral crises during treatment of diabetic ketoacidosis. Diabetes Care 1990;13:22.

Sanson TH, Levin SN: Management of diabetic ketoacidosis. Drugs 1989;38:289.

Hypoglycemia

Arem R: Hypoglycemia associated with renal failure. Endocrinol Metab Clin North Am 1989;18:103.

Arky RA: Hypoglycemia associated with liver disease and ethanol. Endocrinol Metab Clin North Am 1989;18:75.

Cryer PE: Iatrogenic hypoglycemia as a cause of hypoglycemia-associated autonomic failure in IDDM: A vicious cycle. Diabetes 1992;41:255.

Miller SI et al: Hypoglycemia as a manifestation of sepsis. Am J Med 1980;68:649.

Seltzer HS: Drug-induced hypoglycemia: A review of 1418 cases. Endocrinol Metab Clin North Am 1989;18:163.

Yealy DM, Wolfson AB: Hypoglycemia. Emerg Clin North Am 1989;7:837.

Lactic Acidosis

Cohen RD, Woods HF: Lactic acidosis revisited. Diabetes 1983;32:181.

Cooper DJ et al: Bicarbonate does not improve hemodynamics in critically ill patients who have lactic acidosis: A prospective, controlled clinical study. Ann Intern Med 1990;112:492.

Kreisberg RA: Pathogenesis and management of lactic acidosis. Annu Rev Med 1984;35:181.

Mizock BA: Lactic acidosis. Disease-a-Month 1989;35:235.

Narins RG, Cohen JJ: Bicarbonate therapy for organic acidosis: The case for its continued use. Ann Intern Med 1987;106:615.

Alcoholic Ketoacidosis

Miller PD, Heinig RE, Waterhouse C: Treatment of alcoholic acidosis. Arch Intern Med 1978;138:67.

Williams HE: Alcoholic hypoglycemia and ketoacidosis. Med Clin North Am 1984;68:33.

Thyroid Storm

Gavin LA: Thyroid crises. Med Clin North Am 1991;75:179.

Roth RN, McAuliffe MJ: Hyperthyroidism and thyroid storm. Emerg Med Clin North Am 1989;7:873.

Myxedema Coma

Gavin LA: Thyroid crises. Med Clin North Am 1991;75:179.

Hylander B, Rosenqvist U: Treatment of myxedema coma: Factors associated with fatal outcome. Acta Endocrinol 1985;108:65.

Mitchell JM: Thyroid disease in the emergency department: Thyroid function tests and hypothyroidism and myxedema coma. Emerg Med Clin North Am 1989;7:885.

Acute Adrenal Insufficiency (Addison's Disease)

Bosworth DC: Reversible adrenocortical insufficiency in fulminant meningococcemia. Arch Intern Med 1979;139:823.

Burke CW: Adrenocortical insufficiency. Clin Endocrinol Metab 1985;14:947.

Byyny RL: Drug therapy: Withdrawal from glucocorticoid therapy. N Engl J Med 1976;295:30.

Dahlberg PJ, Goellner MH, Pekling GB: Adrenal insufficiency secondary to adrenal hemorrhage: Two case reports and a review of cases confirmed by computed tomography. Arch Intern Med 1990;150:905.

Green LW et al: Adrenal insufficiency as a complication of the acquired immunodeficiency syndrome. Ann Intern Med 1984;101:497.

Rao RH, Vagnucci AH, Amico JA: Bilateral massive adrenal hemorrhage: Early recognition and treatment. Ann Intern Med 1989;110:227.

Rusnak RA: Adrenal and pituitary emergencies. Emerg Clin North Am 1989;7:903.

Seidenwurm DJ et al: Metastases to the adrenal glands and the development of Addison's disease. Cancer 1984;54:552.

Tucker WS Jr et al: Reversible adrenal insufficiency induced by ketoconazole. JAMA 1985;253:2413.

Pheochromocytoma (Catecholamine Crisis)

Bravo EL, Gifford RW Jr: Pheochromocytoma: Diagnosis, localization and management. N Engl J Med 1984;311:1298.

Modlinger RS, Ertel NH, Hauptman JB: Adrenergic blockade in pheochromocytoma. Arch Intern Med 1983;143:2245.

Newell KA et al: Pheochromocytoma multisystem crisis: A surgical emergency. Arch Surg 1989;123:956.

Shapiro B, Fig LM: Management of pheochromocytoma. Endocrinol Metab Clin North Am 1989;18:443.

Van Heerden JA et al: Pheochromocytoma: Current status and changing trends. Surgery 1982;91:367.

Inappropriate Secretion of Antidiuretic Hormone (SIADH)

Anderson RJ: Hospital-associated hyponatremia. Kidney Int 1986;29:1237.

Arieff AI: Osmotic failure: Physiology and strategies for treatment. Hosp Pract (May) 1988;23:173.

Ayus JC, Krothapalli RK, Arieff AI: Changing concepts in treatment of severe symptomatic hyponatremia: Rapid correction and possible relation to central pontine myelinolysis. Am J Med 1985;78:897.

Cluitmans FHM, Meinders AE: Management of severe hyponatremia: Rapid or slow correction? Am J Med 1990;88:161.

Laureno R, Karp BI: Pontine and extrapontine myelinolysis following rapid correction of hyponatremia. Lancet 1988;1:1439.

Nairns RG: Therapy of hyponatremia: Does haste make waste? (Editorial.) N Engl J Med 1986;314:1573.

Sterns, RH: The treatment of hyponatremia: First do no harm. Am J Med 1990;88:557.

Vitting KE et al: Frequency of hyponatremia and nonosmolar vasopressin release in the acquired immunodeficiency syndrome. JAMA 1990;263:973.

Vokes TJ, Robertson GL: Disorders of antidiuretic hormone. Endocrinol Metab Clin North Am 1988;17:281.

Votey SR, Peters AL, Hoffman JR: Disorders of water metabolism: Hyponatremia and hypernatremia. Emerg Clin North Am 1989;7:749.

Zerbe R, Stropes L, Robertson G: Vasopressin function in the syndrome of inappropriate antidiuresis. Annu Rev Med 1980;31:315.

Diabetes Insipidus

Cobb WE, Spare S, Reichlin S: Neurogenic diabetes insipidus: Management with dDAVP (1-desamino-8-D-arginine vasopressin). Ann Intern Med 1978;88:183.

Robertson GL: Differential diagnosis of polyuria. Annu Rev Med 1988;39:425.

Vokes TJ, Robertson GL: Disorders of antidiuretic hormone. Endocrinol Metab Clin North Am 1988;17:281.

Votey ST, Peters AL, Hoffman JR: Disorders of water metabolism: Hyponatremia and hypernatremia. Emerg Med Clin North Am 1989;7:749.

Pituitary Apoplexy

Reid RL, Quigley ME, Yen SSC: Pituitary apoplexy: A review. Arch Neurol 1985;42:712.

Rusnak R: Adrenal and pituitary emergencies. Emerg Med Clin North Am 1989;7:903.

Veldhuis JD, Hammond JM: Endocrine function after spontaneous infarction of the human pituitary: Report, review, and reappraisal. Endocr Rev 1980;1:100.

Wakai S et al: Pituitary apoplexy: Its incidence and clinical significance. J Neurosurg 1981;55:187.

Fluid, Electrolyte, & Acid-Base Emergencies

36

Michael H. Humphreys, MD

I. DIAGNOSIS OF FLUID & ELECTROLYTE DISORDERS

Variations in Body Fluid Volume

Variations in body fluid volume can usually be identified on the basis of the physical examination.

A. Volume Excess: Volume excess is manifested as (**1**) peripheral edema or (**2**) circulatory over- load (jugular venous distention, pleural effusion, cardiac gallop).

B. Volume Depletion: Volume depletion is shown by (**1**) poor skin turgor or (**2**) dry mucous membranes.

C. Circulatory Compromise and Decreased Intravascular Volume: Compromised circulation and decreased intravascular volume are manifested by (**1**) resting tachycardia, (**2**) narrowed pulse pressure, or (**3**) orthostatic hypotension or shock.

Variations in Electrolyte Concentration

Disordered electrolyte concentrations produce

vague symptoms that are referable chiefly to the neuromuscular system and are therefore often mistaken for primary neurologic or metabolic abnormalities.

Detection of electrolyte abnormalities requires laboratory measurement of blood constituents (sodium, potassium, chloride, bicarbonate, hydrogen ion, calcium, magnesium, and phosphorus). These tests are indicated for any patient with even vague neuromuscular symptoms.

Approach to the Patient

A. Normal Values: Evaluation and treatment are based on (1) assessment of total body water and its distribution and (2) electrolyte concentrations.

1. Body water–Table 36–1 lists the normal volumes of various body fluid compartments both as fractions of body weight and as amounts in liters in a hypothetical man or woman.

2. Electrolytes–Table 36–2 presents the normal ranges of serum electrolyte concentrations.

3. Osmolality–The osmolality of fluid in any one compartment is identical to that in all other compartments; normally, it is about 290 mosm/kg.

B. History: The history should include information about the following:

1. Salt and water retention–
a. Retention or loss of fluid.
b. Symptoms of heart failure.
c. Recent increase in weight.
d. Edema or ascites.

2. Volume depletion–
a. Gastrointestinal losses from vomiting or diarrhea.
b. Urinary losses associated with renal disease, administration of diuretics, or diabetes insipidus.
c. Excessive insensible loss from skin associated with fever or sweating.

C. Physical Examination: The physical examination supports the historical data by demonstrating significant volume depletion or excess; particularly helpful in this regard are any documented changes in body weight that have occurred over a short time. A decrease in blood pressure and an increase in pulse rate when the patient changes from the supine to an upright (sitting or standing) position is a sensitive measure of intravascular hypovolemia.

D. Laboratory and X-Ray Examinations: Lab-

Table 36–2. Normal serum electrolyte concentrations.

Sodium (Na$^+$)	136–146 meq/L
Potassium (K$^+$)	3.5–5 meq/L
Chloride (Cl$^-$)	96–106 meq/L
Bicarbonate (HCO$_3^-$)	24–28 meq/L
Calcium (Ca^{2+})	8.5–10.5 mg/dL (4.2–5.2 meq/L)
Magnesium (Mg^{2+})	1.8–3 mg/dL (1.5–2.5 meq/L)
Phosphate (PO$_4^{3-}$)	3–4.5 mg/dL (1–1.5 mmol/L)

oratory measurements and radiologic evaluation provide corroboration and quantification of abnormalities.

II. MANAGEMENT OF SPECIFIC DISORDERS

DISORDERS OF SERUM SODIUM CONCENTRATION

HYPONATREMIA
(See algorithm.)

General Considerations

Hyponatremia is commonly associated with many disease processes (Table 36–3) and use of certain drugs (Table 36–4). It is characterized by a serum sodium concentration under 130 meq/L. Symptoms of hyponatremia vary but relate primarily to alterations in central nervous system function: delirium, drowsiness, and lethargy progressing to coma and seizures. These symptoms may coexist with those caused by concurrent volume depletion: faintness and dizziness,

Table 36–3. Conditions causing hyponatremia.

True hyponatremia
  Hypervolemic:
    Heart failure
    Liver failure
    Kidney failure
    Nephrotic syndrome
  Normovolemic:
    Adrenal corticosteroid insufficiency
    Inappropriate secretion of antidiuretic hormone
    Hypothyroidism
    Drugs (Table 36–4)
    Poisons (methanol, ethylene glycol)
    Psychogenic polydipsia
  Hypovolemic:
    Renal salt loss (diuretics, mineralocorticoid deficiency)
    Extrarenal salt loss (sweating, vomiting, diarrhea, peritonitis, burns, muscle trauma)
Spurious hyponatremia
  Hyperglycemia
  Hyperlipidemia
  Hyperproteinemia

Table 36–1. Volume of body fluid compartments.

	Fraction of Body Weight	Typical Volume	
		Woman (120 lb [55 kg])	Man (154 lb [70 kg])
Total body water	0.5–0.6	28 L	42 L
Intracellular fluid	0.35–0.4	20 L	28 L
Extracellular fluid	0.15–0.2	8 L	14 L
Plasma volume	0.05–0.07	3 L	5 L

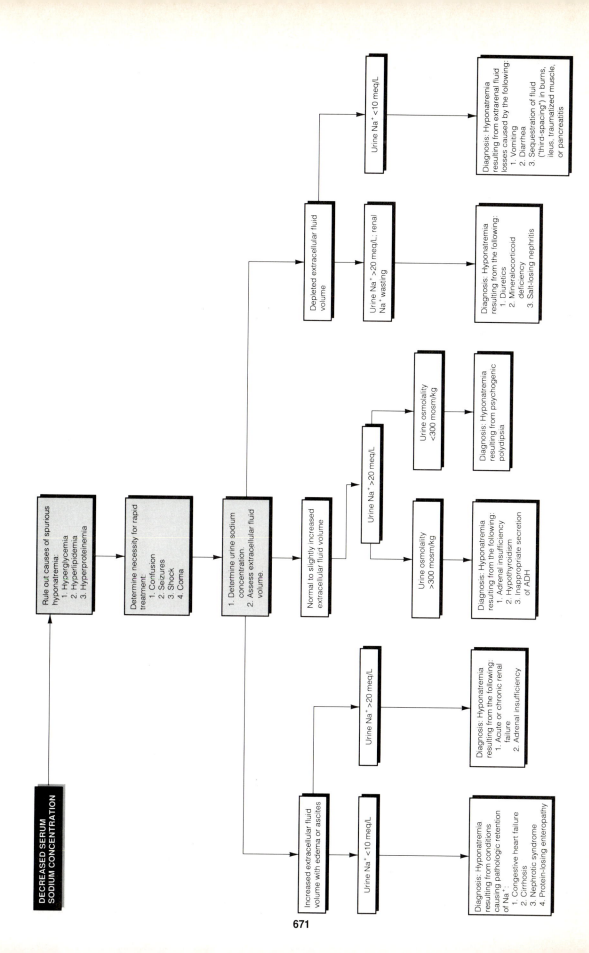

DECREASED SERUM SODIUM CONCENTRATION

Rule out causes of spurious hyponatremia:
1. Hyperglycemia
2. Hyperlipidemia
3. Hyperproteinemia

Determine necessity for rapid treatment:
1. Confusion
2. Seizures
3. Shock
4. Coma

1. Determine urine sodium concentration.
2. Assess extracellular fluid volume.

Normal to slightly increased extracellular fluid volume

Urine Na⁺ >20 meq/L

Urine osmolality <300 mosm/kg

Diagnosis: Hyponatremia resulting from psychogenic polydipsia

Urine osmolality >300 mosm/kg

Diagnosis: Hyponatremia resulting from the following:
1. Adrenal insufficiency
2. Hypothyroidism
3. Inappropriate secretion of ADH

Depleted extracellular fluid volume

Urine Na⁺ <10 meq/L

Diagnosis: Hyponatremia resulting from extrarenal fluid losses caused by the following:
1. Vomiting
2. Diarrhea
3. Sequestration of fluid ("third-spacing") in burns, ileus, traumatized muscle, or pancreatitis

Urine Na⁺ >20 meq/L; renal Na⁺ wasting

Diagnosis: Hyponatremia resulting from the following:
1. Diuretics
2. Mineralocorticoid deficiency
3. Salt-losing nephritis

Increased extracellular fluid volume with edema or ascites

Urine Na⁺ >20 meq/L

Diagnosis: Hyponatremia resulting from the following:
1. Acute or chronic renal failure
2. Adrenal insufficiency

Urine Na⁺ <10 meq/L

Diagnosis: Hyponatremia resulting from conditions causing pathologic retention of Na⁺:
1. Congestive heart failure
2. Cirrhosis
3. Nephrotic syndrome
4. Protein-losing enteropathy

Table 36–4. Drugs implicated in the development of hyponatremia.

Hypoglycemic agents
  Phenformin
  Sulfonylureas (chlorpropamide, tolbutamide)
Antineoplastic compounds
  Vincristine
  Cyclophosphamide
Tricyclic compounds
  Carbamazepine
  Amitriptyline
  Thioridazine
Thiazide diuretics
Others
  Acetaminophen
  Clofibrate
  Indomethacin
  Morphine

orthostatic hypotension, tachycardia, dry mucous membranes, poor skin turgor, oliguria, and thirst.

Rule out spurious hyponatremia arising from the following conditions:

A. Hyperlipidemia and Hyperproteinemia: In hyperlipidemia and hyperproteinemia, the markedly increased amounts of lipid or protein occupy an increased portion of the plasma volume, resulting in decreased volume of water for electrolytes and other solutes, so that the sodium concentration in total plasma volume is decreased; however, if sodium concentration in plasma water is measured, it is normal.

The plasma is turbid and milky if hyperlipidemia is present. The presence of excess plasma proteins can be detected quickly in the laboratory using a protein refractometer. In each of these cases, a normal sodium concentration can be expected if serum osmolality is normal despite the measured hyponatremia. No emergency treatment is required for hyperlipidemia and hyperproteinemia.

B. Hyperglycemia: The increase in extracellular fluid osmolality produced by excess glucose molecules causes the transfer of water from the intracellular to the extracellular compartment, thereby increasing the volume of water there. Since sodium is confined principally in the extracellular space, serum sodium concentration falls. Correction of hyperglycemia usually corrects hyponatremia by approximately 1.6 meq/L of sodium for every fall in glucose concentration of 100 mg/dL (p 689). For example, in a patient with a blood glucose concentration of 1200 mg/dL and serum sodium concentration of 120 meq/L, the serum sodium concentration would be expected to rise to about 138 meq/L if glucose concentration were lowered to 100 mg/dL. Correction of hyperglycemia only shifts water between the intracellular and the extracellular spaces, so that the total body sodium does not change.

Preliminary Evaluation

A. Assess Urgency of Treatment:

1. Serious symptoms–Prompt therapy is indicated if lethargy, confusion, delirium, psychotic behavior, coma, seizures, muscle weakness and cramps, myoclonus, or increased deep tendon reflexes are associated with laboratory evidence of severe hyponatremia (serum sodium < 120 meq/L). Hyponatremia should be presumed to be the cause of symptoms until proved otherwise.

2. Rapidity and intensity of treatment–These factors depend on the severity of hyponatremia and any complications (seizures, altered mental status). Slowly developing hyponatremia is well tolerated even to a serum sodium concentration as low as 120 meq/L. An *abrupt* fall in serum sodium concentration, even though it is of lesser degree, may be poorly tolerated.

B. Assess Extracellular Fluid Volume: The history and physical examination may suggest increased or decreased extracellular fluid volume. This finding—as well as determination of the sodium concentration in a urine specimen obtained *before treatment has been started*—provides a basis for diagnosis.

1. HYPONATREMIA WITH HYPOVOLEMIA

Diagnosis

Hyponatremia with hypovolemia occurs because losses of water and salt have been partially replaced with water only. Patients show signs of hypovolemia (postural hypotension or tachycardia; oliguria) and (occasionally) frank shock.

A. With Renal Sodium Conservation: (Urine sodium < 10 meq/L unless diuretics have been given.) Hyponatremia is due to extrarenal losses of sodium with continued intake of water. Usual causes include gastrointestinal losses (vomiting or diarrhea), severe sweating, or increase in volume of fluid sequestered from extracellular fluid ("third-spacing") (burns, pancreatitis, intestinal obstruction, crush injuries, etc).

B. With Renal Sodium Wasting: (Urine sodium > 20 meq/L.) Hyponatremia is due at least in part to renal sodium wasting such as occurs with diuretic therapy or in patients with adrenal insufficiency. Patients with chronic renal disease may also present with this picture.

Treatment

Restore depleted extracellular fluid volume with infusions of isotonic saline solutions (eg, normal saline or lactated Ringer's injection). Give at a rate of 1 L every 3–4 hours. Hypertonic saline is rarely necessary to treat this form of hyponatremia.

Disposition

The need for hospitalization depends on the underlying cause and the need for prolonged treatment.

2. HYPONATREMIA WITH FLUID OVERLOAD

Diagnosis

Hyponatremia with fluid overload occurs because of pathologic retention of sodium with impaired ability to excrete water. Total body sodium is greater than normal. Signs of fluid overload (jugular venous distention, sacral or peripheral edema, pulmonary edema or pleural effusions, ascites, or anasarca) are present. Evidence of the underlying disease (eg, heart failure, cirrhosis) is usually apparent. The urine sodium concentration is characteristically less than 10 meq/L unless the patient has been taking diuretics, in which case it is higher.

Treatment

A. Water Restriction: Restrict salt and water intake (eg, 2 g of sodium; 1–2 L of water daily). Water restriction is necessary so that insensible water losses will produce slow correction of hyponatremia.

B. Diuretics: Loss of water may need to be accelerated in some patients (eg, those with pulmonary edema) by giving diuretics (eg, furosemide [Lasix], 0.5–1 mg/kg intravenously). If diuretics aggravate renal hypoperfusion, hyponatremia may actually worsen.

C. Hypertonic Saline: It may be advisable to administer small amounts of hypertonic saline (100–200 mL of 5% sodium chloride solution) to patients who already have expanded extracellular fluid volume if they have profound hyponatremia (serum sodium < 110 meq/L) with serious manifestations (eg, coma or seizures). In such cases, monitoring of central venous pressure or pulmonary capillary wedge pressure is advisable, and concomitant administration of furosemide (as above) is usually necessary.

D. Dialysis: In patients with concurrent renal failure, emergency dialysis may be necessary to help correct severe hyponatremia.

Disposition

Hospitalization is required in most cases.

3. HYPONATREMIA WITH ISOVOLEMIA

Diagnosis

Occasionally, hyponatremia develops in patients who show neither surfeit nor deficiency of extracellular fluid volume on physical examination. In this setting, evaluation of urine osmolality in addition to determination of urine sodium may be helpful.

A. Deficiency of Potassium: The uncommon occurrence of hyponatremia resulting from a deficiency in total body potassium (equation 4 [p 689]) has been reported in patients who have taken diuretics without potassium supplementation.

B. Inappropriate Antidiuretic Hormone (ADH) Secretion: In the syndrome of inappropriate secretion of ADH, mild hyponatremia is universal, and urine osmolality is usually over 300 mosm/kg. Drugs other than diuretics have also been associated with hyponatremia; a list of agents producing this side effect is given in Table 36–4. The mechanisms by which these drugs cause hyponatremia is not firmly established but may include inappropriate secretion of ADH.

C. Hypothyroidism: Hypothyroidism may also be associated with isovolemic hyponatremia.

D. Psychogenic Polydipsia: Psychogenic polydipsia may produce mild to moderate hyponatremia caused by excess free water intake. Euvolemia is maintained through the renal excretion of sodium. Urine sodium is typically elevated (> 20 meq/L), and urine osmolality is low (< 300 mosm/kg).

Treatment

Treatment depends entirely on the underlying cause. In patients with precarious hemodynamic status, monitoring of central venous pressure is essential.

A. Inappropriate secretion of ADH is treated primarily by water restriction (eg, 1–2 L/d).

B. Hypokalemic hyponatremia is corrected by restoring body potassium stores. Replace potassium by intravenous infusion at a rate not to exceed 5 meq/kg/24 h, preferably less except in severe deficiencies. Concentrations of solutions should seldom exceed 40 meq/L. If the patient's condition permits oral therapy, this is preferable to parenteral administration of potassium. The usual dose for an adult is 40–120 meq/d.

C. Drugs associated with hyponatremia should be stopped, if possible; the hyponatremia invariably reverses spontaneously.

D. Severe hyponatremia ([Na] < 120 meq/L) without life-threatening symptoms may be treated by administration of isotonic saline with concomitant administration of potent diuretics (eg, furosemide, 0.5–1 mg/kg intravenously). Profound hyponatremia ([Na] < 110 meq/L) or severe hyponatremia with life-threatening manifestations (coma, seizures) can be corrected more rapidly by the infusion of 100–200 mL of hypertonic (5%) sodium chloride solution (adult dose) along with a diuretic.

Disposition

Most patients with isovolemic hyponatremia require hospitalization. Abrupt hyponatremia may be associated with permanent neurologic damage, as may overly rapid correction.

HYPERNATREMIA

Hypernatremia is much less common than hyponatremia but may also cause serious neuromuscular symptoms and signs. It may arise either from excessive water losses or from excessive sodium intake.

Causes

The causes of hypernatremia may be classified as follows:

A. Excessive Water Loss: (Thirst mechanism often deficient.)

1. Nonrenal–Protracted fever and burns.

2. Renal–

a. Tube feeding syndrome (more water than sodium is lost in relation to intake of water and sodium; osmotic diuresis).

b. Diabetes insipidus.

c. Hypercalcemia.

d. Renal failure.

e. Drugs: demeclocycline, lithium.

B. Inadequate Water Intake:

1. Coma.

2. Loss of thirst mechanism.

C. Excessive Sodium Intake: Massive salt ingestion (psychosis; drinking sea water).

D. Dialysis: Peritoneal dialysis or hemodialysis performed with hypertonic saline.

Diagnosis

A. Symptoms and Signs: Hypernatremia is characterized by a serum sodium concentration over 150 meq/L. Symptoms and signs include thirst, weight loss, lethargy, flushed skin, and dehydrated appearance (dry mucous membranes, poor skin turgor). Tachycardia, low blood pressure, and oliguria may be present. Fever, confusion, delirium, hyperpnea, and coma are manifestations of severe hypernatremia. Signs of severe loss of volume may be seen. Elevated levels of blood urea nitrogen and elevated hematocrit may occur.

B. Renal Conservation of Water: The approach to the patient with hypernatremia depends primarily on the results of an assessment of renal conservation of water, most easily done by checking urine osmolality.

1. Urine osmolality greater than 400 mosm/kg–If urine osmolality is greater than 400 mosm/kg, renal water-conserving mechanisms are operating.

a. Nonrenal losses–Hypernatremia is due to nonrenal losses of water from skin, lungs, gut, or burn areas, with attendant failure of water intake to keep pace with water losses. In this situation, total body sodium deficits may also be present despite the hypernatremia.

b. Tube feedings–Hypernatremia with concentrated urine also occurs with high-protein tube feedings with limited water intake. The increased urine urea concentration results in osmotic diuresis, with loss of more water than sodium.

c. Diabetes mellitus–Osmotic diuresis from glycosuria in patients with diabetes mellitus may also result in hypernatremia (after correction for the elevated glucose concentration).

2. Urine osmolality less than 250 mosm/kg–

a. Diabetes insipidus–Hypernatremia accompanied by a urine osmolality of less than 250 mosm/kg is characteristic of diabetes insipidus.

b. Pituitary injury–Impaired secretion of ADH from the pituitary may occur following damage or disease of the pituitary gland or the hypothalamus.

c. Nephrogenic diabetes insipidus–Nephrogenic diabetes insipidus results from insensitivity of the renal distal tubule and collecting duct to ADH; acquired nephrogenic diabetes insipidus may occur in patients treated with lithium or demeclocycline or after relief or prolonged urinary tract obstruction.

3. Urine osmolality approximately equal to plasma osmolality–Hypernatremia may also develop when urine osmolality is about the same as plasma osmolality. In this case, hypernatremia results from impaired renal water conservation, as may occur in the diuretic phase of acute renal failure; in certain cases of postobstructive diuresis, with severe potassium depletion or prolonged hypercalcemia; or in some cases of chronic renal disease.

Treatment

Because of the risk of brain damage and because the ability to regulate water intake is frequently impaired in patients with hypernatremia, they must be treated immediately and with vigor.

A. Hypovolemia: Hyponatremia in the presence of severe hypovolemia should be treated initially with isotonic saline to correct the volume deficit; followed by 5% dextrose in water to replace the free water deficit. A mild volume deficit may be initially treated with 0.45% saline in 5% dextrose in water.

B. Water Deficit: Replace water deficit with intravenous dextrose solutions, eg, 5% dextrose in water.

The amount of sodium excess and the amount of water required to restore serum sodium concentration to normal can be estimated from equations 6 and 7 (p 689). For example, a 70-kg man with a serum sodium concentration of 155 meq/L has an estimated total body water of 35 L and excess sodium of 525 meq (15 meq/L × 35). It would take 3.75 L of water to restore serum sodium to 140 meq/L. In general, the rate of correction of hypernatremia should not exceed 1–2 meq/L/h.

C. Body Deficit of Sodium: Because total body sodium deficits often exist with hypernatremia, fluid therapy often must include sodium in hypotonic replacement solutions.

Disposition

Patients with serum sodium over 150 meq/L require hospitalization. Patients with lesser degrees of hypernatremia may be discharged from the emergency department but should be examined at a clinic or by a private physician within 1 week.

DISORDERS OF SERUM POTASSIUM CONCENTRATION

General Considerations

Potassium is the principal intracellular electrolyte, with over 95% of the body's potassium being stored within cells. The potassium content of the body is set forth in Table 36–5. Disorders of *serum* potassium concentration may not reflect accurately the condition of *body* potassium stores for the following reasons:

A. Serum pH alters the distribution of potassium between cells and plasma: acidosis promotes transfer of potassium from intracellular to extracellular fluid, causing hyperkalemia; alkalosis does the reverse, causing potassium to enter the cells.

B. Extensive cell injury (eg, burns, crush injuries) may release large amounts of potassium into the extracellular fluid and cause hyperkalemia, since tissue cells contain most of the body's potassium.

C. Body potassium content and serum concentrations of potassium are regulated by the kidney; however, the ability of the kidneys to adjust to alterations in serum potassium is slower and less efficient than is the case with sodium.

D. Diuretic-induced potassium loss is one of the major causes of hypokalemia. Diminished food intake alone is rarely a cause of hypokalemia, since most foods contain large amounts of potassium.

HYPOKALEMIA

Hypokalemia is an especially common complication of diuretic therapy. Other causes are set forth in Table 36–6. Most cases of hypokalemia result from excessive potassium wasting.

Diagnosis

Hypokalemia is characterized by a serum potassium concentration under 3.2 meq/L and muscle weakness leading in extreme cases to impaired ventilation. Weakness of smooth muscle causes ileus and flaccid paralysis. Hypokalemia may exacerbate digitalis toxicity and may be associated with cardiac arrhythmias.

Table 36–5. Potassium content of the body.[1]

Body Compartment	Body Potassium (%)
Plasma	0.4
Interstitial fluid and lymph	1
Cartilage and dense connective tissue	0.4
Bone	7.6
Transcellular	1
Intracellular	89.6

[1]Modified and reproduced, with permission, from Ganong WF: *Review of Medical Physiology,* 13th ed. Appleton & Lange, 1987.

Table 36–6. Causes of hypokalemia.[1]

Poor intake
  Starvation, alcoholism
  Prolonged use of intravenous fluids lacking potassium
Reduced absorption
  Malabsorption
  Small bowel bypass; short bowel
Increased loss
  Gastrointestinal: Vomiting, gastrointestinal suction, obstruction, small bowel fistula, diarrhea, villous adenoma, laxative abuse
  Renal: Diuresis (diuretics, osmolar); congenital tubular defects (renal tubular acidosis, Fanconi's syndrome); renal failure; acidosis (especially diabetes); metabolic alkalosis; corticotropin or glucocorticoid excess (Cushing's syndrome); mineralocorticoid excess (aldosterone-renin); licorice abuse; Bartter's syndrome; some antibiotics (amphotericin B, aminoglycosides, sodium load with carbenicillin or ticarcillin); magnesium depletion
  Skin: Burns; excessive sweating
Hypokalemia with no deficit (shift into cells)
  Insulin; beta-adrenergic agonists
  Athletic training; testosterone (anabolic agent) therapy
  Respiratory alkalosis
  Familial periodic paralysis
  Treatment of megaloblastic anemia

[1] Modified and reproduced, with permission, form Schroeder SA et al (editors): *Current Medical Diagnosis & Treatment 1991.* Appleton & Lange, 1991.

Electrocardiographic abnormalities include T wave depression, prolonged QT interval, U waves, and sagging ST segments (Fig 36–1).

Treatment

A. Hypokalemia Due to Alkalosis: If hypokalemia is not associated with depletion of body stores of potassium and is due solely to alkalosis (ie, if it conforms to the relationship expressed in ¶H, p 690), it does not require specific therapy. The initial goal of treatment is to correct the alkalosis or the condition causing it. Hypokalemia, however, may cause or exacerbate metabolic alkalosis (eg, prolonged gastric suction), and potassium repletion is necessary.

B. Hypokalemia Associated With Depletion of Body Potassium Stores: Treat hypokalemia arising from depleted body potassium stores with oral or intravenous administration of potassium salts, depending on severity and associated symptoms.

1. Estimation of deficit–The magnitude of the potassium deficit can be estimated from the nomogram in Fig 36–2 and Table 36–7. Total body potassium concentration (estimated from the patient's nutritional state) is multiplied by the patient's weight in kilograms to provide an estimate of total body potassium capacity. This figure represents the amount of potassium in the body when the patient is in normal potassium balance. Serum potassium concentration and arterial blood pH are used to determine the percentage of total body depletion of potassium in Fig 36–2; this percentage is then used to calculate the estimated potassium deficit. For example, in a moderately wasted 70-kg man, total body potassium

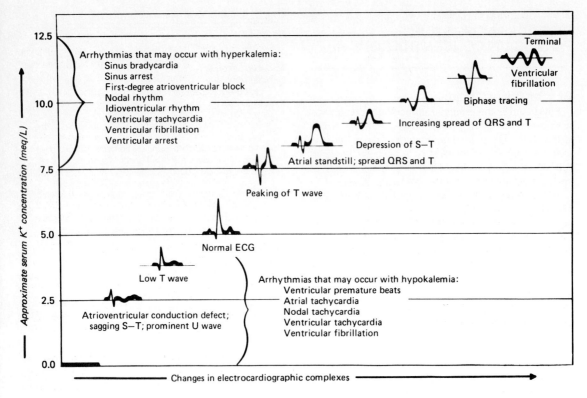

Figure 36–1. Correlation between serum potassium concentration and electrocardiographic findings. Note that correlation is approximate and depends on serum pH and concentrations of other ions (Na+, Ca2+). (Reproduced, with permission, from Krupp MA, Chatton MF [editors]: *Current Medical Diagnosis & Treatment 1974.* Lange, 1974.)

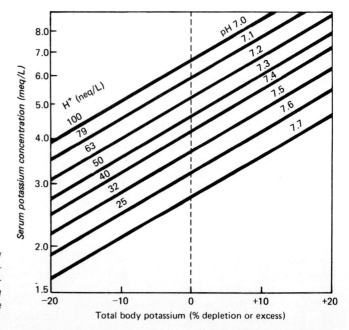

Figure 36–2. Nomogram for determining body potassium stores from serum potassium concentration and arterial blood pH. (Reprinted, with permission, from *University of Washington Teaching Syllabus for the Course on Fluid and Electrolyte Balance.* Edited by B. Scribner, MD.)

Table 36–7. Body potassium concentration according to nutritional state.

	Man (meq/kg)	Woman (meq/kg)
Normal	45	40
Moderate tissue wasting	38	33
Severe tissue wasting	30	26

stores are estimated to be 2660 meq (38 meq/kg × 70 kg). If serum potassium is 2.5 meq/L at normal blood pH, estimated depletion based on Fig 36–2 is 20%. Twenty percent of 2660 meq is 532 meq, the estimated potassium deficit in this patient.

2. Potassium replenishment–Intravenous emergency replenishment of potassium stores is indicated in the patient with severe hypokalemia (serum potassium < 2.5 meq/L), especially if neuromuscular or electrocardiographic manifestations are present.

The concentration of infused potassium should never exceed 40 meq/L, and potassium should be given into a peripheral vein, *not* a central vein. Careful monitoring, with frequent measurement of serum potassium, should be performed to avoid causing hyperkalemia resulting from continued infusion of high potassium concentrations. Greater caution in administering potassium is necessary if renal insufficiency is present. In general, the overall rate of intravenous potassium replacement should not exceed 5 meq/kg/24 h (0.2 meq/kg/h).

If patients are able to take fluids orally, they can be given oral potassium, which is safe and rapidly absorbed. Give K⁺ solution, 40 meq orally every 3–4 hours, until hypokalemia is corrected. High doses of potassium-containing tablets or capsules should be avoided for rapid potassium repletion, as esophageal injury has been reported if stricture is present.

Occasional patients may have hypokalemia and potassium depletion that are refractory to administration of potassium salts. Magnesium deficiency may contribute to this abnormality, and repletion of magnesium will be necessary to bring about full correction of the potassium depletion and hypokalemia.

Disposition

Patients with severe hypokalemia (serum potassium < 2.5 meq/L) require hospitalization for proper diagnosis and correction. Patients with lesser degrees of hypokalemia may be discharged from the emergency department but should be examined at a clinic or by a private physician within 1 week.

HYPERKALEMIA
(See Fig 36–3.)

Hyperkalemia is uncommon; most cases are spurious or are a result of acidosis (Table 36–8).

Diagnosis

A. Symptoms and Signs: Hyperkalemia is characterized by a serum potassium concentration over 5 meq/L. Although symptoms are rare, they may include neuromuscular abnormalities (weakness and paralysis), a metallic taste in the mouth, abdominal distention, and diarrhea. Characteristic electrocardiographic abnormalities include peaked T waves, widened QRS complexes, and flattened P waves; ventricular fibrillation and cardiac arrest may occur (Fig 36–1).

B. Spurious Hyperkalemia: Rule out spurious hyperkalemia caused by the following conditions:

1. Hemolysis of erythrocytes after venipuncture–If serum in the sample appears hemolyzed (pink), draw a new blood sample. Hemolysis is also associated with markedly elevated serum lactate dehydrogenase concentrations.

2. Marked thrombocytosis–Platelet counts over 1 million/μL may result in liberation of significant amounts of potassium as clotting occurs. This effect may be avoided by measuring potassium concentrations on heparinized plasma rather than serum.

3. Fist clenching during antecubital phlebotomy–This action can raise serum potassium concentration in the sample (but not in the body) by

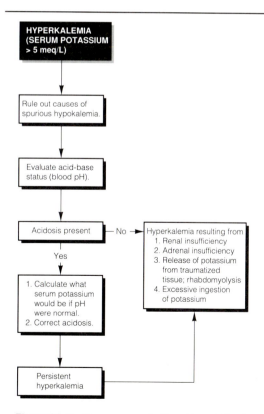

Figure 36–3. Emergency evaluation of hyperkalemia.

Table 36–8. Causes of hyperkalemia.

True hyperkalemia
Acidosis (movement of potassium from cells into extracellular fluid)
Impaired renal potassium excretion:
　Renal disease; oliguria due to severe dehydration
　Mineralocorticoid deficiency
　Drugs (triamterene, spironolactone, amiloride)
Increased potassium load:
　Tissue death (eg, crush injury), burns, severe infections
　Potassium ingestion (eg, salt substitutes)
Spurious hyperkalemia (true serum potassium concentration is normal)
Thrombocytosis (potassium release from platelets during clotting)
Hemolysis during clotting
Delayed separation of serum from clot (diffusion of potassium from erythrocytes)
Fist clenching during phlebotomy (loss of potassium from exercising muscle)

---

releasing potassium from the exercising forearm muscles.

C. True Hyperkalemia: If hyperkalemia is still present after acidosis has been corrected, the cause of hyperkalemia must be determined and treatment instituted accordingly.

1. Renal disease–Renal disease associated with hyperkalemia is always manifested by decreased creatinine clearance and elevated serum creatinine.

2. Mineralocorticoid deficiency–Mineralocorticoid deficiency (eg, Addison's disease, acute adrenal insufficiency) may be manifested by hyperkalemia and hyponatremia. In severe cases, orthostatic hypotension or shock may also be present.

In certain cases of renal insufficiency and type IV renal tubular acidosis, hyporeninemic hypoaldosteronism may also be associated with hyperkalemia. In either case, serum sodium is usually low, which is unusual in other causes of hyperkalemia; renal insufficiency will also be present.

3. Drug-induced hyperkalemia–Drug-induced hyperkalemia (eg, ingestion of aldosterone antagonists or large amounts of potassium) may be diagnosed from the history. Penicillin G, administered as a potassium salt in high doses, may be an iatrogenic cause of hyperkalemia. The use of potassium-containing salt substitutes in patients with sodium-retaining disorders may also predispose to hyperkalemia.

4. Crush injuries or burns–Crush injuries or burns sufficient to produce hyperkalemia are grossly apparent in most cases.

Treatment

The speed with which treatment must be started depends on the degree of hyperkalemia and on symptoms, signs, and electrocardiographic abnormalities consistent with a diagnosis of hyperkalemia.

A. Correction of Acidosis: In hyperkalemia associated with acidosis, intracellular potassium shifts to the extracellular space. The effect of correction of acidosis on serum potassium can be estimated using the nomogram in Fig 36–2 or the general rule that each increase in pH of 0.1 unit may be expected to produce a decrease in serum potassium concentration of 0.6 meq/L.

Correct metabolic acidosis by treating the underlying condition and, in some cases, by giving sodium bicarbonate, 1 meq/kg intravenously over 5 minutes, and correct respiratory acidosis by assisted ventilation.

B. Persistent Hyperkalemia: If life-threatening hyperkalemia is still present after acidosis has been corrected, estimate the degree of hyperkalemia. Immediate action is necessary in 2 situations: (**1**) if serum potassium is over 6 meq/L *and* if there is widening of the QRS complexes on the ECG, or (**2**) if serum potassium is over 7 meq/L, even with no electrocardiographic abnormalities. *Caution:* If hyperkalemia is due to adrenal crisis, give saline and hydrocortisone intravenously (Chapter 35).

C. Immediate-Acting Treatment: (Seconds to minutes.)

1. Give sodium bicarbonate solution, 1 meq/kg intravenously over 5 minutes, to facilitate transfer of potassium from extracellular fluid into the cells.

2. Give calcium (chloride, 5%; or gluconate, 10%), 1–2 ampules intravenously over 5–10 minutes (adult dose). (Do not mix calcium in the same solution with sodium bicarbonate, since insoluble calcium carbonate will precipitate.) Although calcium does not alter serum potassium concentration, it does counteract the cardiac and neuromuscular effects of hyperkalemia.

D. Rapid-Acting Treatment: (Minutes to hours.) As an adjunct to the above treatment for life-threatening hyperkalemia, or when hyperkalemia is not as severe, give glucose, 1–2 mL of a 50% solution per kilogram; and regular insulin, 10 units intravenously over 5 minutes to force potassium into the cells from extracellular fluid.

E. Slow-Acting Treatment: (Hours.) Although the measures described below are not as useful in the emergency department, they are able to induce depletion of total body potassium stores (unlike the regimens discussed above). Such depletion is necessary for long-term control of hyperkalemia in certain settings (crush injury, renal failure).

1. Give potassium exchange resin (sodium polystyrene sulfonate; Kayexalate), 0.3–0.6 g/kg orally or as a retention enema in 150 mL of 25% sorbitol, 3 times a day as needed.

2. Perform peritoneal dialysis or hemodialysis with low-potassium dialysate. In cases of life-threatening hyperkalemia, especially those due to renal insufficiency, dialysis may be required as soon as the more rapidly acting measures described above have been started.

Disposition

Patients with hyperkalemia require hospitalization.

DISORDERS OF SERUM CALCIUM CONCENTRATION

Serum calcium is composed of 2 major fractions. About 45% of total serum calcium is bound to serum proteins (chiefly albumin) or complexed to organic anions such as citrate; the other 55% exists as free, or ionized, calcium. Symptoms and signs of disordered serum calcium concentration are due to changes in the ionized fraction. Proper interpretation of serum calcium concentration requires measurement of serum albumin concentration (p 689). Serum calcium is usually reported in mg/dL; this unit is easily converted to meq/L by dividing by 2. The ionized calcium level in plasma is controlled chiefly by the action of parathyroid hormone and is related to the acid-base status of the patient. Acidosis increases the fraction of total calcium in the ionized form by displacing it from albumin, whereas alkalosis decreases it. As a result, symptomatic hypocalcemia may develop in patients who hyperventilate or in those in whom metabolic acidosis has been rapidly corrected with infusion of sodium bicarbonate.

HYPOCALCEMIA

Hypocalcemia may result from decreased intake or decreased absorption of calcium (eg, vitamin D deficiency, malabsorption syndromes) or from a number of other conditions, eg, renal failure, diuretic therapy, hypoparathyroidism, hypomagnesemia, or hyperphosphatemia (Table 36–9). Hypocalcemia is common but rarely life-threatening.

Diagnosis

The manifestations of hypocalcemia are the same, regardless of the cause. Hypocalcemia is present when the serum calcium concentration is under 8 mg/dL (after correction for the patient's serum albumin concentration by adding 0.8 mg/dL of Ca^{2+} for every gram of albumin below 4 g/dL). Many patients with mild hypocalcemia are asymptomatic. Symptoms and signs of more severe hypocalcemia include tetany, abdominal and muscle cramps, carpopedal spasm, convulsions, diplopia, urinary frequency, and stridor and dyspnea due to laryngospasm. Positive Trousseau's and Chvostek's signs and fasciculations of skeletal muscle also occur. Cataracts may also occur with long-standing hypocalcemia. A prolonged QT interval may be noted on the ECG without U waves (Fig 36–4).

Obtain arterial blood gas samples to rule out (1) hypoventilation secondary to severe hypocalcemia and (2) alkalosis as a cause of tetany. It is important

Table 36–9. Causes of hypocalcemia.[1]

Decreased intake or absorption
Malabsorption
Small bowel bypass, short bowel
Vitamin D deficit (decreased absorption, decreased production of 25-hydroxyvitamin D or 1,25-dihydroxyvitamin D)
Increased loss
Chronic renal insufficiency
Diuretic therapy
Endocrine disease
Hypoparathyroidism (genetic, acquired)
Pseudohypoparathyroidism
Calcitonin secretion with medullary carcinoma of the thyroid
Physiologic causes
Associated with decreased serum albumin
Decreased end organ response to vitamin D
Hyperphosphatemia
Induced by aminoglycoside antibiotics, mithramycin, loop diuretics

[1]Reproduced, with permission, form Schroeder SA et al (editors): *Current Medical Diagnosis & Treatment 1991.* Appleton & Lange, 1991.

to determine serum potassium and magnesium concentrations (coexisting abnormalities are common and may require treatment).

Treatment

Hypocalcemia is rarely life-threatening, although severe hypocalcemia can cause laryngeal stridor and grand mal seizures. Because of the severe potential symptoms, even mild symptoms attributable to hypocalcemia should be treated. Asymptomatic patients do not require treatment in the emergency department.

For initial treatment in an adult, give calcium chloride (5%) or calcium gluconate (10%), one to three

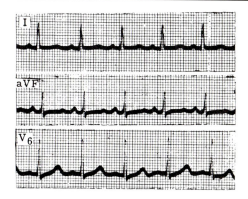

Figure 36–4. The ECG in hypocalcemia. T waves are upright, but the QT is prolonged. This is 0.4 s (corrected for RR of 0.66 s, $QT_c = 0.48$ s) and is abnormal. The lengthening of the QT interval is due to a lengthening of the ST segment and not to any abnormality in the T wave itself. Blood calcium at the time the above recording was made was 6.8 mg/dL. (Reproduced, with permission, from Goldman MJ: *Principles of Clinical Electrocardiography,* 12th ed. Lange, 1986.)

10-mL ampules by intravenous infusion. Then give 1 ampule in 500 mL of normal saline intravenously over 8 hours to provide 100–500 mg of calcium and maintain the serum calcium concentration at 7–8 mg/dL, the level at which symptoms are usually alleviated. Long-term treatment of chronic hypocalcemia requires oral calcium supplements and vitamin D. Treat hypomagnesemia, if present (see below).

Caution: Rarely, hypocalcemia requiring treatment is accompanied by markedly elevated phosphorus concentration (> 6 mg/dL); To prevent metastatic calcification, correct hyperphosphatemia before, or concomitant to, giving calcium. Give intravenous glucose and insulin (see Hyperphosphatemia, below).

Disposition

Patients with acute symptomatic hypocalcemia require hospitalization. Patients with less severe disease may be discharged from the emergency department but should be seen at a clinic or by a private physician within 1 week.

HYPERCALCEMIA

Hypercalcemia is commonly associated with numerous conditions (Table 36–10) and unlike hypocalcemia may have life-threatening consequences.

Diagnosis

Hypercalcemia is characterized by a serum calcium concentration that is over 11 mg/dL (may be as high as 20 mg/dL). Symptoms of hypercalcemia are nonspecific, and the diagnosis may be missed unless serum calcium is measured. Central nervous system depression, stupor, somnolence, weakness, and coma may occur. Psychologic changes include psychosis. Anorexia, vomiting, constipation, and abdominal pain may also be seen.

Renal damage may occur in chronic cases, as shown in impaired concentration ability of the kidney that sometimes leads to polyuria, dehydration, hypernatremia, thirst, and finally azotemia. Band keratopathy may occur in long-standing hypercalcemia. Electrocardiographic abnormalities include prolonged PR interval, shortened QT interval, and flattened T waves.

Parathyroid hormone may facilitate renal bicarbonate excretion as well as phosphate excretion. Therefore, the finding of increased serum bicarbonate levels and a ratio of serum chloride concentration to serum phosphorus concentration of less than 32 suggest that hypercalcemia is not due to increased levels of parathyroid hormone.

Hypercalcemia reflects an increase in the concentration of the ionized fraction of calcium, since elevated levels of calcium-binding serum proteins (chiefly albumin) do not occur except in cases of extreme dehydration.

Table 36–10. Causes of hypercalcemia.[1]

Increased intake or absorption
  Milk-alkali syndrome
  Vitamin D or vitamin A excess
Endocrine disorders
  Primary hyperparathyroidism (adenoma, hyperplasia, carcinoma)
  Secondary hyperparathyroidism (renal insufficiency, malabsorption)
  Acromegaly
  Adrenal insufficiency
Neoplastic disease
  Tumors producing PTH-like peptides (ovary, kidney, lung)
  Metastases to bone
  Lymphoproliferative disease, including multiple myeloma
  Secretion of prostaglandins and osteolytic factors
Miscellaneous causes
  Thiazide diuretic-induced
  Sarcoidosis
  Paget's disease of bone
  Hypophosphatasia
  Immobilization
  Familial hypocalciuric hypercalcemia
  Complications of renal transplantation
  Iatrogenic

[1]Reproduced, with permission, from Schroeder SA et al (editors): *Current Medical Diagnosis & Treatment 1991.* Appleton & Lange, 1991.

Treatment

Any serum calcium concentration above 12 mg/dL requires prompt treatment, especially if symptoms are present. The goal of treatment is to lower serum calcium by general measures and by measures appropriate to the specific cause of hypercalcemia. Avoid immobilization if at all possible.

A. Promote Excretion of Calcium by the Kidney:

1. Fluids–Volume expansion with isotonic saline to increase urinary excretion of calcium is the first step in treating all hypercalcemic patients with normal renal function. Infuse the same amount of intravenous crystalloid solution as is lost by urinary excretion. Such patients may also require monitoring of central venous or pulmonary capillary wedge pressure.

2. Diuretics–Furosemide is also effective in increasing excretion of calcium in patients in whom volume expansion with isotonic saline has been achieved and in whom replacement or urinary volume and electrolyte losses has also occurred. Do not use thiazide diuretics, since they may aggravate hypercalcemia. Give furosemide, 0.5–1 mg/kg intravenously, and monitor fluid status closely, since hypovolemia induced by furosemide will diminish calcium excretion and therefore prolong hypercalcemia.

B. Increase Deposition of Calcium in Bone: Another treatment approach is to promote deposition of calcium into bone or decrease the rate of resorption of calcium from bone.

1. Mithramycin–Given in an intravenous dose of 25 µg/kg, mithramycin lowers serum calcium concentration within 8–12 hours, and this effect may last several days. It is particularly useful for hypercalcemia associated with cancer.

2. Indomethacin–It has recently been suggested that some tumors that metastasize to bone may cause hypercalcemia through a mechanism involving prostaglandin synthesis. In adults with such tumors, indomethacin (an inhibitor of prostaglandin synthesis), 25–50 mg orally 3 times a day, is effective in correcting hypercalcemia. Indomethacin is mainly useful for chronic cases, however, and is of little use in the emergency department.

3. Phosphate–*Caution:* Excessively rapid infusion of phosphate, given to promote deposition of calcium salts into bone, carries a significant risk of producing potentially fatal metastatic or extraosseous calcification. Do *not* give phosphate to any patient with renal insufficiency or in whom hypercalcemia is already associated with hyperphosphatemia.

4. Calcitonin–Salmon calcitonin may be effective in some cases of hypercalcemia; it should be reserved as adjunctive rather than primary therapy. Give 50 Medical Research Council (MRC) units intramuscularly or subcutaneously every 12–24 hours, or 3–6 MRC units/kg/24 h intravenously for adults.

C. Decrease Absorption of Calcium by the Intestine:

1. Corticosteriods reduce any increase in gastrointestinal absorption of calcium, such as occurs in vitamin D intoxication and sarcoidosis. Hydrocortisone, 3–4 mg/kg/d orally or intravenously, should cause a fall in serum calcium concentration within 1–2 days.

2. Dietary intake of calcium should be restricted as an adjunctive measure.

D. Perform Hemodialysis: In patients with renal insufficiency or in whom the above measures are ineffective, hemodialysis with calcium-free dialysate effectively removes calcium from the extracellular fluid.

Disposition

Patients with a serum calcium concentration over 12 mg/dL should be hospitalized. Those with lower levels may be discharged from the emergency department but should be seen at a clinic or by a private physician within 1 week.

DISORDERS OF SERUM PHOSPHORUS CONCENTRATION

HYPOPHOSPHATEMIA

Hypophosphatemia is a common condition with diverse causes (Table 36–11).

Table 36–11. Causes of hypophosphatemia.

Alcoholism
Primary hyperparathyroidism
Phosphorus-deficient parenteral nutrition
Treatment with phosphate-binding antacids
Metabolic or respiratory alkalosis
Uncontrolled diabetes mellitus
Starvation

Diagnosis

Hypophosphatemia is characterized by a serum phosphorus concentration under 2 mg/dL. Diagnosis of hypophosphatemia depends on laboratory measurement of serum phosphorus concentration, since clinical symptoms are usually vague and nonspecific. Acute respiratory alkalosis may lead to hypophosphatemia. Fatigue, neuromuscular weakness, irritability, paresthesias, dysarthria, confusion, convulsions, and coma may occur. At serum levels below 1 mg/dL, hemolysis and impaired neutrophil phagocytosis become evident. Erythrocyte 2,3-diphosphoglycerate is lowered, resulting in decreased delivery of oxygen to the tissues. Rhabdomyolysis may occur.

Treatment

Treatment consists of replacing phosphorus by intravenous or oral phosphate supplements. All patients with a serum phosphorus concentration under 2 mg/dL should receive supplements. Aluminum phosphate gel (Phosphaljel) or neutral phosphate salts, 0.5–1 g/d (of phosphate) orally, can be given (adult dose) (eg, Fleet enema taken orally). Oral phosphate supplements, however, frequently cause constipation.

Phosphates (often given as potassium phosphate), 20–30 mg of elemental phosphorus per kilogram of body weight, may be infused intravenously over 12 hours. Alternatively, potassium phosphate may be added to intravenous solutions in place of potassium chloride for hospitalized patients (maximum concentration of 40 meq/L; infused at a rate of 100–150 mL/h).

Disposition

Hospitalization is invariably necessary for patients with a serum phosphorus concentration under 1 mg/dL and is strongly advised for those whose serum phosphorus is under 2 mg/dL. Patients for whom hospitalization is not indicated should be seen by a physician within 1 week.

HYPERPHOSPHATEMIA

Hyperphosphatemia may result from chronic or acute renal disease, hypoparathyroidism, growth hormone excess, cytolysis (rhabdomyolysis or chemotherapy of lymphoproliferative tumors), excessive enemas with phosphate-containing solutions, or ingestion of large amounts of phosphate, vitamin D, or laxatives.

Diagnosis

Hyperphosphatemia is characterized by a serum phosphorus concentration over 7 mg/dL. No signs are directly referable to hyperphosphatemia. However, hypocalcemia may develop because of tissue deposition of calcium phosphate.

Treatment

A. Glucose and Insulin: Administer 50% glucose and regular insulin as described above (see Hyperkalemia) to produce an initial fall in serum phosphorus.

B. Volume Expansion: Infuse isotonic saline to achieve volume expansion and promote excretion of phosphate by the kidneys in patients with normal renal function. Acetazolamide (Diamox) will also facilitate urinary phosphate excretion. Give 500 mg every 6 hours, but monitor fluid balance closely.

C. Phosphate-Binding Antacids: Oral phosphate-binding antacids such as aluminum hydroxide will cause binding of phosphate in the gut and reduce phosphate absorption.

D. Dialysis: Dialysis is required to lower serum phosphorus concentration in patients with renal failure.

Disposition

Indications for hospitalization usually depend on factors other than hyperphosphatemia itself, eg, renal insufficiency, rhabdomyolysis.

DISORDERS OF SERUM MAGNESIUM CONCENTRATION

HYPOMAGNESEMIA

Hypomagnesemia is commonly associated with several conditions (Table 36–12). It is frequently associated with hypocalcemia and should be sought in all patients with hypocalcemia.

Diagnosis

Hypomagnesemia is characterized by a serum magnesium concentration under 1 meq/L (< 1.2 mg/dL). Hypocalcemia may also occur and may contribute to symptoms.

Carpopedal spasm, tetany, athetoid movements, jerking, coarse and flapping tremors, and hyperexcitability may occur. A positive Babinski's sign, seizures, and weakness are seen. Tachycardia, ventricular arrhythmias, hypertension, and vasomotor

Table 36–12. Causes of hypomagnesemia.[1]

Diminished absorption or intake
  Malabsorption, chronic diarrhea, laxative abuse
  Prolonged gastrointestinal suction
  Small bowel bypass
  Malnutrition
  Alcoholism
  Parenteral alimentation with inadequate Mg^{2+} content
Increased loss
  Diabetic ketoacidosis
  Diuretic therapy
  Diarrhea
  Hyperaldosteronism, Bartter's syndrome
  Associated with hypercalciuria
  Renal magnesium wasting
Unexplained
  Hyperparathyroidism
  Postparathyroidectomy
  Vitamin D therapy
  Induced by aminoglycoside antibiotics, cisplatin

[1]Reproduced, with permission, from Schroeder SA et al (editors): *Current Medical Diagnosis & Treatment 1991*. Appleton & Lange, 1991.

changes occur as well as confusion, disorientation, and psychotic behavior.

Treatment

Hypocalcemia associated with hypomagnesemia is characteristically resistant to calcium supplementation but responds quickly to magnesium replacement.

A. Oral Replacement: The oral route is preferred in patients with long-standing magnesium deficiency. For adults, give magnesium oxide, 250–500 mg 4 times a day.

B. Parenteral Replacement: Reserve parenteral administration of magnesium for patients with severe hypomagnesemia, usually those who have evidence of neuromuscular dysfunction.

1. Intramuscular route–Give magnesium sulfate, 0.1–0.4 mL of 50% solution per kilogram every 6 hours.

2. Intravenous route–Give magnesium chloride as an intravenous infusion at a rate no greater than 0.1–0.2 meq/kg/h.

3. Estimation of amount of magnesium needed–The extracellular magnesium deficit can be estimated by multiplying extracellular fluid volume (~0.2 body weight in kg) times the desired increase in serum magnesium concentration. This amount can then be infused over a 48-hour period.

When magnesium is given parenterally, the serum magnesium concentration must be monitored frequently, and patellar reflexes, which diminish with increasing serum magnesium concentrations, must be checked to safeguard against the development of hypermagnesemia.

Disposition

Patients with symptomatic hypomagnesemia require hospitalization. Patients with less severe magnesium depletion may require hospitalization because of associated conditions.

HYPERMAGNESEMIA

Hypermagnesemia is usually due to renal failure (acute or chronic) that is often associated with excessive magnesium intake (magnesium-containing antacids, magnesium sulfate).

Diagnosis

Hypermagnesemia is characterized by a serum magnesium concentration over 3 meq/L (3.6 mg/dL).

A. Symptoms and Signs: Symptoms and signs vary depending on the severity of hypermagnesemia.

1. Serum concentration of 3—5 meq/L–Peripheral vasodilatation may result in hypotension; nausea and vomiting may also occur.

2. Serum concentration of 5—7 meq/L–Drowsiness, confusion, and lethargy develop, and deep tendon reflexes are depressed or absent.

3. Serum concentration above 10 meq/L–Coma and death occur, preceded by progressive weakness and skeletal muscle paralysis, with depression of the centers of respiration.

B. Electrocardiographic Findings: Electrocardiographic changes include a prolonged PR interval, widened QRS complexes, and elevated T waves.

Treatment

A. Patients with Renal Insufficiency: In patients with severe renal insufficiency, significant hypermagnesemia must be treated by dialysis using a magnesium-free dialysate.

B. Patients With Normal Renal Function:

1. Infusion of isotonic saline solution for volume expansion promotes urinary excretion of magnesium.

2. Potent diuretics such as furosemide (0.5–1 mg/kg intravenously) may also be effective.

3. Intravenous infusion of calcium will temporarily neutralize the neuromuscular effects of hypermagnesemia.

Disposition

All patients with hypermagnesemia require hospitalization.

ACID-BASE DISTURBANCES

Hydrogen ions produced in the process of normal intermediary metabolism must be buffered in the body and then stoichiometrically excreted by the kidneys to avoid accumulation of acid. Table 36–13 shows the relationship of pH to concentration of hydrogen ion.

Bicarbonate-CO_2 System

Quantitatively, the most important buffering agent is the bicarbonate-CO_2 system. The kidneys are responsible for maintaining the concentration of the bicarbonate portion of the buffer pair, while the respiratory system regulates the other half of the buffer pair by controlling the partial pressure of CO_2 (PCO_2) in blood.

A. Arterial Blood Gases: Assessment of acid-base status rests on measurement of arterial blood pH and PCO_2; plasma bicarbonate concentration can be calculated from these measurements.

B. Total CO_2 Concentration: Plasma bicarbonate plus the small amount of CO_2 dissolved in plasma as carbonic acid (H_2CO_3) constitutes the total CO_2 concentration. Normally, the plasma concentration of carbonic acid is low (1.2 mmol/L) compared to the plasma concentration of bicarbonate (24 mmol/L).

Total CO_2 concentration can be directly measured with a simple automated procedure available in any clinical laboratory. The result normally correlates closely with plasma bicarbonate levels calculated by a blood gas machine.

C. Hydrogen Ion Concentration: The equation initially described by Henderson that relates hydrogen ion concentration to the concentrations of the buffer system is shown on p 689 (equation 11). Knowledge of any 2 of the 3 variables in this equation (hydrogen ion, bicarbonate, carbon dioxide) permits determination of the third. Hasselbalch subsequently altered the Henderson equation by transcribing it into units of pH, which have become the standard for reporting hydrogen ion concentration in clinical medicine (p 689, equation 10). In order to use equation 11, the measured pH must be converted to hydrogen ion concentration (Table 36–13). Once pH has been converted to hydrogen ion concentration, it can easily be substituted into equation 11 for analysis of the buffer relationships in any given acid-base disturbance.

Classification of Acid-Base Disorders

Acid-base disorders are first characterized as either acidosis (pH < 7.35; hydrogen ion > 45 neq/L) or alkalosis (pH > 7.45; hydrogen ion < 35 neq/L). Then the primary disturbance and the degree of compensation are assessed using equation 11 (p 689).

A. Primary Disturbances: Acid-base disorders are characterized as either metabolic or respiratory, depending on the cause of the disturbance.

1. Metabolic–When the underlying abnormality is reflected in a change in plasma bicarbonate concentration, the primary disturbance is metabolic.

a. Metabolic acidosis results when excess hydrogen ions are buffered by bicarbonate in plasma, as

Table 36–13. Conversion of pH to hydrogen ion concentration.

pH	H+ (neq/L)
7.00	100
7.10	79
7.15	71
7.20	63
7.25	58
7.30	50
7.40	40
7.50	32
7.55	29
7.60	26

shown by acid pH and lowered bicarbonate concentration (equation 11).

b. Metabolic alkalosis occurs either through loss of hydrogen ion from the body or from retention of alkali and is indicated by an alkaline pH and elevated bicarbonate concentration.

2. Respiratory–Respiratory disorders occur as a result of changes in ventilation and are reflected in primary abnormalities in PCO_2 (equation 11).

a. In **respiratory acidosis,** impaired ventilation leads to an increase in PCO_2 and an acid pH.

b. In **respiratory alkalosis,** hyperventilation decreases PCO_2, and an alkaline pH results.

B. Compensatory Mechanisms: Any primary acid-base disturbance is accompanied by changes in the other element of the bicarbonate-CO_2 buffer system that tend to minimize the effects of the primary disturbance on arterial blood pH. For example, metabolic acidosis stimulates hyperventilation; the lowered PCO_2 then blunts the severity of the decrease in pH (equation 11). Primary respiratory acidosis leads to enhanced reabsorption of bicarbonate by the kidneys and an elevation in plasma bicarbonate concentration. Such compensatory changes are only partial and never entirely restore pH to normal levels.

C. Mixed Disorders: When normal arterial blood pH occurs in combination with abnormal bicarbonate concentration or PCO_2 levels, then a mixture of 2 (or more) primary disturbances is present in which each element cancels the other out to produce normal pH. Such mixed disturbances may also exist when pH is abnormal (see below).

D. Acid-Base Nomogram: A nomogram (Fig 36–5) is helpful in assessing disturbances of acid-base metabolism. In this nomogram, hydrogen ion (top) or pH (bottom) is plotted against plasma bicarbonate concentration. The curved isopleths indicate the values that are seen for PCO_2 at any given hydrogen ion and bicarbonate concentrations. The range of normal values is represented by the circle in the center of the nomogram. The shaded bars represent the 95% confidence limits for 4 common acid-base disturbances. The nomogram may be used to analyze a given patient's disorder and assess the results of treatment.

The response to changes in acid-base balance depends on the severity of the disturbance, the length of time during which compensatory mechanisms operate, and the presence of mixed disturbances. The nomogram can be helpful in sorting out these variables. The shaded areas on the nomogram represent acid-base values that may be found in patients with compensated simple disorders; values falling outside the shaded areas are by definition associated with mixed disorders. The expected degree of compensation for each primary abnormality can also be estimated from the general principles given on p 689.

RESPIRATORY ACIDOSIS

Respiratory acidosis may be caused by pulmonary insufficiency of diverse causes or by neurogenic hypoventilation.

Diagnosis

Respiratory acidosis is characterized by arterial blood hydrogen ion concentration over 45 neq/L, pH under 7.35, PCO_2 over 44 mm Hg, and plasma bicarbonate concentration that varies depending on the duration of the abnormality. Symptoms and signs include fatigue, weakness, irritability, headache, agitation, confusion, lethargy, and coma. Hypoxemia and cyanosis may be present.

A. Acute Respiratory Acidosis: Acute respiratory acidosis results from an abrupt impairment in ventilation that causes an increase in PCO_2 and a consequent rise in hydrogen ion concentration, as shown in equation 11. Because the abnormality is acute, there is little change in the plasma bicarbonate concentration. As shown by shaded area I in Fig 36–5, the increase in PCO_2 is accompanied by a direct increase in hydrogen ion concentration. As a rule of thumb, a 10-mm Hg increase in PCO_2 will be accompanied by a decrease in pH of 0.08 unit (p 689).

B. Chronic Respiratory Acidosis: Chronic respiratory acidosis results when impaired ventilation from chronic respiratory failure causes a sustained elevation of PCO_2. Renal compensatory mechanisms in the form of increased net excretion of hydrogen ion come into play and raise plasma bicarbonate to the extent illustrated by shaded area III in Fig 36–5. Because of renal compensatory mechanisms, marked elevation in PCO_2 produces only small changes in hydrogen ion concentration. Chronic respiratory acidosis is generally well tolerated until severe pulmonary insufficiency leads to hypoxemia, after which the long-term prognosis is poor. As a rule of thumb, an increase of 10 mm Hg in the PCO_2 will be accompanied by a decrease in pH of 0.025 unit.

Treatment

Patients with chronic lung disease and compensated respiratory acidosis may require vigorous treat-

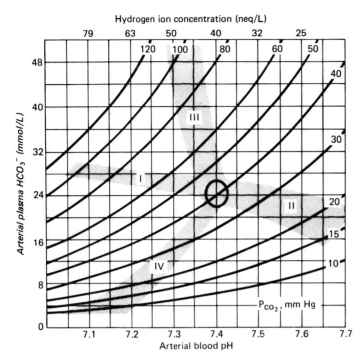

Figure 36–5. Acid-base nomogram for use in assessing acid-base disturbances. The shaded areas represent the 95% confidence limits of values found in 4 common acid-base disorders, and the curved lines are isopleths of varying P_{CO_2} in mm Hg. The circle in the center represents the range of normal values. I = acute respiratory acidosis; II = acute respiratory alkalosis; III = chronic respiratory alkalosis; IV = sustained metabolic acidosis. See text for further details. (Courtesy of A. Sebastian, MD.)

ment if hypercapnia worsens acutely because of intercurrent illness.

A. Acute Respiratory Acidosis: Treatment involves immediate restoration of adequate ventilation. Tracheal intubation with assisted ventilation, or controlled ventilation with morphine sedation, must be used in comatose patients or those with asthma and CO_2 retention.

B. Chronic Respiratory Acidosis: Treatment focuses primarily on improving ventilation. Rapid correction of chronic respiratory acidosis—as may occur if the patient is placed on controlled ventilation—can be dangerous, since P_{CO_2} is lowered rapidly and compensated respiratory acidosis may convert to severe metabolic alkalosis. Initial treatment should aim at normalizing the pH. It is not unusual, however, to see P_{CO_2} levels in the 60–100 mm Hg range in patients with chronic lung disease who are well compensated.

Disposition

Patients with acute (uncompensated) respiratory acidosis require hospitalization; patients with chronic (compensated) respiratory acidosis may require hospitalization if acidosis is associated with worsening hypoxemia.

RESPIRATORY ALKALOSIS

Acute respiratory alkalosis is usually caused by acute hyperventilation brought on by anxiety, septi-

cemia, pulmonary embolism, pleurisy, salicylate toxicity, or other conditions. Chronic alkalosis may be due to chronic pulmonary or liver disease.

Diagnosis

A. Respiratory Alkalosis: Respiratory alkalosis is characterized by arterial blood hydrogen ion concentration under 35 neq/L, pH greater than 7.45, and P_{CO_2} under 35 mm Hg. Acute respiratory alkalosis may cause symptomatic hypocalcemia with paresthesias, tetany, carpopedal spasm, and positive Chvostek and Trousseau signs.

With chronic respiratory alkalosis, headache, apprehension, and irritability occur. The threshold for seizure activity is lowered, and hypophosphatemia may occur.

B. Differentiation of Acute and Chronic Respiratory Alkalosis:

1. Acute hyperventilation lowers P_{CO_2} without concomitant changes in plasma bicarbonate concentration and thereby lowers plasma hydrogen ion concentration, as shown by area II in Fig 36–5. The rule of thumb for predicting pH is the reverse of that used for respiratory acidosis: an acute change of 10 mm Hg in P_{CO_2} will cause a change in pH of 0.08 unit in the opposite direction.

2. Chronic respiratory alkalosis is associated with a decrease in tubular reabsorption of filtered bicarbonate that increases bicarbonate excretion, with consequent lowering of plasma bicarbonate. As bicarbonate concentration falls, chloride concentration rises. This is the same pattern seen in hyperchloremic acidosis, and the 2 conditions can only be distinguished by arterial blood gas and hydrogen ion concentration measurements. Renal compensation for respiratory alkalosis may result in normal blood concentration of hydrogen ion, ie, compensation may be complete.

Treatment

Chronic respiratory alkalosis in itself generally does not require treatment, and attention should be turned instead to the underlying disorder. In certain patients with psychogenic hyperventilation, a rebreathing bag may be helpful in alleviating symptoms, and a mild tranquilizer may reduce the anxiety that often causes the hyperventilation. In all cases of acute respiratory alkalosis, a search should be made for underlying causes (eg, sepsis).

Disposition

The disposition of patients with respiratory alkalosis is determined by the underlying circumstances leading to hyperventilation.

METABOLIC ACIDOSIS

General Considerations

Metabolic acidosis commonly results from an increase in hydrogen ion concentration resulting from a diminution in plasma bicarbonate (equation 11). This diminution occurs either as a result of loss of bicarbonate through titration with excess hydrogen ion or as a result of loss of bicarbonate itself.

A. Increased Anion Gap: When loss of bicarbonate is associated with accumulation of other acidic anions, the anion gap (normally < 12 meq) increases as a result of the accumulation of organic acids not measured by routine laboratory tests. The anion gap may be calculated as follows:

$$\text{Anion gap} = [Na^+] - ([HCO_3^-] + [Cl^-]) = \ < 12 \text{ meq/L}$$

An increased anion gap is associated with the following conditions: (**1**) diabetic ketoacidosis or alcoholic ketoacidosis, (**2**) lactic acidosis or starvation, (**3**) acidosis associated with renal failure, and (**4**) poisoning (aspirin, oxalic acid, ethylene glycol, methanol).

B. Normal Anion Gap: When acidosis results from loss of bicarbonate, there is usually a reciprocal increase in serum chloride concentration (hyperchloremic metabolic acidosis), so that the anion gap remains normal or nearly normal. A normal anion gap is associated with the following conditions: (**1**) renal tubular acidosis, (**2**) administration of excessive ammonium chloride (NH_4Cl), (**3**) protracted diarrhea, (**4**) ureteroenterostomies, (**5**) treatment with carbonic anhydrase inhibitors (acetazolamide), and (**6**) rapid expansion of extracellular fluid with chloride-containing solutions.

Diagnosis

Metabolic acidosis is characterized by arterial blood hydrogen ion concentration over 45 neq/L, pH under 7.35, and plasma bicarbonate concentration under 22 mmol/L. PCO_2 varies depending on the effectiveness of respiratory compensatory mechanisms. There is usually evidence of increased minute ventilation and, in severe cases, Kussmaul breathing. Decreased consciousness, lethargy, disorientation, stupor, and coma accompany severe acidosis. Tachycardia, hypotension, ketonuria, and shock occur, and an odor of acetone may be noted on the breath in cases of diabetic ketoacidosis.

Associated electrolyte disorders may be present (eg, hyperkalemia) or may develop during treatment (hypomagnesemia, hypophosphatemia, hypokalemia, hypocalcemia).

Treatment

Hyperventilation is a compensatory mechanism in metabolic acidosis. At its peak, it lowers PCO_2 to no less than about 15 mm Hg. Serum bicarbonate concentration under 8 meq/L is uniformly associated with severe metabolic acidosis that requires vigorous treatment.

There are 2 goals in the treatment of metabolic acidosis.

A. First, correct the cause of excess hydrogen ion production or bicarbonate loss as rapidly as possible.

1. Diabetic acidosis–Give insulin in an attempt to bring carbohydrate metabolism to normal (Chapter 35).

2. Lactic acidosis–Start measures to improve tissue perfusion depending on the cause, eg, plasma or extracellular fluid volume expansion, and give cardiotonic agents such as dopamine or isoproterenol (Chapter 3). In a minority of cases, lactic acidosis may be due to disorders of production (eg, neoplastic disease) or metabolism (eg, hepatic failure).

B. Second, treat the acidosis itself if arterial pH is 7.2 or less or if respiratory compensatory mechanisms are limited.

1. Parenteral infusions of bicarbonate–Because intracellular buffering is hard to quantitate, replacement therapy with bicarbonate is largely empiric. Initial treatment should attempt to bring serum bicarbonate concentration up to 12 meq/L or to increase it by 5 meq/L, whichever is greater.

The amount of bicarbonate to be administered is determined by multiplying the desired increase in bicarbonate concentration × 0.5 × body weight in kilograms (equation 12). Severe acidosis may require infusion of greater amounts of bicarbonate to achieve desired results. Bicarbonate may be infused intravenously over 5–10 minutes. *Caution:* Infusion of more than this amount may result in overly rapid correction of acidosis, with subsequent transformation into metabolic alkalosis; significant volume expansion may also occur and cause circulatory overload; and hyperosmolality may occur. Also, bicarbonate administration can result in a rapid rise in the PCO_2, and since CO_2 is rapidly diffusible across cell membranes, intracellular acidosis may be worsened. This is particularly important in myocardial cells and in the brain and may lead to myocardial dysfunction and neurologic injury.

a. Contraindications–Recent studies suggest that infusion of bicarbonate may be deleterious in patients with lactic acidosis. Bicarbonate infusions in patients with diabetic ketoacidosis are seldom necessary unless arterial blood pH and plasma bicarbonate concentration are low (< 7.1 and < 5 meq/L, respectively). Studies to date have failed to show an improved survival rate in patients with diabetic ketoacidosis given bicarbonate, and, in fact, the opposite may be true. The use of bicarbonate in the treatment of cardiac arrest has also recently been called into question, and bicarbonate administration has been deemphasized in the algorithms for cardiac arrest resuscitation drawn up by the American Heart Association.

b. Complications–Treatment of metabolic acidosis may change serum potassium and calcium concentrations.

(1) Hypokalemia– As acidosis is corrected, potassium will move into the cells from the extracellular fluid, and hypokalemia may develop.

(2) Hypocalcemia–Rapid correction of metabolic acidosis may decrease the concentration of ionized calcium and produce symptomatic hypocalcemia with tetany and carpopedal spasm.

Give supplemental potassium or calcium intravenously as necessary.

2. Peritoneal dialysis–When infusion of bicarbonate is contraindicated because of fluid overload, peritoneal dialysis may be an acceptable alternative.

METABOLIC ALKALOSIS

General Considerations

Metabolic alkalosis may result either from loss of hydrogen ion (primarily from the stomach) or from retention of bicarbonate (Table 36–14). The pathophysiology of metabolic alkalosis includes at least 3 separate factors.

A. Loss of Hydrogen Ion: Loss of hydrogen ion is the initial cause of metabolic alkalosis. Loss occurs from vomiting of gastric juice, which is rich in hydrochloric acid, or from increased renal excretion of hydrogen ion caused, for example, by mineralocorticoid excess states.

Gastric acid is lost, volume depletion occurs and the ability of the kidney to excrete excess bicarbonate becomes limited, further contributing to alkalosis.

B. Volume Depletion: Chloride depletion (eg, from diuretics) results in a relative increase in bicarbonate (so-called contraction alkalosis).

C. Potassium Depletion: A variable but usually

Table 36–14. Causes of metabolic alkalosis.[1]

Acid loss
  Acid gastric juice (vomiting, suction)
  Chloride excertion with increased reabsorption of HCO_3^- from potent diuretics (furosemide, thiazide, ethacrynic acid)
  Renal acid excretion from excess mineralocorticoid (especially aldosterone)
  K^+ deficiency with H^+ secretion in distal nephron
  Chloride-losing diarrhea (rare)
Bicarbonate gain
  Excessive intake of bicarbonate or precursors (alkalizing salts). Usually requires some degree of renal insufficiency.
  Milk-alkali syndrome
  Metabolism of acetoacetic acid, β-hydroxybutyric acid, ketones, and lactic acid to bicarbonate
  Abrupt decrease of arterial PCO_2 during treatment of chronic hypercapnia (compensated respiratory acidosis)
  Contraction alkalosis (body fluid volume depletion)

[1]Reproduced, with permission, from Schroeder SA et al (editors): *Current Medical Diagnosis & Treatment 1991.* Appleton & Lange, 1991.

significant degree of hypokalemia contributes to alkalosis by facilitating reabsorption of bicarbonate by the kidney.

D. Respiratory Compensation: The degree of hypoventilatory respiratory compensation in metabolic alkalosis is limited by the development of hypoxemia. In a patient with normal lungs, a PCO_2 of 65 mm Hg produces a PO_2 of 60 mm Hg, a level of hypoxemia that may in itself stimulate respiration. Studies in normal subjects have suggested that the usual maximum level of compensation is a PCO_2 of 55–60 mm Hg. Values above this level suggest primary CO_2 retention.

Diagnosis

Metabolic alkalosis is characterized by arterial blood hydrogen ion concentration under 35 neq/L, pH over 7.45, and plasma bicarbonate concentration over 28 mmol/L. PCO_2 is greater than 40 mm Hg. Symptoms and signs are variable. Severe metabolic alkalosis may cause symptomatic hypocalcemia. Volume depletion is usually present.

A. Early Stages: Initially, the kidneys are able to compensate for alkalosis by excreting some of the excess bicarbonate into the urine, and a relatively alkaline urine (pH > 6.5) then results.

Because obligatory excretion of cations accompanies excretion of bicarbonate, concentrations of sodium and potassium in the urine are elevated out of proportion to the degree of volume depletion that may exist. In this circumstance, the chloride concentration in urine may be used to assess the severity of volume depletion: a urine chloride concentration under 10 meq/L indicates avid renal tubular reabsorption of filtered chloride, pointing to significant volume depletion.

B. Later Stages: As volume depletion becomes more severe and as potassium depletion occurs, most or all of the filtered bicarbonate is reabsorbed. Sodium is exchanged for hydrogen ion in the distal tubule. The result is an acid urine (pH < 6.0) with low concentrations of sodium, potassium, and chloride—the so-called paradoxical aciduria of metabolic alkalosis.

Treatment

Caution: Avoid acidifying agents such as ammonium chloride, arginine hydrochloride, or hydrochloric acid, which may correct the alkalosis but do nothing to correct volume depletion and are therefore not recommended.

A. Volume Repletion: Volume expansion with solutions containing sodium chloride is the mainstay of treatment. In the face of ongoing loss of hydrogen ion through continued vomiting or gastric suction, the kidneys can only maintain normal acid-base balance if given sufficient fluid volume with which to adjust the composition of urine. Give normal saline solutions intravenously to all patients with metabolic alkalosis at a rate of infusion determined by the severity of volume depletion; for adults, it should be at least 150 mL/h. Often, administration of saline solutions alone is sufficient to correct the abnormality.

B. Potassium Replacement: In most patients, significant potassium depletion exists along with the metabolic alkalosis, and full correction of alkalosis may not result until potassium loss has also been corrected. Potassium must be given as the chloride salt so as to replace the chloride deficit.

Disposition

A. Mild Metabolic Alkalosis: Patients with mild metabolic alkalosis do not require hospitalization if the underlying cause is clearly defined and corrective treatment can be undertaken on an outpatient basis.

B. Severe Metabolic Alkalosis: Patients with severe metabolic alkalosis require hospitalization for administration of parenteral fluids and close monitoring of electrolyte and acid-base status.

MIXED ACID-BASE DISORDERS

Mixed disorders of acid-base balance occur often. The presence of a mixed disorder must be suspected when an acid-base disturbance causes no shift of arterial blood pH from normal; the unchanged pH indicates complete compensation, which by definition never occurs with a simple or primary disorder. The one exception is chronic respiratory alkalosis, in which full compensation can occur.

The presence of a mixed disorder is confirmed if acid-base values fall outside one of the shaded areas when they are plotted on the nomogram (Fig 36–5). These data only apply to the diagnosis of acute and chronic respiratory acidosis, respiratory alkalosis, and metabolic acidosis, the 4 shaded areas on the nomogram. Although points lying outside the shaded areas indicate mixed disorders, points lying *within* the shaded areas do not conclusively prove that the disorder is a simple primary disturbance, since mixed disturbances may occasionally display characteristics that fall within the shaded areas.

Combined Respiratory & Metabolic Acidosis

Combined respiratory and metabolic acidosis is a medical emergency occurring in patients in acute cardiorespiratory arrest. The 2 objectives of treatment are prompt improvement in ventilation and circulation concomitant with infusion of sodium bicarbonate to correct metabolic acidosis. Careful and frequent monitoring of arterial blood gases and pH status is mandatory.

Metabolic Acidosis & Respiratory Alkalosis

Metabolic acidosis superimposed on respiratory alkalosis commonly arises in patients with septic shock or hepatorenal syndrome. Since the 2 acid-base disorders tend to cancel each other, the disturbance in hydrogen ion concentration is small.

Respiratory Acidosis & Metabolic Alkalosis

Respiratory acidosis combined with metabolic alkalosis commonly occurs in patients with chronic respiratory acidosis who develop a superimposed metabolic alkalosis from antacid or alkali therapy for peptic ulcer disease or from diuretics for cor pulmonale. Since these 2 disturbances tend to cancel each other, the actual abnormality in hydrogen ion concentration is small.

Combined Respiratory & Metabolic Alkalosis

Combined respiratory and metabolic alkalosis usually occurs after prompt and overly vigorous correction of chronic compensated respiratory acidosis through improved ventilation or correction of metabolic acidosis through administration of sodium bicarbonate.

Three Primary Disturbances

Patients may present with 3 primary disturbances simultaneously, eg, respiratory alkalosis resulting from hyperventilation due to liver disease, metabolic alkalosis from protracted vomiting or volume depletion, and metabolic acidosis from severe volume depletion and poor tissue perfusion. This disorder is suggested when a metabolic acidosis/respiratory acidosis mixed acid-base disorder is present and the "potential bicarbonate concentration" (actual serum bicarbonate concentration plus the anion gap) is greater than 26 meq/L.

III. APPENDIX: USEFUL EQUATIONS & FORMULAS

Osmolality

Equation 1

$$P_{osm} = 2[Na^+]_{serum} + \frac{[Glucose]}{18} + \frac{[Blood\ urea\ nitrogen]}{2.8}$$

P_{osm} is in mosm/L, $[Na^+]$ in meq/L, and [glucose] and [blood urea nitrogen] in mg/dL.

When measured osmolality exceeds calculated osmolality by more than 10 mosm/L, an osmolal gap exists owing to the presence of significant quantities of unmeasured solute:

Equation 2

$$Osmolal\ gap = P_{osm\ (measured)} - P_{osm(calc)}$$

If the solute is alcohol, the blood alcohol concentration can be estimated:

Equation 3

Blood alcohol above concentration (mg/dL)
= 4.6 × Osmolal gap

Hyponatremia

To determine whether the cause of the serum sodium concentration ($[Na^+]_{serum}$) abnormality is due to total body sodium, potassium, or water abnormality, equation 4 may be helpful.

Equation 4

$$[Na^+]_{serum} = \frac{[Na^+_e] + [K^+_e]}{TBW}$$

where TBW = total body water (in L), $[Na^+_e]$ = total body Na^+ (in meq), and $[K^+_e]$ = total body K^+ (in meq). TBW may be estimated using equation 5. (See also Table 36–1.) For example, if $[Na^+]_{serum}$ is low and TBW is estimated to be normal, total body sodium or potassium must be decreased, and sodium or potassium replacement is the necessary treatment. However, if TBW is increased and $[Na^+]_{serum}$ is low, diuresis is the necessary treatment.

Equation 5

TBW in L = 0.6 × Body weight in kg

Equation 6

Na^+ deficit above in meq
= 0.6 × (Body weight in kg) (140 − [Na⁺]$_{serum}$)

Equation 7

Water excess in L
$$= \frac{0.6 \times (Body\ weight\ in\ kg)\ (140 - [Na^+]_{serum})}{140}$$

The relationship between serum sodium concentration and serum glucose concentration is as follows: For each increase in serum glucose concentration of 100 mg/dL, there will be a reciprocal decrease of 1.6 meq/L in serum sodium concentration.

Hypernatremia

Equation 8

Na^+ excess in meq = ([Na⁺]$_{serum}$ − 140) (TBW)

Equation 9

Water deficit in L
$$= \frac{0.6 \times (Body\ weight\ in\ kg)\ ([Na^+]_{serum} - 140)}{140}$$

Plasma Calcium Concentration & Plasma Albumin Concentration

For every fall in serum albumin of 1 g/dL, plasma calcium will fall about 0.8 mg/dL. Since this reduction does not reflect a change in free Ca2+ (ionized) concentration, this does not represent true hypocalcemia.

Acid-Base Disturbances

Equation 10

$$ph = 6.1 + log\frac{[HCO_3^-]}{0.03\ PCO_2}$$

Equation 11

$$[H^+] = 24 \times \frac{PCO_2}{[HCO_3^-]}$$

Conversion of pH to $[H^+]$: See Table 36–13.
Calculation of $[H^+]$ from pH:
For each increase in pH of 0.1 unit, multiply normal $[H^+]$ by 0.8. For example,

pH of 7.6 = 40 × 0.8 × 0.8 = 26 neq/L

For each decrease in pH of 0.1 unit, multiply normal $[H^+]$ by 1.25:

pH of 7.3 = 40 × 1.25 = 50 neq/L

If pH and either PCO_2 or HCO_3^- are known, the other variable can be calculated without the use of logarithms by using equation 11.

Rules of thumb for bedside interpretation of acid-base disorders include the following:

A. Metabolic Acidosis: PCO_2 should fall by 1–1.5 mm Hg for every fall in plasma HCO_3^- of 1 meq/L.

B. Metabolic Alkalosis: PCO_2 should rise about 0.5–1 mm Hg for every rise in plasma HCO_3^- of 1 meq/L.

C. Acute Respiratory Acidosis: Plasma HCO_3^- should rise by 1 meq/L for every rise in PCO_2 of 10 mm Hg. Plasma HCO_3^- concentration over 30 meq/L cannot be attributed to acute respiratory acidosis alone. In addition, for every 10-unit change in PCO_2, the pH should change 0.08 units in the opposite direction.

D. Chronic Respiratory Acidosis: Plasma HCO_3^- should rise by 3.5 meq/L for every rise in PCO_2 of 10 mm Hg.

E. Acute Respiratory Alkalosis: Plasma HCO_3^- should fall by 2.5 meq/L for every fall in PCO_2 of 10 mm Hg. Plasma HCO_3^- concentration under 18 meq/L cannot be attributed to acute respiratory alkalosis alone. In addition, for every 10-unit change in PCO_2, the pH should change 0.08 units in the opposite direction.

F. Chronic Respiratory Alkalosis: Plasma HCO_3^- should fall by 5 meq/L for every fall in PCO_2 of 10 mm Hg. Plasma HCO_3^- concentration under 12 meq/L cannot be attributed to chronic respiratory alkalosis alone.

G. Calculation of HCO_3^- Deficit and Excess:

Equation 12

$$HCO_3^-\ deficit\ (acidosis)$$
$$= 0.5^* \times Body\ weight \times (24 - HCO_{3\ plasma}^-)$$

Equation 13

$$HCO_3^-\ excess\ (alkalosis)$$
$$= 0.4 \times Body\ weight \times (HCO_{3\ plasma}^- - 24)$$

In addition, for every 0.10 change in pH units, base deficit will change in the opposite direction by approximately 7 meq/L. Bicarbonate deficit can be calculated by

Equation 14

$$HCO_3^-\ deficit\ (meq)$$
$$= Base\ deficit\ (meq/L) \times Body\ weight\ (kg)/4$$

H. Plasma K^- and pH Concentration: For each change in pH of 0.1 unit, there will be a reciprocal change of about 0.6 meq/L in plasma K^+ concentration. When pH falls, plasma K^+ concentration rises, and vice versa.

REFERENCES

Adrogué HJ et al: Determinants of plasma potassium levels in diabetic ketoacidosis. Medicine 1986;65:163.

Adrogué HJ, Madias NE: Changes in plasma potassium concentration during acute acid-base disturbances. Am J Med 1981;71:456.

Allon M, Dunlay R, Copkney C: Nebulized albuterol for acute hyperkalemia in patients on hemodialysis. Ann Intern Med 1989;110:426.

Alvo M, Warnock DG: Hyperkalemia. (Medical Staff Conference, University of California, San Francisco.) West J Med 1984;141:666.

American Heart Association: Standards and guidelines for cardiopulmonary resuscitation (CPR) and emergency cardiac care (ECC). JAMA 1986;255:2905.

Anderson RJ: Hospital-associated hyponatremia. Kidney Int 1986;29:1237.

Arieff AI: Hyponatremia, convulsions, respiratory arrest, and permanent brain damage after elective surgery in healthy women. N Engl J Med 1986;314:1529.

Arieff AI, DeFronzo RA (editors): *Fluid, Electrolyte, and Acid-Base Disorders.* (2 vols.) Churchill Livingstone, 1985.

Cohen JJ, Kassirer JP: *Acid-Base.* Little, Brown, 1982.

De Rubertis FR: Recognition and reversal of hypocalcemia. Hosp Med 1990;26(4):125.

Don BR et al: Pseudohyperkalemia caused by fist clenching during phlebotomy. N Engl J Med 1990;322:1290.

Feig PU, McCurdy DK: The hypertonic state. N Engl J Med 1977;297:1444.

Fulop M: Serum potassium in lactic acidosis and ketoacidosis. N Engl J Med 1979;300:1087.

Gabow PA: Disorders associated with an altered anion gap. Kidney Int 1986;29:752.

Gabow PA et al: Acid-base disturbances in the salicylate-intoxicated adult. Arch Intern Med 1978;138:1481.

Garella S et al: Severity of metabolic acidosis as a determinant of bicarbonate requirements. N Engl J Med 1973;289:121.

Jamieson MJ: Hypercalcaemia. Br Med J 1985;290:378.

Knochel JP: The clinical status of hypophosphatemia. N Engl J Med 1985;313:447.

Madias NE: Lactic acidosis. Kidney Int 1986;29:752.

Moran SM, Jamison RL: The variable hyponatremic response to hyperglycemia. West J Med 1985;142:49.

Narins RG, Cohen JJ: Bicarbonate therapy for organic acidosis: The case for its continued use. Ann Intern Med 1987;106:615.

Narins RG, Emmett M: Simple and mixed acid-base disorders: A practical approach. Medicine 1980;59:161.

Narins RG et al: Diagnostic strategies in disorders of fluid, electrolyte and acid-base homeostasis. Am J Med 1982;72:496.

Schrier RW (editor): *Renal and Electrolyte Disorders,* 4th ed. Little, Brown, 1991.

Whang R et al: Magnesium depletion as a cause of refractory potassium repletion. Arch Intern Med 1985;145:1686.

Wren K: The delta Δ gap: An approach to mixed acid-base disorders. Ann Emerg Med 1990;19:1310.

Wren K, Slovis BS, Slovis CM: The ability of physicians to predict electrolyte disturbances from the ECG. Ann Emerg Med 1990;19:580.

Yu GC, Lee DB: Clinical disorders of phosphorus metabolism. West J Med 1987;147:569.

---

*In severe acidosis, may be 0.8 or 0.9 × body weight.

Burns & Smoke Inhalation

37

Anthony A. Meyer, MD, PhD, & Patricia R. Salber, MD, FACEP, FACP

IMMEDIATE MANAGEMENT OF LIFE-THREATENING PROBLEMS (See algorithm.)

Begin CPR If Needed

See Chapter 1.

Establish an Adequate Airway

Severe burns to the lower face and neck may be associated with upper airway and laryngeal edema that can cause airway obstruction. Inhalation of super-heated air or steam in a confined space may also cause significant upper airway edema. Full-thickness chest wall burns, especially if they are circumferential, may limit chest wall movement and cause respiratory failure. Consider early endotracheal intubation in all patients with such injuries. If endotracheal intubation is impossible, cricothyrotomy may be necessary. Cricothyrotomy or tracheostomy in burn patients is associated with significant early and late complications. These procedures should be used only as a last resort in burn patients.

Support Ventilation & Oxygenation

Obtain a sample of arterial blood to assess oxygen-ation and to measure carboxyhemoglobin levels (see below). Monitor oxygen saturation by pulse oximetry. (Note that the actual oxygen saturation can be obtained by subtracting the percent of carboxyhemoglobin from the measured value.) Give oxygen, 2–10 L/min, by nasal prongs; *if smoke inhalation may have occurred, give 100% oxygen by tight-fitting reservoir face mask or endotracheal tube.* Burn patients with inhalation injuries require frequent reevaluation because of possible progressive respiratory compromise.

Gain Intravenous Access

Any patient with deep burns covering more than 15% of body surface area (Fig 37–1) requires intravenous fluid resuscitation. Insert 1 or 2 large-bore (≥ 16-gauge) peripheral intravenous catheters, preferably inserted through nonburned skin. If this is not possible, catheters can be placed through eschar, but insertion sites are then changed within 24 hours. Central intravenous catheters should be avoided, if possible, because they are associated with high rates of infection. They are usually not necessary unless the patient has significant underlying cardiac disease.

Draw Samples of Venous Blood

Submit venous blood samples to the laboratory for complete blood count, electrolyte and glucose determinations, renal function tests, coagulation tests, and typing and cross-matching. Arterial blood gas deter-

691

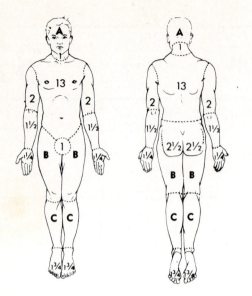

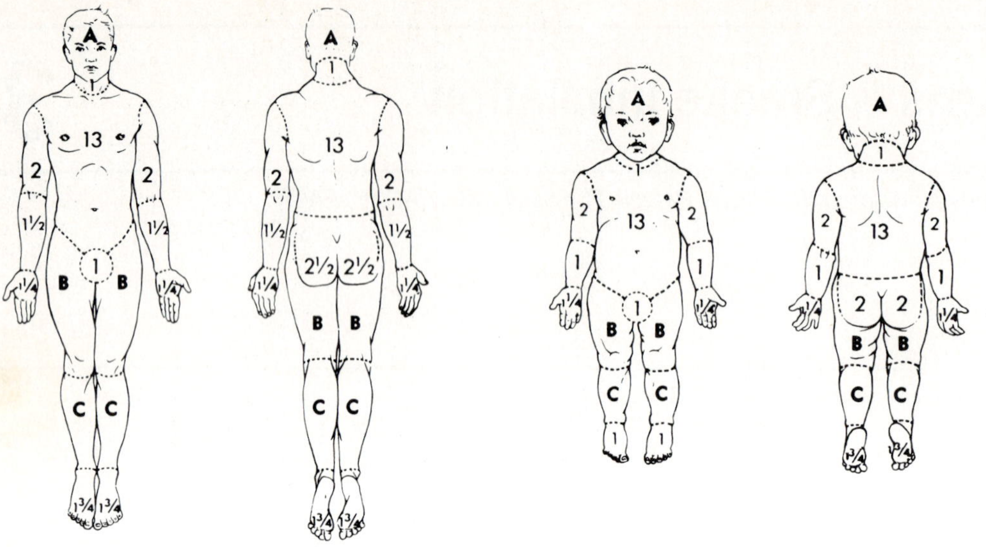

Relative Percentages of Areas Affected by Growth

Area	Age		
	10	15	Adult
A = half of head	5½	4½	3½
B = half of one thigh	4¼	4½	4¾
C = half of one leg	3	3¼	3½

Relative Percentages of Areas Affected by Growth

Area	Age		
	0	1	5
A = half of head	9½	8½	6½
B = half of one thigh	2¾	3¼	4
C = half of one leg	2½	2½	2¾

Figure 37–1. Burn size may be estimated using an age-adjusted burn chart. (Reproduced, with permission, from Way LW [editor]: *Current Surgical Diagnosis & Treatment,* 9th ed. Appleton & Lange, 1991.)

mination and carboxyhemoglobin level should be obtained if smoke inhalation may have occurred.

Begin Fluid Resuscitation

Burns are associated with the loss of large volumes of intravascular fluid, electrolytes, and protein through capillaries with increased permeability. Loss begins soon after injury and is maximal during the first 6–8 hours. Several formulas may be used as guidelines to fluid resuscitation (Table 37–1). Most burn centers use only crystalloid for the first 18–24 hours and use either the Parkland or the modified Brooke formula. These formulas should be individualized for each patient on the basis of the patient's response to therapy. Indices of successful resuscitation are set forth in Table 3–4. In general, infusion rates should be adjusted to maintain urine output at 0.5 mL/kg/h for adults and 1.0 mL/kg/h for children under 10 kg.

Obtain 12-Lead ECG, & Monitor Cardiac Rhythm

Hypoxemia, shock, electrolyte disturbances, or carbon monoxide poisoning in a burn patient may predispose to development of myocardial ischemia or cardiac arrhythmias.

Evaluate for Possible Associated Injuries

Burn patients frequently have other injuries in addition to the burn. Patients who have been burned in motor vehicle accidents or explosions should be evaluated as described in Chapter 4. Search for fractures and injuries of the head, cervical spine, chest, and abdomen in patients who may have jumped or fallen from a burning building or been burned in a motor vehicle crash.

Insert a Urinary Catheter

Insert an indwelling urinary catheter (eg, Foley) to monitor urinary output and to obtain urine for urinalysis (including myoglobin determination if the patient has sustained an electrical burn). Patients with full-thickness burns of the penile glans or shaft may require suprapubic cystostomy. An indwelling urinary catheter is the most important monitoring device in burn patients.

Insert a Nasogastric Tube

Patients with deep burns covering more than 20% of their body surface area will develop ileus. A nasogastric tube will decrease the risk of emesis and possible aspiration. If the patient is to be transported

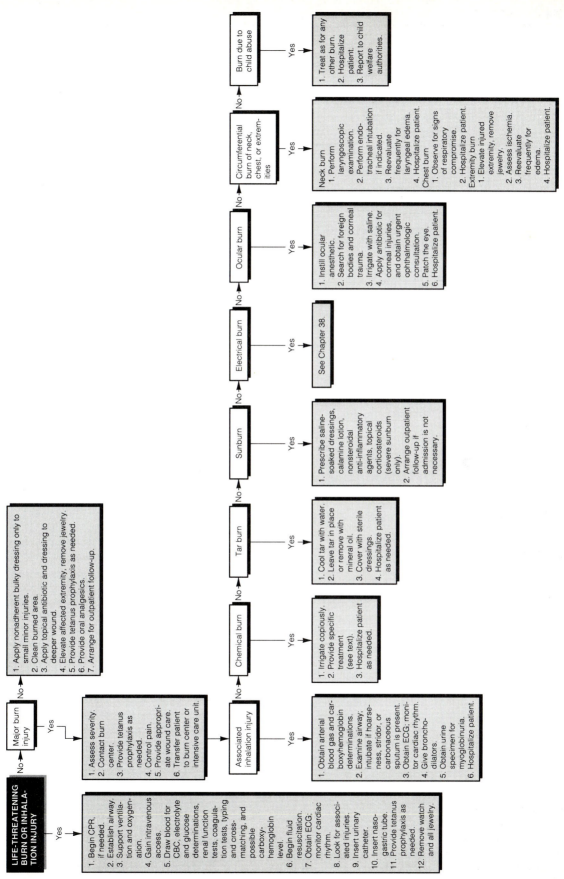

LIFE-THREATENING BURN OR INHALATION INJURY

Yes
1. Begin CPR, if needed.
2. Establish airway.
3. Support ventilation and oxygenation.
4. Gain intravenous access.
5. Draw blood for CBC, electrolyte and glucose determinations, renal function tests, coagulation tests, typing and crossmatching, and possible carboxyhemoglobin level.
6. Begin fluid resuscitation.
7. Obtain ECG; monitor cardiac rhythm.
8. Look for associated injuries.
9. Insert urinary catheter.
10. Insert nasogastric tube.
11. Provide tetanus prophylaxis as needed.
12. Remove watch and all jewelry.

No → Major burn injury

No → Apply nonadherent bulky dressing only to small minor injuries.
1. Apply nonadherent bulky dressing only to small minor injuries.
2. Clean burned area.
3. Apply topical antibiotic and dressing to deeper wound.
4. Elevate affected extremity, remove jewelry.
5. Provide tetanus prophylaxis as needed.
6. Provide oral analgesics.
7. Arrange for outpatient follow-up.

Yes
1. Assess severity.
2. Contact burn center.
3. Provide tetanus prophylaxis as needed.
4. Control pain.
5. Provide appropriate wound care.
6. Transfer patient to burn center or intensive care unit.

Associated inhalation injury
No → Chemical burn
Yes
1. Obtain arterial blood gas and carboxyhemoglobin determinations.
2. Examine airway; intubate if hoarseness, stridor, or carbonaceous sputum is present.
3. Obtain ECG; monitor for cardiac rhythm.
4. Give bronchodilators.
5. Obtain urine specimen for myoglobinuria.
6. Hospitalize patient.

No → Tar burn
Yes (Chemical burn)
1. Irrigate copiously.
2. Provide specific treatment (see text).
3. Hospitalize patient as needed.

No → Sunburn
Yes (Tar burn)
1. Cool tar with water.
2. Leave tar in place or remove with mineral oil.
3. Cover with sterile dressings.
4. Hospitalize patient as needed.

No → Electrical burn
Yes (Sunburn)
1. Prescribe saline-soaked dressings, calamine lotion, nonsteroidal anti-inflammatory agents, topical corticosteroids (severe sunburn only).
2. Arrange outpatient follow-up if admission is not necessary.

No → Ocular burn
Yes (Electrical burn)
See Chapter 38.

No → Circumferential burn of neck, chest, or extremities
Yes (Ocular burn)
1. Instill ocular anesthetic.
2. Search for foreign bodies and corneal trauma.
3. Irrigate with saline.
4. Apply antibiotic for corneal injuries, and obtain urgent ophthalmologic consultation.
5. Patch the eye.
6. Hospitalize patient.

No → Burn due to child abuse
Yes (Circumferential burn)
Neck burn
1. Perform laryngoscopic examination.
2. Perform endotracheal intubation if indicated.
3. Reevaluate frequently for laryngeal edema.
4. Hospitalize patient.
Chest burn
1. Observe for signs of respiratory compromise.
2. Hospitalize patient.
Extremity burn
1. Elevate injured extremity, remove jewelry.
2. Assess ischemia.
3. Reevaluate frequently for edema.
4. Hospitalize patient.

Yes (Burn due to child abuse)
1. Treat as for any other burn.
2. Hospitalize patient.
3. Report to child welfare authorities.

693

Table 37–1. Formulas for fluid resuscitation in burn patients.

| Formula | Day 1[1] | | Day 2 | |
	Crystalloid	Colloid	Crystalloid	Colloid
Parkland (Baxter)	Lactated Ringer's injection, 4 mL/kg per percentage of body surface area burned	None	5% dextrose in water, 2 L/24 h	40–60% of circulating volume
Modified Brooke	Lactated Ringer's injection **Adult:** 2 mL/kg per percentage of body surface area burned **Child:** 3 mL/kg per percentage of body surface area burned	None	Dextrose in saline, or normal saline to maintain adequate urine output	0.3 mL/kg per percentage of body surface area burned
Evans	Normal saline, 1 mL/kg per percentage of body surface area burned **plus** 5% dextrose in water, 2 L/24 hr	1 mL/kg per percentage of body surface area burned	One-half of first 24-hour requirement **plus** 5% dextrose in water, 2 L/24 hr	One-half of first 24-hour requirement

[1]One-half of the calculated volume is given in the first 8 hours; the remainder is given over the next 16 hours.

by air to a burn facility, a nasogastric tube is mandatory, because decreased cabin pressure may cause gastric distention and vomiting. The tube should be on suction or open to air and not clamped during transport.

Provide Tetanus Prophylaxis
See Chapter 24.

Remove Jewelry
Remove all rings, watches, and other jewelry, which could act as a tourniquet when edema develops.

FURTHER EVALUATION OF THE PATIENT WITH BURNS OR INHALATION INJURY

Obtain a History
Ask the patient, witnesses, and relatives about the mechanism of injury (explosion, spilled liquid, house fire, etc) and about the possible presence of combustibles known to be toxic. Find out whether the patient was burned in an open space or in an enclosed space; the latter increases the risk of inhalation injury. Also ask about underlying medical problems, tetanus immunization status, and medication allergies.

Determine the Severity of Injury
An accurate estimate of the severity of injury is crucial in determining the need for hospital admission or referral to a burn center and in guiding initial fluid resuscitation and establishing a prognosis.

Table 37–2 lists several important determinants of burn severity. Table 37–3 is the American Burn Association's classification of burns according to severity. In general, patients with minor burns may be managed as outpatients; patients with moderate uncomplicated burns should be hospitalized; and patients with major burns should be transferred to a burn center. If local personnel or facilities do not have experience in caring for burn patients, any patient with moderate or major burns should be referred to a burn center.

A. Burn Size: Accurate measurement of the burned area, expressed as percentage of body surface area, should be performed in all burn patients. Burn size may be estimated by using an age-adjusted surface area chart (Fig 37–1) or by using the "rule of nines" for adults or the "rule of fives" for infants and children (Table 37–4). The size of scattered small burns can be estimated by comparing them with the size of the patient's hand, which constitutes about 1¼% of body surface area. The extent of all burns should be recorded on a drawing (front and back views) on the patient's chart.

B. Burn Depth: Burns are typically described as first-, second-, or third-degree. A more useful description, based on the wound's ability to heal, is **partial-thickness** (heals spontaneously) and **full-**

Table 37–2. Determinants of burn severity.

Burn size
Burn depth
Burn site
Presence of circumferential burns
Inhalation injury
Electrical injury
Age of patient
Associated injuries
Major underlying medical problems

Table 37–3. Summary of American Burn Association burn severity categorization.

Major burn injury
    Second-degree burn of > 25% body surface area in adults.
    Second-degree burn of > 20% body surface area in children.
    Third-degree burn of > 10% body surface area.
    Most burns involving hands, face, eyes, ears, feet, or peri-
      neum.
    Most patients with the following:
      Inhalation injury.
      Electrical injury.
      Burn injury complicated by other major trauma.
    Poor-risk patients with burns.
Moderate uncomplicated burn injury
    Second-degree burn of 15–25% body surface area in adults.
    Second-degree burn of 10–20% body surface area in chil-
      dren.
    Third-degree burn of < 10% body surface area.
Minor burn injury
    Second-degree burn of < 15% body surface area in adults.
    Second-degree burn of <10% body surface area in children.
    Third-degree burn of < 2% body surface area.

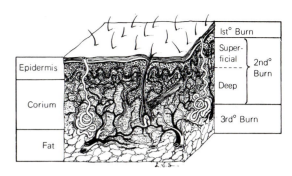

Figure 37–2. Layers of the skin, showing depth of first-, second-, and third-degree burns. (Reproduced, with permission, from Way LW [editor]: *Current Surgical Diagnosis & Treatment,* 9th ed. Appleton & Lange, 1991.)

thickness (requires skin grafting). Deep partial-thickness burns usually require grafting to expedite healing and decrease contractures and hypertrophic scar. Fig 37–2 shows the level of skin involved with each type of burn. Table 37–5 outlines the physical findings usually associated with each type of burn. The depth of the burn should be recorded accurately on a drawing (front and back views) on the patient's chart.

Several principles must be kept in mind when the physician considers burn depth. First, since it is difficult to distinguish deep partial-thickness burns from full-thickness burns, these burns should be assumed to be full-thickness injuries and should be treated accordingly. Second, burn wounds change over 48–72 hours, and what may appear to be superficial injury on initial examination may progress to a deeper-level injury, especially if the patient has poor perfusion or the wound becomes desiccated or infected.

C. Burn Site: Burns in the following areas are considered major injuries:

Table 37–4. Rule of nines (rapid means of estimating body surface area burned in adult patients) and rule of fives (rapid means of estimating body surface area burned in infants and children).

Area	Percentage		
	Adult	**Infant**	**Child**
Head and neck	9	20	15
Arm			
Right	9	10	10
Left	9	10	10
Torso			
Front	18	20	20
Back	18	20	20
Leg			
Right	18	10	15
Left	18	10	15
Genitalia and perineum	1	...	...
Total	100	100	≈ 100

1. Hands and feet–Deep burns of the hands or feet cause scarring and may produce permanent disability.

2. Face–Partial- or full-thickness facial burns may cause severe scarring, with profound physical and emotional impact. They are also often associated with inhalation injury and compromised airway.

3. Eyes–Burns of the eyes may cause corneal scarring and eyelid dysfunction that may ultimately lead to blindness. *Note:* Patients with possible eye burns should be examined as quickly as possible, preferably in the emergency department, because massive periorbital edema often develops and hinders later examination.

4. Ears–Deep burns of the ears predispose to development of pressure deformity and infection. Remember to examine the tympanic membrane in patients with external ear injuries caused by hot liquids or chemicals.

5. Perineum–Burns of the perineum are difficult to manage on an outpatient basis and are more susceptible to infection.

D. Circumferential Burns: Any deep circumferential burn is a potential major injury. Circumferential deep burns of the neck may cause lymphatic and venous obstruction that leads to laryngeal edema and airway obstruction. Circumferential burns of the extremities may restrict blood flow, causing an increase in tissue pressure and ischemia. Circumferential chest wall injuries may impede chest wall movement and lead to respiratory failure.

E. Inhalation Injury: Inhalation injury (burn sustained in a confined space, singed nasal nares, soot around the nares, carbonaceous sputum, hoarseness, stridor, symptoms of respiratory distress, carboxyhemoglobin level > 10%) signifies a major burn. Diagnosis and management of inhalation injuries are discussed below.

F. Electrical Injury: Damage from electrical injury may be extensive even though the outward signs of injury are minimal. Cardiac arrhythmias and renal

Table 37–5. Characteristics of burns of different depth.

	Depth of Burn	Color and Appearance	Skin Texture	Capillary Refill	Pinprick Sensation	Healing
First-degree	Superficial epidermis	Red	Normal	Yes	Yes	5–10 days; no scar
Second-degree	Superficial partial-thickness	Red; may be blistered	Edematous	Yes	Yes	10–21 days; no or minimal scar
	Deep partial-thickness	Pink to white	Thick	Possibly	Possibly	25–60 days; dense scar
Third-degree	Full-thickness	White, black, or brown	Leathery	No	No	No spontaneous healing

failure from myoglobinuria are possible complications. All electrical injuries should be considered major injuries.

G. Age of Patient: The mortality rate from burn injury is increased in very young or very old patients; these are also the age groups in which burns most commonly occur. Burns in a child under age 5 years or in an adult over age 55 years are more likely to be serious.

H. Associated Injuries: Burns may occur in patients who suffer other injuries, such as fractures or internal injuries due to vehicular accidents, falls, or explosions. The associated injuries often place the patient at increased risk of serious complications or death even though the burns themselves are small.

I. Underlying Medical Problems: Major preexisting medical problems in a burn patient are associated with an increased rate of serious complications and death. Patients with a history of myocardial infarction, angina, significant pulmonary disease, diabetes mellitus, or renal failure are considered poor-risk patients even if their burns are not serious. Burned patients with a history of alcohol or other drug abuse are also at higher risk for complications following burn injury.

Provide Tetanus Prophylaxis

See Chapter 24.

Control Pain

Patients with minor burns, especially of the extremities, may relieve pain by immersing the burned part in cool water; do not use this method in patients with larger burns, because of the risks of inducing hypothermia. Oral, subcutaneous, or intramuscular administration of narcotic analgesics may provide adequate pain relief for outpatients; however, intravenous morphine (in increments of 1–3 mg for adults or 0.1–0.2 mg/kg for children) should be used to control pain in patients with moderate or major burn injuries. Take care to avoid precipitating respiratory failure in a burn patient with compromised respiration. Ventilatory support may be required in some patients to permit administration of adequate amounts of analgesics safely.

Provide Appropriate Wound Care

Gently remove clothing, dirt, and other foreign materials adhering to the burn; irrigation with sterile saline (at room temperature) may be helpful. Do not scrub wounds or use harsh detergents or chemical disinfectants (eg, benzalkonium chloride, povidone-iodine). Little or no debridement of moderate or major wounds should be performed in the emergency department. Redundant skin from ruptured blisters of minor superficial partial-thickness burns may be removed, but *intact blisters should be left alone.* The wounds of patients with moderate or major burns, especially those who will be transferred to a burn facility, should not be treated with topical ointments or complex dressings in the emergency department, since these will have to be removed for evaluation upon arrival at the receiving facility. A simple nonadherent dressing such as petrolatum-impregnated gauze or sterile saline-soaked dressings should be applied instead. Management of outpatients with minor burns is discussed in the section on management of specific types of burns.

Transfer the Patient to a Burn Center

All major burns and many moderate burn injuries are best treated in a burn center, which has the personnel, equipment, and experience needed to treat major burns effectively. When a patient with a serious burn is first evaluated, the closest burn center should be contacted immediately, so that recommendations for care can be obtained and plans made for transfer, if indicated. Transfer should be coordinated with the physician at the burn center, and unnecessary delays should be avoided. If transfer can be carried out quickly, escharotomy may be performed at the receiving facility in patients with circumferential burns of the extremities, chest, or neck who do not have signs of respiratory compromise or tissue ischemia (p 701). Fluid resuscitation and all other supportive measures should be continued during transport, and the patient should be kept warm. Complete medical records should be sent with the patient.

EMERGENCY TREATMENT OF SPECIFIC TYPES OF BURNS

SMOKE INHALATION

Mechanism of Injury

The mechanisms of injury in smoke inhalation may be divided into 3 categories: (**1**) thermal injury of the airways, (**2**) chemical injury of airways and lung parenchyma, and (**3**) systemic chemical poisoning. Although one type of injury may predominate in some patients, most patients have a combination of injuries. All victims of smoke inhalation should be examined carefully for the presence of any of these injuries.

A. Thermal Injury: Patients who have been trapped in a fire in a confined space inhale superheated gases and may also suffer from direct flame injury of the face and neck, which is associated with development of marked upper airway edema and possible airway obstruction. Because of the efficient thermal exchange system of the upper airway, direct thermal injury to the lower respiratory tract is very unusual; rarely, exposure to water or steam in the heated gas mixture may produce thermal damage in the lower trachea and bronchi.

B. Chemical Injury: Chemical injury to the airways and lung parenchyma may be caused by noxious products of combustion of flammable materials (Table 37–6). Some of these products are directly toxic to the airways and lung parenchyma. Only the most commonly produced toxins are discussed below.

1. Acrolein–Acrolein is a highly reactive aldehyde that results from combustion of wood and petroleum products. It rapidly reacts with lung and airway tissues, causing injury by protein denaturation. Prolonged inhalation or exposure to high concentrations (> 150 parts per million) for short periods of time (minutes) can be fatal. Lesser exposure causes pulmonary edema due to alveolar capillary leakage; bronchorrhea and bronchospasm, which may be severe; and ventilation-perfusion disturbances which cause hypoxemia that may persist even after the person is no longer exposed to smoke. Acrolein also causes conjunctivitis and ocular tearing even at low concentrations.

2. Hydrochloric acid–Hydrochloric acid is one of the main products of combustion of polyvinyl chloride, a material commonly found in the structural components of houses and high-rise buildings as well as in furnishings and plastics. Hydrolysis occurs when hydrochloric acid comes in contact with the mucosa of the upper airway and tracheobronchial tree, causing protein denaturation and cell death.

Table 37–6. Common toxic products of combustion.

Material Burned	Toxic Product
Wood, paper, cotton	Acrolein, acetaldehyde, formaldehyde, acetic acid, formic acid, nitrogen dioxide, carbon monoxide
Polyvinyl chloride	Hydrochloric acid, phosgene, chlorine
Polyurethane	Hydrocyanic acid, isocyanates (eg, toluene diisocyanate), carbon monoxide
Petroleum products	Acrolein, acetic acid, formic acid
Agricultural wastes, automobile exhaust	Nitrogen dioxide and other oxides of nitrogen; acetic acid; formic acid; carbon monoxide

Even limited exposure may cause marked ocular irritation and tearing, although individuals with repeated or prolonged exposure may become desensitized to this effect. More severe exposure is associated with dyspnea, chest pain, and irritation of mucous membranes. Onset of pulmonary edema may be delayed for 2–12 hours after exposure, and the patient may appear asymptomatic in the interim. Toxic levels of hydrochloric acid gas may persist for as long as 1 hour after a fire has been extinguished. Patients exposed to products of combustion of polyvinyl chloride may also demonstrate premature ventricular contractions and may be at risk for development of lethal cardiac arrhythmias.

3. Toluene diisocyanate–Toluene diisocyanate is a product of combustion of polyurethane, a synthetic material found in almost all homes and offices, where it is used in seat cushions, mattresses, and carpet backing. Toluene diisocyanate is also found in insulation material. Toluene diisocyanate may cause severe bronchospasm, especially in persons with underlying obstructive lung disease, and is also an ocular irritant.

4. Nitrogen dioxide–Nitrogen dioxide is produced in fires involving automobiles or agricultural wastes. It is an uncommon though important toxin, since even brief exposures to high concentrations may cause severe bronchospasm, laryngospasm, and pulmonary edema. If the patient survives, late development of bronchiolitis fibrosa obliterans and chronic interstitial lung disease may occur.

5. Other noxious products–Particulate matter in smoke may stimulate irritant receptors in the large airways and cause bronchoconstriction.

C. Systemic Chemical Poisoning:

1. Carbon monoxide–(See Chapter 39.) The most widely recognized and most common complication of smoke inhalation is carbon monoxide poisoning. Carbon monoxide is a product of incomplete combustion and is produced in varying amounts in all fires. Carbon monoxide binds to hemoglobin with an affinity that is 260 times greater than that of oxygen, forming carboxyhemoglobin. The presence of even small amounts of carboxyhemoglobin drastically alters the affinity of the remaining unbound hemoglobin. Thus, even small concentrations of carbon monoxide may markedly reduce the binding of oxygen to hemoglobin, and the carbon monoxide that is bound is not easily displaced by oxygen. The presence of carboxyhemoglobin shifts the oxyhemoglobin dissociation curve to the left, making it more difficult for hemoglobin to release bound oxygen to the tissues. The net result is tissue hypoxia and lactic acidosis due to cellular anaerobic metabolism. Carbon monoxide also binds to the cytochromes interfering with intracellular energy production, but this binding is 9 times weaker than that to oxygen. In high concentrations, carbon monoxide is also bound to myoglobin; rhabdomyolysis with myoglobinuria and renal failure may occur. The half-life of carboxyhemoglobin is about 4 hours, which can be reduced to 40–50 minutes by administration of 100% oxygen.

2. Cyanide—(See Chapter 39.) Reports have documented the presence of cyanide in the smoke of residential fires. Because of the difficulties in measuring cyanide levels in patients and because of underrecognition and underreporting of smoke-related cyanide poisoning, the clinical relevance of cyanide poisoning in smoke inhalation is uncertain. Because there are risks associated with treating cyanide poisoning—which involves the production of methemoglobin by infusion of sodium nitrite—in a patient who also demonstrates carboxyhemoglobinemia, empiric therapy for cyanide poisoning is not recommended. The diagnosis and treatment of cyanide poisoning are discussed in Chapter 39.

Diagnosis

A. Thermal Injury: Thermal injury to the upper airway should be suspected in any patient who has been in a fire occurring in a confined space, in patients with obvious face or neck burns, and in patients with soot around the nares and soot-tinged sputum or burned nasal or facial hairs. Patients may complain of dyspnea; there may be stridor, drooling, or dysphonia. The diagnosis is confirmed by direct visualization of the larynx by laryngoscopy or in some cases bronchoscopy.

B. Chemical Injury: Chemical injury to the airways and lung parenchyma is difficult to diagnose in the emergency department. Direct laryngoscopy or flexible fiberoptic bronchoscopy may reveal mucosal friability and edema of the airways. Initially, the chest x-ray is often normal; noncardiogenic pulmonary edema may develop hours after exposure. Xenon lung scans, pulmonary function tests, and nitrogen washout studies have all been used to document the extent of pulmonary involvement, but they seldom provide more information than is obtainable by bronchoscopy.

C. Carbon Monoxide Poisoning: Systemic chemical poisoning due to carbon monoxide should be suspected in every victim of fire and may be confirmed by measuring the serum carboxyhemoglobin level. The often-described cherry-red skin color is *not* a frequent or reliable finding in patients with carbon monoxide poisoning. Similarly, arterial blood gas measurements are not reliable determinants of carbon monoxide poisoning, since PO_2 and the *calculated* percentage of oxygen saturation of hemoglobin (the value that is routinely reported by clinical laboratories) are *not* affected by carboxyhemoglobin. The oxygen saturation measured by pulse oximetry does not distinguish oxyhemoglobin from carboxyhemoglobin. Hence, the actual saturation is obtained by subtracting the percent of carboxyhemoglobin from the measured saturation obtained from the pulse oximeter.

Typical nonexposed, nonsmoking individuals may have serum carboxyhemoglobin levels of up to 1%; smokers usually have levels of 4–6%. Levels above 10% signify significant exposure and may be associated with symptoms as outlined in Table 39–16. Patients may be asymptomatic when carboxyhemoglobin levels are below 10–15%. Levels higher than 50–60% are associated with a high incidence of coma and seizures, and levels higher than 70% are frequently fatal. Myocardial ischemia or infarction and cardiac arrhythmias occur frequently, especially in patients with underlying atherosclerotic heart disease. Some patients who may initially appear to have recovered may experience delayed onset of a neurologic syndrome characterized by dementia, ataxia, and other sensory and motor abnormalities. This syndrome may be due to infarcts in the globus pallidus.

Treatment

A. For the critically ill patient, proceed as outlined on p 691. If there are signs of thermal injury to the airway, endotracheal intubation is necessary. In patients with major burns, even if the airway is patent initially, edema frequently occurs minutes or hours later. Prophylactic intubation prevents later urgent, difficult intubation.

B. Obtain arterial blood gas and carboxyhemoglobin determinations in all patients with possible smoke inhalation. While waiting for the results, give 100% oxygen by tight-fitting reservoir mask or, if indicated, by endotracheal tube. Avoid alkalosis and hypothermia, which decrease the dissociation of carbon monoxide from hemoglobin. Indications for hyperbaric oxygen therapy have been described as a carboxyhemoglobin level greater than 25%, neurologic symptoms, seizures, or depressed consciousness. The efficacy of hyperbaric oxygen in clinical management remains unproved. Although therapy shortens the half-life of carboxyhemoglobin to less than 30 minutes, the hazards and the length of time involved in transporting a critically ill patient to the nearest hyperbaric oxygen facility and the limits of resuscitating the patient in the chamber may outweigh the benefits of treatment. Hyperbaric oxygenation may be useful, however, in the severely poisoned patient who fails to respond to therapy with 100% oxygen. If carboxyhemoglobin levels are under 2% and if oxygenation is adequate, the inspired oxygen content can be decreased.

C. In stable patients with suspected thermal or chemical injury of the airway, evaluate mucosal injury using direct laryngoscopy.

D. Obtain an ECG, and monitor cardiac rhythm. Carbon monoxide poisoning is associated with myocardial ischemia and cardiac arrhythmias.

E. Obtain a chest x-ray to look for signs of lung injury if smoke inhalation has occurred and to serve as a baseline for further changes.

F. Give inhaled and parenteral bronchodilators to patients with clinical evidence of bronchospasm (Chapter 27).

G. Obtain a urine specimen for assessment of myoglobinuria. If present, treat as described in Chapter 12.

H. No evidence supports the use of prophylactic antibiotics or systemic corticosteroids in the treatment of inhalation injuries. Broad-spectrum antibiotic prophylaxis may be harmful, since it encourages proliferation of resistant strains, and some studies have reported increased mortality rates after the use of systemic corticosteroids in burn patients.

Disposition

Because victims of smoke inhalation may develop late respiratory failure, these patients should be hospitalized for 24 hours for observation. All patients with carboxyhemoglobin levels higher than 25% should be hospitalized. Patients who present to the emergency department with respiratory compromise or respiratory failure should be hospitalized in an intensive care unit.

CHEMICAL BURNS

Most chemical burns result from exposure of the skin to strong acids or alkalis. Other chemicals that may cause skin damage include phosphorus and phenol. Because full development of chemical burns is slower than that of other types, the size of chemical burns is usually underestimated during initial evaluation.

Diagnosis

Definitive diagnosis of chemical burns depends on the history. The physician should try to ascertain both the type of chemical involved and its concentration. Physical examination of a patient unable to give a history may aid in diagnosis. Alkali burns are frequently full-thickness injuries, appear pale, and feel leathery and slippery. Acid burns are usually partial-thickness injuries and are accompanied by erythema and erosion. Skin is stained black by hydrochloric acid, yellow by nitric acid, and brown by sulfuric acid.

Treatment

The mainstay of treatment of any chemical burn is copious irrigation with large amounts of tap water. To be most effective, treatment should be started immediately after exposure, preferably before arrival in the emergency department.

Remove any contaminated clothing. Do not attempt to neutralize the burn with weak reciprocal chemicals (acids for alkali burns and alkali for acid burns), because the heat generated from the chemical reaction may cause severe thermal injury. Occasionally, the leathery skin of an alkali burn may make it difficult to completely wash off the alkali, and injury may continue; further irrigation and emergency excision of burned tissue by a surgeon experienced in this procedure may be indicated.

After copious irrigation *with water,* the following treatment for specific types of chemical burns may be used:

A. Hydrofluoric Acid: Cover burns with dressings soaked in iced calcium gluconate solution (10%) or magnesium sulfate (25%). In fingertip burns, the fluoride ion often penetrates under the nail bed and matrix, so that it is usually wise to remove the nail or make a large wedge. For persistent pain or more severe burns, the treatment of choice is subcutaneous and intradermal injections of calcium gluconate (10%), 0.5 mL/cm^2 of burned area by a 30-gauge needle. Magnesium sulfate (10%), 0.5 mL/cm^2 of burned area by 30-gauge needle, has also been successful. Larger volumes should not be used, especially in the fingers, because further damage may occur from compartment pressure or the intrinsic toxicity of calcium. In extremely severe burns, some authors recommend intra-arterial perfusion of calcium.

B. Phenol: After copious irrigation with water, enhance the removal of phenol by applying polyethylene glycol, which increases the solubility of phenol. Follow with additional water irrigation.

C. Phosphorus: Phosphorus, a potent oxidizing agent, ignites and melts on air contact and often leaves embedded deposits on the skin. Immersion in cool water is recommended, followed by attempts to debride embedded material. Some authors recommend applying a solution of copper sulfate (3%) in hydroxycellulose (1%) to inactivate the phosphorus and aid in this removal, but few studies of this treatment have been made, and systemic toxicity from copper absorption may occur if copper is used repeatedly or over large areas.

Fluid resuscitation in the patient with large chemical burns is the same as that for patients with similar-sized thermal burns. Because the size of chemical burns may be underestimated initially, the patient should be reevaluated after 24–48 hours.

Disposition

The choice between hospitalization or outpatient management of chemical burns should be made using the same criteria as for thermal burns. However, the physician must remember that the full extent of skin injury may not be readily apparent during the initial emergency department evaluation.

TAR BURNS

Roofing tar usually varies in temperature from 51.1 to 80 °C (124–176 °F). The hands, arms, head, and neck are the most commonly burned areas.

Treatment

Cool the tar immediately with water, which often separates the tar from the skin. If the tar continues to adhere, either leave it in place or apply one of the commercially available cream- or oil-based solvents specially made for this purpose. If these are not available, use mayonnaise or mineral oil. Do not use hydrocarbon solvents, such as paint thinner, since they may further injure burned skin. Cover the wound with sterile dressings. When dressings are changed after 12–24 hours, much of the tar will have separated and will be removed with the dressing.

Initial stabilization of the patient with large tar burns should follow the procedures outlined for thermal burns.

Disposition

The criteria for admission or transfer to a burn center for patients with tar burns are the same as for patients with thermal burns.

SUNBURN

Most sunburn is a first-degree (erythema) or superficial partial-thickness (blisters) burn. Skin changes from sunburn are maximal about 12–24 hours after exposure. Patients usually present to the emergency department for pain relief. Occasionally, a patient with extensive superficial partial-thickness burns will require fluid resuscitation and parenteral analgesics for pain control.

Diagnosis

Diagnosis is based on a history of exposure to the sun (or to ultraviolet light in tanning booths) and physical findings of erythema and blistering.

Treatment

Sunburn can be difficult to treat. Saline-soaked dressings or calamine lotion may provide some relief from pain and itching. Aspirin or other nonsteroidal anti-inflammatory agents (eg, indomethacin, 25–50 mg orally 3–4 times a day) work by blocking the production of prostaglandins that are thought to be important mediators of pain in sunburned skin. More severe burns may benefit from the application of topical corticosteroid preparations such as triamcinolone acetonide, 0.1% (see Table 40–6 for a listing of the relative efficacy of various topical corticosteroids), or a short course of systemic corticosteroids (prednisone, 40 mg orally to start, with the dose tapered over 3–5 days). Patients with extensive partial-thickness sunburn should be treated according to the guidelines described for other thermal burns.

Disposition

Almost all patients with sunburn may be treated on an outpatient basis. If there are large blisters, the patient should be seen again in 2–3 days to make sure that secondary infection has not developed. Patients should be advised to avoid prolonged exposure to the sun in the future and to use a sunscreen (eg, over-the-counter preparations containing PABA [p-aminobenzoic acid] or dioxybenzone) before exposure. Patients requiring fluid resuscitation or parenteral analgesics should be hospitalized.

ELECTRICAL BURNS

See Chapter 38.

OCULAR BURNS
(See also Chapter 25.)

Patients with facial burns may also suffer burns to the eyelid and the eye itself. Such burns are associated with the development of massive periorbital edema that makes delayed examination difficult. It is therefore important that patients with suspected ocular burns be examined promptly, preferably in the emergency department and by an ophthalmologist.

Diagnosis

Instill tetracaine, 0.5%, or proparacaine, 0.5%, in the conjunctival sac to decrease pain during examination. Retract the eyelids, and look for foreign bodies. Remove contact lenses to prevent injury to the cornea due to pressure from edematous lids. Corneal abrasions and thermal injury may be detected by instilling fluorescein in the conjunctival sac and examining the eye using the blue light on an ophthalmoscope, or, if the patient's condition permits, a slit lamp.

Treatment

Irrigate any suspected chemical burn of the eye with large amounts (2 L) of sterile normal saline. Treat corneal abrasions and thermal injuries by instilling an ophthalmic antibiotic in the conjunctival sac and placing an eye patch over the eye. Alkali burns may require larger amounts of irrigating fluid, and irrigation should continue until the effluent pH is normal. Alkali burns usually require emergent ophthalmologic consultation.

Disposition
Burns of the eyes are major injuries. Hospitalize the patient immediately, and obtain urgent ophthalmologic consultation.

CIRCUMFERENTIAL BURNS OF NECK, CHEST, & EXTREMITIES

Circumferential deep burns of the neck may cause lymphatic and venous obstruction leading to laryngeal edema and airway obstruction. Circumferential chest wall injuries may impede chest wall movement and lead to respiratory failure. Circumferential burns of the extremities may restrict blood flow, causing increased tissue pressure with resultant ischemia.

Diagnosis
Patients with deep circumferential neck wounds should undergo direct visualization of the larynx by laryngoscopy. Because laryngeal edema may develop hours after initial examination, frequent reevaluation may be necessary.

Monitor patients with circumferential chest wounds for signs of respiratory compromise (tachypnea, dyspnea, deteriorating arterial blood gas levels); measurement of forced vital capacity or peak airway pressure may be useful.

Carefully examine the extremity distal to the wound in patients with circumferential burns of the extremities. Look for evidence of ischemia (diminished pulses, poor capillary refill, anesthesia); loss of vibratory sense is an early sign. If available, a Doppler ultrasound device is useful to assess distal blood flow. Because edema continues to develop during the first 6–8 hours after burn injury of the extremities, frequent reevaluation is important.

Treatment
Patients with deep circumferential burns of the neck are candidates for early endotracheal intubation.

Elevate the injured extremity of patients with circumferential wounds of the extremities in order to minimize development of edema. Remove rings or other jewelry that could act as a tourniquet when edema develops. If evidence of distal ischemia develops, escharotomy is indicated. Ideally, this should be performed in a burn center by a surgeon experienced in this procedure. Occasionally, escharotomy must be performed in the emergency department before the patient is transported to a burn center for definitive care. Sterilize the overlying skin (Chapter 46), and make medial and lateral incisions through the eschar using a No. 20 scalpel. Incise deeply enough to cut entirely through the burned skin and release the constricting eschar (typically, this occurs at the level of the subcutaneous fat). No anesthesia is required. Blood loss is seldom significant but can be controlled by cautery or suture if necessary.

Patients with a circumferential chest wall burn may require escharotomy in the emergency department. Using sterile technique, incise the eschar along the anterior axillary line bilaterally to the costal margins, and then join these incisions with incisions along the costal margins and just below the clavicles. This releases a segment of chest wall eschar that can move with respiratory excursion.

Disposition
All patients with deep circumferential burns of the neck, extremities, or chest wall should be hospitalized, preferably in a burn center.

BURNS DUE TO CHILD ABUSE

Burns represent 8–14% of child abuse injuries seen in the USA; about 15% of abused children have been intentionally burned at some time.

Diagnosis
Suspect child abuse if there is a delay in seeking medical care, if there is a history of other injuries, or if there is a discrepancy between the history and the physical findings. The injuries most commonly encountered in the emergency department are burns of the perineum caused by immersion in hot water in children who are being toilet-trained, and cigarette burns in children of any age.

Treatment & Disposition
The treatment of burns in children is the same as that of a burn of comparable size in any other patient, but if there is any suspicion that the injury was due to abuse, the child *must be hospitalized and the attending physician informed of the emergency physician's suspicions.* By law, suspected child abuse must be reported to the appropriate child welfare authorities (Chapters 42 and 45). Obtain consultation with appropriate personnel as soon as possible (social worker, nurse, psychologist, pediatrician, etc).

OUTPATIENT MANAGEMENT OF MINOR BURNS

Burns that meet the criteria for outpatient management (described above) may be treated initially in the emergency department, after which arrangements should be made for close follow-up on an outpatient basis.

Treatment
First-degree burns (erythema only) are best treated

with application of nonadherent dressings (eg, petrolatum-impregnated gauze). Clean deeper burns by gently irrigating them with sterile normal saline solution. Blisters should be left intact, and only minimal debridement should be performed. Wounds may be covered with a topical antibiotic such as silver sulfadiazene cream or bacitracin ointment and wrapped in a bulky dressing. Instruct the patient to keep the wound clean and to change dressings and apply topical antibiotic cream twice a day at home. A nonadherent, semipermeable, polyurethane dressing (eg, Epi-Lock), which is left in place for 5–7 days, may be an acceptable alternative for some patients. Such dressings should be covered with roll gauze, which is changed daily. Have the patient elevate affected extremities to minimize development of edema. All patients should receive tetanus prophylaxis as outlined in Chapter 24. Prophylactic systemic antibiotics are not indicated. Control pain with oral analgesics (codeine, oxycodone, etc).

Disposition

Patients should be seen on an outpatient basis in 1–2 days. Ruptured blisters or dead tissue may be debrided at that time. Promptly treat any minor infection with oral antistaphylococcal drugs (eg, dicloxacillin, 250–500 mg orally 4 times a day [children < 40 kg, 25–50 mg/kg/d orally divided into 4 equal doses]; or a first-generation cephalosporin such as cephalexin or cephradine, 250–500 mg orally 4 times a day [children, 25–50 mg/kg/d orally divided into 2 or 4 equal doses]). Patients who develop infections (fever, extensive cellulitis, lymphadenitis), poor-risk patients (diabetics), and unreliable patients must be hospitalized for administration of parenteral antibiotics and continued wound care.

REFERENCES

Coleman DL: Smoke inhalation. West J Med 1981;135:300.

Demling RH: Burns. N Engl J Med 1985;313:1389.

Demling RH: Fluid resuscitation after major burns. JAMA 1983;250:1438.

Fein A, Leff A, Hopewell P: Pathophysiology and management of the complications resulting from fire and the inhaled products of combustion. Crit Care Med 1980;8:94.

Fitzpatrick KT, Moylan JA: Emergency care of chemical burns. Postgrad Med (Oct) 1985;78:189.

Frontiers in understanding burn injuries: Proceedings of a conference, National Institutes of Health, September 1983, Bethesda, Md. J Trauma 1984;24(Suppl 9):S1.

Gerding RL et al: Outpatient management of partial-thickness burns: Briobrane versus 1% silver sulfadiazine. Ann Emerg Med 1990;19:121.

Goodwin CW: Current burn treatment. Adv Surg 1984;18:145.

Herndon DN et al: Treatment of burns in children. Pediatr Clin North Am 1985;32:1311.

Luterman A, Curreri PW: Burn wounds. Chapter 17 in: *Management of Wilderness and Environmental Injuries.* Auerbach PS, Geehr EC (editors). Macmillan, 1983.

Mani MM, Stackhouse SI: Ambulatory management of thermal injuries. Compr Ther 1985;11:24.

Moylan JA: Smoke inhalation and burn injury. Surg Clin North Am 1980;60:1533.

Stair TO et al: Polyurethane and silver sulfadiazine dressings in treatment of partial-thickness burns and abrasions. Am J Emerg Med 1986;4:214.

Stratta RJ et al: Management of tar and asphalt injuries. Am J Surg 1983;146:766.

Vance MV et al: Digital hydrofluoric acid burns: Treatment with intra-arterial calcium infusion. Ann Emerg Med 1986;15:890.

Wiener SL, Barrett J: Burn injury and management. Chapter 5 in: *Trauma Management for Civilian and Military Physicians.* Saunders, 1986.

Disorders Due to Physical & Environmental Agents

38

Paul S. Auerbach, MD

I. IMMEDIATE MANAGEMENT OF LIFE-THREATENING PROBLEMS (See Chapters 1 and 3.)

Accidental Systemic Hypothermia
A. Begin CPR for cardiac arrest due to profound hypothermia (or occurring as a complication of rewarming) (Chapter 1). Start core rewarming procedures (see below). Continue CPR until core temperature exceeds 33 °C (91.4 °F).
B. Treat hypovolemic shock (Chapter 3).
C. Prevent further heat loss with blankets (passive rewarming).
D. Administer oxygen, 6–10 L/min, by mask or nasal prongs, and monitor arterial blood gases and pH.

Heat Stroke
A. Reduce body temperature promptly when hyperpyrexia is extreme (over 41 °C [105.8 °F] rectally) by using ice packs, cooling blanket, and circulating fans. Consider core cooling.
B. Administer oxygen, 6–10 L/min, by mask or nasal prongs.

Lightning Strike
Begin CPR and advanced life support, and continue resuscitation even in the presence of fixed, dilated pupils (the latter may be due to the lightning itself).

Electrical Injuries
A. Remove the victim from the source of the electric current. Protect rescuers from the current with proper insulation.
B. Begin CPR and advanced life support for cardiac or respiratory arrest.

Drowning
A. Begin CPR and advanced life support for cardiac or respiratory arrest.
B. Ensure optimal ventilation and oxygenation.
C. Treat hypothermia.

Decompression Sickness
A. Administer oxygen, 6–10 L/min, by mask.
B. Gain intravenous access, and begin moderate volume expansion with intravenous fluids.
C. Arrange for immediate transfer of the victim to the nearest hyperbaric chamber for recompression therapy.

Arterial Gas Embolism
A. Administer oxygen, 6–10 L/min, by mask.
B. Position the patient on the left side, head down.
C. Arrange for immediate transfer of the victim to the nearest hyperbaric chamber for recompression therapy.

High-Altitude Sickness
A. Administer oxygen, 6–10 L/min, by mask.
B. Transport the victim to a lower altitude (below 1500 m [5000 ft]) as soon as possible.

Venomous Snakebite
A. Immobilize the bitten part.
B. Apply a compression dressing with an elastic wrap.
C. Transport the victim to the nearest emergency department for antivenin therapy.

Bee or Wasp Sting
A. Administer oxygen, 6–10 L/min, by mask.
B. Administer aqueous epinephrine, 1:1000 subcutaneously, 0.3–0.5 mL in adults, 0.01 mL/kg in children.
C. Gain intravenous access and begin moderate volume expansion with intravenous crystalloid.

Puffer Fish or Paralytic Shellfish Poisoning
A. Administer oxygen, 6–10 L/min, by mask.
B. Be prepared to provide mechanical ventilatory assistance.

Stingray, Scorpion Fish, Sea Urchin Envenomation
Soak the wound in hot water to tolerance (45 °C [113 °F]).

Portuguese Man-of-War Sting
Irrigate the wound with acetic acid, 5% (vinegar).

II. EMERGENCY TREATMENT OF SPECIFIC DISORDERS

DISORDERS DUE TO COLD

Individuals vary considerably in their response to environmental cold. Factors that increase the possibility of injury due to cold include poor general physical condition, nonacclimatization, childhood or advanced age, systemic illness, anoxia, and the use of alcohol and other sedative drugs. High wind velocity (windchill factor) and moisture may markedly increase the propensity for cold injury at low temperatures.

SYSTEMIC HYPOTHERMIA

Etiology

A. Healthy Persons: Accidental systemic hypothermia may result from exposure (atmospheric or immersion) to prolonged or extreme cold. Hypothermia may occur in otherwise healthy individuals during occupational or recreational exposure to cold or as a result of accidents or other misfortunes. Alcohol abuse is a common predisposing cause.

B. Persons With Predisposing Factors: Systemic hypothermia may follow exposure to even slightly lowered temperatures when there is preexisting altered homeostasis as a result of debility or disease. Accidental hypothermia is more likely to occur in elderly or inactive people and those with cardiovascular, dermatologic, or cerebrovascular disease; mental retardation; myxedema; or hypopituitarism. The use of sedative-hypnotic or antidepressant drugs may be a contributing factor.

Diagnosis

Lowered body temperature is the sole finding in some patients brought to the emergency department, so that making the diagnosis often depends upon awareness of the possibility of hypothermia.

A. Temperature: The internal (core) body temperature in accidental hypothermia may range from 25 to 35 °C (77–95 °F). Oral and axillary temperatures are useless, and a special rectal or tympanic membrane thermometer that registers temperatures as low as 25 °C (77 °F) is required.

B. Symptoms and Signs: Weakness, easy fatigability, drowsiness, lethargy, and impaired coordination may be early findings. At rectal temperatures below 32 °C (89.6l °F), the patient may become delirious, with progression to coma occurring at lower temperatures. Bradycardia, hypotension, and hypoventilation may occur. Shivering may be minimal and generally is absent at temperatures below 33 °C (91.4 °F). Absence of shivering indicates impending failure of the thermoregulatory mechanism. At rectal temperatures below 30–32 °C (86–89.6 °F), the patient soon becomes unresponsive, the pulse becomes slow and faint or undetectable, and fixed pupils may develop. The patient may appear to be in a state of rigor mortis. Ventricular fibrillation and asystole may occur spontaneously at core temperatures below 28 °C (82.4 °F). *For this reason, a hypothermic patient should not be considered dead until all reasonable resuscitative measures have failed. No one is dead until he or she is "warm and dead."*

C. Laboratory Findings: Several laboratory findings are unique to hypothermia. The ECG may demonstrate prolongation of any conduction interval;

atrial fibrillation is common. A pathognomonic positive deflection in the RT segment is known as a J, or Osborne, wave (Fig 38–1).

Hypoglycemia, hypomagnesemia, and hypophosphatemia are common in hypothermia, particularly in alcoholic individuals. Hyperglycemia may be associated with pancreatic dysfunction. Sodium and potassium levels may be elevated or depressed. Arterial blood gas samples drawn at cold temperatures are generally analyzed at 37 °C (98.6 °F), which causes lowering of pH and elevation of PO_2 and PCO_2 readings.

The temperature-corrected pH of arterial blood may be calculated as follows:

Actual arterial blood pH = Blood pH at 37 °C + (0.015 × 1 °C for every 1 °C below 37 °C)

When correction has been made for temperature, the PO_2 and PCO_2 are elevated 7.2% and 4.4%, respectively, for each 1 °C (Table 38–1). However, clinical therapy is based on uncorrected determinations.

D. Complications: Metabolic acidosis, pneumonia, pancreatitis, renal failure, sepsis, and ventricular fibrillation may occur. Death due to systemic hypothermia usually results from cardiac arrest associated with ventricular fibrillation, which may occur during rewarming.

E. Underlying Conditions: Obtain a brief history from witnesses or relatives of a patient with hypothermia, and perform a general physical and laboratory examination to detect underlying conditions that might predispose to hypothermia. Examination should include an evaluation of renal function (uremia), thyroid function (myxedema), and adrenal function (Addison's disease). If sepsis is a diagnostic possibility, obtain blood for culture.

Treatment

Bundle the victim of suspected hypothermia in dry, warm blankets at the scene of discovery, and transport the person to the nearest hospital as soon as possible. *Transport should be as gentle as possible because of the risk of cardiac arrhythmias due to increased myocardial irritability.* Hospitalization and monitoring in an intensive care unit are required for all victims with initial core temperatures below 32 °C (89.6 °F) or those with complications of hypothermia.

A. CPR: Adequacy of ventilation and circulation must be ensured by careful clinical observation, continuous electrocardiographic monitoring, and serial determinations of arterial blood gases. If cardiac arrest occurs, start CPR (Chapter 1). Do not begin closed chest compression until a careful check has been made for detectable arterial pulses; unnecessary brisk closed chest compression may induce ventricular fibrillation. Because of the protective effects of

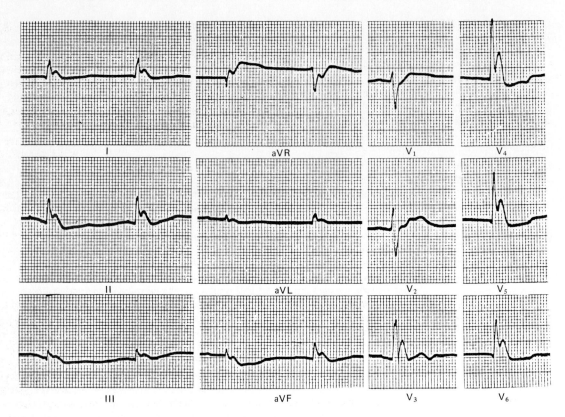

Figure 38–1. Hypothermia. The ventricular rate is 50/min. Atrial activity is not seen. The QRS complexes are narrow and are deformed at their terminal portions by a slurred wave occurring prior to the inscription of the ST–T waves; this is the J (Osborne) wave. The QT interval is prolonged. (Courtesy of R Brindis. Reproduced, with permission, from Goldschlager N, Goldman M: *Principles of Clinical Electrocardiography,* 13th ed. Appleton & Lange, 1989.)

hypothermia, bradycardia and hypotension are generally well tolerated.

1. Establish an airway. Intubation of the unprotected airway and frequent suctioning may be required.

2. Give warm, humidified oxygen. Depression of the respiratory center of hypothermia causes hypoxemia or hypercapnia requiring controlled ventilation and supplemental oxygen. Avoid hyperventilation, since a rapid fall in PCO_2 may trigger ventricular fibrillation.

3. If arterial blood pH is below 7.1, cautiously give bicarbonate (Chapter 3). Do not try to attain neutral pH, as sudden changes in acid-base equilibrium

may cause cardiac arrhythmias. Mild acidosis (pH 7.25–7.35) due to hypothermia in the absence of sepsis is generally well tolerated. *Management should be based on arterial blood gas measurements recorded at 37 °C (98.6 °F).* Recorrection of pH for temperature does not take into account a major blood buffer system, the imidazole ring of histidine residues present in numerous serum proteins. This buffer is less temperature-dependent than the bicarbonate-CO_2 system; hence, the uncorrected pH measured at 37 °C is the best approximation of true blood pH at any body temperature. Manipulation of acid base balance (with controlled respiration or administration of bicarbonate) based on "corrected values" is artificial and potentially hazardous.

4. Correct ventricular fibrillation. Electrical defibrillation is rarely successful at core temperatures below 30 °C (86 °F). Lidocaine and atropine are frequently ineffective in the hypothermic individual. Bretylium tosylate has been used successfully to manage intractable ventricular fibrillation in hypothermic patients. Isoproterenol is also effective and may be used to correct profound, life-threatening bradycardia. However, it should be used with ex-

Table 38–1. Effect of body temperature on arterial blood gases.

	Increased Temperature (for each 1 °C)	Decreased Temperature (for each 1 °C)
pH	↓0.015	↑0.015
PCO_2	↑4.4%	↓4.4%
PO_2	↑7.2%	↓7.2%

treme caution in elderly victims with atherosclerotic heart disease.

5. Correct fluid, electrolyte, and glucose abnormalities. Give thiamine, 100 mg intravenously, naloxone, 2.0 mg intravenously, and dextrose, 25 g intravenously, to all patients with altered mental status who are thought to be hypothermic. Volume expansion with warmed fluid generally helps the rewarming process.

B. Treatment of Underlying Conditions: Treat underlying and predisposing conditions as necessary, eg, heart disease, hypoglycemia, malnutrition, adrenocortical insufficiency (hydrocortisone, 200 mg intravenously), hypothyroidism (levothyroxine, 400 µg intravenously; plus hydrocortisone, 100 mg intravenously).

C. Rewarming: Rewarming is essential but potentially harmful, because peripheral vasodilatation may divert blood flow from internal organs to the skin and shunt cooled blood to the central circulation, causing a brief drop in core temperature. *Rapid rewarming may be hazardous, because hypothermic patients are particularly vulnerable to lethal cardiac arrhythmias.* Core rewarming should be undertaken only if hypothermia is severe and the patient shows cardiovascular instability (cardiac arrest, ventricular fibrillation).

1. Mild hypothermia (core temperature ≥ 33 °C [91.4 °F])–Passive rewarming to prevent further heat loss is sufficient for most patients with mild hypothermia, since their thermoregulatory mechanism is intact, and many of these patients are able to generate heat by shivering. Most patients should be wrapped in dry, heated blankets and carefully monitored. Patients with mild hypothermia who are otherwise healthy usually respond well to heated blankets and the administration of heated (45 °C [113 °F]) intravenous solutions. Another conservative approach—often used to treat elderly or debilitated patients—is to wrap the patient in an electric blanket kept at 37 °C (98.6 °F). Patients must be carefully monitored when any of these rewarming methods are used.

2. Moderate or severe hypothermia (core temperature < 33 °C [91.4 °F])–Moderate to severe hypothermia often requires additional rewarming measures, since thermoregulation is altered or absent. Individualized supportive care is mandatory, since active rewarming is hazardous. As previously mentioned, active core rewarming is necessary only for patients with cardiovascular instability.

a. Active external rewarming methods–Heated blankets, alcohol-circulating blankets, or warm baths have been used, with a rate of rewarming of about 1–2 °C/h (up to 600 kcal/h using hydraulic pads at 45 °C). Because it is easier to monitor the patient and to carry out diagnostic and therapeutic procedures when heated blankets rather than warm baths are used for active rewarming, heated baths are not widely recommended. There is some potential risk with active external rewarming, since marked vasodilation may occur, leading to a drop in blood pressure during rewarming. Some argue against this technique for that reason. If it is used, the patient should be carefully monitored and supported hemodynamically. The application of commercial heat packs directly to hypothermic skin may cause serious burns.

b. Active internal (core) rewarming methods–Internal rewarming is suggested for patients with profound hypothermia of long duration in which there is suspected underlying debilitation, for patients with complications of cardiovascular or respiratory insufficiency, and for patients in cardiac arrest.

(1) Repeated peritoneal dialysis may be performed using warm (45 °C [113 °F]) potassium-free dialysate solution. Up to 68 kcal/h of heat gain is possible. Two liters of solution should be exchanged at intervals of 10 minutes until the rectal temperature reaches 35 °C (95 °F).

(2) Warm fluids (crystalloid solutions) administered by gastrointestinal, colonic, or bladder lavage may be employed. Placement of a nasogastric tube is less invasive but may run the risk of stimulating ventricular dysrhythmias owing to the irritability of the hypothermic heart.

(3) Administration of heated intravenous fluids contributes only 17 kcal/h, which accounts for an increase in body temperature of less than 1/3 °C per liter. Microwave rewarming of crystalloid solutions to 40–42 °C (104–107.6 °F) may be safely accomplished in about 2–3 minutes. This technique causes some hemolysis of erythrocytes, however. Blood may be rewarmed by administering it through a water-coil rewarmer or by reconstituting refrigerated packed red cells with normal saline warmed to 42 °C (107.6 °F).

(4) Heated humidified oxygen, 20 L/min, contributes 30–40 kcal/h.

(5) Thoracic cavity lavage may achieve rapid rewarming with the added advantage of warming the heart more quickly. Two thoracostomy tubes are inserted, and fluid warmed to 41 °C is continuously infused through one and drained through the other.

(6) Extracorporeal blood rewarming methods (eg, with femoral arteriovenous shunts) are necessarily limited to medical centers with an available bypass pump team and surgeons skilled in the technique.

D. Antimicrobials: Patients with severe hypothermia—especially those who are comatose—are at high risk for development of aspiration pneumonia; subsequent pulmonary, urinary tract, or intraperitoneal infections; and sepsis. If severe infection is suspected—and in all urban patients who present with hypothermia and underlying alcoholism—obtain samples of blood and urine for culture, and take material for culture from any other appropriate sites (eg, cerebrospinal fluid). If there is a high likelihood of sepsis, administer broad-spectrum antibiotics (see

Table 34–1). Prophylactic antimicrobial drugs are unnecessary if infection is unlikely.

E. Complications of Rewarming: Observe the patient for signs of metabolic acidosis, cardiac arrhythmias, adult respiratory distress syndrome, pancreatitis, ischemic bowel, pneumonia, or myoglobinuria with renal failure.

Disposition

Hospitalize all patients presenting with core temperatures below 33 °C (91.4 °F), especially if the sensorium is altered. Patients with coexisting illness and core temperatures under 35 °C (95 °F) should also be hospitalized. The mortality rate in healthy patients who suffer severe hypothermia is about 5%. If there are underlying predisposing factors, the rate may exceed 50%.

COLD INJURY OF THE EXTREMITIES

In the normal person, exposure of the extremities to cold produces immediate intense localized vasoconstriction followed by reflex generalized vasoconstriction. When skin temperature falls to 25 °C (77 °F), tissue metabolism is slowed but the relative demand for oxygen exceeds the supply from diminished circulation; thus, the area becomes cyanotic. At 15 °C (59 °F), tissue metabolism is markedly decreased and the dissociation of oxyhemoglobin is reduced, which may give a pink, well-oxygenated appearance to the skin. Tissue damage occurs at this temperature. Tissue death may be caused either by ischemia and thrombosis in capillaries or by actual freezing. Freezing (frostbite) does not occur until the skin temperature drops to –10 to –4 °C (14–24.8 °F); the incidence depends on such factors as wind, moisture, mobility, venous stasis, trauma, malnutrition, and occlusive arterial disease.

1. CHILBLAINS (Pernio)

Diagnosis

Chilblains are red or violaceous pruritic skin lesions, usually on the face or extremities, caused by exposure to cold and humidity without actual freezing of tissues. Lymphocytic vasculitis is common. Chilblains may be associated with edema or blistering and are subsequently aggravated by excessive warmth. With continued exposure, ulcerative or hemorrhagic lesions may appear and progress to scarring, fibrosis, and atrophy.

Treatment & Disposition

Elevate the affected part on pillows or sheepskin, and allow it to warm gradually at room temperature.

Do not rub or massage injured tissues or apply ice or heat. Protect the area from trauma and secondary infection. Refer the patient to a primary-care physician or clinic for follow-up.

2. FROSTBITE

Diagnosis

A. Classification: Frostbite is injury of the tissues due to freezing. It may be divided into 4 grades of severity (similar to the grading system for burns).

1. First-degree–Freezing without blistering; peeling is occasionally present.

2. Second-degree–Freezing with clear blistering.

3. Third-degree–Freezing with death of skin, hemorrhagic blisters, and subcutaneous involvement.

4. Fourth-degree–Freezing with full-thickness involvement (including bone); ultimate loss or deformity of body part.

B. Symptoms and Signs: Frostbitten tissue appears white or blue-white, is firm or hard (frozen), cool to the touch, and generally insensitive. Because cold injury produces anesthesia, many symptoms are not apparent until rewarming begins or the part is closely inspected. In patients with mild frostbite, the symptoms are numbness, paresthesias, and pruritus. With increasing severity, decreased range of motion and prominent swelling are noted. Thawing unmasks local tenderness and burning pain. The tissue becomes discolored, loses its elasticity, and becomes immobile. Profound edema, hemorrhagic blisters, necrosis, and gangrene may occur.

Treatment

A. Systemic Hypothermia: Treat moderate or severe associated systemic hypothermia before managing frostbite.

B. Rewarming:

1. Superficial frostbite–Extremities affected by superficial frostbite (frostnip) should be rewarmed by applying constant warmth, which can be accomplished by exerting gentle pressure with a warm hand (without rubbing); by placing affected fingers in the axilla; and, if toes or heels are involved, by removing footwear, drying feet, and rewarming the parts by covering them with adequate dry socks or other properly fitted protective footwear.

2. Full-thickness frostbite–Rapid thawing at temperatures slightly above body heat may significantly decrease tissue necrosis caused by full-thickness frostbite. Such rewarming is best accomplished by immersing the frozen portion of the body for 15–30 minutes in water heated to 40–42 °C (104–107.6 °F). At this temperature, water feels warm but not hot to the normal hand. Avoid dry heat (eg, stove or open fire), since heat from such a source is more difficult to regulate. After thawing has occurred and the part has returned to normal temperature (usually in about 30 minutes), discontinue the application of heat. *Caution:* Rewarming attempted by exercise may increase tissue damage. Rubbing a frostbitten part with snow or immersing it in ice water is absolutely contraindicated.

3. Possible refreezing–*If there is any possibility of refreezing, the frostbitten part should not be thawed, even if this might mean prolonged walking on frozen feet.* Refreezing results in increased tissue necrosis.

C. Protection of Injured Part: Avoid trauma, eg, pressure or friction. Early physical therapy should not involve tissues with uncertain viability. Keep the patient at bed rest with the affected parts elevated; uncovered, or loosely dressed in sterile bandages; and at room temperature. Blisters may be left intact or debrided. If left intact, they should be covered with *Aloe vera* cream applied every 6 hours; if debrided, they should be covered with silver sulfadiazine (Silvadene) cream applied every 12 hours. Unless contraindicated, give ibuprofen in low doses (400–600 mg for adults, 60–120 mg for children) every 8–12 hours for 72 hours. Avoid tight occlusive bandages or immobilization with plaster casts.

D. Anti-infective Measures: It is important to prevent infection after rewarming. Maintain a sterile environment. Protect skin blebs from physical contact. Local infections may be treated with applications of dilute (5–10%) organic iodine disinfectants (eg, povidone-iodine). Whirlpool therapy at temperatures of 32.2–37.8 °C (90–100 °F) twice daily for 30 minutes for a period of 3 or more weeks helps to cleanse the skin and debride superficial dead tissue. Antimicrobials may be required for deep infections; some authorities recommend prophylactic penicillin for most cases of second- and third-degree frostbite. Tetanus prophylaxis is required.

E. Anticoagulants: Consistent benefit from anticoagulation has not been demonstrated.

F. Dextran: Consistent benefit from administration of low-molecular-weight dextran has not been demonstrated.

G. Reserpine: Intra-arterial administration of reserpine may be of benefit as a chemical sympatholytic agent. Although reserpine appears to provide immediate benefit in the resolution of vasospasm, randomized prospective evaluation is necessary to demonstrate long-term benefits. The author does not currently recommend this therapy.

H. Surgery: *Amputation or debridement should not be considered until it is definitely established that tissues are dead.* The line of demarcation between injured and normal tissue may not appear until 3–5 weeks after injury; mummification of the injured extremity may require the same length of time. Technetium Tc99m pyrophosphate scanning accurately predicts the level of ultimate amputation.

Regional sympathectomy performed 36–72 hours after injury has reportedly ameliorated the early sequelae of frostbite, but the value of this measure with respect to long-term benefits is controversial.

Disposition

Hospitalize all patients with second- and third-degree frostbite and patients with extensive areas of first-degree frostbite.

3. IMMERSION SYNDROME (Immersion Foot; Trench Foot)

Diagnosis

Immersion foot (or hand) is caused by prolonged immersion in cool or cold water or mud that causes alternating arterial vasospasm and vasodilatation. The affected parts are first cold and anesthetic. Hyperemia follows after 24–48 hours, and the parts become warm, with intense burning and tingling pain. Blistering, swelling, redness, ecchymoses, and ulceration are noted. The posthyperemic phase occurs after 2–6 weeks and causes the limbs to become cyanotic, with increased sensitivity to cold. Complications include lymphangitis, cellulitis, thrombophlebitis, and wet gangrene.

Treatment & Disposition

Treatment is best started during or before the stage of reactive hyperemia.

Immediate treatment consists of protecting the extremities from trauma and secondary infection.

Rewarm the injured areas gradually by exposing them to air (not to ice or extreme heat). Do not soak or massage the skin. The patient should remain at bed rest until all ulcers have healed. Keep the affected parts elevated to aid in removal of edema fluid, and protect pressure sites (eg, heels) with pillows or booties lined with cotton batting. Give antimicrobials only if infection occurs.

Hospitalize all patients with immersion syndrome.

DISORDERS DUE TO HEAT

The 5 main disorders due to environmental heat stress are (1) heat edema, (2) heat syncope, (3) heat cramps, (4) heat exhaustion, and (5) heat stroke.

Acclimatization usually results after 8–10 days of exposure to high temperatures, but even a fully acclimatized person may suffer a heat disorder when heat exposure is combined with excessive fatigue, severe infection, alcohol intoxication, use of anticholinergic drugs, or failure to maintain hydration, salt intake, or caloric intake. Elderly or obese persons and those with chronic debilitating diseases are most suscepti-ble to heat disorders due to circulatory failure or fail-ure of the sweating mechanism.

HEAT EDEMA

Nonacclimatized individuals, particularly the el-derly, may develop swelling of the feet and ankles that is generally associated with periods of prolonged sitting or standing. The edema is not complicated by manifestations of congestive heart failure or lym-phatic disease. The cause of heat edema is muscular and cutaneous vasodilation combined with venous stasis. Interstitial fluid then accumulates in the lower extremities. Because the problem is self-limited, treatment involves use of support hose and simple el-evation of the lower limbs. Diuretics are not indi-cated.

HEAT SYNCOPE

Simple fainting may occur suddenly after exertion in the heat. Cutaneous and muscular vasodilation re-distributes intravascular volume to the periphery of the body. Volume loss and prolonged standing (pool-ing in the lower extremities) also contribute to the de-velopment of inadequate central venous return and insufficient cerebral perfusion. The patient's skin is cool and moist, the pulse is weak, and there is tran-sient hypotension. In general, core temperature is normal or mildly elevated. The patient usually re-sponds promptly to rest in a recumbent position, cooling, and oral rehydration. Evaluate elderly peo-ple who suffer syncopal episodes for hypoglycemia, arrhythmias, and fixed myocardial or cerebrovascular lesions.

HEAT CRAMPS

Diagnosis

Heat cramps are due primarily to salt depletion and are manifested by painful spasms of the voluntary muscles of the abdomen and extremities. The skin may be moist or dry, and cool or warm. Muscle fas-ciculations may be present. The core temperature is normal or only slightly elevated. Laboratory studies (rarely indicated) may reveal hemoconcentration and low serum sodium levels, although this is variable, and normal serum sodium levels are frequently noted. Hypokalemia occurs occasionally.

Treatment & Disposition

Give sodium chloride, 1 g orally every 45–60 min-utes (repeated 4–6 times) with large amounts of water; or give physiologic saline solution intrave-nously. Give supplementary potassium as dictated by measured serum levels. Replace glucose if needed. An alternative therapy for mild symptoms is a com-mercial electrolyte solution, eg, Gatorade. These measures usually relieve the attack promptly. Place the patient in a cool place, and massage sore muscles gently.

The patient should rest for 1–3 days depending upon the severity of the attack. Hospitalization is usu-ally not required.

HEAT EXHAUSTION

Heat exhaustion is a systemic reaction to pro-longed heat exposure (hours to days) and is due to sodium depletion, dehydration, accumulation of me-tabolites, or a combination of these factors. It is a pre-monitory syndrome that rapidly evolves to heat stroke.

Diagnosis

A. Water Depletion: When heat exhaustion is due predominantly to water depletion (usually when the water supply is inadequate), intense thirst and weakness occur, with marked central nervous system symptoms, including muscular incoordination, psy-chosis, delirium, and coma. Hyperthermia may occur.

If circulatory failure or seizures occur, the condi-tion may rapidly progress to heat stroke (see below).

B. Salt Depletion: Individuals not acclimatized to heat may develop symptoms as a result of salt de-pletion. This condition occurs when thermal sweating is replaced by an adequate intake of water but insuffi-cient salt. Symptoms include muscle cramps, nausea and vomiting, diarrhea, weakness, pale skin, tachy-cardia, and hypotension. Body temperature is usually normal or mildly elevated. Serum sodium levels are low, so replenishing water without salt only aggra-vates the symptoms. The patient may not be thirsty and may or may not be sweating.

Measurement of serum electrolytes and renal func-tion is advisable in most patients, since serum sodium concentration may be markedly low in patients suf-fering from heat exhaustion. Myoglobinuria indicates subclinical rhabdomyolysis.

Treatment & Disposition

Initial treatment includes placing the patient in a cool place and giving adequate cool water and salted (< 200 mosm/L) fruit drinks or salt tablets according to the estimated amount of water and salt depletion. If the patient is unable to drink fluids, give normal sa-line or lactated Ringer's injection with 5% glucose supplementation intravenously in accordance with clinical and laboratory findings. If there is marked hyponatremia with water intoxication, administration of intravenous hypertonic saline may be required (Chapter 36).

Hospitalize the patient for observation and treat-ment.

HEAT STROKE

Heat stroke is characterized by dysfunction of the heat-regulating mechanism, with altered mental status (ranging from confusion to coma) and elevated core body temperature in excess of 41 °C (105.8 °F). Sweating is variable. The extremely high body temperature rapidly causes widespread damage to body tissues, with significant rhabdomyolysis. Illness and death result from destruction of cerebral, cardiovascular, hepatic, and renal tissue.

Heat stroke usually follows excessive exposure to heat or strenuous physical activity under exceptionally hot environmental conditions, although it may develop in elderly, infirm, or otherwise susceptible individuals in the absence of unusual exposure to heat. Cardiovascular disease, diabetes, cystic fibrosis, alcoholism, obesity, recent febrile illness, and debility are predisposing factors. Anesthetics, paralyzing agents, diuretics, sedatives, antidepressants, and anticholinergic drugs may also be contributing factors.

Diagnosis

A. Symptoms and Signs: Premonitory findings include headache, dizziness, nausea, diarrhea, visual disturbances, confusion, and convulsions. Coma may ensue. The skin is hot, flushed (cyanosis may be present), and usually dry (although sweating may be present). Prior to cardiovascular collapse, the pulse may be strong and rapid. Blood pressure is initially elevated but falls with increasing cardiac failure. The rectal temperature may be as high as 46.5 °C (115.6 °F). Hyperventilation may cause initial respiratory alkalosis, which is generally followed by metabolic acidosis. Stigmas of coagulopathy include hematuria, hematemesis, bruising, petechiae, and oozing at sites of venipuncture.

B. Laboratory Findings: Laboratory findings include hemoconcentration, decreased blood coagulation, and evidence of disseminated intravascular coagulation. Hypoprothrombinemia, hypofibrinogenemia, or thrombocytopenia may also be present. The white blood count is routinely elevated. Hypophosphatemia and hypokalemia are not uncommon. Hyperkalemia is associated with acute renal failure. There is scanty concentrated urine ("machine oil urine") containing protein, tubular casts, and myoglobin. There is enzymatic evidence of liver and muscle damage (elevated CK, ALT [SGPT], AST [SGOT] levels).

Treatment

Act quickly to prevent further injury.

A. Maintain an adequate airway and ventilation; monitor arterial blood gas levels. Give supplemental oxygen, 6–10 L/min, by mask or nasal prongs.

B. *Reduce body temperature promptly.* As a first aid measure, place the patient in a shady, cool place, and remove clothing. Sprinkle the patient's entire body with water, and cool by fanning. Alcohol sponging is unnecessary and potentially dangerous (alcohol intoxication). If the victim is near a cold stream, cautiously immerse the trunk in cool water.

In the emergency department, place the patient on a cooling blanket, and place ice packs on the axilla, posterior neck, and inguinal areas (do not apply ice directly to the skin). Evaporative heat loss may be maximized by suspending the nude patient in a mesh net, spraying atomized water at a temperature of 15 °C (59 °F) over the subject, and blowing air at a temperature of 45–48 °C (113–118.4 °F) in such a way that it reaches the skin at a temperature of 33 °C (91.4 °F) and a flow rate of 30 m/min. If the temperature cannot be rapidly lowered or if the victim is unresponsive and the initial core temperature exceeds 42 °C (107.6 °F), begin peritoneal lavage with cold potassium-free dialysate, 2 L every 10–15 minutes. When the rectal temperature drops to 38 °C (100.4 °F), discontinue active measures to lower temperature, but continue temperature monitoring. If the temperature starts to rise again, resume the cooling process. Iced gastric, rectal, or bladder lavage has not yet been prospectively evaluated in humans.

Chlorpromazine, 10–25 mg slowly intravenously, may be given as needed to control shivering.

C. Maintain adequate urinary output (30–50 mL/h). Insert an indwelling urinary catheter to monitor urine output. If myoglobinuria is present, alkalize the urine with intravenous administration of bicarbonate, and consider the use of mannitol, 0.25 g/kg intravenously, to promote diuresis. Maintain blood pressure and urine output with intravenous infusion of crystalloid solutions and inotropic agents as necessary (monitoring of central venous pressure or pulmonary capillary wedge pressure may be required). Dobutamine may be preferable to dopamine as an inotropic agent, since it does not have the alpha-adrenergic renal effects associated with dopamine at rapid rates of infusion. Aspirin and acetaminophen are of no value in lowering body temperature in exertional heat stroke, since these agents block the effects of endogenous pyrogens that act upon the hypothalamus during a febrile episode.

Disposition

Hospitalize all patients whose core temperature has exceeded 41 °C (105.8 °F) for treatment of possible complications (disseminated intravascular coagulation, renal failure, hepatic failure, rhabdomyolysis, cardiac arrhythmias, myocardial infarction, and coma).

With early diagnosis and proper care, 80–90% of previously healthy patients should survive. Extreme hyperpyrexia (rectal temperature > 42 °C [107.6 °F]), persistent coma after cooling, markedly elevated ALT (SGPT) and AST (SGOT) levels, and hyperkalemia associated with extensive rhabdomyolysis are unfavorable prognostic signs.

ELECTRICAL INJURIES

LIGHTNING INJURIES

Lightning associated with thunderstorms strikes the earth more than 120 times per second. Although the number of lightning strikes in human beings is low, at least 200–400 people are killed each year as a result of injuries caused by lightning.

A stroke of lightning travels from a thundercloud to the ground at a speed of 10,000 km/s (10^7 m/s), and it briefly attains voltages over 100 million V and temperatures of up to 3000 °C (5432 °F). Lightning is direct current (DC). The most common form of lightning is streak lightning. Injuries are caused by a direct strike, splash (from trees, buildings, fences, etc), step voltage, or blunt trauma. In step voltage, ground surface current is transmitted through a circuit created by the victim's legs (pathway of least resistance).

Diagnosis

Suspect lightning injury in a person found dazed, unconscious, or injured in the vicinity of a thunderstorm. Certain pathognomonic clinical signs help to establish the diagnosis.

A. Burns: Although enormous levels of electrical energy are generated in a lightning strike, burns are frequently superficial. The **flashover phenomenon** channels most of the current along the outside of the body (over the skin) rather than through the victim, as occurs in other types of electrical injury. As the current races over the body, it vaporizes moisture on the skin and may destroy clothing in an explosive manner. Burns of unusual patterns may be noted.

1. Linear burns–Linear burns are first- and second-degree burns that begin at the head and neck and course in a branching pattern down the chest and legs. They tend to follow areas with a heavy concentration of sweat.

2. Punctate burns–Punctate burns are clusters of discrete, circular, partial- or full-thickness burns that form starburst patterns on the skin.

3. Feathering burns–Feathering burns are not true burns but rather cutaneous imprints from electron showers that track through the skin. They create a fernlike pattern with delicate branching. These patterns are also called **ferning, keraunographic markings,** and **Lichtenberg's flowers** or **figures.**

4. Thermal burns–Thermal burns from clothing or heated metal are typical second- and third-degree burns. Cranial burns (direct or indirect head strike) and leg burns (ground current) are associated with increased death rates.

B. Altered Mental Status: Victims of lightning strike are usually disoriented, combative, or comatose. Rarely, they are alert, but they typically have amnesia for the event.

C. Cardiac Arrest: Cardiac arrest is a result of sudden cardiac standstill induced by the massive DC countershock of the lightning strike. Spontaneous resumption of normal cardiac function is the rule if cardiac standstill is not complicated by simultaneous respiratory arrest (brain stem shock or contusion). Both asystole and ventricular fibrillation have been associated with lightning strike. Myocardial infarction is a potential acute complication.

D. Neurologic Injuries: Central nervous system injuries include epidural and subdural hematomas, subarachnoid hemorrhage, coagulation burn injuries of brain, intraventricular hemorrhage, and respiratory paralysis. Seizures, loss of consciousness, and peripheral neurovascular instability are common. Anterograde amnesia and confusion are noted in most patients.

E. Musculoskeletal Injuries: Victims of lightning strike are frequently thrown to the ground by tetanic muscle contractions, or they may be injured by falls from heights. Fractures of the skull, spine, ribs, and extremities may occur. Intrathoracic and abdominal injuries result from blunt trauma.

F. Eye and Ear Injuries: Eye injuries associated with lightning strike include cataracts, corneal abrasions, hyphema, uveitis, vitreous hemorrhage, and iridocyclitis. *Dilated pupils should never be the sole criterion for termination of resuscitative efforts, since they may merely reflect transient autonomic sympathetic discharge or parasympathetic inhibition.* Temporary sensorineural hearing loss with or without rupture of the tympanic membrane may result from the loud noise and physical shock wave.

Treatment

A. Maintain the Airway, and Begin CPR: Respiratory arrest is the most common cause of death in persons who have been struck by lightning. Artificial respiration should be continued until spontaneous respiration resumes or the rescuer cannot continue because of exhaustion. Begin closed chest compression if no pulse (carotid or femoral) is present (Chapter 1). Victims struck by lightning and apparently dead have been successfully resuscitated after prolonged efforts.

B. Anticipate Traumatic Injury: Management of the victim of lightning strike is the same as that for a person who has sustained severe blunt trauma. Examine the entire body for evidence of significant skeletal, muscular, or internal injury. Obtain x-rays of the cervical spine and chest, an ECG, and appropriate laboratory tests (urinalysis; CBC; blood urea nitrogen and serum electrolyte and creatinine measurements; and CK-MB, LDH, and AST [SGOT] enzyme determinations). If the patient's level of consciousness deteriorates, if focal neurologic signs are present, or if coma is prolonged, obtain a CT scan of the brain. Fasciotomy of paralyzed or pulseless extremities should be guided by measurement of intracompartmental tissue pressures in order to avoid unnecessary surgery on limbs that are apparently pulseless as the result of transient sympathetic overactivity.

C. Begin Burn Therapy and Fluid Replacement: Management of burn wounds follows standard procedures (Chapter 37). Rhabdomyolysis and myoglobinuria are rarely caused by lightning strike unless there has been severe thermal injury or blunt trauma to muscle. Administration of intravenous fluids should therefore be adjusted according to blood pressure readings and urine output. Alkalization of the urine and administration of mannitol are not necessary unless myoglobinuria is present. If there is significant brain injury, intracranial and pulmonary artery pressure monitoring may be necessary for proper evaluation of fluid replacement.

Disposition

All patients who have been struck by lightning should be hospitalized with cardiac monitoring for 24 hours. Obtain serial cardiac isoenzyme determinations and ECGs. Screen the urine regularly for evidence of myoglobinuria. Results of visual acuity and hearing tests should be recorded to establish a baseline measurement.

If the victim has suffered cardiopulmonary arrest and resuscitation efforts have been successful (resumption of spontaneous *cardiac* activity), allow a minimum of 12–24 hours before weaning the patient from the ventilator to see if spontaneous *respiratory* activity resumes. Electroencephalographic abnormalities are not uncommon and may clear over 24–72 hours. Dilated pupils cannot be used as an early diagnostic criterion for brain death.

ELECTRIC SHOCK & BURNS

Electric shock may result from carelessness or ignorance in working with electricity, faulty appliances and equipment, or severed electric power lines, or it may be an accident of nature (lightning). Dry skin offers high resistance to passage of ordinary levels of electric current. However, skin moistened with water, sweat, saline solution, or urine offers greatly reduced resistance to electric current. The amount and type of current, the duration and area of exposure, and the pathway of the current through the body determine the degree of damage. When current passes through the heart or the brain, death may be rapid.

Direct current (DC) is much less dangerous than alternating current (AC), although electrochemical skin burns have been reported from DC current as low as 3 V. High-voltage AC current with a high number of cycles per second (hertz, Hz) may be less dangerous than low-voltage current with fewer cycles per second.

Alternating current of 25–300 Hz and 25–220 V, a range that includes house current in most locales, tends to cause ventricular fibrillation if the pathway includes the heart. With voltages over 1000 V, respiratory paralysis often occurs. With intermediate voltages (220–1000 V), a mixed picture of respiratory insufficiency and arrhythmias is noted.

Diagnosis

A. Electric Shock: Electric shock may produce momentary or prolonged loss of consciousness. Ventricular fibrillation is the most serious immediate arrhythmia. Respiration may continue for a few minutes after injury or be absent, with immediate respiratory paralysis. When respiratory failure occurs, the patient becomes unconscious. Although a pulse can be felt, the patient is cyanotic, with cool, clammy skin and marked hypotension.

After recovery from mild to moderate electric shock, muscular pain, fatigue, headache, and generalized or focal nervous irritability occur. Physical signs vary according to the sites of action of the current.

B. Electrical Burns: There are 3 distinct types of electrical burns: (**1**) flash (arc) burns, (**2**) flame burns, and (**3**) direct burning of the tissues by electric current. The latter cause entry wounds that are usually sharply demarcated, round or oval, painless gray areas with a surrounding inflammatory reaction. The exit wounds are more ragged-looking, with an "exploded" appearance. Initial examination of the surface wound is often misleading, since the injury may appear relatively innocuous despite extensive deep tissue destruction. Little destruction may be evident for the first 7–10 days; ischemia and sloughing then occur slowly in severely affected areas. The temperature generated in an arc burn from household electric current (110–220 V) may reach 3000 °C (5432 °F).

Common complications include cardiac arrhythmias or cardiac failure, circulatory shock, hemorrhage, and myoglobinuria.

Treatment

A. Electric Shock:

1. Free the victim from the current at once. This may be done in many ways, but the rescuer must be protected. Turn off the power, sever the wire with a dry wooden-handled axe, make a proper ground to divert the current, or drag the victim carefully away using dry clothing, a leather belt, rubber, or other dry nonconductive materials.

2. Check cardiac and ventilatory function. If the patient is apneic or pulseless, began artificial ventilation or CPR (Chapter 1).

B. Electrical Burns: Treat tissue burns conservatively. The direction and extent of tissue injury may not be apparent for 7–10 days. Treat circulatory shock, if present, with intravenous infusion of crystalloid solutions. Locate entrance and exit wounds to help determine the pathway of the current. If current has passed through the chest, obtain an ECG. Serum CK-MB isoenzyme levels may be falsely elevated immediately after high-voltage electrical injuries and should not be considered a reliable indicator of myocardial damage. Monitor cardiac rhythm to detect rhythm disturbances in unconscious victims, those who have presented with cardiac arrhythmias, or those with an abnormal ECG. If myoglobinuria is present, monitor arterial blood pH at regular intervals to detect acidosis, which requires intravenous bicarbonate therapy to alkalize the urine and maintain blood pH above 7.35. Use intravenous mannitol, 0.25 g/kg, to promote moderate diuresis.

The need for fasciotomy should be assessed by measurement of intracompartmental tissue pressures. In children who have bitten electrical cords, be alert for delayed (up to 3 weeks) erosion of the labial artery.

Disposition

Hospitalize all small children and patients who have lost consciousness or suffered cardiac or respiratory arrest, as well as those with ischemic chest pain, myoglobinuria, or significant burn wounds.

RADIATION INJURIES

The effects of radiation have been observed in the clinical use of x-rays and radioactive agents, after occupational or accidental exposure, and following the use of atomic weapons. The harm derived depends on the quantity of radiation delivered to the body, the type of radiation (x-rays, neutrons, gamma rays, or alpha or beta particles), the site of exposure, and the duration of exposure.

Tolerance to radiation is difficult to define, and there are no absolute standards for all types and levels of radiation. In the USA, the National Committee on Radiation Protection has set the maximum permissible limits of radiation exposure for occupationally exposed workers over the age of 18 years at 0.1 rem* per week for the whole body (not to exceed 5 rems per year) and 1.5 rems per week for the hands. (For purposes of comparison, routine chest x-rays deliver

---

*In radiation terminology, a "rad" is the unit of absorbed dose and a "rem" is the unit of dose of any radiation to body tissue in terms of its estimated biologic effect. The amount of radiation dose delivered to the body is expressed in roentgens. For x-ray or gamma radiation, rems, rads, and roentgens are virtually the same; for particulate radiation emitted from radioactive materials, these units may differ greatly (eg, for neutrons, 1 rad = 10 rems). One gray (Gy) = 100 rads. One sievert (Sv) = 100 rems.

0.1–0.2 rem). If recommended limits are exceeded, radiation injury may occur.

Death after acute lethal radiation exposure is usually due to destruction of hematopoietic organs, gastrointestinal tract mucosal damage, central nervous system damage, or widespread vascular injury. Vomiting within 1 hour after radiation exposure is often a sign of lethal exposure.

A. 4—6 Gy (400—600 Rads): Doses of 4–6 Gy (400–600 rads) of x-ray or gamma radiation applied to the entire body at one time will kill more than half of exposed persons within 60 days; death is usually due to hemorrhage, anemia, and infection secondary to injured hematopoietic cells.

B. 10—30 Gy (1000—3000 Rads): Doses of 10–30 Gy (1000–3000 rads) to the entire body are associated with a death rate of 100%. Destruction of gastrointestinal tract mucosa and bone marrow leads to death within 2 weeks. Bloody diarrhea begins with 4–5 days and is followed by hemorrhage and sepsis.

C. 30 Gy (3000 Rads) and Above: Doses above 30 Gy (3000 rads) to the entire body cause widespread vascular damage, cerebral anoxia with seizures, ataxia, coma, hypotensive shock, and death within a few days.

Diagnosis

A. Injury to Skin and Mucous Membranes: Irradiation causes erythema, epilation, destruction of fingernails, or epidermolysis, depending upon the dose.

B. Injury to Deep Structures:

1. Hematopoietic tissues–Injury to bone marrow may cause a decrease in production of blood elements. Lymphocytes are most sensitive, PMNs next most sensitive, and erythrocytes least sensitive. Damage to blood-forming organs may vary from transient depression of one or more blood elements to pancytopenia.

2. Cardiovascular system–Pericarditis with effusion or constrictive pericarditis may occur many months after exposure to ionizing radiation. Myocarditis is less common than pericarditis. Smaller vessels (capillaries and arterioles) are more readily damaged than larger blood vessels. If injury is mild, recovery of function occurs.

3. Gonads–In males, small single doses of radiation (2–3 Gy; 200–300 rads) cause transient aspermatogenesis, and larger doses (6–8 Gy; 600–800 rads) may cause sterility. In females, single doses of 2 Gy (200 rads) may produce sterility. Moderate to heavy irradiation of the embryo in utero results in injury to the fetus or causes embryonic death and abortion.

4. Respiratory tract–High or repeated moderate doses of radiation may cause delayed pneumonitis (weeks or months).

5. Mouth, pharynx, esophagus, and stomach–Mucositis with edema and painful swallowing of food may occur within hours to days after exposure to radiation. The salivary glands are relatively radioresistant. Gastric secretion may be temporarily (occasionally permanently) inhibited by moderately high doses of radiation.

6. Intestines–Loss of mucosa with ulceration and inflammation may follow moderately large doses of radiation.

7. Viscera and endocrine glands–Hepatitis and nephritis may be delayed complications of therapeutic irradiation. Normal thyroid, pituitary, pancreas, adrenals, and bladder are relatively resistant to low or moderate doses of radiation.

8. Nervous system–High doses of radiation may damage the brain and spinal cord by impairing their blood supply. Peripheral and autonomic nerves are highly resistant to radiation.

C. Systemic Reaction (Radiation Sickness): Common symptoms are anorexia, nausea and vomiting, weakness, exhaustion, and lassitude. Prostration may occur in some cases.

Radiation sickness associated with x-ray therapy is most likely to occur when the therapy is given in large dosage to large areas over the abdomen, less often when given over the extremities.

Treatment

There is no specific treatment for the biologic effects of ionizing radiation. Safe and effective radioprotective drugs are not available.

A. Local Treatment: The success of treatment of local radiation injury depends upon the extent, degree, and location of tissue injury. A victim exposed to more than 0.25–0.5 Gy (25–50 rads) of radioactive iodine should receive potassium iodide, 130 mg (65 mg for children) orally every day for 10 days, to prevent uptake in the thyroid gland. The drug should be given in the first hour after exposure, since it is only 50% effective after a delay of 3 hours.

B. Systemic Treatment: Treatment of the systemic reaction following irradiation is symptomatic and supportive. No truly effective antiemetic is available for the distressing nausea that frequently occurs. When irradiation levels are sufficient to cause damage to the gastrointestinal tract mucosa, bone marrow, and other vital organs, prolonged hospitalization with supportive medical and nursing care is frequently necessary. Bone marrow transplantation should be considered for all victims with exposures exceeding 3 Gy (300 rads).

Disposition

All patients with signs or symptoms of radiation exposure must be hospitalized. Advice may be obtained from the Radiation Emergency Assistance Center/Training Site (REAC/TS) in Oak Ridge, Tennessee ([615] 576–3131). The 24-hour emergency network telephone number is (615) 481–1000.

DROWNING

The asphyxia associated with drowning is usually due to aspiration of fluid, but it may result from airway obstruction caused by laryngeal spasm that occurs while the victim is gasping under water. About 10% of victims develop laryngospasm after the first gulp and never aspirate water ("dry drowning"). The rapid sequence of events after submersion—hypoxemia, laryngospasm, fluid aspiration, ineffective circulation, brain injury, and brain death—may occur within 5–10 minutes. This sequence may be delayed for longer periods if the victim, especially a child, has been submerged in very cold water or if the victim has ingested significant amounts of barbiturates. Immersion in cold water can also cause a rapid fall in core temperature, so that systemic hypothermia and death may occur before actual drowning.

The differences in the pathophysiology of aspiration of fresh water (hypotonic) and seawater (hypertonic) usually have little clinical significance in humans, since the amount of fluid aspirated in most patients is small. The primary effect in both instances is disruption of the vascular endothelium and dilution of pulmonary surfactant, with resulting atelectasis and perfusion of poorly ventilated alveoli (large physiologic shunt). Foreign materials such as sand, algae, microorganisms, oil, or chemicals in the aspirated fluid may cause additional pulmonary injury. Fresh water, when absorbed, may produce hemodilution and intravascular hemolysis. Aspiration of large amounts of seawater may result in hypovolemia and hemoconcentration. Clinical features in both types of drowning are similar, and prompt ventilatory management is mandatory.

A number of initial factors may precede neardrowning and may need to be considered in management: (**1**) use of alcohol or other drugs (a contributing factor in an estimated 25% of adult drownings), (**2**) extreme fatigue, (**3**) intentional hyperventilation just prior to diving or swimming under water ("shallow water blackout"), (**4**) sudden acute illness (eg, epilepsy, myocardial infarction), (**5**) head or spinal cord injury sustained in platform diving or surfing accidents, (**6**) venomous stings by aquatic animals, and (**7**) decompression illness or air embolism associated with scuba diving.

Hypoxemia, acidosis, and hypoperfusion of vital organs are common factors accounting for the high incidence of illness and death associated with drowning. Other problems include variations in vascular volume, cardiac failure, renal insufficiency, electrolyte abnormalities, hematologic disturbances, and infection.

Diagnosis

The victim of near-drowning may present with a wide range of clinical manifestations. Spontaneous return of consciousness often occurs in otherwise healthy individuals when submersion is brief. Other patients respond promptly to immediate artificial ventilation. Vomiting is common. Patients with more severe near-drowning may suffer frank pulmonary failure, pulmonary edema, shock, anoxic encephalopathy, cerebral edema, and cardiac arrest. A few patients may be deceptively asymptomatic during the recovery period, only to deteriorate as a result of acute respiratory failure in the ensuing 6–24 hours.

A. Symptoms and Signs: The patient may be unconscious, semiconscious, or awake and apprehensive. Cyanosis, trismus, apnea, tachypnea, and wheezing may be present. A pink froth from the mouth and nose indicates pulmonary edema. Cardiovascular manifestations may include tachycardia, arrhythmias, hypotension, shock, and cardiac arrest.

B. Laboratory Findings: Urinalysis may show proteinuria, hemoglobinuria, and ketonuria. The white blood cell count is elevated because of leukocyte demargination induced by stress. The PO_2 is usually decreased and the PCO_2 increased or decreased. Metabolic acidosis is always present.

C. X-Ray Findings: Chest x-rays may show pneumonitis or pulmonary edema. It is important to remember that preliminary x-rays may appear normal in patients with mild symptoms.

Treatment

Begin resuscitation immediately! Do not waste any time attempting to drain water from the victim's lungs or stomach. (If, however, a tense, water-filled *stomach* prevents adequate lung expansion, place the victim supine, perform the Heimlich maneuver [Chapter 1], clear the victim's mouth with a finger sweep, and resume artificial ventilation.) Place the patient in a slightly head-down position (15 degrees) to allow fluid to drain from the mouth.

A. Open the airway and ventilate the patient. If the victim is not breathing, clear the mouth and pharynx with the fingers, open the victim's airway, and institute immediate mouth-to-mouth or mouth-to-nose breathing (Chapter 1). Give oxygen in high concentrations by continuous positive airway pressure.

B. Perform endotracheal intubation for assisted ventilation as soon as possible, and begin positive end-expiratory pressure breathing. *Consider the possibility of cervical spine injury, particularly in a diving or surfing accident.*

C. Establish circulation. Check for a carotid or femoral pulse. If a pulse cannot be detected, start CPR without delay (Chapter 1). External chest compression cannot be effectively performed in the water; therefore, bring the victim ashore or out of the water as quickly as possible in order to attempt resuscitation. Monitor the effectiveness of CPR with arterial blood gas measurements.

D. Measure the patient's core temperature and treat systemic hypothermia. Hypothermia improves the chances for survival. If the patient is in full cardiac arrest (ventricular fibrillation or pulseless ventricular tachycardia, asystole, or mechanical dissociation), use core rewarming techniques (see Systemic Hypothermia, above) to attain a core temperature of 33–35 °C (91.4–95 °F) before discontinuing CPR. If the patient shows signs of life (spontaneous respirations, detectable pulse), core rewarming techniques may not be necessary. Complete recovery has been reported after prolonged resuscitative efforts, even when victims have had dilated, fixed pupils. This is particularly true of infants and children, in whom the brain is protected by hypothermia.

Disposition

Hospitalize all victims of near-drowning with or without aspiration for at least 24 hours for observation, chest x-rays, and serial arterial blood gas determinations. Pneumonitis or pulmonary edema may not become evident for 12–24 hours.

DISORDERS DUE TO ATMOSPHERIC PRESSURE CHANGES

DECOMPRESSION SICKNESS (Caisson Disease, "Bends")

Decompression sickness has long been recognized as an occupational hazard for professional divers. In recent years, the popular sport of scuba diving has exposed a large number of variably trained individuals to the hazards of decompression sickness.

Divers using conventional diving gear (scuba: self-contained underwater breathing apparatus) breathe air or other oxygen-containing gas mixtures that are at the same pressure as that of the surrounding water. Water pressure increases by 1 atmosphere (atm) for every 10 m (33 ft) below the surface. The increased pressure increases the amount of gas dissolved in plasma and other body fluids. During ascent, as external pressure decreases, the dissolved gases (predominantly nitrogen) escape from tissues as gas bubbles. A similar disorder occurs in persons who rapidly ascend to altitudes above 2000 m (6600 ft) in unpressurized aircraft. The size and number of gas bubbles escaping from the tissues are functions of the depth and duration of the dive, the degree of physical exertion (exercise increases the amount of dissolved nitrogen), and the speed of ascent. It is the release of gas bubbles and the site of release that determine the symptoms.

Diagnosis

Symptoms begin to appear within 30 minutes in half of patients; most demonstrate symptoms within 6 hours. Although the clinical picture varies, certain symptoms typically occur. These include severe pain in and near large joints ("bends"), prickling or burning sensations in the skin, skin rashes or mottling, and the "chokes" (cough, shortness of breath, and substernal discomfort caused by bubble formation in the pulmonary arterial circulation). Other manifestations include visual disturbances (scotomas), weakness or paralysis (bubble formation in the epidural venous plexus of the spinal cord), vertigo, headache, aphasia, and coma. Diffuse capillary involvement may lead to accumulation of fluid in the interstitial space, hemoconcentration, and, in severe cases, hypotension.

Treatment

A. Early Measures:
1. Give oxygen, 6–10 L/min, by mask.
2. Give mild analgesics as needed.
3. In the absence of congestive heart failure, give intravenous fluids (5% dextrose in normal saline or lactated Ringer's injection) to correct dehydration and maintain normal hydration.

B. Recompression: Immediate recompression is the *only* effective treatment. Rapid transport to a treatment facility for immediate recompression is necessary not only to relieve symptoms but also to prevent permanent impairment. Patients with persistent symptoms may be treated with hyperbaric oxygen successfully up to 7 days after the onset of serious decompression sickness. All emergency department physicians should know the location of the nearest hyperbaric chamber. The local public health department or nearest naval facility may be able to provide such information. In the USA, clinical advice may be rapidly obtained by telephoning the National Diving Accident Network (DAN) at Duke University ([919] 684–8111). A patient who is transported to a hyperbaric chamber by aircraft must not be exposed to a cabin altitude higher than 300 m (1000 ft).

C. Complications: Further measures may be necessary to relieve some of the complications associated with the "bends," eg, shock, spinal cord injury, bladder paralysis, hemoconcentration, and disseminated intravascular coagulation.

Disposition

Transport the patient immediately to the nearest recompression center (hyperbaric chamber) for evaluation and treatment. *Never attempt recompression in the water.*

ARTERIAL GAS EMBOLISM

Diving regulators maintain the pressure of the gas being breathed and thereby enable the diver to descend and maintain lung expansion against the pressure of the surrounding water. Because of the pressure/volume relationship (Boyle's law: $P_1 V_1 = P_2 V_2$), greater volume changes for a given change in depth occur near the surface than at a greater depth.

If the breath is held on ascent (by closure of the glottis) or if air is trapped in the lung by bronchospasm during ascent, the volume of gas in the lung expands. When a pressure differential of about 80 mm Hg is reached, air will be forced from the alveoli through the pulmonary alveolocapillary membrane. The result will be air in the interstitial space (creating pneumothorax or mediastinal emphysema) or formation of bubbles in the pulmonary venous circulation. These bubbles travel through the left side of the heart into the systemic arterial circulation, where they may be trapped in smaller arteries and cause coronary artery or cerebrovascular occlusion.

Diagnosis

A. Arterial Embolism: Patients usually present with dramatic symptoms. If the symptoms occur more than 10 minutes after the diver has surfaced, they are *not* due to air embolism.

1. If air bubbles enter the cerebral circulation, the victim becomes unconscious or suffers a seizure during ascent or immediately upon surfacing. Other symptoms include blindness, confusion, or an apparent acute stroke.

2. If the bubbles have entered the coronary arteries, the person presents with symptoms similar to those of acute myocardial infarction, with chest pain, arrhythmias, and collapse.

B. Pneumothorax: Signs of pneumothorax or mediastinal emphysema develop more slowly and are not as life-threatening; signs include shortness of breath, hyperresonance of the chest to percussion and decreased breath sounds on the affected side, and subcutaneous crepitus that may extend into the neck.

Treatment

A. Early Measures:
1. Give oxygen, 6–10 L/min, by mask.
2. Position the victim head down (15–30 degrees) on the left side in the Trendelenburg position.
3. Give 5% dextrose in normal saline or lactated Ringer's injection intravenously to maintain urine output at 1–2 mL/kg/h.

B. Recompression: Immediate recompression is the *only* effective treatment; the patient should be transported to a hyperbaric chamber immediately (see Decompression Sickness, above).

Disposition

Transport the patient immediately to the nearest recompression center (hyperbaric chamber) for evaluation and treatment. *Never attempt recompression in the water.*

HIGH-ALTITUDE SICKNESS
(Mountain Sickness)

Rapid means of modern transportation have increased the number of unacclimatized people who are exposed to the effects of high altitude. Lack of sufficient time for acclimatization, increased physical activity, and varying degrees of ill health may be responsible for the acute and chronic disturbances that result from hypoxemia at altitudes greater than 2000 m (6600 ft). Marked individual differences in tolerance to hypoxemia exist. Acclimatization involves a variety of changes that affect the respiratory, circulatory, hematopoietic, renal, and pulmonary systems.

1. ACUTE MOUNTAIN SICKNESS

Diagnosis

Symptoms and signs include headache (the commonest and usually the most prominent symptom), lassitude, difficulty in concentrating, sleep disturbances, drowsiness, dizziness, insomnia, anorexia, nausea and vomiting, dyspnea on exertion, and palpitations.

Symptoms are often worse on the second and third day after ascent but usually clear completely within 5–7 days. Serious illness is rare; deaths from mountain sickness do not occur, by definition.

Treatment

The most effective treatments are descent to lower altitude and administration of oxygen. Headache responds to analgesics. Narcotics should be used judiciously to avoid distorting sleep patterns or masking signs of altered mental status, which accompany impending high-altitude encephalopathy. Recent studies show that severe or rapidly progressive mountain sickness may respond favorably to dexamethasone, 4–6 mg orally every 6 hours, until signs of improvement occur; the dose is then tapered over 3–5 days.

Prevention

Preventive measures include gradual ascent, adequate rest, avoidance of alcohol and tobacco, and avoidance of strenuous exercise until acclimatization has been achieved. Acetazolamide has been shown to decrease the severity of mountain sickness; however, the side effects of diuresis and acral paresthesias are annoying to many patients. Give 250 mg orally 2–3 times daily, the day before and for several days during and after ascent.

Disposition

If symptoms persist, returning to lower altitude is curative.

2. ACUTE HIGH-ALTITUDE PULMONARY EDEMA

Diagnosis

Acute high-altitude pulmonary edema (HAPE) is a serious disorder usually occurring at levels above 2400 m (8000 ft). High-altitude pulmonary edema is associated with exercise and rapid ascent and is commonly noted in young, previously healthy individuals who have not become properly acclimatized. Known risk factors for development of high-altitude pulmonary edema are previous episodes of the disease; congenital absence of one pulmonary artery; and brief sojourn at low altitude—and return to high altitude—by persons acclimatized to living at high altitudes.

A. Symptoms and Signs: Early symptoms of high-altitude pulmonary edema may appear within 6–36 hours after arrival at high altitude and include dry, incessant cough; dyspnea at rest; and substernal discomfort. Later symptoms include wheezing, orthopnea, and hemoptysis.

Physical signs include tachycardia, tachypnea, cyanosis, rales, rhonchi, and confusion that progresses to coma. Death may occur in untreated individuals.

B. Laboratory Findings: The white blood cell count and hematocrit are often slightly elevated. The erythrocyte sedimentation rate is usually normal. Fluid collected by bronchoalveolar lavage shows high protein and cellular content associated with the high-permeability vascular leak due to hypoxia and increased pulmonary vascular pressure.

C. X-Ray Findings: Findings on chest x-ray are variable. In mild disease, patchy infiltrates in a solitary lung field (commonly the right middle lobe) are noted. The infiltrates rarely coalesce and generally do not involve the base of the lungs. The central pulmonary arteries are dilated, but the cardiac shadow is of normal size. In severe illness, infiltrates are more generalized, but no left atrial enlargement or Kerley lines are noted. Unilateral pulmonary edema is consistent with unilateral atresia of the pulmonary artery.

D. Electrocardiographic Findings: Transient, nonspecific electrocardiographic changes (tachycardia, right ventricular strain) may occur.

Treatment

Early recognition of the disease is crucial. Persistent dry cough and dyspnea in a person who has recently arrived at high altitude should be considered high-altitude pulmonary edema until proved otherwise.

A. Rest: Limit the patient's physical activity as much as possible. The sitting or semi-Fowler position is usually the most comfortable.

B. Oxygen: Give oxygen, 6–10 L/min, by mask; otherwise, deliver the maximum amount possible with the equipment at hand.

C. Continuous Positive Pressure Ventilation: Application of continuous positive pressure during spontaneous ventilation (which can be achieved with a portable apparatus) relieves symptoms and improves oxygenation in patients with high-altitude pulmonary edema and is a useful temporizing measure during descent.

D. Descent: Development of high-altitude pulmonary edema is an automatic indication for descent to lower altitude as quickly as possible (a descent of 500–1000 m [1650–3300 ft] is usually sufficient), although it is best to descend below an altitude of 1500 m [5000 ft]). Supplemental oxygen and descent to a lower altitude should bring about marked improvement within 12–72 hours.

E. Avoidance of Drugs: Avoid ineffective (and possibly dangerous) drugs (including digitalis, morphine, and powerful diuretics). Acetazolamide does not have a place in the management of established high-altitude pulmonary edema.

Prevention

Preventive measures include (**1**) education of prospective mountaineers about the possibility of serious pulmonary edema, (**2**) gradual ascent to permit acclimatization, and (**3**) rest and avoidance of strenuous exercise for 1–2 days after arrival at high altitudes. Medical attention should be sought promptly if respiratory symptoms develop.

Patients with a history of high-altitude pulmonary edema who develop tachycardia and cough at high altitude should be transported to lower altitudes for proper evaluation and hospitalization if necessary.

Mountaineering parties climbing at 2400 m (8000 ft) or higher should carry a supply of oxygen and equipment sufficient for several days if hospital facilities are not available.

People with symptomatic cardiac or pulmonary disease should avoid high altitudes.

Disposition

Hospitalization is generally recommended if symptoms persist for more than a few hours after return to lower altitudes.

3. HIGH-ALTITUDE CEREBRAL EDEMA

Diagnosis

Acute high-altitude cerebral edema (HACE) is a syndrome related to hypoxemia and occurs at elevations above 2400 m (8000 ft). Like its counterpart high-altitude pulmonary edema, it is more common in unacclimatized individuals. Although certain clinical findings are related to cerebral edema (papilledema, retinal hemorrhages, increased cerebrospinal fluid pressure), there may well be other causative factors.

Early symptoms include severe headache, ataxia, confusion, incoordination, and drunken behavior.

Neurologic examination may demonstrate focal abnormalities or weakness of the extremities. Because high-altitude pulmonary edema commonly accompanies high-altitude cerebral edema, the patient may be lethargic and short of breath and may demonstrate tachycardia. Later symptoms include seizures and coma. Cerebral venous thrombosis is a rare and potentially catastrophic complication.

Treatment

It is crucial to recognize early manifestations. Because the symptoms of early high-altitude cerebral edema are similar to those of acute mountain sickness, anyone with headache and fatigue at high altitude must be watched closely for signs of deterioration. Inability to walk a straight line is a fairly sensitive test for incipient high-altitude cerebral edema.

A. Oxygen: Give oxygen, 6–10 L/min, by mask. If at all possible, keep the patient in a sitting position, with the head elevated.

B. Descent: Development of high-altitude cerebral edema is an automatic indication for descent to lower altitude as quickly as possible (a descent of 500–1000 m [1650–3300 ft] is usually sufficient, although it is best to descend below an altitude of 1500 m [5000 ft]). Recent studies show that high-altitude cerebral edema may respond favorably to dexamethasone, 4–6 mg orally every 6 hours, until improvement occurs; the dose is then tapered over 3–5 days.

Disposition

Hospitalization is generally recommended if symptoms persist for more than a few hours after return to lower altitudes.

VENOMOUS ANIMALS

SNAKES

Snakes bite at least 50,000 humans each year in the USA. Most snakebites are from nonpoisonous snakes. There are 2 main types of poisonous snakes: crotalids, or pit vipers (rattlesnakes, cottonmouths [water moccasins]), and elapids (coral snakes, cobras). Among venomous bites in the USA, 95% are from pit vipers (mostly rattlesnakes). Envenomation occurs in only 15–20% of venomous bites.

Snake venom is a complex mixture of proteolytic enzymes and toxic proteins. In general, crotalid venom is mainly cytolytic, whereas elapid venom is mainly neurotoxic. Cytolytic venom lyses cells, enhances local spread of venom, and causes hemolysis, increased capillary permeability, and altered hemostasis. Neurotoxic venom can disrupt neuromuscular activity, causing paresthesias, weakness, and respiratory paralysis.

Diagnosis

Identify the snake if at all possible. Pit vipers have large triangular heads with pits between the eyes and the nose. Coral snakes have black and red circumferential bands separated by narrower yellow bands ("red on yellow, kill a fellow; red on black, venom lack"). If the identity of a snake is not obvious, obtain help from a herpetologist or a poison control center.

Collect the snake, if possible, for positive identification; take care to avoid being bitten. Remember that the head of a decapitated snake may exhibit reflex actions for as long as 1 hour after it has been severed from the body.

Elapids and the Mojave green rattlesnake may produce few or no early local signs of envenomation, but neurologic symptoms (paresthesias, blurred vision, dysphagia, hypersalivation, ptosis, respiratory depression) may appear after a delay of 2–6 hours.

Treatment

A. Emergency First Aid Measures: The best management is to transport the patient to the nearest hospital. Immobilize the bitten part as if it were a fracture, and hold it below the level of the heart. Remove rings or other constrictive items. If at all possible, the patient should avoid exertion. If an elastic wrap (eg, Ace bandage) is available, wrap it firmly around a cloth or gauze pad (6–8 × 6–8 × 2–3 cm) placed directly over the site of the bite, but not so tightly as to impede venous return. Alternatively, apply a venolymphatic occlusive constriction band proximal to the bite on the affected extremity. *Do not* use a tourniquet; *do not* apply ice; *do not* incise or apply suction to the wound. Incision and suctioning of the wound are indicated only if the snake is large and has been positively identified as venomous; if the victim is young, elderly, or infirm; and if the nearest source of antivenin is more than 2 hours distant. Commercial venom extractors used without incision of the wound and applied within 5 minutes of the bite may remove as much as 25–30% of the venom.

B. Hospital Measures:

1. Monitor vital signs.

2. Insert 2 intravenous catheters, and send blood for typing and cross-matching; coagulation panel; CBC and platelet count; and blood urea nitrogen, creatinine, total protein, albumin, and electrolyte measurements. Obtain urine for urinalysis (note the presence of myoglobin or heme pigments).

3. Treat hypotension or shock by intravenous infusion of crystalloid solution. If the hematocrit falls below 30%, packed red cells should also be given.

4. Measure the circumference of the bitten extremity frequently, and note any spread of swelling.

5. Identify the species of snake, if possible.

6. Evaluate the presenting symptoms and signs. Pay particular attention to a history of snakebite (and snakebite treatment); note presence of perioral and scalp paresthesias (early signs of envenomation) and allergy to animal products. Decide if antivenin is needed (Table 38–2).

7. If antivenin is used, give in accordance with the following principles:

a. Perform a skin test for horse serum sensitivity. *This should be done only if antivenin is to be used.* Inject antivenin, 0.02 mL of a 1:10 dilution intradermally, with 0.02 mL of normal saline injected elsewhere as a control. Erythema and a wheal reaction within 30 minutes constitute a positive reaction. A positive reaction does not contraindicate the administration of antivenin but reinforces the need for greater caution in its use. A negative reaction is no guarantee against anaphylaxis. Antivenin should be administered in an intensive care unit, and personnel and equipment for resuscitation should be readily available.

Adults who develop anaphylaxis should receive a 0.1-mg bolus of aqueous epinephrine, 1:1000, diluted in 10 mL of normal saline and infused over 10 minutes. An epinephrine infusion may be prepared by adding 1 mg of aqueous epinephrine, 1:1000, to 250 mL of normal saline for a concentration of 4 µg/mL. The infusion should be started at a rate of 1 µg/min and increased to 4–5 µg/min as required. In children, start infusion at 0.1 µg/kg/min, not to exceed 1.5 µg/kg/min.

b. Give antivenin by slow intravenous drip only. *Do not* give it intramuscularly or inject it into the bite area. Be prepared to administer epinephrine and diphenhydramine at the same time to control hypersensitivity reactions. Premedication with corticosteroids may be of some value. The development and use of newer purified antibodies (IgG) may diminish the risk of anaphylaxis currently associated with the use of antivenin products.

Table 38–2. Classification and treatment of crotalid or rattlesnake bite.

Symptoms	Degree of Envenomation	Dose[1]
None (either local or systemic)	None	None
Local swelling, pain; no systemic symptoms	Minimal	3–5 vials
Progressive swelling with mild systemic symptoms (paresthesias, nausea)	Moderate	8–10 vials
Severe swelling, pain, and ecchymosis; marked systemic symptoms (hypotension, fasciculations, or clotting deficit)	Severe	15–20 vials

[1]Polyvalent Crotalidae antivenin; available from Wyeth Laboratories ([215] 688–4400 days; [215] 644–8000 or [215] 878–9500 nights and emergencies); help in locating antivenin may be obtained from the Arizona Poison and Drug Information Center ([602] 626–6016).

c. Give adequate amounts of antivenin (Table 38–2), since undertreatment is the most common cause of treatment failure. The dose should be sufficient to reverse the signs and symptoms of envenomation. Polyvalent crotalid antivenin is effective against all pit vipers found in the USA. For severe envenomation, more than 20 vials may be necessary. If the snake has been identified as a Mojave rattlesnake, the initial dose should be 10 vials. For coral snake (Eastern or Texas variety) bites, give 3–6 vials of Eastern coral snake antivenin. Coral snake antivenin is not effective against the bites of the Arizona or Sonoran coral snake.

8. Administer appropriate tetanus prophylaxis. If the bite wound is severe, administer a broad-spectrum antibiotic (eg, cefazolin, 100 mg/kg/d intravenously in 3 divided doses).

9. The decision to perform fasciotomy (surgical decompression) should be guided by the measurement of compartment pressures with a pressure transducer, slit plastic catheter, needle, or wick.

10. If antivenin is used, anticipate and be prepared to treat serum sickness.

Disposition

Hospitalize all patients who have been bitten by poisonous snakes.

BEES & WASPS

Bees, wasps, and ants are members of the order Hymenoptera. In the USA, domesticated honeybees, feral bumblebees, paper wasps, yellow jackets, and fire ants are the most common attackers. These insects inject venom through a stinger connected to a venom reservoir supplied by venom glands. Stings from flying Hymenoptera are generally single unless a swarm or nest is encountered. Stings are common in summer months. The head and neck are followed by the extremities in frequency of stings.

Diagnosis

A sting in an unsensitized individual causes immediate pain, erythema, and edema. A mildly sensitive person suffers hives, wheezing, malaise, conjunctivitis, rhinitis, fever, and nausea. A severely sensitive individual suffers diffuse urticaria, facial swelling and laryngeal edema, bronchospasm, cyanosis, vomiting, abdominal pain, arrhythmias, and hypotension. Persons who suffer multiple stings or who are under treatment with beta-adrenergic blocking drugs may experience more severe reactions.

Treatment

Severe reactions, such as anaphylaxis, must be treated promptly, as they may cause rapid systemic decompensation and death. The effectiveness of first aid measures is largely related to the rapidity with which they are undertaken.

A. For a Severe Reaction, Administer Epinephrine: At the first indication of severe hypersensitivity, administer aqueous epinephrine 1:1000 subcutaneously, 0.3–0.5 mL in adults and 0.01 mL/kg in children. These doses may be repeated every 20–30 minutes as necessary. Aqueous epinephrine by aerosol is not an adequate first aid measure against systemic anaphylaxis. In the event that the victim does not respond to subcutaneously administered epinephrine, the adult patient should receive a 0.1-mg (0.1-mL) bolus of 1:1000 aqueous epinephrine diluted in 10 mL of normal saline infused over 10 minutes. A mixture for continuous infusion should be prepared by adding 1 mg (1 mL) of 1:1000 aqueous epinephrine to 250 mL of normal saline (4 μg/mL). This infusion should be started at a rate of 1 μg per minute and increased to 4 μg per minute depending on the clinical response. In children, the rate of infusion is 0.1 μg/kg/min, up to a maximum of 1.5 μg/kg/min. *Note:* Infusion rates in excess of 0.5 μg/kg/min may be associated with cardiac ischemia and arrhythmias.

B. Manage the Airway: If orofacial swelling is present and airway obstruction is a possibility, perform early endotracheal intubation, before vocal cord and pharyngeal edema preclude this approach and mandate creation of a surgical airway. Administer supplemental oxygen by face mask at a flow rate of 6–10 L/min. If bronchospasm is present, consider the use of aerosolized albuterol or metaproterenol.

C. Obtain Intravenous Access, Manage Hypotension: Early in management, place at least one large-bore intravenous line through which epinephrine and crystalloid can be administered. Maintain intravascular volume with normal saline or lactated Ringer's solution. If necessary, judiciously administer a dopaminergic pressor agent. In a critical situation, a brief augmentation of blood pressure may be achieved by application of Military Antishock Trousers (MAST), which contribute to increased systemic vascular resistance (Chapter 46).

D. Initiate Adjunctive Measures: Remove stings or fragments by scraping, not with forceps. Apply topical ice packs with or without a paste of papain (unseasoned meat tenderizer). In lesser envenomations, administer diphenhydramine, 50–100 mg (1 mg/kg in children) intravenously, intramuscularly, or orally. In moderate or severe envenomations, an intravenous corticosteroid such as hydrocortisone, 2 mg/kg, should be administered at the earliest opportunity. Appropriate tetanus prophylaxis should be completed.

Disposition

Patients with cardiovascular or respiratory compromise should be admitted to an intensive care unit. Patients with mild or local reactions can be sent home with oral diphenhydramine.

BLACK WIDOW SPIDER
(Latrodectus mactans)

Diagnosis

The female black widow spider is shiny black, with a red hourglass marking on its abdomen. Only the female is dangerous. This spider is common in California and other parts of the USA. Other *Latrodectus* species may be found in other countries. The venom is a neurotoxin that acts on the myoneural junction.

The bite itself is minor and often unnoticed at first. Characteristic symptoms of envenomation occur within 10–60 minutes, including severe pain in the bitten extremity and muscle spasms of the abdomen and trunk. Diffuse paresthesias are noted. Headache, nausea and vomiting, hyperactive deep tendon reflexes, and ptosis may be noted. Victims are in agonizing pain; the rigidity of abdominal muscles may mimic a surgical emergency. Severe hypertension may occur. Deaths are rare; at greatest risk are small infants or older patients with preexisting cardiovascular disease. Symptoms peak at 2–3 hours after the bite and may last up to 24 hours.

Treatment

Most patients respond to narcotic analgesics. Calcium gluconate, 0.1–0.2 mL/kg slowly intravenously, is often effective in alleviating muscle spasm. Methocarbamol, 1 g intravenously, infused at a rate no faster than 100 mg/min, is less effective. Local applications of ice should be used judiciously. Antivenin should be reserved for use in seriously ill infants and older patients and should be preceded by horse serum sensitivity testing (see ¶B7, above). One vial of antivenin is sufficient for most patients; give 1 ampule (2.5 mL) in 10–50 mL of normal saline by slow intravenous infusion.

Disposition

All patients who have been bitten by a black widow spider should be observed for 12–24 hours, since hypertension and muscle spasm commonly recur. Hospitalization is necessary for all patients under 14 years of age, those older than 65 years of age, those with a history of hypertension, and those who present with severe symptoms.

BROWN RECLUSE SPIDER
(Loxosceles reclusa;
Other Loxosceles Species)

Diagnosis

The brown recluse spider has a dark, violin-shaped area on its back. It is found in old woodpiles, attics, closets, and clothes piles and prefers dark, undisturbed places. The venom, which contains sphingomyelinase D, is chiefly cytotoxic, causing local tissue destruction; it also has a hemolytic component, but this is rarely of clinical significance.

The bite initially seems mild and often goes unnoticed. Pain at the site begins 1–4 hours later, and an erythematous area with a central pustule or hemorrhagic vesicle may be seen. The typical bull's-eye lesion is created when the red blister is encircled by a pale, irregularly shaped and ischemic halo, which in turn is surrounded by extravasated blood. The pustule may gradually grow to form a craterlike lesion over 3–4 days, with associated lymphadenopathy and low-grade fever. Healing is slow, and large lesions may occasionally require skin grafting. Rarely, there is a generalized systemic reaction 24–48 hours after the bite, with fever, malaise, arthralgias, rash, and hemolysis. Rare fatalities have occurred in small children, who have shown massive intravascular hemolysis, accompanied by hemoglobinuria, jaundice, hypotension, renal failure, pulmonary edema, and disseminated intravascular coagulation.

The bites of many other insects may be mistaken for brown recluse spider bites and lead to unnecessary treatment. One helpful clue (although not absolutely reliable) is that spiders tend to bite only once, whereas other insects leave multiple bites.

Treatment

Authorities previously recommended early wide excision of the crater lesion, intralesional injections of corticosteroids, or high doses of systemic corticosteroids. Clinical studies at Vanderbilt University Hospital have developed another treatment approach. If a brown recluse spider bite is strongly suspected or confirmed, obtain a glucose-6-phosphate dehydrogenase (G6PD) screen, and immediately give dapsone, 50 mg (adult dose) orally twice daily for 10 days. (The efficacy of dapsone in children has not been studied and is not currently recommended.) If G6PD enzyme deficiency is documented, discontinue dapsone in order to avoid hemolysis. Also give erythromycin, 250 mg orally 4 times daily for 10 days. Ice and elevation may also be beneficial. Avoid exercise or application of heat, which may increase the activity of sphingomyelinase D. This treatment appears superior to previous therapeutic regimens. An antivenin product derived from rabbits is currently under investigation. If injected directly into the wound within 48 hours of envenomation, it appears to be markedly effective. Many brown recluse spider bites are minor and heal without specific treatment other than tetanus prophylaxis (Chapter 46) and local wound care.

Disposition

Most patients with brown recluse spider bites can be treated on an outpatient basis. Patients with large or infected wounds or those who have signs of a systemic reaction should be hospitalized.

SCORPIONS
(Centruroides exilicauda)

Most scorpions are relatively harmless, producing only local envenomation reactions. However, *Centruroides exilicauda [sculpturatus]* may produce severe systemic toxicity.

This arthropod is small and yellowish, has a small tubercle (telson) at the base of its stinger, and is 2.5–7.5 cm (1–3 in) long. It is found mostly in the southwestern USA (Arizona, New Mexico, Texas, and along the Colorado River) but may rarely be transported in freight to distant states. Related arthropods are found in many other parts of the world.

The venom of *C exilicauda* contains a neurotoxin that may produce severe systemic symptoms. Other scorpion stings generally produce only local reactions.

Diagnosis

The initial sting is intensely painful with little or no erythema or swelling. Light percussion of the wound causes intense pain. Although pain and paresthesias generally resolve within 4 hours, local symptoms may persist for several days.

Generalized reactions may occur within 60 minutes and include extreme restlessness, uncontrollable jerking, nystagmus, diaphoresis, diplopia, incontinence, hypersalivation, confusion, seizures, hypertension, and occasionally wheezing or stridor.

Children under 10 years of age are more likely to have severe or prolonged reactions; older children and adults usually recover within 10–12 hours.

Treatment

Periodic applications of ice may relieve local pain; avoid intense cooling. Immobilize the affected part. *Do not* apply a tourniquet.

Most children recover with supportive care alone but should be observed in an intensive care unit. Strong depressants or tranquilizers do not appear to shorten the duration of symptoms and may produce respiratory depression; specifically, opiate analgesics seem to potentiate the toxicity of the venom. Diazepam or phenobarbital may be used to control seizures; sympatholytic antihypertensive agents may be required to control hypertension.

Goat serum antivenin is available in Arizona (Arizona Poison and Drug Information Center [602] 626-6016) but has not yet been approved by the US Food and Drug Administration. It is effective only for stings from *C exilicauda* and is not of benefit for stings from scorpions from South America, Asia, or the Middle East.

Disposition

Hospitalize all patients with *C exilicauda* stings for supportive care.

HAZARDOUS MARINE LIFE

Many ocean-dwelling animals are potentially harmful to humans because of their ability to traumatize, envenom, or otherwise poison their victims with bites or stings. Most human injuries result from envenomation.

1. STINGRAY

Stingrays (Fig 38–2) are the fish most commonly responsible for human envenomations; at least 2000 stings occur annually in the USA. Stingrays are usually encountered in the waters off coastal regions, where they lie partially submerged in the sand. When they are disturbed, they lash upward with a muscular tail, which carries 1–4 venomous stings. Each sting is a retroserrate vasodentin spine containing multiple venom glands surrounded by an integumentary sheath. Injury due to stingrays therefore involves both a traumatic wound (which can be quite severe) and envenomation. The most common sites of injury are the lower extremities, followed by the upper extremities, abdomen, and chest. Wound necrosis is not uncommon.

Diagnosis

The sting is followed by immediate intense local pain and moderate swelling with bleeding. The pain radiates centrally and can be so severe that it causes disorientation. Systemic symptoms occur within 30 minutes of the sting and include nausea and vomiting, weakness, diaphoresis, vertigo, tachycardia, and muscle cramps. If envenomation has been severe, syncope, paralysis, hypotension, cardiac arrhythmias, and death may occur.

Treatment
A. Irrigate the Wound: Irrigate the wound with whatever diluent is at hand (preferably sterile saline

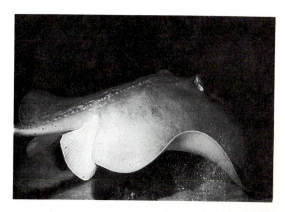

Figure 38–2. Stingrays rise rapidly from the sand to inflict a painful sting with their barbed tails.

or water). Remove any obvious pieces of foreign matter.

B. Anesthetize the Wound: Soak the wound in hot water to tolerance (45–50 °C [113–122 °F]) for 30–60 minutes. If heat fails to relieve the pain, infiltrate the wound with lidocaine, 1–2% without epinephrine; or perform regional nerve block. *Do not apply ice to the wound.*

C. Explore the Wound: Exploration and debridement should be performed in a proper operative facility with loupes or a microscope, so that all tissue fragments may be removed. Close the wound loosely around drains, or pack it open.

D. Give Antibiotics: Administer standard tetanus prophylaxis (Chapter 46), and start treatment with trimethoprim-sulfamethoxazole (160 mg and 800 mg, respectively, twice a day), ciprofloxacin (500 mg twice a day), or tetracycline (500 mg 4 times a day) for 7 days.

Disposition

Any patient with significant envenomation from a stingray sting should be observed for 4–6 hours for appearance of systemic side effects. Patients who are discharged should have close outpatient follow-up for wound care.

2. PORTUGUESE MAN-OF-WAR

The Portuguese man-of-war (Fig 38–3) is a freefloating animal having a sail that is filled with carbon monoxide and nitrogen and from which are suspended tentacles laden with nematocysts. These tentacles may reach lengths of 15 m (50 ft) (Pacific) and 30 m (100 ft) (Atlantic), and they carry hundreds of thousands of nematocysts. When anything touches the tentacles, the nematocysts are discharged into the victim by means of a venom-charged needle. Brokenoff tentacles washed up onto beaches may remain capable of discharging venom for weeks.

Diagnosis

A mild sting causes instantaneous burning pain, paresthesias, and a typical red or violaceous rash distributed in a whiplike pattern. Moderate envenomation causes additional blistering, local edema, and more severe pain, which may radiate centrally from the extremities. Severe envenomation causes the typical skin reaction as well as a host of systemic symptoms that usually appear within the first 4–8 hours: headache, lethargy, vertigo, ataxia, syncope, seizures, coma, vomiting, dysphagia, muscle spasm, anaphylaxis, hemolysis, cardiac arrhythmias, conjunctivitis, corneal ulceration, bronchospasm, respiratory failure, and death. Rarely, a delayed reaction resembling erythema nodosum affects both the site of the envenomation and tissue distant from the wound; immune sensitization has been implicated as a possible cause.

Treatment

Systemic symptoms and dysfunction are managed supportively. There is no effective antivenin for a Portuguese man-of-war sting. Limit envenomation by prompt management of the dermatitis.

A. Rinse the Wound: Rinse the wound immediately with seawater or saline, *not* with fresh water. Do not rub the wound with ice, towels, or sand.

B. Detoxify the Venom: Irrigate the wound with acetic acid (vinegar), 5%; or isopropyl alcohol (rubbing alcohol), 40–70%. Alternative irrigants (which have met with varying success) include urine, diluted household ammonia, or a paste made of papain (unseasoned meat tenderizer) and water. For the Chesapeake sea nettle, use a slurry of baking soda.

C. Remove the Nematocysts: Gently apply a lather of shaving cream or paste of baking soda, flour, or talc. Shave the area with a razor blade. Reapply acetic acid or isopropyl alcohol.

D. Soothe the Skin: Apply a thin layer of hydrocortisone lotion, 1%.

E. Treat the Allergic Reaction: Give prednisone, 60 mg orally, and taper the dose over 10–14 days.

Disposition

Any victim who has sustained a severe Portuguese man-of-war sting should be observed for 6–8 hours for development of systemic symptoms. Elderly or very young victims should be hospitalized for 24 hours for observation.

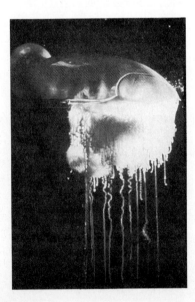

Figure 38–3. Portuguese man-of-war. Note the "stinging battery" of nematocysts directly under the gas-filled sail. (Courtesy of L Madin.)

3. SCORPION FISH

Scorpion fish are divided into 3 groups on the basis of appearance and structure of the venom organ: zebra fish (lionfish [Fig 38–4]), scorpion fish, and stonefish. The venom apparatus consists of 12 or 13 dorsal spines, 3 anal spines, and 2 pelvic spines, all of which can be erected upon stimulation. The venom can be highly toxic (stonefish) and contains chemical fractions analogous to those contained in stingray venom.

Diagnosis
Scorpion fish stings vary in intensity depending upon the species. Most cause immediate pain, with central radiation of discomfort. Local ischemia at the wound site progresses over days to marked swelling, erythema, and cellulitis. Prolonged indolent wound infections are not uncommon. Systemic symptoms occur within the first few hours and include vomiting, weakness, diarrhea, delirium, seizures, paresthesias, fever, arthritis, hypertension, cardiac arrhythmias, respiratory failure, hypotension, and death.

Treatment
Systemic symptoms and dysfunctions are managed supportively. An antivenin is available in Australia for management of stings by the Indo-Pacific stonefish. It is manufactured by Commonwealth Serum Laboratories, Melbourne, Australia. For scorpion fish stings occurring in coastal waters surrounding the USA, institute the following regimen:

A. Provide Pain Relief: Immerse the wound in hot water to tolerance (45–50 °C [113–122 °F]) for 30–60 minutes. If heat fails to relieve the pain, infiltrate the wound with lidocaine, 1–2% without epinephrine; or perform regional nerve block. Pain from a stonefish sting may be so severe that it causes delirium requiring parenteral narcotic analgesics for relief.

B. Manage the Wound: Debride and explore the wound, and remove all foreign material. If there is a chance that a spine may have entered a joint, these procedures should be performed in the operating room, and the surgeon should use magnifying loupes to explore the joint. Do not suture wounds tightly; allow adequate drainage.

C. Give Antibiotics: Administer standard tetanus prophylaxis (Chapter 46), and start treatment with trimethoprim-sulfamethoxazole (160 mg and 800 mg, respectively, twice a day), ciprofloxacin (500 mg twice a day), or tetracycline (500 mg 4 times a day) for 7 days.

Disposition
A patient who has sustained significant envenomation from a scorpion fish sting should be observed for 4–6 hours for development of systemic symptoms. All patients should be seen frequently on an outpatient basis for wound care once they have been discharged.

4. SEA URCHIN

Sea urchins (Fig 38–5) are egg-shaped, globular, or flattened echinoderms found in areas ranging from the shallow intertidal zone to great oceanic depths. Some species are covered with sharp, brittle, venom-filled spines that readily break off. Most sea urchin venom contains several toxic fractions that may include cholinergic compounds and potent neurotoxins. Envenomation occurs when a victim inadvertently handles or falls on a sea urchin and the spines penetrate the skin.

Diagnosis
Injuries caused by sea urchin spines are associated with immediate intense burning pain, followed by erythema, edema, and aching. One or more spines typi-

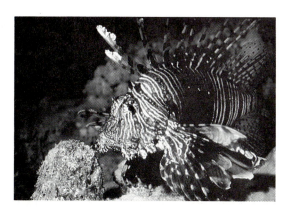

Figure 38–4. The zebra fish (lionfish) remains well camouflaged and uses its dorsal, pelvic, and anal fins to envenomate its victims. The pectoral plumes are not connected to venom glands.

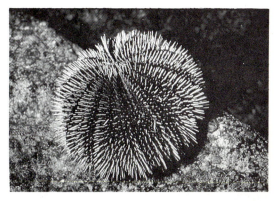

Figure 38–5. The multiple sharp, venom-filled spines of the sea urchin are readily detached from the animal and easily penetrate the skin of its victim.

cally break off in the skin. A purplish discoloration indicates penetration of the skin but does not necessarily mean that a spine remains. Multiple wounds may cause a systemic reaction, including nausea and vomiting, intense pain, paralysis, aphonia, respiratory distress, and death. Pain may subside within the first 2 hours, but paralysis may remain for 6–8 hours.

Treatment

Systemic symptoms and dysfunctions are managed supportively. No antivenin is available for sea urchin venom.

A. Relieve Pain: Immerse the wound in hot water to tolerance (45–50 °C [113–122 °F]) for 30–60 minutes. If heat fails to relieve the pain, infiltrate the wound with lidocaine, 1–2% without epinephrine; or perform regional nerve block.

B. Remove Embedded Spines: Halt the envenomation process by carefully removing the spines (avoid fragmentation). Although some thin spines may be absorbed over 2–3 weeks, as many as possible should be removed. Remove all thick spines, because of the potential for foreign body reactions and infections. Many spines are radiopaque and can be visualized using soft tissue x-ray techniques. Obtain surgical consultation if there is a chance a spine may have entered a joint, if a spine is near a significant neurovascular structure, or if a spine has been lost in a closed space in the hand. In these cases, the spine should be removed in the operating room with the aid of magnifying loupes. Do not suture the wounds tightly; allow adequate drainage.

Disposition

Any patient with significant sea urchin envenomation should be observed for 4–6 hours for appearance of systemic effects. Patients who are discharged should have frequent outpatient follow-up for wound care.

INGESTION OF POISONOUS FISH

The more intensive harvesting of marine plants and animals for food has increased the number of poisoning episodes due to ingestion of such items. Emergency physicians should obtain a dietary history from any patient who presents with gastroenteritis, respiratory compromise, confusing neurologic signs, or sudden unexplained systemic illness.

1. CIGUATERA TOXIN POISONING

Ciguatera fish poisoning is caused by tropical and semitropical marine coral reef fish whose tissues accumulate toxins that originate in the toxic dinoflagellate *Gambierdiscus toxicus.* The toxin is ingested by small herbivorous fishes, which are eaten by larger carnivorous fishes, with humans as the final consumer. Larger and older fish are more toxic in ciguatera-endemic areas. The most frequently implicated fishes in the USA include barracuda, jack, snapper, and grouper.

Diagnosis

Symptoms usually occur within 15–60 minutes of ingestion—almost always within 12 hours—and increase in severity over the next 4–6 hours. Symptoms include abdominal pain, nausea and vomiting, diarrhea, chills, paresthesias, pruritus, dysphagia, odontalgia, pathognomonic reversal of the sensation of hot and cold, fatigue, athetosis, ataxia, vertigo, headache, myalgias, bradycardia, hypotension, central respiratory failure, and coma, with an overall death rate of 0.1–12%. More severe reactions often occur in persons previously poisoned by the toxin. Untreated, the gastroenteritis usually resolves in 24–48 hours, whereas the neurologic syndrome may last for weeks. The diagnosis is made on the basis of clinical findings; there is currently no test that indicates the presence of ciguatoxin in human blood.

Treatment and Disposition

Treatment is largely supportive and symptomatic. Gastric emptying (gastric lavage or emesis), catharsis, and instillation of activated charcoal may be of limited value if performed within 3 hours after ingestion. Magnesium-based cathartics should be avoided. Hypotension should be treated with intravenous infusion of crystalloid solutions and vasopressors. Mannitol infusion, 1 g/kg intravenously, has been reported to reverse cardiac depression and severe neurologic symptoms. Bradyarrhythmias generally respond well to atropine. Treat persistent myocardial failure with judicious administration of calcium gluconate, 1–3 g intravenously over 24 hours; the rationale is that the toxin occupies calcium receptor sites that affect the permeability of the pores in neural and myocardial membranes to sodium. Although many other drugs have been recommended, none is as yet of proven benefit.

Patients with cardiovascular symptoms should be admitted for observation.

2. SCOMBROID POISONING

Scombroid poisoning follows the ingestion of toxic fish of the families Scomberesocidae and Scombroidea, which include albacore, tuna, mackerel, bonito, kingfish, and wahoo. Scombroid poisoning can also be caused by nonscombroid fish such as dolphin, sardine, anchovy, amberjack, and ocean salmon. In Hawaii, the dolphin *Coryphaena hippurus* is a common cause; in the northeastern USA, it is the bluefish *(Pomatomus saltatrix).* This pseudoallergic syndrome results from the improper preservation or refrigeration of dark-fleshed fish. Muscle tissue undergoes bacteria-induced degradation that transforms histidine to histamine. Histamine levels higher than 20–50 mg/100 mL are noted in toxic fish. It has been suggested that histamine alone is unlikely to be the sole toxin, since oral histamine is converted in the bowel to N-acetyl histamine.

Diagnosis

Symptoms occur within 15–90 minutes of ingestion and are the same as those caused by histamine, eg, flushing of the face, neck, and upper torso; sensation of warmth; urticaria; pruritus; angioneurotic edema; epigastric pain; abdominal cramps; diarrhea; nausea and vomiting; headache, thirst; pharyngitis; tachycardia; palpitations; bronchospasm; and hypotension. Untreated mild or moderate scombroid poisoning resolves within 6–12 hours.

Treatment and Disposition

Treatment is directed at reversing the effects of histamine. Patients with minor poisoning without respiratory distress should receive diphenhydramine, 25–75 mg orally. If the reaction is severe, give epinephrine, 0.3–0.5 mL of 1:1000 solution subcutaneously. Nausea and vomiting are usually controlled by the antihistamine; in refractory cases, the H_2 antagonists cimetidine (300 mg intravenously) or ranitidine (50 mg intravenously) may be given. Oral cimetidine (300 mg every 6 hours) may be used to combat persistent headache. If the patient presents in the emergency department within 1 hour of consuming a large amount of scombroid fish, it may be helpful to empty the stomach (gastric lavage or emesis) and administer activated charcoal, 50–100 g in sorbitol.

Patients with serious illness should be admitted for observation.

3. PUFFER FISH (TETRODOTOXIN) POISONING

Tetrodotoxin is one of the most potent nonprotein poisons found in nature and is characteristic of the order Tetraodontiformes. The poison is found in puffer fish, also known as toadfish, blowfish, globefish, swellfish, balloonfish, and porcupine fish. Some of these tropical and subtropical fish are prepared as delicacies ("fugu") in Japan by trained and licensed chefs. Tetrodotoxin is believed to be chemically identical to toxins isolated from certain North American newts, Central American frogs, and the Australian blue-ringed octopus. The toxin is distributed throughout the entire fish, with the greatest concentrations in the liver, gonads, intestine, and skin. The poison interferes with central and peripheral neuromuscular transmission, causing depression of the medullary respiratory mechanism, intracardiac conduction, and myocardial and skeletal muscle contractility. The

toxin is water-soluble but very difficult to remove from the fish by cooking.

Diagnosis

The onset of symptoms can be as rapid as 10 minutes or can be delayed for up to 4 hours. Victims initially develop paresthesias, followed by hypersalivation, diaphoresis, lethargy, headache, nausea, vomiting, abdominal pain, diarrhea, weakness, ataxia, tremor, paralysis, respiratory failure, coma, and hypotension. Sixty percent of victims die, most within the first 6 hours.

Treatment

A. Manage the Airway: If the victim is obtunded or there is evidence of dysphagia or respiratory insufficiency, endotracheal intubation should be performed and supplemental oxygen administered, guided by serial arterial blood gas measurements. Prompt ventilatory support in the setting of rapid paralysis is the most important intervention to prevent anoxic brain damage.

B. Perform Gastric Emptying: If the victim shows any neurologic signs that indicate impending paralysis or respiratory difficulty, gastric emptying should be preceded by endotracheal intubation. The toxin is gastric acid-stable and partially inactivated in alkaline solutions. If treatment is within 3 hours of ingestion, perform gastric lavage with at least 2 L of 2% sodium bicarbonate solution in 200-mL aliquots, followed by intragastric placement of 50–100 g of activated charcoal in 70% sorbitol solution.

C. Provide Symptom-Based Life Support: Hypotension may necessitate administration of crystalloid solutions or, rarely, the addition of a pressor agent. Bradyarrhythmias generally respond to atropine; heart block may necessitate temporary placement of a transvenous or transcutaneous pacemaker.

Disposition

Patients with respiratory difficulties, cardiovascular symptoms, or paralysis should be hospitalized in an intensive care unit. Patients with symptoms of a minor intoxication, which may be limited to paresthesias and mild dysphagia, should be observed in the emergency department or intensive care unit for at least 8 hours to detect deterioration.

4. PARALYTIC SHELLFISH POISONING

Bivalve mollusks filter large quantities of water unselectively to gather plankton and extract oxygen. This action leads to concentration of bacteria, viruses, biologic toxins, and other substances in the tissues of such shellfish. Paralytic shellfish poisoning is induced by ingesting any of a variety of clams, oysters, scallops, mussels, chitons, limpets, murex, starfish, and sandcrabs. The source of toxicity is the toxin elaborated by various planktonic dinoflagellates and protozoan organisms. The most common dinoflagellates are *Protogonyaulax* (or *Alexandrium*) and *Ptychodiscus* species, which are responsible for colored "tides" and enormous mortality in bird and marine populations. Saxitoxin, elaborated by *Protogonyaulax,* is found in greatest concentrations in the digestive organs, gills, and siphon. No physical characteristic distinguishes the carrier animal. A toxin concentration of greater than 75–80 µg/100 g of shellfish tissue is considered hazardous. The toxin blocks sodium conductance, inhibiting neuromuscular transmission at the axonal and muscle membrane levels. In humans, a lethal dose of purified saxitoxin is 0.1 mg.

Diagnosis

Within minutes to a few hours of ingestion of contaminated shellfish, intraoral and perioral paresthesias ensue. These rapidly involve the neck and distal extremities. Other symptoms include dizziness, incoordination, weakness, incoherence, dysarthria, sialorrhea, dysphagia, diarrhea, nausea, vomiting, dysmetria, headache, loss of vision, and tachycardia. Flaccid paralysis and respiratory insufficiency may follow. Unless there is a period of anoxia, the victim will often remain awake and alert, although paralyzed. Death due to respiratory arrest occurs in up to 25% of victims within the first 12 hours.

Treatment

A. Manage the Airway: If the victim is obtunded or there is evidence of dysphagia or respiratory insufficiency, endotracheal intubation should be performed and supplemental oxygen administered, guided by serial arterial blood gas measurements. Prompt ventilatory support in the setting of rapid paralysis is the most important intervention to prevent anoxic brain damage.

B. Perform Gastric Emptying: If the victim shows any neurologic signs that indicate impending paralysis or respiratory difficulty, gastric emptying should be preceded by endotracheal intubation. The toxin is gastric acid-stable and partially inactivated in alkaline solutions. If treatment is within 3 hours of ingestion, perform gastric lavage with at least 2 L of 2% sodium bicarbonate solution in 200-mL aliquots, followed by intragastric placement of 50–100 g of activated charcoal in 70% sorbitol solution.

C. Provide Symptom-Based Life Support: Hypotension may necessitate administration of crystalloid solutions or, rarely, the addition of a pressor agent. Bradyarrhythmias generally respond to atropine; heart block may necessitate temporary placement of a transvenous or transcutaneous pacemaker.

Disposition

Patients with respiratory difficulties, cardiovascular symptoms, or paralysis should be hospitalized in an intensive care unit. Patients with symptoms of a minor intoxication, which may be limited to paresthesias and mild dysphagia, should be observed in the emergency department or intensive care unit for at least 8 hours to detect deterioration.

REFERENCES

General
Auerbach PS, Geehr EC (editors): *Management of Wilderness and Environmental Emergencies,* 2nd ed. Mosby, 1989.

Disorders Due to Cold
Hall KN, Syverud SA: Closed thoracic cavity lavage in the treatment of severe hypothermia in human beings. Ann Emerg Med 1990;19:204.

Johnson L: Hypothermia. In: *Principles and Practice of Emergency Medicine,* 2nd ed. Schwartz GR et al (editors). Saunders, 1986.

Leaman PL, Martyak GG: Microwave warming of resuscitation fluids. Ann Emerg Med 1985;14:876.

Lloyd EL: *Hypothermia and Cold Stress.* Aspen, 1986.

Maningas PA et al: Regional blood flow during hypothermic arrest. Ann Emerg Med 1986;15:390.

McCauley RL et al: Frostbite injuries: A rational approach based on the pathophysiology. J Trauma 1983;23:143.

Mehta RC, Wilson MA: Frostbite injury: Prediction of tissue viability with triple phase bone scanning. Radiology 1989;170:511.

Morris DL et al: Hemodynamic characteristics of patients with hypothermia due to occult infection and other causes. Ann Intern Med 1985;102:153.

Page RE, Robertson GA: Management of the frostbitten hand. Hand 1983;15:185.

Pozos RS, Wittmers LE (editors): *The Nature and Treatment of Hypothermia.* Univ of Minnesota Press, 1983.

Shields CP, Sixsmith DM: Treatment of moderate to severe hypothermia in an urban setting. Ann Emerg Med 1990;19:1093.

Wong KC: Physiology and pharmacology of hypothermia. West J Med 1983;138:227.

Zell SC, Kurtz KJ: Severe exposure hypothermia: A resuscitation protocol. Ann Emerg Med 1985;14:339.

Disorders Due to Heat
Carter BJ, Cammermeyer M: Emergence of real casualties during simulated chemical warfare training under high heat conditions. Milit Med 1985;150:657.

Graham BS et al: Nonexertional heatstrokes: Physiologic management and cooling in 14 patients. Arch Intern Med 1986;146:87.

Khogali M, Hales JRS (editors): *Heat Stroke and Temperature Regulation.* Academic Press, 1983.

Syverud SA et al: Iced gastric lavage for treatment of

heatstroke: Efficacy in a canine model. Ann Emerg Med 1985;14:424.

Electrical Injuries

Amy BW et al: Lightning injury with survival in five patients. JAMA 1985;253:243.

Chilbert M et al: Measure of tissue resistivity in experimental electrical burns. J Trauma 1985;25:209.

Cwinn AA, Cantrill SV: Lightning injuries. J Emerg Med 1985;2:379.

Hammond J, Ward CG: Myocardial damage and electrical injuries: Significance of early elevation of CPK-MB isoenzymes. South Med J 1986;79:414.

Purdue GF, Hunt JL: Electrocardiographic monitoring after electrical injury: Necessity or luxury. J Trauma 1986;26:166.

Radiation Injuries

Geiger HJ: The accident at Chernobyl and the medical response. JAMA 1986;256:609.

A Guide to the Management of Injuries Arising From Exposure to or Involving Ionizing Radiation. American Medical Association, 1984.

Drowning

Bierens JJLM et al: Submersion cases in the Netherlands. Ann Emerg Med 1989;18:366.

Karch SB: Pathology of the lung in near-drowning. Am J Emerg Med 1986;4:4.

O'Carrol PW, Alkon E, Weiss B: Drowning mortality in Los Angeles County, 1976–1984. JAMA 1988;260:380.

Ornato JP: The resuscitation of near-drowning victims. JAMA 1986;256:75.

Disorders Due to Atmospheric Pressure Changes

Balk M: Alveolar hemorrhage as a manifestation of pulmonary barotrauma after scuba diving. Ann Emerg Med 1990;19:930.

Calder IM: Autopsy and experimental observations on factors leading to barotrauma in man. Undersea Biomed Res 1985;12:165.

Davis JC: *Hyperbaric Oxygen Therapy: A Committee Report.* Undersea Medical Society, 1983.

Dickey LS: Diving injuries. J Emerg Med 1984;1:249.

Johnson TS, Rock PB: Acute mountain sickness. N Engl J Med 1988;319:841.

Larson EB: Positive airway pressure for high-altitude pulmonary oedema. Lancet 1985;1:371.

Myers RAM, Bray P: Delayed treatment of serious decompression sickness. Ann Emerg Med 1985;14:254.

Schoene RB et al: High-altitude pulmonary edema and exercise at 4400 meters on Mount McKinley: Effect of expiratory positive airway pressure. Chest 1985;87:330.

Zell SC, Goodman PH: Acetazolamide and dexamethasone in the prevention of acute mountain sickness. West J Med 1988;148:541.

Venomous Animals

Auerbach PS: Bee, wasp, and spider envenomation. In: *Current Therapy in Emergency Medicine.* Callaham ML (editor). B. C. Decker, 1987.

Auerbach PS: Hazardous marine animals. Emerg Med Clin North Am 1984;2:531.

Barach EM et al: Epinephrine for treatment of anaphylactic shock. JAMA 1984;251:2118.

Burnett JW, Rubinstein H, Calton GJ: First aid for jellyfish envenomation. South Med J 1983;76:870.

Christopher DG, Rodning CB: Crotalidae envenomation. South Med J 1986;79:159.

Exton D, Williamson J (editors): *The Marine Stinger Book.* The Surf Life-Saving Association of Australia, 1985.

Grainger CR: Sting ray injuries. Trans R Soc Trop Med Hyg 1985;79:443.

Jurkovich GJ et al: Complications of Crotalidae antivenin therapy. J Trauma 1988;28:1032.

King LE, Rees RS: Dapsone treatment of a brown recluse bite. JAMA 1983;250:648.

Kizer KW, Auerbach PS: Marine envenomations: Not just as problem of the tropics. Emerg Med Rep 1985;6:129.

Kizer KW, McKinney HE, Auerbach PS: Scorpaenidae envenomation: A five-year poison center experience. JAMA 1985;253:807.

Likes K, Banner W, Chavez M: *Centruroides exilicauda* envenomation in Arizona. West J Med 1983;141:634.

Maretic Z: Latrodectism: Variations in clinical manifestations provoked by *Latrodectus* species of spiders. Toxicon 1983;21:457.

Wagner CW, Golladay ES: Crotalid envenomation in children: Selective conservative management. J Pediatr Surg 1989;24:128.

Ingestion of Poisonous Fish

Hokama Y: A rapid, simplified enzyme immunoassay stick test for the detection of ciguatoxin and related polyethers from fish tissues. Toxicon 1985;23:939.

Mills AR, Passmore R: Pelagic paralysis. Lancet 1988;1:161.

Prescott BD Jr: "Scombroid poisoning" and bluefish: The Connecticut connection. Conn Med 1984;48:105.

Torda TA, Sinclair E, Ulyatt DB: Puffer fish (tetrodotoxin) poisoning: Clinical record and suggested management. Med J Aust 1973;1:599.

Yentsch CM: Paralytic shellfish poisoning: An emerging perspective. In: *Seafood Toxins.* Ragelis EP (editor). American Chemical Society, 1984.

39

Poisoning

Kent R. Olson, MD, FACEP, & Charles E. Becker, MD

IMMEDIATE MANAGEMENT OF LIFE-THREATENING CONDITIONS

Victims of Poisoning With Coma, Seizures, or Marked Obtundation

A. Keep Airway Open: Establish and maintain an adequate airway and ventilation. Begin supplemental oxygen, 5–10 L/min, by nasal prongs or mask. If the patient has no gag reflex, intubate the trachea with a cuffed endotracheal tube as soon as possible to protect the airway, facilitate oxygenation and removal of airway secretions, and permit assisted ventilation if necessary.

B. Obtain Arterial Blood Gas Measurements: Obtain arterial blood for blood gas and pH measurements to determine adequacy of ventilation and perfusion.

C. Gain Intravenous Access: Insert a large-bore ($\geq$ 18-gauge) peripheral or central intravenous catheter, and draw blood for complete blood count, serum electrolyte and blood glucose measurements, and tests of renal and hepatic function.

D. Treat Coma Promptly: (See Chapter 10.)
1. Give glucose, 50 mL of a 50% solution (25 g of glucose) intravenously over 3–4 minutes.
2. Give naloxone (Narcan, others), 0.4–2 mg intravenously. If the patient's response is weak or if narcotic overdose is suspected, give repeated doses of 2 mg every 1–2 minutes up to a total dosage of 10–20 mg. *Note:* The duration of action of naloxone (2–3 hours) is shorter than that of many of the narcotics it reverses. Patients responding to naloxone must be observed for at least 3 hours after the last dose of naloxone.
3. If alcoholism or malnutrition is suspected, give thiamine, 100 mg intramuscularly or in intravenous solution.

E. Maintain Circulation: Maintain circulation, and treat shock by restoring intravascular volume with intravenous infusion of crystalloid solutions (Chapter 3). *Caution:* Fluid overload and pulmonary edema may occur with overvigorous hydration. If administration of more than 20–30 mL/kg of crystalloid solution and usual doses of dopamine (ie, 5–15 µg/kg/min intravenously) fail to restore blood pressure, insert a pulmonary artery catheter to obtain pressure readings and help guide further therapy with fluids or pressor agents.

F. Treat Seizures: (See Chapter 11.) If the patient is experiencing seizures, give diazepam, 0.1–0.2 mg/kg intravenously over 1–2 minutes. If this is not effective, give phenobarbital, 15 mg/kg intravenously at a rate no faster than 50 mg/min, or phenytoin, 15–18 mg/kg intravenously at a rate no faster than 50 mg/min, or both.

G. Start Electrocardiographic Monitoring: Start cardiac monitoring. Obtain a 12-lead ECG, and note especially the rate, rhythm, presence of arrhythmias, and PR, QRS, and QT intervals. If overdose of tricyclic antidepressants is suspected, obtain serial ECGs.

H. Perform Gastric Lavage: Perform gastric lavage with a large-bore orogastric or nasogastric tube (Ewald tube) for any potentially lethal ingestion and in any patient with altered mental status who might have ingested a toxic substance (see section on decontamination, below).

I. Search for Associated Illness: Look for other causes of coma or seizures (Chapters 10 and 11). In particular, look for (**1**) head trauma (focal neurologic deficits or asymmetric seizures), (**2**) other trauma causing hemorrhage or shock, (**3**) infection (generalized or central nervous system), (**4**) metabolic disorders (hyponatremia, hyperglycemia), (**5**) hypothermia (use a rectal thermometer that can measure temperatures lower than 32 °C [89.6 °F], or (**6**) hyperthermia.

Victims of Poisoning With Intact Gag Reflex & Lethargy

Management is the same as that outlined above for patients with absent gag reflex, except that endotracheal intubation may not be necessary before gastric lavage. The airway may be adequately protected by placing the patient in the lateral decubitus position with the head and trunk slightly lower than the feet (Trendelenburg position).

FURTHER MANAGEMENT OF VICTIMS OF POISONING

For assistance in identifying drugs and poisons and access to expert toxicologic consultation, contact a local regional poison control center (Table 39–1). Experts at the poison center can provide immediate assistance in selecting appropriate laboratory or toxicity tests, recommending preferred methods of gut decontamination, using antidotes, and advising on patient disposition.

Obtain Brief History

Obtain as much information as possible from paramedics, bystanders, police, family, and friends. Ask about recent use of drugs or medications, and find out whether there were any empty pill bottles, medications, or drug paraphernalia at the scene. If several patients present with similar symptoms of poisoning, consider carbon monoxide poisoning, food poison-

Table 39–1. AAPCC-certified regional poison centers in the USA.[1]

State	Poison Center	Telephone Number
Alabama	Children's Hospital of Alabama, Birmingham	(800) 292-6678 (205) 939-9201
Arizona	Arizona Poison and Drug Information Center, Tucson	(800) 362-0101 (AZ only) (602) 626-6016
	Samaritan Regional Poison Center, Phoenix	(602) 253-3334
California	Fresno Regional Poison Control Center, Fresno	(800) 346-5922 (CA only) (209) 445-1222
	San Diego Regional Poison Center, University of California, San Diego	(800) 876-4766 (CA only) (619) 543-6000
	San Francisco Bay Area Regional Poison Center, San Francisco	(800) 523-2222 (CA only) (415) 476-6600
	Santa Clara Valley Regional Poison Center, San Jose	(800) 662-9886 (CA only) (408) 299-5112
	UC Davis Medical Center Regional Poison Center, Sacramento	(800) 342-9293 (CA only) (916)734-3692
Colorado (also Montana, Las Vegas)	Rocky Mountain Poison Center, Denver	(303) 629-1123 (800) 525-5042 (MT only) (800) 969-6179 (Las Vegas)
Florida	Florida Poison Information Center, Tampa	(800) 282-3171 (FL only) (813) 253-4444
Georgia	Georgia Poison Control Center, Atlanta	(800) 282-5846 (GA only) (404) 589-4400
Indiana	Indiana Poison Center Indianapolis	(800) 382-9097 (317) 929-2323
Kentucky	Kentucky Regional Poison Center, Louisville	(800) 722-5725 (KY only) (502) 629-7275
Maryland	Maryland Poison Center, Baltimore	(800) 492-2414 (MD only) (301) 328-7701
Massachusetts	Massachusetts Poison Control System, Boston	(800) 682-9211 (MA only) (617) 232-2120
Michigan	Blodgett Regional Poison Center, Grand Rapids	(800) 632-2727 (MI only)
	Poison Control Center, Children's Hospital Detroit	(313) 745-5711
Minnesota	Hennepin Regional Poison Center, Minneapolis	(612) 347-3141
	Minnesota Regional Poison Center, St Paul	(612) 221-2113
Missouri	Cardinal Glennon Children's Hospital Regional Poison Center, St Louis	(800) 366-8888 (314) 772-5200
Montana	See Colorado	
Nebraska (also Wyoming)	The Poison Center, Omaha	(800) 955-9119 (402) 390-5555
New Jersey	New Jersey Poison Information and Education System, Newark	(800) 962-1253 (NJ only) (201) 923-0764
New Mexico	New Mexico Poison and Drug Information Center, Albuquerque	(800) 432-6866 (NM only) (505) 843-2551
New York	Long Island Regional Poison Control Center, East Meadow	(516) 542-2323
	New York City Poison Center, New York City	(212) 340-4494 (212) 764-7667

(continued)

Table 39–1. AAPCC-certified regional poison centers in the USA.[1] (continued)

State	Poison Center	Telephone Number
Ohio	Central Ohio Poison Center, Columbus	(800) 682-7625 (OH only) (614) 228-1323
	Regional Poison Control System and Drug and Poison Information Center, Cincinnati	(800) 872-5111 (513) 558-5111
Oregon	Oregon Poison Center, Portland	(800) 452-7165 (OR only) (503) 494-8968
Pennsylvania	Pittsburgh Poison Center, Pittsburgh	(412) 681-6669
	The Poison Control Center, Philadelphia	(215) 386-2100
Rhode Island	Rhode Island Poison Center, Providence	(401) 277-5727
Texas	North Texas Poison Center, Dallas	(800) 441-0040 (TX only) (214) 590-5000
Utah	Intermountain Regional Poison Center, Salt Lake City	(800) 456-7707 (UT only) (801) 581-2151
Washington, DC (also Northern Virginia)	National Capital Poison Center, Washington, DC	(202) 625-3333
Virginia	Blue Ridge Poison Center, Charlottesville	(800) 451-1428 (804) 925-5543
West Virginia	West Virginia Poison Center, Charleston	(800) 642-3625 (WV only) (304) 348-4211
Wyoming	*See* Nebraska	

[1]American Association of Poison Control Centers. (AAPCC) Regional Certification Committee, April 1992.

ing, or other toxin that can affect multiple victims simultaneously. Correlate the history with physical findings and results of laboratory tests, but do not be misled by the history. What the patient or friends say was ingested may differ from what was actually swallowed, especially in suicide attempts.

Decontaminate as Soon as Possible

A. Inhaled Poisons: Remove the patient from the source of poison, and give oxygen by mask. Inhalation of a water aerosol may help to dilute inhaled irritants in the nasopharynx. Check for hoarseness and singed nasal hairs (eg, after smoke inhalation), and be alert for delayed development of upper airway obstruction or pulmonary edema.

B. Contaminated Eyes: (See Chapter 25.) Wash the eyes immediately with copious amounts of plain water or normal saline; *do not* use neutralizing solutions. Hang a bottle containing 500–1000 mL of normal saline above the patient, and dribble the solution slowly into the corner of the injured eye through the intravenous tubing.

If the contaminating material was acidic or basic, tears may be checked with pH paper after the eyes have been washed to make sure that all toxic material has been removed. A careful eye examination is indicated following irrigation (Chapter 25).

C. Contaminated Skin: Wash the skin immediately with plenty of water and dilute soap solution.

Discard contaminated clothes in a marked plastic bag. Certain toxins, such as organophosphates, are well absorbed through the skin and are difficult to remove.

Hydrofluoric acid burns are particularly penetrating and corrosive. Prompt immersion of the burn into Epsom salts solution or 10% calcium gluconate solution or 2.5% gel, or subcutaneous injection of calcium gluconate deep to the burn (0.5 mL of 10% solution per square centimeter of burn area) may be helpful. A plastic surgeon (or hand surgeon) should be consulted for injuries involving the fingers.

D. Ingested Poisons: The traditional approach has been to remove ingested toxins by emesis or gastric lavage, followed by activated charcoal and catharsis. However, recent evidence suggests that gastric emptying (particularly emesis) may have limited efficacy, especially if initiated more than 1 hour after the ingestion, and may delay the administration of charcoal. Gastric lavage is the preferred method of gastric emptying, particularly in patients who have taken a rapid-acting convulsant or those with a rapidly declining level of consciousness.

1. Emesis–Emesis is most useful if initiated at home within a few minutes of the ingestion, and it is of questionable value when given in the emergency department for most ingestions. Emesis is still recommended for emergency department treatment of drugs not adsorbed to charcoal (eg, iron, lithium).

Do not induce vomiting in a patient in coma or

with a depressed gag reflex. Do not induce vomiting if caustics or low-viscosity hydrocarbons (see Hydrocarbons, below) have been ingested, or if rapid-acting convulsants (Table 39–2) have been ingested. When induction of vomiting is appropriate, induce emesis even if the patient claims to have already vomited spontaneously—the amount vomited may not have been sufficient to empty the stomach.

To induce emesis, give syrup of ipecac, 15 mL orally for children, 30 mL for adults. Following ipecac, most clinicians give 2–3 glasses of plain water. Recent evidence, however, suggests that ipecac is equally effective with or without water. If vomiting does not occur in 20 minutes, repeat the dose once. If ipecac is still ineffective, proceed with gastric lavage.

Do not use apomorphine. Although induction of emesis is more rapid and predictable with apomorphine, this drug is difficult to use and may cause respiratory depression and hypotension.

2. Gastric lavage–Perform gastric lavage for suspected serious ingestions when attempts to induce emesis fail, when patients are uncooperative or lethargic, when the gag reflex is markedly depressed, or in patients who have ingested rapid-acting convulsants (Table 39–2). The patient should be placed in the left lateral decubitus position with the head down, and if the gag reflex is depressed, the airway must be protected with a cuffed endotracheal tube.

Gastric lavage is performed with a large-bore (at least 36F for adults) orogastric or nasogastric tube. (Pill fragments cannot be removed through standard-sized nasogastric tubes.) Use tap water or saline at body temperature in 250-mL increments, and continue lavage until fluid returns clear or free of pill fragments.

3. Activated charcoal–Following emesis or lavage, give activated charcoal, 50–100 g as a slurry obtained by mixing the charcoal with an equal amount of water. Activated charcoal may also be given both before and after gastric lavage. For oral administration, charcoal can be made more palatable by adding a small amount of cherry, licorice, or chocolate flavoring just before administration. Mixing the charcoal with 1 mL/kg of 70% sorbitol improves taste and also provides cathartic action. Recent studies suggest that in patients with minor ingestions administration of oral activated charcoal alone without prior gut emptying is just as effective as traditional use of emesis or lavage before charcoal.

Charcoal has great adsorptive properties and can bind most poisons (exceptions include alcohols, potassium, lithium, and iron). If the ingested dose of poison is known, attempt to give at least 10 times that weight of charcoal, in divided doses if necessary.

4. Whole bowel irrigation–Recently, whole bowel irrigation has been used successfully for removal of iron tablets and sustained-release and enteric-coated preparations. This technique utilizes a balanced electrolyte–polyethylene glycol solution (Colyte, Golytely) to flush out the entire intestinal tract. It is given by nasogastric tube, 1–2 L/h (400–500 mL/min in children), until the rectal effluent is clear (3–5 hours or more).

Perform Complete Physical Examination

Look for characteristic physical signs of various kinds of poisoning while immediate treatment measures are being started. Physical signs associated with specific poisons are listed in Tables 39–3 and 39–4. Table 39–5 lists common exposures in several occupations or industries.

Order Laboratory & X-Ray Studies

A. Obtain arterial blood gas and pH measurements to determine adequacy of ventilation and circulation.

B. Draw blood for measurement of serum electrolytes, blood urea nitrogen, blood glucose, and serum osmolality. Calculate anion and osmolar gaps (Tables 39–6 and 39–7).

C. Obtain an ECG, and look for widened QRS complexes or QT intervals, atrioventricular block, ventricular tachyarrhythmias, or evidence of ischemia (Table 39–8).

D. Obtain a chest x-ray to look for pulmonary edema (caused by narcotics, barbiturates, salicylates, etchlorvynol, or corrosive chemicals) or infiltrates (due to aspiration of gastric contents, inhalation of certain metal fumes, or hydrocarbon aspiration).

E. Obtain an abdominal x-ray to look for radiopaque pills or toxins (Table 39–9).

F. Obtain urine for toxicologic screening and routine analysis, and look for calcium oxalate crystals (ethylene glycol poisoning); positive test for occult blood (myoglobinuria, hemolysis); or positive test for phenylpyruvic acid (eg, Phenistix) in phenothiazine or salicylate overdose (may be negative in patients with acid urine).

G. Request toxicologic studies. Results of toxicologic studies may be useful in later confirmation of the diagnosis but are rarely helpful in the emergency department. It is more cost-effective to save serum and urine samples in the laboratory and analyze them later only if necessary. For certain types of poisoning, however, obtaining estimates of drug concentration quickly is valuable in determining the need for spe-

Table 39–2. Examples of rapid-acting convulsants.

Amphetamines	Isoniazid
Camphor	Lindane
Chlordane	Nicotine
Cocaine	Strychnine
Cyclic antidepressants	

Table 39–3. Physical findings associated with various types of poisons.

Altered vital signs
  Hypertension: amphetamines, phencyclidine, phenylpropanolamine, anticholinergics, cocaine, nicotine
  Hypotension: sedative-hypnotics, narcotics, antihypertensives, theophylline, clonidine, beta-blockers, tricyclic antidepressants
  Hyperthermia: salicylates, amphetamines, cocaine, phencyclidine, anticholinergics, seizures due to any cause
  Hypothermia: narcotics, barbiturates, ethanol, other sedative-hypnotics, clonidine, phenothiazines
  Hyperpnea: salicylates or other agents causing metabolic acidosis
Ocular signs
  Miosis (pinpoint pupils): narcotics, clonidine, organophosphates, phenothiazines, severe sedative-hypnotic overdose, pilocarpine
  Mydriasis (dilated pupils): anticholinergics, amphetamines, cocaine, LSD, glutethimide
  Nystagmus: phenytoin, phencyclidine (especially vertical nystagmus), alcohol, many sedative-hypnotics
  Ophthalmoplegia: botulism, sedative-hypnotics
  Oculogyric crisis: haloperidol, other antipsychotics
  Optic neuritis: methanol
Breath odors
  Smoke: fire-associated toxins (see section on inhalants)
  Garlic: arsenic, arsine gas, organophosphates
  Bitter almond or silver polish: cyanide
  Wintergreen: methyl salicylate
  Pearlike: chloral hydrate
  Rotten eggs: hydrogen sulfide
  Acetone: diabetic ketoacidosis, isopropanol
  Typical odors of ethanol, ammonia, tobacco, disinfectants, camphor, glue, paraldehyde
Skin signs
  Cyanosis: ergotamine, agents causing hypoxemia, hypotension, or methemoglobinemia
  Flushed, red: carbon monoxide (rare), cyanide (rare), anticholinergics, boric acid
  Acneiform rash: bromides, chlorinated aromatic hydrocarbons
  Bullae: nonspecific for sedative-hypnotic overdose, carbon monoxide, and other causes of coma
Altered muscle tone
  Increased: amphetamines, phencyclidine, antipsychotics
  Flaccid: sedative-hypnotics, narcotics, clonidine
  Fasciculations: organophosphates, lithium
  Rigidity: haloperidol, phencyclidine, strychnine
  Dystonic posturing: antipsychotics, phencyclidine
  Tremor: lithium, nicotine, or stimulant overdose; alcohol or sedative-hypnonotic withdrawal
  Asterixis (flapping tremor): agents causing hepatic encephalopathy
  Seizures: tricycline antidepressants, theophylline, amphetamines, cocaine, phencyclidine, phenothiazines, isoniazid, lindane, other chlorinated hydrocarbons and pesticides

cific therapy (Table 39–10). When overdose with any of these drugs is suspected, request urgent concentration measurements for the specific drugs.

Accelerate Elimination of Poisons

A. Toxicokinetics: The rational management of drug overdose requires an understanding of the absorption, distribution, and elimination of the toxin. Most published kinetic parameters have been determined at normal doses, whereas pharmacokinetics in victims of poisoning are often more complex.

Dissolution and absorption of toxin or gastric emptying time may be altered in poisoned patients, so that the peak effects may be delayed (as occurs with anticholinergics). The gastrointestinal tract may be injured, allowing increased absorption of certain materials (eg, iron). If the finite capacity of the liver to metabolize a drug is exceeded, an increased amount of the drug may be delivered to the systemic circulation. If the concentration of the toxin in the bloodstream increases dramatically, protein binding may be saturated (eg, salicylate), so that the fraction of free toxin increases. Circulatory insufficiency, hypothermia, and electrolyte and acid-base imbalance influence the metabolism and excretion of ingested drugs. Any of these factors may drastically alter "normal" kinetics and confuse calculations. Despite these limitations, pharmacokinetic principles may be useful in the management of drug overdose. Definitions of some commonly used terms in toxicology are set forth below.

1. Half-life—The half-life of a toxin is the time required to eliminate one-half of the toxin from the body. This parameter is most meaningful for the many drugs (eg, barbiturates, theophylline) that exhibit **first-order kinetics,** in which a fixed *percentage* of the toxin is removed per unit of time. Other drugs (eg, alcohol) have **zero-order kinetics,** in which a fixed *amount* of toxin is removed per unit of time. In an overdose, pathways of elimination are often saturated, and first-order kinetics are replaced by fixed or zero-order elimination.

2. Volume of distribution (V_d)—The volume of distribution is the "apparent" volume into which the toxin is distributed after absorption. If a drug is sequestered outside the blood and is highly tissue-bound, it will have a very large volume of distribution. Table 39–11 gives the volume of distribution for several common drugs.

3. Clearance—Clearance is the volume of plasma that can be cleared of toxin per unit of time. Clearance includes both renal and metabolic components, and the proportion that each contributes to total clearance is important; eg, a toxin may be 95% metabolized and 5% renally excreted, in which case doubling the renal clearance of the toxin will not significantly enhance its total elimination from the body.

Knowledge of these parameters is helpful when measures to increase drug elimination—eg, forced alkaline diuresis, hemodialysis, or hemoperfusion—are under consideration. For example, toxins with very large volumes of distribution are present in only minute quantities in plasma and are not efficiently removed by dialysis or diuresis. Measures to enhance elimination of drugs with rapid intrinsic clearance rates will not contribute significantly to the overall elimination rate.

B. Methods to Enhance Drug Elimination: The decision to use measures to improve drug elimi-

Table 39–4. Common toxic syndromes associated with major drug groups.[1]

Antidepressants (eg, amitriptyline, doxepin, amoxapine) Anticholinergic features common: dilated pupils, tachycardia, hot dry skin, decreased bowel sounds. The "three Cs": Coma, convulsions, and cardiac problems are the most common causes of death. A major diagnostic feature is widening of the QRS complex greater than 0.1 s on ECG (*not* seen with amoxapine). Hypotension and ventricular arrhythmias are common.	**Opioid drugs (cont'd)** Skin cool; may show signs of intravenous drug abuse with asssociated infectious disease complications. Bowel sounds decreased. Muscle tone flaccid; occasionally see twitching, rigidity. Clonidine may present with identical syndrome.
Key interventions: Control seizures, correct acidosis with ventilation and HCO_3. Avoid use of ipecac and physostigmine.	**Key interventions:** Airway support. Frequent use of naloxone may be necessary because of its short half-life.
Antimuscarinic drugs (eg, atropine, scopolamine, antihistamines, tricyclic antidepressants, jimsonweed, *Amanita muscaria* mushrooms) Hallucinations, delirium, coma. Seizures may occur with tricyclic antidepressants, antihistamines. Tachycardia, hypertension. Hyperthermia with hot, dry skin. Mydriasis. Decreased bowel sounds, urinary retention.	**Salicylates** Confusion, lethargy, coma, seizures. Hyperventilation, hyperthermia. Anion gap metabolic acidosis. Dehydration, potassium loss; hyper- or hypoglycemia. Acute overdose: 6-hour level over 100 mg/dL (1000 mg/L) very serious. Chronic or accidental overdose: level not reliable; more severe toxicity; often mistakenly diagnosed as upper respiratory infection or gastroenteritis.
Key interventions: Control hyperthermia. Physostigmine is of limited value.	**Key interventions:** Make the diagnosis; correction of acidosis and fluid and electrolyte abnormalities; hemodialysis if pH or CNS symptoms cannot be controlled.
Cholinomimetic drugs (eg, organophosphate and carbamate insecticides) Anxiety, agitation, seizures, coma. May see bradycardia (muscarinic effect) or tachycardia (nicotinic effect). Pinpoint pupils. Excessive salivation, sweating. Bowel sounds hyperactive, with abdominal cramping, diarrhea. Muscle fasciculations and twitching followed by flaccid paralysis. Death due to respiratory muscle paralysis.	**Sedative-hypnotics** (eg, barbiturates, diazepam, ethanol) Highly variable depending on stage of intoxication; initially disinhibition and rowdiness, later lethargy, stupor, coma. With deep coma: hypotension, somewhat small pupils. Nystagmus common with moderate intoxication. Bowel sounds decreased in deep coma. Muscle tone usually flaccid; if increased, suspect PCP, methaqualone. May be associated with hypothermia (do not administer room temperature fluid).
Key interventions: Respiratory support, atropine, pralidoxime (2-PAM). Remove clothes, wash skin, follow ECG, check other workers.	**Key interventions:** Airway and repiratory support. Avoid fluid overload.
Opioid drugs (eg, morphine, heroin, meperidine, codeine, methadone) Sleepiness, lethargy, or coma, depending on dose. Blood pressure and heart rate usually decreased. Hypoventilation or apnea. Pinpoint pupils.	**Stimulant drugs** (eg, amphetamines, cocaine, PCP) Agitation, psychosis, seizures. Hypertension, tachycardia, arrhythmias. Mydriasis (usually). Vertical and horizontal nystagmus are common with PCP poisoning. Skin warm and sweaty. Muscle tone increased: muscle necrosis is possible. Hyperthermia may be major complication.
	Key interventions: Control seizures, blood pressure, and hyperthermia.

[1]Reproduced, with permission, from Katzung BG (editor): *Basic & Clinical Pharmacology,* 4th ed. Appleton & Lange, 1989.

nation should be based on a rational understanding of the drug's properties and the clinical condition of the patient. Most patients respond satisfactorily to appropriate supportive care. The risks, time, and expense involved in hemodialysis or hemoperfusion must be weighed against the possible benefits. In some patients, the severe potential toxicity of the poison warrants immediate hemodialysis (Table 39–12). With other poisons, dialysis is of no theoretic or proved benefit.

1. Diuresis and pH manipulations–Since many toxins are weak acids or bases, they can be ionized in solutions of varying pH. In the ionized state, they are less likely to cross cell membranes, and their reabsorption by the renal tubular epithelium is decreased. The clinical significance of these measures depends on the contribution of renal elimination to

total body clearance. It is also important to consider the possible adverse effects of overhydration, alkalemia, or acidemia. *Most studies have failed to show a significant effect of forced diuresis or pH manipulation on the outcome of poisoning.*

a. Weak acids such as salicylate and phenobarbital are more fully ionized in basic solutions, so that alkalizing the urine may serve to trap them in the tubular lumen, thus increasing excretion of the drug in the urine.

b. Weak bases such as amphetamines, strychnine, and phencyclidine are more ionized in an acid medium; acidification of the urine has been proposed to enhance their removal. However, acidification may promote myoglobinuric renal failure in patients with rhabdomyolysis (a common complication of poisoning by these agents).

Table 39–5. Selected occupations and specific exposures.[1]

Occupation or Industry	Exposures (Syndrome)
Baker	Flour, fungi, grain dust (asthma)
Battery maunfacturing or repair	Lead
Butcher	Vinyl plastic fumes (asthma)
Carpenter	Wood dust, wood preservatives (skin problems, nasal cancer)
Cement worker	Potassium chromate, dichromate (asthma)
Coal miner	Dust, silica (lung disease)
Dentist	Mercury, waste anesthetic gases
Dry cleaner	Solvents (liver, skin, and neurologic disease [neuropathy])
Electronics worker	Toluene diisocyanate (asthma); solvent exposure, hydrofluoric acid (skin burns)
Electroplating	Cyanide, chromium, nickel
Explosives manufac-turing	Nitrates (headache and rebound vasoconstriction)
Farm worker	Pesticides; infectious agents; NO_2, pentachlorophenol, H_2S
Felt maker	Mercury (neuropathy)
Fire fighter	Carcinogens, smoke products (eg, CO, CN, asbestos)
Foundry worker	Silica (lung disease)
Fumigator	Methyl bromide (encephalopathy, neuropathy), sulfuryl fluoride (pulmonary edema), organophosphates and carbamates
Hospital worker	Infectious agents, radiation, cleansers, ethylene oxide
Insulation industry	Formaldehyde, asbestos, fiberglass
Insulators	Asbestos, fiberglass
Jackhammer operator	Vibration (vascular disease)
Meat packing or weighing	Polyvinylchloride or papain (asthma, Q fever)
Miner	Dust (lung disease)
Office worker	Poorly designed workplace (joint and eye problems)
Painter	Solvents, lead, isocyanates
Pathology technician	Fluorocarbons (palpitations)
Petroleum industry	Benzene (leukemia), NH_3 and H_2S, polycylic aromatic hydrocarbons
Pottery industry	Silica, lead
Poultry worker	Asthma, psittacosis
Radiator repair	Lead
Rubber manufacturing	Ethylenediamine (asthma, bladder cancer)
Sausage maker	Garlic powder (asthma)
Seaman	Asbestos
Sewer worker	H_2S (hydrogen sulfide)
Shoe repair	Benzene (leukemia), benzidine (bladder cancer)

(*continued*)

Table 39–5 (cont'd). Selected occupations and specific exposures.[1]

Spelunker	Histoplasmosis, rabies
Sterilizer operator	Ethylene oxide (polyneuropathy)
Vintner	Arsenic (cancer and dermatitis)
Welder	Metal and polymer fume fever, ultraviolet radiation (skin and corneal burns), lead
Woodworker	N-Hexane (neuropathy), dust (asthma)

[1]Reproduced, with permission, from Olson KR et al (editors): *Poisoning & Drug Overdose.* Appleton & Lange, 1990.

2. Hemodialysis–During hemodialysis, toxin is removed from the blood into a dialysate solution across a semipermeable membrane. The toxin must be relatively water-soluble and not highly protein-bound. It should have a small volume of distribution and slow rate of intrinsic elimination (a long half-life). Hemodialysis is effective in removing methanol, ethylene glycol, salicylates, and lithium, among other drugs (Table 39–12). It is also of value in correcting pH and electrolyte imbalances, especially in anuric patients.

3. Peritoneal dialysis is much less efficient than hemodialysis in removing most drugs.

4. Hemoperfusion–In hemoperfusion, blood is pumped through a column of adsorbent material (charcoal or resin) and returned to the patient's circulation. Vascular access similar to that for hemodialysis is required. The kinetic conditions required are the same as in hemodialysis—ie, the drug should have a small volume of distribution and a slow rate of intrinsic clearance. Hemoperfusion has the advantage that the drug or toxin is in direct contact with the adsorbent material; therefore, high molecular weight, poor water solubility, and even plasma protein binding are not limiting factors as they are in hemodialysis. Hemoperfusion is commonly associated with thrombocytopenia. Hemoperfusion will not correct pH or electrolyte imbalances.

5. Repeated doses of activated charcoal– Repeated doses of charcoal given orally or via gastric tube (20–30 every 3–4 hours) may enhance elimination of some drugs and toxins from the bloodstream

Table 39–6. Drugs causing metabolic acidosis associated with an elevated anion gap.[1]

Direct causes of acidosis
  Alcohols: methanol, ethanol, ethylene glycol
  Salicylates
  Paraldehyde
  Phenformin
Indirect causes of acidosis
  Seizures (eg, isoniazid)
  Hypotension (eg, barbiturates)
  Hypoxemia (eg, carbon monoxide, cyanide)

[1]Anion gap = $(Na^+ + K^+) - (HCO_3^- + Cl^-)$ = 12–16 meq/L.

Table 39–7. Calculation of the osmolar gap in toxicology.

The olmolar gap (Δosm) is determined by subtracting the calculated serum osmolality from the measured serum osmolality. Calculated osmolality:

$$osm = 2(Na^+) + \frac{Glucose}{18} + \frac{BUN}{2.8}$$

Osmolar gap:

$$\Delta osm = \text{measured osm} - \text{Calculated osm}$$

Serum osmolality may be increased by contributions of circulating alcohols and other low-molecular-weight substances. Since these substances are not included in the calculated osmolality, there will be a gap proportionate to their serum concentration and inversely proprotional to their molecular weight:

$$\text{Serum concentration (mg/dL)} \approx \Delta osm \times \frac{\text{Molecular weight}}{10}$$

For ethanol (the commonest cause of Δosm), a gap of 30 mosm/L indicates an ethanol level of

$$30 \times 46/10 = 138 \text{ mg/dL}$$

	Molecular Weight	Lethal Concentration (mg/dL)	Corresponding Δosm (mosm/L)
Ethanol	46	350	75
Methanol	32	80	25
Ethylene glycol	62	200	35
Isopropanol	60	350	60

Note: Most laboratories use the freezing point method for calculating osmolality. If the vaporization point method is used, alcohols are driven off and their contribution to osmolality is lost.

Table 39–8. Electrocardiographic manifestations of poisoning.

Sign	Examples of Causes
Prolonged QT interval	Hypocalcemia (ethylene glycol) Tricyclic antidepressants Type I antiarrhythmic agents
Prolonged QRS interval	Phenothiazines (selected) Tricyclic antidepressants Type I antiarrhythmic agents
Atrioventricular block	Beta-adrenergic blockers Calcium channel–blocking agents Digitalis glycosides Tricyclic antidepressants Type I antiarrhythmic agents
Ventricular tachyarrhythmias	Amphetamines, cocaine Digitalis glycosides Theophylline Tricyclic antidepressants Type I antiarrhythmic agents
Ischemic pattern or current of injury	Cellular asphyxiants (cyanide, carbon monoxide) Hypoxemia (pneumonia) Hypotension

Table 39–9. Drugs and toxins that may be radiopaque.[1]

Chloral hydrate Heavy metals (iron, arsenic) Iodide Psychotropics (phenothiazines, tricyclic antidepressants) Sodium Enteric-coated tablets	Mnemonic is CHIPS

[1]**Caution:** Recent studies suggest that these drugs are *not* routinely visible on x-ray. If tablets have dissolved, false-negative x-ray results may occur. Abdominal x-rays are therefore useful only if positive findings are seen.

by a type of "gut dialysis." Drugs for which this may be useful include theophylline, phenytoin, salicylate, dapsone, nadolol, carbamazepine, and phenobarbital.

C. Antidotes: Table 39–13 sets forth several common useful antidotes. Their indications and dosages are discussed in the sections on specific toxins. The half-life of the antidote relative to that of the toxin must be considered. Most importantly, antidotes should not be used indiscriminately and without regard for the clinical condition of the patient. They may have serious side effects and in some cases may be more toxic than the poison. *Always treat the specific symptoms manifested by the patient, not those known to be associated with a certain poison.*

Caution: The "universal antidote" consisting of burnt toast, magnesium oxide, and tannic acid is not of value and may be potentially harmful. Other ineffective or dangerous remedies are described in Table 39–14.

MANAGEMENT OF CONDITIONS ASSOCIATED WITH POISONING

Management of Airway

It is essential to protect the lungs from aspiration and maintain adequate ventilation and oxygenation.

Table 39–10. Drugs for which serum levels are useful in guiding treatment of poisoning.

Drug or Toxin	Therapy (Contingent on Drug Level)
Acetaminophen	Acetylcysteine
Carboxyhemoglobin	Oxygen (100%)
Digoxin	Digoxin-specific antibodies
Ethylene glycol	Ethanol infusion; hemodialysis
Iron	Deferoxamine
Lithium	Hemodialysis
Methanol	Ethanol infusion; hemodialysis
Salicylate	Hemodialysis
Theophylline	Hemoperfusion

Table 39–11. Volumes of distribution for some common drugs.

Drugs With Large Volumes of Distribution		Drugs With Small Volumes of Distribution	
Chlorpromazine	10–20 L/kg	Acetaminophen	0.8 L/kg
Haloperidol	20–30 L/kg	Digitoxin	0.5 L/kg
Amitriptyline	> 40 L/kg	Ethanol	0.6 L/kg
Imipramine	10–20 L/kg	Isoniazid	0.6 L/kg
Digoxin	6–10 L/kg	Lithium	1.1 L/kg
Meperidine	4 L/kg	Phenytoin	0.6 L/kg
Methadone	5 L/kg	Salicylate	0.2 L/kg
		Theophylline	0.5 L/kg

In the patient with a depressed gag reflex, gastric lavage and spontaneous vomiting or emesis induced by syrup of ipecac may result in significant aspiration if the airway is unprotected. Some guidelines to airway management follow.

A. Need for Endotracheal Intubation:

1. Patients in coma or with markedly depressed gag reflex–Endotracheal intubation should always be performed in these patients, especially before gastric lavage.

2. Awake patient with normal gag reflex–Gastric intubation and lavage may be performed without special precautions.

3. Lethargic patient–The lethargic patient with fluctuating mental status and a variable gag reflex poses a more difficult problem in management. If the gag reflex is intact, cautious gastric lavage may be performed with the patient in the left lateral decubitus position and with the head of the bed or gurney tilted down at an angle of 10–20 degrees. *If there is any doubt about the patient's ability to protect the airway with a gag or cough reflex, gastric lavage must be*

Table 39–12. Indications for hemodialysis (HD or hemoperfusion (HP) in the management of common types of poisoning.

Indicated immediately if intoxication is significant
  Methanol (HD)
  Ethylene glycol (HD)
  Lithium (HD)
  Paraquat (HP)
  Salicylate (HD)
  Theophylline (HP preferred over HD)
Indicated if supportive measures are unsuccessful or if prolonged coma is expected
  Phenobarbital (HP preferred over HD)
  Ethchlorvynol (HP)
  Digitoxin (HP)
  Tricyclic antidepressants (HP)
Not indicated
  Digoxin
  Benzodiazepines (diazepam, chlordiazepoxide)
  Glutethimide
  Narcotics
  Short-acting barbiturates
  Amphetamines, phencyclidine, cocaine
  Quinidine, procainamide
  Chlorpromazine, haloperidol, and other antipsychotics

Table 39–13. Some poisons for which there are specific antidotes.

Poison	Specific Antidote
Acetaminophen	Acetylcysteine
Anticholinergics	Physostigmine
Anticholinesterases (organophosphates, carbamates, physostigmine)	Atropine Pralidoxime (2-PAM)
Benzodiazepines	Flumazenil
Beta-blockers	Glucagon
Calcium channel blockers	Calcium
Carbon monoxide	100% Oxygen
Cyanide	Sodium nitrite Sodium thiosulfate Vitamin B_{12A} (not yet approved for use in the USA)
Digoxin	Digoxin-specific antibodies
Heavy metals (Table 39–19)	Chelating agents
Isoniazid	Pyridoxine (vitamin B_6)
Methanol, ethylene glycol	Ethanol, folate, 4-methyl pyrazole (not approved for use in the USA)
Narcotics	Naloxone
Tricyclic antidepressants	Sodium bicarbonate

preceded by intubation with a cuffed endotracheal tube.

If intubation is not immediately performed, it is crucial to monitor the status of the airway closely and to position the patient so as to prevent aspiration. An initially responsive patient may rapidly become more obtunded. Significant swelling and upper airway obstruction may be late developments after thermal, chemical, and caustic burns.

B. Choice of Intubation Technique: (See Chapter 46.)

1. Orotracheal intubation–This technique is useful for the comatose patient, since it is rapid and the location of the endotracheal tube can be verified by direct vision. It is difficult to perform in patients

Table 39–14. Examples of ineffective or dangerous "antidotes."

"Antidote"	Application	Problems
Amphetamines, caffeine, or doxapram	Nonspecific arousal, eg, sedative overdose	Cardiac arrhythmias, seizures
Mineral oil	Petroleum distillate ingestion	Lipoid pneumonia
Physostigmine	Nonspecific arousal, eg, diazepam overdose, tricyclic antidepressants	Bradycardia, asystole, seizures
"Universal antidote" (burnt toast, tea)	Absorbent in gut	Ineffective; aspiration; wastes time
Vinegar, other weak acids	Neutralization of alkali burns	Ineffective; may worsen injury

who are awake or can be easily aroused, and in patients with spasm of the masseter muscle (trismus).

2. Nasotracheal intubation–This technique is slower than orotracheal intubation because the tube is not directed into the trachea under direct vision. However, jaw relaxation is not required, and insertion is easier in the agitated patient. Nasotracheal intubation also has the advantage of not requiring neck manipulation in a patient who may have cervical spine injury. It should generally be performed only in patients capable of spontaneous respiration.

Seizures
(See Chapter 11.)

A. General Measures: Management of drug-induced seizures is generally the same as that for seizures due to other causes, ie, protection of the airway, use of anticonvulsants, and correction of acidosis, hypoxemia, electrolyte abnormalities, and hyperthermia. Seizures unrelated to poisoning may also occur as a result of intracranial bleeding from trauma, hypoglycemia, or hyponatremia. Seizures caused by poisoning are rarely focal, nor are they associated with asymmetric neurologic findings. Meningitis may mimic metabolic or toxic encephalopathy and must be ruled out by lumbar puncture (Chapter 46).

B. Specific Therapy: In certain types of poisoning, refractory seizures may require specific therapy.

1. Seizures occurring as a result of theophylline, lithium, or salicylate overdose usually require hemodialysis or hemoperfusion to accelerate removal of the drug.

2. In isoniazid poisoning with seizures refractory to diazepam, administer pyridoxine, 5 g (or 1 g per gram of isoniazid ingested) intravenously.

3. Seizures due to organophosphate poisoning may respond to atropine and pralidoxime. (See Organophosphates & Other Cholinesterase Inhibitors, below.)

Hypotension
(See Chapter 3.)

Hypotension is a common associated condition in victims of poisoning. The mechanism of hypotension may be direct cardiac depression, peripheral vasodilatation, or fluid deficits or shifts that result in hypovolemia. Concurrent hypothermia may aggravate hypotension. Be alert for possible concurrent trauma with occult internal bleeding or concurrent infection with septic shock.

In the absence of associated pulmonary edema, a fluid challenge should be given with intravenous boluses of normal saline, 200 mL every 15 minutes to an average maximum of 1 L (for adults). A central venous or pulmonary artery catheter may need to be inserted to monitor fluid needs and response to therapy. Monitoring of urine output with an indwelling catheter is recommended. If hypotension and hypoperfusion are severe and unresponsive to administration of fluids and temperature correction, vasopressors may be of benefit (Inside Front Cover).

Thermodysregulation

See Chapter 38 for further details of the management of hypothermia and hyperthermia.

A. Hyperthermia: Many drugs cause hyperthermia, either by direct toxic effects on temperature-regulating mechanisms or through associated hyperactivity or seizures.

1. Salicylate intoxication causes hyperthermia by uncoupling of oxidative phosphorylation, resulting in inefficient (and therefore heat-generating) production of ATP.

2. Phenothiazines inhibit the autoregulatory ability of the central nervous system, leading to environmentally induced hypothermia or hyperthermia.

3. Hyperthermia may result from seizures or extreme hyperactivity (particularly if the patient has to be forcibly restrained) following poisoning by phencyclidine or amphetamines.

4. The anticholinergic properties of many drugs (eg, antihistamines, tricyclic antidepressants) can aggravate hyperthermia by inhibiting sweating.

For dangerous core temperatures above 41 °C (105.8 °F), cool the patient rapidly by immersion in cool water, gastric lavage, or sponge bathing with evaporation accelerated by fanning; treat seizures. Muscular hyperactivity is most effectively treated with neuromuscular paralysis and assisted ventilation. Acidification of the urine (eg, for amphetamine overdose) should be avoided, as it may increase the deposition of myoglobin in the kidney and heighten the risk of renal failure.

B. Hypothermia: Hypothermia may be caused by certain drugs, exposure to cold, hypoglycemia, sepsis, or hypothyroidism. The diagnosis may be missed if a rectal thermometer capable of reading temperatures in the range of 24–32 °C (75.2–89.6 °F) is not used.

For severe hypothermia, rapidly restore normal body temperature with warm intravenous fluids, warm gastric or peritoneal lavage, or ventilation with warmed, humidified air. Slow passive rewarming by external means is usually sufficient in milder cases.

Delayed Severe Toxicity

Initial evaluation may fail to reveal the seriousness of poisoning with some drugs. Severe, potentially preventable hepatic damage may occur after acetaminophen overdose unless the physician determines acetaminophen levels and administers the antidote acetylcysteine, when appropriate, early in treatment. Other poisons with characteristically delayed severe toxicity are listed in Table 39–15.

The development of **sustained-release preparations** has increased the chances of nearly normal results on initial evaluation. The possibility that a sustained-release preparation has been used must be

Table 39–15. Selected examples of poisons with delayed severe toxicity.

Poison	Delayed Effect
Acetaminophen	Hepatic necrosis
Amanita mushrooms	Hepatic necrosis
Carbon tetrachloride	Hepatic and renal damage
Methanol	Blindness
Paraquat	Pulmonary fibrosis
Super-warfarins	Bleeding
Thallium	Peripheral neuropathy, hair loss

considered in theophylline or salicylate poisoning, because with these drugs, serum or blood concentrations are used to evaluate the severity of intoxication. Under these circumstances, it is prudent to observe the patient longer and obtain a second blood level reading before deciding on further treatment and disposition.

EMERGENCY TREATMENT OF SPECIFIC POISONINGS

ACETAMINOPHEN

General Considerations

Acetaminophen is an ingredient in numerous over-the-counter and prescription preparations. Because it is frequently combined with codeine and propoxyphene, the more dramatic symptoms caused by these opiates may overshadow the potential toxicity of acetaminophen.

One of the products of the normal metabolism of acetaminophen is hepatotoxic; at toxic levels, it saturates the glutathione detoxification system in the liver and accumulates, causing delayed hepatic injury (24–72 hours after ingestion). The toxic dose of acetaminophen is considered to be over 140 mg/kg. This margin of safety is probably lower in patients who are chronic alcohol abusers, those with liver disease, and those with induced microsomal enzymes.

Diagnosis

Caution: Shortly after ingestion of acetaminophen there may be no symptoms or only anorexia or nausea; hepatic necrosis may not become clinically apparent until 24–48 hours later, when nausea, jaundice, and markedly elevated results on liver function tests may appear. Hepatic failure may follow.

Treatment

A. General Management: Provide intensive supportive care and gastrointestinal decontamination as described on p 733. Activated charcoal should be administered regardless of the possibility that acetylcysteine may be administered (see ¶C, below).

B. Estimate Severity: Obtain a 4-hour postingestion acetaminophen serum concentration measurement, and use the nomogram (Fig 39–1) to predict the range of severity. If the 4-hour level is over 150 µg/mL, begin treatment with acetylcysteine. Because acetaminophen and salicylate are often ingested simultaneously, a measurement of serum salicylate concentration should also be obtained immediately.

C. Start Acetylcysteine Therapy: Acetylcysteine (Mucomyst) substitutes for glutathione and binds the toxic metabolite of acetaminophen, thus inactivating and detoxifying it. Give 140 mg/kg orally of a 10% or 20% solution diluted to 5% with citrus juice or soda. Follow with 70 mg/kg orally every 4 hours for 18 doses or until the serum acetaminophen level is 0. If the patient vomits a dose within 1 hour, it should be repeated; slow drip by nasogastric tube and administration of an antiemetic (eg, metoclopramide, 10–20 mg intravenously) may be helpful. Although intravenous use of acetylcysteine is not yet approved in the USA, it has been successful in Europe.

The effectiveness of acetylcysteine depends on its use early in treatment; it must be given within 12–16

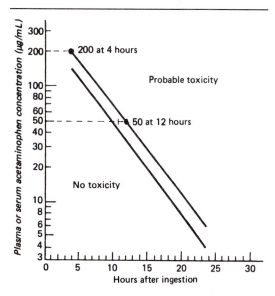

Figure 39–1. Nomogram for prediction of acetaminophen hepatotoxicity following acute overdosage. The upper line defines serum acetaminophen concentrations known to be associated with hepatotoxicity; the lower line defines serum levels 25% below those expected to cause hepatotoxicity. To give a margin for error, the lower line should be used as a guide to treatment. (Modified and reproduced, with permission, from Rumack BM, Matthew M: Acetaminophen poisoning and toxicity. Pediatrics 1975;55:871.)

hours of ingestion of acetaminophen and preferably within 8–10 hours. If there is a history of significant acetaminophen ingestion and if rapid determination of serum acetaminophen levels is not possible, start treatment with acetylcysteine empirically while awaiting the results of laboratory tests.

In the past, activated charcoal was not used with oral acetylcysteine, since the charcoal adsorbs up to 30% of the antidote. Currently, most toxicologists do not consider this a contraindication to use of charcoal. Some give an increased loading dose (190 mg/kg) of acetylcysteine.

Disposition

Use serum concentration of acetaminophen as a guide to the severity of poisoning, and hospitalize all patients requiring acetylcysteine therapy and those with evidence of hepatotoxicity.

AMPHETAMINES & OTHER RELATED STIMULANTS

General Considerations

Amphetamine and other stimulants are widely available, primarily through street sales of illicit drugs but also in the so-called "legal high" diet preparations. These drug combinations may contain varying amounts of methamphetamine, methylenedioxyamphetamine (MDA), caffeine, ephedrine, and phenylpropanolamine. Illicitly obtained stimulants may also contain phencyclidine (p 758). Cocaine is discussed on p 747.

All of these drugs are central nervous system stimulants and cause sympathetic hyperactivity. Some may produce significant vasoconstriction, causing hypertension and bradycardia. Since most of these drugs have short half-lives and since their peak effect and toxicity occur within the first 1–2 hours, serum drug level measurements are of little value, and measures to enhance elimination generally do not alter the outcome.

Diagnosis

Significant amphetamine poisoning is always accompanied by symptoms. Euphoria, mydriasis, and restlessness progress in severe cases to toxic psychosis and seizures. Hypertension may be accompanied by bradycardia or tachycardia, and ventricular arrhythmias may occur. Seizures and hyperthermia may produce rhabdomyolysis and myoglobinuria. Recently, reports have documented severe toxic encephalopathy and even cerebrovascular accidents following relatively moderate doses of phenylpropanolamine.

Treatment

A. Provide intensive supportive care and gastrointestinal decontamination as described on p 733. For severe agitation or psychotic behavior, diazepam, 0.1–0.2 mg/kg intravenously over 1–2 minutes, may be helpful; repeat every 5–10 minutes until sedation has been achieved. Midazolam, 0.05–0.1 mg/kg intravenously (slowly) or 0.1–0.2 mg/kg intramuscularly, or haloperidol, 0.1–0.2 mg/kg intramuscularly, is also effective.

B. Treat seizures with diazepam, followed by phenobarbital or phenytoin or both. (Chapter 11.)

C. If diastolic blood pressure is over 120 mm Hg or if hypertensive encephalopathy is present, give nitroprusside, 0.5–5 μg/kg/min. Alternatively, give phentolamine, 0.1 mg/kg intravenously slowly. Measure blood pressure every 5–10 minutes; the dose may be repeated every 10–20 minutes if necessary.

D. Tachycardia and ventricular tachyarrhythmias may respond to administration of propranolol, 0.05–0.1 mg/kg intravenously.

E. Monitor temperature, and start cooling measures (see p 740 and Chapter 38) if hyperthermia occurs. Check the urine for myoglobin.

F. Acidification of the urine theoretically accelerates elimination of amphetamine but is not recommended, because the efficacy of this mechanism has not been documented, and acidification may accelerate myoglobinuric renal failure.

G. If chest pain is present, perform an ECG, and consider hospitalization to rule out myocardial ischemia/infarction.

H. Patients with seizures may require CT scanning to rule out intracranial hemorrhage.

Disposition

Hospitalize patients with complications (psychotic behavior, hypertension, hyperthermia) or those with prolonged symptoms.

ANTICHOLINERGICS

General Considerations

Atropine, scopolamine, belladonna, many antihistamines, and tricyclic antidepressants are anticholinergics. Many plants (jimsonweed [*Datura stramonium*], nightshade, *Amanita muscaria* mushrooms) also contain anticholinergic compounds.

Diagnosis

These drugs block cholinergic receptors both centrally and peripherally. Significant poisoning is always accompanied by some symptoms or signs, including delirium, blurred vision, mydriasis, hallucinations, coma, dry mucous membranes, inhibition of sweating, hyperthermia, tachycardia, and decreased gastric and bladder motility. Peak effects may be delayed. Convulsions have been attributed to anticholinergics, but no causative relationship has been established. Antihistamines and tricyclic antidepressants cause seizures, but by mechanisms different from their anticholinergic effects.

Treatment

A. Provide intensive supportive care and gastrointestinal decontamination as described on p 733.

B. Physostigmine, 0.01–0.03 mg/kg slowly intravenously, is a specific antidote for anticholinergics; however, it should be reserved for patients with severe symptoms, eg, hyperthermia or tachyarrhythmias. Because of its toxicity (bradycardia, seizures), it generally *should not* be used for hallucinations or as a diagnostic test. Atropine must be readily available when physostigmine is given, and electrocardiographic monitoring is required. Physostigmine is contraindicated in patients with tricyclic antidepressant overdose, asthma, or mechanical bowel or bladder obstruction.

Disposition

Hospitalize patients who have incapacitating signs or symptoms of anticholinergic poisoning.

BETA-ADRENERGIC BLOCKING AGENTS

General Considerations

Beta-adrenergic blocking agents are widely used in clinical medicine to treat hypertension, arrhythmias, angina pectoris, migraine headache, and thyrotoxicosis. Beta-blockers act by competing with catecholamines for a finite number of β_1 and β_2 receptor sites. The β_1 receptors are responsible for increasing the force and rate of cardiac contraction; β_2 receptors mediate vasodilation, bronchial smooth muscle dilation, and a number of metabolic effects, including glycogenolysis. Excessive beta blockade can therefore cause hypotension, bradycardia, bronchoconstriction, and hypoglycemia. In overdose, β_1 and β_2 selectivity is lost, and generalized beta blockade is seen. Some agents (eg, pindolol) possess partial beta agonist activity and may cause hypertension and tachycardia in overdose.

Diagnosis

The main features of massive beta-blocker overdose are hypotension and bradycardia. Pulmonary edema or bronchospasm may also occur, especially in patients with preexisting congestive heart failure or asthma. Hypoglycemia and hyperkalemia are sometimes seen. Convulsions are common with propranolol and other agents (eg, oxprenolol) with high lipid solubility and marked membrane-depressant effects. Seizures have not been reported with atenolol, pindolol, or practolol. The ECG may show sinus bradycardia, first-degree atrioventricular block, prolonged QRS interval, or advanced atrioventricular block. Death is usually due to profound myocardial depression, with advanced atrioventricular block or asystole. The heart may not respond to attempts at pacing, even with high currents.

Blood concentrations of beta-blockers may assist in confirming the diagnosis, but they are not useful in determining the severity of intoxication or the prognosis.

Treatment

A. General management of overdose, including airway protection, treatment of hypoglycemia, and gastrointestinal decontamination should be undertaken as outlined on pp 731–734.

B. Treat hypotension initially with fluids as outlined on pp 731 and 740. If this is unsuccessful, use glucagon, 5–10 mg (100–150 μg/kg) as an intravenous bolus, followed by an infusion of 2–5 mg/h. Glucagon increases intracellular cAMP by a mechanism different from that of beta receptors.

C. Advanced atrioventricular block or bradycardia resulting in hypotension may be treated initially with atropine 0.01–0.03 mg/kg intravenously, or isoproterenol, 0.05–0.3 μg/kg/min by intravenous infusion. Glucagon is also useful. If these are unsuccessful, cardiac pacing may be necessary.

D. Enhance elimination. Because of the relatively large volume of distribution and extensive protein binding, dialysis is not likely to be of value for propranolol overdose. Less lipophilic agents (eg, atenolol, nadolol) have much smaller volumes of distribution and may be eliminated by dialysis or hemoperfusion, but they are less likely to cause profound toxicity.

Disposition

Patients should remain under observation for at least 6–8 hours after ingestion. Patients with significant beta-blocker intoxication (eg, profound bradycardia, conduction abnormalities, hypotension, shock) should be hospitalized.

CALCIUM CHANNEL–BLOCKING AGENTS

General Considerations

Calcium channel blockers are being used with increasing frequency for coronary artery spasm, classic angina pectoris, as well as for systemic and pulmonary hypertension and heart failure. Four calcium channel blockers are currently available: verapamil, nitrendipine, nifedipine, and diltiazem. These agents block the slow calcium channels and have the following cardiovascular effects: they depress sinus node activity, slow atrioventricular nodal conduction, cause coronary and peripheral vasodilatation, and depress myocardial contractility. Verapamil and diltiazem are especially dangerous when there is sinus or atrioventricular nodal disease, Wolff-Parkinson-White syndrome, digitalis therapy, or in patients receiving beta-blockers, quinidine, disopyramide, or other myocardial depressant drugs. Nifedipine is especially dangerous in patients receiving nitrates or beta-blockers and in patients with obstructive valvular heart disease. Nifedipine is more likely to be associated with increased heart rate and vasodilatation than verapamil or diltiazem. Calcium channel blockers may also block insulin release, placing patients who require insulin or oral hypoglycemic agents at special risk for hypoglycemia.

Diagnosis

The main manifestations of calcium channel blocker overdose are hypotension, bradycardia, depressed mental function, and metabolic acidosis. The bradycardia results from varying degrees of atrioventricular block, junctional rhythm, asystole, or sinus bradycardia. The manifestations of an overdose are proportionate to the amount of drug ingested. Analysis of the blood for calcium channel blocker concentrations may assist in confirming a diagnosis but is not useful in quickly determining the severity of the overdose. Hyperkalemia and seizures, which are sometimes observed in overdoses of beta-blockers, are not prominent in overdoses of calcium channel blockers. The ECG shows evidence of bradyarrhythmia with atrioventricular block. Death results from severe myocardial depression leading to asystole.

Treatment

A. General management includes airway protection and gastrointestinal decontamination as outlined on pp 731–734. Induction of emesis may be potentially hazardous, leading to increased vagal tone and worsening of bradyarrhythmias.

B. Constant cardiac monitoring is essential. Appropriate pharmacologic management in seriously ill patients may require placement of central intravenous lines.

C. Leg elevation, Trendelenburg positioning, and fluid management, as outlined on pp 731 and 740, may be required.

D. Advanced atrioventricular block and bradycardia resulting in hypotension may be treated initially with atropine 0.01–0.03 mg/kg intravenously, or isoproterenol, 0.05–0.3 µg/kg/min as an intravenous infusion). Cardiac pacing may be required.

E. In hypotensive patients not responding to the therapy outlined above, calcium solutions have sometimes been successful. Administer 10% calcium chloride, 5–10 mL (adult) or 0.1–0.2 mL/kg (child) intravenously, or 10% calcium gluconate, 10–20 mL (adult) or 0.2–0.4 mL/kg (child). Calcium administration is most beneficial for decreased myocardial contractility and less effective for atrioventricular nodal block and peripheral vasodilatation. Special research drugs that facilitate calcium entry into cells have been used experimentally in the treatment of calcium

channel blocker overdose but are not yet available in the USA.

Disposition

Asymptomatic patients should be observed for at least 8–10 hours. Patients with significant calcium channel blocker overdose should be hospitalized for monitoring and observation.

CARBON MONOXIDE

General Considerations

Carbon monoxide is produced by incomplete combustion of organic materials and is found in engine exhaust, gas heaters, burning charcoal briquettes, and solid alcohol (Sterno Canned Heat, many others). Any fire may also produce large quantities of carbon monoxide.

Carbon monoxide binds to hemoglobin with an affinity about 200 times greater than that of oxygen. The resulting carboxyhemoglobin complex cannot transport oxygen, causing tissue hypoxia that can lead to death or permanent neurologic damage if untreated. Hemoglobin saturation and blood oxygen content are dangerously low despite adequate (or elevated) arterial PO_2 levels.

Diagnosis

Significant poisoning is always accompanied by symptoms, and severity of symptoms usually (but not always) correlates with carboxyhemoglobin levels (Table 39–16). The earliest reliable diagnostic symptom is headache. Usually, PO_2 is normal, although there may be metabolic acidosis due to tissue hypoxia. Using oxygen saturation calculated from PO_2 (based on assumption of normal hemoglobin) or measured by pulse oximetry will provide an incorrect estimate of oxygen-carrying capacity. Blood may be cherry-red, but the patient rarely appears pink. The ECG may show ischemia or infarction in a person with coronary disease. Delayed central nervous system effects such as parkinsonism, memory loss, and personality changes can occur after recovery.

Treatment

Act quickly: Delay in treatment may worsen neurologic damage.

A. Administer 100% oxygen by nonrebreathing face mask or endotracheal tube, *not* by nasal prongs or loose-fitting face mask. Oxygen competes with carbon monoxide for hemoglobin binding sites. The half-life of carboxyhemoglobin in a person breathing room air is 5–6 hours; in 100% oxygen, it is only 1 hour. Hyperbaric 100% oxygen lowers the carboxyhemoglobin level even more rapidly, but it is seldom readily available and its superiority over 100% oxygen has not been proved.

Table 39–16. Clinical findings in carbon monoxide poisoning.

Estimated Carbon Monoxide Concentration (parts per million)	Carboxyhemoglobin (% of Total Hemoglobin)	Symptoms
Less than 35 ppm (cigarette smoking)	5	None, or mild headache.
0.005% (50 ppm)	10	Slight headache, dyspnea on vigorous exertion.
0.01% (100 ppm)	20	Throbbing headache, dyspnea with moderate exertion.
0.02% (200 ppm)	30	Severe headache, irritability, fatigue, dimness of vision.
0.03–0.05% (300–500 ppm)	40–50	Headache, tachycardia, confusion, lethargy, collapse.
0.08–0.12% (800–1200 ppm)	60–70	Coma, convulsions.
0.19% (1900 ppm)	80	Rapidly fatal.

B. Obtain arterial blood for measurement of carboxyhemoglobin content and arterial blood gases.

C. If carbon monoxide poisoning is associated with smoke inhalation, a chest x-ray should be obtained and consideration given to hospitalization and monitoring for development of noncardiogenic pulmonary edema.

D. The use of corticosteroids and mannitol for cerebral edema has been recommended, but their value in preventing late neurologic sequelae remains unproved.

Disposition

All patients with significant carbon monoxide poisoning (chest pain or other evidence of cardiac ischemia, neurologic signs, or carboxyhemoglobin concentrations above 25%) must be hospitalized and given oxygen. Oxygen may be administered in a hyperbaric chamber if it is readily available.

CARDIAC GLYCOSIDES
(Digitalis, etc)

General Considerations

Digoxin, digitoxin, foxglove *(Digitalis purpurea)*, oleander, lily of the valley, and some rodenticides are sources of digitalis and cardiac glycosides.

Cardiac glycosides have multiple effects on cardiac tissue; they enhance cardiac contractility, slow atrioventricular conduction, and enhance automaticity. These effects mediate the severity of toxicity in high doses. Digoxin has a large volume of distribution (6–10 L/kg) and a half-life of about 40 hours; for the most part, it is excreted unchanged in the urine. Digitoxin, on the other hand, has a small volume of distribution, is highly protein-bound, and undergoes extensive enterohepatic recirculation; its half-life is 7 days.

Diagnosis

Most patients with clinically significant cardiac glycoside poisoning exhibit symptoms, although their appearance may be delayed for a few hours after ingestion. Common symptoms include anorexia, nausea and vomiting, diarrhea, and abdominal discomfort. Blurred vision, color vision disturbance (chromatopsia), and neurologic symptoms may also occur. The most serious toxic effects are those that cause rhythm and conduction disturbances in the heart, eg, third-degree atrioventricular block, bradycardia, ventricular ectopy, and paroxysmal atrial tachycardia with atrioventricular block. In patients with chronic atrial fibrillation, digitalis toxicity may cause nonparoxysmal junctional tachycardia, which is characterized by a regular rhythm with narrow QRS complexes and a heart rate of 90–120 beats/min (Chapter 29). Although hypokalemia may aggravate digitalis toxicity in the patient on chronic therapy, acute ingestion of an overdose is often associated with hyperkalemia. Hyperkalemia is probably a better measure of severe toxicity than the serum digoxin level. Therapeutic serum levels of digoxin are 0.5–2 ng/mL; for digitoxin, 18–22 ng/mL.

Treatment

A. General Management: Provide intensive supportive care and gastrointestinal decontamination as described on p 733.

B. Electrolyte Abnormalities: If hypokalemia is present, replace potassium (Chapter 36). For severe hyperkalemia, measures to reduce the potassium level may be necessary (Chapter 36). Avoid the use of calcium, which may potentiate the cardiac toxicity of digitalis. Magnesium replacement may be beneficial.

C. Arrhythmias: (See also Chapter 29.)

1. For symptomatic bradycardia or second- or third-degree atrioventricular block, atropine, 0.5–0.6 mg intravenously, repeated every 5 minutes if there is no response, may be helpful. The total dose should not exceed 2 mg. A transcutaneous pacemaker may be used.

2. For ventricular ectopic beats, both lidocaine and phenytoin are effective, although lidocaine is easier to use. Give 1 mg/kg as an intravenous bolus, followed by 1–4 mg/min by continuous infusion. Phenytoin is often effective in low doses. Start with 5 mg/kg given slowly intravenously (no faster than 0.5 mg/kg/min), and repeat as necessary up to 15 mg/kg.

3. Avoid DC countershock, because it may cause serious conduction and rhythm disturbances in patients with digitalis toxicity. If countershock is unavoidable, use the lowest voltage that is effective.

D. Drug Removal: Dialysis or hemoperfusion is of no value for digoxin because of its large volume of distribution. Digitoxin may be effectively removed by hemoperfusion and by repeated doses of activated charcoal or cholestyramine, which interrupt enterohepatic recirculation.

E. Digitalis Antibodies: Digitalis-specific Fab fragment antibodies are extremely effective and are indicated for patients with serious arrhythmias or severe hyperkalemia. Each vial of Digibind binds 0.6 mg of digoxin. Toxicity usually is reversed within 5–10 minutes, and the digoxin-antibody complex is excreted in the urine. After Digibind administration, serum digoxin levels are elevated owing to cross-reaction of the complex in the assay. For information on use and how to calculate the dosage, call a local regional poison control center (Table 39–1), or consult *Poisindex* or the *Physicians' Desk Reference.*

Disposition

All patients with digitalis and other cardiac glycoside poisoning require hospitalization in a cardiac-monitored unit for observation and treatment. Onset of cardiac toxicity may be delayed 6–12 hours after acute ingestion.

CAUSTICS & CORROSIVES

General Considerations

Corrosive agents include strong acids, alkalis (caustics), oxidizing agents, and other chemicals. They are commonly used in household cleaners (Table 39–17).

A. Acids: Toilet bowl cleaners, bleaches, battery acid, soldering flux (zinc chloride), and many industrial sources contain acids.

B. Alkalis: Lye (drain cleaners, reagent tablets used to detect glucose in urine [Clinitest, many others]), ammonia, and industrial-grade detergents contain caustic alkalis.

The mechanism of toxicity is tissue destruction resulting from coagulative (acids) and liquefactive (alkali) necrosis and heat injury during neutralization of the chemical by water in body tissues. Most household bleaches and detergents are dilute and do not cause severe corrosive burns. Concentrated alkalis are common in the household, especially in granular form or strongly concentrated liquids (pH > 12.5), and these cause severe tissue damage. Corrosive burns may lead to airway or intestinal edema and obstruction, mucosal perforation, and (later) stricture formation.

Diagnosis

Symptoms are almost always present with significant ingestion and include mouth and throat pain, dysphagia, drooling, and substernal or abdominal pain. However, significant gastric or esophageal burns may be present without oral lesions. Skin and eye burns may also occur (Chapters 25 and 37).

Treatment

A. Dilute the corrosive material with plenty of water, normal saline, or milk. *Do not* give neutralizers, since they may increase the heat of hydration and worsen subsequent tissue destruction.

B. *Do not* induce vomiting, as this may produce further tissue damage.

C. After liquid corrosive ingestion, careful insertion of a nasogastric tube and gastric lavage is recommended by some gastroenterologists.

D. Diagnostic endoscopy should be performed in any symptomatic patient with or without oral burns. Whether to perform endoscopy in the asymptomatic patient without oral burns is controversial.

E. No studies support the efficacy of corticosteroids in preventing stricture formation, and the authors do not recommend them. Esophageal or gastric perforation is a contraindication to their use.

F. Prophylactic antibiotics in the absence of overt esophageal or gastric perforation are of unproved value and are not recommended by the authors.

Disposition

Hospitalize all patients known or thought to have ingested or inhaled (aspirated) caustic or corrosive agents with a potential for tissue damage. Skin burns may be managed on an outpatient basis if they are of mild to moderate severity (Chapter 37). Eye injuries should be copiously irrigated and evaluated by an ophthalmologist (Chapter 25).

Table 39–17. Common corrosive agents.

Type	Examples	Injury
Concentrated alkali	Clinitest tablets Drain cleaners Ammonia Lye Oven cleaners	Penetrating liquefaction necrosis
Concentrated acids	Pool disinfectants Toilet bowl cleaners	Coagulation necrosis
Weaker cleaning agents	Cationic detergents (dishwasher detergents) Household bleach	Superficial burns and irritation; deep burns (rare)

COCAINE & LOCAL ANESTHETICS

General Considerations

Cocaine is a natural extract from coca leaves. It is a local anesthetic that also has sympathomimetic effects. Overdoses of all local anesthetics are manifested by initial excitement and seizures, followed by depression of the central nervous system. Peak effects occur rapidly, usually in less than 1 hour.

A. Cocaine: All significant overdoses are associated with symptoms. Intravenous injection of cocaine and inhalation (smoking) of free base, or "crack," cocaine may result in very high levels. Cocaine causes euphoria, excitement, and restlessness; toxic psychosis, seizures, hypertension, tachycardia, dysrhythmias, and hyperthermia may follow absorption of toxic amounts. Myocardial infarction has occurred. The average toxic dose varies, and tolerance develops; a safe dose is probably less than 2–3 mg/kg.

B. Local Anesthetics: Common local anesthetics such as lidocaine, mepivacaine, and procaine have no toxic effects in usual doses. With excessive doses, they cause tremors, anxiety, and restlessness, followed by seizures and then cardiorespiratory depression. Toxic doses for these drugs vary and depend on the route and duration of administration. Maximum recommended doses for infiltration anesthesia in adults are lidocaine, 300 mg; mepivacaine, 400 mg; and procaine, 1000 mg (see Table 24–1). Larger doses may be tolerated if epinephrine has been included in the preparation.

Treatment

A. General Management: Provide intensive supportive care and gastrointestinal decontamination as described on p 733.

B. Cocaine Overdose: Treat manifestations of sympathetic hyperactivity in the same way as for amphetamine overdose. Since effects peak rapidly, measures to enhance elimination of the drug from the body are unnecessary.

Patients with chest pain suggestive of ischemia should be evaluated with a 12-lead ECG and considered for admission to rule out myocardial infarction. Myocardial infarction may be present even with a normal ECG. Patients with a new onset of seizures may need CT scanning to rule out intracranial hemorrhage.

C. Overdose With Common Local Anesthetics: Treatment consists of supportive measures with particular attention to respiratory depression and hypotension. Seizures are usually brief and do not require anticonvulsant therapy.

Disposition

Hospitalize patients with cocaine or local anesthetic poisoning manifested by multiple seizures, hyperthermia, ischemic chest pain, or severe hypertension.

CYANIDE

General Considerations

Fumigants, hydrocyanic acid gas used in industry, amygdalin (Laetrile) in fruit pits (eg, apricot, cherry, peach), and burning plastics and fabrics are sources of cyanide. Cyanide poisoning has also resulted from metabolism of ingested acetonitrile in an artificial nail–removing solution.

Cyanide is a rapidly absorbed cellular asphyxiant that acts by inhibiting the cytochrome oxidase system for oxygen utilization in cells. Death may occur within minutes after a dose of 200 mg. In fatal poisoning, blood levels usually exceed 1–2 µg/mL. Cyanide gas is much more toxic than salt forms because of its rapid absorption.

Diagnosis

Significant poisoning is associated with rapidly developing symptoms, including headache, nausea and vomiting, anxiety, confusion, and collapse. Initial hypertension and bradycardia progress to hypotension, tachycardia, and apnea. The smell of bitter almonds is present occasionally. The skin may appear pink. The measured oxygen saturation of venous blood may be elevated as a result of failure of oxygen uptake by the tissues.

Treatment

Note: *Act quickly. Treatment must be started within 5–10 minutes in cases of severe poisoning in order to be successful.* In witnessed cases of cyanide poisoning, begin therapy without waiting for symptoms. If activated charcoal is available, administer it at once—although its binding affinity for cyanide is low, it can adsorb a lethal dose.

Every emergency department should have a prepackaged cyanide antidote kit containing sodium nitrite, 300 mg in 10-mL ampules (2); sodium thiosulfate, 12.5 g in 50-mL ampules (2); amyl nitrite inhalant, 0.3 mL (12 aspirols); plus syringes and stomach tube (Table 39–18).

A. Nitrites: Nitrites produce methemoglobin, which binds free cyanide.

1. Break a capsule of amyl nitrite under the patient's nose for deep inhalation while starting an

Table 39–18. Prepackaged cyanide antidote kit.[1]

Antidote	How Supplied	Dose
Amyl nitrite	0.3 mL (aspirol inhalant)	Break 1–2 aspirols under patient's nose
Sodium nitrite	3 g/dL (300 mg in 10 mL [vials])	6 mg/kg intravenously (0.2 mL/kg)
Sodium thiosulfate	25 g/dL (12.5 g in 50 mL [vials])	250 mg/kg intravenously (1 mL/kg)

[1]In USA, manufactured by Eli Lilly & Co.

intravenous infusion of sodium nitrite and thiosulfate.

2. Give sodium nitrite, 300 mg (10-mL ampule) intravenously for adults; for children, start with 6 mg/kg. *Caution:* Do not overtreat; fatal methemoglobinemia has resulted from overzealous use of nitrites. After initial therapy, guide subsequent treatment by monitoring symptoms and signs. The goal of nitrite therapy is a methemoglobin level of 25–30%.

B. Thiosulfate: Sodium thiosulfate is a cofactor in the rhodanese enzyme conversion of cyanide to thiocyanate, which is less toxic and readily excreted. Give thiosulfate, 1 mL/kg of 25% solution intravenously.

C. Vitamin B_{12A} (hydroxocobalamin) has been successfully used in Europe and is now available at some poison centers as part of a national study.

Disposition

All patients with suspected or documented cyanide poisoning should be hospitalized.

DRUG-INDUCED METHEMOGLOBINEMIA

General Considerations

Hemoglobin becomes methemoglobin when iron is oxidized from the ferrous to the ferric form. Methemoglobin is a dark chocolate color and can no longer bind oxygen or carbon dioxide. Conversion of hemoglobin to methemoglobin decreases both delivery of oxygen to the tissues and removal of carbon dioxide, and tissue hypoxia may result.

Methemoglobin is produced endogenously in small quantities and is reduced by methemoglobin reductase; normally, less than 1–2% of hemoglobin is methemoglobin. Methemoglobinemia is caused by various oxidant drugs and poisons: nitrites (nitroglycerin, butyl nitrite, amyl nitrite), nitrates (food preservatives, some well water), nitrous gases, chloroquine and primaquine, phenazopyridine (Pyridium, others), sulfonamides, sulfones, aniline dye derivatives, phenacetin, dapsone, benzocaine, prilocaine, and nitrobenzenes.

Diagnosis

Symptoms correlate with the degree of methemoglobinemia. When the level of methemoglobin exceeds 15% of hemoglobin, blood appears chocolate-brown when it is dripped onto filter paper. The exact concentration of methemoglobin in the blood may be determined spectrophotometrically. However, the PO_2 and calculated oxyhemoglobin on routine arterial blood gases are falsely normal, and the measured saturation by pulse oximetry is unreliable.

Conversion of up to 25% of normal hemoglobin to methemoglobin is usually not associated with clinical findings other than peripheral and perioral cyanosis.

At conversion levels of 35–40%, patients experience lassitude, fatigue, and dyspnea. At conversion levels exceeding 60%, coma and death may occur as a result of severe central nervous system depression.

Treatment

A. General Management: Provide intensive supportive care and gastrointestinal decontamination as described on p 733.

B. Give Oxygen: Oxygen per se does not affect the methemoglobin level, but it should be given to improve tissue oxygenation pending the start of specific therapy. Give oxygen, 5–10 L/min, by mask or nasal prongs; in comatose or severely acidotic patients, give 100% oxygen by rebreathing mask or endotracheal tube. Continue oxygen therapy for 1–2 hours after giving methylene blue. Always give oxygen if the percentage of methemoglobin is higher than 40% or if the patient has severe symptoms.

C. Give Methylene Blue: Methylene blue is a specific antidote for methemoglobinemia. The dose is 1–2 mg/kg, or 0.1 mL/kg of a 1% solution, given intravenously over 5 minutes. The dose may be repeated once after 1 hour, but the amount specified should not be exceeded, because an overdose of methylene blue can also cause methemoglobinemia. Patients with glucose-6-phosphate dehydrogenase (G6PD) deficiency may not respond to methylene blue and may experience hemolysis.

D. Remove Source: Discontinue the offending drug or chemical.

Disposition

Patients with methemoglobinemia who show symptoms should be hospitalized for treatment. Some agents (eg, dapsone) may produce prolonged or recurrent methemoglobinemia over several days.

ETHANOL & OTHER ALCOHOLS

Methanol, ethylene glycol, and even isopropanol have been used as cheap substitutes for ethanol, although this practice is less common now than formerly. These alcohols may also be ingested accidentally or in suicide attempts. All are capable of causing intoxication similar to that produced by ethanol, and all can widen the osmolar gap (Table 39–7); however, additional toxic effects occur as a result of the metabolic process.

1. ETHANOL

General Considerations

Ethanol is a central nervous system depressant. It is metabolized by alcohol dehydrogenase (in most cases by fixed-rate, zero-order kinetics) at a rate of about 7–10 g/h, resulting in a decrease in blood alcohol concentration of 20–30 mg/dL/h. The rate of elimination among individuals varies, as does tolerance. In the USA, legal impairment for purposes of driving is generally defined as blood (or breath) ethanol concentrations above 100 mg/dL; coma usually occurs with levels exceeding 300 mg/dL, except in chronic ethanol abusers who have developed tolerance.

Diagnosis

Symptoms of alcohol intoxication include ataxia, dysarthria, depressed sensorium, and nystagmus. The breath may smell of alcohol, but this is neither sensitive nor specific. Coma and respiratory depression with subsequent pulmonary aspiration and trauma are common causes of associated illness and death. Laboratory diagnosis may be aided by direct determination of the blood ethanol concentration or by its estimation from the calculated osmolar gap (Table 39–7).

Treatment

A. Provide intensive supportive care and gastrointestinal decontamination as described on p 733. Supportive care is the primary mode of therapy. Special care should be taken to prevent aspiration.

B. Give glucose and thiamine as needed.

1. Give thiamine, 100 mg intramuscularly or intravenously, to prevent Wernicke's syndrome.

2. Check for hypoglycemia, since ethanol inhibits gluconeogenesis, and give glucose, 50 mL of a 50% solution (25 g of glucose) intravenously over 3–4 minutes, if needed.

C. Diagnose and correct associated disorders such as hypovolemia, hypothermia, infection, trauma, or gastrointestinal tract bleeding.

D. *Do not* use fructose therapy or forced diuresis.

Disposition

Hospitalize patients with ethanol poisoning if ethanol intoxication has caused abnormalities that would of themselves require hospitalization (eg, obtundation, seizures, hypoglycemia).

Complications of Alcoholism

Since many patients who present with symptoms of poisoning are users or abusers of alcohol and other sedative-hypnotics, it is important to distinguish between overdose and withdrawal and complications of alcoholism. The alcohol withdrawal syndrome is well described and usually consists of severe anxiety and tremulousness.

A. Withdrawal Seizures: Seizures generally occur early (6–48 hours after abstinence) and are few in number, brief, generalized, and self-limited. They do not require anticonvulsant therapy.

B. Delirium Tremens: Hyperthermia, tachycardia, disorientation, and hallucinations characteristically occur late (72 hours after abstinence) and are usually not accompanied by seizures. This syndrome of autonomic hyperactivity may be life-threatening and requires specific treatment. Give diazepam, 5 mg intravenously slowly every 5 minutes, until relief of symptoms or mild sedation occurs.

These time patterns are rough estimates, and some degree of overlap often occurs. For withdrawal from other sedative-hypnotics, the time course may be longer.

C. Other Complications:

1. Nutritionally associated complications of alcoholism include vitamin deficiencies (thiamine, folate, and cyanocobalamin) and starvation ketoacidosis (alcoholic ketoacidosis).

2. Hepatic encephalopathy may be confused with alcohol withdrawal syndrome. In hepatic encephalopathy, there is usually evidence of chronic liver disease, lethargy or stupor, and asterixis. Hepatic encephalopathy is commonly associated with gastrointestinal tract bleeding and sepsis and may be aggravated by sedatives.

3. Meningitis may mimic delirium tremens or hepatic encephalopathy.

2. METHANOL

General Considerations

Methanol is found in solid alcohol (Sterno Canned Heat, many others), paint strippers, automobile windshield washer fluid, and many other readily available products. It is metabolized by alcohol dehydrogenase to formaldehyde and formic acid. An osmolar gap and metabolic acidosis with an anion gap result. Optic neuritis (caused by formate) that results in blindness has been described after overdose. Early diagnosis is essential, because permanent blindness or death may result if methanol intoxication is left untreated.

Diagnosis

Early symptoms of intoxication are similar to those caused by ethanol ingestion. As the methanol is metabolized to formic acid (this may be delayed 6–12 hours if ethanol has also been ingested), visual disturbances invariably occur (blurred vision or hazy, snowlike patterns), along with hyperemia of the optic disk, headache, dizziness, and breathlessness. In severe toxicity, seizures and coma may occur.

Examination shows variable degrees of central nervous system dysfunction (agitation and intoxication to coma). The retinas may appear suffused and bright red. Early after ingestion, the only finding may be inebriation with an elevated osmolar gap. Later, severe metabolic acidosis occurs.

Treatment

If serious intoxication is suspected, begin therapy

even before receiving the results of blood methanol concentration determinations.

A. Provide intensive supportive care and gastrointestinal decontamination as described on p 733.

B. Begin infusion of ethanol. Ethanol is metabolized in preference to methanol by alcohol dehydrogenase, thus blocking further metabolism of methanol. The loading dose of ethanol for an average 70-kg adult is 0.7 g/kg (2 mL/kg of 100-proof [50%] ethanol orally; or 7 mL/kg of 10% ethanol intravenously).

Maintain continuous infusion of 0.07–0.1 g/kg/h to keep blood concentration of ethanol between 100 and 200 mg/dL. These levels are sufficient to produce clinically evident intoxication. Ethanol may be given intravenously or orally, but intravenous solutions must be at concentrations of 10% or less to prevent hypertonicity of the solution. Monitor and maintain adequate ventilation during the infusion of ethanol.

A new drug, 4-methylpyrazole, blocks alcohol dehydrogenase and may replace ethanol when it becomes available in the USA (not yet approved).

C. Correct metabolic acidosis with sodium bicarbonate; keep the pH at 7.2 or higher.

D. Folate deficiency increases the toxicity of methanol (in animals), so folate replacement may be helpful.

E. Hemodialysis is indicated for methanol blood concentrations higher than 50 mg/dL and should be started as soon as possible. The ethanol infusion must be adjusted to replace ethanol lost in dialysis (increase ethanol to 0.15–0.2 g/kg/h).

Disposition

Hospitalize all patients with suspected or documented methanol poisoning. If the osmolar gap and anion gap are both normal 1 hour after suspected ingestion, serious intoxication is very unlikely.

3. ETHYLENE GLYCOL

General Considerations

Ethylene glycol is a common ingredient of deicers and antifreeze products. It is sweet-tasting, and some preparations are attractively colored. Following ingestion, it is metabolized by alcohol dehydrogenase to oxalic acid. Symptoms may occur within 30 minutes or after a delay of several hours as calcium oxalate crystals are deposited in various tissues, including the central nervous system, myocardium, and kidneys.

Diagnosis

Nausea and vomiting and headache may progress to stupor, seizures, coma, and renal failure. There are usually no visual symptoms, and the ocular fundi appear normal (as distinguished from their appearance in methanol poisoning). An osmolar gap is present,

and after metabolism to toxic products there is usually a severe acidosis, and crystals of calcium oxalate may be seen in the urine. The urine may be fluorescent under an ultraviolet lamp owing to the fluorescein often added to commercial antifreeze products.

Treatment

Treatment is the same as for methanol intoxication. Hemodialysis is indicated for severe intoxication (serum level over 100 mg/dL, or severe metabolic acidosis).

Disposition

Hospitalize all patients with suspected or documented ethylene glycol intoxication.

4. ISOPROPANOL

General Considerations

Isopropanol is a common ingredient in many household products, especially rubbing alcohol. It causes intoxication with central nervous system depression; blood concentrations of 150 mg/dL are frequently associated with deep coma. It is metabolized by alcohol dehydrogenase to acetone. Both the alcohol and its metabolite cause an elevated osmolar gap. The odor—and acetonemia without acidosis—is characteristic of isopropanol intoxication.

Treatment

Treatment is primarily supportive and similar to that for ethanol intoxication.

Disposition

Hospitalize patients with isopropanol intoxication who have significant signs (eg, stupor or coma).

HEAVY METALS

1. IRON

General Considerations

Iron poisoning results primarily from ingestion of mineral supplements containing divalent iron: ferrous sulfate (20% elemental iron), ferrous fumarate (33%), and ferrous gluconate (12%).

Absorption of iron is dose-related and may increase dramatically with overdose levels, especially when the corrosive action of iron has damaged the intestinal mucosal barrier. Iron also causes vasodilatation and disruption of cellular electron transport. The elemental iron equivalent should be used when toxic doses are being estimated; an amount higher than 20–30 mg/kg causes toxicity, and amounts over 60 mg/kg are potentially lethal. Blood concentrations of iron may assist in the diagnosis of acute toxicity but may be unreliable owing to concurrent absorption of iron and distribution in the tissues. A peak concentration in serum often occurs 4–5 hours after ingestion. Serum concentrations over 400 μg/dL are potentially serious, and levels over 1000 μg/dL are associated with severe poisoning.

Diagnosis

Four stages of intoxication are commonly described:

A. Severe nausea and vomiting and abdominal pain occur within 1–4 hours. Hyperglycemia and leukocytosis are common. In severe cases, hemorrhagic gastroenteritis, shock, acidosis, and coma may follow. A plain film of the abdomen may show radiopaque iron tablets.

B. During the next period, which lasts 6–12 hours and sometimes up to 24 hours, the patient may appear relatively well or may even improve.

C. A third stage of shock, acidosis, and hypoglycemia may occur 12–24 hours after ingestion of significant amounts of iron and reflects a severe course and poor outlook. Serum iron concentrations at this stage may be deceptively low, because most absorbed iron has been taken up by tissues.

D. Late sequelae such as pyloric stenosis, hepatic failure, and residual neurologic damage may occur.

Treatment

A. Provide intensive supportive care and gastrointestinal decontamination as described on p 733. Empty the stomach by induced emesis with syrup of ipecac or gastric lavage. For serious or massive ingestion, enhance removal of iron from the gastrointestinal tract with whole bowel irrigation (p 734). Activated charcoal is not effective.

B. Intravenous chelation with deferoxamine is the treatment of choice when symptoms of iron poisoning are evident or when the serum iron level is over 400 μg/dL (Table 39–19). The iron-deferoxamine complex is excreted in the urine and has a pink color. If urinary output is inadequate, the complex may be removed by peritoneal dialysis or hemodialysis. If iron poisoning is suspected, a trial dose of deferoxamine (80 mg/kg intravenously over 5–6 hours, maximum 1 g) is recommended pending the arrival of results of serum iron level determinations. Pink urine (due to the iron-deferoxamine complex) after this test dose confirms the presence of free iron and indicates the need for further therapy.

C. Observe the patient for several hours when ingestion of significant amounts of iron is suspected, since symptoms in the initial phase may be deceptively mild.

Disposition

Hospitalize all patients with suspected or documented cases of iron poisoning. If patients remain asymptomatic, with a negative abdominal x-ray and no elevation of white blood cell count or blood glucose 6 hours after ingestion, they may be discharged to home care.

2. LEAD

General Considerations

Lead is found in paint in older homes, pottery glazes containing lead (not used commercially in the USA), and fumes from welding, smelting, and battery manufacturing. Gasoline may contain organic lead (tetraethyl lead). Most adult cases of lead poisoning are due to inhalation exposure; chronic ingestion is the most common cause of lead poisoning in children.

Lead is well absorbed from the respiratory tract and usually poorly absorbed from the gastrointestinal tract; target organs are bone, kidney, bone marrow, and the nervous system. Lead toxicity usually occurs with chronic absorption of more than 0.5 mg/d; a single chip of lead-based paint may contain 50–100 mg of lead. Most lead poisoning results from chronic, subacute exposure rather than acute exposure to large amounts.

Diagnosis

Early symptoms of lead poisoning are nonspecific,

Table 39–19. Chelating agents for heavy metal poisoning: indications, dosages, and toxicities.

Metal	Chelating Agent	Dose	Side Effects
Iron	Deferoxamine	10–15 mg/kg/h until serum iron levels fall to less than 400 μg/dL or until urine no longer has characteristic pink color. Higher doses have been used in massive over-doses—consult a poison control center.	Hypotension with rapid intravenous route of administration.
Lead	Edetate calcium disodium (EDTA)	15 mg/kg/dose every 4–5 hours (60–75 mg/kg/d) intramuscularly in 3–6 divided doses for 5 days. Should be started *after* first dose of BAL (see below). May also be given by slow intravenous drip at concentrations no greater than 0.5% (5 mg/mL.).	Reversible acute tubular necrosis; zinc and vitamin B_6 depletion. Do not give orally.
Lead, arsenic, mercury	Dimercaprol (BAL)	3–5 mg/kg/dose intramuscularly every 4 hours for 5 days.	Hypertension, lacrimation, burning lips, nausea and vomiting.
	Penicillamine	100 mg/kg/d (maximum dose 1 g) orally in 4 divided doses on an empty stomach.	Nephrotic syndrome, loss of sense of taste.

eg, listlessness, irritability, headache, abdominal pain, and constipation. Subtle behavioral changes and intellectual impairment may occur in children. With severe toxicity, lethargy, clumsiness, ataxia, seizures, and coma occur. Peripheral neuropathy (lead palsy)—characterized chiefly by extensor muscle weakness with minimal sensory loss—occurs after prolonged chronic exposure. Exposure to organic lead compounds produces a more dramatic acute encephalopathy than does exposure to inorganic lead. Delirium and hallucinations are associated symptoms.

The best standard diagnostic tool is the concentration of lead in the blood. (The concentration in the hair is not useful.) Up to 25 µg/dL is considered normal but may in fact be toxic over long periods, especially in children. Over 70 µg/dL is serious and usually requires hospitalization. Plain films of the abdomen may show radiopaque (ingested) lead in the gastrointestinal tract. Microcytic anemia may be present, and when it is associated with basophilic stippling of red blood cells on the peripheral blood smear, it strongly suggests lead poisoning.

Treatment

A. General Management: Provide intensive supportive care and gastrointestinal decontamination as described on p 733.

B. Chelation Therapy: (See Tables 39–19 and 39–20.) Treatment depends on blood lead concentration; if the hematocrit is less than 20%, adjust the lead level as shown in the following equation:

$$\frac{\text{Normal hematocrit}}{\text{Patient's hematocrit}} \times \text{Blood lead level} = \frac{\text{Corrected blood}}{\text{lead level}}$$

Proceed with treatment as outlined in Table 39–20. The use of dimercaprol (BAL) for treatment of severe

Table 39–20. Treatment of chronic lead poisoning.

Blood Lead Concentration	Treatment
< 25 µg/dL	None. No evidence of recent significant exposure to lead.
25–50 µg/dL	Stop further exposure to lead, and monitor blood lead levels monthly.
50–70 µg/dL	Symptomatic patients: Give dimercaprol (BAL) and EDTA (Table 39–19).
	Asymptomatic patients: Perform EDTA mobilization test. Give EDTA, 500 g/m² or 25 mg/kg (maximum 1 g) intramuscularly or intravenously over 1 hour, and obtain 24-hour urine lead determination. If urine/lead concentration is greater than 1 µg/mg of EDTA, give full course of EDTA chelation therapy (Table 39–19).
> 70 µg/dL	Give dimercaprol (BAL) and EDTA (Table 39–19).

lead poisoning is widely accepted but of unproved benefit.

A new chelating agent, 2,3-dimercaptosuccinic acid (2,3-DMSA), can be given orally and is highly effective.

Disposition

Hospitalize patients with symptoms of severe lead poisoning or blood lead concentrations higher than 70 µg/dL.

3. ARSENIC

General Considerations

Many insecticides, rodenticides, and wood preservatives are sources of trivalent arsenic. The much less toxic pentavalent organic arsenic found in shellfish and other foods produces positive urine screens for arsenic but is not associated with clinical toxicity. Highly toxic arsine gas is produced by burning arsenic-containing ores and is used in the electronics industry.

Arsenic is well absorbed by the respiratory and gastrointestinal tracts, binds avidly to tissue proteins, and accumulates in tissue. The lethal dose of trivalent arsenic is about 100–300 mg in an adult; the pentavalent form is rapidly excreted and less toxic.

Diagnosis

A. Arsenic Salt Ingestion:

1. Acute poisoning–Symptoms include crampy abdominal pain, vomiting, profuse watery diarrhea, a burning sensation in mucous membranes, conjunctivitis, tremor, and seizures. A garlic odor is sometimes noted on the breath. Abdominal plain films may show radiopaque material in the gut. Periorbital edema may occur after 1–2 days.

2. Chronic poisoning–Symptoms include peripheral sensory and motor neuropathy, malaise, anorexia, alopecia, anemia, and stomatitis. These symptoms are also noted during recovery from an episode of acute poisoning.

B. Arsine Gas Inhalation: Arsine gas is highly toxic and causes rapid intravascular hemolysis and renal failure. Other characteristics of arsenic toxicity are often not seen.

C. Laboratory Studies: Measurement of 24-hour urinary arsenic excretion levels is useful but can be misleading, since ingestion of shellfish containing nontoxic forms of arsenic may cause transient elevation of arsenic levels. The chief usefulness of this measurement lies in monitoring the response to chelation therapy. In chronic poisoning, arsenic concentrations are elevated in the hair and nails.

Treatment

A. Acute Poisoning: Provide intensive supportive care and gastrointestinal decontamination as described on p 733. Perform gastric lavage. Give dimercaprol (Table 39–19), and continue until the urine arsenic level is less than 50 µg/24 h.

B. Chronic Poisoning: Although it is of unproved benefit, many toxicologists administer oral penicillamine (Table 39–19). Reversal of neurologic symptoms may be incomplete.

C. Arsine Gas Inhalation: Blood transfusion may be necessary for severe hemolysis. Give adequate fluids to prevent renal hemoglobin deposition. Chelation therapy is of no value for acute exposure to arsine gas.

Disposition

Hospitalize all patients with suspected or documented arsenic poisoning.

4. MERCURY

General Considerations

Elemental mercury vapor is produced in the course of various manufacturing procedures, during repair of mercury-containing instruments, and when the liquid metal is heated (eg, home ore processing). Inorganic mercury salts are present in disinfectants and older cathartics and diuretics. Organic mercury is found in fungicides used in seed grain and in environmentally contaminated seafood.

Mercury is avidly bound to sulfhydryl groups and disrupts cellular enzyme and membrane function.

Diagnosis

A. Elemental Mercury: Liquid mercury is nontoxic if swallowed, but mercury vapor is well absorbed by inhalation and rapidly enters the central nervous system. With large exposure, encephalopathy, gingivitis, and pneumonitis may occur. The predominant manifestations of chronic mercury poisoning are various neuropsychiatric symptoms (erethism): tremor, anxiety, incapacitating shyness, and irritability.

B. Inorganic Mercury: Salts of inorganic mercury are corrosive and irritating to the gastrointestinal tract. Mercurous salts (eg, calomel) are poorly absorbed and generally less toxic than mercuric salts, which cause gastroenteritis with bloody emesis and diarrhea. The target organ is the kidney; acute tubular necrosis is common. Chronic intoxication may cause gingivitis, salivation, dysarthria, intention tremor (mainly of the fingers, eyes, and tongue), nervousness, emotional outbursts, and memory loss.

C. Organic Mercury: Organic mercury (methyl mercury, ethyl mercury) has been implicated in epidemic poisonings resulting from ingestion of seed grain fumigated with mercury compounds or from consumption of heavily contaminated seafood. These compounds are well absorbed and reach high levels in the nervous system. They can also cross the pla-

centa. Tremor and neuropsychiatric symptoms are similar to those occurring with exposure to the vapor of elemental mercury, but the development of peculiar sensory deficits is unique to this type of mercury poisoning. These distinctive symptoms include paresthesias, constriction of visual fields, and loss of hearing, smell, and taste. Incoordination, choreoathetosis, stupor, and incontinence may occur. Uncontrollable crying and laughter are also seen. The developing fetus may concentrate mercury in the central nervous system, with resulting congenital cerebral palsy, mental retardation, and other birth defects.

D. Laboratory Studies: Blood mercury concentrations are helpful; normal levels are less than 5 µg/dL, and symptoms of toxicity are frequent with concentrations over 25 µg/dL. Urine mercury concentrations over 15 µg/L on a 24-hour collection also suggest toxicity.

Treatment

A. General Management: Provide intensive supportive care and gastrointestinal decontamination as described on p 733.

B. Chelation: Dimercaprol (BAL) or penicillamine chelation therapy (Table 39–19) should be used in patients with a history of significant mercury ingestion or chronic toxicity. The prognosis for improvement of neuropsychiatric symptoms is unpredictable, since irreversible neuronal damage may have occurred. A new oral chelating agent, 2,3-DMSA, has recently been approved for use in the USA.

C. Supportive Treatment: Renal failure—a common occurrence after poisoning with inorganic mercuric salts—is treated with general supportive measures, which may include dialysis.

Disposition

Hospitalize all patients with suspected or documented mercury poisoning.

HYDROCARBONS

General Considerations

Hydrocarbons—a large group of compounds that includes petroleum distillates—exert various toxic effects. They are classified by 2 characteristics: viscosity (low-viscosity products are more likely to cause chemical aspiration pneumonia) and their potential for systemic toxicity (central nervous system or cardiac toxicity). These properties are summarized in Table 39–21.

A. High-Viscosity Lubricants: Motor oil, white petrolatum, etc. These are not toxic.

B. Low-Viscosity Compounds With No Known Systemic Toxicity: Furniture polish, mineral spirits, lighter fluid, kerosene, gasoline.

C. Low-Viscosity Compounds With Un-

Table 39-21. Clinical features of hydrocarbon poisoning.

Type	Examples	Risk of Pneumonia	Risk of Systemic Toxicity	Treatment
High-viscosity	Vaseline Motor oil Gasoline	Low	Low	None.
Low-viscosity, nontoxic	Furniture polish Mineral spirits Kerosene Lighter fluid	High	Low	Observe for pneumonia. *Do not* induce emesis.
Low-viscosity, unknown systemic toxicity	Turpentine Pine oil	High	Variable	Observe for pneumonia. *Do not* induce emesis if less than 1-2 mL/kg was ingested.
Low-viscosity, known systemic toxicity	Camphor Phenol Chlorinated insecticides Hydrocarbons (benzene, toluene, etc)	High	High	Induce emesis, or perform lavage. Give activated charcoal.

known or Unproved Systemic Toxicity: Pine oil, turpentine.

D. Low-Viscosity Compounds With Established Systemic Toxicity: Halogenated or aromatic hydrocarbons (benzene, toluene), camphor, phenol, and insecticides.

The major complication following ingestion of petroleum distillates is aspiration pneumonitis, which may occur with poisoning caused by any of the low-viscosity compounds.

Most cases of poisoning are accidental, and exposure is rarely more than a taste (5–10 mL). As little as 1–2 mL of low-viscosity compounds may produce severe chemical pneumonitis if aspirated into the tracheobronchial tree.

Accidental or intentional inhalation of hydrocarbon vapors may produce irritation, nausea, and headache. Exposure to volatile vapors in an enclosed area may result in hypoxia owing to displacement of oxygen from the atmosphere. Inhalation of aromatic (eg, toluene) or halogenated (eg, freons, trichloroethylene) hydrocarbon solvents may cause euphoria, confusion, hallucinations, coma, and cardiac arrhythmias. Chronic exposure to toluene may cause myopathy, hypokalemia, renal tubular acidosis, and neuropathy.

Diagnosis

Symptoms suggesting aspiration are choking, coughing, or gasping immediately following ingestion of a toxic compound. Physical signs of aspiration are often present but may be delayed for up to 4–6 hours; eg, chest x-ray may reveal infiltrates before physical signs appear. Systemic signs of toxicity include narcosis, delirium, and (for certain compounds) seizures. Some of these effects may result from hypoxemia due to pneumonitis. Hydrocarbons may sensitize the myocardium to the arrhythmogenic effects of endogenous catecholamines.

Treatment

Although emesis or gastric lavage of any ingested hydrocarbon may increase the chances of aspiration, ingestion of even small amounts of low-viscosity compounds with known significant systemic toxicity requires either induced emesis or gastric lavage. For example, the camphor contained in 10 mL of Campho-Phenique is sufficient to cause seizures in a child. The toxic dose of benzene or toluene is unknown but may be less than 10 mL.

A. High-Viscosity Lubricants: No treatment is required.

B. Low-Viscosity Compounds With No Known Systemic Toxicity: If there are unequivocal signs of aspiration pneumonitis, protect the airway if necessary to prevent further aspiration, and give oxygen (see Pulmonary Aspiration Syndrome in Chapter 27). There is no evidence that systemic corticosteroids or prophylactic antibiotics are of benefit in aspiration syndrome.

If the patient is asymptomatic and has no history of coughing or choking after ingestion, aspiration is unlikely. *Do not induce emesis,* since it may increase the risk of aspiration. Observe the patient closely for 4–6 hours to detect signs of possible aspiration, and x-ray only those patients who are symptomatic or develop cough or dyspnea while under observation.

C. Low-Viscosity Compounds With Unknown or Unproved Toxicity: It is unclear whether these compounds have inherent systemic toxic effects apart from chemical pneumonitis, and controversy exists regarding the use of lavage or induced emesis to clear a compound of this group from the body. Many authorities currently recommend emesis if more than 1 mL/kg has been ingested, although it is unlikely that most patients could ingest this amount accidentally. Evaluate the patient, and treat for possible pulmonary aspiration, as described above.

D. Low-Viscosity Compounds With Known

Systemic Toxicity: Induced emesis is generally recommended if more than 15–30 mL has been ingested and the child is at home and ipecac is available. However, do not use ipecac with camphor or other agents known to cause rapid onset of seizures. Alternatively, perform lavage with activated charcoal immediately, which may be more effective than emesis in limiting absorption. Activated charcoal is especially useful if the toxin (eg, camphor) is known to produce coma or seizures abruptly. If lethargy, coma, or seizures are present, intubate the patient with a cuffed endotracheal tube, and perform gastric lavage. Evaluate the patient for possible pulmonary aspiration.

Disposition

Hospitalize patients who have ingested low-viscosity petroleum distillates if there are symptoms or signs of systemic toxicity (eg, lethargy, seizures) or pneumonitis (coughing, choking, abnormal findings on chest x-ray). Since delayed onset of pulmonary complications may occur after hydrocarbon poisoning, it is prudent to observe patients for 4–6 hours before discharging them from the emergency department.

INHALANTS
(Toxic Gases & Vapors)

General Considerations

Many toxic inhalants are produced by combustion of household or industrial products in accidental fires (eg, carbon monoxide, phosgene) or as by-products of work activity (eg, welding). Many toxic chemicals exist in gaseous form (chlorine, arsine), and exposure occurs during an accidental spill or leak. Toxic gases can be classified as (**1**) simple asphyxiants, (**2**) chemical asphyxiants and systemic poisons, and (**3**) irritants or corrosives (Table 39–22).

A. Simple Asphyxiants: Methane, propane, and inert gases cause toxicity by lowering the ambient oxygen concentration.

B. Chemical Asphyxiants and Systemic Poisons: Examples include carbon monoxide, cyanide, and hydrogen sulfide. These substances possess intrinsic systemic toxicity that is manifested after absorption into the circulation.

C. Irritants or Corrosives: These substances cause cellular destruction and inflammation when they come in contact with the tracheobronchial tree, usually by producing acids or alkali upon contact with moisture. Gases that are highly water-soluble (eg, chlorine, ammonia) cause immediate irritation, mainly of the upper airway and conjunctiva, whereas gases that are poorly soluble in water (eg, nitrogen dioxide) may be more deeply inhaled, producing delayed lower airway destruction with chemical pneumonitis and pulmonary edema.

Diagnosis

Symptoms and signs vary depending on the toxin. In an accidental fire, combinations of all classes of toxic inhalants may be responsible for symptoms of toxicity, eg, a burning sensation in the eyes and mouth, sore throat, brassy cough, dyspnea, and headache. Look for singed nasal hairs, carbonaceous deposits on the nose and face, upper airway swelling or obstruction, wheezing or signs of pulmonary edema, and manifestations of systemic toxicity. Obtain arterial blood gas determinations, carboxyhemoglobin level measurements, and chest x-ray.

Treatment

A. Remove the patient from the source of toxic gases, and begin supplemental oxygen, 10 L/min, by mask. For victims of smoke inhalation or carbon monoxide poisoning (p 744), give 100% oxygen.

B. Treatment of poisoning caused by chemical asphyxiants and systemic toxins depends on the specific toxin. For cyanide, see p 747; for hydrogen sulfide poisoning, use sodium nitrate, as outlined in the cyanide section. (Although unproved, nitrite therapy may decrease sulfide toxicity by binding it with methemoglobin. Thiosulfate *should not* be used for hydrogen sulfide intoxication, since the enzyme rhodanese is not involved in elimination of sulfide.)

C. For upper airway irritation, humidified oxygen is often effective. Carefully observe the patient for stridor and other signs of progressive airway obstruction that would require endotracheal intubation.

D. For bronchospasm, give nebulized bronchodilators (see Asthma in Chapter 27).

Disposition

Hospitalize all patients with significant symptoms or signs of poisoning caused by inhalation of toxic gases for observation and treatment. Patients exposed briefly to high-solubility irritant gases whose symptoms have resolved can be safely discharged; however, those exposed to low-solubility irritants such as nitrogen oxides or phosgene may experience delayed onset pulmonary edema or chemical pneumonitis and should be admitted for 16–24 hours' observation.

ISONIAZID
(INH)

General Considerations

Isoniazid (INH) is a common antituberculosis drug that is often prescribed in amounts sufficient to provide a 3- to 6-month supply.

The principal manifestations of isoniazid overdose are seizures, metabolic acidosis, and coma. Seizures may be due to depression of gamma-aminobutyric acid (GABA) levels in the central nervous system. Severe metabolic acidosis accompanies recurrent seizure activity. The estimated acute toxic dose is be-

Table 39–22. Clinical features of toxic gases and fumes.

Class of Toxin	Toxin	Source	Clinical Features	Treatment
Simple asphyxiants	Propane	Cooking gas.	All displace normal air and lower F_{IO2}. Symptoms of hypoxemia, without airway irritation.	Remove patient from source; give oxygen.
	Methane	Cooking gas.		
	Carbon dioxide	All fires.		
	Inert gases (nitrogen, argon)	Industry (especially welding).		
Chemical asphyxiants	Carbon monoxide	Fires.	Forms carboxyhemoglobin; inhibits oxygen trasport. Headache is earliest symptom.	100% oxygen.
	Hydrocyanic acid	Industry; burning plastics, furniture, fabrics.	Highly toxic cellular asphyxiant (see section on cyanide).	Use cyanide antidote (Table 39–18).
	Hydrogen sulfide	Liquid manure pits, decaying organic materials.	Highly toxic cellular asphyxiant similar to cyanide; sudden collapse; ability to smell characteristic odor of rotten eggs is rapidly fatigued.	Use sodium nitrite as for cyanide (makes sulmethemoglobin). *Do not* use thiosulfate.
Irritants High solubility in water	Chlorine gas Hydrochloric acid	Industry; swimming pool chemical; bleach mixed with acid at home.	Early onset of lacrimation, sore throat, stridor, tracheobronchitis; with heavy exposure, may progress to pulmonary edema in 2–6 hours.	Humidified oxygen; bronchodilators; airway management.
	Ammonia	Industry; burning fabrics.		
Low solubility in water	Nitrogen dioxide	Burning cellulose; fabrics. Grain silos (acrid red gas).	Has sweet "electric" smell. Delayed onset (12–24 hours) of tracheobronchitis, pneumonitis, and pulmonary edema. Late chronic bronchitis.	Oxygen; observation for 24–48 hours; steroids (controversial).
	Ozone	Inert gas arc welding industry.		
	Phosgene	Burning of chlorinated organic material.		
Allergenic	Toluene diisocyanate	Manufacture of polyurethanes.	Reactive bronchoconstriction; may have long-term effects (chronic obstructive pulmonary disease) in susceptible persons.	Bronchodilators.
Metal fumes	Zinc Copper Tin Teflon	Welding (especially galvanized metal welding).	"Metal fumes fever." Chills, fever, myalgias, headache, nonproductive cough, leukocytosis (4–8 hours after exposure).	Self-limited (12–24 hours).
	Arsine	Burning arsenic-containing ores; electronics industry.	Highly toxic. Hemolysis, pulmonary edema, renal failure; chronic arsenic toxicity.	Exchange transfusion; use dimercaprol (BAL) for chronic arsenic toxicity only.
	Mercury Lead	Industry, welding.	See specific metals.	

tween 80 and 100 mg/kg, although this range may be lower in patients with preexisting seizure disorders, vitamin B_6 deficiency, or chronic alcoholism.

Diagnosis

Symptoms occur one-half to 3 hours following ingestion and include nausea and vomiting, slurred speech, dizziness, lethargy progressing to stupor, hyperreflexia, seizures, metabolic acidosis, hyperglycemia, and cardiovascular and respiratory depression. Symptoms and signs occur promptly after significant poisoning.

Treatment

A. General Management: Provide intensive supportive care and gastrointestinal decontamination as described on p 733.

B. Seizures: Treat seizures with diazepam, as described in Chapter 11. If diazepam is not effective, give pyridoxine (vitamin B_6) in doses equivalent to the amount ingested (gram for gram). If the amount ingested is unknown, start with 5 g (0.1 g/kg) intravenously given over 3–5 minutes, and repeat every 10–15 minutes until seizures are controlled.

C. Drug Elimination: Since the half-life of isoniazid is normally 1–3 hours, measures such as forced diuresis, dialysis, or perfusion are unlikely to be of benefit.

Disposition

Hospitalize all patients who have ingested more

than 80 mg/kg of isoniazid and those who have signs or symptoms suggesting isoniazid poisoning.

LITHIUM

General Considerations

Lithium is frequently used for manic-depressive illness and other psychiatric disorders. It is a monovalent cation like sodium and potassium; unlike these cations, however, it has only a small gradient of distribution across cell membranes and cannot maintain membrane potentials. It is rapidly absorbed into extracellular fluid, with an initial volume of distribution of 0.1–0.2 L/kg. Its distribution into selected tissues then occurs slowly over several hours. Its final volume of distribution is about 1 L/kg. It is excreted unchanged in the urine and actively reabsorbed, with a half-life of approximately 22 hours (with normal renal function). Sodium and water depletion lead to marked increases in the reabsorption of lithium and to elevation of blood concentrations of lithium.

Diagnosis

Symptoms of lithium overdose include apathy, lethargy, tremor, slurred speech, ataxia, and fasciculations, which may progress in severe overdose to choreoathetosis, seizures, coma, and death. Persistent neurologic sequelae may occur. Toxicity is frequently accidental and occurs secondary to chronic sodium depletion, diuretic therapy, and dehydration; in these cases, the serum lithium level is a more reliable index to the severity of overdose, since there has been adequate time for distribution into the central nervous system. In such circumstances, blood concentrations of lithium higher than 2 meq/L are usually associated with toxicity.

In acute overdose, in contrast, initially elevated serum lithium concentrations may be misleading, since distribution into tissues occurs over several hours. For example, an initial "toxic level" of 4 meq/L may easily fall to 1 meq/L with final distribution. Thus, in acute overdose, repeated measurements of serum lithium levels and assessment of mental status (eg, every 4 hours) are more helpful than a single assessment in evaluating toxicity.

Treatment

A. Provide intensive supportive care and gastrointestinal decontamination as described on p 733.

B. The treatment of choice for serious intoxication is hemodialysis. The specific indications for hemodialysis have not been well defined by careful studies, but dialysis should be considered in any patient with obtundation, seizures, or coma, or when serum levels at equilibrium exceed 4 meq/L. However, many patients with high levels do not have serious clinical toxicity. Dialysis is the only route of elimination in patients with renal failure. Hemoperfusion is not effective.

C. Because the drug is reabsorbed in the kidney when sodium and fluids are depleted, administration of intravenous saline may promote lithium excretion. Normal urine flow rates are adequate; the value of forced saline diuresis using large fluid volumes is unclear, and the authors do not recommend it.

D. Activated charcoal does not adsorb lithium and is of no value.

E. In order to prevent chronic (accidental) toxicity, frequent assessment of fluid and sodium balance and lithium levels is recommended in patients treated with lithium.

Disposition

Hospitalize all patients with serum lithium concentrations above 2–3 meq/L and all who show objective signs of lithium intoxication.

OPIATES

General Considerations

Codeine, propoxyphene, and other opiates with varying potencies and durations of action are found in a wide range of prescription analgesic preparations; some, such as dextromethorphan, are found in nonprescription drugs.

The opiates act on central nervous system receptors and cause sedation, hypotension, bradycardia, hypothermia, and respiratory depression. Most opiates have a half-life of 3–6 hours; the major exceptions are methadone (15–20 hours) and propoxyphene (12–15 hours).

Diagnosis

Opiate intoxication should be considered in any comatose or lethargic patient, especially when the clinical findings listed above are present. Pinpoint pupils are a typical sign, although in mixed overdoses, pupils in mid position may be found. Signs of parenteral drug abuse may or may not be apparent. Pulmonary edema may occur. The diagnosis is confirmed if toxic concentrations of opiates are found in blood or urine or if the patient regains consciousness after administration of naloxone.

Clonidine (an antihypertensive agent) overdose may be associated with identical findings, but patients fail to respond to naloxone.

Treatment

A. Provide intensive supportive care and gastrointestinal decontamination as described on p 733. Maintain adequate airway and ventilation.

B. Give naloxone (a specific narcotic antagonist) to all patients with suspected opiate overdose. Start with 0.4–2 mg intravenously. Repeat 3 or 4 times if no response occurs and narcotic overdose is suspected. Some authorities recommend up to 10–20 mg to treat suspected narcotic overdose. Propoxyphene poisoning seems to be particularly resistant to the usual doses of naloxone. Because naloxone has a half-life of 1 hour and effects lasting only 2–3 hours (shorter than many opiates), its effects may wear off before those of the narcotic, permitting the patient to lapse into coma again. If relapse occurs after the first response to naloxone, a naloxone continuous infusion may be started, using approximately the dose required to initially awaken the patient given over each hour.

C. Watch carefully for withdrawal symptoms caused by naloxone. Chronic narcotic abusers who have developed tolerance to opiates may develop acute narcotic withdrawal when naloxone is given. Although this syndrome is not life-threatening, it is a management problem in the emergency department if the patient becomes combative or uncooperative or signs out of the hospital before adequate treatment can be given. Careful titration of the naloxone dose may help to prevent narcotic withdrawal syndrome.

Disposition

Hospitalize and observe all patients thought or known to have ingested significant amounts of opiates and those who relapse after the initial response to naloxone. Patients with heroin overdose who respond to naloxone may be safely discharged if they are asymptomatic 3 hours after the last dose.

ORGANOPHOSPHATES & OTHER CHOLINESTERASE INHIBITORS

General Considerations

Cholinesterase inhibitors are found in a wide variety of insecticides (organophosphates and carbamates) available for home and commercial use (crop sprays, bug bombs, flea collars). Some chemical warfare agents ("nerve gases") are also cholinesterase inhibitors.

These compounds inhibit acetylcholinesterase and therefore allow accumulation of acetylcholine at muscarinic and nicotinic receptors in nerve endings. Organophosphates bind irreversibly with the enzyme, whereas carbamates are considered reversible inhibitors. All are rapidly absorbed from the skin, gastrointestinal tract, and respiratory tract. Toxicity and potency vary widely. Workers constantly exposed to organophosphates and infants with underdeveloped cholinesterase activity are at greater risk for intoxication.

Diagnosis

Miosis, excessive salivation, bronchospasm, hyperactive bowel sounds, and lethargy typically occur shortly after exposure. Either bradycardia (musca-

rinic effect) or tachycardia (nicotinic effect) may be observed. Symptoms of toxicity are easily remembered with the aid of the mnemonic DUMBELS (*D*iarrhea; *U*rination; *M*iosis; *B*ronchorrhea, *B*radycardia, *B*ronchospasm; *E*xcitation with muscle fasciculation, anxiety, and seizures; *L*acrimation; and *S*alivation). Death is usually caused by respiratory depression.

Measurement of the plasma or red blood cell cholinesterase level is helpful in confirming acute toxicity; cholinesterase levels become low soon after exposure.

Treatment

A. Provide intensive supportive care and gastrointestinal decontamination as described on p 733. Careful management of the airway is important, because significant bronchial secretions, bronchospasm, and hypoventilation may occur. Position the patient so as to avoid aspiration, and provide suction as required. Give supplemental oxygen, 5 L/min, by mask or nasal prongs. Intubation may be required.

B. Remove and isolate the patient's clothing, and carefully wash the skin with soap and water. Medical personnel should be careful to avoid cross-contamination.

C. Atropine is a symptomatic treatment for muscarinic signs (salivation, bronchorrhea, bronchospasm, sweating). Large doses may be required. Start with 1–2 mg intravenously (0.5 mg in children), followed by repeated doses of 2–4 mg every 5–10 minutes until signs of atropinization occur: flushing, mydriasis, drying of secretions, and tachycardia. The use of up to 50 mg in 24 hours is not unusual.

D. Pralidoxime (Protopam, 2-PAM) competitively inhibits binding of organophosphates to acetylcholinesterase and should be given to all patients with significant intoxication. It is not required for carbamate poisoning, since the toxicity of carbamate is transient. The dose is 1–2 g (children: 25–50 mg/kg) in saline intravenously over 5–10 minutes. The dose may be repeated every 3–4 hours or given as a constant infusion. Adequate renal function is a prerequisite for use of pralidoxime, since it is excreted in the urine.

Disposition

Hospitalize all patients with suspected or documented serious organophosphate poisoning. Poisoning by carbamates is usually transient, and patients experiencing rapid recovery may be discharged.

PHENCYCLIDINE (PCP)

General Considerations

Phencyclidine (PCP)—a common adulterant of marihuana, amphetamines, and street hallucinogens—is also called "angel dust" or "crystal." It may be smoked, snorted, ingested, or injected.

Phencyclidine is a sympathomimetic, hallucinogenic, dissociative agent originally used as a veterinary anesthetic. It has a rapid onset of action when smoked or snorted, causing euphoria and hallucinations. Serious overdose does not usually occur with smoking, since users can titrate the dose to achieve the desired effect. Ingestion of 20–25 mg of phencyclidine can cause severe intoxication. Phencyclidine has a very large volume of distribution (2–4 L/kg), with a half-life of several hours to days. As a weak base, it is ionized in acidic media such as the stomach and acidic urine. It is eliminated primarily by metabolism. Since only about 10% is excreted in the urine, increasing urinary output or urinary acidification (to cause ion trapping) is unlikely to increase elimination of the drug significantly.

Diagnosis

Symptoms typically fluctuate, with patients alternating unpredictably from severe agitation to quiet stupor. Bizarre, paranoid behavior and extreme violence may occur unexpectedly. Both vertical and horizontal nystagmus are common. The pupils may be large or small. Hypertension, tachycardia, and hyperthermia are common. Marked muscle rigidity, dystonias, and seizures may occur. Hyperthermia and rhabdomyolysis resulting in myoglobinuria and renal failure are a major cause of subsequent illness. The diagnosis is made primarily on clinical grounds but may be confirmed by demonstrating phencyclidine in urine or gastric aspirate. Serum phencyclidine concentrations are not of value in emergency management.

Treatment

A. General Management: Provide intensive supportive care and gastrointestinal decontamination as described on p 733. Most instances of phencyclidine intoxication are mild and self-limited, and patients need no specific treatment other than to be in a quiet and supportive environment.

B. Moderate to Severe Poisoning: Diazepam, 2–5 mg intravenously every 30 minutes until sedation is achieved, is effective in controlling moderate agitation or anxiety.

Haloperidol, 5–10 mg intravenously, may also be effective in controlling toxic psychosis. The goal of treatment is to prevent complications stemming from muscular hyperactivity and subsequent hyperthermia and rhabdomyolysis.

C. Rhabdomyolysis or Myoglobinuria: If the patient has rhabdomyolysis or myoglobinuria, maintain urine output with intravenous fluids and mannitol. Alkalization of urine is recommended in order to minimize renal deposition of myoglobin. (See also Chapter 12.)

D. Enhanced Elimination: Because phencyclidine has a large volume of distribution, dialysis procedures are not useful. Acidification of the urine with ammonium chloride or hydrogen chloride has been used, but it does not significantly increase the total elimination rate, and it is not recommended. There is also evidence that aciduria may worsen myoglobinuric renal toxicity.

Disposition

Hospitalize patients with moderate to severe phencyclidine poisoning, particularly if hyperthermia, severe muscular rigidity, or evidence of rhabdomyolysis is an accompanying manifestation.

PHENOTHIAZINES & OTHER ANTIPSYCHOTICS

General Considerations

Chlorpromazine (Thorazine, many others), prochlorperazine (Compazine), haloperidol (Haldol, others), and many other phenothiazines and butyrophenones are antipsychotic drugs.

The mechanism of toxicity of the antipsychotics is complex. Antiadrenergic properties cause sedation and hypotension; anticholinergic effects are manifested by dry mouth and tachycardia; and antidopaminergic properties may produce extrapyramidal side effects (most commonly seen with haloperidol). The contribution of each of these effects in cases of drug overdose depends on the specific drug and on the individual patient. Most of these compounds have large volumes of distribution (10–30 L/kg) and long half-lives (12–30 hours); dialysis is not effective.

Diagnosis

Extrapyramidal side effects may occur even at therapeutic doses and include dystonic posturing, spasm of orofacial muscles, cogwheel rigidity, and spasticity. With acute overdose, sedation, miosis, and hypotension are common. Coma and seizures may occur with very large ingestions. Prolongation of the QT interval and ventricular arrhythmias may occur. Disruption of the temperature-regulating mechanism may lead to hyperthermia or hypothermia. Abdominal x-rays may show radiopaque tablets in the gut.

Treatment

A. General Management: Provide intensive supportive care and gastrointestinal decontamination as described on p 733. Treat hypotension with intravenous crystalloid solution; if a vasopressor is needed, norepinephrine is preferable.

B. Extrapyramidal Reactions: Diphenhydramine (Benadryl, many others), 0.5–1 mg/kg intravenously slowly; or benztropine (Cogentin), 1–2 mg intramuscularly for adults, is recommended for extrapyramidal reactions. Relapse may occur; dispense oral anticholinergics for 2–3 days. Sophisticated drug-seeking patients have been known to simulate dystonias in order to receive these medicines.

Disposition

Hospitalize patients with suspected or documented poisoning due to antipsychotics. Indications of significant poisoning include (1) a large number of pill fragments found in the stomach or intestines by means of lavage, emesis, or abdominal plain film; (2) rapidly worsening clinical findings; and (3) obtundation. Patients with extrapyramidal reactions who respond to anticholinergic therapy may be discharged.

POISONOUS MUSHROOMS

General Considerations

There are over 5000 varieties of mushrooms in the USA, about 100 of which can be toxic. Most poisonous mushrooms act as gastrointestinal irritants. Table 39–23 lists the 6 major types of poisonous mushrooms, symptoms, and treatment. The most significant are *Amanita phalloides* and other mushrooms containing amatoxin, which may produce fatal hepatic necrosis.

Assistance with identification of specimens can often be obtained from a university biology department or mycology society. *Poisindex* and regional poison control centers may also help with identification. However, since accurate identification of mushrooms is difficult without an experienced mycologist and impractical because many types of mushrooms are often ingested at one time, the best approach to mushroom ingestion is to assume that the most toxic types have been consumed. *Delayed* onset (6–12 hours) of gastrointestinal symptoms suggests amatoxin or monomethylhydrazine poisoning.

Treatment

A. Provide intensive supportive care and gastrointestinal decontamination as described on p 733.

B. When it is not known what kinds of mushrooms have been consumed, induce emesis. Nasogastric tubes are too small to remove segments. Give activated charcoal after emesis has occurred.

C. If poisoning with amanitin toxin (amatoxin) is suspected, hospitalize the patient for observation, and obtain baseline hepatic and renal function measurements. Although a variety of potential antidotes have been recommended, including corticosteroids, penicillin G, thioctic acid, silibinin, and other drugs, none has been proved to work. More important than specific antidotes is supportive care, including aggressive fluid replacement for massive gastroenteritis, supplemental glucose, and supportive treatment for hepatic encephalopathy. Several patients with massive hepatic necrosis have been successfully treated with hepatic transplantation.

D. Specific treatment for various kinds of mushroom poisoning is set forth in Table 39–23.

Disposition

Hospitalize patients thought or known to have ingested mushrooms known to cause serious poisoning (Table 39–23).

POISONOUS PLANTS

General Considerations

There are several hundred species of plants in the USA that contain toxic compounds. Some examples of nontoxic and toxic plants are set forth in Tables 39–24 and 39–25. Details about identification, mechanism of toxicity, and treatment are best obtained

Table 39–23. Poisonous mushrooms.[1]

Toxin	Genus	Symptoms and Signs	Onset	Treatment
Amatoxin	*Amanita (A phalloides, A verna, A virosa)*	Severe gastroenteritis, followed by delayed hepatic and renal failure after 48–72 hours.	6–24 hours	Supportive. Correct dehydration. Thioctic acid is of unproved benefit.
Muscarine	*Inocybe, Clitocybe*	Muscarinic (salivation, miosis, bradycardia, diarrhea).	30 minutes to 1 hour	Supportive. Give atropine, 0.5–2 mg intravenously, for severe cholinergic symptoms and signs.
Ibotenic acid, muscimol	*Amanita muscaria* ("fly agaric")	Anticholinergic (mydriasis, tachycardia, hyperpyrexia, delirium).	30 minutes to 2 hours	Supportive. Give physostigmine, 0.5–2 mg intravenously, for severe anticholinergic symptoms and signs.
Coprine	*Coprinus*	Disulfiramlike effect occurs with ingestion of ethanol.	30 minutes to 2 days	Supportive. Abstain from ethanol for 3–4 days.
Monomethyl-hydrazine	*Gyromitra*	Gastroenteritis; occasionally hemolysis, hepatic and renal failure.	6–12 hours	Supportive. Correct dehydration. Pyridoxine, 2.5 mg/kg intravenously, may be helpful.
Psilocybin	*Psilocybe*	Hallucinations.	15–30 minutes	Supportive.
Gastrointestinal irritants	Many species	Nausea and vomiting, diarrhea.	30 minutes to 2 hours.	Supportive. Correct dehydration.

[1]Modified and reproduced, with permission, from Becker CE et al: *West J Med* 1976;125:100.

Table 39–24. Some nontoxic plants.

African violet (*Saintpaulia ionantha*)
Baby tears (*Helxine soleirolii*)
Bridal veil (*Genista monosperma pendula*)
Coleus species
Fuchsia species
Gardenia (*Gardenia radicans*)
Jade plant (*Crassula argentea*)
Piggyback Begonia (*Begonia hispida cucullifera*)
Piggyback plant (*Tolmiea menziesii*)
Rubber plant (*Ficus elastica "Decora"*)
Spider plant (*Chlorophytum comosum*)
Swedish ivy (*Plectranthus australis*)
Wandering Jew (*Tradescantia albiflora, T fluminensis, Zebrina pendula*)
Zebra plant (*Calathea zebrina*)

Table 39–25. Some poisonous plants.[1]

Plant name	Type of Toxin
Azalea (*Rhododendron* species)	Andromedotoxin (nicotinelike and cardiotoxic)
Black nightshade (*Solanum nigrum*)	Solanine
Caladium	Oxalates
Castor bean (*Ricinus communis*)	Toxalbumin (ricin)
Deadly nightshade (*Atropa belladonna*)	Anticholinergic
Delphinium	Nicotinelike
Dumb cane (*Dieffenbachia*)	Oxalates
Elderberry (*Sambucus*)	Cyanogenic (ripe berries nontoxic)
Foxglove (*Digitalis purpurea*)	Cardiac glycosides
Hydrangea	Cyanogenic
Jequirity bean, rosary bean (*Abrus precatorius*)	Toxalbumin (a lectin)
Jerusalem cherry (*Solanum pseudocapsicum*)	Solanine
Jimsonweed (*Datura stramonium*)	Anticholinergic
Lantana	Anticholinergic
Lily of the valley (*Convallaria majalis*)	Cardiac glycosides
Lobelia	Nicotinelike
Mistletoe (*Viscum album, Phoradendron flavescens*)	Tyramine (hypertension; gastroenteritis)
Mountain laurel (*Kalmia latifolia*)	Andromedotoxin (nicotinelike and cardiotoxic)
Oleander (*Nerium oleander*)	Cardiac glycosides
Philodendron	Oxalates
Pits (of cherry, apricot, peach)	Cyanogenic (amygdalin)
Poison hemlock (*Conium maculatum*)	Nicotinelike
Poinsettia (*Euphorbia pulcherrima*)	Oxalatelike
Tobacco (*Nicotiana tabacum*)	Nicotine
Water hemlock (*Cicuta maculata*)	Cicutoxin (seizures)
Yew (*Taxus* species)	Taxine (gastroenteritis, cardiac toxicity)

[1]This short list is for illustrative purposes only. Consult other sources (eg, regional poison control center) for information on specific plants.

from a local poison control center or from *Poisindex.* When the identity of a plant is unknown, it is helpful to take along a sample to a local nursery or to a botanist. Gardening books are also useful sources of identification.

It is important to treat the specific symptoms manifested by the patient, not those thought to be associated with the type of poisonous plant believed to have been ingested. Many similar species of plants have widely varying potencies and combinations of toxins; the age of the plant, soil condition, and other factors all influence the severity of toxic symptoms.

Classes of Toxins

Some of the more common plant toxins are described below. The list is not complete.

A. Oxalates: Insoluble calcium oxalate crystals in the leaves and stems of some plants irritate the mucous membranes and can cause edema of the mouth, throat, and tongue. In rare severe reactions, drooling, dysphagia, and airway obstruction may occur. Renal failure may occur if sufficient amounts of oxalates are absorbed.

B. Amygdalin and Cyanogenic Glycosides: Cyanide is produced by the gastrointestinal hydrolysis of chewed-up fruit pits or seeds. (*Prunus* species: cherry, apricot, peach) or leaves and stems (*Hydrangea,* elderberry). Severe poisoning is uncommon. See the section on cyanide poisoning for details of symptoms and therapy.

C. Cardiac Glycosides: Digitalis and similar compounds are present in varying amounts in certain plants. Death after consumption of only one oleander leaf has been reported (see Cardiac Glycosides).

D. Anticholinergics: The typical anticholinergic syndrome of dry mouth, tachycardia, delirium, urinary retention, and mydriasis is seen. Most poisonings are mild, and supportive treatment is sufficient (see Anticholinergics).

E. Nicotinelike Toxins: These toxins include nicotine, coniine, and aconitine. Symptoms include nausea and vomiting, salivation, diarrhea, restlessness, and seizures. Mydriasis may also occur. Fol-

lowing an initial phase of excitement, respiratory depression and hypotension may occur.

F. Solanine: Solanine has effects similar to those of nicotine. In addition, plants containing solanine often have significant amounts of atropinic alkaloids, so that the net effect is unpredictable. Onset of symptoms may be delayed several hours.

G. Toxalbumins: These highly toxic compounds (eg, abrin, ricin, phallin) can cause acute gastroenteritis, dehydration, and shock. Convulsions, hemolysis, and renal and hepatic injury can also occur. Oral and esophageal irritation or burns may be seen.

Treatment

In general, emesis is recommended after ingestion of any unidentified plants or those with known potentially serious toxic effects. Follow emesis with activated charcoal, a cathartic, and symptomatic treatment as needed. Keep the patient under observation. Begin specific treatment as indicated for the specific toxins involved.

Disposition

Disposition depends on the plant ingested and the symptoms experienced.

SALICYLATES

General Considerations

Salicylates are present in numerous prescription and nonprescription medications, eg, analgesics, bismuth subsalicylate (Pepto-Bismol, many others), or oil of wintergreen (methyl salicylate).

The mechanism of toxicity with salicylate poisoning is complex and includes direct central nervous system stimulation, uncoupling of oxidative phosphorylation, inhibition of Krebs cycle enzymes, and interference with hemostatic mechanisms. The volume of distribution is dose-dependent and usually small; with significant ingestion, however, redistribution of the drug into the central nervous system occurs. Because salicylate is a weak acid, acidemia increases its penetration of the central nervous system. The half-life may increase from 2 to 20 hours at overdose levels as a result of saturation of liver metabolism. The elimination of salicylate is increased in alkaline urine. The minimum acute toxic dose is 150 mg/kg, with severe toxicity occurring at doses over 300–500 mg/kg. However, many cases of toxicity are a result of prolonged overtreatment of minor illnesses ("subacute" or "accidental" overdose). The chronically ill and the elderly are at greater risk for subacute toxicity because of relative hypoalbuminemia and renal insufficiency.

Diagnosis

Early manifestations of overdose include nausea and vomiting, tinnitus, listlessness, and hyperventilation. Loss of fluid and electrolytes is common. Initial respiratory alkalosis is followed by severe metabolic acidosis, hypokalemia, and hypoglycemia. Seizures, hyperpyrexia, and coma occur as toxicity becomes more severe. Measurement of the blood salicylate concentration is essential for effective management, although it is not as reliable an indicator of the severity of illness if subacute toxicity is present. In cases of acute salicylate ingestion, the Done nomogram (Fig

39–2), combined with a 6-hour blood salicylate concentration reading, helps to predict toxicity if serum pH is normal. In the presence of acidosis, toxicity occurs with considerably lower levels. Salicylate determinations should be repeated every 4–6 hours. Repeated measurements are especially important for ingestion of sustained-release or enteric-coated preparations, which are absorbed slowly and which may result in delayed peak levels.

With subacute ("accidental") toxicity, severity of poisoning does not correlate well with serum salicylate concentration, but levels above 30 mg/dL (300 mg/L) are significant. Patients with subacute toxicity are frequently very young or very old, and they usually present with dehydration, obtundation, and acidosis. The diagnosis is often missed while the physician concentrates on the more prominent secondary complications. Cerebral and pulmonary edema and death are more common in patients with subacute toxicity.

A Phenistix test of urine may be positive (purple or purple-brown) with salicylate toxicity, but false-negative results have been reported in patients with acid urine.

Treatment

A. Provide intensive supportive care and gastrointestinal decontamination as described on p 733. After acute overdose, give adequate charcoal to bind ingested salicylate; several doses of 50–100 g may be

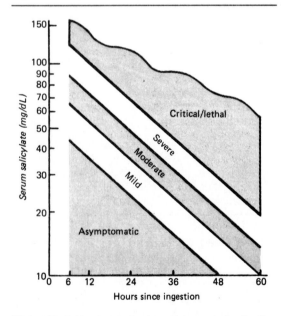

Figure 39–2. Nomogram for determining severity of salicylate intoxication. Absorption kinetics assume acute (1-time) ingestion of non–enteric-coated preparation. ***Note:*** Units are in mg/dL; many laboratories now report serum levels in mg/L, which are 10-fold higher. (Redrawn and reproduced, with permission, from Done AK: Salicylate intoxication: Significance of measurement of salicylate in blood in cases of acute ingestion. Pediatrics 1960;26:800.)

necessary to achieve a goal of 10:1 ratio of charcoal:salicylate.

B. Correct dehydration, hypoglycemia, hypokalemia, and acidosis. For significant dehydration, start with 20 mL/kg of an intravenous crystalloid solution given over 1–2 hours, and then give 3–5 mL/kg/h. To correct acidosis and promote excretion of salicylate in the urine, give sodium bicarbonate, 1 meq/kg/h. Concurrent correction of potassium deficit is mandatory. Urine pH should be maintained at 7–7.5. Alkalization of the urine is often unsuccessful in critically ill patients (especially the elderly), and it may aggravate pulmonary and cerebral edema.

C. Hemodialysis is recommended for critically ill patients with persistent seizures, acidosis that fails to respond to treatment, or high salicylate concentrations (eg, > 120 mg/dL [1200 mg/L] at 6 hours). Hemodialysis is efficient in removing salicylate and can help to correct pH and electrolyte abnormalities. Consider early hemodialysis in ill patients with subacute overdose. Although there are no proved guidelines, elderly patients with serum salicylate levels over 60 mg/dL and those with significant neurologic toxicity should probably receive immediate hemodialysis.

D. Obtain measurements of serum salicylate every 4–6 hours to monitor adequacy of treatment.

E. If there is evidence of salicylate-induced hypoprothrombinemia, give vitamin K, 10 mg intramuscularly.

F. Rehydration and rapid correction of acidemia are essential. Give glucose, and replace potassium deficits.

Disposition

Hospitalize all patients with known or suspected severe salicylate poisoning. Patients who have ingested enteric-coated tablets (eg, Ecotrin) may remain asymptomatic for several hours or even days; repeated blood levels and abdominal x-rays or even endoscopy may be necessary if a massive ingestion is suspected.

SEDATIVE-HYPNOTICS

General Considerations

Sedative-hypnotics include a broad range of drugs used to treat anxiety or insomnia. They can induce tolerance and can cause a withdrawal syndrome similar to that associated with ethanol withdrawal (except for time of onset and duration). These agents are found singly and in various drug combinations.

Absorption, distribution, and elimination of sedative-hypnotics vary. Brief descriptions of the kinetic parameters of several common sedative-hypnotics are listed in Table 39–26. In general, the mechanism of toxicity of these drugs is depression of the central nervous system similar to that caused by ethanol.

Diagnosis

Clinical manifestations of overdose include nystagmus, ophthalmoplegia, ataxia, dysarthria, lethargy, somnolence, respiratory depression, hypotension, and hypothermia. With the onset of deep coma, oculocephalic reflexes are lost, and the pupils become nonreactive to light. The initial EEG may be flat, although the patient may subsequently recover completely. Serum drug levels may be misleading, since levels of intoxication and rate of elimination vary enormously from person to person, depending on prior drug use and the patient's physical state.

Table 39–26. Pharmacokinetic data on common sedative-hypnotic drugs.

	Volume of Distribution (V_d)(L/kg)	Disappearance Half-Time ($t_{1/2}$)		Maximum Therapeutic Level (µg/mL)	Treatment	Comments
		Normal (hours)	Overdose (hours)			
Chloral hydrate (Noctec, many others)	0.6	4–8	10–20	15	Supportive.	Gastritis; arrhythmias; pills are radiopaque.
Diazepam (Valium, Valrelease, many others)	1–2	30–70	50–140	5	Supportive.	Severe overdose uncommon unless combined with other drugs.
Ethchlorvynol (Placidyl)	3–4	10–20	20–100	100	Supportive. Hemoperfusion in severe poisoning.	Pink or green gastric aspirate with pungent odor; prolonged coma with overdose.
Glutethimide (Doriden, many others)	20–25	8–12	24–40	0.5	Supportive.	Cyclic variation in mental status; mydriasis.
Pentobarbital (Nembutal, others)	1–2	20–30	50	50	Supportive.	More lipid-soluble and shorter-acting than phenobarbital.
Phenobarbital (Luminal, many others)	0.75	60–100	70–120	30	Supportive. Hemoperfusion in severe poisoning.	Avoid fluid overload. Repeated doses of charcoal by gastric tube may hasten elimination.

Treatment

A. Provide intensive supportive care and gastro-intestinal decontamination as described on p 733. Treat shock and hypotension with an initial bolus (p 740) of 200–1000 mL of intravenous crystalloid solution (Chapter 3). Restore the patient's core temperature to normal levels, since hypothermia will worsen hypotension. Monitoring the pulmonary capillary wedge pressure is helpful in avoiding fluid overload and determining the need for pressor agents. Vasopressors should be used only if adequate fluid replacement is ineffective (as determined by pulmonary capillary wedge pressure measurements).

B. Reserve hemodialysis or hemoperfusion for those patients who remain hypotensive or otherwise unstable despite aggressive supportive care. These measures successfully remove only a few sedative-hypnotics (eg, phenobarbital, meprobamate, ethchlorvynol).

C. The benzodiazepine antagonist flumazenil (Mazicon) is now available: the dose is 0.2 mg IV slowly repeated every 5–10 minutes as needed, up to a maximum 3–5 mg. Effects wear off in 1–3 hours and resedation is common. Contraindications include known seizure disorder, benzodiazepine addiction, and tricyclic antidepressant overdose.

Disposition

Hospitalize patients with sedative-hypnotic drug poisoning resulting in depression of vital reflexes (eg, respiration, gag reflex).

THEOPHYLLINE & METHYLXANTHINES

General Considerations

Theophylline causes bronchodilatation; gastric, central nervous system, and cardiac stimulation; and vasodilation. The half-life is between 4 and 8 hours. The half-life is shortened in chronic smokers and prolonged in patients with congestive heart failure or cirrhosis. In acute overdose, the half-life may be markedly prolonged (up to 50 hours).

The minimum acute toxic dose is over 10 mg/kg, or 700 mg, in the average adult. Since metabolism of the drug varies markedly depending on the clinical status of the patient, careful monitoring of patients receiving therapeutic doses is necessary to avoid iatrogenic toxicity.

Diagnosis

Mild symptoms of toxicity are nausea and vomiting, abdominal cramps, tremor, and anxiety. Arrhythmias and seizures occur with more serious intoxication. Seizures are often refractory to treatment with standard anticonvulsants. Acute single overdose has different characteristics from chronic, subacute overmedication: **(1) Acute overdose** is characterized by hypotension, tachycardia, and hypokalemia. Seizures and serious arrhythmias are common with levels over 100 mg/L but rare with levels under 90 mg/L; and **(2) chronic intoxication** may result in seizures and arrhythmias with much lower serum levels (ie, 20–70 mg/L). Hypotension and hypokalemia are uncommon.

Sustained-release theophylline preparations are now commonly used, so that after acute overdose, early blood concentrations of the drug may be low and gastrointestinal symptoms may be absent.

Treatment

A. General Management: Provide intensive supportive care and gastrointestinal decontamination as described on p 733.

B. Gastrointestinal Decontamination: If a significant dose has been ingested, induce emesis or perform lavage even if spontaneous emesis has already occurred. Consider whole bowel irrigation.

C. Treat Seizures: Seizures (Chapter 11) are usually very difficult to control with standard drugs. Start with diazepam, 0.1–0.2 mg/kg as an intravenous bolus, followed by phenobarbital, 15 mg/kg, intravenously over 20–30 minutes. Perform hemoperfusion immediately if seizures are not controlled.

D. Hypotension: Treat hypotension with intravenous fluids. Propranolol, 0.02–0.05 mg/kg, or esmolol, 25–50 µg/kg/min, intravenously, may successfully reverse hypotension and tachycardia, which are both mediated by excessive beta-adrenergic stimulation.

E. Arrhythmias: Ventricular tachyarrhythmias and rapid atrial fibrillation may be controlled with propranolol or esmolol (same dosage as in ¶D, above) intravenously, or standard antiarrhythmics.

F. Hemoperfusion: Hemoperfusion is the treatment of choice for severe poisoning (intractable seizures; acute overdose with serum level over 90–100 mg/L). Guidelines for hemoperfusion in subacute overdoses are not clear. Repeated doses of activated charcoal (p 737) may be very effective at lowering theophylline levels, obviating hemoperfusion.

Disposition

Hospitalize patients with significant theophylline poisoning (serum concentrations above 30 µg/mL or signs or symptoms of toxicity).

TRICYCLIC ANTIDEPRESSANTS

General Considerations

Major tricyclic antidepressants include amitriptyline (Elavil, many others), imipramine (Tofranil, many others), and doxepin (Adapin, Sinequan). Maprotiline (Ludiomil) is a tetracyclic antidepressant with similar properties.

The antidepressants are analogs of phenothiazines, with complex effects, including anticholinergic, alpha-adrenergic receptor-blocking, and quinidinelike activity on the heart. They are well absorbed and highly tissue-bound, with volumes of distribution of 10–40 L/kg. These drugs are eliminated primarily by metabolism in the liver, and the half-lives are 10–30 hours. The average toxic dose is more than 5 mg/kg, with severe poisoning occurring at doses of 10–20 mg/kg.

Diagnosis

Many symptoms are the result of the anticholinergic activity of these drugs, eg, mydriasis, dry mouth, tachycardia, agitation, and hallucinations. The onset of coma may be rapid, even precipitous. Twitching and myoclonic jerking have been noted, and seizures occur frequently and may be difficult to treat.

Cardiovascular manifestations are the most dramatic and life-threatening (Fig 39–3). Quinidinelike slowing of conduction is reflected by widening of the QRS complex (> 100 ms) and prolonged QT and PR intervals. Varying degrees of atrioventricular block and ventricular tachycardia are common. Atypical ("torsade de pointes") ventricular tachycardia may occur. Profound hypotension resulting from decreased contractility and vasodilatation may occur and is a frequent cause of death. Hypoxemia and acidosis aggravate the cardiovascular toxicity of tricyclic antidepressants.

Diagnosis is generally based on history, relevant physical findings, widened QRS complexes, and prolonged QT intervals (3 Cs: *C*ardiac abnormalities, *C*onvulsions, and *C*oma). The diagnosis may be confirmed by qualitative or quantitative tests for these drugs in the blood. Plasma concentrations over 1000 ng/mL are consistent with symptoms of severe toxic-

ity, but correlation of blood levels of the drug with severity of symptoms is not well established.

Note: Newer cyclic antidepressants (amoxapine) and antipsychotics (loxapine) can cause seizures and coma without associated cardiovascular toxicity or electrocardiographic changes.

Treatment

A. Provide intensive supportive care and gastrointestinal decontamination as described on p 733. Much controversy exists about the appropriate management of overdose of tricyclic antidepressants. Basic guidelines to treatment follow.

B. Do not induce emesis because of the well-established risk of seizures and coma.

C. Perform gastric lavage, administering activated charcoal at the beginning and again at the end of the procedure.

D. Constant monitoring of the ECG for at least 6 hours is mandatory. Progressive widening of the QRS complex indicates worsening toxicity.

E. Seizures should be treated with diazepam and phenytoin (Chapter 11). Physostigmine *should not* be used for seizures (in spite of common recommendations to the contrary), because it may itself cause seizures and other complications as described below.

F. Sinus tachycardia is benign and usually does not require treatment. Physostigmine and propranolol may aggravate conduction abnormalities and should not be used.

G. Ventricular arrhythmias and conduction defects may respond to sodium bicarbonate, 50–100 meq (1–2 meq/kg) as an intravenous bolus. It is not clear whether the improvement is merely a result of correction of acidosis, a result of transient hypernatremia, or a result of a shift in the protein-binding of the drug with alkalosis. Lidocaine, 1–2 mg/kg as an intravenous bolus (Chapter 28), is frequently effective. Phenytoin (15–18 mg/kg intravenously over 20–30 minutes) is the logical drug of choice because it enhances conduction while decreasing automaticity, but there is no proof that it is more effective. Quinidinelike drugs (eg, quinidine, procainamide, disopyramide) are contraindicated, because they worsen cardiotoxicity.

H. Hypotension should be treated initially with intravenous infusion of sodium bicarbonate (50–100 meq, 1–2 meq/kg) and crystalloid solutions. If the patient fails to respond after 1–2 L have been infused, further therapy should be guided by measurement of pulmonary artery wedge pressures and cardiac output.

I. Hemoperfusion has been reported anecdotally to reduce cardiotoxicity, although it is theoretically useless because of the huge volume of distribution of the tricyclic antidepressants.

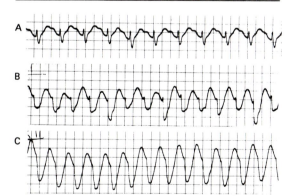

Figure 39–3. Cardiac arrhythmias resulting from tricyclic antidepressant overdose. ***A:*** Delayed intraventricular conduction results in prolonged QRS interval (0.18 s). ***B*** and ***C:*** Supraventricular tachycardia with progressive widening of QRS complexes mimics ventricular tachycardia. (Reproduced, with permission, from Benowitz NL, Goldschlager N: Cardiac disturbances in the toxicologic patient. Page 71 in: *Clinical Management of Poisoning and Drug Overdose.* Haddad LM, Winchester JF [editors]. Saunders, 1983.)

Disposition

Hospitalize all symptomatic patients with overdose of tricyclic antidepressants. Observe asymptomatic patients for a minimum of 6–8 hours, taking repeated measurements of the vital signs and QRS interval.

WARFARIN & OTHER ANTICOAGULANTS

General Considerations

Dicumarol and other natural anticoagulants are found in sweet clover. Warfarin and other synthetic coumarinlike anticoagulants are used therapeutically and as rodenticides.

Warfarin and other coumarinlike compounds inhibit blood clotting by interfering with the synthesis of vitamin K–dependent clotting factors (II, VII, IX, X). Only the synthesis of new factors is affected, and the anticoagulation effect is delayed until currently circulating factors have degraded. Thus, effects may be seen within 8–12 hours after ingestion, since factor II has only a 6-hour half-life, but peak effects are usually not observed until 1–2 days after ingestion because of the longer half-lives (24–60 hours) of the other clotting factors.

The potency and pharmacokinetics of various coumarin anticoagulants vary. Warfarin is highly bound to albumin and has a half-life of 35 hours. It is metabolized by the liver. Multiple drug interactions are known to increase or decrease the anticoagulation effect (Table 39–27).

A single overdose with warfarin does not usually cause significant bleeding, because the half-life of warfarin is shorter than that of some of the clotting factors. Chronic warfarin administration carries a greater risk of excessive anticoagulation and bleeding. However, some newer, extremely potent and long-acting anticoagulants (brodifacoum, indanediones) may produce severe bleeding disturbance for several weeks to months following a single overdose.

Diagnosis

Excessive anticoagulation may result in ecchymoses, hematuria, uterine bleeding, melena, epistaxis, gingival bleeding, hemoptysis, or hematemesis. Hematomas may result in compression neuropathy or compartment syndrome. Life-threatening cardiac tamponade and intracranial hemorrhage have been reported. Such complications can be prevented if the prothrombin time is carefully monitored and kept

Table 39–27. Interactions of warfarin and oral anticoagulants with selected drugs.

Increased Anticoagulation Effect	Decreased Anticoagulation Effect
Allopurinol	Barbiturates
Chloral hydrate	Carbamazepine
Cimetidine	Cholestyramine
Disulfiram	Glutethimide
Indomethacin	Oral contraceptives
Quinidine	Rifampin
Salicylates	
Sulfonamides	

within the desired therapeutic range; if interacting drugs are avoided; and if antidotal therapy is begun promptly when necessary.

Treatment

A. Provide intensive supportive care and gastrointestinal decontamination as described on p 733. Treatment is rarely required for acute single overdose of warfarin, because the dose involved (eg, from typical rodenticide) is small, and any anticoagulation effect is usually brief and mild. However, caution and careful follow-up are indicated after ingestion of newer "super-warfarins" (brodifacoum, indanediones). Obtain a baseline prothrombin time, and repeat the measurement after 24 and 48 hours.

B. For hemorrhage or other bleeding complications, give vitamin K_1, 1–2 mg intravenously, which will begin to restore clotting factor levels within about 6–8 hours. If a more rapid reversal is required, fresh-frozen plasma may be given. For patients with asymptomatic mild prolongation of the prothrombin time, simply withholding warfarin is usually satisfactory; or vitamin K may be given, 10 mg every 3–5 days, orally, intramuscularly, or subcutaneously. *Note:* Do not give vitamin K prophylactically, since it may mask symptomatic exposure by preventing prolongation of prothrombin time.

Disposition

Hospitalize all patients with significantly prolonged prothrombin times, evidence of bleeding, or history of ingestion of massive amounts of anticoagulants. Patients who have documented anticoagulant effect after ingestion of newer "super-warfarin" rodenticides will need close follow-up and repeated vitamin K dosing for up to several weeks.

REFERENCES

General

Albertson TE et al: Superiority of activated charcoal alone compared with ipecac and activated charcoal in the treatment of acute toxic ingestions. Ann Emerg Med 1989;18:56.

Doull J, Klaassen C, Amdur M (editors): *Casarett and Doull's Toxicology: The Basic Science of Poisons,* 3rd ed. Macmillan, 1990.

Ellenhorn M, Barceloux D: *Medical Toxicology.* Elsevier, 1988.

Gilman AG, Goodman LS, Gilman A (editors): *Goodman and Gilman's The Pharmacological Basis of Therapeutics,* 8th ed. Macmillan, 1990.

Goldfrank L et al (editors): *Goldfrank's Toxicologic Emergencies,* 4th ed. Appleton-Century-Crofts, 1990.

Gosselin RE et al: *Clinical Toxicology of Commercial Products,* 6th ed. Williams & Wilkins, 1988.

Haddad LM, Winchester JF (editors): *Clinical Management of Poisoning and Drug Overdose,* 2nd ed. Saunders, 1990.

Olson KR et al (editors): *Poisoning and Drug Overdose.* Appleton & Lange, 1990.

Proctor NH, Hughes JP, Fischman M: *Chemical Hazards of the Workplace,* 2nd ed. Lippincott, 1988.

Rumack BH (editor): *Poisindex: An Emergency Poison Management System.* Micromedex. [Published quarterly.]

Acetaminophen

Seeff LB et al: Acetaminophen hepatotoxicity in alcoholics: A therapeutic misadventure. Ann Intern Med 1986;104:399.

Smilkstein MJ et al: Efficacy of oral N-acetylcysteine in the treatment of acetaminophen overdose: Analysis of the National Multicenter Study (1976 to 1985). N Engl J Med 1988;319:1557.

Amphetamines & Other Stimulants

Derlet RW et al: Amphetamine toxicity: Experience with 127 cases. J Emerg Med 1989;7:157.

Pentel P: Toxicity of over-the-counter stimulants. JAMA 1984;252:1898.

Anticholinergics

Fahy P et al: Serial serum drug concentrations and prolonged anticholinergic toxicity after benztropine (Cogentin) overdose. Am J Emerg Med 1989;7:199.

Klein-Schwartz W, Oderda GM: Jimsonweed intoxication in adolescents and young adults. Am J Dis Child 1984;138:737.

Beta-Adrenergic Blocking Agents

Agura ED, Wexler LF, Witzburg RA: Massive propranolol overdose: Successful treatment with high-dose isoproterenol and glucagon. Am J Med 1986;80:755.

Weinstein RS: Recognition and management of poisoning with beta-adrenergic blocking agents. Ann Emerg Med 1984;13:1123.

Calcium Channel Blockers

Henry M, Kay MM, Viccellio P: Cardiogenic shock associated with calcium-channel and beta blockers: Reversal with intravenous calcium chloride. Am J Emerg Med 1985;3:334.

Horowitz BZ, Rhee KJ: Massive verapamil ingestion: A report of two cases and a review of the literature. Am J Emerg Med 1989;7:624.

Ramoska EA, Spiller HA, Myers A: Calcium channel blocker toxicity. Ann Emerg Med 1990;19:649.

Carbon Monoxide

Olson KR: Carbon monoxide poisoning: Mechanisms, presentation, and controversies in management. J Emerg Med 1984;1:233.

Sloan EP et al: Complications and protocol considerations in carbon monoxide–poisoned patients who require hyperbaric oxygen therapy: Report from a ten-year experience. Ann Emerg Med 1989;18:629.

Cardiac Glycosides (Digitalis, etc)

Shumaik GM et al: Oleander poisoning: Treatment with digoxin-specific antibody fragments. Ann Emerg Med 1988;17:732.

Wenger TL et al: Treatment of 63 severely digitalis-toxic patients with digoxin-specific antibody fragments. J Am Coll Cardiol 1985;5:118A.

Caustics

Rothstein FC: Caustic injuries to the esophagus in children. Pediatr Clin North Am 1986;33:665.

Vance MV et al: Digital hydrofluoric acid burns: Treatment with intra-arterial calcium infusion. Ann Emerg Med 1986;15:890.

Cocaine & Local Anesthetics

Derlet RW, Albertson TE: Emergency department presentation of cocaine intoxication. Ann Emerg Med 1989;18:182.

Ernst AA, Sanders WM: Unexpected cocaine intoxication presenting as seizures in children. Ann Emerg Med 1989;18:774.

Mueller PD et al: Cocaine. Emerg Med Clin North Am 1990;8:481.

Roth D et al: Acute rhabdomyolysis associated with cocaine intoxication. N Engl J Med 1988;319:673.

Tokarski GF et al: An evaluation of cocaine-induced chest pain. Ann Emerg Med 1990;19:1088.

Cyanide

Caravati EM, Litovitz TL: Pediatric cyanide intoxication and death from an acetonitrile-containing cosmetic. JAMA 1988;260:3470.

Marrs TC: Antidotal treatment of acute cyanide poisoning. Adverse Drug React Acute Poisoning Rev 1988;7:179.

Drug-Induced Methemoglobinemia

Curry S: Methemoglobinemia. Ann Emerg Med 1982;11:214.

Linakis JG et al: Recurrent methemoglobinemia after acute dapsone ingestion in a child. J Emerg Med 1989;7:477.

Ethanol & Other Alcohols

Becker CE: Methanol poisoning. J Emerg Med 1983;1:51.

Bobbitt WH et al: Severe ethylene glycol intoxication with multisystem failure. West J Med 1986;144:225.

Ekins BR et al: Standardized treatment of severe methanol poisoning with ethanol and hemodialysis. West J Med 1985;142:337.

Heavy Metals

Aronow R et al: Mercury exposure from interior latex paint—Michigan. Morbid Mortal Weekly Rep 1990;39(8):125.

Proudfoot AT, Simpson D, Dyson EH: Management of acute iron poisoning. Med Toxicol 1986;1:83.

Rempel D: The lead-exposed worker. JAMA 1989;262:532.

Saady JJ et al: Estimation of the body burden of arsenic in a child fatally poisoned by arsenite weed killer. J Anal Toxicol 1989;13:310.

Schneitzer L et al: Lead poisoning in adults from renovation of an older home. Ann Emerg Med 1990;19:415.

Tenenbein M: Whole bowel irrigation in iron poisoning. J Pediatr 1987;111:142.

Hydrocarbons

Brook MP et al: Pine oil cleaner ingestion. Ann Emerg Med 1989;18:391.

Machado B et al: Accidental hydrocarbon ingestion cases telephoned to a regional poison center. Ann Emerg Med 1988;17:804.

Inhalants (Toxic Gases & Vapors)

Hedberg K et al: An outbreak of nitrogen dioxide–induced respiratory illness among hockey players. JAMA 1989;262:3014.

Langford RM, Armstrong RF: Algorithm for managing injury from smoke inhalation. Br Med J 1989;299:902.

Isoniazid (INH)

Wason S, Lacouture PG, Lovejoy FH Jr: Single high-dose pyridoxine treatment for isoniazid overdose. JAMA 1981;246:1102.

Lithium

Dyson EH et al: Self-poisoning and therapeutic intoxication with lithium. Hum Toxicol 1987;6:325.

Simard M et al: Lithium carbonate intoxication: A case report and review of the literature. Arch Intern Med 1989;149:36.

Opiates

Moore RA et al: Naloxone: Underdosage after narcotic poisoning. Am J Dis Child 1980;134:156.

Goldfrank L et al: A dosing nomogram for continuous infusion intravenous naloxone. Ann Emerg Med 1986;15:566.

Organophosphates & Other Cholinesterase Inhibitors

Clifford NJ, Nies AS: Organophosphate intoxication from wearing a laundered uniform previously contaminated with parathion. JAMA 1989;262:3035.

Namba T: Poisoning due to organophosphate insecticides: Acute and chronic manifestations. Am J Med 1971;50:475.

Zweiner RJ, Ginsberg CM: Organophosphate and carbamate poisoning in infants and children. Pediatrics 1988;81:121.

Phencyclidine (PCP)

McCarron MM et al: Acute phencyclidine intoxication: Clinical patterns, complications, and treatment. Ann Emerg Med 1981;10:290.

Patel R et al: Myoglobinuric acute renal failure in phencyclidine overdose: Report of observations in eight cases. Ann Emerg Med 1980;9:549.

Phenothiazines & Other Antipsychotics

Barry D, Meyskens FL Jr, Becker CE: Phenothiazine poisoning: A review of 48 cases. Calif Med (Jan) 1973;118:1.

Niemann JT et al: Cardiac conduction and rhythm disturbances following suicidal ingestion of mesoridazine. Ann Emerg Med 1981;10:585.

Poisonous Mushrooms

Klein AS et al: *Amanita* poisoning: Treatment and the role of liver transplantation. Am J Med 1989;86:187.

Pond SM et al: Amatoxin poisoning in northern California, 1982–1983. West J Med 1986;145:204.

Poisonous Plants

Arena JM: Plants that poison. Emerg Med (June 15) 1989:20.

Kingsbury JM: *Poisonous Plants of the United States and Canada*. Prentice-Hall, 1964.

Salicylates

Dugandzic RM et al: Evaluation of the validity of the Done nomogram in the management of acute salicylate intoxication. Ann Emerg Med 1989;18:1186.

McGuigan MA: A two-year review of salicylate deaths in Ontario. Arch Intern Med 1987;147:510.

Sedative-Hypnotics

Goodman JM et al: Barbiturate intoxication: Morbidity and mortality. West J Med 1976;124:179.

Hojer J et al: Benzodiazepine poisoning: Experience of 702 admissions to an intensive care unit during a 14-year period. J Intern Med 1989;226:117.

Pond SM et al: Randomized study of the treatment of phenobarbital overdose with repeated doses of activated charcoal. JAMA 1984;251:3104.

Theophylline & Methylxanthines

Gaar GG et al: The effects of esmolol on the hemodynamics of acute theophylline toxicity. Ann Emerg Med 1987;16:1334.

Gaudreault P, Guay J: Theophylline poisoning: Pharmacological considerations and clinical management. Med Toxicol 1986;1:169.

Olson KR et al: Theophylline overdose: Acute single ingestion versus chronic repeated overmedication. Am J Emerg Med 1985;3:386.

Tricyclic Antidepressants

Boehnert MT, Lovejoy FH Jr: Value of the QRS duration versus the serum drug level in predicting seizures and ventricular arrhythmias after an acute overdose of tricyclic antidepressants. N Engl J Med 1985;313:474.

Callaham M, Kassel D: Epidemiology of fatal tricyclic antidepressant ingestion: Implications for management. Ann Emerg Med 1985;14:1.

Shannon M, Merola J, Lovejoy FH Jr: Hypotension in severe tricyclic antidepressant overdose. Am J Emerg Med 1988;6:439.

Warfarin & Other Anticoagulants

Lipton RA, Klass EM: Human ingestion of a "super-warfarin" rodenticide resulting in a prolonged anticoagulant effect. JAMA 1984;252:3004.

Smolinske SC et al: Superwarfarin poisoning in children: A prospective study. Pediatrics 1989;84:490.

Dermatologic Emergencies

40

Steven A. Davis, MD

IMMEDIATE MANAGEMENT OF LIFE-THREATENING PROBLEMS

ANAPHYLACTIC SHOCK

Anaphylactic shock may present with dermatologic signs or symptoms (itching, urticaria, etc). If the patient manifests systemic signs (dyspnea, confusion, or shock), assume that anaphylaxis is present, and give appropriate treatment immediately (Chapter 3).

INTENSE PRURITUS (Itching)

Pruritus may be classified as either itching associated with skin lesions or itching without skin lesions.

A. Pruritus With Skin Lesions: Causes of itching associated with skin lesions include:
1. Contact dermatitis, allergic or irritant.
2. Urticaria.
3. Infestations or bites.
4. Allergic reactions to drugs.
5. Anaphylaxis.
6. Miscellaneous other dermatitides.

B. Pruritus Without Skin Lesions: Causes of itching without skin lesions include:
1. Dry skin (eg, excessive use of soap).
2. Psychogenic factors.
3. Hepatic and biliary disease, especially if associated with obstructive jaundice.
4. Endocrinopathies (eg, hyperthyroidism, diabetes mellitus, carcinoid syndrome).
5. Malignant neoplasms (especially Hodgkin's disease and other lymphomas).
6. Uremia.

Diagnosis

A. History: Important diagnostic clues may be obtained by asking the patient about the following points:

1. Precise timing of onset–Sudden or simultaneous appearance of lesions, especially in the morning, suggests an exogenous cause, eg, bites.

2. Intake of drugs–Ask about the patient's use of nonprescription over-the-counter drugs such as vitamins, aspirin, and laxatives as well as prescribed medications.

3. Application of topical preparations–Ask about the use of nonprescription creams, salves, or lotions; soaps; perfumes; cosmetics, including hair color or hair treatments; or shaving preparations.

4. Progression of lesions– Ask whether some lesions appear while others regress, eg, urticaria.

B. Examination: Have the patient undress completely, and examine both clothing and hair (seams of clothing may contain lice).

1. Interdigital, pubic, axillary, or nipple lesions– Scabies.

2. Grouped papules–Bites.

3. Generalized morbilliform (measleslike) eruptions–Drug reaction.

4. Discrete weeping patches, often with vesicles, that may be scattered–Allergic or irritant contact dermatitis (eg, *Rhus* dermatitis [poison oak]).

5. Raised, evanescent plaques–Urticaria.

6. Lesions usually confined to areas of direct contact with skin–Contact dermatitis from clothing, dyes, jewelry, or watchbands.

Treatment

A. General Measures: Although it may seem a trivial symptom, severe generalized itching is disabling, and treatment should be started in the emergency department.

1. Systemic antipruritics–Antihistamines cause drowsiness, and the patient should be cautioned against drinking alcohol, driving, or operating heavy equipment. Any of the following may be tried:

a. Diphenhydramine (Benadryl, many others), 25–50 mg orally 2–4 times a day.

b. Chlorpheniramine (Chlor-Trimeton, Phenetron, many others), 4 mg orally 2–4 times a day.

c. Hydroxyzine (Atarax, Vistaril, many others), 10–25 mg orally 2–4 times a day, is probably the most effective antihistamine for itching in general.

d. Cyproheptadine (Periactin), 4 mg orally 2–4 times a day, is primarily effective in urticaria.

e. Terfenadine (Seldane), 60 mg orally twice daily, or astemizole (Hismanal), 10 mg once daily, causes drowsiness less frequently than other antihistamines in some patients.

2. Topical antipruritic measures–

a. Emollients (eg, white petrolatum) may be used for dry skin. Tub baths to which a capful of bath oil has been added may be soothing, but baths should be short, should use water that is not extremely hot, and should be followed by application of an emollient.

b. Drying agents (eg, calamine lotion) may be used for lesions that are oozing or weeping.

B. Specific Measures:

1. Scabies and lice–Infestations with mites or lice may be treated with topical insecticides. Since a diagnosis of scabies may be difficult to confirm, empiric treatment is often undertaken (see Scabies & Pediculosis, below).

2. Drug reactions–Adverse reactions to drugs are common. The suspected offending agent should be discontinued.

3. Contact dermatitis–Systemic corticosteroids may be indicated for contact dermatitis (see Poison Ivy, Oak, & Sumac [*Rhus* Dermatitis], below).

Disposition

A. Pruritus With Skin Lesions: Patients who are acutely ill with generalized lesions that are exfoliating or moist should be hospitalized for supportive care, definitive diagnosis, and treatment. Patients who are not acutely ill may be discharged from the emergency department for follow-up within a few days. Patients with persistent symptoms may benefit from dermatologic consultation.

B. Pruritus Without Skin Lesions: Provide antipruritic medication and advice, and refer the patient to a primary care physician or dermatologist for evaluation if other systemic illness is suspected or if symptoms persist. Hospitalization is rarely indicated.

EXFOLIATION & ERYTHRODERMA

Exfoliation denotes sloughing of epidermal cells in a profuse and generalized manner. In some cases, the skin may be dry and show fine scaling; in others, the skin may be more moist, and peeling may be manifested as sloughing off of sheets of blistered skin. Severe sloughing may be associated with marked fluid loss through the skin that occasionally progresses to shock.

Erythroderma includes widespread or generalized abnormal redness. The skin will feel warm to hot, and the patient may be febrile or hypotensive. Tachycardia may be present. Erythroderma may rapidly progress to exfoliation.

Causes of exfoliation and erythroderma are set forth in Table 40–1.

Diagnosis

A. History:

1. Previous skin disease–Exfoliation commonly denotes exacerbation of a chronic preexisting skin condition. Withdrawal of systemic corticosteroids may precipitate onset of symptoms (eg, pustular

Table 40–1. Causes of exfoliation and erythroderma.

Psoriasis	Toxic shock syndrome
Toxic eipidermal necrolysis	Lymphomas (including myco-
Atopic dermatitis	sis fungoides)
Drug eruptions	Seborrheic dermatitis
Dermatophytosis (eg, ringworm)	Sézary syndrome
Pityriasis rubra pilaris	Contact dermatitis
Staphylococcal scalded skin	Idiopathic
syndrome	Lichen planus

psoriasis). Atopic dermatitis may be associated with a long history of "rashes" or "childhood eczema."

2. Relationship to drug use–Onset of symptoms with a history of drug intake within the previous 14 days usually signifies drug eruption. Onset 2–14 days after application of topical medication or some other over-the-counter remedy or cosmetic (especially products containing benzocaine or neomycin) points to a diagnosis of contact dermatitis. Worsening of rash with application of topical corticosteroids may occur in dermatophytosis or may be an allergic reaction to propylene glycol in the corticosteroid preparation.

3. Systemic signs or symptoms of prior or concurrent infection– Systemic signs may be noted in staphylococcal scalded skin syndrome or toxic shock syndrome.

4. Systemic signs or symptoms of malignant neoplasms–Weight loss and other symptoms are associated with lymphomas, especially T cell lymphomas (mycosis fungoides and Sézary syndrome).

B. Physical Examination:
1. Generalized findings–
a. Fever, toxicity, skin tenderness–Staphylococcal scalded skin syndrome or toxic shock syndrome.
b. Generalized redness and severe itching–Sézary syndrome.
2. Specific local lesions–
a. Plaques on elbows or knees–Psoriasis.
b. Pitting or dystrophic changes of nails–Psoriasis.
c. Fungal thickening of nails (onychomycosis)–Dermatophytosis.
d. Flexural thickening–Atopic dermatitis.
e. Scaling of scalp, central face (around the nose and mouth), chest, and back–Seborrheic dermatitis.
f. Waxy (carnauba wax–like) thickening of palms and soles–Pityriasis rubra pilaris.

Treatment

A. Emergency Measures: Treat shock (Chapter 3). Weeping exfoliative dermatitis may be associated with severe hypotension or shock, either from fluid loss or from the toxin causing the skin disease (eg, toxic shock syndrome). To reiterate—
1. Obtain complete vital signs.
2. Insert a large-bore (≥ 16-gauge) intravenous catheter.

3. Draw blood for CBC, serum electrolyte and blood glucose determinations, and tests of renal and hepatic function. Obtain 2 blood cultures if the patient is febrile.
4. Begin rapid (1 L/h for an adult) infusion of crystalloid solution to increase blood pressure.
5. Obtain emergency dermatologic consultation.
B. Specific Measures:
1. Cover weeping or open lesions with saline-soaked dressings.
2. Begin antimicrobials if staphylococcal disease is suspected, eg, nafcillin or oxacillin, 150 mg/kg/d orally in 4–6 divided doses.
3. Narcotic analgesics may be needed for pain.

Disposition

All patients with extensive exfoliative dermatitis or diffuse erythroderma should be hospitalized and may need intensive care unit admission for management of shock.

PURPURA & VASCULITIS

Purpura is a condition characterized by bleeding into the skin. Small punctate purpuric lesions are called petechiae, while larger purpuric lesions are called ecchymoses. The clinical hallmark of purpuric lesions is failure to blanch when pressure is applied. The diagnosis may be confirmed by **diascopy** (a glass slide is pressed against the lesion thought to contain extravascular hemoglobin or its breakdown products. Lesions with an intact underlying vasculature will blanch; purpuric lesions will not).

Vasculitis is an inflammatory change in blood vessels that may lead to purpura because of destruction of the vessel wall, with subsequent hemorrhage into surrounding tissues.

A purpuric lesion that feels perfectly smooth to the touch implies simple bleeding into the tissues, and the causes vary; they include trauma and blood dyscrasias. A *palpable* purpuric lesion that is slightly papular or vesiculopustular is a classic sign of underlying necrotizing vasculitis. Such lesions may have an infectious or immunologic origin.

Some causes of purpura are listed in Table 40–2.

Diagnosis
A. History: There may be a history of systemic symptoms (urinary tract or abdominal manifestations, fever, arthritis) suggesting systemic vasculitis (Henoch-Schönlein syndrome, polyarteritis, infections [eg, meningococcemia]). There may also be a history of use of drugs known to cause purpura or vasculitis (barbiturates, thiazide diuretics, quinidine, chlorpromazine, and sulfonamides). Digitoxin, phenytoin, heparin, methyldopa, PAS (*p*-aminosalicylic acid), and rifampin may also cause vasculitis.
B. Symptoms and Signs: Purpura in an acutely

Table 40–2. Causes of purpura.

Blood disorders
 Platelet deficiency syndromes
  Idiopathic thrombocytopenic purpura
  Drug-induced thrombocytopenia
  Thrombotic thrombocytopenic purpura
  Disseminated intravascular coagulopathy
  Platelet and coagulation disorders
  Wiskott-Aldrich syndrome
  Thrombocytopenia associated with myeloproliferative disorders
Vascular changes
 Necrotizing vasculitis
  Idiopathic
  Collagen vascular diseases
  Drug eruptions
  Systemic infections (meningococcal, gonococcal, rickettsial infection)
  Immune complex disease
  Hereditary hemorrhagic telangiectasia (Rendu-Osler-Weber disease)
  Pseudoxanthoma elasticum
  Wegener's granulomatosis
Other causes
 Drug-induced (especially corticosteroids)
 Trauma
 Scurvy
 Ehlers-Danlos syndrome
 Senile purpura
 Dysproteinemia

ill patient with fever and hypotension suggests sepsis with disseminated intravascular coagulation. Altered mental status may occur in thrombotic thrombocytopenic purpura, meningococcal infections, or collagen vascular disease with central nervous system involvement. Differentiate between palpable (vasculitic) and flat (nonvasculitic) purpura.

C. Laboratory Findings:

1. Coagulation tests–Coagulation abnormalities occur, eg, thrombocytopenia, prolonged prothrombin time and partial thromboplastin time, positive Hess capillary test for capillary fragility (tourniquet test), etc.

2. Urinalysis–Hematuria suggests renal vasculitis but may occur as the result of renal purpura.

3. Smear and culture–Aspirate purpuric lesions to obtain material for staining with Gram's stain, and obtain blood cultures to determine whether infection is present.

Treatment

A. Obtain the following in all patients with unexplained purpuric lesions before they leave the emergency department: CBC and differential and coagulation panel (platelet count, partial thromboplastin time, prothrombin time).

B. If purpura is palpable, send urine for urinalysis and microscopic examination, and obtain an erythrocyte sedimentation rate.

C. If the patient is acutely ill or if infection is suspected, obtain 2 blood cultures, and aspirate a sample

of material from skin lesions. Obtain material from other potential sites of infection for culture and Gram-stained smear.

D. Treat shock (Chapter 3).

E. Establish a tentative causative diagnosis. Helpful diagnostic clues and organisms that commonly cause purpura include the following:

1. Meningococci (patient may have meningitis).

2. Gonococci (lesions are often pustular; patient may have tenosynovitis).

3. Staphylococci (lesions are often pustular).

4. Rickettsiae (rickettsiae are endemic in the area).

5. Viruses (arboviruses are endemic in the area).

F. Begin empiric antimicrobial therapy (see Table 3–6).

G. Additional specific measures depend on the cause.

Disposition

A. Diffuse Purpura: Patients with diffuse purpura, systemic symptoms and signs, coagulation abnormalities, or nephritis should be hospitalized for evaluation and treatment.

B. Localized Purpura: Patients with localized purpura without systemic symptoms or signs or abnormalities on laboratory tests may be discharged with follow-up within 1 week.

EMERGENCY TREATMENT OF SPECIFIC DISORDERS

POISON IVY, OAK, & SUMAC (*Rhus* Dermatitis)

Rhus dermatitis occurs as poison oak dermatitis in the western USA and poison ivy and poison sumac dermatitis in the rest of the USA. It is a delayed hypersensitivity reaction to an oleoresin in these plants. Primary sensitization is usually followed by an eruption 1–2 weeks after exposure. Reexposure typically results in eruptions 12–48 hours after exposure. The resin is reasonably stable when dry and may be carried in smoke from burning leaves and on the coats of animals.

Diagnosis

A. History: There is a history of exposure to *Rhus* species 24–48 hours previously. There may be a history of previous sensitivity to these plants. The patient should be asked about visits to parks or outdoor areas 24–48 hours before eruption of the lesions and also about exposure 1–2 weeks before (because of the possibility of delayed eruption following primary sensitization). Inquire also about contact with pets or other animals that might have been exposed to these plants.

B. Symptoms and Signs: Lesions may be acute and disabling or (more commonly) low-grade and persistent. Lesions erupting in linear streaks corresponding to areas of contact with vines or stems are helpful diagnostic clues. Severe reactions include puffiness and swelling about the eyes, face, and genitalia. In some patients, lesions spread to new locations over a period of weeks. The spread of lesions is not due to blister fluid or scratching but rather to systemic sensitization to the allergen. Patients often cannot sleep or work because of the intense and intractable pruritus. The skin rash consists of patchy erythema or linear streaking, often with edema or clear vesicles. Secondary bacterial infection may occur as a result of repeated traumatization of the skin by scratching.

Treatment

A. Systemic (Oral) Corticosteroids: Although most patients with significant *Rhus* dermatitis do not respond to topical corticosteroids or other topical treatment, they usually respond dramatically to oral corticosteroids. Corticosteroid therapy should be started and then tapered over a 12- to 14-day period (Table 40–3). Shorter treatment periods, especially those under 1 week or less, often result in rebound flare of the hypersensitivity reaction, with eruption of new lesions. Patients should be instructed to complete the full course of medication even if the rash has completely subsided in the meantime. Oral corticosteroids are often preferred to parenteral preparations because of the ease with which the dose can be modified or discontinued if side effects occur.

Patients with one or more of the following findings associated with *Rhus* dermatitis are candidates for systemic corticosteroids. Table 40–4 sets forth relative contraindications to the use of systemic corticosteroids.

(1) Progressive lesions or pruritus unresponsive to topical therapy.

Table 40–3. Representative short-course systemic corticosteroid regimens for adults.

2-Week Tapered Course of Oral Prednisone	
Week 1	**Week 2**
Day 1 60 mg	Day 8 30 mg
Day 2 60 mg	Day 9 20 mg
Day 3 50 mg	Day 10 20 mg
Day 4 50 mg	Day 11 20 mg
Day 5 40 mg	Day 12 20 mg
Day 6 40 mg	Day 13 10 mg
Day 7 30 mg	Day 14 10 mg

3-Week Tapered Course of Oral Corticosteroids	
Prednisone	**Triamcinolone**
Week 1 60 mg/d	48 mg/d
Week 2 30 mg/d	24 mg/d
Week 3 20 mg/d	16 mg/d

Table 40–4. Relative contraindications to use of systemic corticosteroids.

Tuberculosis (active or previously active)
Hypertension
Glaucoma
Pregnancy
Diabetes
Previous adverse reaction to systemic corticosteroids
Cataracts
Peptic ulcer
Ophthalmic herpes simplex
Psychosis

(2) Intractable pruritus that prevents the patient from sleeping or functioning normally.

(3) Swelling and edema of face or genitalia.

(4) Large patches of vesicles or bullae.

B. Topical Treatment: Weeping, edematous areas or areas with broken vesicles or bullae may be dressed 3 times a day for 15 minutes with compresses that have been soaked in appropriate astringent solutions (Table 40–5). A 24- to 48-hour trial of the superpotent topical corticosteroid agent augmented betamethasone dipropionate (Diprolene ointment) can be undertaken for limited disease or when systemic corticosteroids are contraindicated. Other potent topical agents may also be tried (Table 40–6). Creams are preferable to ointments on exudative lesions.

C. Antipruritics: Antipruritics are often needed (see Intense Pruritus, above).

Table 40–5. Common topical dermatologic preparations for the treatment of weeping dermatoses.

Preparation	Use and Comments
Astringent and antiseptic solutions	
Aluminum acetate (Burow's) solution Typically diluted to 1:40 (available premixed from the pharmacy). Alternatively, dissolve 1 tablet or package of Domeboro or Pedi-Boro in 1 pint of water.	For oozing or weeping lesions. Soak dressing in solution beforehand, or apply directly to compress over the lesion. Keep dressing moist for 10–15 minutes. Apply every 15–30 minutes for 48 hours. Do not use with plastic wrap or other impervious material.
Acetic acid (vinegar) Dilute ordinary white vinegar 1:10 with water.	Same as for aluminum acetate solution.
Antiseptic and drying paints	
Carbol-fuchsin solution (Castellani's paint) Contains fuchsin, 0.3%; phenol, 4.5%; resorcinol, 10%; acetone, 1.5%; and alcohol, 13%	Same as for aluminum acetate solution. Use twice a day to dry up lesions and prevent bacterial or fungal infection. Stains skin and clothing red. Do not apply to large denuded areas for extended treatment, because systemic absorption of phenol may be nephrotoxic.
Gentian violet, 1% solution	Drying agent with antibacterial and antimycotic properties. Contains no phenol. Stains skin and clothing purple.

Table 40–6. Relative efficacy of topical corticosteroids in various formulations.[1]

Lowest efficacy	
0.25%–2.5%	Hydrocortisone
0.25%	Methylprednisolone acetate (Medrol)
0.04%	Dexamethasone[2] (Hexadrol)
0.1%	Dexamethasone[2] (Decaderm)
1.0%	Methylprednisolone acetate (Medrol)
0.5%	Prednisolone (Meti-Derm)
0.2%	Betamethasone[2] (Celestone)
Low efficacy	
0.01%	Fluocinolone acetonide[2] (Fluonid, Synalar)
0.01%	Betamethasone valerate[2] (Valisone)
0.025%	Fluorometholone[2] (Oxylone)
0.05%	Aclometasone dipropionate (Aclovate)
0.025%	Triamcinolone acetonide[2] (Aristocort, Kenalog, Triacet)
0.1%	Clocortolone pivalate[2] (Cloderm)
0.03%	Flumethasone pivalate[2] (Locorten)
Intermediate efficacy	
0.2%	Hydrocortisone valerate (Westcort)
0.1%	Mometasone furoate (Elocon)
0.1%	Hydrocortisone butyrate (Locoid)
0.025%	Betamethasone benzoate[2] (Benisone, Flurobate, Uticort)
0.025%	Flurandrenolide[2] (Cordran)
0.1%	Betamethasone valerate[2] (Valisone)
0.05%	Desonide (Tridesilon, Desowen)
0.025%	Halcinonide[2] (Halog)
0.05%	Desoximetasone[2] (Topicort L.P.)
0.05%	Flurandrenolide[2] (Cordran)
0.1%	Triamcinolone acetonide[2]
0.025%	Fluocinolone acetonide[2]
High efficacy	
0.05%	Betamethasone dipropionate[2] (Diprosone)
0.1%	Amcinonide[2] (Cyclocort)
0.25%	Desoximetasone[2] (Topicort)
0.5%	Triamcinolone acetonide[2]
0.2%	Fluocinolone acetonide[2] (Synalar-HP)
0.05%	Diflorasone diacetate[2] (Florone, Maxiflor)
0.1%	Halcinonide[2] (Halog)
0.05%	Fluocinonide[2] (Lidex, Topsyn)
Highest efficacy	
0.05%	Betamethasone dipropionate[2] in optimized vehicle (Diprolene)
0.05%	Diflorasone diacetate[2] in optimized vehicle (Psorcon)
0.05%	Clobetasol propionate[2] (Temovate)

[1]Modified and reproduced, with permission, from Katzung BG (editor): *Basic & Clinical Pharmacology,* 4th ed. Appleton & Lange, 1989.
[2]Fluorinated steroids.

Disposition

Hospitalize patients with severe, disabling contact dermatitis, and obtain emergency dermatologic consultation.

Patients who are given systemic corticosteroids or who have other medical conditions should be scheduled for follow-up in 3 days. Advise the patient to learn to recognize the plants and avoid them, since the best therapy is prevention.

Antigen-specific hyposensitization to poison oak is of potential value for severely and recurrently affected individuals, although side effects limit its reasonable use to those individuals with persistent, eg, occupational exposure.

URTICARIA & ANGIOEDEMA (Hives)

Urticaria (hives) may appear suddenly and for the first time at any age and on any part of the body and is usually associated with pruritus. Angioedema is characterized by swelling in the subcutaneous or submucosal tissue (often of the face) but without pruritus. In most acute cases, the cause is not readily apparent, and the condition clears spontaneously. About 15–20% of individuals will suffer at least one attack of urticaria during their lifetime. Some causes of urticaria and angioedema are shown in Table 40–7. There is also a hereditary form of angioedema that is often associated with upper airway and gastrointestinal tract symptoms.

Diagnosis

A. Urticaria: Hives are localized swellings in the skin that produce raised lesions that are often gyrate or polycyclic and sharply demarcated, with an erythematous or blanched base and border. They are usually intensely itchy. Multiple lesions in various states of development and resolution occur. Single lesions fade within hours and seldom last longer than 1 day.

Table 40–7. Common causes of urticaria and sporadic angioedema.

Foods	Physical agents (less commonly)
Shellfish	Pressure
Citrus fruits	Sunlight
Berries	Cold
Eggs	Heat
Nuts	**Intercurrent illness** (occasionally)
Chocolate	Infections (infectious mononucleosis, hepa-
Pollens	titis B)
Drugs	Endocrinopathies
Penicillin	Malignant neoplasms (especially lymphoma)
Sulfonamides	Collagen vascular disease (systemic lupus
	erythematosus, dermatomyositis)
	Autoimmune thyroiditis
	Mastocytosis
	C1q esterase inhibitor deficiency

In urticaria caused by foodstuffs, lesions usually erupt within minutes after eating (rarely more than 24–48 hours after ingestion).

Since swelling results from edema within the dermis, the epidermis may be taut but is not otherwise affected. Evaluation of the patient with urticaria should include a general history and physical examination to discover possible underlying disease.

B. Angioedema: The lesions of angioedema are large wheals (swollen and nonpitting), often of the eyelids, lips, or other parts of the face and extremities. Involvement of mucous membranes or the pharynx and larynx may cause airway obstruction. Urticaria or angioedema may herald the onset of systemic anaphylaxis, which is characterized by shortness of breath (caused by laryngeal or pulmonary edema) and hypotension progressing to shock (Chapter 3).

Treatment

A. Emergency Measures:

1. Treat anaphylactic shock–See Chapter 3.

2. Protect airway–Protect the airway if upper airway obstruction is present (Chapter 3).

3. Medicate to reduce obstructive swelling–

a. Epinephrine–For severe acute urticaria or angioedema, give epinephrine, 0.3–0.5 mL of 1:1000 solution subcutaneously. In the absence of cardiovascular or other contraindications, the dose may be repeated again in 30–60 minutes.

b. Antihistamines–Histamine is one of several mediators producing the vascular changes observed in urticaria. For this reason, a trial of antihistamines (p 770) may be effective in reducing the number of lesions or their frequency of occurrence.

When antihistaminic drugs of the H_1 receptor type (eg, hydroxyzine hydrochloride; diphenhydramine) are ineffective, the addition of an H_2 receptor-selective antihistamine (eg, ranitidine or cimetidine) may help. A typical regimen is hydroxyzine hydrochloride, 25 mg orally 2–4 times a day; plus cimetidine, 300 mg orally 4 times a day.

Since oral antihistamines are quickly absorbed into the bloodstream, the intramuscular route of administration offers no real advantage. These drugs may cause drowsiness, and patients should be cautioned against drinking alcohol, driving, or operating heavy equipment while taking them.

4. Provide reassurance–If itching is not incapacitating and if the patient is willing to let the lesions abate spontaneously, medication need not be given. Reassurance that hives are a benign process and that they typically disappear within hours to days may be adequate.

5. Avoid corticosteroids–The use of systemic corticosteroids for *acute* urticaria is rarely justified. Systemic corticosteroids are occasionally justified for *chronic* urticaria (lasting longer than 4–6 weeks)

when all other treatment has failed. Such therapy should not be started in the emergency department.

6. Treat C1q esterase inhibitor deficiency– C1q esterase inhibitor deficiency (hereditary angioedema) requires replacement of C1q esterase inhibitor. Give C1q esterase inhibitor concentrate, in 5% dextrose over 10–45 minutes. If C1q esterase inhibitor concentrate is unavailable, fresh-frozen plasma may be administered.

B. Avoidance or Removal of Causative Agents: Offending agents should be avoided. If aspirin is identified as the causative agent, avoidance of other salicylates and salicylate-containing foods (see Noid reference) may be helpful.

Disposition

Hospitalize patients with diffuse, severe urticaria if systemic symptoms (eg, upper airway obstruction, bronchospasm) do not resolve completely. Patients with localized urticaria without systemic symptoms may be discharged after treatment in the emergency department and should be seen in follow-up within a few days if lesions persist.

SCABIES & PEDICULOSIS

Etiology

A. Scabies: Scabies is a common infestation caused by *Sarcoptes scabiei,* a virtually invisible (0.1-mm) mite transmitted by intimate but not necessarily sexual contact. Mites survive several days at the most when separated from the host; therefore, close physical contact is a more important mode of transmission than is exposure to contaminated clothing or bedding.

B. Pediculosis (Lice):

1. Pediculosis pubis–Infestation with *Pthirus pubis,* a barely visible (2-mm) louse in the pubic region and sometimes the eyelashes or axillas. Infection is spread by intimate contact, often sexual. The lice survive for about 1 day off the host.

2. Pediculosis capitis–Infestation in the scalp with *Pediculus humanus* var *capitis,* visible (3-mm) lice. The small grayish-white cocoonlike nits may be seen attached to hair shafts. The disease is easily spread through casual contact and by fomites such as shared combs or hats. The lice usually survive only a few days off the host.

3. Pediculosis corporis–Infestation with *Pediculus humanus* var *corporis.* The louse is usually found on clothing, particularly in seams around warm areas, eg, waist, and comes onto the skin only to feed.

Diagnosis

A. Scabies: Scabies is characterized by dozens to hundreds of tiny, punctate excoriations, papules, and nodules and a few superficial burrows. Interdigital areas, the penis and scrotum, umbilical and pubic regions, ankles, and breasts are classic sites of involvement. Inflammatory nodules and papules occurring on both the penis and the scrotum are a particularly helpful diagnostic sign in males; similar lesions occur on the nipples and areolae in females.

Pruritus is intense and often seems worse at night; the patient often gives a history of itching for 1–3 weeks.

No organisms or nits can be seen with the naked eye. Burrows or papules may be scraped with a No. 15 blade, the scrapings applied to a glass slide along with drops of oil or water, and the preparation examined under low power. Intact mites, eggs, or waste material may be seen.

Intimate contacts of the infested person may also be infested.

B. Pediculosis:

1. Pediculosis pubis–Infestation with pubic lice should be considered if the patient complains of perineal pruritus, especially if there is a history of exposure. Examination shows adult lice attached to the skin and nits attached to hair shafts. Blue macules around the thighs or pubic area may occur at sites where the organisms are feeding.

2. Pediculosis corporis–Infestation with body lice should be considered if the patient complains of diffuse pruritus, especially if there is evidence of generally poor hygiene. Examination reveals erythematous macules, wheals, and excoriations, often with superinfection (eg, impetigo, cellulitis). Lice are found mostly in clothing (especially the seams) rather than on the body.

3. Pediculosis capitis–Infestation with head lice should be considered if the patient complains of itching of the scalp or eyelashes. Examination shows adult lice in the hair, with nits at the base of the hair shafts. Macules, wheals, and excoriations are present.

C. Coexisting Sexually Transmitted Diseases: Since both scabies and pediculosis may be sexually transmitted, examination for other sexually transmitted diseases should be performed and a serologic test for syphilis (VDRL or other) obtained.

Treatment

A. Scabies:

1. Adults (except pregnant or lactating women) and older children–

a. Permethrin 5% cream (Elimite)–After an evening shower or bath, the patient should apply permethrin 5% cream to the body from the neck down, taking care to include all creases, folds, and perineal surfaces. The following day (ie, after about 8–12 hours), the patient should shower or bathe thoroughly to remove the medication. One tube of permethrin 5% cream (60 g) should be sufficient to treat 1 or 2 persons. One application is credited with curing uncomplicated scabies infestations in 90% of those treated.

Underclothing, bedding, and towels should be laundered in hot water or dry-cleaned to destroy possible residual organisms.

Household pets (cats and dogs) may be infested with scabies ("canine scabies"). Failure to treat such animals may result in reinfection of previously treated human hosts.

b. Lindane cream or lotion (Kwell, many others)–This is a time-honored remedy for scabies infestation, with a published cure rate approximately that of permethrin 5%, although some pockets of lindane-resistant scabies mites have been documented during the last decade. Because lindane is a hydrocarbon (hexachlorobenzene), it is capable of eliciting central nervous system or other side effects when used repeatedly or in elderly or immunocompromised individuals. Many dermatologists now relegate lindane to a backup role, to be used when permethrin 5% cream fails.

c. Crotamiton (Eurax) cream, 10%–This is another alternative therapy for scabies infestation and one that is relatively free from side effects. It is applied as a cream to the entire body from the neck down nightly for 2 nights and thoroughly washed off 24 hours after the second application.

d. Sulfur in petrolatum, 6%– This is another alternative treatment without systemic toxicity. Apply to the entire body from the neck down nightly for 3 nights. Patients may bathe before reapplying the drug and should bathe 24 hours after the final application. This medication has an unpleasant odor and should be used only if other therapy is contraindicated.

2. Infants and children under 10 years of age; pregnant or lactating women–Use permethrin 5%, crotamiton, or sulfur in petrolatum as described above.

Relief of itching usually begins within a few days after treatment with scabicides. However, some itching may persist for several weeks after adequate therapy. Patients should be told that much of the itching is due to an allergic reaction to the mite and its products and that it often takes 1–3 weeks for all itching to disappear. A *single* re-treatment after 1 week may be appropriate if the patient fails to respond to the first application. Multiple, frequent applications of scabicides for persistent pruritus are not indicated and may cause skin irritation or skin sensitization.

3. Adjunctive measures—Various antipruritic agents may be used after initial treatment with the regimens described above.

a. A shake lotion (eg, calamine) or Eucerin cream (containing 50% water-in-oil emulsion of petrolatum, mineral oil, mineral wax, and wool wax alcohols) may be applied after lindane has been washed off.

b. Systemic antipruritic agents—See p 770.

c. Moderate-strength topical corticosteroids (Table 40–6) may be used on papules or nodules that persist for weeks to months in the absence of continued infection.

It may be necessary to inject triamcinolone (Kenalog, many others), 10 mg/mL subcutaneously, into persistent papules, or to apply potent topical corticosteroids or a coal tar gel (Estar, many others).

B. Pediculosis:

1. Pediculosis corporis, pubis, and capitis– Permethrin 1% cream rinse (Nix) can be applied to the groin, axillas, and scalp for 10 minutes and then washed off. Alternatively, lindane 1% shampoo can be applied to the same areas, left overnight (about 8 hours), and washed off on the following day. Alternatively, lindane 1% can be used as a shampoo, left on for 4 minutes, and then thoroughly washed off. Lindane should not be used on pregnant or lactating women or children under 10 years of age.

Over-the-counter synergized pyrethrins (RID, R & C Shampoo, A-200, and others) appear equally effective in the treatment of head lice. Follow the label directions.

2. Pediculosis of the eyelashes–Apply occlusive ophthalmic ointment (eg, petrolatum) to the eyelid margins twice daily for 10 days to smother lice and nits. Lindane or other drugs should not be applied to the eyes.

3. Adjunctive measures–Bedding and clothing should be washed in hot water or dry-cleaned. Hats, combs, and brushes should be thoroughly cleaned before being reused. Sexual contacts of patients should also be treated, and close contacts of patients with pediculosis capitis and corporis should be examined for lice. Patients should be told that empty or dead nits may remain on hair shafts for long periods of time after treatment and that only demonstrable living adult organisms are an indication for re-treatment.

Disposition

Patients who do not experience significant relief from symptoms within a week after treatment has begun should be referred to a dermatologist.

IMPETIGO

Bacterial infection of the skin may be primary (impetigo) or secondary to preexisting dermatosis (impetiginization). The colonizing agent is usually *Staphylococcus aureus.*

Impetigo can begin on the face, particularly in proximity to the nose or moist corners of the mouth, or any other part of the body. Initial lesions typically are small, itchy, or vesicular patches that later become encrusted (honey-colored). Lesions commonly spread to contiguous areas over a period of a few days, and scattered, generalized lesions may appear.

Symptoms of impetigo range from mild to intense itching. Fever is absent in all but the most serious cases. Lesions of impetigo are not always honey-colored crusts; they range from indolent-appearing, moist, tumid pink plaques to frankly vesicular or bullous lesions. Bullous impetigo is particularly common in children and may be intensely itchy. Lesions that are thick or deep (ecthyma) can lead to permanent scarring.

Diagnosis

The rapid development of multiple lesions, accompanying pruritus, and presence of honey-colored crusts suggest the diagnosis of impetigo. Gram's stain of fluid from lesions showing the presence of gram-positive cocci may aid in diagnosis but does not exclude underlying dermatosis with secondary impetiginization. When the diagnosis is in doubt, a bacterial culture may be taken immediately prior to the empiric use of antibiotics. Treatment can be adjusted on the basis of culture results, or a new diagnosis can be entertained in cases of treatment failure.

Treatment

The surest effective treatment is with oral antibiotics active against *S aureus.* Dicloxicillin or erythromycin, 250–500 mg orally 4 times daily (in children, 12.5–50 mg/kg/d in 4–6 divided doses or 30–50 mg/kg/d in 4 divided doses, respectively) for 5–7 days usually is sufficient. Because in vitro cultures of impetiginized areas may show resistance to erythromycin, many practitioners prefer dicloxicillin.

Mupirocin (Bactroban) is a recently approved topical antibiotic that is efficacious in the treatment of impetigo. It is applied to affected areas twice daily for 5–10 days. When impetigo is widespread, aggressive, or potentially scarring or when infectious spread to others is a possibility, oral antibiotics are preferred.

Disposition

Impetigo treated as outlined above typically begins to subside in 24–48 hours, and a follow-up examination may be unnecessary. Patients should be provided with instructions for follow-up care with a primary care physician or dermatologist if lesions do not respond to treatment. Patients who have lesions on parts of the body where organisms may be easily spread to others (eg, on the hands) should be told that the threat of spread is small though real. Food handlers in particular should not prepare food for others unless lesions are adequately covered or are dried and resolving.

ERYTHEMA MULTIFORME & STEVENS-JOHNSON SYNDROME

Erythema multiforme and Stevens-Johnson syndrome are considered to be "reaction patterns," for which the most commonly documented triggers include concurrent herpes simplex infections and systemic medications. Frequently, however, no specific precipitating cause for these eruptions can be found.

Diagnosis

The patient with erythema multiforme (EM) classically presents with painful or burning erythematous or violaceous patches on the palms and soles. Oval or circular lesions may have dusky, concentric centers ("target lesions"). Not infrequently, erythematous plaques or papules are present on the extremities or trunk, mucous membrane patches or erosions are present, and palmar/plantar lesions may be absent.

Stevens-Johnson syndrome (SJS) is a severe and potentially life-threatening variant of erythema multiforme. Oral and genital mucosal lesions may be severe, bullous, and erosive. Truncal lesions may also be widespread, and the patient can become critically ill from fluid and electrolyte imbalance and intercurrent bacterial infection.

Treatment

Erythema multiforme is typically self-limited, with pain and lesions abating within 10–20 days. Severe erythema multiforme and Stevens-Johnson syndrome are often treated with systemic corticosteroids, beginning in the high-dose range (prednisone, 60–200 mg/d), although universal proof of efficacy is lacking.

Emergency treatment consists of the following:

A. Elimination of ongoing etiologic triggers, such as herpes simplex infection (see acyclovir, below), or discontinuation of intercurrent medication that may have precipitated the eruption.

B. Treatment of secondary infection in eroded areas due to *Staphylococcus aureus, Candida,* or other organisms.

C. Referral to a dermatologist for definitive diagnosis or biopsy and to distinguish Stevens-Johnson syndrome from other erosive conditions such as toxic epidermal necrolysis, staphylococcal scalded skin syndrome, toxic shock syndrome, and septicemia with cutaneous stigmata.

D. When symptoms are severe and diagnosis of Stevens-Johnson syndrome is strongly suspected, the commencement of intravenous empiric corticosteroid therapy, equivalent to 80–120 mg of prednisone per day, pending confirmation of the diagnosis.

TOXIC EPIDERMAL NECROLYSIS

Etiology

Toxic epidermal necrolysis (TEN) occurs without apparent provocation and as a reaction to a variety of known agents, including infections, neoplasms, and drugs such as butazones, barbiturates, hydantoins, and sulfonamides. Toxic epidermal necrolysis occurs mainly in adults and is associated with a death rate of 25–30%.

In addition, 2 conditions are characterized by epidermal necrosis that mimic toxic epidermal necrolysis and are related to staphylococcal infection.

Staphylococcal scalded skin syndrome is associated with clinical findings similar to those of toxic epidermal necrolysis, but the cause, patient profile, and prognosis of the disease are different. Staphylococcal scalded skin syndrome occurs mostly in children under 5 years of age and is caused by an exotoxin released during infection with phage group 2 staphylococci. The death rate in staphylococcal scalded skin syndrome is low (2–3%).

Toxic shock syndrome is also caused by a staphylococcal toxin but has clinical features different from staphylococcal scalded skin syndrome. It can have a high death rate.

Diagnosis

A. Toxic Epidermal Necrolysis: The acute prodrome of toxic epidermal necrolysis includes fever, malaise, arthralgias, and skin tenderness. Within a few hours to a few days, a morbilliform rash appears, becomes vesiculobullous, and eventually desquamates. Mucous membrane involvement is often marked.

B. Staphylococcal Scalded Skin Syndrome: The patient is also systemically ill and may have widespread desquamation and significant cutaneous tenderness, but the mucous membranes are spared or minimally involved.

C. Toxic Shock Syndrome: (See also Chapters 3 and 34.) Fever and a diffuse erythematous rash with mucositis (pharyngitis, vaginitis) are present. Hypotension and shock are common. Most cases have occurred in menstruating women and are associated with tampon usage and heavy vaginal colonization by *S aureus.* Occasional cases result from other types of staphylococcal infection (abscesses, etc).

Skin biopsy has proved helpful in distinguishing between toxic shock syndrome and toxic epidermal necrolysis; such immediate differentiation can be critical, since treatment for the 2 conditions is significantly different.

Treatment

A. Treat shock (Chapter 3).

B. Insert a large-bore intravenous catheter, and draw blood for CBC with differential, serum electrolyte determinations, and renal function tests.

C. Obtain cultures of blood and material from the skin, vagina, and any other possible sites of infection.

D. If staphylococcal scalded skin syndrome or toxic shock syndrome is suspected, begin nafcillin or oxacillin, 150 mg/kg/d intravenously in 4–6 divided doses. Clindamycin, 40 mg/kg/d orally or intravenously in 3 divided doses; or vancomycin, 20 mg/kg/d intravenously in 2 divided doses, may be used in patients allergic to penicillin.

E. If toxic epidermal necrolysis is suspected, high doses of corticosteroids (prednisone, 150–250 mg/d orally or intravenously in 4 divided doses) may be lifesaving.

F. Cover open lesions with saline-soaked dressings.

G. Obtain emergency general medical and dermatologic consultation for definitive diagnosis.

Disposition

Patients with toxic epidermal necrolysis, toxic shock syndrome, or staphylococcal scalded skin syndrome should be hospitalized immediately and emergency general medical and dermatologic consultation obtained.

GENERALIZED PUSTULAR PSORIASIS

Generalized pustular psoriasis has a variety of presentations and causes, and the prognosis varies accordingly. Pustular psoriasis with systemic symptoms is rare. It may arise spontaneously from typical plaquelike psoriasis or after infection or drug use (especially after withdrawal of systemic corticosteroids).

Diagnosis

Patients with severe, acute generalized pustular psoriasis may or may not present with the plaquelike lesions or other common signs of psoriasis. Findings may range from widespread, fiery erythema with sheets of pustules to more indolent, annular lesions or milder generalized erythema with scattered pustules.

In the most fulminant form of generalized pustular psoriasis, the patient has severe systemic symptoms, including tachycardia, high fever, chills, and generalized discomfort.

Widespread erythema and tachycardia in older patients or in those with compromised cardiovascular function may precipitate cardiac failure resulting from high output demands.

Treatment
A. Patients With Systemic Symptoms:
1. Maintain oral and intravenous hydration.
2. Give aspirin or acetaminophen for fever.
3. Obtain emergency dermatologic consultation to confirm the diagnosis and to determine therapy (corticosteroids, methotrexate, etretinate [Tegison], etc).
B. Patients Without Systemic Symptoms:
Patients who do not require systemic therapy may be treated with astringents, compresses, and baths to dry up oozing areas (Table 40–5). Medium- and high-strength topical corticosteroid creams (Table 40–6) may be applied 3 times a day.

Disposition

Patients with acute generalized pustular psoriasis with systemic symptoms should be hospitalized immediately and emergency dermatologic consultation sought. In doubtful cases, the dermatologist should evaluate the patient in the emergency department to determine the need for hospitalization. Patients with subacute or chronic psoriasis without systemic symptoms may be discharged to be seen by a dermatologist or primary care physician within a few days.

ZOSTER

Zoster (shingles) is caused by reactivation of latent neuronal infection by varicella-zoster virus, the agent causing chickenpox. Although it occurs in all age groups, it is more common in older people. One attack appears to confer immunity, and recurrences are rare.

Diagnosis
(See Table 40–8.)
A. Pain: Pain may begin before, during, or after the onset of lesions; rarely, it is absent. It is often deep, aching, or lancinating and, if present before the onset of lesions, may be confused with pain associated with other organic disease, eg, pulmonary embolism or myocardial infarction (when a thoracic dermatome is involved).

B. Lesions are usually found on the trunk or in the area innervated by the ophthalmic division of the trigeminal nerve. Lesions occur in a unilateral dermatomal distribution and do not cross the midline. Lesions begin as erythematous maculopapules but rapidly develop a vesicular center ("dewdrop on a rose petal"). The vesicles may be tiny or may be large bullae. New crops of lesions, which may continue to appear for several days after onset of the rash, eventually dry up, crust over, and disappear entirely over 3–4 weeks, usually without substantial scarring. In some patients, limited dissemination of the virus may occur, and lesions may be found distant from the involved dermatome.

C. Zoster is self-limited, although treatment may be indicated to reduce pain, the duration of the illness, and the likelihood of postherpetic neuralgia, the chief complication of the disease, which is seen more often in elderly patients. Residual pain, itching, or aching may follow an acute eruption and persist for months or indefinitely.

Treatment

Major goals in the treatment of zoster are the following:

A. Alleviating Pain: Aspirin or acetaminophen with codeine (30 mg) is sufficient for pain relief, although severe pain may occasionally require more potent narcotic analgesics. Saline compresses may be helpful.

Oral acyclovir (Zovirax), 800 mg 5 times daily for 10 days, significantly shortens the period of viral shedding, accelerates healing time by 50%, and decreases acute pain. Initiation of treatment more than 4–7 days after lesions appear may be ineffective, except for herpes zoster ophthalmicus, for which later treatment may still reduce ocular complications.

Given in this manner, acyclovir has shown few adverse effects. The most common involve the gastrointestinal tract, with about 2–5% of patients experiencing flatulence, constipation, diarrhea, or nausea.

Table 40–8. Diagnosis of cutaneous herpesvirus infection (herpes simplex or varicella-zoster).

Diagnostic Method	Comments
Viral culture Aspirate vesicle fluid with 27-gauge needle and 1-mL syringe. Alternatively, swab open lesions with small cotton or Dacron swab. Place swab in virology holding medium, refrigerate, and culture within 24–48 hours.	Herpes simplex virus can usually be identified in 2–4 days. Fairly sensitive, highly specific test. Now widely available.
Direct immunofluorescence or immunoperoxidase staining Puncture roof of lesion with needle or scalpel, and swab vigorously with cotton or Dacron swab to obtain cells from base of vesicle. Swab 2 circles (3/16 in [0.5 cm]) onto a clean microscope slide. After specimen has dried, submit for testing.	Results available in 4–8 hours under optimal conditions. Fairly sensitive and specific test. Now widely available.
Tzanck test Unroof fresh vesicle or bulla with fine sharp scissors. Carefully blot fluid with gauze so as not to disturb underlying cells. Scrape cloudy material from floor of lesion with dull edge of scalpel blade, and smear material onto glass slide. Air dry, stain with Giemsa's stain, and cover with coverslip for microscopic examination. Cells infected with herpes simplex or varicella-zoster are multinucleate, with intranuclear inclusions; such findings are absent in other conditions causing vesicular eruptions, such as vaccinia and pemphigus vulgaris.	Moderately sensitive, nonspecific test; does not differentiate between herpes simplex and varicella-zoster.

B. Preventing Postherpetic Neuralgia: Persistent pain after cutaneous lesions have healed, postherpetic neuralgia, rarely occurs in patients under age 40 years but is found in more than half of untreated patients over age 60 years. While oral acyclovir has been shown to decrease acute pain in zoster, it is unclear to what extent it decreases the occurrence of postherpetic neuralgia.

Capsaicin (Axsain, Zostrix) applied topically 3–4 times daily may be helpful in alleviating postherpetic cutaneous pain. It is derived from red (cayenne) pepper and is thought to reduce local pain by depleting and preventing reaccumulation of substance P from peripheral sensory neurons. Capsaicin may cause itching or irritation when first applied, but the discomfort usually subsides.

Systemic corticosteroids given early in the disease can reduce the incidence of postherpetic neuralgia in patients over age 50. One recent study suggests that in patients treated with oral acyclovir, oral corticosteroid therapy did not alter the frequency of postherpetic neuralgia. Thus, compared with the benefits and risks of high-dose oral acyclovir, oral corticosteroid therapy, while of some potential value in severely affected patients, will no longer be the preferred drug therapy for alleviating acute zoster pain and preventing postherpetic neuralgia.

C. Preventing Secondary Bacterial Infection: Crusting or weeping vesicles and open areas may be soaked or bathed in tap water twice daily, or compresses soaked in astringent solutions (Table 40–5) may be applied twice daily. Areas that appear to be at risk for bacterial superinfection can be treated with topical mupirocin (Bactroban) twice daily.

D. Preventing Scarring: Patients should be cautioned to avoid manipulating eschars, since this may cause scarring if dermis adheres to the eschars. Patients with eschars may apply white petrolatum twice daily to aid in reepithelization.

E. Minimizing Ocular Complications: Lesions on the tip of the nose suggest involvement of the nasociliary branch of the ophthalmic division of the trigeminal nerve. Patients with lesions in this location should be treated with oral acyclovir to reduce ocular complications, even if lesions have been present more than 2–3 days. The eye should be carefully examined using a slit lamp. Systemic corticosteroid use is contraindicated. Ophthalmologic consultation should be obtained.

Patients with lesions and pain severe enough to require treatment with oral acyclovir, narcotic analgesics, or systemic corticosteroids should be seen in follow-up in 4–7 days and less often thereafter as needed to monitor healing and possible adverse effects of medications.

Disposition

Hospitalization is not required unless dissemination has occurred in an immunocompromised patient.

HERPES SIMPLEX INFECTION

Herpes simplex virus is a major cause of recurrent orofacial and genital lesions and causes other types of illness as well (keratitis, encephalitis). Infection is spread by direct contact. Primary infection is often the most severe, although it may be asymptomatic. After the primary lesion has healed, the virus remains latent in paraspinal ganglia, where it periodically reactivates in response to diverse stimuli.

Herpes simplex virus type 1 tends to be associated with oral lesions and is spread by contact with saliva from an affected person, whereas herpes simplex virus type 2 causes mainly genital lesions and is spread primarily by sexual contact.

Diagnosis

A. Primary Herpes Simplex Infection: The first clinical attack of herpes simplex virus infection is usually the most severe. Patients may present with fever, malaise, and arthralgias. Infection is characterized at first by grouped vesicles and later by denudation, erosions, or punctate lesions on a swollen, tender, painful erythematous base. Local pain and regional adenopathy are usually marked. Gingivostomatitis is the most common manifestation of herpes simplex type 1 infection; patients with herpes simplex type 2 infection usually present with genital lesions (vulva, vagina, penis, anus, perineum). Patients (especially women) with genital herpes may have aseptic meningitis. The primary illness usually disappears in 2–3 weeks but may last as long as 6 weeks.

B. Recurrent Herpes Simplex Infection: Recurrence of infection is common and may be triggered by fever, exposure to ultraviolet light, friction or trauma associated with sexual intercourse, menstruation, and possibly stress or fatigue. Focal itching, pain, or aching may precede the appearance of vesicles by hours to a few days in some patients. Vesicles usually rupture spontaneously within a few days and heal within a week without scarring. The virus may be recovered as long as lesions are moist; until the area is completely dry and healed, the patient should avoid direct skin-to-skin contact with others.

C. Specific Diagnosis: For either primary or recurrent herpes, especially genital herpes, the diagnosis should be confirmed by culture or antigen detection (Table 40–8).

Treatment

A. Primary Infection:

1. Antipyretics or analgesics may help to relieve systemic symptoms.

2. Acyclovir should be given to all patients with primary infection. Severely ill patients should be hospitalized for administration of intravenous acyclovir (15 mg/kg/d in 2–3 divided doses). Other patients should receive oral acyclovir, 200 mg 5 times a day for 10 days. Treatment of herpes proctitis requires a higher dose, 400 mg 5 times a day for 10 days.

3. Antibiotics are not necessary unless local purulence or cultures or Gram-stained smears positive for bacteria suggest concomitant bacterial infection. *Candida* vaginitis occurs frequently in women with primary genital herpes (Chapter 34).

4. Bathe exposed affected areas, or apply compresses every 4 hours, and apply astringent solutions as long as lesions are moist (Table 40–5).

5. Apply topical anesthetics such as viscous lidocaine or diphenhydramine elixir for severe local pain. Apply to the skin or inside the mouth as needed.

6. Rinses with antiseptics such as benzalkonium chloride, 1:1000 solution; or hydrogen peroxide may soothe and clean the oral mucosa.

B. Recurrent Infection:

1. Patients should not touch or manipulate lesions and should avoid physical contact with others around the area of moist or active lesions.

2. Acyclovir, 200 mg orally 5 times a day for 5 days, will somewhat reduce healing time and the duration of virus shedding if it is started within a day of onset of lesions. A regimen of 800 mg twice daily for 5 days appears equally effective.

3. The following preparations may help to dry lesions, prevent secondary infection, and provide symptomatic relief:

  a. Castellani's paint (contains fuchsin, 0.3%; phenol, 4.5%; resorcinol, 10%; acetone, 1.5%; and alcohol, 13%).

  b. Gentian violet, 1%.

  c. Campho-Phenique (contains phenol, 4.7%; and camphor, 10.8%).

  d. Blistex (contains camphor, 1%; phenol, 0.4%; peppermint oil; lanolin; and petrolatum).

4. Compresses or soaks may help to soothe weeping lesions (Table 40–5).

C. Smallpox Vaccination: Smallpox vaccination is not indicated for preventing herpes simplex infection, because it has not been proved to reliably prevent recurrent herpes simplex infection, and it has caused severe and even fatal generalized vaccinia.

Disposition

A. Hospitalization is often indicated for patients with primary genital herpes, who may have severe pain, systemic symptoms, and other complications (aseptic meningitis, neuropathic bladder). Hospitalization is also required for patients with large or rapidly progressive lesions, especially if the patient is immunocompromised.

B. Patients with newly diagnosed or recurrent herpes simplex infections may suffer both physically and psychologically because of the present epidemic of genital herpes infections in the USA. Patients are often frightened and confused about the nature of the disease and its mode of transmission. Counseling should be provided in the emergency department to explain the disease, answer any questions, and provide information on various treatment methods so that the patient can make an informed evaluation of efficacy, risks, and side effects. Patients should be referred for follow-up with primary care providers in 1–2 weeks.

C. Pregnant patients with newly diagnosed genital herpes should be referred to an obstetrician.

D. Obtain a serologic test for syphilis (eg, VDRL) in all patients to rule out coexisting syphilis.

PEMPHIGUS VULGARIS

Pemphigus vulgaris is a chronic, severe blistering disease usually seen in patients who are middle-aged or older. If the disease is left untreated, death usually occurs in 12–18 months. Corticosteroids and immunosuppressive agents may dramatically reduce the death rate.

Diagnosis

The disease typically begins insidiously with a few groups of lesions or scattered erosions or bullae, often on the oral mucosa. Generalized spread of lesions usually occurs months later. Bullae rupture easily, and the epidermis of apparently normal skin may be easily denuded with pressure from a fingertip (Nikolsky sign). Erosions, especially those in the mouth, may be painful.

Unless lesions are complicated by secondary bacterial infection, patients are not usually febrile.

Confirmation of the diagnosis is not basically an emergency department procedure. The differentiation of pemphigus vulgaris from other bullous diseases is important so that appropriate systemic therapy can be started quickly, usually in a matter of days.

Differential Diagnosis

A. Pemphigus lesions tend not to be dermatomal in distribution; those of zoster are.

B. Pemphigus often involves the oral mucosa; zoster does not.

C. The bullae associated with pemphigus appear gradually, occur on normal-appearing skin, and are flaccid in comparison with the tense vesicles with an erythematous base that characterize early zoster infections. The lesions of pemphigus are usually not acute, inflamed, or itchy like those of herpes simplex or varicella-zoster infections, bullous impetigo, or contact dermatitis.

D. Pemphigus lesions may be present for weeks to months before the patient seeks medical attention, whereas the usual severe, acute onset of many other vesiculobullous diseases usually brings patients to the emergency department earlier in the course of the disease.

Treatment

A. Corticosteroids: Since the dose of systemic corticosteroids initially used to treat severe pemphigus may be very high (prednisone, 200–400 mg orally per day) and the diagnosis is seldom certain in the emergency department, treatment with corticosteroids should not be started in the emergency department.

B. Other Measures: Patients thought to have pemphigus may be given nonnarcotic analgesics and astringents for weeping cutaneous and oral lesions (Table 40–5).

Disposition

Refer all patients thought to have pemphigus vulgaris to a dermatologist within 1–2 days. The patient should be hospitalized immediately if infection, fever, or other systemic findings are present.

PURPURA FULMINANS

Purpura fulminans has generally been understood to mean sudden onset of ecchymoses accompanying meningococcal and other septicemias. More recently, the use of the term has been reserved more for the acute, purpuric sequelae to streptococcal infections, scarlet fever, or varicella that are usually seen in children and are associated with disseminated intravascular coagulation, fever, and shock.

Diagnosis

The chief diagnostic features are extensive ecchymoses (purpura) with a predilection for the distal extremities, accompanied by systemic toxicity with high fever, often in a child. The disorder appears concurrently with or following an infection, which may be mild, and quickly progresses to shock, which may be due to hypovolemia, endotoxemia, or addisonian crisis from adrenal hemorrhage (Waterhouse-Friderichsen syndrome). Laboratory examination shows severe disseminated intravascular coagulation (thrombocytopenia, prolonged partial thromboplastin and thrombin times, elevated levels of fibrin degradation products).

Treatment

A. Treat Shock: (See Chapter 3.)

1. Insert a large-bore (≥ 16-gauge) intravenous catheter.

2. Draw blood for CBC and differential, serum electrolyte and blood glucose determinations, tests of renal and hepatic function, and coagulation panel (platelet count; thrombin, prothrombin, and partial thromboplastin times; fibrin degradation products; and fibrinogen level).

3. Begin rapid infusion of crystalloid solution to support blood pressure.

4. Give hydrocortisone, 100 mg intravenously every 6 hours.

B. Treat Bacteremia:

1. Obtain 1–2 blood cultures as well as material from other appropriate body fluids (urine, cerebrospinal fluid, skin lesions) for culture.

2. Begin empiric antimicrobial therapy with one of the following: **(a)** penicillin, 300,000 units/kg/d intravenously in 6 divided doses; or **(b)** chloramphenicol, 60 mg/kg/d intravenously in 4 divided doses, for patients allergic to penicillin. (See also Table 3–6.)

C. Treat Disseminated Intravascular Coagulation: Specific therapy for disseminated intravascular coagulation is discussed in Chapter 33.

Disposition

Hospitalize all patients with purpura fulminans, preferably in the intensive care unit if shock is present or sepsis is suspected.

DRUG ERUPTIONS

Cutaneous eruptions have been associated with almost all medications, including those that patients themselves do not often consider "medicines," eg, vitamins, aspirins, and laxatives.

A variety of immunologic mechanisms have been associated with drug eruptions. The timing and extent of sensitization may be unpredictable. Patients may suddenly react to drugs they have taken without reaction for years. A drug-related rash may subside while the patient is still taking the medication. A drug eruption may or may not recur when the offending drug is reintroduced, and a rash may begin as long as 2 weeks after a drug has been discontinued.

Diagnosis

Manifestations of drug-related skin eruptions are set forth in Table 40–9.

Skin conditions that may simulate drug eruptions include syphilis, pityriasis rosea, lichen planus, sarcoidosis, leprosy, and dermatitis due to physical agents, such as ultraviolet light or contactants. In contrast to secondary syphilis, in which itching is usually absent or mild, itching is common and often marked in drug eruptions.

Acute urticarial reactions may be accompanied by signs of systemic anaphylaxis; see Chapter 3 for emergency treatment. Drugs may also be implicated as a cause of toxic epidermal necrolysis (p 778).

Treatment

A. Evaluate the Course of Lesions: Whether or not to discontinue a drug or to switch drugs depends on the severity of the eruption and on the necessity for the medication; in critical illness, benefits may outweigh the side effects. A mildly pruritic eruption that appears stable or is progressing slowly (over a period of days) might not necessarily be a criterion for discontinuing a critical medication. Also, some drug eruptions disappear even though the patient continues to take the drug.

B. Discontinue the Drug If Required: Severe signs that may require discontinuing or switching a medication include rapid progression of lesions, intractable and disabling pruritus, mucous membrane involvement, cutaneous erosions, or vesiculobullous lesions.

Table 40–9. Clinical manifestations of drug eruptions.

Urticaria	Vasculitis
Morbilliform rash	Toxic epidermal necrolysis
Fixed eruptions	Acneiform eruptions
Erythema multiforme	Vesiculobullous lesions
Alopecia	Exfoliative dermatitis
"Lichenoid" reactions	Lupus erythematosus-like lesions
Eczematous reactions	Pityriasis rosea-like lesions
Pigmentary changes	Granulomatous lesions
Photodermatitis	

C. Discontinue All Nonessential Drugs: When a drug eruption is suspected, all medications that are not absolutely essential should be discontinued.

D. Treat Symptoms: Following discontinuation of the offending agent, drug eruptions usually resolve spontaneously over a few days, although topical corticosteroids (eg, hydrocortisone cream, 1%; or triamcinolone cream, 0.025–0.1%, twice daily) may speed resolution of pruritic and eczematous lesions. A shake lotion (eg, calamine lotion) twice daily may also relieve itching. A simple emollient such as white petrolatum or Eucerin lotion (containing mineral oil, isopropyl myristate, PEG-40, glycerin ester, aluminum stearate, and other ingredients) may relieve itching and drying while the eruption gradually resolves.

E. Test for Syphilis: Since drug eruptions may simulate signs of secondary syphilis, a serologic test for syphilis should be ordered when the cause of a drug-related or other cutaneous eruption is not known with certainty.

Disposition

Hospitalization is indicated for patients with fever or signs of severe systemic involvement and for those with diffuse erythroderma or exfoliation.

If a supposed drug eruption fails to begin clearing in 1–2 days after discontinuation of the suspected agent, the patient should see a dermatologist within a few days.

Advise the patient that drug allergy may exist and that the patient should inform physicians of this in the future. If the drug reaction was major (urticarial or anaphylactoid), the patient should consider wearing a Medic-Alert tag or bracelet.

PITYRIASIS ROSEA

Symptoms and Signs

Pityriasis rosea is a common, benign, and self-limited condition. It typically begins with a "herald patch," a 1- to 3-cm oval, red, raised, and slightly scaly patch on the torso or proximal extremities that is commonly confused with ringworm. Typically, a few days later, multiple other ovoid patches appear. When profuse, these lesions may assume a fir tree–like pattern on the back, so called because they are aligned parallel to skin folds.

There is great variation in the way pityriasis rosea presents, however, and many cases do not have the classic appearance. Itching is typically present and is roughly proportionate to the number of lesions.

Differential Diagnosis

Pityriasis rosea can be confused with tinea corporis (ringworm), secondary syphilis, psoriasis, nummular dermatitis, viral exanthems, and drug eruptions. A serologic test for syphilis may be advisable.

Treatment

The only uniformly successful treatment for this condition is administration of systemic corticosteroids, which are indicated only if the itching is so intense as to prevent sleeping or working. If deemed necessary, and with appropriate regard for contraindications, a 7- to 10-day tapered course of prednisone, beginning with 30–50 mg/d (adult) may be helpful. Although pityriasis rosea is suppressed with corticosteroids, its natural history may not be altered; the condition may recur when corticosteroids are withdrawn.

Intense sun exposure may help in some cases but cannot be recommended as otherwise safe; topical corticosteroids are not generally of consistent benefit.

Prognosis

With or without treatment, this disorder lasts between 1 and 3 months. Many cases reach a peak at 3–4 weeks and have resolved by 6 weeks. There are no systemic sequelae.

TINEA CORPORIS
(Ringworm)

Symptoms and Signs

The classic "ringworm" is a 1- to 2-cm red, raised, scaly round patch with a relatively flat or smooth center. It may, however, be irregular, flat, and vague in outline. Ringworm is commonly seen on the trunk and extremities and can occur on the face (tinea faciale), hands (tinea manuum), feet (tinea pedis), and groin (tinea cruris). It is almost invariably itchy. Administration of topical corticosteroids alleviates the itching somewhat while making the eruption itself appear unchanged or worse.

Treatment

Several topical antifungal agents, (eg, econazole nitrate and ciclopirox olamine applied once or twice daily) may be effective against lesions of tinea corporis that previously may have responded only to systemic therapy. For widespread tinea corporis or lesions unresponsive to topical treatment, griseofulvin ultramicrosize, 250–500 mg/d, may be given until clearing is demonstrated by microscopic examination of a scraping prepared with potassium hydroxide that shows no hyphae or spores.

Prognosis

Effective treatment typically reduces itching dramatically within 2 to 4 days. Established cases may require 2–6 weeks of therapy before complete resolution occurs. Resolution of lesions on the scalp and on the soles of the feet may take longer.

MOLLUSCUM CONTAGIOSUM

Symptoms and Signs

The classic lesions are 1- to 3-mm, shiny, dome-shaped, umbilicated papules. In adults they typically appear on the waist, buttocks, or perineum; in children, they are commonly seen on the face and chest. Genital lesions in children should be evaluated within an overall context relating to the possibility of intimate or sexual contact with an affected adult.

Lesions not infrequently become inflamed, and some may become large (3–5 mm in diameter). They may be mistaken clinically for furuncles, amelanotic melanomas, and infected moles.

Treatment

Light application of liquid nitrogen is the treatment most likely to achieve a cure. Most adults and some children tolerate these painful sessions well. An alternative treatment, though not as uniformly successful, is a once-daily application of a prepared salicylic acid/lactic acid in collodion solution (Occlusal, Duofilm).

Prognosis

Without treatment, the lesions of molluscum contagiosum often spread to unaffected areas on the patient's skin or to other persons in close contact with the patient. When evaluating children it may be preferable to defer treatment, since the methods noted above may be painful and spontaneous remission can occur within 6–24 months.

TINEA VERSICOLOR

Symptoms and Signs

Lesions consist of usually asymptomatic, brown or tan circular patches that may become confluent. Typical distribution is over the shoulders, back, chest and arms, though this fungal condition may also be seen in other areas including the face, groin, and legs. Examination of scales under the microscope with potassium hydroxide will reveal numerous short hyphae and spores ("spaghetti and meatballs"). This condition may be chronic and is exacerbated by a hot, humid climate.

Treatment

Selenium sulfide lotion 2.5% is effective when applied to all affected areas at bedtime, left on overnight, and washed off in the morning. Application once a week for 4 weeks is recommended. Alternatively, numerous antifungal creams or lotions (eg, econazole nitrate, ciclopirox olamine, miconazole, and clotrimazole) are also effective when applied to all affected areas once daily for 1 week.

REFERENCES

Arndt KA: *Manual of Dermatologic Therapeutics,* 4th ed. Little, Brown, 1988.

Arndt KA, Jick H: Rates of cutaneous reactions to drugs: A report from the Boston Collaborative Drug Surveillance Program. JAMA 1976;235:918.

Baker H, Ryan T: Generalized pustular psoriasis: A clinical and epidemiological study of 104 cases. Br J Dermatol 1968;80:771.

Callen JP, Cooper MA (guest editors): Symposium on dermatologic emergencies. Emerg Med Clin North Am 1985;3:641. [Entire issue.]

Cobo M: Reduction of the ocular complications of herpes zoster ophthalmicus by oral acyclovir. Am J Med 1988; 85(Suppl 2A):90.

Douglas JM et al: A double-blind study of oral acyclovir for suppression of recurrences of genital herpes simplex virus infection. N Engl J Med 1984;310:1551.

Epstein WL, Byers VS, Frankart W: Induction of antigen-specific hyposensitization to poison oak in sensitizied adults. Arch Dermatol 1982;118:630.

Esman V et al: Prenisolone does not prevent post-herpetic neuralgia. Lancet 1987;2:126.

Fitzpatrick TB et al (editors): *Dermatology in General Medicine: Textbook and Atlas,* 3rd ed. McGraw-Hill, 1987.

Goldberg LH et al: Oral acyclovir for episodic treatment of recurrent genital herpes: Efficacy and safety. J Am Acad Dermatol 1986;15:256.

Heng-Leong C et al: The incidence of erythema multiforme, Stevens-Johnson syndrome, and toxic epidermal necrolysis. Arch Dermatol 1990;126:43.

Hodge SJ: Purpura fulminans. Cutis 1978;21:830.

Huff JC et al: Therapy of herpes zoster with oral acyclovir. Am J Med 1988;85(Suppl 2A):84.

Hurwitz RM et al: Toxic shock syndrome or toxic epidermal necrolysis? J Am Acad Dermatol 1982;7:246.

Jacobson KW, Branch LB, Nelson HS: Laboratory tests in chronic urticaria. JAMA 1980;243:1644.

Keczkes K, Basheer AM: Do corticosteroids prevent postherpetic neuralgia? Br J Dermatol 1980;102:551.

Lever WF, Schaumburg-Lever G: Treatment of pemphigus vulgaris. Arch Dermatol 1984;120:44.

Leznoff A et al: Association of chronic urticaria and angioedema with thyroid autoimmunity. Arch Dermatol 1983;119:636.

Meinking TL et al: Comparative efficacy of treatments for pediculosis capitis infestations. Arch Dermatol 1986; 122:267.

Miller DA, Freeman GL, Akers WA: Chronic urticaria. Am J Med 1968;44:68.

Monroe EW et al: Combined H_1 and H_2 antihistamine therapy in chronic urticaria. Arch Dermatol 1981;117:404.

Noid HE, Schulze TW, Winkelmann RK: Diet plan for patients with salicylate-induced urticaria. Arch Dermatol 1974;109:866.

Orkin M, Maibach HI: Scabies in children. Pediatr Clin North Am 1978;25:371.

Parker CW: Drug allergy. (3 parts.) N Engl J Med 1975; 292:511, 732, 957.

Robboy SJ et al: The skin in disseminated intravascular coagulation: Prospective analysis of thirty-six cases. Br J Dermatol 1973;88:221.

Rosenbaum MM, Roenigk HH: Treatment of generalized pustular psoriasis with etretinate (Ro 10–9359) and methotrexate. J Am Acad Dermatol 1984;10:357.

Strom B et al: A population-based study of Stevens-Johnson syndrome. Arch Dermatol 1991;127:831.

Taplin D, Meinking TL: Pyrethrins and pyrethroids in dermatology. Arch Derm 1990;126(2):213.

41 Psychiatric Emergencies

Jerome A. Motto, MD

EMERGENCY MANAGEMENT OF HOSTILE, ABUSIVE, VIOLENT, OR ASSAULTIVE BEHAVIOR

Physical violence is seldom a manifestation of psychiatric disorder. Instead, most violent acts reflect the perpetrator's low frustration tolerance or life-style and cultural values combined with the temporary influence of unbearable stress or the relaxation of inhibition and distortion of reality brought about by alcohol or other drugs.

Psychiatric conditions in which violent behavior may be a problem are those associated with persecutory ideas, schizophrenic disorders, or manic states. Such violent behavior may result in part from a false sense of security in the emergency department staff, who may be misled by the patient's innocuous appearance, subdued demeanor, or seemingly good spirits and who therefore may not take care to reassure the patient about the safety of the setting and the benevolent intentions of the staff.

A history of violent behavior is the best predictor of potential violence. *If a patient is brought to the emergency department in restraints, do not remove the restraints until a careful evaluation has been completed, even though the patient appears relaxed and cooperative.* Try to perform the evaluation away from the mainstream of emergency department traffic. Police officers, the sight of guns, the presence of injured or weeping patients, or staff members hurrying by who are calling to each other or even laughing together can be extremely disturbing to a highly charged patient.

Take time with potentially violent patients. Though it may try the patience of a busy staff, there is no substitute for allowing the patient to set the pace. Psychiatric disturbances call for an accepting, nonjudgmental, supportive attitude and demeanor on the part of helping persons. The physician must maintain a deliberate and methodical manner, avoiding power struggles and any attempt at heroic measures to control the situation. Use the patient's family or other trusted persons, if present, for standby support and assistance. Give continuous reassurance, explain the need for any planned procedure (physical examination, giving medication, etc), and ask repeatedly whether the patient is able to cooperate with the next step to be taken. Dealing with psychiatric emergencies requires readiness to be guided by subjective impressions to a greater extent than in other disorders. Adequate assessment of psychiatric conditions is often time-consuming, but good practice allows no alternatives.

Initial Management of Violent or Severely Agitated Patients

A. Restraints: If the patient is violent to the extent that evaluation and treatment are not possible, ask security personnel to physically restrain the patient. Search the patient for weapons. Do not leave the patient alone to "cool off."

B. Sedation: If the patient is too agitated to evaluate, give lorazepam, 1–2 mg orally or intramuscularly, or diazepam, 5–10 mg orally every 30 minutes until the patient is able to cooperate, to a maximum of 4 doses. Keep in mind that benzodiazepines can have a disinhibiting as well as sedating effect.

C. Antipsychotics: For agitated psychotic or delirious patients who are not calmed by sedation within 1 hour, add haloperidol, 5 mg intramuscularly every 30 minutes, until the patient becomes manageable. For elderly patients, use only incremental doses of 1–2 mg. With a history or present evidence of extrapyramidal symptoms, add benztropine mesylate, 1–2 mg orally or intramuscularly every 8 hours as needed to minimize such symptoms.

Diagnosis

A. Principal Symptom Complex: In the emergency department, precise diagnosis is often less important than determining the principal symptom complex and initiating management of symptoms. Furthermore, psychiatric conditions frequently occur in various combinations and with atypical patterns, so that standard diagnostic terms are often inadequate to clearly characterize a given condition.

B. Medical Examination and Evaluation: A detailed medical history usually makes the diagnosis obvious (eg, drug ingestion), but supplemental sources of information may be necessary (family, friends, police, employer, therapist, or physician).

1. Perform a brief physical examination–Pay special attention to findings characteristic of disorders that may be associated with violent behavior. These include the following:

a. Head injury.

b. Evidence of drug use, eg, needle tracks, pupillary constriction or dilatation.

c. Hypertension and nystagmus in young people, suggesting phencyclidine (PCP) abuse.

d. Hyperplasia of the gums, suggesting long-term use of phenytoin and a possible postictal state.

e. Stigmas of long-term alcohol abuse—enlarged liver, capillary distention, spider angiomas, etc.

f. Medic-Alert tag (possible diabetes).

2. Exclude organic disease–Almost every known behavioral aberration can be brought about by an organic process or toxic condition. This should be kept in mind and reconsidered frequently, especially if the patient's condition when first seen (eg, acute paranoid psychosis) precludes full medical evaluation. See Chapter 14 for details.

Most organic diseases can be ruled out as a cause of psychiatric abnormalities if results on the following examinations and tests are normal:

a. Vital signs, including temperature.

b. Serum electrolytes.

c. Serum calcium.

d. Liver and renal function tests.

e. Blood glucose.

f. Thyroid function tests.

g. Toxicology screen (for phencyclidine, amphetamines, etc).

3. Perform a brief mental status examination–An adequate examination can be condensed into an evaluation of intellectual function and inquiries designed to disclose a thought disorder, mood disorder, or personality disorder.

a. Intellectual function–Intellectual function will often be evident from the medical history but can be briefly assessed in terms of orientation (to time, place, and person), memory (short-term and long-term), concentration, and judgment. Use the patient's own experience for this assessment: times, dates, current events, telephone numbers, addresses, names, sequences of events, relationships, and actions taken in recent life situations.

b. Thought disorder–Thought disorder is evaluated by a matter-of-fact inquiry about "strange" or "unusual" experiences, such as hearing or seeing things when nothing is there, being controlled by others, thinking that others are trying to do one harm, or getting messages through unusual means, eg, via television or mental telepathy.

c. Mood disorder–Mood disorder is usually manifested by depression. Specific inquiry should be made about despondency, crying, insomnia, anorexia, feelings of discouragement, and suicidal or homicidal ideas.

Mania is evaluated by asking about periods of feeling elated, powerful, free of usual concerns, or "too happy" or about making elaborate plans, needing little sleep, or spending money more freely than usual. The expression of any powerful feeling (guilt, anger, anxiety, fear, etc) should be elicited, and the patient should be encouraged to discuss the feeling openly.

d. Personality disorder–Personality disorder is identified by determining whether the violent behavior is the person's usual way of responding to stress (ie, antisocial personality), an occasional unpredictable outburst (ie, intermittent explosive disorder), a reflection of ongoing morbid suspiciousness or ideas of reference (ie, paranoid personality), an impulsive overreaction (ie, histrionic or borderline personality), or otherwise a manifestation of personality structure rather than a superimposed acute or chronic psychiatric illness.

C. Psychiatric Examination and Evaluation: Psychiatric evaluation can proceed as soon as there is evidence that organic disease is not causing the patient's symptoms. Of immediate concern are any suicidal or homicidal tendencies and the patient's capacity for ordinary self-care. The emergency physician must also search for life-threatening illnesses or conditions resulting from the psychiatric disturbance, such as dehydration or malnutrition.

The evaluation and management of specific psychiatric disorders are discussed in the next section. Regardless of diagnosis, the characteristics most often associated with violent behavior tend to have the following patterns:

(1) Angry, irrational, paranoid, deluded.
(2) Overactive, assaultive, violent, combative.
(3) Unmanageable, uncooperative, hostile, abusive.
(4) Disturbed, hallucinating.

The following observations have been found useful in relating to patients who have been violent or who threaten violence in the emergency department (adapted from Renshaw, 1972):

1. Use a matter-of-fact yet friendly approach in making a personal introduction that identifies the role as well as the speaker: "Mr Allen, I'm Dr Gonzalez of the emergency department staff."

2. Indicate a function as helper: "I understand you need some assistance, and I'd like to help you if I can."

3. Indicate an interest in the patient as a person by continuing to use the patient's surname: "Mrs Carson."

4. Define the problem: "I'm told the police brought you here because you were threatening to hurt someone."

5. Express perception and understanding of the patient feelings: "What was making you so angry?"

6. Try quiet persuasion: "Just wait a while and try to get your control back." Most people recognize and respond to a desire to help.

7. Resist any impulse to take over. The cardinal principle is to evaluate what is going on first and then take action.

8. Accept personal limitations in interacting with the patient. If no response has been elicited to this point, proceed as follows:

9. Try to help the patient with external controls:

a. Direct command–If the patient is shouting, a direct verbal command to stop shouting is sometimes enough.

b. Verbal threat–"If you don't come with us, we'll have to carry you."

c. Close supervision–Stay with the patient. Have an aide or relative accompany the patient at all times.

d. Direct physical restraint–Holding the patient in a controlled way can be reassuring.

e. Mechanical restraint–Wristlets, blanket wrapping, or leather restraints are seldom required but may be needed on occasion.

f. Chemical restraint–Neuroleptics are the most often used chemical restraint but should not be relied on as the sole means of restraint.

g. Legal restraint–Use appropriate documents for temporary involuntary detention. Be sure they are filled out accurately and completely. (See Involuntary Procedures, p 800.)

10. When the patient is under control, explain exactly what is planned: "We are going to take an elevator to the ward, where you can get some sleep. As soon as you have calmed down and can be up comfortably, we'll take off the restraints."

Treatment

Emergency care of any organic disorder (eg, drug overdose, hypoglycemia) has first priority. Use an antipsychotic such as haloperidol, 2–5 mg intramuscularly, to facilitate this care if necessary. Family members may also be able to provide assistance.

Disposition

Disposition is dictated by the results of medical and psychiatric assessment and requirements for continued care. If the physical problem is not life-threatening and the risk of suicide or homicide does not seem serious, it may be best to allow a resistant, hostile, or combative patient to leave the emergency department without further treatment and to hope for another opportunity to be of service at a later time under better circumstances. This does not apply to a psychotic patient or a patient with a grossly disturbed sensorium due to an organic state (eg, delirium), for whom hospitalization is essential. In doubtful cases, it is probably wise to err on the side of hospitalization. (See Involuntary Procedures, p 800.) In any case, be sure to make an entry in the patient's chart that details the rationale for the final disposition.

EMERGENCY TREATMENT OF SPECIFIC DISORDERS

The psychiatric conditions that most commonly present as emergencies are discussed below. The disorders themselves do not always constitute an emergency, yet an emergency can arise from any one of them. It is the effect of the actual or potential behavior *associated* with a disorder that generates the need for immediate attention—eg, starvation in anorexia nervosa or exhaustion in mania.

ORGANICALLY INDUCED DISORDERS

The frequency with which psychiatric symptoms are produced by organic dysfunction cannot be overstressed. Acute alcoholic intoxication is the most common and is discussed below. Three conditions are occurring with increasing frequency in the emergency department and must be part of the differential diagnosis in ruling out a physical disorder.

1. AIDS ENCEPHALOPATHY

In encephalopathy due to acquired immunodeficiency syndrome (AIDS), aberrations of mood, thinking, cognitive function, or behavior either precede or follow the diagnosis of AIDS. Hospitalization for complete assessment is required. Treatment focuses on psychologic and social support.

2. COCAINE PSYCHOSIS

Greater use of the free base form of cocaine ("crack") has resulted in an increasing number of cocaine-related psychotic states. Paranoid symptoms are the most common manifestations, but a wide range of other symptoms occurs. These are characterized by their diversity and unpredictability and include despondency, euphoria, delusions, hallucinations, and delirium. Hospitalization for appropriate management and detoxification is required.

3. NEUROLEPTIC MALIGNANT SYNDROME

This condition is a potentially lethal complication of antipsychotic drug therapy and is characterized by fever, muscular rigidity, altered consciousness, elevated creatine phosphokinase (CK), and autonomic nervous system dysfunction. After other organic causes (eg, central nervous system infection, focal brain lesion, metabolic disorder) have been ruled out, this diagnosis must be considered in any patient receiving neuroleptics who develops fever and central nervous system abnormalities. The relationship of neuroleptic malignant syndrome to malignant hyperthermia is not clear. Hospitalization is indicated. Definitive treatment, beyond immediate withdrawal of all psychotropic medications and prompt supportive care, is not yet clearly established.

ACUTE ALCOHOLIC INTOXICATION
(See Chapters 14 and 39 for complications and withdrawal syndromes.)

Diagnosis
Acute alcoholic intoxication may be manifested by the following characteristics: combative, hostile, abusive, or belligerent behavior; a staggering, ataxic gait; the odor of alcohol on the breath; flushed facies; and perhaps ecchymoses. A somnolent or comatose patient may be severely intoxicated.

A. General Measures:

1. If the patient is boisterous or aggressive, advise security personnel that assistance may be needed.

2. Approach the patient in a nonthreatening manner. Listen carefully to what the patient says, despite verbal abuse. Do not sustain eye contact (this is threatening).

3. Offer the patient food (eg, coffee, cookies), and arrange to talk quietly in an unconfined area. Acknowledge any fear aroused by the patient's behavior.

B. Specific Measures:

1. Estimate blood alcohol level (breath, blood, or urine sample), and perform a complete examination, including a careful neurologic examination, because head injuries are common in alcohol abusers.

2. Rule out pneumonia, hypoglycemia, hypovolemia, diabetes mellitus, Wernicke's syndrome, acidosis, and gastrointestinal tract bleeding.

Treatment
A. If sedation is indicated, the first choice is diazepam, 10 mg orally, repeated hourly until the patient is calm enough to lie down. If the patient is unable to take medication orally, give 5 mg slowly intravenously. With significant liver disease, lorazepam, 1 mg, can be substituted for 5 mg of diazepam.

B. In very belligerent patients, use haloperidol, 2–5 mg orally or 5 mg intramuscularly every 30 minutes, until the patient is manageable.

C. Give thiamine, 100 mg intramuscularly or intravenously.

D. Let the patient sleep. Guard against aspiration of vomitus by having the patient lie on one side rather than be supine.

Disposition

In uncomplicated cases, refer the patient to an outpatient detoxification program. If another serious disorder is present, hospitalization may be necessary. The emergency physician is responsible for appropriate disposition of the intoxicated patient. Therefore, be sure that the patient is not allowed to leave the emergency department prematurely. A subsequent accident may not only injure the patient or others but may also expose the physician and the hospital to liability for those injuries. Be sure to give instructions and information about the patient's condition to a responsible friend or family member. If the patient belongs to Alcoholics Anonymous, that organization may be able to provide someone to help carry out the plans for disposition. If in doubt, transfer the patient to an inpatient detoxification setting. If there is no transportation, the police will assist with transfer in some communities.

PANIC ATTACKS

Patients with acute panic attacks commonly present to the emergency department. Such attacks may create severe distress in the patient and the family and must be taken seriously in order to avert precipitous behavior.

Emergency Factors

The most serious potential factor in a panic attack is that it may lead to incapacitation and, in some instances, suicide. This is especially true when the patient has a low pain threshold, becomes exhausted, loses hope, and becomes so desperate that anything that offers relief will be considered.

Diagnosis

Rapid pulse and respiration, insomnia, anorexia, profuse sweating, dry mouth, and dilated pupils occur. The patient may also be described as frightened, apprehensive, agitated, distracted, giddy, panicky, or tremulous.

The onset of an acute anxiety attack is usually sudden. The patient experiences intense cardiovascular and respiratory response, with constriction of the muscles of the chest and throat that produces feelings of choking, inability to get enough air into the lungs, and chest pain. The patient has difficulty breathing, feels close to fainting, and may be convinced that a heart attack is in progress. The belief that a heart attack is occurring often complicates that problem by generating even more anxiety, which intensifies the end-organ responses frightening the patient still more. This in turn creates even more anxiety, until the patient panics.

Differential Diagnosis

The most important organic conditions that must be considered in the differential diagnosis are amphetamine or cocaine poisoning, intoxication with cannabis or hallucinogens, mitral valve prolapse, hyperthyroidism, hypocalcemia, hypoglycemia, pheochromocytoma, and pulmonary embolism. If chest pain or shortness of breath is present, exclude organic disease (Chapters 5 and 6). Fear of infection with the AIDS virus is an increasingly frequent precipitant of anxiety and panic attacks.

Treatment

A. Perform a brief but careful physical examination not only to rule out organic causes of severe anxiety but also to be able to offer verbal reassurance about the patient's physical condition. When the patient fears a heart attack, an ECG should be obtained.

B. For the hyperventilating patient, increasing arterial PCO_2 by rebreathing into an airtight bag can be useful in reducing some of the secondary somatic signs—muscle twitching, numbness and tingling of the extremities—caused by the respiratory alkalosis associated with hyperventilation.

C. Reassure the patient about the benign nature and limited duration of the episode, and repeat the reassurance as often as necessary.

D. Review with the patient in a calm and quiet setting the period preceding the onset of symptoms to determine whether the panic episode is due to identifiable stressors. Panic attacks usually last less than 1 hour, so any procedure may appear effective and lead the clinician to underestimate the seriousness of the disorder.

E. For acute anxiety, alprazolam (Xanax), 0.5–1 mg orally 3 times a day, lorazepam (Ativan), 1–2 mg sublingually or orally 2–4 times a day, or oxazepam (Serax), 15–30 mg orally 4 times a day, usually provides relief. For severe panic attacks requiring immediate control, lorazepam, 1–2 mg intramuscularly or intravenously, or diazepam (Valium, others), 5–10 mg intravenously, can be used. Owing to the risk of respiratory depression, the intravenous route of administration should be used only when a physician familiar with these agents is present and resuscitation equipment is available. Respiratory depression can usually be avoided by giving intravenous doses slowly (eg, for diazepam, not more than 5 mg/min). For longer term treatment without risking benzodiazepine dependence, good results have been obtained with tricyclic agents (eg, nortriptyline, 75 mg on retiring, or desipramine, 75–125 mg on retiring), especially when supplemented with lithium, 300 mg 2 or 3 times a day.

Disposition

A. Refer the patient for outpatient follow-up, monitoring, continued evaluation, and maintenance medication. Provide for interim medication in case anxiety recurs before follow-up can be implemented.

B. Give instructions about rebreathing into an airtight bag if symptoms of hyperventilation recur.

DEPRESSIVE STATES

A depressed patient often presents to the emergency department because of weight loss or a suicide attempt.

Emergency Factors

Suicide is the commonest risk in depressed patients, although malnutrition may also become an emergency. Families of severely depressed patients may be subject to extreme stress and turmoil. The patient with psychotic depression in whom homicide is a strong possibility represents the most urgent situation.

Diagnosis

Intense feelings of sadness, guilt, or hopelessness are common. The patient is preoccupied, distracted, and tense and may sit motionless, staring into space. Sleeplessness and withdrawal from the activities of daily life occur frequently. The patient is pessimistic and may be suicidal as well as being self-critical, irritable, and indecisive, with fits of crying and morbid thoughts. On the other hand, symptoms opposite to those classically associated with depression may be seen: inability to cry, excessive sleeping, overeating, and agitation rather than lethargy.

Poorly defined organic complaints (eg, headache, backache) may be manifestations of depression but should not be accepted as such without at least a brief evaluation for organic disease (Chapters 13 and 15).

Different age groups tend to experience depression in different ways. A child or adolescent may act out in a destructive manner such as drug abuse, truancy, or fire setting. Older patients may become irritable and preoccupied with vague somatic complaints.

Psychotic depression is characterized by somatic delusions: "My blood is turning to water," "My insides are rotting away," "I have sawdust in my intestines." Psychosis also takes the form of persecutory ideas, often with grandiose expressions of guilt, eg, "I am responsible for the war," or "I have infected the world with syphilis."

Treatment

Treat metabolic disorders, drug ingestion, or other potentially life-threatening medical conditions first. Depressed patients usually do not require medication in the emergency department. If the patient manifests destructive behavior, haloperidol, 5 mg intramuscularly, may help to reduce agitation.

Disposition

Hospitalize all patients with severely incapacitating depressive states—especially if they are suicidal or homicidal—and obtain psychiatric consultation immediately. See below for evaluation of the potential for suicide. Depressed patients who are able to function on a day-to-day basis and who are not suicidal or homicidal may be referred for psychiatric evaluation.

SUICIDAL STATES

The management of suicidal states in the emergency department incorporates 3 steps: recognition, assessment of risk, and treatment. These steps follow and often overlap medical procedures.

Diagnosis

A. Recognition of Potential Suicide: When a patient presents in the emergency department because of the threat of suicide or an actual attempt, the suicidal state has already been defined. The potential for suicide may be obscured if the patient presents with chronic, intractable, or ambiguous complaints (eg, insomnia, pain, fatigue, diabetes, epilepsy, unchangeable life circumstances) or if the person is not actually a patient but is in the emergency department because of involvement in a stressful situation, eg, the driver of a car involved in an accident that has killed someone, or the mother of a severely burned child.

Direct inquiry is an appropriate means of screening for potential suicide, even if it is limited to a simple "How are you managing emotionally?" or "Do you think you can handle this okay?" or "Are you discouraged about how things are going?" If the response is not reassuring, patients with chronic, recurring, or progressive problems require a systematic review of signs and symptoms of depression, eg, insomnia, anorexia, crying spells, despondency, apathy, or inability to work.

The final focus in questioning is on feelings of hopelessness and suicidal ideas: "Does it get so bad that you think it is not worth going on—that you think of suicide?" Any acknowledgment of suicidal thoughts or impulse requires that the physician proceed to assess the risk of suicide.

B. Assessment of Risk: The immediate goal is to decide whether hospitalization is required either because of a severe risk of suicide or because of an underlying psychiatric disorder.

1. Direct questioning–The direct question is a useful initial approach to estimating the degree of risk: "How do you feel *now* about killing yourself?" or "You must have felt pretty low to take those pills—do things look any different now?" or "If you leave the hospital in the next few hours do you think this will happen again?" Any reassuring response should be questioned gently but firmly—"What is different now?" or "Why wouldn't you do it again if nothing has changed?" The patient's tone, manner, attitude, and verbal responses usually enable the physician to make an intuitive estimate of the risk of suicide.

2. Specific risk factors–

a. Age–The older the patient is, the more seriously the physician must regard any suicidal behavior. Middle-aged and especially elderly persons do not use suicidal gestures as often as patients in their late teens and 20s. On the other hand, suicidal gestures by children or young teenagers should also be viewed as a sign of serious disturbance.

b. Race–Asian and Caucasian persons have a higher risk of suicide than people of other ethnic backgrounds. A non-Caucasian patient who is well integrated into a predominantly Caucasian culture has the same risk of suicide as a Caucasian.

c. Prior suicide attempt–The greater the number of suicide attempts, the greater the likelihood of further attempts and, eventually, successful suicide.

d. Violence of attempt–Patients who attempt suicide by physically active or violent means (guns, jumping) are generally more serious in their intent to commit suicide than are those who use drugs.

e. Detailed suicide plan–A patient who threatens or has attempted suicide in a carefully planned manner must be considered at high risk. This risk factor is especially significant if the means to be used are readily available or already at hand, such as a gun or supply of drugs.

f. Psychosis–A psychotic state, eg, delusional or bizarre behavior or hallucinatory experience, is a special high-risk factor regardless of other considerations.

g. Hopelessness–An end-of-the-rope feeling ("I just can't go on anymore") or expressions of futility ("It's no use") indicate a very high degree of risk.

h. Motivation to seek help–The patient's willingness and ability to accept assistance do not alter the immediate degree of risk of a suicidal act, but they do allow more treatment alternatives if competent personnel are available, eg, a day treatment or outpatient program.

i. Capacity to relate to others–The patient's ability to relate to others in a meaningful way may make possible some alternatives besides hospitalization.

j. Resources–Supportive family members or friends, a job, a place to live, etc, contribute to a support system that may obviate the need for hospitalization.

Treatment

Unless the physician's assessment dictates otherwise, the patient who has presented to the emergency department with a suicide threat or attempt must be considered at high risk of suicide while in the emergency department. The following are the mainstays of treatment:

A. Observation: If possible, situate the patient in sight of the nursing station. Use family or friends as companions when staff members are not available. If the patient is taken from the emergency department for x-rays or other procedures, instruct an attendant to remain with the patient until they both return to the emergency department. When possible, have someone accompany the patient to the bathroom.

B. Environmental Safety Check: If the emergency department is not on the first floor, avoid using a bed near a window that can be opened. See that sharp implements, drugs, belts, and highly toxic cleaning supplies (eg, toilet bowl cleaner) are not readily accessible.

C. Emotional Support: Staff members should provide repeated verbal reassurance of their desire to help in order to reduce the chance of problems in handling suicidal patients.

One of the most important contributions of the emergency department staff is to treat suicidal persons with empathic concern and respect. Suicidal patients are especially vulnerable to any sign of irritation or contempt and tend to seize on the slightest clue that others are rejecting them as meaning they do not deserve the care of others and are better off dead. On the other hand, a feeling of acceptance when their emotions are so openly exposed can favorably change their outlook on the potential of human relationships and of their own lives.

D. Pharmacologic Support: An anxiolytic or antipsychotic drug (eg, diazepam, 10 mg orally; or haloperidol, 2–5 mg intramuscularly every 30 minutes as needed, respectively) should be given if the patient's psychologic state and degree of agitation require it.

Disposition

The final decision about hospitalization is based on the risk factors involved, the physician's intuitive sense of the severity of risk, and the strength of the support system available outside the hospital. Follow-up arrangements that are as complete as possible should be made by the emergency department and as little as possible left to the patient. If hospitalization is voluntary, be sure to inform the patient about locked wards and other circumstances that may be encountered. Involuntary hospitalization is discussed on p 800. For optimal care, a follow-up telephone call should be made to find out whether the plans made in the emergency department have been carried out and whether responsibility for continuing care has been assumed by an appropriate person or agency. If medication is needed, discharge the patient with only the minimum amount necessary until the next appointment to avoid the possibility of suicide by drug overdose. Trazodone (Desyrel), bupropion (Wellbutrin), and fluoxetine (Prozac) are relatively safe in this regard.

Medicolegal Issues

Though the best legal protection is afforded by optimal care, potential legal liability can be greatly reduced by 5 simple steps:

A. Document the assessment of risk.

B. Document the plans made in view of that risk.

C. Document implementation of the plans.

D. Put a psychiatric consultation note in the chart that is consistent with the actions taken.

E. Provide family members with as much empathic support and opportunity to provide input as circumstances allow.

THOUGHT DISORDERS

1. SCHIZOPHRENIC DISORGANIZATION

Schizophrenia is common. Most people with schizophrenia are not institutionalized but go about their daily lives with varying degrees of effectiveness. The cause is unknown, but the disorder probably represents a combination of genetic, organic, psychologic, and environmental factors. When a patient with this disorder presents in the emergency department, it usually implies that the grossly defective ability to test and evaluate the reality of perceptions inherent in this disorder has precipitated responses that either the patient or other persons cannot tolerate.

Emergency Factors

Depending on the thought content and resulting feelings and behavior, the patient experiencing schizophrenic disorganization must be considered at risk for suicide; self-mutilation; assaultive behavior; destruction or damage to property; potential incapacity for self-care, as manifested by starvation, malnutrition, or deliberate exposure to traffic hazards; and disruption of social tranquility by intrusive, bizarre, loud, or offensive behavior (eg, public nudity or masturbation).

Diagnosis

Delusions, hallucinations, or bizarre or infantile speech or behavior should suggest schizophrenia. Organic brain disorders (eg, steroid toxicity, alcohol withdrawal, encephalitis, AIDS encephalopathy) must be ruled out to diagnose schizophrenia with confidence. Common manifestations of disorganization of thought and behavior are many and include the following:

A. Social withdrawal, often with poor personal hygiene.

B. Preoccupation with inner thoughts, often sexual or religious in nature.

C. Generally "flat" (emotionless) affect, with quick mood shifts that do not correlate with the circumstances.

D. "Distancing," or giving the examiner the impression of being separated from and not communicating with the patient.

E. Loose or incongruous associations in thought or speech sequences.

F. Hallucinations, often derogatory to the patient.

G. Delusions, often grandiose or persecutory.

H. Psychomotor retardation with catatonia.

I. A belief that external events have personal significance (eg, that voices, laughter, a horn honking are directly related in some way to the patient).

J. Anxiety and impaired concentration.

K. Bizarre or infantile behavior.

Treatment

A. Hospitalization: The key to emergency management of schizophrenia is a supportive setting combined with an antipsychotic medication for control of grossly disruptive behavior. If the patient is cooperative and able to tolerate preliminary psychiatric evaluation without disrupting the emergency department staff or patients, it is best to withhold antipsychotics until the patient has been transferred to a definitive treatment facility. Such a delay enables the psychiatric treatment staff to better assess the patient's baseline condition and begin the antipsychotic regimen they prefer.

B. Drugs: If the patient's behavior is violent or otherwise disrupts the emergency department and requires pharmacologic intervention, haloperidol, 5–10 mg intramuscularly (start with 2 mg in elderly patients), can be used in most cases. The dose can be repeated every 30–60 minutes until the situation is under control. Other high-potency neuroleptics (eg, perphenazine, thiothixene) can also be used to control disruptive behavior and may be usefully combined with benzodiazepines as discussed above under Initial Management of Violent or Severely Agitated Patients. Clozapine is not generally suitable for emergency use owing to current procedural requirements.

Disposition

Obtain immediate psychiatric consultation. Patients who are suicidal, homicidal, disruptive, or otherwise unable to care for themselves should be hospitalized without delay. Others should be referred to a psychiatric facility for further evaluation and treatment planning.

2. PARANOID STATES

Emergency Factors

Caution: The frequent association of paranoid states with extreme fear and anger generates a maximum potential for violence. The physician must carefully evaluate the suicidal as well as the homicidal expression of these feelings. Socially disruptive behavior such as locking oneself in a room and sealing up the doors and windows to prevent poison gas from entering, or loud, abusive behavior in a public place (which often leads to altercations with the police) can also create an emergency. Refusing to eat and drink for fear of being poisoned can result in severe malnutrition. On the other hand, many sweet-tempered, gentle, often elderly persons may have florid paranoid symptoms that do not create an emergency.

Diagnosis

A. Symptoms and Signs: Paranoid states are among the most common kinds of thought disorders, and they merit close attention, because they are potential emergencies. They are characterized chiefly by the presence of well-organized persecutory delusions or grandiose ideas. Be aware that organic disease or drugs (eg, amphetamine abuse, corticosteroid excess, or alcohol withdrawal) may cause paranoid symptoms, but these should not be confused with a paranoid state.

The patient is often hyperalert and seems to have increased memory for details both in the immediate situation and in the recent and remote past.

Alcohol withdrawal is the condition most commonly associated with persecutory ideas. Other causes include amphetamine overdose and depressive psychosis or mania. It is helpful to remember that extreme suspiciousness and distrust do not necessarily imply a paranoid pattern but may reflect the patient's culture, life pattern, or experience.

Patients with paranoid disorders often appear remarkably composed, articulate, well-dressed, informed, and educated, and they function at a rather high level of competence. Such patients often have considerable strength of personality, which may lead the physician to overlook the underlying psychosis. The presenting complaint may be somewhat unusual, eg, a tingling sensation of the arms or several ecchymoses on the legs. Only when the patient explains to the interviewer that symptoms have been caused by a "radar beam" or that people are maliciously administering "shots" to cause torment and physical illness does it become clear that there is an underlying psychiatric disorder requiring attention.

B. Interview Technique: The following guidelines may be useful in interviewing patients with paranoid disorders:

1. The interview should be unpressured. Give the patient plenty of time and space to evaluate the interviewer before any effort is made to enlist the patient's cooperation.

2. Stand or sit a comfortable distance away (1.5–3 m [5–10 ft]) from the patient, and do not block the door to the room.

3. Start with a personal introduction ("I'm Dr Chang"), and let the patient know that the staff is aware of the patient's situation and knows why the patient is in the emergency department. Emphasize that discussion of any topic by the patient will be welcomed and is of interest.

4. Be as candid as possible. Efforts at subterfuge or half-truths are sensed immediately and can make the patient suspect the interviewer of playing a part in the general persecutory scheme. This feeling may cause the patient to leave abruptly or become even more hostile and resistant.

5. Maintain a responsive and matter-of-fact approach in the face of what may be an angry, demanding, and accusing manner on the part of the patient.

6. Do not argue with the patient. If the physician is challenged to comment on the patient's delusional ideas, it should be made clear in a matter-of-fact way that the interviewer's view of the matter differs from that of the patient. Smiling or laughing on the interviewer's part tends to be seen as mocking and inappropriate.

7. Make any reasonable concession to assure the patient of an unequivocal desire to help as much as possible.

Treatment & Disposition

The key to emergency management of paranoid states is to defuse any immediate threat of violence and to transfer the patient to a psychiatric unit for longer-term planning and treatment. These goals may be difficult to accomplish. Some measures that may be helpful in handling paranoid patients follow, although they must not be assumed to apply to all such patients. Most patients are compliant as long as staff members are responsive and demonstrate that they can be trusted.

A. Explain and evaluate previously applied physical restraints. Restraints should not be removed until the physician has had a chance to get acquainted with the person and the situation. Discuss with the patient the reason restraints were used and ask whether the patient is more in control now than before. If in doubt, leave the restraints on.

B. Check for weapons. Ask direct questions, and search the patient's belongings to make sure that the patient is not armed. A policy that requires all patients to change into hospital clothing facilitates this procedure.

If the patient is armed and refuses to relinquish the weapon voluntarily, try to find someone whom the patients trusts—family member, spouse, religious adviser, social worker, friend—to persuade the patient to do so. Candor is important: "Everyone is too frightened to help you when you have a weapon."

C. Be patient. Take time to listen, to repeat, and to respond to the patient's fears; a few extra hours are time well spent. Trying to rush the process may scare away the patient for a prolonged period or even precipitate a violent act. If the patient demands some concession as a condition for cooperating, accept it if at all possible without undue concern about "bargaining" or "being manipulated." However, do not make a promise that clearly cannot be kept in order to elicit cooperative behavior.

D. Use restraints with skill and caution. If all else

fails, ask security personnel to intercede. Medical staff members are generally not able to restrain a physically healthy man, especially if he is frightened. Heroic measures are not helpful. A physician with no choice but to personally restrain a patient should have the assistance of at least twice the number of persons thought to be required (eg, 6–8 people) before confronting the patient. The patient usually acquiesces quietly in the face of such a display. If a resisting patient must be moved, the ideal number of people required is 5, one for each limb and one to open doors and assist. Three is the minimal number acceptable to safely escort a potentially resistant or violent patient.

E. Give drugs judiciously. The use of medications for management of paranoid patients is the same as for those with schizophrenic disorganization (p 793). It is preferable to determine the best institution or hospital for definitive treatment (inpatient facility, day care, etc) and transfer the patient there *before* starting antipsychotics. Antipsychotics should be given if the patient is being disruptive, however.

3. CATATONIC STATES (Withdrawn Type)

This section discusses only the withdrawn type of catatonia, since the excited type can be considered a form of schizophrenic disorganization (discussed above). Catatonic states may be seen as the patient's response to a flood of anxiety of paralyzing proportions. Since verbal interchange is often impossible, the presence of hallucinations or delusional ideas can generally only be inferred from behavioral clues.

Emergency Factors

Severe malnutrition, dehydration, and pneumonia may become life-threatening. Unpredictable alternation between catatonia and excitement may cause major social disruption, with the potential for injury to self or others. Gastric hyperacidity with fatal aspiration have also been described.

Diagnosis

Although many clinical variants are seen, the patient is usually brought to the emergency department because the inhibition of movement, speech, eating, or other activities has aroused concern in others. Onset of symptoms may be either acute or gradual. Specific criteria are as follows:

A. Severe motor retardation, varying from relative immobility to apparent unresponsiveness to all stimuli.

B. Absence of organic cause of symptoms (Chapters 10 and 12).

C. Absence of another concurrent thought disorder (eg, severe depressive psychomotor retardation).

D. Mutism, immobility, unresponsiveness, "waxy flexibility" (the patient's limbs retain any position in

which they are placed), and a history of similar episodes are diagnostic if organic disorders and drug intoxication have been ruled out.

E. Some speech or a visible effort to phonate may be present. Communication, even slight, may often be achieved by asking the patient to blink or nod for an affirmative reply to yes/no questions. Such communication may help to clarify whether delusional ideas or hallucinations are present. Amobarbital given intravenously may enable the patient to communicate freely but should be administered by personnel familiar with its use.

F. Patients may be hyperalert and gaze intently at the interviewer or may sit with eyes closed as though in a coma ("catatonic stupor"). Unlike comatose patients, however, catatonic patients are aware of what goes on around them and are affected by it (eg, comments by the medical staff).

G. Episodes of excitement alternating with periods of withdrawal reflect the characteristic absence of impulse control that marks the excited catatonic state.

Differential Diagnosis

Midbrain and brain stem abnormalities and many toxic agents can cause catatonic symptoms (Chapter 10). It is important to determine the presence and quality of any psychotic thinking in order to differentiate a catatonic state from depressive conditions with accompanying severe psychomotor retardation. If the patient has a history of conversion reactions, the possibility of hysterical psychosis must be considered. A patient with akinetic mutism usually does not show posturing. Furthermore, the patient is amnestic for the episode of mutism and fails to improve after administration of amobarbital. Neuroleptic malignant syndrome may also present as catatonia (see above, under Organically Induced Disorders).

Treatment & Disposition

A. Evaluate the patient's physical and metabolic status (ie, perform a physical examination, and obtain blood glucose levels and tests of renal and hepatic function).

B. Give an antipsychotic agent (eg, haloperidol, 5 mg intramuscularly) only if the patient has periods of excitement or must be transferred to a distant facility; otherwise, such agents should *not* be given in the emergency department.

C. Explain the proposed plan of treatment to the patient, with repeated verbal reassurance at each step.

D. Transfer the patient to an inpatient psychiatric unit. Be sure to provide all pertinent data (including laboratory data) and suggestions for physical care if needed.

MOOD DISORDERS

1. MANIC STATES

Mania is an uncommon disorder with a strong genetic element (60% concordance in monozygotic twins). Most patients with manic states have a bipolar affective disorder, in which manic episodes alternate with depressive episodes. Some patients have a unipolar illness with episodes of mania alone, although unipolar illness with depression alone is much more common. Patients are characterized as hypomanic when symptoms are less severe and reality testing is better preserved, although the transition to full-blown mania is such that the distinction is often difficult to discern. Hypomania can be difficult to recognize, because it is characterized by behavior patterns similar to those sanctioned by society; it may be hard to believe that an attractive, pleasant, and energetic patient—albeit talkative, jocular, and overly friendly—is so disordered that psychiatric hospitalization must be seriously considered. *Caution: Manic states are as serious as other major psychiatric dysfunctions, although they may outwardly appear to be less severe.*

Emergency Factors
A. Overactivity: Days or weeks of overactivity without adequate eating, drinking, or sleeping may result in dehydration and exhaustion progressing to a moribund state and death if the cycle is not interrupted.

B. Behavioral Excesses: Impaired judgment and lack of discretion may lead to impulsive excessive spending or sexual behavior that creates havoc. The patient may demonstrate irrepressible energy in insisting on telephone calls to the mayor, the governor, or other officials.

C. Hostility: The undercurrent of hostility associated with manic states may cause loud altercations, social turmoil, or automobile accidents and may lead to suicidal behavior. Homicidal or assaultive actions may also occur.

Diagnosis
The predominance of an infectious, inappropriate euphoria; hyperactivity; and talkativeness with sharply decreased need to eat or sleep suggest a diagnosis of bipolar disorder, manic type. Inappropriate singing, dancing, joking, punning, "clang association" (association of disconnected ideas resulting only from similarity of sounds), and flight of ideas are classic findings.

An episode of depression frequently precedes the manic phase, and even during the manic episode, momentary lapses into a depressive state with tears and despondency may occur.

Other patients may have bursts of angry or aggressive behavior. In severe manic states, outspoken ideas of persecution and expansive grandiosity may raise the question of a possible schizophrenic process. When disordered thought processes are prominent, a diagnosis of schizoaffective disorder must be considered, and the most effective management in the emergency department is the same as that for schizophrenia.

Differential Diagnosis
A useful criterion in differentiating manic states from schizophrenic hyperactivity or catatonic excitement is the infectiousness of the mood. If the observer is moved to laugh or be sad along with the patient, the illness is more likely to be a mood disorder (eg, mania), whereas if the patient's behavior produces no such impulse in the observer, the illness is more probably a thought disorder (eg, schizophrenia). The patient may be using various medications, drugs, or alcohol that may cloud the clinical picture. Observation for up to 24 hours may be necessary before the diagnosis can be made with confidence and treatment can proceed. A toxicology screen may be helpful.

Treatment & Disposition
A. Hospitalize the Patient: *Do not underestimate the need for hospitalization.* Despite behavior that is seemingly within normal limits, almost all manic patients who present in the emergency department require hospitalization. Repeated reassurance may be helpful, but manic patients are notoriously uncooperative and resistant to hospitalization. It is often necessary to use involuntary measures, such as police assistance, in apprehending and transporting the patient, or authorization for an emergency psychiatric "hold" (p 800), permitting short-term involuntary detention in a psychiatric setting. Family members and friends can be helpful in providing continued reassurance, observation, transportation, and participation in the plans for discharge.

B. Reduce Activity: In acute manic states the goals of emergency treatment are to reduce the level of manic behavior without delay and to transfer the patient to an inpatient setting where adequate nutrition and sleep are assured and where the patient may be evaluated for treatment with lithium or carbamazepine.

C. Give Drugs: Any of the antipsychotics will suffice for immediate management, eg, haloperidol, 5–10 mg intramuscularly every 30–60 minutes, until the patient is able to travel or cooperate. If the inpatient unit is in the same building as the emergency department, haloperidol may be given after the transfer. *Do not begin lithium treatment in the emergency department,* because it does not bring manic symptoms under control as rapidly as haloperidol, and the dosage is harder to regulate. If lithium is subsequently given, the haloperidol should be gradually tapered to minimize the risk of an adverse reaction to the lithium-haloperidol combination. This is of special concern if environmental temperatures are high.

D. Prevent Outbursts of Underlying Hostility: Keep in mind that underlying the immense amount of energy expended in manic states are intense negative feelings that may surface only as episodes of irritability. Be careful in trying even gently physical persuasion, eg, taking the patient's arm to lead him or her to an elevator, since a violent upsurge of hostility may occur. Outbursts of hostility and violence may emerge despite the surface euphoria, so it is wise to retain a police escort or have ample attendants present until the patient is in a controlled setting.

2. DEPRESSIVE STATES

See p 791.

ANOREXIA NERVOSA

Anorexia nervosa is one of the few psychiatric conditions that can lead to death by means other than suicide. In the emergency department, it is usually encountered in persons whose chief complaint gives no indication of anorexia nervosa. The patient is often brought (or coerced into coming) to the hospital by concerned family or friends who recognize the seriousness of the severe weight loss. The chief complaint may be a minor physical problem or a secondary complication such as fatigue or amenorrhea. Depression is common and may be manifested as such or as a suicide attempt. Descriptions such as "passive aggressive personality" or "emotionally labile personality" are common in the medical history.

Emergency Factors
Inanition is potentially life-threatening. Persistent vomiting, often self-induced (bulimia), can result in loss of tooth enamel and profound electrolyte disturbance. In spite of remarkable bursts of energy, the avitaminosis, metabolic imbalance, and cachexia predispose the patient to serious complications such as cardiac arrhythmias and life-threatening infections. Suicide must also be considered, especially if the patient is faced with a coercive feeding program.

Diagnosis
The key to diagnosis of anorexia nervosa is severe weight loss to the point of cachexia and emaciation in a person who seems unconcerned about the obvious emaciation. The patient also appears to have an aversion for food and persistently refuses to accept a dietary regimen designed to correct the weight loss. Anorexia nervosa is seen mostly in young women (ratio 10:1) and is characterized by the following findings:

A. Onset before age 25 years.

B. Absence of other disease that could cause the same clinical picture (eg, Simmonds' disease, hypothalamic tumor, severe depression, paranoid fear of poisoning).

C. Failure to respond to admonitions, threats, promises, or reassurance to eat.

D. Amenorrhea.

E. Absence of hunger.

F. Periods of hyperactivity without feeling subsequent fatigue.

G. Self-induced vomiting (bulimia) or cathartic abuse, especially after an eating binge.

H. History of being overweight, episodic hyperphagia, or interest in fad diets.

I. Morbid fear of fat or obesity.

Treatment & Disposition
The primary management problem is persuading the patient to voluntarily accept hospitalization for restoration of normal nutritional status (parenteral nutrition may be required) and psychotherapy. If the patient is so weak that mental function is severely impaired, this may not be difficult. In other situations, it may take the concerted efforts of family, friends, and physicians to persuade the patient to accept hospitalization. When the disease is clearly life-threatening, involuntary measures are justified (p 800).

The patient is usually transferred from the emergency department to a psychiatric unit, but a medical ward is acceptable if psychiatric facilities are not adequately staffed. Hospitalization in a medical ward is also preferred if life-threatening organic complications are present (eg, pneumonia, avitaminosis). Combined nutritional, pharmacologic, and psychotherapeutic treatment can be carried out until the patient's physical condition permits transfer to a psychiatric ward or an outpatient facility.

CONVERSION DISORDERS & HYSTERICAL STATES

Since the days of Janet, Charcot, and Bernheim, clinicians have observed that relatively unsophisticated and impressionable persons are the most vulnerable to conversion disorders (loss of or alteration of physical functioning suggesting a physical disorder). Motor or sensory dysfunction as a purely psychologic symptom is uncommon, but the question whether a psychiatric problem exists is frequent in the emergency department. When a young person under emotional stress presents with acute onset of dramatic symptoms (eg, aphonia, paralysis of both legs, loss of memory, complete blindness), conversion disorder is one of the first diagnoses to come to mind, but such a clear-cut situation is rare. On the other hand, the emergence of symptoms owing to suggestibility or the *intensification* of existing symptoms as a result of emotional factors ("psychogenic overlay") is common. In these instances, the task of the emergency physician is not to distinguish between the familiar "organic versus functional" dichotomy but rather to assess the *degree* to which an organic problem is being distorted by psychologic factors.

Emergency Factors

Unlike some other psychologic disorders, conversion disorders have no inherent emergency characteristics such as the risk of suicide or self-mutilation, but there are some associated hazards.

A. A diagnosis of conversion disorder may blind the emergency department staff to accurate diagnosis of some acute organic conditions amenable to treatment, especially if the pathologic mechanism of the organic disease is not clearly evident and if the emergency department staff is too busy to perform a thorough evaluation of the patient. Patients with Guillain-Barré syndrome or botulism have been misdiagnosed as having hysterical weakness.

Patients with viral encephalitis, tuberculous meningitis, and cervical fracture have also been erroneously referred from the emergency department to a psychiatric service with a mistaken diagnosis of "hysterical paralysis" (Chapter 12). Similarly, patients with pulmonary emboli or pulmonary vascular disease have been said to have "hysterical" dyspnea and hyperventilation (Chapter 5).

B. On the other hand, if conversion disorder is not considered as a possible diagnosis, the emergency staff may be tempted to carry out elaborate and unnecessary procedures.

Diagnosis

A. Presence of Sensory or Motor Dysfunction: Sudden onset of dramatic sensory or motor dysfunction in a young person under known psychologic stress and with no corroborating history or results on physical examination or laboratory tests (Chapter 12) warrants a presumptive diagnosis of conversion disorder. The diagnosis is strengthened by a history of episodes of acute, transitory loss of sensorimotor function involving different sensory modalities or muscle groups. Dysfunction with a fluctuating pattern, a pattern of involvement that does not conform to known neuroanatomic relationships, a striking absence of concern about the sudden disability ("la belle indifférence"), absence of any self-injury (eg, from "fainting"), and intact sphincter control help to confirm the diagnosis. A maneuver that helps to differentiate hysterical paralysis of one leg from genuine paralysis is to ask the supine patient to lift the affected leg from the bed. Counterpressure with the heel of the other (unaffected) leg is absent in conversion states and malingering (Hoover's sign).

Although conversion disorder is the most dramatic form of psychologically induced physical disability, other syndromes are recognized under the rubric of "somatoform disorders," specifically,

1. Somatization disorder–Somatization disorder takes the form of a multiplicity of nonspecific symptoms of several years' duration that have no organic explanation.

2. Hypochondriasis–Hypochondriasis represents an anxious preoccupation with physical signs or sensations that are misinterpreted as manifestations of serious disease.

3. Somatoform pain disorder–Somatoform pain disorder is seen as complaints of severe and prolonged pain inconsistent with nerve distribution or known pathology and serving an identifiable psychologic purpose. Disappearance of the pain by suggestion, hypnosis, or amobarbital interview suggests this disorder.

4. Undifferentiated somatoform disorder–Undifferentiated somatoform disorders include unexplainable physical complaints linked to psychologic factors but not fitting any of the categories above.

B. History: The history of the patient and an understanding of the total personality may be helpful, especially if the patient is middle-aged or older. A person's mechanisms for coping with adversity tend to remain similar throughout life. If a conversion disorder has not been noted as a reaction to stress in the past, it is unlikely that such a reaction will appear for the first time in middle age or later. "Psychogenic overlay" is suggested by a certain histrionic quality in the patient, with a tendency to overstate or exaggerate symptoms and to acquire new symptoms by suggestion.

C. Physical Examination and Laboratory Studies: The absence of physical and laboratory findings that might account for presenting signs and symptoms is not in itself a sound basis for diagnosis of a psychiatric disorder; psychiatric findings consistent with conversion reaction must be noted as well.

D. Use of Amobarbital: Intravenous administration of amobarbital as a means of confirming the diagnosis and providing clues for further management should be used by persons experienced in this procedure.

Treatment & Disposition

Keep the patient separated from friends and family during the interviewing and testing procedures. If symptoms are disabling and persist throughout the emergency evaluation, referral to an inpatient psychiatric unit is indicated. It is appropriate to reassure family members that such disability usually lasts only hours to days. The dysfunction often disappears on the way to the ward or shortly after admission. If the diagnosis is uncertain, medical or neurologic consultation is indicated.

For symptoms such as dysphonia that are not disabling, referral to an outpatient setting such as a speech clinic is appropriate. Psychiatric resources then can be used to assist with definitive treatment.

PSYCHOGENIC FUGUE

Psychogenic fugue is the most commonly encountered dissociative state in the emergency department. It is characterized by abrupt onset after a specific stressful situation, eg, psychologically catastrophic accident, rejection by a person of great importance in the patient's life, or threat of severe loss. Psychogenic fugue may be considered a homeostatic mechanism that effectively protects the patient from perceiving unbearable circumstances.

A number of organic diseases and drug intoxications may also cause prolonged periods of amnesia and may mimic psychogenic fugue. The most common is alcohol abuse, which may produce blackouts that last for days or weeks, during which time the person continues purposeful behavior, such as working, talking, or driving. If such symptoms are found in a person subject to criminal charges and awaiting trial, Ganser syndrome (simulated psychosis) or other forms of malingering must be considered.

Diagnosis

Abrupt loss of memory is temporally associated with a high-stress situation. The patient is apparently in good health and alert; communicates readily but is unable to answer ordinary questions about name, address, and events preceding arrival at the hospital; and exhibits concern and cooperation in assessment procedures. The patient often travels long distances without recall, and it is often the patient's confusion in a bus or train station that attracts the attention of others. Occasionally, the patient presents to a police officer or to the emergency department, asking for assistance. The amnesia may be incomplete, and the patient may be able to recall a few memories vaguely, as though from a dream, eg, "Are you married?" "I think so, but I'm not really sure." Recovery occurs spontaneously within a few hours to several weeks. When the patient recovers, there is amnesia for the period of dissociation. Organic amnestic states must be excluded (Chapter 14).

Emergency Factors

Patients in this dissociative state are vulnerable to social and economic disruption. This vulnerability and an attempt to allay concerns of family members are the primary reasons for urgent treatment.

Treatment

Reassure the patient and concerned persons that the episode is not indefinite and that it will resolve in hours to weeks. Direct encouragement and emotional support may help to dispel amnesia, in which case these measures should be pursued as long as they produce results.

Intravenous administration of amobarbital to confirm the diagnosis and provide clues to further management by restoring the patient's memory should be performed by persons experienced in this procedure.

Disposition

Hospitalization is necessary until the patient has recovered sufficient memory to permit care and follow-up on an outpatient basis. Hospitalization is also required if the use of amobarbital is contemplated.

BORDERLINE STATES WITH MULTIPLE ADMISSIONS (Recurrent Drop-Ins)

Patients who are apparently resistant to help but who persist in seeking assistance from the emergency department staff pose a special problem. Clinical findings vary but usually include lacerations, infections, complications of drug and alcohol abuse, emotional lability, transient psychotic episodes, and suicide attempts or gestures. These patients tend to demand and complain, cooperate unpredictably with hospital staff, and frequently leave impulsively against medical advice. They are also called "borderline personalities," and the constellation of symptoms is often labeled "borderline state" or "borderline syndrome." Because of their many visits to the hospital, these patients have extensive medical records, and they may generate considerable tension between the medical and the psychiatric services.

Treatment

The following measures have proved useful in the treatment of borderline conditions in the emergency department:

A. Provide whatever medical or surgical care is required, eg, suturing, hydration.

B. If the patient is undergoing psychiatric treatment at the time, contact the therapist immediately, and provide a summary of the immediate situation. It may be possible to arrange for disposition immediately, depending on the therapist's knowledge of and relationship with the patient. Consider putting the patient on the telephone to discuss directly with the therapist the best course of action.

C. Investigate new sources of support. If the patient has no therapist or if the therapist is on vacation (which sometimes precipitates the crisis), explore the possibility of using family or friends as sources of information and temporary support, with full knowledge that such persons are often as frustrated as emergency department personnel and may themselves precipitate a crisis.

D. Carefully assess the situation in order to determine the best course of treatment, eg, reassurance, antipsychotic drugs, sedative-hypnotics, follow-up visits, referral, or hospitalization.

E. Assign a therapist. If the patient repeatedly causes serious disruption of the emergency department, it may help to assign responsibility for that patient's emergency care to one person on each shift of both the psychiatric and the emergency department staff. That staff person is notified whenever the patient presents. The rapport and knowledge of the patient that develop from such an arrangement may facilitate efficient management and disposition. The medical-surgical emergency department staff may be able to be more supportive if they know that they can always call on a person who is familiar with the patient's history. The designated staff member can focus on the issues of low self-esteem, dependency needs, strivings for independence, impulsive behavior, and low frustration tolerance that underlie crises.

F. It is important to respond to these patients with persistent concern, viewing their abrasiveness as a chronic symptom over which they have limited control. Rebuffing or rejecting the patient often leads to escalating demands, which may culminate in a suicidal act.

INVOLUNTARY PROCEDURES
(See also Chapter 45.)

Involuntary procedures include restraint, detention, and diagnostic or treatment measures performed without first securing the patient's informed consent. When appropriately used, these procedures are simply one facet of good medical care, but their philosophic and legal implications should prompt the physician to consider the following guidelines:

In a dire and obviously life-threatening emergency (eg, serious self-injury), act promptly to secure the patient's well-being, without regard for legal issues. Administration of psychotropic medications may be included in lifesaving measures. An exception to this principle may occur if the patient's next of kin actively intervenes, but even in this instance, the physician cannot be held liable for improper conduct if the action taken reflects the physician's best judgment and is carried out in good faith.

In circumstances that are not life-threatening, assess the patient's ability to (1) understand the situation and (2) form a reasoned judgment based on that understanding. Such an assessment is the clinical basis for determining the patient's capacity to give informed consent. Consent cannot be given if the patient is unable to exercise this understanding in order to form a reasoned judgment. Careful and repeated explanation and questioning may be necessary. Interpreters may be required if the physician and the patient do not speak the same language. The decision about the capacity to give consent must be based on the physician's judgment. A patient may be deemed able to consent to some procedures (eg, blood transfusion) and not to others (eg, lumbar puncture).

If a psychiatric consultant is available, a formal mental status examination in the medical record provides valuable documentation of this assessment. The psychiatrist cannot determine a patient's competence in a legal sense but can judge whether intellectual dysfunction precludes understanding of the illness and of the consequences of suggested treatment.

Even though the law may be clear on the issue of obtaining informed consent, the judgment about the patient's capacity to give it is subjective. Since there is no way to circumvent this problem, it is appropriate (required in some states in the USA) to obtain the written concurrence of another (preferably senior) physician and the patient's next of kin (preferably a parent, spouse, or oldest child, if available) for any procedure carried out without the patient's informed consent.

Obtain consent from available family members whenever possible, and document in writing that they understand the need for and risks of the planned procedure. This policy applies whether or not the patient is able to give consent but is especially important when the patient resists treatment or hospitalization.

If the patient in non–life-threatening circumstances is unable to understand the situation but needs hospital care (eg, severe alcohol intoxication), both restraint and detention without the patient's informed consent may be used as necessary, and psychotropic medication may be given as needed.

When an involuntary procedure is required by a *psychiatric* disorder, commitment measures that vary from state to state in the USA provide for psychiatric assessment and treatment. The considerations most commonly used in assessing the need for involuntary procedures are (1) danger posed to oneself, (2) danger posed to others, or (3) severe disability (inability to provide for one's food, clothing, shelter, or daily needs). Emergency physicians must know the requirements and procedures for instituting involuntary measures in the area where they practice.

Note: Medical and surgical procedures (eg, drawing blood, suturing) are usually not included in commitment provisions and require a specific court order if the patient refuses them. The hospital's legal department is responsible for expediting necessary action to secure such court orders. Special rules usually apply for minors.

Suicidal patients constitute a management problem because they often resist hospitalization. Involuntary measures are definitely indicated if the person is (1) psychotic, (2) delirious, (3) panicked, or (4) severely depressed, or if the person has another severe psychiatric disorder. When a person deliberately chooses suicide after careful consideration of life and its prospects, the physician may offer to counsel the patient in whatever way may be helpful, but it is difficult to justify an involuntary procedure as a deterrent. Philosophic differences about the extent to which a physician should intervene to prevent suicide engender controversy, and legal rulings on this issue are also controversial. When forced to a decision about involuntary measures, many clinicians forego ethical considerations and pragmatically remember that legal suits for "wrongful death" actions (allowing the person to leave) are more numerous than those for "assault" or "violation of civil rights" (detention). However, involuntary detention may separate the suicidal person from sources of help and psychologic support and may worsen the long-term prognosis.

Hospitalization—whether voluntary or involuntary—should be considered more readily for suicidal states in adolescents than in other age groups.

PSYCHOTROPIC DRUGS IN THE EMERGENCY DEPARTMENT

Two classes of drugs are commonly used for psychiatric patients in an emergency setting: antipsychotics (major tranquilizers) and sedative-hypnotics (minor tranquilizers). Lithium, tricyclic antidepressants, monoamine oxidase inhibitors, and central nervous system stimulants (eg, dextroamphetamine, methylphenidate) should generally not be administered in the emergency department.

Antipsychotic Drugs (Major Tranquilizers)

When agitation, excitement, hostility, uncooperativeness, or disorganization of thought processes is due to functional psychosis, prompt administration of an antipsychotic will rapidly produce improvement.

Familiarity with the use of only 2 agents of the many available is usually sufficient: chlorpromazine (Thorazine, others) and haloperidol (Haldol). Thioridazine (Mellaril, others) may be substituted for chlorpromazine; and perphenazine (Trilafon, others), trifluoperazine (Stelazine, others), fluphenazine (Prolixin, others), prochlorperazine (Compazine), or thiothixene (Navane, others) may be substituted for haloperidol. Select only 2 or 3 of these drugs (eg, chlorpromazine plus one of the high-potency drugs [eg, haloperidol, fluphenazine]) to become well acquainted with in order to be able to use them confidently and efficiently. If good results have previously been obtained with a particular drug, consider starting with that one if it is available.

As well as its antipsychotic effect, chlorpromazine provides more sedation but also produces more hypotension than haloperidol, especially in older patients.

Haloperidol is more likely to cause dystonia. (See Chapter 39 for treatment of phenothiazine toxicity.) The oral route is preferred, but intramuscular administration may be necessary for resistant patients. Intravenous haloperidol, in doses similar to those for intramuscular injection, has been described as effective and free of extrapyramidal side effects or other adverse reactions. Table 41–1 shows comparable oral and intramuscular doses.

Adequate control of disruptive symptoms can usually be achieved by repeating the intramuscular dose of these drugs every 30–60 minutes until the patient is calm enough to permit necessary procedures to be performed. If the patient is not disruptive and will be hospitalized, administration of medication should be deferred until the patient has been admitted to the hospital.

Observe precautions regarding possible drug allergies, and monitor both the rate and the quality of respiration (or arterial blood gases) as well as blood pressure. There have been a few reports of sudden death associated with rapid tranquilization as well as with prolonged high-dosage phenothiazine therapy. The cause of death has presumably been drug-induced ventricular fibrillation.

Drugs for Treatment of Parkinsonian Side Effects

The muscular and autonomic dysfunctions produced by antipsychotics range from blurring of vision and a mild rhythmic tremor to severe bodily contortions and opisthotonos, and they may be dramatic and disabling. Compulsive motor activity (akathisia), facial twitching, upturning gaze, and involuntary biting and chewing movements that may lacerate the tongue and inner aspect of the cheeks also occur. These side effects and the reaction they produce in patients are sometimes bizarre enough to be mistaken for psychiatric symptoms.

Benztropine mesylate (Cogentin, others), 2–4 mg

Table 41–1. Equivalent oral and intramuscular dosages for some common antipsychotic medications.

	Oral (mg)	Intramuscular (mg)
Chlorpromazine (Thorazine, many others)	100	25
Thioridazine (Mellaril, Millazine)	100	Not available
Haloperidol (Haldol)	2	3–5
Fluphenazine (Permitil, Prolixin)	5	2.5–5
Perphenazine (Trilafon)	8	5
Trifluoperazine (Stelazine, Suprazine)	5	2–4
Prochlorperazine (Chlorazine, Compazine)	5	5–10
Thiothixene (Navane)	5	4

intramuscularly or intravenously; or diphenhydramine (Benadryl, many others), 50–100 mg intramuscularly or intravenously, provides rapid and marked relief of symptoms. Other effective antiparkinsonian medications are trihexyphenidyl (Artane), procyclidine (Kemadrin), and amantadine (Symmetrel). Akathisia may be resistant to these agents but will often respond to propranolol or to benzodiazepines. These drugs are generally not effective in the treatment of tardive dyskinesias, which are resistant to drug modification and are not appropriately treated in the emergency department.

Sedative-Hypnotics
(Minor Tranquilizers)

For agitation or for organically induced disturbances (eg, alcohol withdrawal syndromes), the following are the most useful: chlordiazepoxide (Librium, others), diazepam (Valium, others), clorazepate (Tranxene, others), alprazolam (Xanax), lorazepam (Ativan, others), prazepam (Centrax), and oxazepam (Serax, others). Barbiturates and exotic tranquilizers (eg, glutethimide [Doriden, Doriglute], methaqualone [Mequin, Parest, Quaalude; all now withdrawn from the market]) are not more effective than diazepam, are substantially more toxic, and have a higher potential for abuse.

Give diazepam, 5–10 mg orally or intravenously; repeat in doses of 5–10 mg every 1–2 hours until the patient's tension is reduced to a tolerable level. Intramuscular administration is not recommended, because it is associated with erratic absorption. Intravenous administration should be slow (5 mg/min). The drug should be given with caution to the elderly or alcohol or barbiturate abusers because of the risk of apnea or cardiac arrest. Unless combined with other agents, the toxicity of diazepam is low, and there are no serious side effects beyond drowsiness, although in long-term use, physical and psychologic dependence, tolerance, and withdrawal symptoms must be considered. These issues are not a consideration in the emergency use of diazepam.

For patients with severe liver disease, oxazepam may be preferable, since unlike diazepam, it is not metabolized by the liver. Give 15–30 mg orally every 1–2 hours until the patient is calm. Lorazepam, 1 mg orally every 6 hours, also puts less demand on the liver. Lorazepam can be administered sublingually if oral intake is not feasible.

The specificity of a given anxiolytic agent for a particular clinical problem is not yet clear. As with the antipsychotic medications discussed above, it is appropriate to become thoroughly familiar with only 2 or 3 of these compounds in order to develop confidence in their use.

A sleep medication may be required when patients are referred to another facility or must wait over a weekend before seeing a therapist. Another benzodiazepine, flurazepam (Dalmane, others), 30–60 mg orally, is a commonly prescribed sedative-hypnotic for psychiatric patients. This drug is effective and safe. Diazepam, 10–20 mg orally, is also useful for inducing sleep. Benzodiazepines with much shorter half-lives are also available, such as temazepam (Restoril, others) or triazolam (Halcion), although anecdotal evidence raises questions about retrograde amnesia and other adverse reactions to the latter agent. Chloral hydrate, 1–2 g orally, is also effective, but it is not as safe as the benzodiazepines because it has more potential for abuse and may cause gastritis.

THE FAMILY IN THE EMERGENCY DEPARTMENT

The presence of the patient's family in the emergency department poses problems in addition to those encountered in caring for the patient. The guidelines provided below may prove useful.

Distraught Family

When an individual has an acute, unexpected, and potentially lethal disorder such as myocardial infarction, automobile accident, unexpected suicide attempt, or severe burn or gunshot wound, one important role of the emergency department staff is to provide emotional support for the patient's family until they are better able to cope with the situation.

A. Find a quiet place for family members to be together where they can support each other, cry openly without embarrassment, pace up and down, and discuss the emergency privately with the medical staff.

B. Keep the family as informed as possible, and provide new information as soon as it is available: "Dr Gonzalez is examining your son now." "The x-rays show a severe fracture of the tibia." "Vital signs are not very good—we've started a transfusion." "Your son Carlos is still in surgery; I'm sorry, but the chances of saving his leg are only fair." "You can see Marilyn as soon as she is awake—in about an hour."

C. Provide a channel of communication for the family to ask questions of the medical staff and to permit access to treatment rooms or surgery areas. An emergency department volunteer worker can be designated for this purpose. The responsible physician should provide at least a final summary if possible.

D. Encourage family members to provide information about the situation, even though the medical problem seems clear-cut. Family members will feel that they are being helpful, and valuable data may be obtained at times.

E. Offer whatever amenities are available, eg, helping with phone calls, obtaining coffee or snacks, calling the hospital chaplain if desired, and providing information about hospital procedures, visiting hours, etc.

F. If a family member seems unable to cope with the situation, offer a sedative, eg, diazepam, 5 mg orally every 2 hours, until a calming effect is achieved.

G. Some family members who may feel directly or indirectly responsible for the course of events may feel guilty. The emergency department staff should be prepared to listen in a nonjudgmental way, should urge the family to accept doing whatever can be done at the moment to deal with what has happened (rather than dwelling on the past: "I shouldn't have . . ." or "If only we had done that."), and should encourage hope that the future will bring resolution of problems and a chance to make a fresh start.

H. The emergency department staff should be prepared to provide referral to a grief counseling program in the event of a death or severely incapacitating injury. A local suicide prevention and crisis center often provides such a service.

I. When a psychiatric patient is accompanied by family members to the emergency department, it is likely that the underlying difficulty involves a family-related conflict. It is not easy to refer families to a treatment resource, but in appropriate cases, family therapy may be the most effective method of treatment over both the short and long term.

Angry, Exasperated, Rejecting Family

In the case of patients who have chronic behavioral problems such as repeated suicide threats and attempts, drug abuse, and alcohol abuse, the task in dealing with the family is to offer support and at the same time salvage as much as possible of the patient's own support system.

A. The guidelines discussed above may also prove helpful in dealing with angry families.

B. Try to contact family members as soon as possible, since they sometimes disappear shortly after delivering the patient to the emergency department.

C. Empathize with family members about the frustration inherent in the situation. Family members tend to feel that they have sincerely tried to help the patient for a long time but that their efforts have been unappreciated and even exploited.

D. Be prepared for animosity toward health care personnel, who may be blamed by family members for failing to deal effectively with the problem in the past and who are thus held responsible for the present situation. The family may also resentfully believe that health care personnel are implying that family members are responsible both for causing the problem and for finding a solution for it.

REFERENCES

General

Bassuk EL, Birk AW (editors): *Emergency Psychiatry.* Plenum Press, 1984.

Guggenheim FG, Weiner MF (editors): *Manual of Psychiatric Consultation and Emergency Care.* Jason Aronson, 1984.

Hillard J (editor): *Manual of Clinical Emergency Psychiatry.* American Psychiatric Association Press, 1990.

Hyman S (editor): *Manual of Psychiatric Emergencies,* 2nd ed. Little, Brown, 1988.

Mezzich J, Zimmer B (editors): *Emergency Psychiatry.* International Universities Press, 1990.

Violent Behavior

Dubin WR: Evaluating and managing the violent patient. Ann Emerg Med 1981;10:481.

Dubin R, Wilson S, Mercer C: Assaults against psychiatrists in outpatient settings. J Clin Psychiatry 1988;49:338.

Gray G: Assaults by patients against psychiatric residents at a public psychiatric hospital. Academic Psychiatry 1989;13:81.

Hyman S: The violent patient. Chapter 5 in: *Manual of Psychiatric Emergencies,* 2nd ed. Hyman S (editor). Little, Brown, 1988.

Jacobs D: Evaluation and management of the violent patient in emergency settings. Psychiatr Clin North Am 1983;6:259.

Renshaw D: Psychiatric first aid in an emergency. Am J Nursing 1972;72:497.

Tupin JP: The violent patient: A strategy for management and diagnosis. Hosp Community Psychiatry 1983;34:37.

Organically Induced Disorders

Adler L et al: A controlled assessment of propranolol in the treatment of neuroleptic-induced akathisia. Br J Psychiatry 1986;174:477.

Bierer B, Bierer M: Psychiatric symptoms of medical illness and drug toxicity. Chapter 20 in: *Manual of Psychiatric Emergencies,* 2nd ed. Hyman S (editor). Little, Brown, 1988.

Dubin WR, Weiss KJ, Zeccardi JA: Organic brain syndrome: The psychiatric imposter. JAMA 1983;249:60.

Jefferson J, Marshall J: *Neuropsychiatric Features of Medical Disorders.* Plenum, 1981.

Lazarus A: Neuroleptic malignant syndrome. Hosp Community Psychiatry 1989;40:1224.

Levinson DF, Simpson GM: Neuroleptic-induced extrapyramidal symptoms with fever: Heterogeneity of the "neuroleptic malignant syndrome." Arch Gen Psychiatry 1986;43:839.

Perry S: Organic mental disorders caused by HIV: Update on early diagnosis and treatment. Am J Psychiatry 1990;147:696.

Rund DA, Summers WK, Levin M: Alcohol use and psychiatric illness in emergency patients. JAMA 1981;245:1240.

Anxiety & Panic States

Camara E: Lithium potentiation of antidepressant treatment in panic disorder. (Letter.) J Clin Psychopharmacol 1990;10:225.

Sheehan DV: Monoamine oxidase inhibitors and alprazolam in the treatment of panic disorder and agoraphobia. Psychiatr Clin North Am 1984;8:49.

Tesar G, Rosenbaum I: Successful use of clonazepam in patients with treatment resistant panic. J Nerv Ment Dis 1986;174:477.

Suicidal States

Fauman B: Consultations in emergency medicine: Suicidal patients in the emergency department. Ann Emerg Med 1981;10:389.

Feinstein R, Plutchik R: Violence and suicide risk assessment in the psychiatric emergency room. Compr Psychiatry 1990;31:337.

Jacobs D: Evaluation and care of suicidal behavior in emergency settings. Int J Psychiatry Med 1982;12:295.

Motto J: Identifying and treating suicidal patients in a general medical setting. Resident Staff Physician (March) 1983;29:79.

Acute Psychotic & Agitated States

Bodkin JA: Emerging uses for high-potency benzodiazepines in psychotic disorders. J Clin Psychiatry 1990;51–5(Suppl):41.

Easton M, Janicak P: The use of benzodiazepines in psychotic disorders. Psychiatr Ann 1990;20:535.

Ellison JM: Emergency treatment of acute psychosis, agitation, and anxiety. Hosp Community Psychiatry 1985;36:351.

Garza-Treviño E et al: Efficacy of combinations of intramuscular antipsychotics and sedative hypnotics for control of psychotic agitation. Am J Psychiatry 1989;146:1598.

Anorexia Nervosa

American College of Physicians Health and Public Policy Committee: Eating disorders: Anorexia nervosa and bulimia. Ann Intern Med 1986;105:790.

Herzog DB, Copeland PM: Eating disorders. N Engl J Med 1985;313:295.

Pryor T, McGilley B, Roach N: Psychopharmacology and eating disorders: Dawning of a new age. Ann Psychiatry 1990;20:711.

Conversion Disorders & Hysterical States

Chodoff P: The diagnosis of hysteria: An overview. Am J Psychiatry 1974;131:1073.

Raskin M, Talbott J, Meyerson A: Diagnosis of conversion reactions. JAMA 1966;197:530.

Borderline States With Multiple Admissions

Ellison JM, Blum N, Barsky AJ: Repeat visitors in the psychiatric emergency service: A critical review of the data. Hosp Community Psychiatry 1986;37:37.

Purdie FR, Honigman B, Rosen P: The chronic emergency department patient. Ann Emerg Med 1981;10:298.

Geriatric Psychiatric Emergencies

Herst L: Emergency psychiatry for the elderly. Psychiatr Clin North Am 1983;6:271.

Maletta G: Pharmacologic treatment and management of the aggressive demented patient. Psychiatr Ann 1990;20:682.

Martin R: Geriatric psychopharmacology: Present and future. Psychiatr Ann 1990;20:682.

Waxman HM et al: Geriatric psychiatry in the emergency department. 2. Evaluation and treatment of geriatric and nongeriatric admissions. J Am Geriatr Soc 1984;32:343.

Psychotropic Drugs

Jacobs D: Psychopharmacologic management of the psychiatric emergency patient. Gen Hosp Psychiatry 1984;6:203.

The Family in the Emergency Department

Perlmutter RA: Family involvement in psychiatric emergencies. Hosp Community Psychiatry 1983;34:255.

Involuntary Procedures

Segal S et al: Civil commitment in the psychiatric emergency room. 1. The assessment of dangerousness by emergency room clinician. 2. Mental disorder indicators and three dangerousness criteria. 3. Dispositions as a function of mental disorder and dangerousness indicators. Arch Gen Psychiatry 1988;45:748, 753, 759.

Amobarbital (Amytal) Interview

Kwentus J: The drug-assisted interview. Chapter 33 in: Manual of Psychiatric Consultation and Emergency Care. Guggenheim F, Weiner M (editors). Jason Aronson, 1984.

Perry JC, Jacobs D: Overview: Clinical applications of the Amytal interview in psychiatric emergency settings. Am J Psychiatry 1982;139:552.

The Decision to Hospitalize

Boren C, Zeman P: Psychiatric triage. Conn Med 1985;49:570.

Murphy JG, Fenichel GS, Jacobson S: Psychiatry in the emergency department: Factors associated with treatment and disposition. Am J Emerg Med 1984;2:309.

Nursing in Psychiatric Emergencies

Yoder L, Jones SL: The emergency room nurse and the psychiatric patient. J Psychosoc Nurs Ment Health Serv 1982;20:22.

Pediatric Emergencies

42

Ronald A. Dieckmann, MD, MPH, FAAP, FACEP, & Kevin Coulter, MD, FAAP

General Considerations

A. Epidemiology: Children constitute the most diverse and challenging patient population facing the emergency physician. They represent approximately 10% of prehospital and 30% of emergency department patients. Critical illness and injury in children are less frequent than in the adult population and occur in only about 5% of emergency department pediatric patients.

The epidemiology of pediatric emergency medicine changes with the clinical setting. In the prehospital environment, the common presenting complaints are trauma, seizures, respiratory distress, and toxicologic emergencies. In the emergency department, the commonest complaints are either **infections,** including upper respiratory infections, gastroenteritis, and otitis media, or **trauma.**

Injury is the leading cause of pediatric morbidity and mortality between the age of 1 year and adulthood. Illness also exacts a terrible toll from the childhood population, especially in the youngest age groups, even though many childhood maladies are preventable or their complications could be reduced through preventive measures or earlier recognition of distress.

B. Assessment: Assessment of the pediatric patient in the emergency department requires an age-specific approach. The important actions in a developmentally appropriate examination are summarized in Table 42–1. A calm, reassuring, and gen-

Table 42–1. Actions in a developmentally appropriate examination of children.[1]

Age Group	Developmental Characteristics	Actions
Infants	Often experience separation anxiety after 6 months of age.	Have parent hold baby for most of examination.
		Distract infant with brightly colored toys or by talking. Small stuffed animals that clip onto stethoscopes are effective for distracting infants and toddlers while assessing breath sounds.
Toddlers	Eager to please.	Explain what pleases you (eg, "Holding still will make it easier for me to listen to you.").
		Show pleasure when child cooperates.
	Need to feel autonomous.	Have child help to unbutton shirt.
	Fantasies are prevalent.	Use child's fantasies to elicit cooperation (eg, "I'm going to listen to you with my stethoscope to hear if you have any ducks quacking inside.").
	Fear separation from parents.	Have parent hold child while you listen to child's chest.
	Learn through sensorimotor experiences.	Explain what you will do with child in short sentences using sensory terms.
		Allow child to play with equipment (eg, have child "blow out the light" from otoscope, listen to own heartbeat with stethoscope).
Preschoolers	Ask lots of questions.	Give child opportunity to ask questions.
		Answer with simple, short, responses.
		Answer only what is asked.
	Attempt to cope with new situations.	Encourage play to help child relate to emergency department experience.
	Have prominent fears of castration.	Tell child which part of body you will examine.
School-aged children	Are absorbed with concrete aspects of siutations.	Supply child with technical explanations about what occurs.
		Use simple drawings such as an upside-down tree to explain pulmonary anatomy.
	Understand body mechanics.	Use examination time as an opportunity to teach about health.
	May need privacy.	Ensure privacy while listening to child's chest; parents may need to leave room momentarily.
	Feel peers are important.	Emphasize emergency department experience as a unique event to share with friends.
Adolescents	Definitely need privacy.	Decide who will be present during physical examination before examination.
	Think logically and concretely.	Be straightforward in your approach; do not be condescending.
	Have concerns about results of their treatment.	Advise adolescents of their response to aerosols and other treatments.
		Keep them informed of expected outcomes of treatment.
		Report evidence of normal physical examination findings as well as abnormal ones.

[1]Modified and reproduced, with permission, from Wabschall J: Nursing management of children during a mild to moderate asthma attack. J Emerg Nurs 1986;12:137.

tle manner on the part of the physician will facilitate information collection and encourage patient cooperation in examination and testing.

Often, the diagnosis, management, and disposition of the pediatric emergency department patient require knowledge of the child's growth and development. There are simple guidelines for estimation of weight, height, and head circumference for children of different ages (Table 42–2). Assessment of growth is most accurate when considered in terms of prior growth in the same individual. For rapid developmental evaluation, use the standard Denver Developmental Screening Test (Fig 42–1).

Severity of acute pediatric illness and injury is often difficult to discern. In contrast to the direct anatomic examination that underlies physical evaluation of the adult, in children, observational methods of assessment may be more sensitive to illness and injury acuity (Table 42–3). Such observations appear to be more predictive of serious illness than anatomic physical examination using standard palpation, percussion, and auscultation techniques.

Assessment and management of the distressed pediatric patient require appropriately sized equipment. Emergency department equipment and supplies for children are itemized in Table 42–4. Table 42–5 provides equipment sizes for invasive procedures in children of different age groups.

Vital signs vary by age (Table 42–6). A rapid formula for estimating systolic blood pressure is 80 + (2 × age [in years]). The maximum effective heart rate in infants is 200/min; in young children, 150/min; and in school-aged children, 120/min. Respiratory rate decreases with advancing age, ranging from 50/min in the newborn period to 40 at 1 year, 30 at 2 years, 20 at 3 years, and 16 throughout school ages. *Utilization of vital signs to assess vital functions in pediatrics, however, is hazardous.* Appropriate-sized measuring equipment is imperative, techniques must be careful, and interpretation must be age-related. Furthermore, even accurately obtained, age-adjusted vital signs may be insensitive. Instead, other objective measures of cardiopulmonary function—such as

the pediatric observational scale (Table 42–3)—and simple physical signs—such as skin color, temperature, and capillary refill—are often better triage and assessment tools.

C. Concept of the "Distressed Family": The emergency department physician must appreciate the intimate relationship of the child to the family. Acute pediatric illness and injury are inextricably part of the family environment and dynamics. Not only the child but also the entire nuclear and extended family may experience major psychologic, emotional, and financial consequences of pediatric emergencies. Effective care requires appropriate consideration of child within the "distressed family," enlistment of parent assistance in evaluation and management, and provision of psychologic support.

D. Pain and Sedation: Too often, the inexperienced physician neglects pain control or conscious sedation because of misunderstanding about the significance of pain in the young child, unwarranted fear of addicting children to narcotic agents, or ignorance of appropriate agents. When a painful procedure is necessary, an effective approach integrates careful explanation directly to the child and enlistment of parental understanding and assistance. Sometimes a restraint apparatus will facilitate the procedure.

The following are guidelines for a variety of clinical situations:

1. For wound repair, use a formulation of cocaine, 11.8%; epinephrine, 1:2000; and tetracaine, 0.5%, as a topical anesthetic. Place the solution, soaked into sterile gauze pads, directly in the wound, and hold in place for 10 minutes. Blanched wound edges indicate that anesthesia is present. This formulation will usually achieve complete local anesthesia on the face and scalp and partial anesthesia on the extremities. Supplemental lidocaine infiltration may also be necessary. Do not allow the solution to get in the nose or onto mucosal surfaces, since *seizures or death may result from systemic cocaine absorption and toxicity.*

2. For most patients who require pharmacologic pain management, use a combination of intramuscular meperidine, 2 mg/kg, and hydroxyzine, 1 mg/kg.

Table 42–2. Typical patterns of physical growth.[1]

Weight	Birth weight (BW) is regained by 10th–14th day. Average weight gain per day: 0–6 mo = 20 g; 6–12 mo = 15 g. BW doubles at ~ 4 months, triples at ~ 12 months, quadruples at ~ 24 months. During second year, average weight gain per month = ~0.25 kg. After age 2 years, average annual gain until adolescence = ~ 2.3 kg.
Length/height	By end of first year, birth length increases by 50%. Birth length doubles by 4 years, triples by 13 years. Average height gain during second year = ~ 12 cm. After age 2 years, average annual growth until adolescence ≥ 5 cm.
Head circumference	Average head growth per week: 0–2 months = ~0.5 cm, 2–6 months = ~0.25 cm. Average total head growth from 0–3 months = ~5 cm, 3–6 months = ~4 cm, 6–9 months = ~2 cm, 9 months–1 year = ~1 cm

[1]Reproduced, with permission, from Overby KJ: Pediatric health supervision. Page 17 in: *Rudolph's Pediatrics,* 19th ed. Rudolph AM. Appleton & Lange, 1991.

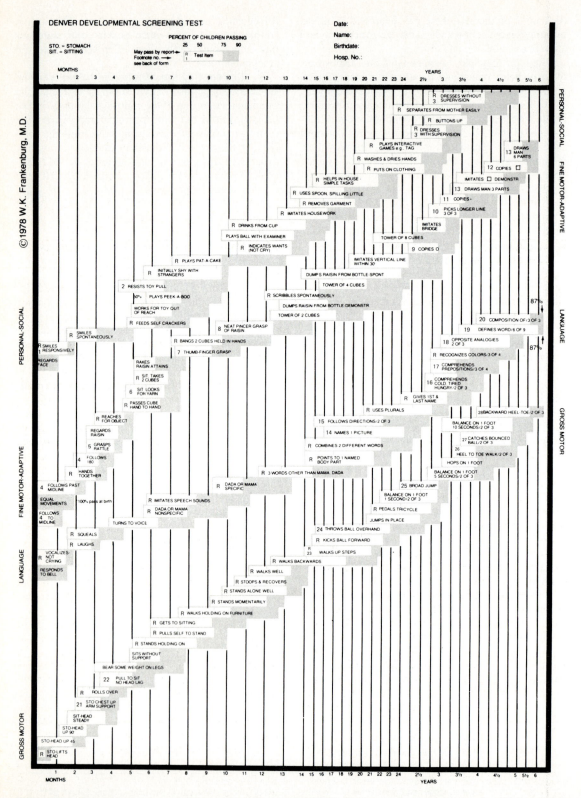

Figure 42–1. Denver Developmental Screening Test, Revised (DDST-R). (Reproduced, with permission, from Hathaway WE et al: *Current Pediatric Diagnosis & Treatment*, 10th ed. Appleton & Lange, 1991.)

Table 42–3. Predictive model: Acute illness observational scale.[1]

Observation Item	1 Normal	2 Moderate Impairment	3 Severe Impairment
Quality of cry	Strong with normal tone or content and not crying	Whimpering or sobbing	Weak or moaning or high pitched
Reaction to parent stimulation	Cries briefly then stops or content and not crying	Cries off and on	Continual cry or hardly responds
State variation	If awake, stays awake or if asleep and stimulated, wakes up quickly	Eyes close briefly, awake or wakes with prolonged stimulation	Falls to sleep or will not rouse
Color	Pink	Pale extremities or acrocyanosis	Pale or cyanotic or mottled or ashen
Hydration	Skin normal, eyes normal and mucous membranes moist	Skin, eyes are normal and mouth slightly dry	Skin doughy or tented and dry mucous membranes or sunken eyes
Response (talk, smile) to social overtures	Smiles or alerts ($\leq$ 2 mo)	Brief smile or alerts briefly ($\leq$ 2 mo)	No smile, face anxious, dull, expressionless or no alerting ($\leq$ 2 mo)

Score: < 10, only 2.7% had a serious illness; 11–15, 26.2% had a serious illness; > 16, 92.3% had a serious illness.

[1]Reproduced, with permission, from McCarthy PL et al: Observational scales for febrile children. Pediatrics 1982;70:806.

Despite previous practice, chlorpromazine must not be administered concurrently, since *it may increase the child's perception of pain as well as heighten risk for respiratory depression and hypotension.*

3. For painful procedures requiring both sedation and analgesia, employ a combination of morphine sulfate, 0.1 mg/kg intravenously, and midazolam, 0.05 mg/kg intravenously. Monitor the child's respiratory status after administration with pulse oximetry.

4. For individuals requiring imaging studies such as CT scan or MRI, use pentobarbital, 5 mg/kg intramuscularly.

5. Two other drugs are used for painful procedures: **(a)** inhaled nitrous oxide, although administration requires a reliable scavenging system to avoid exposure to staff as well as a careful regulatory method for oxygen delivery in the oxygen–nitrous oxide mix; **(b)** ketamine, 4 mg/kg intramuscularly, for procedural situations involving children under 10 years, especially burn debridement, foreign body removal, deep wound care, abscess incision and drainage, sexual abuse evaluation, and interventions such as lumbar puncture or orthopedic reductions. Use atropine, 0.01 mg/kg (maximum, 0.5 mg), as part of the same intramuscular injection to avoid hypersalivation. Intravenous administration is better for longer procedures. Ketamine may elevate intracranial pressure, induce emesis, and occasionally precipitate laryngospasm; it may also cause an adverse behavioral reaction upon emergence from sedation in children over 10–12 years. Nonetheless, it is an effective drug when used by trained personnel and with appropriate cardiopulmonary monitoring including vital signs and continuous pulse oximetry.

6. Outpatient analgesia should ordinarily include a nonsteroidal, anti-inflammatory drug such as ibuprofen, which is available in a flavored liquid preparation. This drug can also be used in combination with oral narcotic agents for treatment of severe pain. Aspirin, 10–20 mg/kg/dose every 4–6 hours, and acetaminophen, 10–15 mg/kg/dose every 4-6 hours, are essentially equivalent analgesic drugs for treatment of mild pain on an outpatient basis.

E. Drug and Fluid Administration: *All parenterally and orally administered agents must be given strictly on a per kilogram basis,* until maximum adult doses and volumes are reached. Overdosing and overhydration are dangerous errors in emergency pediatrics. Underdosing is also frequent, especially in the infant or small child. Both physician and nurse must meticulously review drug and fluid orders to ensure that they are age- and weight-corrected. (See also the appendix to this chapter.)

Vascular access is often the rate-limiting step in provision of lifesaving therapy to critically ill and injured children. The emergency department physician must be familiar with a variety of techniques for access into the cardiopulmonary system.

1. Endotracheal tube—In critically ill, intubated patients, the endotracheal route is an effective conduit for administration of a variety lifesaving drugs, including epinephrine, atropine, lidocaine, naloxone, and diazepam. Epinephrine is by far the most commonly used. When administered through the endotracheal tube, higher doses must be employed to achieve adequate serum concentrations. The pharmacokinetics of endotracheal epinephrine administration may be optimized by delivering the drug directly into the highly vascular trachea and proximal tracheobronchial tree instead of directly into the endotracheal tube. The preferred technique requires insertion of a nasogastric tube or a size 5F umbilical catheter past the distal tip of the endotracheal tube with direct instillation of drugs through the tube. Since endotra-

Table 42–4. Emergency department equipment and supplies for children.[1]

Emergency cart or other system to house all supplies, equipment, and drugs for a designated pediatric resuscitation area

Monitoring devices
ECG monitor-defibrillator/cardioverter with pediatric and adult-sized paddles and hard-copy recording capability
Otoscope/ophthalmoscope/stethoscope
Pulse oximeter with pediatric adapter
Sphygmomanometer and Doppler ultrasound blood pressure devices
Arterial and venous pressure monitoring equipment immediately available to emergency department
Rectal temperature probe
Hypothermia thermometer
Blood pressure cuffs
  Neonatal, infant, child
  Adult: arm, thigh
End-tidal P_{CO_2} monitor
Blood gas kit

Vascular access supplies and equipment
CVP (central venous pressure) kits, 18–22 gauge (4)
Catheter over-the-needle devices, 16, 18, 20, 22, 24 (2 each)
Butterflies, 18, 21, 23 (4 each)
Intraosseous needles, 16 gauge (4)
Tourniquets (3), rubber bands
Sponges, 10 cm × 10 cm
Providone-iodine swabs (10)
Alcohol swabs (10)
Tape, waterproof, 1 cm, 2.5 cm, 5 cm (1 roll each)
Stopcocks (2)
T-connectors (3)
IV tubing, 80 cm (2)
Armboards (2 each size)
Tincture of benzoin
Providone prep solution
Betadine ointment (2)
IV fluid/blood warmer
Infusion pumps, drip or volumetric, with microinfusion capability
IV administration sets and extension tubing
IV solutions
  Normal saline
  10% dextrose in normal saline
  Ringer's lactate
  Mannitol, 20%
  Albumin, 5%, 25%

Respiratory equipment and supplies
Bag-valve-mask resuscitator, self-inflating, pediatric and adult sizes
Suction devices
Laryngoscope handle
Laryngoscope blades
  Curved: 2, 3
  Straight or Miller: 0, 1, 2, 3
Stylets for endotracheal tubes, infant, adult (1 each)
Magill forceps
Endotracheal tubes
  Uncuffed sizes: 2.5, 3.0, 3.5, 4.0, 4.5, 5.0 (2 each)
  Cuffed sizes: 5.5, 6.0, 6.5, 7.0, 7.5, 8.0, (2 each)
Tracheostomy tubes
  Shiley tube sizes: 00, 1, 2, 3, 4, 6
Oral airways
  Sizes: 0, 1, 2, 3, 4, 5

Nasopharyngeal airways
  Sizes: 12, 16, 20, 24, 28, 30F
Clear oxygen masks
  Standard and nonrebreathing, neonatal, infant, child, and adult sizes
Nasal cannulas, child and adult sizes (2 each)
Oxygen cylinder, flow meter, tubing
Suction catheters
  Sizes: 6F, 8F, 10F, 14F (2 each)
Yankauer suction tip (4)
T-nasogastric tubes
  Sizes: 6F, 8F, 10F, 12F, 14F, 16F (2 each)
Tongue blades (5)
Lubricant jelly (4)

Medications (unit dose prepackaged, 2 of each)
Atropine, 0.1 mg/mL, 10 mL
Calcium chloride, 10%, 10 mL
Dextrose, 25%, 10 mL
Diazepam, 5 mg/mL
Lorazepam, 2 or 4 mg/mL
Epinephrine, I:10,000, 10mL
Lidocaine, 1%, 10 mL
Naloxone, 0.4 mg/mL
Phenobarbital, 65 mg/mL
Phenytoin, 50 mg/mL
Sodium bicarbonate, 7.5%, 50 mL
Sodium bicarbonate, 4.2%, 10 mL
Related supplies/ equipment
  Medication chart, tape, or other system to ensure ready access to information on proper per-kilogram dose for resuscitation drugs and equipment sizes
  Syringes: TB, 3 mL, 5 mL, 10 mL, 20 mL, 30 mL, 60 mL (5 each)
  Needles: 21 gauge, 23 gauge, 25 gauge (5 each)
  Feeding tubes (for endotracheal drugs): 3.5F, 5F, 8F (2 each)

Specialized pediatric trays for the following procedures:
Tube thoracostomy and water seal drainage
Thoracotomy tray with chest tubes, 8F–40F
Cricothyrotomy including needle cricothyrotomy
Peritoneal lavage
Venous cutdown
Lumbar puncture
Umbilical vessel cannulation
Catheterization: Foley catheter, 5F–12F (2 each)
Obstetric pack
Intracranial pressure monitoring
Newborn kit

Fracture management devices
Spine board, child and adult sizes
Femur splint (Hare traction), child and adult sizes
Spine board
Semirigid neck collars, child and adult sizes
Sandbags
Extremity splints, various sizes

Miscellaneous equipment
Infant scale
Heating source, overhead warmer preferred
Cardiac backboard
MAST trousers, toddler, child, and adult sizes

[1]Adapted and reproduced, with permission, from Schafermeyer RW, Pons PT: *Pediatric Equipment Guidelines.* American College of Emergency Physicians, 1992.

Table 42–5. Equipment and sizes available for invasive procedures.

Age	Inner Diameter Endotracheal Tube (mm)	Laryngoscope Blade	Chest Tube (F)	Nasogastric/Foley (F)
Newborn	2.5–3	0–1	8–12	5
1 month	3.5	1	12	8
6 months	3.5	1	16	8
1 year	4	1	20	8
2–3 years	4.5	1	24	8
4–5 years	5–6	2	28	10
6–8 years	6–6.5	2	32	10
10–12 years	7	2–3	32	12
14 years	7.5	3	40	12

cheal drugs may be more effective if aerosolized, dilute the drug with normal saline to a maximum volume of 0.5–1 mL/kg, then inject rapidly to achieve a partially aerosolized form.

2. Intravenous access–In infants, the scalp is an ideal site for cannulation; use a size 25 butterfly needle. In children past the neonatal period, the dorsal veins of the hand, antecubital fossa, or dorsum of the foot are usually accessible with a 24- or 22-gauge over-the-needle catheter. The external jugular vein is a large vein, usually easily visualized and readily cannulated with a 20-gauge over-the-needle catheter if the child is properly restrained and the head is held in a dependent position.

3. Intraosseous infusion–(See also Chapter 46.) For patients under 5 years of age in extremis and requiring lifesaving drug and fluid administration, this is an alternative method of administration. A short, thick needle with trocar tip is inserted into the intramedullary space of the bone. The richly vascularized intramedullary space allows for direct entry of drugs and fluids into the central circulation through emissary veins. The easiest insertion sites are the medial proximal tibia (Fig 42–2) or the distal midline femur. Intraosseous infusion is a rapid and effective technique of achieving therapeutic serum concentrations of almost all important drugs; moreover, a large fluid volume can be rapidly administered in injured or dehydrated patients. When necessary, insert multiple intraosseous lines. The commonest complication of this procedure is osteomyelitis.

F. Medicolegal Considerations: Most exposure to legal liability derives from the patient's status as a minor. While state laws protecting children vary significantly, there are some common legal principles.

Consent issues are frequent and often vexing problems in the emergency department. Consent may be difficult to obtain either because of the absence of the legal guardian or because the actual caretaker of the child may be neither the legal guardian nor a legally authorized surrogate. *If the child's legal guardian is unavailable, it is essential that the health provider make and clearly document every effort to communicate directly with the child's legal representative.*

When the child's condition allows, informed consent must be obtained from the legal representative. If

Table 42–6. Age-related vital signs.

Age	Mean Weight (kg)	Minimum Systolic Blood Pressure	Normal Heart Rate	Normal Respiratory Rate
Premature	2.5	40	120–170	40–60
Term	3.5	50	100–170	40–60
3 months	6	50	100–170	30–50
6 months	8	60	100–170	30–50
1 year	10	65	100–170	30–40
2 years	13	65	100–160	20–30
4 years	15	70	80–130	20
6 years	20	75	70–115	16
8 years	25	80	70–110	16
10 years	30	85	60–105	16
12 years	40	90	60–100	16

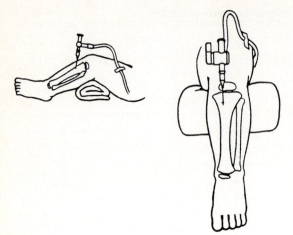

Figure 42–2. Technique for insertion of a tibial intraosseous line. (Reproduced, with permission, from Dieckmann RA: Emergency procedures. Page 649 in: *Pediatric Emergency Medicine: A Clinician's Reference.* Grossman M, Dieckmann RA [editors]. Lippincott, 1991.)

the condition is life-threatening and permanent harm or physical disability will result from delay of appropriate medical interventions, treatment must be implemented under the concept of "implied consent," including appropriate analgesia. If the characteristics of this legal action are not clearly spelled out by emergency department policy, consultation with the hospital's legal authority is prudent. Whenever treatment is instituted without formal consent, the reasons for such action must be documented on the patient's medical record.

Another dilemma occurs when a child presents to the emergency department with acute serious injury or illness and the legal representative refuses appropriate medical assistance. When the condition is such that permanent impairment or death may result from failure to treat, emergency legal recourse through the local juvenile court system may be required, especially when the legal representative is incompetent owing to substance abuse or other debilitating mental conditions.

In some circumstances, parental consent is not needed for emergency care. This list includes "emancipated minors," who by law are able to act as adults and consent to medical care, although they have not obtained legal age of maturity. Emancipated minors include individuals who are married, pregnant, in active duty in the armed services, or declared emancipated by the Superior Court. Moreover, many states recognize "mature minors," a status whereby a minor also has the power to consent to medical care. Such situations include substance abuse, mental disease, sexually transmitted disease, or pregnancy.

G. Death in the Emergency Department: The sudden and unexpected death of an infant or child in

the emergency department constitutes one of the most difficult situations in emergency practice. Careful and compassionate dialogue between the physician and parents, and between the physician and emergency department staff, is essential for minimizing chaos in the clinical setting and for reducing confusion and anger among bereaved families and department personnel. An emergency department death protocol for children is suggested in Table 42–7. Debriefing for health care workers may also be appropriate within 48–72 hours to alleviate stress that may impair work performance or cause psychologic disability.

CARDIOVASCULAR EMERGENCIES

Evaluation of cardiopulmonary function in children, especially in infants and younger children, requires special techniques. Vital signs are generally insensitive and nonspecific. Blood pressure poorly reflects volume status. When perfusion is mistakenly equated with blood pressure, early signs of hypovolemia can be missed. Fig 42–3 demonstrates the relationship of a child's blood volume to blood pressure during acute blood loss. In children, hypovolemia triggers compensatory tachycardia and intense peripheral vasoconstriction, which effectively main-

Table 42–7. Emergency department death protocol for children.[1]

Establish primary family liaison for consistent communication. Limit family access to medical information to liaison and attending physician.
Place family in private room, with drinks and telephone.
Ensure family support services: clergy (minister, priest, rabbi); key family members (other parent, children); psychologist when necessary.
Monitor friends and family members to ensure supportive environment for parents.
Contact primary physician and enlist his or her assistance.
Notify coroner about death. Establish necessity for autopsy before speaking to family about death.
After the body is cleaned and the room restored to order, encourage the parents to view the body and touch the child.
Explain to family the purpose of lines and tubes before they view the child.
Ensure complete chart documentation.
Administer rights of baptism to the Roman Catholic child. This can be done by any person of any faith: "I baptize you in the name of the Father, Son, and Holy Ghost. Amen."
Consider organ and tissue donation.
Give the family names and telephone numbers of the attending physician, coroner, and funeral home.
Encourage follow-up with primary physician.

[1]Reproduced, with permission, from Dieckmann RA: Death of a child in the emergency department. In: *Pediatric Emergency Medicine: A Clinician's Reference.* Grossman M, Dieckmann RA (editors). Lippincott, 1991.

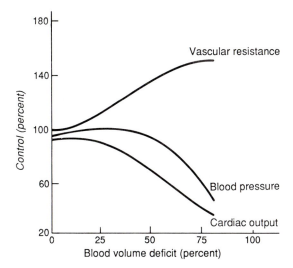

Figure 42–3. Relationship of blood volume to blood pressure in children during acute blood loss. (Reproduced, with permission, from Schwaitzberg SD, Bergman KS, Harris BH: A pediatric trauma model of continuous hemorrhage. J Pediatr Surg 1988;23:605.)

tains blood pressure until volume loss exceeds about 50% of intravascular volume.

Tachycardia, while sensitive to cardiopulmonary duress, is nonspecific. Normal heart rate also varies with age, and tachycardia is a common response to many types of stress (eg, fever, anxiety, hypoxia, hypovolemia). In children, assessment of volume status should focus primarily on skin signs (temperature, color, capillary refill, turgor) in combination with heart rate. Feeling the skin at the knee is an excellent first maneuver to assess warmth and skin perfusion. Rate of urine output may be the next best measure of core perfusion. Adequate core blood flow results in 1–2 mL/kg/h of urine production. Therefore, in the unstable child with suspected perfusion abnormalities, *a urinary bladder catheter is imperative to monitor output.*

Cardiac rhythm disturbances in children are unusual. The commonest is bradycardia, usually secondary to hypoxia. Properly applied pulse oximetry, at the triage desk or as part of initial clinical assessment, is an easy and useful method of rapid evaluation of oxygen saturation in patients with slow or rapid heart rates. When a primary tachycardia occurs, it is usually supraventricular in origin. In the distressed child, electrocardiographic monitoring will assist in evaluating cardiovascular status and in judging response to therapy.

DEHYDRATION

Acute dehydration is a common pediatric emergency. Diarrhea and vomiting are the most frequent causes. Other common causes are blood loss, burn wounds, open wounds, fever or hyperthermia, sweating, inadequate fluid intake, polyuria, and poisoning.

Diagnosis

Clinical evaluation of the dehydrated child requires assessment of hydration status. Orthostatic vital signs may be helpful for judging volume status in stable, alert patients (> 10% drop in blood pressure or > 15% increase in heart rate implies dehydration). Comparison of presenting weight with recent weights is likewise useful. Management is dictated by degree of acuity (mild, 3–5% weight loss; moderate, 10%; severe, 15%). Formulate initial treatment on the basis of clinical evaluation of degree of dehydration. Laboratory assessment of type of dehydration assists the physician in later strategies for specific electrolyte replacement. Serum sodium concentration is the most important laboratory parameter. Serum sodium concentration does not indicate degree of hydration but does provide a useful measure for titrating sodium repletion (see below).

Treatment

After rapid assessment of degree of dehydration, management must match severity of illness.

A. For severely dehydrated patients, provide supplemental oxygen, attach pulse oximeter and cardiac monitor, and establish intravenous or intraosseous access with one or 2 secure catheters.

B. For a severely dehydrated infant or young child, rapidly infuse a balanced isotonic solution with dextrose (eg, 5% dextrose in normal saline or lactated Ringer's injection); in the older child or diabetic, use normal saline or a combined electrolyte solution (eg, Plasma-Lyte).

C. Administer a fluid bolus at 20 mL/kg, then repeat boluses at 20 mL/kg until physical signs (heart rate, skin temperature, and capillary refill) indicate improved perfusion. After 60 mL/kg of isotonic fluid have been administered, if vital signs have not normalized, consider administration of packed red blood cells, 10–20 mL/kg, fresh-frozen plasma, or occasionally 5% albuminated saline.

D. After stabilization, slow the intravenous infusion, and devise a therapeutic plan. Insert a urinary bladder catheter if the child has uncertain volume replacement requirements. Send blood for complete blood count (CBC), electrolytes, glucose, blood urea nitrogen (BUN), and creatinine measurements. Arterial blood gas determination is indicated in the child who remains unstable after 60 mL/kg of volume administration.

E. When laboratory data are available, titrate sodium and water repletion accordingly. For hyponatremic and isotonic dehydration, replace the calculated volume deficit over 24 hours, giving 50% of the deficit in the first 8 hours and the remaining 50% over the following 16 hours. *Ongoing losses and maintenance requirements must also be included.* Control fever, since insensitive water losses are significantly increased by temperature elevation. Add small amounts of potassium to the ongoing infusion, once urination is observed, and replace calculated potassium deficits over 48 hours. The minimal daily maintenance requirements for water, sodium, and potassium are noted in Table 42–8. For hypernatremic dehydration, divide fluid and electrolyte replacement evenly over 48 hours to avoid rapid osmolal shifts and central nervous system complications.

F. Use oral rehydration therapy (ORT) in most dehydrated patients. Children can usually take fluids by mouth. Vomiting does not contraindicate use of ORT. Unless there is shock, altered mental status or severe weakness, ORT may be utilized as part of early emergency department and in-hospital management for most dehydrated patients. Other patients not requiring hospitalization can be easily rehydrated using this technique. The composition of ORT as set by the World Health Organization includes 90 meq/L of sodium, 20 meq/L of potassium, 30 meq/L of citrate, and a 1–2% glucose concentration. Commercial preparations that provide approximately these electrolyte constituents include Pedialyte, Lytren, and Resol. If the child can be discharged, prescribe home fluid replacement that is appropriate for the age of the child, the calculated deficit, and ongoing losses.

SHOCK

Diagnosis

Shock is inadequate oxygen delivery to tissues. Most causes of shock in children (eg, gastrointestinal fluid losses, burns, blood loss from acute injury) involve decreased stroke volume usually from hypovolemia (**hypovolemic shock**). **Septic shock,** a form of **distributive shock,** occurs usually in the patient under 2 years of age and must always be considered in the sick-appearing, febrile child. **Anaphylac-**

Table 42–8. Daily maintenance requirements for fluids and electrolytes.

Weight	Water Requirement[1]	Sodium Requirement	Potassium Requirement[2]
1–10 kg	100 mL/kg		
11–20 kg	50 mL/kg + 1000 mL	3 meq/kg	2 meq/kg
> 20 kg	20 mL/kg + 1500 mL		

[1]Assumes child is normothermic. Fever significantly increases insensible water losses.

[2]Do not exceed 0.25 meq/kg/h intravenously. Use oral route when possible. Add KCl to intravenous infusion after urination.

tic shock, another form of distributive shock, may develop after bee stings or after in-hospital use of parenteral drugs or contrast agents. **Cardiogenic shock** is extremely rare in children but may complicate congenital heart disease or toxicologic emergencies.

Shock is not hypotension. Successful management includes early recognition of the compensated, normotensive phase of shock. During the compensated phase of hypovolemic shock, vital signs in the supine patient are usually normal, except for mild tachycardia. Skin signs of hypoperfusion are usually evident, and laboratory testing may disclose metabolic acidosis. Intervention is usually successful during this phase. When the hypotensive, decompensated phase develops in the absence of recognition and effective treatment, irreversible shock and death may result.

Treatment

Rapid clinical assessment should disclose a shock category, so that focused treatment can be immediately instituted (Chapter 3). Failure to act expeditiously and aggressively is a common error and may significantly increase mortality risk. An algorithm for treatment of uncompensated shock in children is shown in Fig 42–4.

A. Consider immediate endotracheal intubation. In the ill-appearing child with signs of shock and sepsis or the frankly hypotensive child, this should be accomplished either immediately or after failure to respond to first-line resuscitation with oxygen and fluids. After intubation, insert a nasogastric tube.

B. Apply supplemental oxygen, attach pulse oximeter and cardiac monitor, establish 2 secure intravenous catheters, and insert urinary bladder catheter.

C. Initiate volume resuscitation if indicated, or begin administration of inotropic agent.

D. When inotropic agents are utilized, adequate intravascular volume must be present. Inotropic infusions can then be titrated at the bedside, often using multiple infusions (dopamine, epinephrine, dobutamine), until perfusion is restored. Start with dopamine at 5–10 μg/kg/min, then add a second drip if cardiovascular response does not occur at 30 μg/kg/min. If physical examination is equivocal for hydration status, a chest x-ray may help: dehydration or overhydration is reflected in the appearance of pulmonary vessels.

E. Obtain arterial blood gases, CBC, electrolytes, platelets, coagulation studies, and blood cultures (if infection is suspected) to help guide secondary treatment after stabilization. A chest x-ray is also necessary in most cases.

CONGESTIVE HEART FAILURE

Diagnosis

Congestive heart failure (CHF) is unusual in childhood. It usually presents in the first year of life in pa-

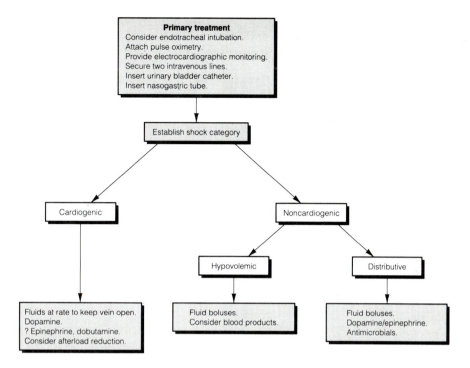

Figure 42–4. Treatment algorithm for pediatric uncompensated shock.

tients with congenital heart disease. The structural conditions causing CHF at different times during infancy are listed in Table 42–9. Myocarditis and other cardiomyopathies, toxicologic conditions, and coronary artery disease are also included in the differential diagnosis of new heart failure in childhood.

Treatment

When congestive heart failure has progressed to frank pulmonary edema, treat as follows:

A. Assess need for immediate endotracheal intubation in the severely distressed, hypotensive, or hypoxic patient (pulse oximetry < 85% on 100% oxygen).

B. Apply 100% oxygen, sometimes with positive pressure ventilation through an endotracheal tube, and attach pulse oximeter and cardiac monitor. Insert urinary bladder catheter.

C. Establish a secure intravenous line with 5% dextrose in water at a rate to keep the vein open.

D. Administer morphine sulfate, 0.1 mg/kg intravenously.

E. Administer furosemide, 1 mg/kg intravenously.

F. Obtain arterial blood gas, CBC, electrolyte, BUN, creatinine, and digoxin levels if appropriate. Obtain an ECG. Order a chest x-ray in the room or with nurse or physician in attendance in the radiology suite.

G. Administer digoxin. Digitalization doses are

Table 42–9. Structural causes of congestive heart failure during infancy.

Newborn period
 Hypoplastic left heart
 Arteriovenous fistula
 Large placental–fetal transfusion
 Regurgitation of the pulmonic or tricuspid valves
 Third-degree atrioventricular block
 Paroxysmal atrial tachycardia
First month
 Aortic coarctation with patent ductus arteriosus
 Ventricular septal defect
 Total anomalous pulmonary venous return
 Tricuspid atresia
 Truncus arteriosus
First 6 months
 Transposition of the great vessels
 Ventricular septal defect
 Patent ductus arteriosus
 Truncus arteriosus with large left-to-right shunt
Six to 12 months
 Ventricular septal defect
 Endocardial fibroelastosis
 Total anomalous pulmonary venous return

[1]Reproduced, with permission, from Hoffman JIE: Congestive heart failure, Page 54 in: *Pediatric Emergency Medicine: A Clinician's Reference.* Grossman M, Dieckmann RA (editors). Lippincott, 1991.

30 µg/kg in premature infants, 45 µg/kg in full-term to 2-year-old patients, and 30 µg/kg in children over 2 years of age. (Digitalization doses should be divided into 3 separate portions.)

H. Occasionally, patients with severe pulmonary edema unresponsive to initial therapy require either dopamine, dobutamine, or both.

CARDIAC DYSRHYTHMIAS

Although uncommon, dysrhythmias sometimes present in children with known congenital heart disease, acquired heart disease (eg, myocarditis), or secondary to other metabolic or toxicologic disorders. Therapy is aimed at the underlying condition. Evaluation of dysrhythmias includes clinical assessment of cardiopulmonary status and interpretation of the ECG. *Key electrocardiographic features are heart rate and width of the QRS complex.* These constituents must be evaluated against age-specific norms.

Treatment
(See Table 42–10.)

A. Apply supplemental oxygen; attach pulse oximeter and cardiac monitor.

B. Establish a secure intravenous line with 5% dextrose in water at a rate to keep the vein open.

C. Obtain an ECG if the patient is hemodynamically stable.

D. *Unstable patients with tachydysrhythmias require immediate electrical DC countershock.* Initial mode (synchronized or asynchronized) and exact energy levels are dictated by the nature of the dysrhythmia.

E. If electrical conversion does not occur with initial shock, double electrical doses until conversion occurs or until the maximum electrical dose is 8 J/kg. If synchronized countershock fails at 4 J/kg, switch to asynchronized mode (defibrillation). Ensure that paddles are held firmly against chest wall and that a good conductive agent is employed. If standard 4.5-cm pediatric paddles are unavailable for sterno-apical placement, use adult paddles in an anteroposterior configuration.

F. Pretreat conscious patients requiring cardioversion with light anesthesia (diazepam, 0.1 mg/kg), and be prepared to perform endotracheal intubation and full cardiopulmonary resuscitation.

Table 42–10. Treatment of common pediatric dysrhythmias.

Rhythm	Rate/min	QRS	Initial Treatment	Drug Therapy
Narrow complex tachycardias Sinus tachycardia	100–250	< 0.10	Oxygen, fluids, warmth, calm manner.	Treatment of primary condition.
Atrial flutter	300–500	< 0.10	If unstable, synchronized electrical DC cardioversion, 0.25 J/kg. If stable, vagal maneuvers (rectal stimulation, ice water to face, Valsalva).	Digoxin, 10 µg/kg intravenously. Procainamide, 15 mg/kg intravenously, over 30 min.
Atrial fibrillation	60–190	< 0.10	As for atrial flutter.	As for atrial flutter.
Supraventricular	120–300	0.10	As for atrial flutter.	Adenosine, 0.1 mg/kg rapid intravenous push. Repeat at 0.2 mg/kg.
Wide complex tachycardias Ventricular tachycardia	150–260	> 0.10	If unstable, synchronized electrical DC cardioversion, 1 J/kg, then double. If stable, lidocaine, 1 mg/kg, then 30–50 µg/kg/min.	Lidocaine, 1 mg/kg, then 30–50 µg/kg/min.
Wolff-Parkinson-White syndrome	150–300	> 0.10	As for ventricular tachycardia.	As for ventricular tachycardia.
Ventricular fibrillation	300–500	Variable	DC cardioversion, 2 J/kg, then double.	Lidocaine, 1 mg/kg, then 30–50 µg/kg/min. Bretylium, 5 mg/kg, then 10–30 mg/kg.
Bradycardia Sinus	Age-related	< 0.10	Oxygen, stimulation.	Atropine, 0.01–0.02 mg/kg (minimum, 0.1 mg). Isoproterenol, 0.05–0.5 µg/kg/min.
Atrioventricular block	Age-related	Variable	Oxygen. If unstable, transcutaneous or transvenous pacing.	As for sinus bradycardia.

RESPIRATORY DISTRESS

In children, normal ventilation and oxygenation occurs with minimal visible effort. Evaluation of respiratory function includes assessment of rate, work of breathing, skin and mucous membrane color, and mental status. Respiratory rate alone is an insensitive indicator of respiratory distress, since rates vary significantly with age, excitement, anxiety, or fever. Tachypnea may be an early manifestation of respiratory distress, or it may result from respiratory compensation for metabolic acidosis caused by shock, diabetic ketoacidosis, inborn errors of metabolism, salicylism, or chronic renal insufficiency. A slow respiratory rate may indicate impending respiratory failure.

Observation alone will usually disclose distress or increased work of breathing. A child with noisy breathing is especially worrisome, especially if inspiratory stridor is present. This denotes upper airway obstruction. Immediate therapy is indicated to relieve obstruction and improve oxygenation and ventilation. Increased work of breathing is also evidenced by nasal flaring and by suprasternal, intercostal, and subcostal retractions. Retractions become more pronounced cephalad to caudad with increasing hypoxia. Grunting is produced by premature glottic closure and usually represents alveolar collapse and loss of lung volume, which develop in patients with pulmonary edema, pneumonia, or atelectasis. Auscultation will provide further differentiation of disease possibilities. Wheezing, rales, or decreased breath sounds may be present. However, auscultation is often inaccurate in the busy, noisy emergency department setting. Cyanosis, when present, represents severe distress and is best seen on mucous membranes of the mouth and nail beds. Peripheral cyanosis is more likely due to circulatory failure than to pulmonary failure. Finally, mental status changes may be a clue to gas exchange abnormalities. Hypoxic patients are restless and agitated; hypercapnic patients are drowsy or even comatose.

Rapid evaluation of respiratory function is imperative in all distressed emergency department pediatric patients. Respiratory failure and respiratory arrest due to a wide spectrum of causes (eg, head trauma, coma, poisoning, pneumonia, asthma, foreign body aspiration) are the commonest causes of cardiac arrest in childhood. Timely, aggressive intervention in early stages as well as meticulous respiratory monitoring by means of pulse oximetry and continuous observation will avert preventable adverse patient outcomes. *Children with respiratory distress should not be sent for imaging studies without qualified personnel in attendance.* Early hospital admission is usually warranted for such patients.

Pulse oximetry must be used liberally in the emergency department setting in order to disclose undetected oxygen desaturation states. Pulse oximetry is noninvasive, simple, and reasonably accurate. Use this assessment modality in all cases of suspected respiratory distress, cardiopulmonary disease, or serious trauma. In selected patients, especially those with significant tachypnea or work of breathing, pulse oximetry may underestimate degree of distress, and it provides no indication of adequacy of ventilation (ie, PCO_2). In such patients, obtain arterial blood gas levels to help measure the severity and nature of the ventilation or oxygenation disturbance.

APNEA

Apnea means cessation of ventilation for 20 seconds or for 10–20 seconds in patients who also manifest bradycardia, cyanosis, or pallor. Ordinary sleep will sometimes cause breathing irregularities easily confused with apnea. Central apnea occurs in newborn infants, often in preterm infants. Infection, metabolic abnormalities, anemia, hypoxia, or central nervous system injury may be associated with newborn apnea. Obstructive apnea occurs in later infancy and childhood and is related to obstructive upper airway conditions.

Treatment
A. In Infants: Apnea in the infant may be symptomatic of life-threatening illness. Such patients ordinarily require hospital admission for observation and full work-up for infections and for central nervous system, metabolic, and feeding problems. In the emergency department,

1. Place child on supplemental oxygen, and apply pulse oximeter and cardiac monitor or apnea monitor.

2. Establish intravenous access with 5% dextrose in quarter- or half-normal saline, at maintenance rate for weight (Table 42–8).

3. Obtain blood for CBC, electrolytes, BUN, creatinine, and cultures. Obtain clean urine for urinalysis, culture, and toxicology studies. Consider spinal fluid analysis in most infants and any young child with meningeal signs, toxicity, or altered mental status. CT scan can usually precede spinal fluid analysis in the child who does not appear acutely infected.

4. Obtain a chest x-ray. Consider an ECG.

5. Admit for observation and further evaluation.

B. In Children: Obstructive apnea in the slightly older patient may be serious. Focus evaluation on obstructive upper pharyngeal lesions such as tonsillitis and pharyngitis or laryngomalacia. Chest x-ray and lateral neck films, along with laryngoscopy, are often necessary. Emergency department evaluation may be insufficient to exclude a serious diagnosis, and hospital admission may be indicated.

UPPER AIRWAY OBSTRUCTION

Diagnosis

Upper airway obstruction is usually readily apparent. *Inspiratory stridor is the hallmark.* The child is dyspneic and shows signs of respiratory distress, including tachypnea, flaring, and supraclavicular, intercostal, and subcostal retractions. Ventilation and sometimes oxygenation abnormalities are present. If obstruction is severe, hypercapnia will be present, usually along with depressed mental status, cyanosis, and decreased air movement. Arterial blood gases will demonstrate carbon dioxide retention and often hypoxemia. Pulse oximetry will be abnormal in most advanced cases, but normal in typical cases.

Differential Diagnosis

In children, the common causes of stridor and upper airway obstruction are croup, epiglottitis, and foreign body aspiration. The epidemiologic and clinical characteristics of these entities are compared in Table 42–11. Other less common conditions producing stridor are bacterial tracheitis (usually *Staphylococcus aureus* or *Haemophilus influenzae* type b), retropharyngeal or peritonsillar abscess, trauma, caustic ingestions, neoplasm, or angioneurotic edema.

Treatment
(See Figure 42–5.)

1. Clear the airway using procedures recommended in Table 42–12 for the patient with complete airway obstruction.

2. Avoid airway clearance maneuvers in the patient with incomplete or partial airway obstruction, since this may worsen obstruction. Allow the child to adopt a position of comfort, usually on the parent's lap.

3. Apply supplemental oxygen, and attach pulse oximeter and cardiac monitor.

A. Epiglottitis:

1. If a child presents with clinical findings suggestive of epiglottitis, *immediately arrange to establish a definitive airway,* preferably by nasotracheal intubation in the operating room.

2. In the rare case in which abrupt airway obstruction occurs, first attempt orotracheal intubation. Usually this technique will succeed. If direct laryngoscopy and orotracheal intubation fails, perform needle cricothyrotomy or surgical cricothyrotomy.

3. Minimize all invasive interventions in order to avert patient agitation and potential precipitous airway obstruction.

4. Administer antimicrobial therapy with cefotaxime, 50 mg/kg, or ampicillin, 100 mg/kg, and chloramphenicol, 25 mg/kg intravenously, after obtaining blood cultures.

5. In a patient with a lower likelihood of epiglottitis, a soft tissue lateral film of the neck may be useful to help demonstrate the swollen epiglottis (see Fig 26–8).

6. *A physician should be at the bedside of the patient at all times,* including in the radiology suite, prepared to perform definitive airway maneuvers.

B. Croup (Laryngotracheobronchitis): If history and clinical assessment, sometimes in combination with lateral neck x-rays and chest x-rays, suggest croup, therapy includes the following:

1. Apply humidified oxygen, and attach pulse

Table 42–11. Differential diagnosis of upper airway obstruction.

	Croup	Epiglottitis	Foreign Body
Age	6 months to 3 years	2–5 years	Under 3 years
Cause	Parainfluenza	*H influenzae*	Foreign body
Season	Fall or winter	Any	Any
Time of day	Night or morning	Any	Daytime
Illness features Onset	Slow	Abrupt	Abrupt
Upper respiratory infection	Yes	No	No
Fever	Low	High	None
Toxic	Mild	Yes	No
Pharyngitis	Possible	Yes	No
Drooling	No	Yes	No
Stridor	Inspiratory + expiratory	Inspiratory	Inspiratory + expiratory
Position	Variable	Sitting	Variable
Hoarseness	Yes	Rare	No
Ancillary tests White blood count	Normal	High	Normal
Chest x-ray	Steepel sign	Normal	Hyperinflation
Lateral neck	Normal	Swollen epiglottis	May show radiopaque body

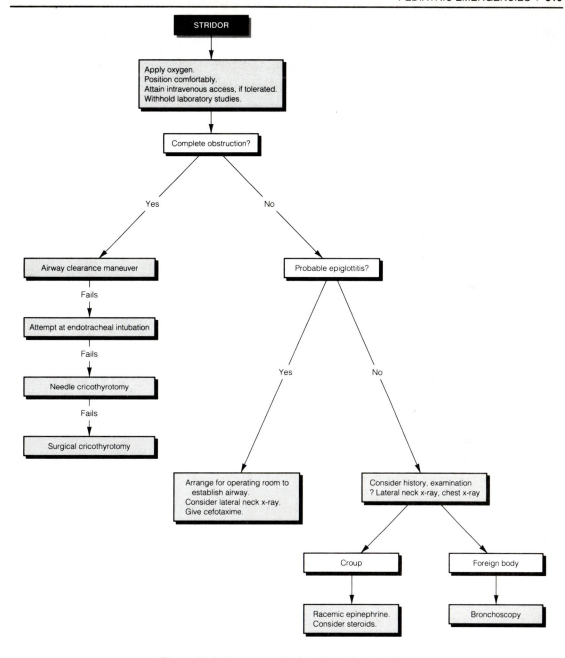

Figure 42–5. Treatment algorithm for pediatric stridor.

oximeter and cardiac monitor. Rarely is immediate endotracheal intubation necessary before attempts at medical management.

2. Keep child in position of comfort, usually on the parent's lap.

3. For moderately to severely distressed children, administer nebulized 2.25% racemic epinephrine to reduce laryngeal edema. Give 0.25 mL in 2.5 mL of normal saline for children weighing up to 20 kg, 0.5 mL in 2.5 mL of normal saline for children weighing 20–40 kg, and 0.75 mL in 2.5 mL of normal saline for children weighing > 40 kg.

4. Since rebound airway edema occurs predictably in 4–6 hours, children receiving racemic epinephrine require hospitalization.

5. For the minimally distressed child with no stridor at rest and pulse oximetry > 92% on room air, consider cool, humidified oxygen with nebulized saline. If this is effective in the emergency department at reducing upper airway obstruction, such patients

Table 42–12. Treatment of foreign body obstruction.[1]

Under 1 Year of Age	Over 1 Year of Age
1. (a) Place the infant face down on the rescuer's forearm in a 60-degree head-down position with the head and neck stabilized. Rest the forearm firmly against the rescuer's body for additional support. (b) For the choking large infant, an alternative method is to lay the infant face down over the rescuer's lap, with the head firmly supported and held lower than the trunk. **2.** Administer 4 back blows rapidly with the heel of the hand high between shoulder blades. **3.** If obstruction is not relieved, turn the infant over to a supine position resting on a firm surface and deliver 4 rapid chest thrusts (similar to external cardiac compressions) over the sternum using 2 fingers. **4.** If breathing is not resumed, open the victims's mouth by grasping both the tongue and the lower jaw between thumb and finger and lifting (the tongue-jaw lift technique); this draws the tongue away from the back of the throat and may help relieve the obstruction. If the foreign body is visualized, it may be manually extracted by a finger sweep. However, blind sweeps may cause further obstruction and thus should be avoided. **5.** If no spontaneous breathing occurs, attempt ventilation with 2 breaths by mouth-to-mouth or mouth-to-mouth-and-nose technique. **6.** Repeat steps 1–5, and persist in performing the above techniques as needed.	**1.** Apply a series of 6–10 abdominal thrusts (the Heimlich maneuver) until the foreign body is expelled. The child should be placed on his or her back. The rescuer should kneel at the child's feet if the child is on the floor, or stand at the child's feet if the child is on a table. The astride position is not recommended for small children. The heel of one hand should be placed in the midline between navel and rib cage and the second hand placed on top of the first and pressed into the abdomen with an upward thrust. In small children, the maneuver must be applied gently. It should consist of a rapid inward and upward thrust. **2.** If the obstruction is not relieved using the Heimlich maneuver, open the airway using the tongue–jaw lift technique, and attempt to visualize the foreign body. No blind finger sweeps should be used. **3.** If no spontaneous respirations result, attempt to ventilate the victim. If unsuccessful, repeat a series of 6–10 abdominal thrusts. **4.** Repeat steps 1–3 and persist in performing the above sequence while rapidly seeking aid from emergency medical services. ***If the Choking Victim is an Older Child*** An older, larger child can be treated as an adult in the standing, sitting, or recumbent (supine) position.

[1]Reproduced, with permission, from Committee on Accident and Poison Prevention, American Academy of Pediatrics: First Aid for the Choking Victim. *Pediatrics* 1988;81:741.

may ordinarily be discharged and may use cool mist therapy at home.

6. Administer dexamethasone, 0.25–0.6 mg/kg intramuscularly, in selected patients with severe croup. Which patients will benefit from corticosteroid therapy is not clear; however, children presenting with pulse oximetry < 85%, severe stridor at rest, and lethargy not relieved by racemic epinephrine may be appropriate candidates.

C. Foreign Body Aspiration: The anatomic level and completeness of airway obstruction will dictate physical findings. The history is usually highly suggestive, with a brief asymptomatic interval, then sudden dyspnea, coughing, and gagging, after the child has handled a small object such as jewelry, toy, pin, peanut, or candy. In 20% of cases, the object is in the upper airway; in 80%, it is in the main stem or lobar bronchus. Stridor is present if the object is lodged high, at the level of the larynx; wheezing and decreased breath sounds occur if is it lodged below the larynx. There may be no findings except mild tachypnea. Lateral neck x-rays may be helpful for radiopaque foreign bodies in the neck. When lower airway occlusion is suspected, chest x-rays taken in decubitus positions bilaterally (preferentially in expiration) will often reveal hyperinflation in the affected lung area. This finding is most visible in the *dependent lung*, which will be more radiolucent when compared with the superior lung in the same decubi-

tus view or with the contralateral dependent lung in the other decubitus view.

1. If obstruction is complete and airway clearance maneuvers (Table 42–12) fail, perform laryngoscopy immediately, and attempt to remove the foreign body with Magill forceps under direct vision. After removal of the foreign body, insert a properly sized endotracheal tube to prevent later inflammatory obstruction.

2. In most patients, obstruction is partial. Apply supplemental oxygen, and attach pulse oximeter and cardiac monitor. Do not attempt endotracheal intubation.

3. Establish venous access and begin 5% dextrose in quarter- or half-normal saline, at maintenance rate (Table 42–8).

4. Allow patient to assume position of comfort, usually on parent's lap.

5. Obtain chest x-rays (see above). Maintain constant observation of patient by nurse or physician.

6. Arrange for rigid bronchoscopy, under general anesthesia, to remove the foreign object.

LOWER AIRWAY DISORDERS

Lower airway disorders are a disparate group of conditions with varying clinical presentations that may affect oxygenation and ventilation. Lower airway disease includes both obstructive conditions and parenchymal or alveolar disease. The clinical hallmarks are dyspnea and tachypnea, often with cough. Wheezing denotes an obstructive process.

In children, the commonest causes of lower airway obstruction are bronchiolitis, asthma, and foreign body obstruction. In infants, congenital anomalies of the airway (tracheal web, cysts, vascular rings, lobar emphysema) must also be considered. Pneumonia is the most frequent pediatric alveolar disorder, although pulmonary edema, inhalation injury, and cystic fibrosis must also be excluded.

Bronchiolitis

A. Diagnosis: Bronchiolitis is a wintertime acute lower airway respiratory disease, usually caused by respiratory syncytial virus, that produces small airway obstruction. It primarily affects children under 12 months of age. Cough, coryza, and upper respiratory symptoms, usually with fever, precede wheezing and dyspnea. Clinical signs of respiratory distress are variable. The white blood cell count is normal, and the chest x-ray shows shifting patterns of hyperaeration and atelectasis. Hypercapnia, hypoxemia, or both may be present.

B. Treatment:

1. Apply supplemental oxygen, and attach pulse oximeter. Keep child on parent's lap.

2. If wheezing is present, bring about bronchodilatation with subcutaneous epinephrine, 0.01 mg/kg of 1:1000 solution, or inhaled albuterol, 0.1 mg/kg/dose of 0.5% solution (0.02 mL/kg/dose) by mask (maximum 2.5 mg).

3. If bronchodilator therapy produces improvement, continue bronchodilator therapy as discussed below for asthma.

Asthma

A. Diagnosis: The commonest pediatric respiratory disease is reactive airway disease, or asthma. Dyspnea, cough, and wheezing are part of the usual presentation. In infancy, wheezing is typically associated with bronchiolitis, caused by the respiratory syncytial virus. The relationship of bronchiolitis in infancy to childhood asthma is not clear, although approximately one-half of infants with bronchiolitis later develop asthma. Bronchiolitis may respond to bronchodilator therapy with albuterol or subcutaneous epinephrine, which indicates reversible smooth muscle spasm. In both conditions, mucus plugging of small airways, edema, and bronchial constriction are key pathophysiologic features. Asthma appears to be increasing in prevalence, and morbidity and mortality rates associated with this condition are worsening.

Peak expiratory flow rate (EFR) is extremely useful in asthma evaluation, and hand-held pediatric-sized devices should be available in the emergency department. Expiratory flow rate is more sensitive than auscultation, pulsus paradoxus, or other physical signs in gauging severity of obstruction and response to therapy. Children at 4–5 years of age can successfully use hand-held peak flow meters. Fig 42–6 provides normal expiratory flow rates for different heights. Comparison of presenting expiratory flow rate with known baseline values is especially helpful. Arterial blood gas measurements and chest x-ray are necessary in severe cases.

B. Treatment: See Fig 42–7.

1. Use continuous undiluted beta-adrenergic agents (usually 0.5% albuterol) for the moderate to severe asthmatic.

2. For the mild asthmatic, give albuterol nebulizer therapy, 0.1 mg/kg/dose of 0.5% solution (0.02 mL/kg/dose) by mask every 1–2 hours. Metered dose inhalers—in combination with spacer devices and with masks for infants—are probably as effective as oxygen-powered nebulizers for most asthma cases, even for children as young as 6 months.

3. For the child who cannot accept the albuterol nebulizer by mask, administer subcutaneous epinephrine, 0.01 mg/kg/dose of 1:1000 solution (0.01 mL/kg/dose).

4. In the child who does not respond to beta agonists or epinephrine, try inhaled anticholinergics (nebulized atropine, 2 mg of 0.1% solution). Ipratrop-

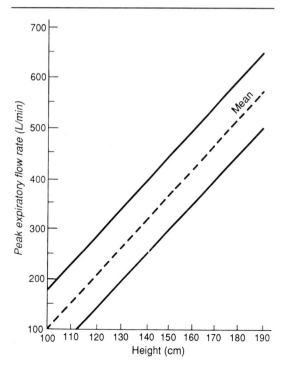

Figure 42–6. Nomogram for normal peak expiratory flow rates. (Modified and reproduced, with permission, from Godfrey S, Kamburoff PL, Nairn JR: Spirometry, using volumes and airway resistance in normal children aged 5 to 18 years. Br J Dis Chest 1970;64:15.)

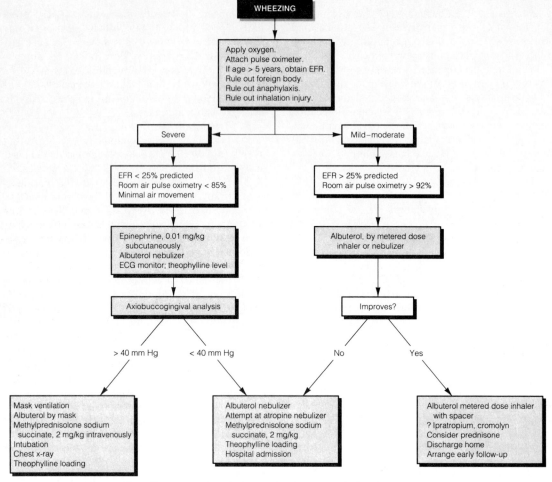

Figure 42–7. Treatment algorithm for pediatric asthma. EFR = Expiratory flow rate.

ium, 1–3 metered doses, in hospital or as home therapy is helpful in such cases, but it has a delayed onset of action and therefore has little role in the emergency department.

5. Theophylline compounds have a more limited place in emergency department management of mild to moderate asthma than previously believed. Intravenous theophylline loading is best reserved for the severely distressed child (eg, expiratory flow rate < 25% predicted for age) or for the child not responding to frequent albuterol and anticholinergic inhalation treatments.

6. When theophylline is prescribed in the emergency department, dosing must be adjusted to reflect changes in metabolism of the drug by certain other agents. Phenobarbital, phenytoin, and rifampin increase theophylline metabolism, whereas erythromycin and cimetidine decrease it.

7. Administer methylprednisolone, 1–2 mg/kg/dose intravenously or orally. Corticosteroid treatment must be initiated early in the moderately to severely distressed child, the individual who is already taking

corticosteroids, or one who has required prior intubation or hospital admission for asthma.

Pneumonia

A. Diagnosis: Pneumonia presents with symptoms of cough and dyspnea, with or without fever. Abdominal pain may be the presenting complaint. There are usually some signs of respiratory distress, including wheezing, rales, rhonchi, or focal absence of breath sounds. Physical evaluation may be nonspecific. Tachypnea and respiratory distress may be present with a clear chest on auscultation or with discrete rales in affected lung segments. Chest x-rays show lobar or peribronchial parahilar patterns of infiltration, sometimes with pleural effusion.

Pediatric pneumonia can be caused by bacteria, viruses, *Mycoplasma,* mycobacteria, or *Chlamydia* (Table 42–13). Certain clinical or laboratory features suggest specific causes: high fever, appearance of illness, significant leukocytosis, and pleural effusion suggest bacteria; afebrile pneumonia with eosinophilia in infancy suggests *Chlamydia;* extreme lym-

Table 42–13. Causes of pneumonia by age.[1]

Age	Infecting Organism

2 weeks	Bacteria
	  Group B streptococcus
	  Gram-negative bacilli
	Viruses

2 weeks to 2 months	*Chlamydia*
	Viruses
	Bacteria
	  S pneumoniae
	  S aureus
	  H influenzae

2 months to 3 years	Viruses
	Bacteria
	  S pneumoniae
	  H influenzae
	  S aureus

3 years to 12 years	Viruses
	Bacteria
	  S pneumoniae
	  M pneumoniae

13 years to 19 years	M pneumoniae Viruses Bacteria S pneumoniae

[1]Reproduced, with permission, from Fleisher G: Infectious disease emergencies. Page 439 in: *Textbook of Pediatric Emergency Medicine*, 2nd ed. Fleisher G. Williams & Wilkins, 1988.

phocytosis in an unimmunized infant with whooping cough suggests pertussis; hilar adenopathy and upper lobe infiltration suggest primary tuberculosis. In younger children, rapid diagnostic testing for respiratory syncytial virus (by immunofluorescent and ELISA antigen techniques performed on nasal or conjunctival specimens) may provide the cause. In older children, sputum Gram staining may guide initial therapy.

B. Treatment: Rapid evaluation of respiratory status, in combination with pulse oximetry and occasionally arterial blood gas determination, will direct the immediate therapy. Patients with documented pneumonia require hospital admission if they are young (< 3 months of age); have preexisting pulmonary disease, probable primary tuberculosis, or significant pleural effusion; are ill-appearing; or have significant respiratory distress.

1. Provide supplemental oxygen, and attach pulse oximeter.

2. Evaluate degree of respiratory distress. Significant respiratory distress is best defined by pulse oximetry < 92% on room air or by an alveolar-arterial oxygen gradient > 35. A rapid determination of the alveolar-arterial oxygen gradient at sea level = 145 − $(PO_2 + PCO_2)$.

3. Consider the probable cause. Obtain a chest x-ray, CBC, sputum Gram staining and culture, and possibly respiratory syncytial virus studies.

4. Administer antimicrobial therapy for the likely pathogen:

a. Immediately administer intravenous cefotaxime, 50 mg/kg/dose every 8 hours, for infants less than 12 months old.

b. Administer cefotaxime or ampicillin, 150 mg/kg/d intravenously in 3 divided doses, for the older child. Nafcillin, 100 mg/kg/d intravenously in 4 divided doses, may be needed for possible staphylococcal disease or failure to respond to cefotaxime or ampicillin alone.

c. In severely distressed children with positive antigen studies for respiratory syncytial virus, ribavirin, a specific antiviral agent, may be indicated if appropriate isolation and staff protection techniques are available in the hospital.

d. Arrange for in-hospital multiple drug therapy with isoniazid, rifampin, and pyrazinamide for children with clinical and epidemiologic evidence of primary pulmonary tuberculosis.

5. Most children do not require hospitalization and can be discharged home, with appropriate follow-up, on the following agents:

a. Prescribe erythromycin, 50 mg/kg/d orally in divided doses every 6 hours for 10 days, for infants 4–12 weeks of age with a picture of *Chlamydia* pneumonia.

b. Prescribe oral amoxicillin, 30–50 mg/kg/d in 3 divided doses, or amoxicillin-clavulanate, for children 3 months old to school age.

c. Prescribe erythromycin, 30–50 mg/kg/d orally in divided doses, for school-aged children with mild disease.

d. Apply an intradermal PPD test and arrange 48 hour follow-up.

NEUROLOGIC EMERGENCY

Objective neurologic evaluation of the emergency department patient involves recognition of age-appropriate differences in cognitive function. For patients with altered mental status, an objective scale, such as the pediatric Glasgow Coma Scale (Table 42–14) will help reduce interobserver differences in assessment and provide a measure for comparison during serial examinations.

SEIZURES

Seizures are common pediatric emergencies in both the prehospital environment and the emergency department. Approximately 5% of all children have one or more seizures before 16 years of age. Epilepsy is a chronic condition of recurrent seizures that develops in only a small portion of patients who have sin-

Table 42–14. Pediatric Glasgow Coma scale.[1]

	Eyes Opening	
Score	> 1 Year	< 1 Year
4	Spontaneously	Spontaneously
3	To verbal command	To shout
2	To pain	To pain
1	No response	No response
	Best Motor Response	
	> 1 Year	< 1 Year
6	Obeys	Spontaneous
5	Localizes pain	Localizes pain
4	Flexion-withdrawal	Flexion-withdrawal
3	Flexion-abnormal (decorticate rigidity)	Flexion-abnormal (decorticate rigidity)
2	Extension (decerebrate rigidity)	Extension (decerebrate rigidity)
1	No response	No response
	Best Verbal Response	
	> 5 Years	2–5 Years	0–23 Months
5	Oriented and converses	Appropriate words and phrases	Smiles, coos appropriately
4	Disoriented and converses	Inappropriate words	Cries, consolable
3	Inappropriate words	Persistent cries or screams	Persistent inappropriate crying or screaming
2	Incomprehensible sounds	Grunts	Grunts, agitated/restless
1	No response	No response	No response

Total 3–15

[1]Reproduced, with permission, from Jennett B, Teasdale G: Aspects of coma after severe head injury. *Lancet* 1977;1:878.

gle seizures. Most seizures in childhood are single, generalized tonic-clonic events lasting a few minutes. Seizures may be generalized or focal (Table 42–15). **Status epilepticus** is defined as continuous seizure activity for 30 minutes or as recurrent seizures without intervening return of consciousness. Seizures may be generalized or focal, or focal with secondary generalization. Focal status epilepticus may present with or without preserved consciousness. Status epilepticus is often the first presentation of seizures in childhood.

The causes of seizures and status epilepticus in children are multiple and age-dependent. Children under 3 years of age presenting with status epilepticus are most likely to have serious conditions, eg, central nervous system infections or vascular disorders, anoxia, trauma, intoxications, or metabolic abnormalities. Many of these conditions are treatable. In older children, however, status epilepticus is usually the result of chronic epilepsy with noncompliance for anticonvulsive medications, chronic progressive encephalopathy, or idiopathic encephalopathy. *The likelihood of serious underlying disease in a child presenting with status epilepticus is inversely correlated with age.*

Febrile seizures are also common in childhood.

Table 42–15. International classification of seizures.[1]

Partial seizures
  Simple partial (consciousness retained)
    Motor
    Sensory
    Autonomic
    Psychic
  Complex partial (consciousness impaired)
    Simple partial, followed by impaired consciousness
    Consciousness impaired at onset
  Partial seizures with secondary generalization
Generalized seizures
  Absences
    Typical
    Atypical
  Generalized tonic-clonic
  Tonic
  Clonic
  Myoclonic
  Atonic
Unclassified seizures

[1]Reproduced, with permission, from: Dreifuss FE et al: Proposal for revised clinical and EEG classification of epileptic seizures. *Epilepsia* 1981;22:489.

The peak age is between 8 and 20 months, although they may occur in children from approximately 6 months to 6 years of age. Often, underlying diseases are simply upper respiratory tract infections or gastroenteritis. Febrile seizures may be simple or complex. A simple febrile seizure typically occurs as a generalized self-limited tonic/clonic seizure of several minutes' duration. Complex febrile seizure denotes a seizure with high-risk features, including focal onset, postictal neurologic abnormalities, or duration greater than 15 minutes. Other high-risk features include prior neurologic or developmental abnormalities or a history of epilepsy in the nuclear family. The simple febrile seizure is usually benign and requires no therapy; however, children presenting with high-risk features are at greater risk for recurrent afebrile features. Furthermore, the child under 1 year of age at the time of the first febrile seizure may be a candidate for ongoing anticonvulsant therapy. When chronic anticonvulsant therapy is deemed appropriate, this decision should ordinarily include consultation and follow-up with the primary physician.

Many children will present in the postictal state. In such patients, search for a specific cause. Obtain a history from the parents beginning with a precise description of the seizure itself, including the nature of onset (focal or generalized), duration, and quality of motor feature. Exclude syncope, hysteria, breath-holding, and night terrors. Other confusional states that may be difficult to distinguish from seizures include migraine headache, hereditary chin trembling, familial choreoathetosis, and narcolepsy. Also exclude head trauma and alcohol or drug intoxication. Certain drugs are well associated with seizure activity. They are cyclic antidepressants, sympathomimetics (cocaine, amphetamine, phencyclidine), theophylline, isoniazid, phenothiazines, camphor, anticholinergics, antihistamines, and lindane. Physical examination should specifically exclude head trauma, bulging fontanelle, papilledema, meningeal irritation, focal neurologic signs, cutaneous lesions, and systemic disease.

Treatment

A well-organized approach to seizure management minimizes the complications of the acute electrical and metabolic derangements and averts iatrogenic complications. Ensure adequate ventilation and oxygenation in the patient with active seizures, then address termination of the seizure and reversal of metabolic imbalances. Finally, attempt to establish the cause in order to implement specific therapy.

A. General:

1. Open the airway, and use suction to clear secretions or foreign bodies, then administer oxygen. Ordinarily, reserve intubation until there is failure of medical management.

2. Protect the child from injury by manually holding the head. Remove tight-fitting clothing.

3. Establish intravenous access, and draw blood for immediate bedside glucose determination and other appropriate laboratory investigations, including CBC; glucose, lead, calcium, and magnesium levels; liver and renal function; and electrolytes, ammonia, and pertinent drug levels. Send urine for toxicologic screening.

4. If rapid bedside glucose determination is less than 90 mg/dL, administer 25% dextrose in water, 2 mL/kg/dose slowly intravenously. In children over 3 years of age, give 50% dextrose in water at 1 mL/kg.

5. Administer naloxone, 2 mg intravenously.

6. If child is febrile, administer rectal acetaminophen, 10–15 mg/kg. If fever fails to respond to acetaminophen, use tepid water baths to reduce temperature.

B. Specific: If seizures continue after first-line supportive care, consider immediate anticonvulsant therapy (Table 42–16). Duration of seizure activity may be related to ultimate neurologic outcome, particularly in patients with severe underlying disease.

1. Alternatives to intravenous diazepam include rectal diazepam, 0.5 mg/kg administered by lubricated tuberculin syringe approximately 5 cm into the rectum, or intramuscular lorazepam, 0.1 mg/kg.

2. Phenytoin or phenobarbital may be also be given intraosseously.

INFECTIOUS DISEASES

FEVER

The evaluation of febrile children is a common problem for the emergency physician. While most of these children will have benign, self-limited viral infections, a few will have invasive disease with bacterial pathogens that may cause significant illness and even death. The ability to identify those children at increased risk for serious disease is the key to management. Because young children are at increased risk for more serious disease, the age of the child frequently determines the extent of the evaluation.

1. FEVER IN INFANTS

General Considerations

Management of fever in the infant under 3 months of age is complicated and controversial. Signs of disease at this age are frequently subtle and nonspecific, and there are multiple sources of infection. Relative to older infants, these infants uncommonly have febrile disease, and when present, it more likely reflects a serious invasive infection. Causes of fever at this

Table 42–16. Drug therapy of status epilepticus in children.[1]

Drug	Dose	Route of Administration[2]	Rate	Complications/Comments
First-Line Agents				
Oxygen	100%	Nasal cannula, mask, ET	Maximum	None with brief use. Clear airway with suction. Use pulse oximetry to evaluate hypoxia.
Dextrose	Children: $D_{50}W$ at 1 mL/kg. Infants: $D_{25}W$ at 2 mL/kg.	IV, IO	Bolus	Hyperosmolality. Use only if blood glucose test strip is < 90 mg/dL. Avoid IO route if possible.
Naloxone	Children: 2 mg. Infants: 0.4 mg.	IV, IM, IO, ET	Bolus	None.
Pyridoxine	Infants: 100 mg.	IV	Bolus	None. Use in neonates with simultaneous EEG if possible.
Diazepam *or* Lorazepam	IV/IO: 0.1–0.3 mg/kg. PR: 0.2–0.5 mg/kg.	IV, IO, PR	1 mg/min Bolus	Respiratory arrest and hypotension. Avoid in neonates.
	IV/IM/SL: 0.1 mg/kg.	IV, IM, SL, PR	Bolus	Respiratory arrest, hypotension, sedation.
Phenytoin	20 mg/kg. Repeat 20 mg/kg to total of 40 mg/kg.	IV, IO	Children: 1 mg/kg/min Infants: 0.5 mg/kg/min	Heart block, bradycardia, hypotension.
Second-Line Agents				
Phenobarbital	20 mg/kg.	IV, IM, IO	1–2 mg/kg/min	Respiratory arrest, hypotension.
Third-Line Agents				
Lidocaine	1 mg/kg.	IV, IO	Bolus, then 20–50 µg/kg/min	Respiratory depression, bradycardia, hypotension.
Pentobarbital	15 mg/kg/h over 1 hour followed with 1–2 mg/kg/h.	IV	Bolus, then 1–2 mg/kg/h	Respiratory arrest, hypotension. Dose must attain EEG burst suppression. Patient must be intubated in intensive care unit.

[1]Reproduced, with permission, from Dieckmann RA: Seizures in childhood. Page 1254 in: *Current Practice of Emergency Medicine*, 2nd ed. Callaham ML. Decker, 1991.

[2]ET = endotracheal; IM = intramuscular; IO = intraosseous; IV = intravenous; PR = rectal; SL = sublingual.

age include (**1**) infections inquired in the household; (**2**) late onset of disease acquired in the nursery, at delivery, or in utero; and (**3**) infections secondary to anatomic or physiologic abnormalities.

Household-acquired infections are the most likely cause of fever in this age group, particularly with an uncomplicated prenatal and delivery history. Respiratory and gastrointestinal infections are most common. The incidence of invasive disease caused by *H influenzae* and *Streptococcus pneumoniae* is significant in the first 2 months of life. Other causes include the late onset of signs of congenital infection, such as rubella, cytomegalovirus, or syphilis. In addition, the delayed onset of infection acquired at delivery, eg, group B streptococcus and *Listeria*, are important infections in this age group. Disease acquired in the nursery before discharge, eg, *S aureus*, may also become manifest during this time. Additionally, infections associated with an underlying anatomic abnormality, particularly those of the urinary tract, are potential sources of infection.

The younger the infant, the greater is the risk of disease. The incidence of bacteremia in febrile infants under 1 month of age is approximately 7–8% and in infants 1–2 months of age, approximately 3–4%. In infants under 3 months of age with temperatures over 40 °C, the incidence of serious disease may be as high as 30–40%.

Diagnosis

Evaluation includes a careful history of the pregnancy, delivery, and nursery course of the infant. Inquire about household infections. Look for general signs of illness, including lethargy and irritability. Otitis media is not uncommon in infants under 2 months of age. Other clues to the source of fever are (**1**) congenital infection (rash, jaundice, hepatosplenomegaly, macrocephaly); (**2**) urinary tract infection (direct hyperbilirubinemia); (**3**) group B streptococcus (pseudoparalysis, cellulitis, meningitis); and (**4**) *Listeria* (meningitis).

The laboratory evaluation of febrile infants under 2 months of age includes the following:

A. CBC and Blood Culture: A white blood cell count < 5000 or > 15,000 increases the probability of sepsis.

B. Peripheral Blood Smear: Toxic granulation and vacuolization of white cells are sensitive indicators for invasive bacterial disease.

C. Lumbar Puncture: Both bacterial and aseptic meningitis may be serious in febrile infants under 2 months of age.

D. Urine Culture: A bagged specimen is not adequate because of the high incidence of contamination. Suprapubic aspiration and bladder catheterization are the preferred methods of obtaining urine.

E. Chest X-ray: Pneumonia may be present even in infants without cough, tachypnea, or rales.

F. Antigen Detection: Send cerebrospinal fluid for counterimmunoelectrophoresis or latex agglutination for group B streptococcus, *H influenzae, S pneumoniae, Neisseria meningitidis.*

Treatment
(See Fig 42–8.)

A. Management must be conservative. If evalua-

tion discloses a local infection, eg, meningitis, pneumonia, or urinary tract infection, hospitalize the infant, and promptly institute intravenous antibiotic therapy.

1. For infants 0–4 weeks of age, if the suspected etiologic organism is group B streptococcus, *Listeria,* or *E coli,* give ampicillin, 100–200 mg/kg/d intravenously in 4 divided doses, and gentamicin, 3–7.5 mg/kg/d intravenously in 3 divided doses.

2. For infants 4–8 weeks of age, if the suspected etiologic organism is group B streptococcus, *Listeria, H influenzae,* or *S pneumoniae,* give ampicillin, 100–200 mg/kg/d intravenously in 4 divided doses, and ceftriaxone, 50–100 mg/kg/d intravenously in 1–2 di-

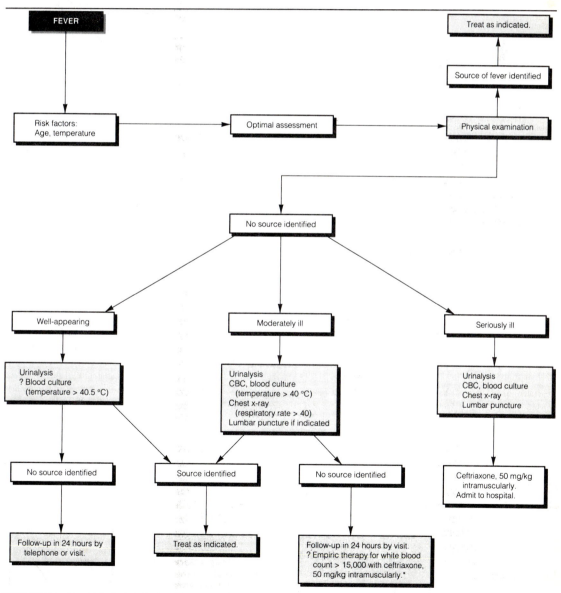

*Blood culture must be obtained prior to treatment.

Figure 42–8. Algorithm for management of febrile children 2–24 months of age.

vided doses, or cefotaxime, 100–200 mg/kg/d intravenously in 3–4 divided doses.

3. The cephalosporins are not active against *Listeria* and thus are not recommended as the sole treatment for presumed sepsis in infants under 8 weeks of age. If there is concern about *S aureus,* ampicillin should be replaced with a penicillinase-resistant antibiotic such as nafcillin, 150 mg/kg/d intravenously in 4 divided doses.

B. The infant with otitis media who clinically appears well may be discharged on antibiotics, with careful follow-up.

C. If there is no focal infection, hospitalize the infant and treat empirically while awaiting culture results. If the infant is older than 6 weeks of age, looks clinically well, and has a completely normal laboratory and radiographic evaluation, and if the physician is comfortable with the parent's ability to watch the child and to return in 12–24 hours, outpatient management without antibiotics may be acceptable.

2. FEVER IN CHILDREN

General Considerations

Fever in the child 2 months to 2 years of age is the chief complaint in almost 20% of all pediatric emergency department visits. The febrile child from 2–24 months of age presents several dilemmas. These children are often not immunologically competent against common encapsulated pathogens *(H influenzae* and *S pneumoniae)* and thus are at increased risk for occult invasive bacterial diseases (eg, pneumonia, urinary tract infection, meningitis, occult bacteremia). Invasive bacterial disease may present as an undifferentiated febrile illness.

Diagnosis

Pneumonia may present in young children without auscultatory findings in the chest, the only clues being a history of cough with fever and tachypnea on physical examination. Urinary tract infections are occult infections in young children because dysuria and urinary frequency are not clinically apparent in this age group. While meningitis may present as a significantly obtunded child, initially children show only high fever and irritability.

Occult bacteremia is the presence of bacteremia in a young child who is only moderately ill-appearing. Risk factors appear to be age of the child and height of the fever at presentation. The incidence is greatest between 2 and 24 months of age. Approximately 6% of children presenting to an emergency department with temperatures over 38.5 °C have bacteremia. The likelihood of bacteremia increases with increasing fever and may exceed 10% in children with temperatures over 40 °C. *S pneumoniae* and *H influenzae* are the commonest pathogens. A white blood cell count of greater than 15,000 is a sensitive test for identify-

ing bacteremic febrile children, but it lacks specificity. Almost 90% of children with occult bacteremia recover spontaneously. The remaining 10% develop a focus of infection (eg, cellulitis, meningitis) usually within 24–48 hours of initial presentation.

Treatment

A. Evaluate the child before administering acetaminophen and then again after the temperature has been lowered. Acetaminophen is equally effective in lowering the temperature in both bacteremic and nonbacteremic febrile children. However, the child with meningitis is more likely not to be clinically improved after the use of antipyretics. If the examination discloses a source of infection, appropriate laboratory work and treatment can be initiated.

B. A recognizable viral syndrome (eg, herpetic gingivostomatitis, hand-foot-and-mouth disease) can qualify as a "source" of a high fever in a child and may require no further ancillary studies. If a virus is suspected, treat the child symptomatically with oral fluids and antipyretics, and follow-up by telephone contact or reexamine within 24 hours.

C. If blood cultures become positive (usually an encapsulated organism; rarely, *Salmonella* or *N meningitidis*), admit the child to the hospital for intravenous therapy regardless of the clinical appearance on return visit.

D. The use of empiric antibiotic therapy in febrile children under 24 months of age with a white blood count greater than 15,000 is controversial. No prospective study has documented efficacy in improving outcome. Consider antibiotic therapy in such patients with ceftriaxone, 50 mg/kg intramuscularly. Alternative therapies include oral amoxicillin or amoxicillin/clavulanate. Obtain a blood culture before giving antibiotics, and ensure close follow-up. Complications of bacteremia usually become apparent within 48 hours, prior to the results of a blood culture. Thus, the moderately ill child should be rechecked within 24 hours.

E. The young febrile child appearing seriously ill requires aggressive diagnostic evaluation and prompt institution of parenteral antibiotic therapy. Obtain cultures of blood, urine, and cerebrospinal fluid, and begin antibiotics. If physical examination or laboratory evaluation does not disclose a source of infection, use a second- or third-generation cephalosporin intravenously (eg, cefuroxime, ceftriaxone). Regardless of whether a source of infection is found, hospitalize seriously ill febrile children for continued antibiotic therapy and observation.

MENINGITIS

General Considerations

Meningitis is an infection of the central nervous system that is characterized by fever, alteration in the level of consciousness, and in some instances a stiff neck. Acute bacterial meningitis is of particular concern to the emergency physician because failure to make a prompt diagnosis and institute antibiotic treatment may result in significant illness and possibly death.

Meningitis occurs following invasion of the subarachnoid space by a pathogenic organism. In children, this occurs most commonly by hematogenous spread but may also occur by direct extension from a contiguous focus of infection such as sinusitis or mastoiditis. Disruption of the normal anatomic barriers to the cerebrospinal fluid secondary to a basilar skull fracture or a congenital sinus tract may also result in infection. Acute meningitis is usually of viral or bacterial origin (Table 42–17). The onset of meningitis in children usually follows one of 2 patterns: **(1)** The illness develops over several days as a nonspecific febrile illness. **(2)** Signs of central nervous infection develop over hours.

Diagnosis

In infants, the clinical findings may be nonspecific: restlessness, irritability, poor feeding, emesis, diarrhea, lethargy, decreased tone, respiratory distress, full fontanelle (late finding), and seizures. Obvious neck stiffness or other signs of meningeal irritation, eg, Kernig's or Brudzinski's signs, are not reliably present in infants under 18 months of age. In children over 18 months of age, headache, nausea, vomiting, signs of increased intracranial pressure, focal neurologic signs, fever, lethargy, and photophobia are common.

The diagnosis is established by evaluation of the cerebrospinal fluid by lumbar puncture. Contraindications to performing a lumbar puncture in children with suspected meningitis include **(1)** hemodynamic instability (child in shock or having respiratory difficulties); **(2)** evidence of mass lesion or increased intracranial pressure, eg, focal neurologic signs (hemiparesis, facial palsy, gaze preference), altered pupillary reactions, bradycardia, hypotension, apnea, posturing; **(3)** a bleeding disorder; **(4)** infection overlying the lumbar puncture site (eg, cellulitis). If a contraindication exists in a patient with clinical suspicion of meningitis, *give intravenous antibiotics immediately.* The lumbar puncture may be performed when the child is stabilized or when the contraindication has resolved.

Diagnostic studies include the following:

A. Cerebrospinal fluid analysis, including cell count, Gram staining, protein and glucose determinations, and culture (Table 42–18). The cell count in the cerebrospinal fluid should be performed quickly because delay over 90 minutes will result in lysis of white blood cells.

B. Peripheral white blood cell count and serum glucose determination. Ideally, these should be done before the lumbar puncture, since both will increase during a lumbar puncture. It takes approximately 30 minutes for serum glucose to equilibrate with spinal fluid.

C. Blood culture.

D. Serum electrolytes. The syndrome of inappropriate secretion of antidiuretic hormone (SIADH) is not uncommon in acute meningitis, with resulting hyponatremia and volume overload.

E. CT scan. If a mass lesion or increased intracranial pressure is suspected, give antibiotics immediately and obtain an emergent CT scan.

Treatment

A. Assess the airway. In a child with significant central nervous system depression who has an impaired gag reflex or is hypoventilating, perform an elective orotracheal intubation.

B. Apply oxygen. Use 100% nonrebreather reservoir bag/mask if child is severely ill. Monitor with pulse oximeter.

C. Attach electrocardiographic monitor, and watch closely for bradycardia.

D. Initiate an intravenous line with 5% dextrose in half-normal saline in the child below 2 years of age and in normal saline for the child older than 2 years. After stabilization, change the intravenous solution to provide calculated fluid and electrolyte needs.

E. Assess the child's intravascular volume by means of blood pressure, heart rate, and capillary refill. Hypovolemia can compromise perfusion of the central nervous system. Aggressive rehydration is indicated if signs of hypovolemia are present. If the child is euvolemic, give fluids at two-thirds of the normal maintenance rate until serum electrolyte results have been obtained. If there is evidence of SIADH, continue the child at two-thirds of the maintenance rate. If no SIADH is present, increase intravenous fluids to the normal maintenance rate.

Table 42–17. Cause of meningitis by age group.

Age	Bacterial Cause	Other Cause
< 1 month	Group B streptococcus Listeria E coli	Enterovirus Candida albicans
1–3 months	Group B streptococcus Listeria E coli H influenzae S pneumoniae N meningitidis	Enterovirus
3 months to 6 years	H influenzae S pneumoniae N meningitidis	Enterovirus Mumps M tuberculosis Cryptococcus Coccidioidomycosis
Older child	S pneumoniae N meningitidis	Enterovirus Mumps M tuberculosis Cryptococcus Coccidioidomycosis

Table 42–18. Cerebrospinal fluid values in normal and disease states.[1]

Diagnosis	White Blood Cell Count (%PMN)	Glucose (% serum) (mg/dL)	Protein (mg/dL)	Gram's Stain	Intracranial Pressure (mm H$_2$O)
Normal	< 6 (0)	> 40 (> 50)	< 35	Negative	< 180
Bacterial meningitis	200–10,000 (80–100)	< 40 (< 50)	100–500	Positive	> 200
Partially treated	200–10,000 (40–100)	< 40 (< 50)	100–500	Positive or Negative	> 200
Viral	25–1000 (< 50)	> 40 (> 50)	50–100	Negative	< 180
Mycobacterial	50–1000 (< 50)	< 40	50–300	Negative	> 200

[1]Adapted from Tureen J: Meningitis. In: *Pediatric Emergency Medicine: A Clinician's Reference.* Grossman M, Dieckmann RA (editors). Lippincott, 1991.

F. Administer dexamethasone, 0.6 mg/kg/d in divided doses every 6 hours for 4 days. This drug decreases neurologic sequelae of bacterial meningitis in young children. Give the first dose when antibiotic therapy is started.

G. Administer antimicrobial therapy based on the child's age and the most likely pathogens (Table 42–19).

H. Treat seizures aggressively with anticonvulsants (Table 42–16).

Disposition

Children with proved or suspected bacterial meningitis require prompt hospitalization, ideally in an intensive care unit.

ACUTE OTITIS MEDIA

General Considerations

After viral upper respiratory infection, otitis media is the commonest infectious pediatric disease. It accounts for up to one-third of pediatric office visits and a high proportion of illness visits to the emergency department.

Acute otitis media results from auditory (eustachian) tube dysfunction, usually following an upper respiratory infection. In infants and children, *S pneumoniae* and *H influenzae* type b are the commonest pathogens. *Moraxella catarrhalis* and *Streptococcus pyogenes* are infrequent causes.

Diagnosis

The history is typically that of an infant or child who has had an upper respiratory infection for a few days and then presents with symptoms of ear pain. The pain of otitis media is typically acute in onset, severe, constant, and associated with hearing loss. Younger, preverbal children tend to have nonspecific symptoms of irritability, lethargy, gastrointestinal disturbances, and frequently poor sleeping. Children with acute otitis media may be afebrile or have only mild temperature elevation. High fever (> 40 °C) should alert the physician to the possibility of a more serious underlying infection, such as meningitis or pneumonia. Older children can accurately describe the source of their pain. Pus may rupture through the tympanic membrane, producing a purulent discharge and a prompt decrease in pain. Otoscopy reveals an opaque white tympanic membrane bulging outward and loss of visible ossicles. Erythema of the tympanic membrane is a common finding but is not nearly as sensitive as loss of normal tympanic membrane landmarks. Decreased movement of the tympanic membrane, demonstrable by pneumatic otoscopy, is sensitive and specific.

Occasionally, facial nerve paralysis develops acutely. Vertigo and sensorineural hearing loss may

Table 42–19. Empiric antibiotic therapy for meningitis.[1]

Age of Patient	Antibiotic	Dose (mg/kg/d)	Emergency Dose (mg/kg)
0–1 month	Ampicillin plus gentamicin	200 7.5	50 2.5
1–3 months	Ampicillin plus ceftriaxone or cefotaxime	200 100 200	50 50 50
3 months to 6 years	Ceftriaxone or Cefotaxime	100 200	50 50
6 years to adult	Penicillin G, benzathine	300,000 U	50,000 U

[1]Adapted from Tureen J: Meningitis. In: *Pediatric Emergency Medicine: A Clinician's Reference.* Grossman M, Dieckmann RA (editors). Lippincott, 1991.

occur if inflammation spreads to the inner ear and causes serous or purulent labyrinthitis. Mastoiditis occurs with infection of the bony structure of these air cells. The mastoid area becomes red, tender, and swollen. Typically the auricle is pushed laterally and downward.

No laboratory tests or x-rays are generally required. The bacteriology of otitis media has been clearly defined. Tympanocentesis is indicated only when unusual organisms may be present (eg, in neonates or immunosuppressed patients) or if acute otitis media is complicated by meningitis. If there is a clinical concern for mastoiditis, CT scan can detect small collections of fluid within the mastoid air cells as well as destruction of the bony septa.

Treatment

A. Begin antimicrobial therapy with amoxicillin, 45 mg/kg/d in divided doses every 8 hours (Table 42–20).

B. Consider alternative antibiotics if a child has been treated for acute otitis media with amoxicillin within the past month, the prevalence of beta-lactamase-producing organisms in the community is high, or the child is at risk for an unusual organism.

C. Treat uncomplicated otitis media for 10 days, and arrange for reevaluation.

D. Treat associated pain and fever with acetaminophen.

E. Hospitalize infants under 8 weeks of age with acute otitis media if fever is present or the infant appears ill. Perform full evaluation for sepsis and meningitis, and treat with intravenous antibiotics active against *S aureus* and gram-negative organisms, eg, cefuroxime, 100–150 mg/kg/d in divided doses every 8 hours.

F. If facial nerve paralysis accompanies acute otitis media, perform myringotomy, administer intravenous antibiotics, and hospitalize.

G. Treat mastoiditis like osteomyelitis. Perform myringotomy, culture, and Gram staining of middle ear fluid, and give antibiotics based on Gram staining. Drainage of the mastoid may be required.

Disposition

A. A repeat ear examination should be performed at the end of therapy.

B. Children should be reexamined if there is no clinical improvement in 48 hours.

PHARYNGITIS

General Considerations

Infections of the pharynx cause mucosal inflammation and ulceration, resulting in pain that is exacerbated by swallowing. The commonest causes of pharyngitis in children are viruses and group A streptococcus. Enteroviruses, particularly coxsackievirus, cause erythematous and vesicular lesions on the soft palate and pharynx. Other viruses associated with pharyngitis include adenovirus, influenza virus, parainfluenza virus, rhinovirus, Epstein-Barr virus, and respiratory syncytial virus. Bacteria other than group A streptococcus occasionally cause pharyngitis. *Corynebacterium diphtheriae* is now a rare cause of membranous pharyngitis in the USA. *Corynebacterium hemolyticum* has been associated with pharyngitis and erythematous rash in adolescents. Sexually active teenagers and victims of sexual abuse may have pharyngeal infection with *Neisseria gonorrhoeae*. *Mycoplasma pneumoniae* may also cause pharyngitis, but this is usually associated with more prominent lower respiratory tract infections. Acute uvulitis has been associated with *H influenzae* type B.

Diagnosis

Children under 3 years of age with tonsillar exudate usually have a viral infection. Children at this age with streptococcal respiratory infections are more likely to have chronic mucopurulent rhinitis with excoriation of nares, low-grade fever, and cervical adenopathy. Abdominal pain and headache are frequent findings in children with streptococcal pharyngitis and may distract the physician from the diagnosis.

Throat cultures remain the most practical and reliable means of diagnosing streptococcal pharyngitis.

Table 42–20. Dosage of antibiotics and activity against usual pathogens in acute otitis media.

Drug	Dosage	*Streptococcus pneumoniae*	*Haemophilus influenzae*	*Moraxella catarrhalis*	*Streptococcus pyogenes*
Amoxicillin	40 mg/kg/d	+	±	±	+
Trimethoprim-sulfamethoxazole	8 mg/kg/d twice daily	+	+	+	–
Erythromycin-sulfisoxazole	40 mg/kg/d 3 times daily	+	+	+	+
Amoxicillin-clavulanate	20 mg/kg/d 3 times daily	+	+	+	+
Cefaclor	40 mg/kg/d 3 times daily	+	+	±	+

± Inactive against strains producing beta-lactamase.

Rapid detection of streptococcal antigen from throat swabs is possible, but these assays lack the sensitivity of throat cultures. Throat cultures are not cost-effective in the following situations: (1) children < 3 years old; (2) children > 3 years old with copious rhinorrhea, cough, and conjunctivitis; (3) children with recognizable viral lesions of the oropharynx (eg, herpetic vesicles, enteroviral exanthem).

The white blood cell count may be elevated with streptococcal pharyngitis, but this is a nonspecific finding. White blood cell count may also be increased with Epstein-Barr virus infection, where the blood smear will show 10–20% atypical lymphocytes and a mononucleosis test (Monospot, many others) is positive. Children over 4 years old with infectious mononucleosis will develop heterophilic antibodies 1–2 weeks into the course of infection in 30% of cases. Heterophilic antibodies are less common in children under 4 years of age.

Tonsillar infections with group A streptococcus may extend into surrounding tissues and result in peritonsillar cellulitis or abscess; the child will usually present with fever, toxicity, muffled voice, tender superior cervical lymphadenopathy, trismus, and drooling. Peritonsillar abscess is commonly unilateral. Initially there is edema and erythema of the soft palate and tonsil and frequently but not invariably a whitish tonsillar exudate. Peritonsillar abscess is characterized by deviation of the tonsil and soft palate on the affected side medially, causing the uvula to point away from the side of the abscess. Retropharyngeal or lateral pharyngeal abscesses may also develop in concert with group A streptococcal pharyngitis and are often associated with stridor and signs similar to those of peritonsillar abscess.

Treatment

A. Use symptomatic therapy to decrease discomfort, including acetaminophen and salt water gargles.

B. Prescribe oral penicillin (or alternative) for suspected streptococcal pharyngitis. If antibiotic therapy is initiated within 7–9 days of onset of illness, acute rheumatic fever can be prevented.

1. Penicillin V, 40,000 U/kg/d orally in 2 or 3 divided doses for 10 days.

2. Erythromycin ethylsuccinate or estolate, 50 mg/kg/d orally in 2 or 3 divided doses for 10 days.

3. Benzathine penicillin G, 600,000 U (1 dose) intramuscularly in children weighing < 27 kg; 1,200,000 U intramuscularly (1 dose) in children weighing > 27 kg.

C. If streptococcal pharyngitis is likely, begin antibiotic therapy at the time of the examination. The duration of symptoms can be decreased if treatment is begun before culture results are available.

D. If the rapid antigen test is positive, begin treatment. A negative rapid antigen test, however, in a patient with strong clinical criteria, should be followed up with a throat culture.

E. If patient compliance is suspect or if the patient is vomiting oral medication, benzathine penicillin G in a single intramuscular dose (600,000 U < 27 kg; 1,200,000 U > 27 kg) is effective. The pain may be lessened if it is used in a mixture with procaine penicillin G. The total dose is still based on the amount benzathine penicillin G.

F. For children who are allergic to penicillin, erythromycin, 40 mg/kg in divided doses 4 times a day, is an effective alternative treatment. It has the additional benefit of efficacy against *M pneumoniae* and *C hemolyticum*.

G. Treat early stages of peritonsillar cellulitis on an outpatient basis with penicillin and follow-up. If the disease has progressed to deviation of the soft palate and uvula, hospitalize the child and initiate intravenous antibiotics with aqueous penicillin G, 250,000 units/kg/d in divided doses every 4 hours, after needle aspiration. Consult an ear, nose, and throat surgeon if the abscess cannot be easily aspirated and for consideration of definitive incision and drainage.

Disposition

A. A repeat examination is indicated if no improvement occurs in 48 hours. Particularly in older children and adolescents, a mononucleosis test should then be done.

B. Children with early signs of peritonsillar abscess must be reexamined in 12–24 hours.

PERIORBITAL CELLULITIS

Diagnosis

Periorbital swelling is a common problem in children. The primary task is to differentiate serious and life-threatening causes of this finding from those that are benign. Cellulitis restricted to the eyelid is preseptal or periorbital. If the infection involves orbital contents posterior to the septum, this is referred to as orbital cellulitis. Differentiation of these 2 entities is essential to management. Table 42–21 lists the differential considerations of periorbital swelling. Periorbital cellulitis can be classified as secondary to sinusitis (group I), secondary to disruption of local skin integrity (group II), or secondary to bacteremia with no apparent predisposing focus (group III).

A. **Group I:** Periorbital swelling from sinusitis is usually subacute in onset, evolves over several days, and is neither tender nor indurated. Fever is typically absent or low grade. This condition can occur at any age, but it is rare in infancy. X-rays show sinus opacification. Blood cultures are almost always negative. This is the commonest form of periorbital cellulitis and is caused by those organisms which commonly cause sinusitis (ie, nontypable *H influenzae*, *S pneumoniae*, *M catarrhalis*, *S pyogenes*).

B. **Group II:** Primary skin infection about the eye

Table 42–21. Differential diagnosis of periorbital swelling.[1]

Diagnosis	Onset	Appearance	Other Features
Periorbital and orbital cellulitis	Rapid	Reddish, violaceous	Usually unilateral Tender swelling with fever
Trauma	Variable	Reddish, blue	Tense or soft nontender Swelling not associated with fever
Insect bite	Variable	Red, no color	Bite may be visible
Allergic reaction	Rapid	No color	Bilateral, nontender, afebrile
Reactive edema	Days	No color	Unilateral or bilateral evidence of sinusitis

[1]Adapted, with permission, from Luten RC: Evaluation of periorbital swelling. In: *The Emergently Ill Child.* Barkin R (editor). Aspen Publishers, 1987.

may result from secondary infection or prior trauma or insect bite. There is rapid onset of tender and indurate preseptal swelling with fever. Blood cultures are typically negative. *S aureus* and group A streptococcus are the commonest pathogens.

C. Group III: Children with idiopathic periorbital cellulitis are generally younger than the previous 2 groups. These children have a history of a mild upper respiratory infection for 1–5 days followed by rapid onset of high fever and preseptal swelling. Swelling is often tender and indurated. Blood cultures are typically positive for *H influenzae* type B or *S pneumoniae*. Because these children are bacteremic, they are at risk for other foci of infection (eg, meningitis, arthritis).

Orbital cellulitis can be distinguished clinically from periorbital cellulitis by the presence of proptosis, ophthalmoplegia, pain on eye movement, and loss of vision. Patients are usually febrile; blood cultures are usually negative. Orbital cellulitis is usually secondary to extension of pus from sinusitis (usually ethmoidal) into the orbit or due to penetrating orbital trauma. The commonest bacterial organisms include *H influenzae, S pneumoniae, M catarrhalis, S aureus,* and anaerobes.

Laboratory findings include leukocytosis. Obtain blood cultures in children with periorbital swelling. Perform a lumbar puncture in ill-appearing children with acute onset of fever and periorbital swelling. Radiographic examination of the sinuses may be helpful to differentiate sinusitis. CT scan is the diagnostic test of choice when orbital cellulitis is suspected. CT scan will clearly define any orbital swelling, the presence of pus in the orbit, and infection in the perinasal sinuses. This information is essential to evaluate the need for surgical drainage.

Treatment

A. Hospitalize any child with periorbital swelling who is febrile and appears ill.

B. Begin intravenous antibiotic therapy. Treat young children whose periorbital cellulitis is not secondary to an external skin infection with cefuroxime, 100–150 mg/kg/d in divided doses every 8 hours.

C. In children whose infection is secondary to an external skin source, use nafcillin, 150 mg/kg/d in divided doses every 6 hours.

D. In a child with an orbital cellulitis secondary to direct extension from a contiguous sinus, use cefuroxime, 150 mg/kg/d in divided doses every 8 hours, and also cover for anaerobic bacteria with clindamycin, 25–40 mg/kg/d in divided doses every 6 hours. Consult an ophthalmologist whenever orbital cellulitis is suspected.

E. Consider ambulatory therapy in the child with early periorbital cellulitis who is afebrile and does not appear ill. Use ceftriaxone, 50 mg/kg intramuscularly, and repeat evaluation in 24 hours. If improvement has occurred, the child can be started on an oral antibiotic regimen such as amoxicillin/clavulanate, 20–40 mg/kg/d for 10 days. If contiguous skin infection is present, continue therapy in 24 hours with dicloxacillin, 50 m/kg/d in divided doses 4 times a day.

Disposition

A. Children with acute onset of fever, toxicity, and periorbital swelling should be promptly hospitalized for intravenous antibiotic therapy.

B. Children less acutely ill who are treated as outpatients should be reexamined in 12–24 hours.

URINARY TRACT INFECTION

General Considerations

Urinary tract infections are relatively common in children. Risk in the first 11 years of life for boys and girls is 1% and 3%, respectively. About 40% of these children will have recurrent infections. Many have vesicoureteral reflux, and some have urinary tract anomalies or renal scarring.

In children, *Escherichia coli* is the predominant pathogen (approximately 95% of initial infections and 80–90% of all infections). Other organisms causing urinary tract infections are *Klebsiella, Proteus mirabilis* (particularly in males), coagulase-negative staphylococci (in adolescent females), adenovirus (hemorrhagic cystitis), *Chlamydia trachomatis* (frequency-dysuria syndrome), and enterococci and *H influenzae* (uncommon). Children with congenital anomalies of the urinary tract are at increased risk for infection. Vesicoureteral reflux is present in 29–50% of children with urinary tract infection. Other abnormalities include obstruction at the level of the urethra, bladder, or ureter and duplication of the urinary tract and ureteroceles. In male infants, increased susceptibility to infection may be related to an uncircumcised penis.

In the first months of life, urinary tract infections are most common in males. By 4 months of age, however, urinary tract infections are 10 times more common in females, and this female predominance continues through childhood and adolescence. Approximately one-third of newborns with urinary tract infection are bacteremic. By 1–3 months of age, the incidence of bacteremia with urinary tract infection is decreased to 18% and by 3–8 months of age to 6%.

Diagnosis

In the neonate, nonspecific symptoms predominate. Poor feeding, irritability, fever, vomiting, diarrhea, and slow weight gain are common symptoms. The neonate may also develop a direct hyperbilirubinemia. In infants from 1 month to 2 years of age, nonspecific symptoms still predominate. Alert parents may note urinary frequency, dribbling, weak stream, and abdominal distress during voiding. Many young infants with urinary tract infection are febrile. In preschool and school-aged children, dysuria is a frequent symptom and may be accompanied by abdominal and flank pain, frequency, urgency, enuresis, and fever. Dysuria is a nonspecific symptom in children, however. Up to two-thirds of children with dysuria will have other causes than urinary tract infection, such as chemical urethritis from strong soaps, diaper rash, or pinworm. In adolescent females, dysuria and frequency are common with urinary tract infection but may also be secondary to vaginitis or the acute urethral syndrome.

The key to diagnosis is demonstration of bacteria in the urine. Methods of collecting urine in children include a urine bag taped to the perineum, clean-catch specimens, bladder catheterization, and suprapubic aspiration. The urine specimen collected by bag is helpful only if it proves to be negative. *Most positive cultures from urine bag specimens in infants and newborns represent contamination.* Febrile infants under 8 weeks of age who are likely to be admitted to the hospital should undergo either bladder catheterization or suprapubic aspiration. Older infants and children should undergo bladder catheterization if the bag urine specimen shows evidence of infection. Midstream clean-catch specimens are acceptable in children who can void on command.

Urine test strips employing a nitrite and leukocyte esterase indicator are helpful. Most urinary pathogens will convert nitrite to nitrate, and false-positive reactions are uncommon. However, false-negative results can occur with urinary pathogens unable to convert nitrite to nitrate (eg, *Staphylococcus saprophyticus,* enterococcus). Therefore, if the urine test strip is negative for nitrite and clinical findings or history suggest possible urinary infection, other tests are still indicated.

Urine collected by the clean-catch method is likely to be infected if there are > 10^4 colonies of a single organism. In urine collected by bladder catheterization or suprapubic aspiration, $\geq 10^3$ colonies of a single organism represents infection. Greater than 5 white blood cells per high-power field of urine sediment in a child who is symptomatic of urinary tract infection is highly suggestive. However, pyuria alone is not a reliable guide for identification of a urinary tract infection. *Any bacterium* present on Gram staining of unspun urine, when viewed under oil immersion, is a sensitive indicator of urinary tract infection.

Obtain a blood culture in neonates, infants, and any child who is highly febrile. Assume that children with fever, back pain, and costovertebral angle tenderness have pyelonephritis. As many as 25% of children, however, with urinary tract infections and no symptoms of pyelonephritis have upper tract disease. At present there is no effective noninvasive means to identify upper tract infections.

Treatment

A. In children who are to be treated as outpatients, use oral antibiotics effective against *E coli.*

1. Trimethoprim-sulfamethoxazole, 6 mg (trimethoprim), 30 mg (sulfamethoxazole)/kg/d.

2. Sulfisoxazole, 150 mg/kg/d.

3. Amoxicillin, 30 mg/kg/d.

4. Cephalexin, 25–50 mg/kg/d.

5. Cephradine, 25–50 mg/kg/d.

B. Hospitalize neonates and young infants with urinary tract infections, and give intravenous antibiotics on the presumption of pyelonephritis. Use ampicillin, 100–200 mg/kg/d in divided doses every 6 hours, and gentamycin, 3–7.5 mg/kg/d in divided doses every 8 hours.

C. Hospitalize any older child with urinary tract infection who is febrile and ill-appearing or who has clear signs of upper tract disease. Administer intravenous ampicillin and gentamicin in combination or a third-generation cephalosporin such as ceftriaxone, 100 mg/kg/d in divided doses every 12 hours.

D. Because of the frequency of urinary tract anomalies in children who have urinary tract infections, evaluation of the urinary tract by sonogram and voiding cystourethrogram are frequently indicated in boys of any age; girls under 3 years of age; and girls over 3 years of age with a history of abnormal voiding pattern, failure to thrive, hypertension, abnormal abdominal findings, clinical pyelonephritis, previous urinary tract infection, or failure to respond promptly to therapy. The sonogram can be done during the acute illness if necessary. Order a voiding cystourethrogram approximately 1 month after diagnosis. Postpubertal females with recurrent uncomplicated cystitis do not require imaging studies.

Disposition

A. Admit febrile children under 2 years of age with urinary tract infection to the hospital for intravenous antibiotic administration. Older children who are ill-appearing or have clinical signs of pyelonephritis should also be hospitalized.

B. Children treated as outpatients will require a repeat urine culture to document cure in 1 week. If there is no clinical improvement in 48 hours, prompt reevaluation is indicated.

GASTROENTERITIS

General Considerations

Diarrhea is a common reason for bringing a child to medical attention. Dehydration frequently complicates diarrhea in children, particularly in young infants who experience a greater net fluid and electrolyte loss. Acute diarrhea in children most commonly results from infectious gastroenteritis. Keys to management include identification of those children who will benefit from antimicrobial therapy, prevention or treatment of dehydration, and identification of those children with diarrhea secondary to other processes (eg, intussusception, hemolytic uremic syndrome). In the USA, rotavirus is the commonest cause of acute diarrhea, particularly in winter months.

Diagnosis

A. Symptoms and Signs: Information regarding the duration of diarrhea, number of stools per day, frequency of urination, presence of tears when crying, and most recent weight of the child are helpful in assessing the risk of dehydration. A history of frequent vomiting, particularly early in the course of the disease, is suggestive of a viral cause. High fever, lack of vomiting, abdominal pain with bowel movements, and the presence of gross blood and mucus in the stool suggest a bacterial cause. A history of recent antibiotic use suggests the possibility of pseudomembranous colitis. A history of recent travel suggests the possibility of a parasitic infection or traveler's diarrhea. Children in day care are particularly susceptible to infections with *Giardia lamblia.* Inquire about a common outbreak of symptoms in family members that may suggest food poisoning. Assess the state of hydration of the child and look for signs of appendicitis or intussusception.

B. Diagnostic Procedures:

1. A stool culture is the most reliable means of identifying a bacterial cause. It is not cost effective, however, to culture the stool of every child with diarrhea. Culture those children at highest risk for bacterial disease. The following children should have their stool cultured for *Shigella, Salmonella,* and *Campylobacter:*

a. Children presenting with obvious symptoms of acute bacterial dysentery, ie, fever, watery stool, fecal leukocytes, and gross blood in the stool.

b. Children who have abrupt onset of frequent stools without the initial vomiting common to viral gastroenteritis. A methylene blue slide examination for the presence of fecal leukocytes should be made of their stool. A positive result is a sensitive indicator of a bacterial pathogen. Trophozoites of *G lamblia* may also be identified.

c. Children with hemoglobinopathies and immunodeficiencies.

2. A peripheral white blood cell count may be helpful, since *Salmonella* and *Shigella* can cause leukocytosis. Some patients with *Shigella* infection may have a low white blood cell count with a marked shift to the left.

3. In any child appearing dehydrated, serum electrolytes, BUN, and creatinine should be checked.

4. Blood cultures are also indicated in young infants with bloody diarrhea and any child who appears significantly ill.

5. Children in day care or with a recent history of travel should have stool examined for parasites.

Treatment

A. The use of oral rehydration solutions for children with mild to moderate dehydration and of intravenous fluids for children with more severe dehydration is critical to prevent severe morbidity and mortality. Breastfeeding infants should continue to breast-feed while taking oral rehydration.

B. Antiemetic and antidiarrheal drugs occasionally worsen symptoms in children with gastroenteritis.

C. The empiric use of antibiotic therapy is indicated for obvious symptoms of bacterial dysentery. Trimethoprim-sulfamethoxazole (trimethoprim, 8–12 mg/kg; sulfamethoxazole, 30–60 mg/kg for 24 hours in divided doses every 12 hours) can be given empirically until culture results are available.

D. Hospitalize young infants who are febrile with bloody diarrhea. They are at increased risk for *Salmonella* bacteremia.

Disposition

A. Hospitalize children with moderate to severe dehydration, particularly if vomiting prohibits oral rehydration, and young infants with fever and bloody diarrhea.

B. Instruct parents about the signs of dehydration and the proper use of oral rehydration solutions.

C. Infants under 6 months of age should be followed up by telephone or be seen in 24 hours. Reevaluate older children if diarrhea persists longer than 3 days.

D. Children with bloody diarrhea should be reexamined in 24 hours.

SEPTIC ARTHRITIS

General Considerations

Septic arthritis is an acute bacterial infection of a joint. Delay in treatment may result in permanent damage and loss of function of the infected joint. Septic arthritis in children usually occurs through hematogenous seeding. It may also result from contiguous spread of osteomyelitis or through a penetrating injury. The bacterial cause is age-related (Table 42–22). Special clinical situations include **(1)** *N gonorrhoeae* joint infections in young children who have been sexually abused. **(2)** Patients with sickle cell disease are at high risk for joint infections with *Salmonella.*

Diagnosis

A. Symptoms and Signs: Almost all patients have fever and malaise. Typically the infected joint is hot, painful, and swollen and has overlying erythema. Early in the disease, the child may present with an unexplained limp. In young infants with hip involvement, the obvious findings of swelling and erythema may be absent. More commonly the infant will not move the leg on the infected side and will choose to keep the leg abducted and externally rotated. Movement of the hip causes pain.

B. Diagnostic Procedures:

1. Definitive diagnosis is established by aspiration of the joint. Joint fluid should be examined for cell count and differential, Gram staining and culture, protein and glucose determinations, and mucin clot. Gram staining of joint fluid is important, since up to 30% of joint aspirates may be sterile.

2. A complete blood count and erythrocyte sedimentation rate are helpful, particularly when considering noninfectious diagnoses.

3. Perform a blood culture, since it may produce a pathogen even with a negative joint aspirate culture.

4. Radiographic studies of the joint are of limited help in the older child with obvious joint infection. They usually demonstrate capsular swelling. Radiographic studies may be helpful in the evaluation of the hip, since the physical examination may not be definitive. Ultrasound may be able to identify small joint effusions.

5. Radionuclide studies may show diffuse uptake within the joint.

Treatment

A. Successful management depends on prompt antibiotic therapy and surgical drainage as indicated (Table 42–22). Gram staining may be helpful in guiding choice of antibiotics.

B. Septic arthritis of the hip is a surgical emergency, and these patients should undergo prompt surgical drainage.

C. Children with sickle cell disease should receive adequate therapy for *Salmonella* until culture results are known.

Disposition

A. Children with suspected septic arthritis should be hospitalized for intravenous antibiotic therapy.

B. Orthopedic consultation should be obtained to evaluate the need for surgical drainage of the involved joint.

ACUTE OSTEOMYELITIS

General Considerations

Acute osteomyelitis is a pyogenic infection of bone that occurs in about 1 in 5000 children before the age of 13 years. Although any bone may be involved, in children the long bones are more frequently infected. Infection usually is the result of seeding although spread from a contiguous focus or through direct traumatic inoculation can also occur.

Over 90% of cases of acute hematogenous osteomyelitis are caused by *S aureus.* Group A streptococci and *H influenzae* are less common causes. In neonates, osteomyelitis may also be caused by group B streptococci and gram-negative enteric organisms. Children with sickle cell disease are at risk for *Salmonella* osteomyelitis. Puncture wounds to the plantar surface of the foot may result in *Pseudomonas aeruginosa* osteomyelitis.

Diagnosis

A. Symptoms and Signs: The clinical hallmarks are fever and well-localized bone tenderness. Chills, malaise, and appearance of illness are frequently present. Lower extremity disease will frequently result in a limp. Point tenderness is usually evident on careful examination. There may also be swelling, warmth, redness, and focal induration at the site of infection. The young infant is usually irritable when the affected extremity is touched or moved.

Table 42–22. Causes and treatment of septic arthritis in infants and children.[1]

Age	Possible Pathogen	Therapy
0–2 months	Group B streptococcus, gram-negative rods	Ampicillin (100 mg/kg/d) plus gentamicin (7.5 mg/kg/d) *or* cefotaxime (100 mg/kg/d)
2 months to 4 years	*H influenzae, S aureus*	Nafcillin (100 mg/kg/d) plus cefotaxime (100 mg/kg/d)
> 4 years	*S aureus*	Nafcillin (100 mg/kg/d)

[1]Adapted, with permission, from Nurico S, Walker WA: Acute diarrhea. In: *Ambulatory Pediatric Care.* Dersheurtz RA (editor). Lippincott, 1980.

Pseudoparalysis is common, and occasionally significant swelling of the extremity will occur.

B. Diagnostic Procedures:

1. Draw blood for culture, CBC, and erythrocyte sedimentation rate. Blood cultures are positive in about 60% of patients with osteomyelitis.

2. Orthopedic consultation should be obtained concerning aspiration of bone at the site of tenderness, since there may be some risk of epiphyseal damage.

3. Obtain plain films of the affected extremity. Radiographic changes occur in 3 stages:

a. Soft tissue swelling around the metaphysis—0–3 days.

b. Swelling of the muscles and obliteration of the fat planes—3–7 days.

c. Bone destruction and periosteal new bone formation—10–21 days.

4. Once the child has been admitted to the hospital, technetium bone scans may be helpful.

Treatment

A. The mainstay of treatment of acute bacterial hematogenous osteomyelitis is parenteral antibiotics. Since culture results are usually not available when the diagnosis is first made, empiric therapy depends on the age of the patient (Table 42–23).

B. In children with puncture wound osteomyelitis of the foot, surgical debridement is an important part of therapy. Parenteral antibiotics active against *Pseudomonas* should be started.

Disposition

Hospitalize children in whom acute osteomyelitis is suspected.

EXANTHEMS
(See Table 42–24).

Important considerations are the age of the child, time of the year, knowledge of illnesses currently present in the community, history of exposure to individuals with rashes, medication history, prodromal symptoms such as fever, and initial appearance and progression of the rash. The physician should note how ill the child appears, the morphology and distri-

Table 42–23. Empiric antibiotic therapy for osteomyelitis.

Age	Possible Pathogen	Therapy
0–2 months	Group B streptococcus, gram-negative rods	Ampicillin (200 mg/kg/d) plus gentamicin (7.5 mg/kg/d)
2 months to 4 years	S aureus, H influenzae	Nafcillin (200 mg/kg/d) plus cefotaxime (100 mg/kg/d)
> 4 years	S aureus, group A streptococcus	Nafcillin (100 mg/kg/d)

bution of the rash, mucous membrane involvement, associated lymphadenopathy, and presence of hepatosplenomegaly.

GASTROINTESTINAL DISORDERS

ABDOMINAL PAIN

General Considerations

Abdominal pain is a common complaint. Causes are many and include both intra-abdominal and systemic illnesses. The child presenting with acute severe abdominal pain may have an acute abdomen requiring immediate surgical intervention. Recognition of the acute abdomen in children may be difficult but is critical in reducing morbidity and mortality.

Abdominal pain can originate from 3 neural pathways. **Visceral pain** originates from distention of a viscus, which stimulates nerves locally that send impulses to the central nervous system through autonomic parasympathetic fibers. Because these nerve fibers from different organs overlap, visceral pain is not specific to the site of the viscus involved. **Somatic pain** is generally intense and well localized. It arises from irritation of the parietal perineum. Frequently there is abdominal muscle reflex spasm over the site of pain. **Referred pain** is somatic or visceral in origin but is felt elsewhere.

Common causes of abdominal pain in infants are colic, constipation, gastroenteritis, intussusception, viral syndrome, and volvulus; in younger children, appendicitis, constipation, gastroenteritis, pneumonia, streptococcal pharyngitis, urinary tract infection, and viral syndrome; and in school-aged children, appendicitis, pregnancy, gastroenteritis, pneumonia, peptic ulcer, and pelvic inflammatory disease.

Diagnosis
(See Table 42–25.)

A. Symptoms and Signs: Note the nature of the pain, including time of onset, duration, severity, and location; associated gastrointestinal symptoms, including anorexia, vomiting, diarrhea, and constipation; associated systemic symptoms, including fever, cough, sore throat, dysuria, rash, and joint pain; and history of significant disease, particularly sickle cell disease, renal disease, and gynecologic disorders (for adolescents).

Obtain accurate vital signs. Observe the child over a period of time. Children with colicky pain may appear quiet and even lethargic and then suddenly develop crampy pain. Perform a complete physical examination, and assess the child's state of hydration and perfusion. Group A streptococcal pharyngitis and

Table 42–24. Exanthems.[1]

Disease (Etiology)	Usual Age	Season	Prodrome	Morphology
Measles (rubeola virus)	Infants to young adults	Winter/spring	High fever, symptoms of upper respiratory infection, conjunctivitis	Erythematous macules and papules, become confluent
Rubella (rubella virus)	Adolescents/young adults	Spring	Absent or low-grade fever, malaise	Rose pink papules, not confluent
Erythema infectiosum (parvovirus B19)	5–15 years	Winter/spring	Usually none	Slapped cheeks; reticular erythema or maculopapular
Enteroviral exanthems (coxsackie, echovirus, other enteroviruses)	Young children	Summer/fall	Fever (occasional)	Extremely variable; maculopapular, petechial, purpuric, vesicular
Hand-foot-mouth syndrome (several coxsackieviruses)	Children	Summer/fall	Fever (occasional), sore mouth	Grey-white vesicles 3–7 mm on normal or erythematous base
Adenovirus exanthems (adenoviruses)	5 months to 5 years	Winter/spring	Fever, symptoms of upper respiratory infection	Rubellaform, morbilliform, roseolalike
Chickenpox (varicellazoster virus)	1–14 years	Late fall/ winter/spring	Usually none	Macules, papules rapidly become vesicles on erythematous base, then crusts
Roseola (?herpesvirus 6)	6 months to 3 years	Spring/fall	High fever for 3–5 days	Maculopapular rash appears *after* fever declines
Lyme disease (Borrelia carried by ticks)	School age	Summer, geographical distribution	None	Erythema chronicum migrans
Rocky Mountain spotted fever (Rickettsia rickettsii carried by ticks)	Any age	Summer	Fever, malaise	Maculopapular and petechial rash
Kawasaki disease	6 months to 6 years	Winter/spring	High fever, irritability	Polymorphous—papular, morbilliform, erythema with desquamation
Gilanotti-Crosti syndrome (hepatitis B, cytomegalovirus coxsackievirus, Epstein-Barr virus, etc.)	1–6 years	Any season	Usually absent	Papules or papulovesicles; may become confluent
Scarlet fever (group B streptococcus)	School age	Fall to spring	Acute onset with fever, sore throat	Diffuse erythema with sandpaper texture
Staphylococcal scalded skin syndrome (*S aureus*/epidermolytic toxin)	Infants	Any season	None	Abrupt onset, tenter erythroderma
Toxic shock syndrome/*Staphylococcus* toxin	Adolescents/young adults	Any season	None	Macular erythroderma
Meningococcemia/meningococcus	< 2 years	Winter/spring	Malaise, fever, symptoms of upper respiratory infection	Papules, petechiae, purpura

[1]Reproduced, with permission, from Williams ML, Friedan IJ: Dermatologic disorders. In: *Pediatric Emergency Medicine.* Grossman M, Dieckmann R (editors). Lippincott, 1991.

Table 42–24. Exanthems.[1] (continued)

Distribution	Associated Findings	Diagnosis	Special Management
Begins on face and moves downward over whole body	Koplik's spots, "toxic" appearance, photophobia, cough, adenopathy, high fever	Usually clinical; acute/convalescent hemagglutinin (HAI) serologic test	Report to public health.
Begins on face and moves downward	Postauricular and occipital adenopathy, headache, malaise	Rubella IgM or acute/convalescent HAI serologic test	Report to public health; check for exposure to pregnant women.
Usually arms/legs, may be generalized	Waxes and wanes for several weeks, occasional arthritis, headache, malaise	Usually clinical; acute/convalescent serologic test	
Usually generalized, may be acral	Low-grade fever, occasional myocarditis, aseptic meningitis, pleurodynia	Usually clinical; viral culture from throat, rectal swabs in selected cases	If petechiae or purpura, *must consider* meningococcemia.
Hands/feet most common, diaper area, occasionally generalized	Oral ulcers, occasional fever, adenopathy	Same as for enteroviral exanthems	
Generalized	Fever, symptoms of upper respiratory infection, occasionally pneumonia	Viral isolation or acute/convalescent seroconversion	
Often begins on scalp or face, more profuse on trunk than extremities	Pruritus, fever, oral lesions, occasional malaise	Usually clinical; Tzanck preparation or direct immunofluorescence	Antihistamines for itching; aspirin contraindicated (Reye's syndrome).
Trunk, neck, may be generalized, lasts hours to days	Cervical and postauricular adenopathy	Clinical	
Trunk, extremities	Fever, later arthritis; cardiac, neurologic complications	Serologic test	Penicillin for children < 9 years of age, tetracycline for older children.
Wrists, ankles, palms, soles, later trunk	Central nervous system, pulmonary, cardiac lesions	Serologic test	Treat on presumptive clinical grounds.
Generalized, often with perineal accentuation	Conjunctivitis, cheilitis, glossitis, peripheral edema, adenopathy	Clinical	Admit to hospital for intravenous gamma globulin, salicylates.
Face, arms, legs, buttocks, spares the torso	Occasional lymphadenopathy, hepatomegaly, splenomegaly	Clinical; hepatitis B and Epstein-Barr serologic test	
Facial flushing with circumoral pallor, linear erythema in skin folds	Exudative pharyngitis, palatal petechiae, abdominal pain	Throat cultures	Intramuscular penicillin or oral erythromycin.
Diffuse with perioral, perinasal scaling	Fever, conjunctivitis, rhintis	Clinical; culture of *S aureus* from systemic site (not skin)	Neonate; if blistering present, hospitalize for intravenous nafcillin and fluid/electrolyte therapy.
Generalized	Hypotension; fever, myalgias, diarrhea/vomiting	Clinical case definition criteria, isolation of *S aureus* from cervix, etc.	Treat hypotension, admit to hospital; antibiotics to eradicate *S aureus*.
Trunk, extremities, palms, soles	Temp > 40 °C, meningism, circulatory collapse	Clinical, blood culture, spinal tap	Immediate intravenous penicillin in emergency department; treat for shock, if present.

Table 42–25. Common nontraumatic causes of abdominal pain.[1]

Clinical Entity	Diagnostic Findings	Comment
Infectious Conditions		
Influenza	Signs and symptoms of viral illness.	Treat symptoms.
Pneumonia	Fever, dyspnea, cough, ± chest pain.	Treat pathogen.
Pyelonephritis or cystitis	More frequent in females, congenital abnormalities common, costovertebral angle tenderness.	Needs urology consultation, intravenous pyelogram.
Inflammatory Conditions		
Appendicitis	Starts as periumbilical pain, then pain in right lower quadrant, followed by anorexia ± emesis.	Needs immediate operation, may rupture early.
Meckel's diverticulitis	Often indistinguishable from appendicitis, recurrent gastrointestinal bleeding.	Similar to above, may need blood.
Salpingitis	Cervical motion tenderness and adnexal tenderness, ± vaginal discharge.	Requires admission and antibiotics.
Obstructive Conditions		
Hirschsprung's disease	Infants do not pass meconium in 24 hours owing to aganglionic colon and rectum, diarrhea ± emesis, abdomen distended, no rectal stool.	Decompress stomach; barium enema, rectal biopsy.
Intussusception	Child usually < 2 years of age, with colicky pain, right upper quadrant mass present, with no bowel in right lower quadrant, currant-jelly stool frequent.	Barium enema imperative: surgical consultation.
Volvulus	Sudden cramps with tenderness and distention, sigmoid volvulus common, gastric, midgut and transverse volvulus less comon, obstruction marked.	Fluids needed; surgical consultation; barium enema.
Masses		
Ectopic pregnancy	Lower quadrant pain and tenderness, with amenorrhea; adnexal tenderness.	Transfuse early; obstetric consultation.
Incarcerated inguinal hernia	Tender mass in inguinal area of infant, erythema suggests strangulation. Bowel gangrene possible.	Surgical consultation.
Tumor	May have minor symptoms or chronic pain; neuroblastoma, Wilms' tumor, and lymphoma are most common.	Oncology consultation.

[1]Modified and reproduced, with permission, from Dieckmann RA: Abdominal pain. In *Pediatric Emergency Medicine: A Clinician's Reference*. Grossman M, Dieckmann RA (editors). Lippincott, 1991.

lower lobe pneumonia are 2 common sources of referred abdominal pain. Inspect the abdomen for signs of generalized distention or visible bowel loops. Auscultate the abdomen to evaluate the nature of the bowel sounds. Decreased or absent bowel sounds may signal an ileus, while sudden rushes of bowel sounds associated with crampy abdominal pain may indicate the presence of an intussusception. Gently seek out the areas of maximal tenderness. Careful percussion will determine areas of rebound pain. Perform a rectal examination. Localized tenderness to digital examination of the rectum may disclose a retrocecal appendicitis. In boys, examine the testicles to rule out epididymitis or testicular torsion. In sexually active girls, rule out pelvic inflammatory disease.

B. Diagnostic Procedures:

1. Urinalysis for evidence of a urinary tract infection.

2. Complete blood count with differential. The white blood cell count may be normal early in appendicitis but frequently will become elevated with continued inflammation. A shift to the left may also be present.

3. Electrolytes, BUN, and creatinine measure-

ments in children who appear dehydrated after protracted vomiting or diarrhea.

4. Blood clot for typing and cross-matching when abdominal surgery is anticipated.

5. Serum pregnancy test in adolescent girls.

6. Chest x-ray in children with abdominal pain and respiratory symptoms (cough and tachypnea). Lower lobe pneumonia in children may frequently result in referred pain to the abdomen that can mimic an acute abdomen.

7. Flat and upright, or decubitus, abdominal films in children with an acute abdomen to demonstrate obstruction, a radiopaque ureteral stone, or free air from a perforated viscus.

8. Abdominal ultrasound to detect inflammation of the appendix.

9. Barium enema to look for intussusception in children with recurrent episodes of cramping abdominal pain, vomiting, and bloody stools. Contraindicated when there are signs of peritonitis.

Disposition

A. Obtain surgical consultation when there is concern about a child with a possible acute abdomen.

B. If surgery is not immediately indicated, ensure close observation and follow-up. Admit the child to the hospital for frequent abdominal examinations.

C. Outpatient management is indicated only when an acute abdomen appears unlikely and the physician is certain that the child will be returned for an examination within 12–24 hours.

VOMITING

General Considerations

Causes of vomiting in children may be categorized as due to direct irritation to the gastrointestinal tract, intestinal or gastric outlet obstruction, effect of a toxin or other noxious stimulus on the central nervous system, or elevated intracranial pressure.

Diagnosis

Look for precipitating factors including trauma, medications, feeding techniques, and recent illness. It is helpful to know the nature of the vomitus (eg, bilious), the relationship to eating and position, and whether it is projectile. The absence of passage of stool or gas implies obstruction. Inspect the abdomen for signs of obstruction, and look for evidence of a systemic illness, eg, otitis media or urinary tract infection.

A. Vomiting in the Newborn: Infants commonly regurgitate a portion of feedings. Nonforceful regurgitation is usually benign. Forceful vomiting, however, often indicates serious disease. Causes of gastrointestinal obstruction in newborns include the following:

1. Intestinal atresia–Vomiting begins shortly after birth. Abdominal films reveal distention of the stomach and duodenum with an absence of colonic air. Early surgical intervention is necessary.

2. Meconium ileus–Antenatal perforation of the intestines secondary to obstruction with meconium results in vomiting shortly after birth; 90% of patients have cystic fibrosis.

3. Meconium plug syndrome–The distal colon becomes obstructed with a plug of meconium. A barium enema shows the plug and usually relieves the obstruction. This entity is suggestive of Hirschsprung's disease.

4. Midgut volvulus–This abdominal emergency usually presents in the first month of life with bile-stained vomiting and abdominal distention. An upper gastrointestinal series usually demonstrates obstruction. Immediate surgical management is essential.

5. Hirschsprung's disease–Delayed passage of meconium associated with abdominal distention and bilious vomiting is suggestive. A barium enema is helpful in diagnosis.

6. Pyloric stenosis–Muscular hypertrophy of the pylorus typically causes obstruction at about 4–8 weeks of age. Infants typically have projectile, non-

bilious vomiting associated with decreased stool production and failure to thrive. Examination of the abdomen may disclose visible peristaltic waves, and a pyloric "tumor" may be palpable.

B. Vomiting in Infants and Children: Most infants and children who vomit have gastroenteritis. More serious causes of vomiting include the following:

1. Gastrointestinal obstruction in the young child, particularly intussusception, should be considered. Examine the abdomen for a sausage-shaped mass in the right upper quadrant and the rectum for "currant-jelly stools" in the child presenting with intermittent crampy abdominal pain followed by vomiting. If there is a history of trauma, duodenal hematoma and traumatic pancreatitis should be considered.

2. Appendicitis may begin with a history of nausea and vomiting prior to the appearance of right lower quadrant abdominal pain.

3. Hepatitis in children is commonly associated with anorexia and vomiting.

4. In children with protracted vomiting and increasing lethargy, consider the diagnosis of Reye's syndrome. Obtain blood for liver function tests and ammonia and glucose measurements.

Treatment
(See Fig 42–9.)

A. Administer fluids if the child is dehydrated or is obstructed.

B. Insert a nasogastric tube if there is a suggestion of obstruction.

C. Obtain upright and supine films if signs of obstruction are present. A barium enema is indicated when considering the diagnosis of intussusception. Perform an upper gastrointestinal series emergently in the infant with bilious emesis who may have a midgut volvulus.

D. Obtain a urinalysis, CBC, platelet count, and electrolyte measurement as indicated by the clinical condition of the child.

BLEEDING

General Considerations

Gastrointestinal hemorrhage in children usually results from ulceration of the bowel mucosal lining secondary to infection or ischemia. Subsequent bleeding into the gastrointestinal tract can present in a number of ways. **Hematemesis** (vomiting of blood) and **melena** (black stool) usually indicate that the site of bleeding is in the stomach or duodenum proximal to the ligament of Treitz. **Hematochezia** (red blood per rectum) usually indicates bleeding in the distal small bowel or colon. In children, however, rapid gastrointestinal transit may result in hematochezia following upper gastrointestinal bleeding.

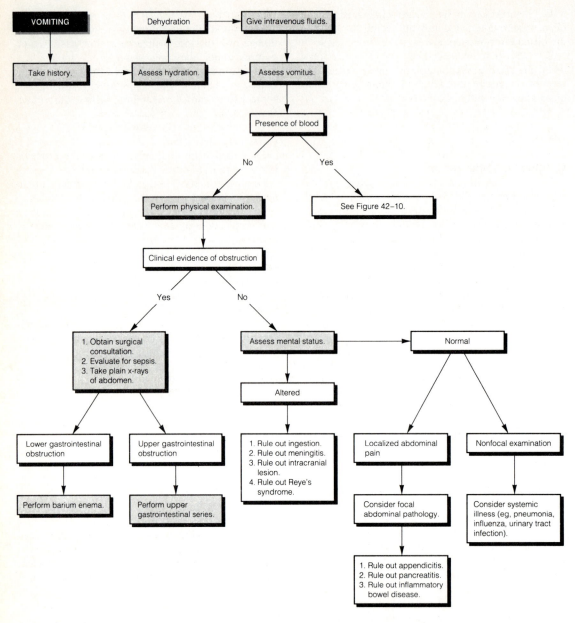

Figure 42–9. Algorithmic approach to vomiting.

Diagnosis

The patient's age and the amount and type of bleeding help determine the most likely cause. Profuse, painless bleeding may indicate Meckel's diverticulum. Bleeding associated with pain may occur with intussusception. Diarrhea associated with bleeding per rectum usually indicates bacterial dysentery.

Obtain vital signs to detect cardiovascular compromise. Clinical signs of liver disease may indicate a coagulopathy of esophageal varices as a possible cause of bleeding.

Occasionally what appears to be gastrointestinal hemorrhage is not truly from the gastrointestinal tract. Epistaxis, nasopharyngeal trauma, and hemoptysis may result in coffee-ground emesis. Some substances may color the emesis or stool red, eg, food colorings, beets, red gelatin, artificial fruit drinks, and antibiotic syrups. The vomitus or stool should be routinely checked with a guaiac test for occult blood.

A. Bleeding in the Newborn:

1. Swallowed maternal blood can result in hematemesis or melena in the newborn. These infants usually appear otherwise healthy. An Apt-Downey test can differentiate infant from maternal blood by identifying fetal hemoglobin.

2. Hemorrhagic disease of the newborn may present with melena or hematochezia. However, there is usually other evidence of a generalized bleeding disorder. Maternal medications such as aspirin or anticoagulants may result in neonatal hemorrhage.

3. In an infant with asphyxia or sepsis, stress ulcers may cause significant gastrointestinal bleeding.

B. Upper Gastrointestinal Tract Bleeding in Infants and Children:

1. The commonest cause is esophagitis or gastric and duodenal ulceration.

2. Esophageal varices are an uncommon cause of bleeding in young children that may develop with severe liver disease.

3. With forceful vomiting, tears of the distal esophagus (Mallory-Weiss) can occur in the esophagus, causing upper gastrointestinal hemorrhage.

C. Lower Gastrointestinal Tract Bleeding in Infants and Children:

1. Anal fissures are the commonest cause of hematochezia in infants.

2. Sensitivity to cow's milk protein can result in severe colitis with bloody stools.

3. Intussusception should always be considered in a child who presents with colicky abdominal pain followed by vomiting. Typically between episodes of vomiting, these children may appear well. Bloody stool helps establish the diagnosis.

4. Meckel's diverticulum may present with the painless appearance of bright red blood per rectum. Sufficient blood may be lost to result in cardiovascular compromise. The gastric mucosa within the diverticulum can be identified on technetium scan.

5. Fever and diarrhea associated with blood per rectum are usually secondary to an invasive bacterial infection of the colon. Culture stool for *Campylobacter, Shigella,* and *Salmonella.*

6. Hemolytic uremic syndrome is characterized by acute renal failure with thrombocytopenia, hemolytic anemia, and bloody diarrhea. These children are usually quite ill and require hospitalization and close observation.

7. Intestinal polyps are not uncommon in young children and may result in bright red blood per rectum. A diagnosis can be established by colonoscopy.

8. Henoch-Schönlein purpura is characterized by small vessel vasculitis of the skin, gastrointestinal tract, and kidneys. These children will at times have palpable purpura of the skin, joint swelling and pain, and colicky abdominal pain. Gastrointestinal bleeding may be secondary to submucosal hemorrhage. These children are also at increased risk for intussusception.

9. Inflammatory bowel disease may present with evidence of gastrointestinal bleeding associated with anemia, poor growth, abdominal pain, and diarrhea.

Treatment
(See Figs 42–10 and 42–11.)

A. Evaluate cardiovascular status. Admit children with acute upper gastrointestinal bleeding to the hospital for stabilization and endoscopic evaluation. Children with lower gastrointestinal bleeding can be evaluated as outpatients as long as they appear well and are hemodynamically stable.

B. Achieve intravenous access if there has been significant blood loss.

C. Send blood for CBC, platelet count, coagulation studies, and typing and cross-matching.

D. Infuse saline or Ringer's lactated injection initially if the child is in shock. Alternatively, infuse type O/Rh⁻ blood.

E. Place a nasogastric tube to determine if the site of bleeding is in the upper gastrointestinal tract.

F. If blood loss is greater than 10 mL/kg/h, emergent surgical intervention may be necessary to control bleeding.

Disposition

1. Admit children with active upper gastrointestinal bleeding to the hospital. Obtain consultation with a gastroenterologist.

2. Children with lower gastrointestinal tract bleeding can be evaluated as outpatients if they are hemodynamically stable.

3. Stabilize a hemodynamically unstable patient before performing diagnostic procedures. Emergent surgical intervention may be necessary to identify the site of bleeding.

FOREIGN BODY

Diagnosis

A. Esophageal Foreign Bodies: Foreign bodies within the esophagus become lodged at the cervical esophagus, aortic arch, or lower esophageal sphincter. Esophageal obstruction secondary to a foreign body may result in substernal chest pain and increased salivation secondary to inability to swallow. The physical examination is usually normal unless perforation has occurred. X-ray examination of the chest will usually disclose the foreign body; in the esophagus it is best seen on an anteroposterior film. A radiolucent foreign body (eg, plastic) may not be visible on x-ray.

B. Gastric and Small Bowel Foreign Bodies: Most foreign bodies that successfully pass through the esophagus will navigate the remainder of the gastrointestinal tract without difficulty. The occasional object that is unable to pass through the stomach after a period of 3 days should be removed by endoscopy. Intestinal obstruction may occur if a foreign body becomes lodged in the region of the ileocecal valve.

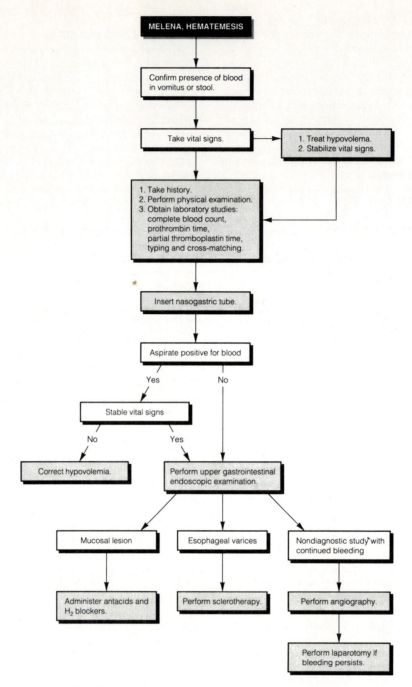

Figure 42–10. Treatment algorithm for melena and hematemesis.

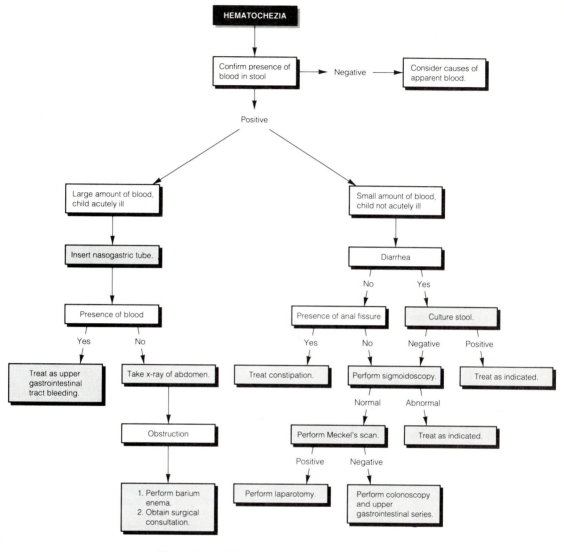

Figure 42–11. Treatment algorithm for hematochezia.

HEMATOLOGIC DISEASES

ANEMIA

General Considerations

In children, over 75% of anemias are due to iron deficiency or thalassemia minor, both of which are characterized by microcytosis. The commonest cause of anemia in children between 6 months and 2 years of age is nutritional iron deficiency. Typically this results from excessive cow's milk intake. Less commonly iron deficiency anemia will occur secondary to chronic blood loss, usually from the gastrointesti-

nal tract (eg, duodenal ulcer, Meckel's diverticulum, and polyps).

Anemias not due to iron deficiency are caused by one of 2 processes: (**1**) Decreased erythrocyte production or release from the bone marrow, eg, transient erythroblastopenia of childhood (TEC). TEC typically occurs in children between 1 and 2 years of age. Severe anemia and reticulocytopenia spontaneously resolve in 1–2 months. (**2**) Increased destruction, sequestration, or acute loss of circulating red cells owing to sickle cell disease, autoimmune hemolytic anemia, or hemolytic uremic syndrome, or blood loss due to trauma, surgery, or peptic ulcer disease.

Diagnosis

With rapid onset of anemia from blood loss or hemolysis, signs of cardiovascular compromise as well as impending cardiac failure may be present. With slow onset of anemia, typically children will show pallor and decreased exercise tolerance but no evidence of cardiovascular compromise even with extremely low levels of hemoglobin. Hemolytic anemias may cause jaundice and splenomegaly. Petechiae may indicate hemolytic uremic syndrome.

Laboratory evaluation should include a complete blood count with hemoglobin, red blood cell indices, white blood cell and platelet counts, peripheral smear, and reticulocyte counts. Anemia with microcytosis in a young child strongly suggests iron deficiency. If the stool is negative for occult blood, further tests are not necessary if the child is not severely anemic.

Treatment

A. Treat iron deficiency with elemental iron at 3–6 mg/kg/d in 1–2 daily doses. Continue iron therapy for 2 months after the anemia is corrected. Restrict cow's milk intake.

B. If anemia has developed slowly, patients can often tolerate remarkably low hemoglobin levels, even to 4–5 g/dL, without the need for transfusion if other effective therapy is available.

C. Transfuse children who experience a rapid decline in hemoglobin to < 7, particularly if there are signs of cardiovascular compromise.

D. In patients with gradual onset of anemia who do require transfusion, slow transfusion is recommended, since these children are at risk for congestive heart failure with rapid transfusion. Administer a diuretic prior to transfusion to prevent circulatory overload (eg, furosemide, 1 mg/kg intravenously).

Disposition

A. Obtain consultation with a hematologist for anemias requiring transfusion, anemias associated with hemolysis, and anemias without an obvious cause.

B. Recheck the hemoglobin level in children receiving iron therapy in 2–4 weeks to document response.

SICKLE CELL DISEASE

Diagnosis

A. Symptoms and Signs: Vaso-occlusive events are associated with severe local pain, fever, leukocytosis, and impaired organ function. Abdominal pain may be severe and suggest appendicitis or cholecystitis. In young children, a common initial vaso-occlusive episode is manifested by hand-foot-and-mouth disease, with acute swelling and pain of one or both hands or feet. Bone and joint pain may be quite severe, and differentiation from skeletal infection may be difficult. Splenic infarcts may cause severe ab-

dominal pain and lead to progressive atrophy of the spleen. Vaso-occlusive crises may involve the central nervous system and produce neurologic symptoms of severe headache, visual disturbances, coma, and seizures. Large vessel thrombosis during these crises may result in stroke. A combination of pulmonary infarcts and infection may lead to the acute chest syndrome manifested by chest pain, dyspnea, and tachypnea. These children may become severely hypoxic. Priapism is another complication of sickling and can be extremely uncomfortable to the child.

B. Diagnostic Procedures:

1. Obtain a complete blood count and reticulocyte count. A decrease in hematocrit from baseline may indicate the need for transfusion. The absence of reticulocytosis indicates an aplastic crisis and heralds an abrupt decrease in the hematocrit.

2. Obtain cultures of blood and urine if fever is present.

3. If bone pain is associated with high fever, chills, toxicity, and leukocytosis, bone aspiration is indicated to diagnose osteomyelitis.

4. Obtain blood for electrolytes and venous pH measurements. Acidosis worsens ischemic crises.

5. Obtain x-rays of the chest if cough, tachypnea, or dyspnea is present.

Treatment

A. Administer oxygen, 5 L/min, by nasal cannula. Oxygenation and vigorous intravenous fluid hydration are important in reversing the sickling process.

B. Begin an intravenous line, and give 5% dextrose in half-normal saline at 3 mL/kg/h.

C. If acidosis is present, administer bicarbonate, 2 mg/kg intravenously every 12 hours until the acidosis is corrected.

D. Treatment of pain in a sickling crisis is important in the recovery of the child. Acetaminophen with or without codeine can be used for mild pain. For severe pain, give intravenous morphine sulfate, 0.1 mg/kg every 2–4 hours, or meperidine, 1 mg/kg every 3–4 hours. Ask the patient to quantitate the pain to guide dosing.

E. Partial exchange transfusion is indicated for the termination of life-threatening vaso-occlusive episodes.

Disposition

A. Children who can maintain adequate oral fluid intake and whose pain is controlled with oral medication can be managed as outpatients with close follow-up.

B. Admit to the hospital those children who require continued parenteral therapy for pain, cannot maintain adequate oral hydration, or have required more than 2 visits for treatment of the same painful crisis.

C. Ask the patient to use an objective scale (eg, 1–10) to grade severity of pain. Use this scale to guide pain management. Do not be hesitant to use parenteral narcotics for adequate pain control because of concerns about drug addiction.

ANEMIC CRISES

General Considerations

Rapid decrease in hemoglobin level can occur in the following circumstances: (**1**) Splenic sequestration producing sudden massive splenic enlargement, hypotension, and death. This is one of the 2 commonest causes of death in young patients with sickle cell disease. (**2**) Bone marrow aplasia following infections, most commonly with parvovirus. The reticulocyte count is usually low. (**3**) Hemolysis due to glucose-6-phosphate dehydrogenase (G6PD) deficiency or transfusion reactions.

Treatment

A. Severe anemic crises should be treated aggressively with immediate transfusion of packed red blood cells. Sequestration crises are particularly dangerous, since the child may die within hours unless transfusion occurs.

B. Children with sickle cell disease have increased susceptibility to sepsis with *S pneumoniae* and *H influenzae*. They are also at increased risk for *Salmonella* osteomyelitis and *Mycoplasma pneumoniae*. Since overwhelming infection in children with sickle cell disease can be rapidly fatal, those who present with high fever without any localizing signs of infection should be immediately treated with an intravenous antibiotic and hospitalized. Blood culture should be obtained. An antibiotic active against *S pneumoniae* and beta-lactamase-producing *H influenzae* is indicated (eg, cefuroxime, 100 mg/kg every 24 hours). In older children with a low-grade fever, outpatient therapy may be considered with oral antibiotics or intramuscular ceftriaxone, 50 mg/kg. Conduct a follow-up examination in 12–24 hours.

IDIOPATHIC THROMBOCYTOPENIC PURPURA

General Considerations

Idiopathic thrombocytopenic purpura (ITP) results from increased destruction of platelets causing severe thrombocytopenia. It commonly follows a viral illness. It is usually benign and self-limited; approximately 75% of cases resolve within 6 months.

Diagnosis

A. Symptoms and Signs: These children usually present with the abrupt appearance of petechiae, purpura, and spontaneous bleeding of the skin and mucous membranes. They may also have epistaxis. Early in the disease, intracranial hemorrhage occurs in approximately 1% of patients. These patients usually manifest severe headache or altered level of consciousness. Children with ITP typically appear in good health. They usually are not febrile and do not have splenomegaly.

B. Diagnostic Procedures:

1. Obtain a CBC, blood smear, and platelet count. Typically the platelet count is < 100,000 platelets/μL and not uncommonly is < 20,000 platelets/μL.

2. A bone marrow examination may be recommended by the hematologist if the presentation is atypical.

Treatment

A. Observation is adequate for children with only moderately severe thrombocytopenia.

B. If the platelet count is < 10,000–20,000/μL or if there is extensive bleeding, corticosteroid therapy is recommended. Corticosteroids will usually cause the platelet count to increase within 48–72 hours.

C. Emergent intervention is needed for severe gastrointestinal bleeding, hematuria, or intracranial hemorrhage. Whole-blood transfusion may be required for severe anemia. Intravenous corticosteroids should be administered as hydrocortisone, 4–5 mg/kg/dose every 6 hours intravenously.

D. Intravenous infusion of gamma globulin will also result in a rapid rise in platelet count.

E. Platelet transfusions are indicated with life-threatening hemorrhage, but the half-life of transfused platelets is brief.

Disposition

A. Admit children with ITP to the hospital when the platelet count is < 10,000/μL or significant bleeding is present, particularly the young child for whom avoidance of traumatic play is difficult.

B. Advise older children to avoid all contact sports and vigorous playground activities during the acute phase of the disease.

C. Obtain emergent neurosurgical consultation for any signs of intracranial hemorrhage.

D. Obtain hematologic consultation and a bone marrow examination before corticosteroid therapy is initiated.

NEWBORN EMERGENCIES

Diagnosis

The need for resuscitation of the newborn infant is based on the Apgar score. Vital signs should be recorded frequently to monitor the success of resuscitation. Physical examination should establish the degree of maturity of the infant as well as the integrity of the respiratory and cardiovascular functions.

Treatment

The key to treatment of the newborn infant is to be prepared and use an organized team approach. A "code card" posted in the emergency department can help guide drug dosing and choice of equipment sizes.

A. If time permits, alert the obstetric service and nursery staff prior to the birth of the baby. Electronic fetal monitoring is helpful if time and equipment availability permit.

B. An overhead radiant warmer should be present and turned on. If one is not available, use heating lamps or warm blankets. Proper equipment should be available and functioning (Table 42–26).

C. At birth the umbilical cord should be quickly clamped and then cut. The infant should be placed under the radiant warmer and immediately assessed, and an Apgar score should be assigned. The heart rate can be monitored by palpation of the umbilical arterial pulse. The oropharynx can be gently suctioned and the infant stimulated by rubbing its back. The infant should be towel-dried. An Apgar score should be assigned at 1 and 5 minutes.

D. Infants who are bradycardic, apneic, or significantly depressed require immediate resuscitative efforts (Fig 42–12).

E. Epinephrine, atropine, or naloxone can be administered endotracheally during resuscitative efforts prior to the establishment of vascular access. When this route is used, double the usual intravenous dosages of these medications.

F. Umbilical vein catheterization can also be used for emergent drug administration or volume expansion. Umbilical artery catheterization can be used for frequent arterial blood gas analysis and blood pressure readings.

G. Continue to assign Apgar scores at 5-minute intervals to determine the need for continued resuscitative efforts. Be alert to complications particular to the newborn when resuscitation does not result in expected improvement (eg, meconium aspiration, respiratory distress syndrome, shock, maternal substance abuse, pneumothorax, choanal atresia, diaphragmatic hernia, tracheoesophageal fistula). As the Apgar score improves, prepare the infant for transport to the nursery for close monitoring and care as indicated.

Table 42–26. Equipment required for neonatal resuscitation.[1]

	Prehospital/ Field	Emergency Department
Blankets (warm)	+	
Heat lamp or radiant warmer		+
Thermometer, temperature probe	±	+
Oxygen source (warm, humid)	+	+
Lighting	+	+
Infant stethoscope	+	+
Suction catheter with syringe	+	
Suction catheter with machine	±	+
Face masks (preterm, term)	+	+
Self-inflating bag, pop-off	+	
Anesthesia bag, manometer		+
Endotracheal tubes (2.5–4mm)	+	+
Stylet	±	±
Sterile needles, syringes, stopcocks	+	+
Oral airways (000–0)	±	±
Laryngoscope (0 and 1 Miller blades)		+
Spare bulbs and batteries		+
Cord tie, clamps	+	+
Hemostat, forceps, scissors, scalpel	+	+
Umbilical catheters (3.5 and 5F)		+
Resuscitation drugs	+	+
Sterile attire, drapes		+
ECG monitor		+
Blood pressure monitor		+
Blood gas machine		+
Glucose reagent sticks	+	+
Defibrillator	±	+
Umbilical catheter tray		+
Thoracostomy tray		+

[1]Reproduced, with permission, from Partridge JC: Neonatal resuscitation. In: *Pediatric Emergency Medicine: A Clinician's Reference.* Grossman M, Dieckmann RA (editors). Lippincott, 1991.

CHILD ABUSE

PHYSICAL ABUSE

General Considerations

Management of possible child abuse is one of the most difficult clinical problems facing the emergency physician. The emergency department is a frequent site for the initial presentation of physical abuse. The

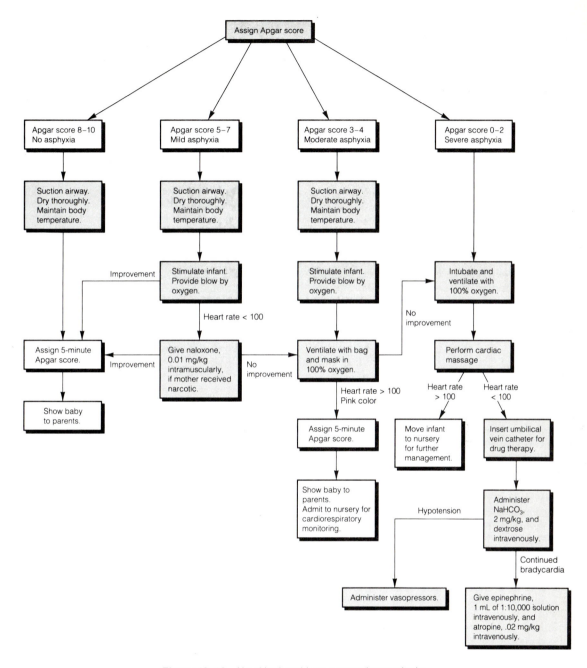

Figure 42–12. Algorithmic guide to neonatal resuscitation.

physician's responsibilities are to **(1)** acknowledge that a problem exists; **(2)** maintain a high index of suspicion; **(3)** discuss concerns with the parents in a sensitive and compassionate manner; **(4)** ensure protection of the child; **(5)** perform a complete medical evaluation of injuries or neglect, including documentation and radiologic imaging if indicated; and **(6)** report suspicions to child protective services.

The key to diagnosis of physical abuse is matching a carefully taken history with the extent of injury. Historical indicators of abuse include **(1)** a history that overestimates or underestimates the injury; **(2)** a history that suggests a lack of proper supervision; **(3)** inconsistencies or changes in the history; and **(4)** a delay in seeking medical care.

Note the quality of the parent-child interaction. Note whether the parents appear to be under the influence of drugs or alcohol.

Consider the motor skills and capabilities of the child when evaluating the worthiness of the history. Injuries that could occur accidentally only in an older child with more advanced motor skills strongly suggest the possibility of nonaccidental injury.

Physical indicators of abuse include **(1)** injuries that do not match the history; **(2)** specific pathognomonic injuries, eg, looped wire marks or cigarette burns; **(3)** multiple injuries in various stages of healing; **(4)** different types of injuries or disease, eg, burns and fractures; **(5)** overall evidence of poor care; and **(6)** evidence of failure to thrive.

Diagnosis

A. Signs and Symptoms:

1. Bruises–The skin is the most commonly injured site. Injuries from physical abuse may be either nonspecific bruises or pathognomonic injuries that clearly reflect the instrument used to strike the child. The specific pattern of bruising may be indicative of nonaccidental trauma. Young children accidentally bruise themselves in predictable ways. A pattern of bruising significantly different from that of accidental bruises should raise suspicion of nonaccidental trauma. Locations of possible accidental cutaneous injuries in the young child are the shins and knees, hips (iliac crests), spinal prominences, chin, forehead, face (facial scratches in infants), lower arms, and elbows. Locations of injuries that probably are not accidental are the buttocks, inner thighs, genitalia, perineum, rectum, abdomen, chest, cheeks, neck, ears, and inner surface of upper arms. Be alert to specific abusive cutaneous injuries, eg, wire loop marks made by extension cords, belt marks, burns from hot objects such as silverware or heat vents, and belt buckle marks.

2. Skeletal trauma–Skeletal trauma occurs in one-fifth to one-third of abuse cases. More than half these fractures occur in children under 1 year of age. Suspicious fractures include

a. Femoral fractures (spiral or transverse) in children under 3 years of age are suspicious. Minor falls, under 30–60 cm, usually do not result in femoral fractures.

b. Epiphyseal metaphyseal fractures in young infants and children are virtually diagnostic of abuse because they usually do not occur with accidental falls. These fractures usually occur as a result of severe pulling, twisting, or shaking of a child's limbs. These activities produce severe acceleration-deceleration forces on the limbs, resulting in metaphyseal chip fractures.

c. Rib fractures in infants under 2 years of age are extremely uncommon because the infant's rib cage is extremely pliant. Rib fractures in these children should always raise the possibility of nonaccidental trauma.

3. Burns–Burn injuries should raise the possibility of abuse in young children when they do not fit the normal accidental pattern. Children may be held down in scalding water as a means of discipline. These immersion burns typically cause injury to the buttocks and to the hands and feet in a stocking-glove distribution. The line of demarcation between burned and normal skin is usually quite abrupt. The flexion creases of the legs are usually spared. Children may also be burned by hot objects such as heater grates, curling irons, or cigarettes. Cigarette burns typically cause a deep circular burn about 5–10 mm in diameter. They may be difficult to differentiate from impetigo or insect bites.

4. Skin lesions–See Table 42–27.

5. Head injuries–Head injuries carry the highest incidence of morbidity and mortality. Abusive head injuries either are due to direct impact with a fist or other object or are secondary to severe rotational forces during vigorous shaking. Many children with abusive intracranial injury suffer a combination of impact and shaking injuries. Both shaking and impact can cause severe acceleration-deceleration forces to the brain, resulting in shearing injury to the bridging vessels that connect the brain to the dura. Subdural hematomas can then occur with resulting cerebral

Table 42–27. Differential diagnosis of skin lesions in child abuse.

Skin Lesion	Diagnostic Procedure
Bruising Trauma	
Hemophilia	Prothrombin time, partial thromboplastin time
von Willebrand's disease	Bleeding time, von Willebrand factor, antigen and ristocetin cofactor
Idiopathic thrombocytopenic purpura	Complete blood count, platelet count
Periorbital ecchymoses secondary to neuroblastoma	CT scan
Mongolian spots	History, location
Coin rubbing	History, location, configuration
Self-inflicted	Depression, mental retardation
Local erythema, bullae Burn	
Impetigo	Culture, Gram staining
Photosensitivity reaction	History of sensitizing agent
Herpes simplex, herpes zoster	Culture, Tzanck smear
Car-seat burn	History
Hair loss Traumatic alopecia	History
Tinea capitis	Fungal culture, KOH slide
Alopecia areata	Clinical appearance
Seborrhea, eczema	Clinical appearance

compression. In addition, these forces can cause direct neuronal injury within the brain. Infants who are severely shaken can present with sudden onset of seizure or coma but have no signs of head trauma. Typically infants who are severely shaken will have bilateral retinal hemorrhages and on CT scan may have bilateral subdural hemorrhages.

6. Abdominal injuries–Nonaccidental abdominal injury may produce severe injury to the viscera, including intramural hematomas of the small bowel, splenic or hepatic lacerations, traumatic pancreatitis, and renal contusions.

B. Diagnostic Procedures:
1. CBC, platelet, and coagulation studies.
2. Serum calcium and phosphorous levels.
3. Serologic test for syphilis (VDRL or rapid plasma reagin [RPR]).
4. Urinalysis.
5. A skeletal x-ray series, if indicated, of the skull, ribs, and long bones.

SEXUAL ABUSE

General Considerations

Sexual abuse is involvement of children and adolescents in sexual activities they cannot comprehend because of their developmental level, activities to which they are unable to give informed consent, or activities that violate social taboos. These activities may physically injure the child and leave detectable patterns of trauma, but often sexual abuse may involve genital touching or fondling that does not cause detectable injury and may even be physically pleasurable to the child. Most victims of sexual abuse are female, and the mean age is approximately 7–8 years. Children are usually molested by males who are well known to them, either as a family member or trusted friend. Adolescents are more commonly molested by strangers.

Diagnosis

Various behavioral reactions may ensue following sexual abuse. In preschool children, these can be fear states (eg, fear of adult males), nightmares, precocious sexual behavior, enuresis, encopresis, or behavior regression. In school-aged children, indicators may be precocious sexual behavior, sexual aggression toward other children, cross-dressing, school failure, truancy, running away, or depression. Adolescents may demonstrate behavioral problems with drugs, promiscuity, prostitution, running away, sexual aggression toward other children, depression, somatic complaints, or school failure.

Disclosures of sexual abuse may many times be incomplete and then later retracted because the perpetrator is typically someone the child feels great allegiance to and is dependent on.

Some children who are sexually abused show signs of abuse, including genital and nongenital trauma as well as the presence of sexually transmitted diseases (STDs). A sexually transmitted disease may be the only indication that a child has been molested (Table 42–28). Direct injuries to hymenal tissue are rarely accidental. Hymenal lacerations should always raise the possibility of sexual abuse. Typical straddle injuries do not cause hymenal lacerations. Anal penetration may result in erythema and swelling of the perianal tissue as well as lacerations, abrasions, and bruising.

Children in whom sexual abuse is being considered should be evaluated at a center where health care providers accustomed to examining sexual abuse victims are located. The goals of the medical evaluation are to (1) treat any medical illness or injuries, (2) provide crisis counseling, (3) provide protection for the child if necessary, and (4) precisely document injuries and collect evidence for use by the legal system.

Approach the child in a compassionate, nonthreatening manner, and ask nonleading questions in an attempt to uncover whether sexual abuse has occurred. The physical examination should be performed immediately if sexual assault has occurred within 72 hours or the child has signs or symptoms of genital injury or infection. Look for both nongenital and genital injuries. Many examiners employ a colposcope with a camera attachment to provide photographic documentation of genital injuries. A speculum examination in a prepubertal child is indicated only when there are symptoms of vaginal injury (eg, vaginal bleeding). This is best done under general anesthesia. Laboratory tests in the diagnosis of sexually transmitted diseases should be obtained routinely, including wet mount and Gram staining of genital or rectal discharge; genital and rectal cultures for *N gonorrhoeae* and *C trachomatis;* pharyngeal culture for *N gonorrhoeae;* culture of lesions suspicious for herpes simplex; serologic studies for hepatitis B and human immunodeficiency virus, if indicated.

If the sexual assault has occurred within 72 hours of the examination, seminal fluid may be present on or within the child. The proper collection of this evidence is essential. Physicians who examine sexual abuse victims must be fully knowledgeable of the protocol for evidence collection in their locale.

Treatment

A. Physical injuries should be treated as necessary. Inspect vaginal lacerations for possible extension into the abdominal cavity. Significant perineal or vaginal lacerations are best examined under general anesthesia in the operating room.

B. Because STDs are relatively uncommon in prepubertal victims of sexual abuse, empiric therapy is recommended only if the child has a vaginal or rectal discharge that on Gram staining is suggestive of gonorrhea. Adolescent victims of sexual assault should be routinely treated for STDs at the time of the

Table 42–28. Sexually transmitted diseases in children.[1]

Organism	Incubation Period	Clinical Features	Nonabusive Transmission	
			Perinatal Transmission	Nonsexual Contact
Neisseria gonorrhoeae	3–7 days	Vaginitis (prepubertal females); profuse discharge Cervicitis, pelvic inflammatory disease (postpubertal females Pharyngitis, proctitis, urethritis Disseminated disease: rash, arthralgias, tenosynovitis, arthritis Asymptomatic carriage: vagina, cervix, pharynx, rectum	Yes, neonatal conjunctivitis	Not documented in children
Chlamydia trachomatis	7–21 days	Vaginitis (prepubertal females) Cervicitis, endometritis (postpubertal females) Urethritis, proctitis, epidymitis, prostatitis, Reiter's syndrome, perihepatitis Asymptomatic carriage: vagina, cervix, rectum	Yes, may have asymptomatic vaginal, rectal carriage for up to 2 years	Not documented in children
Herpes simplex types 1 and 2	5–7 days	Painful vesicles on labia, vagina, anus, rectum	Yes	Documented with type1: autoinoculation from oral to genital sites
Condyloma acuminatum, human papillomavirus	2–3 months average ? over 1 year	Mucosa: red, mulberry-type lesions Skin: verrucous warts common; may be pigmented papules	Yes	Possible
Trichomonas vaginalis	3–28 days	Vaginitis Asymptomatic carriage: urethra	Yes, neonate may carry in the vagina for 3–6 weeks after birth	Not documented in children
Syphilis	Primary: 10–90 days	Primary: chancre Secondary: rash, lymphadenitis, mucous patches, condyloma latum	Yes	Yes

[1]Reproduced, with permission, from Coulter K: Sexual abuse. In: *Pediatric Emergency Medicine: A Clinician's Reference.* Grossman M, Dieckmann RA (editors). Lippincott, 1991.

examination, since the incidence of STDs in this group is significant. Adolescents should be treated empirically for both *Chlamydia* (doxycycline, 100 mg twice a day for 10 days) and gonorrhea (ceftriaxone, 250 mg intramuscularly).

C. After documentation of a negative urine pregnancy test, adolescent girls should be offered prophylaxis against conception with Norgestrel (Ovral), 2 pills at the time of examination and 2 pills 12 hours later orally.

D. Pediatric and adolescent victims of sexual abuse should be offered counseling following the initial evaluation. Many children will require extensive counseling, particularly those who are victims of long-term incestuous relationships.

Disposition

1. Children and adolescents may be discharged home if their medical condition permits and safety can be ensured.

2. If the child is at risk for further sexual abuse, removal from parental custody and placement in shelter care is indicated.

APPENDIX: COMMONLY USED PEDIATRIC DRUGS

Acetaminophen
Orally or rectally: 10–15 mg/kg/dose; or 80 mg/yr to 5 yr, every 4 hours.

Albuterol, 0.5%
Inhaled: 0.1 mg/kg/dose (max. 2.5 mg).
Orally: 0.1–0.2 mg/kg/dose (max. 12 kg) 3 to 4 times daily.

Aminophylline
Orally: 5–6 mg/kg/dose; give every 6 hours.
Intravenously: 5 mg/kg/dose (give every 6 hours); or 1 mg/kg/h as continuous infusion.

Amoxicillin
Orally only:
Child: 50 mg/kg/d in 3 divided doses.
Adolescent: 500 mg every 8 hours.

Ampicillin
Orally: 100 mg/kg/d in 4 divided doses.
Intramuscularly or intravenously:

Newborn: 100–150 mg/kg/d.
Child or older: 150–200 mg/kg/d.

Aspirin
Orally only: 10–20 mg/kg/dose; give every 4 hours.

Atropine
Intravenously, intramuscularly, subcutaneously, orally: 0.01 mg/kg, up to 0.5 mg maximum; minimum: 0.1 mg.

Cefaclor
Orally only:
Child: 45–60 mg/kg/d in 3–4 divided doses.
Adolescent: 250–1000 mg every 8 hours.

Cefazolin
Intramuscularly or intravenously:
Newborn: Do not use.
Child: 100 mg/kg/d in 3 divided doses.
Adolescent: 2–6 g/d in 3 divided doses.

Cefotaxime
Intravenously, intramuscularly: 150 mg/kg/d in 3 divided doses.

Chlorpheniramine
Orally or subcutaneously: 0.1 mg/kg/dose 3 or 4 times daily.

Dexamethasone
Intravenously, intramuscularly, orally: 0.1–0.2 mg/kg/d.

Diazepam
Orally: 0.12–0.8 mg/kg/d in 4 divided doses.
Intravenously: 0.1–0.3 mg/kg up to 10 mg.
Rectally: 0.5 mg/kg, up to 10 mg.

Diphenhydramine
Orally: 4–6 mg/kg/d in 3–4 divided doses.
Intravenously: 1–2 mg/kg/dose.

Epinephrine (Aqueous) 1:1000
Subcutaneously: 0.01 mL/kg/dose (maximum 0.4 mL/dose).

Erythromycin
Orally:
Newborn: 20–40 mg/kg/d in 2 divided doses.
Child: 30–40 mg/kg/d in 4 divided doses.
Intravenously (give over 30–60 minutes):
Newborn: 10 mg/kg/d in 2 divided doses.
Child: 10–20 mg/kg/d in 4 divided doses.
Adolescent: 2–4 g/d in 4 divided doses.

Furosemide
Intravenously, intramuscularly, orally: 1–2 mg/kg/dose every 12–48 hours.

Hydroxyzine
Orally: 0.25–0.5 mg/kg, 4 times daily.
Intramuscularly: 1 mg/kg/dose.

Ibuprofen
Orally: 5–10 mg/kg/dose, 4 times daily.

Ipecac
Orally: 15–30 mL/dose. May repeat once in 20 minutes if vomiting does not occur.

Meperidine
Orally: 2–3 mg/kg/dose every 3–4 hours.
Intravenously or intramuscularly: 1–2 mg/kg/dose.

Morphine
Subcutaneously, intramuscularly, or intravenously: 0.1–0.2 mg/kg/dose every 3–4 hours as needed.

Naloxone
Intramuscularly or intravenously: 0.01–0.03 mg/kg/dose.

Penicillin G, Aqueous (Sodium or Potassium Salt)
Intramuscularly or intravenously:
Newborn (< 7 days old): 200,000 units/kg/d in 4–6 divided doses.
Newborn (≥ 7 days old): 400,000 units/kg/d in 6 divided doses.
Child: 400,000 units/kg/d in 4–6 divided doses.
Adolescent: 5–20 million units/d in 4–6 divided doses.

Penicillin G, Benzathine
Intramuscularly only: 1.2 million units every 1–4 weeks.

Penicillin G, Procaine
Intramuscularly only:
Newborn: 50,000 units/kg/d in 1–2 divided doses.
Child or older: $100–600 \times 10^3$ units every 12–24 hours.

Penicillin V (Phenoxymethyl Penicillin)
Orally only:
Newborn: 100 mg/kg/d in 4 divided doses.
Child or older: 30–100 mg/kg/d in 4 divided doses.

Penicillinase-Resistant Penicillins (Methicillin, Nafcillin, Oxacillin, Cloxacillin, Dicloxacillin)
Orally (dicloxacillin and cloxacillin): 50–100 mg/kg/d in 4 divided doses.
Intravenously (methicillin, oxacillin, nafcillin):
Newborn: methicillin or nafcillin, 100–150 mg/kg/d in 4 divided doses.
Child: 100–150 mg/kg/d.
Adolescent: 150–200 mg/kg/d.

Pentobarbital
Orally: 1–5 mg/kg/dose (repeat once only).
Intravenously: 5 mg/kg/dose.

Phenobarbital
Orally: 6–10 mg/kg/d in 4–6 divided doses.
Intramuscularly or intravenously:
Loading dose: 20 mg/kg.

Phenytoin
Intravenously, orally: 15–20 mg/kg loading dose; administer 1 mg/kg/min in normal saline.

Prednisone
Orally: 1–2 mg/kg/d, up to 60 mg/d maximum.

Sulfamethoxazole
  Orally only:
    Child: 50 mg/kg/d in 2 divided doses.
    Adolescent: 1–3 g/d in 2–3 divided doses.

Sulfisoxazole
  Orally:
    Newborn: Do not use.
    Child: 120–150 mg/kg/d in 4 divided doses.
    Adolescent: 2–4 g/d in 4 divided doses.

Intravenously:
    Child or older: 120 mg/kg/d in 4 divided doses.

Trimethoprim-Sulfamethoxazole
  Orally or intravenously (doses for trimethoprim compo-
    nent only):
  Newborn: Not recommended.
  Infant or older: Bacterial infection: 8–10 mg/kg/d in
    2–3 divided doses. Pneumocystosis: 20 mg/kg/d in
    4 divided doses.

REFERENCES

American Heart Association, American Academy of Pediat-
  rics: *Textbook of Pediatric Advanced Life Support.*
  American Heart Association, 1988.
Fleisher G, Ludwig S: *Textbook of Pediatric Emergency
  Medicine,* 2nd ed. Williams & Wilkins, 1988.
Grossman M, Dieckmann RA (editors): *Pediatric Emer-
  gency Medicine: A Clinician's Reference.* Lippincott,
  1991.
Hathaway WE et al (editors): *Current Pediatric Diagnosis
  & Treatment,* 10th ed. Appleton & Lange, 1991.
Rudolph AM, Hoffman J: *Rudolph's Pediatrics,* 19th ed.
  Appleton & Lange, 1991.

Prehospital Emergency Medical Services

43

Charles E. Saunders, MD, FACEP, FACP, & Thomas Hearne, PhD

The delivery of effective, organized, prehospital emergency medical services (EMS) is a relatively recent development.

When medical emergencies are reported, trained medical personnel can now commonly provide emergency care at the scene within 6–10 minutes. The skills of these personnel range from basic first aid techniques and cardiopulmonary resuscitation (CPR) to advanced life support techniques, including defibrillation, endotracheal intubation, and the use of emergency medications. Patients are stabilized prior to transport to the hospital. Sophisticated radio communications permit ongoing discussion of patient status and treatment between emergency medical personnel at the scene and the supervising physician at the base hospital. Air ambulances (fixed-wing aircraft or helicopters) staffed with medically trained flight crews can rapidly evacuate and transport patients from a remote emergency scene to a regional medical center.

COMPONENTS OF THE EMERGENCY MEDICAL SERVICES SYSTEM

Modern emergency medical services systems consist of several major components: (**1**) professional field personnel trained to provide specific levels or types of care, (**2**) a comprehensive emergency communications network, (**3**) hospital emergency department physicians and nurses who supervise the treatment provided by EMS field personnel, (**4**) hospitals categorized according to their relationship with EMS field personnel and according to the level of care they can provide, and (**5**) EMS administrative officials who manage and coordinate the elements of the system.

Professional EMS Field Personnel

The health professionals and first responders who provide prehospital care are trained to carry out specific levels of care, ranging from basic first aid and cardiopulmonary resuscitation (CPR) provided by first responders, through basic life support given by emergency medical technicians (EMTs), to the advanced life support provided by advanced EMTs (paramedics). These personnel provide care only as extensions or agents of physicians and are not independently licensed to provide medical care. The care they deliver is authorized by standing orders or protocols from physician directors or by orders transmitted by radio from supervisory physicians at the base hospital to EMS personnel at the scene. A critical element in the development of EMS over the past 15–20 years has been the recognition that personnel without prior medical training can be prepared through relatively short courses to provide effective prehospital care. The designations, levels of training, and skills of EMS personnel are now largely standardized according to United States Department of Transportation (DOT) curriculum and formal categories established in 1983 by the National Registry of Emergency Medical Technicians. Types of EMS field personnel and their training are described below and summarized in Table 43–1.

A. First Responders: First responders may include law enforcement officers, rescue squad members, fire fighters, or volunteers EMS personnel. First-responder courses usually consist of about 40 hours of classroom instruction and clinical training in basic first aid and CPR. First responders are equipped with basic emergency care equipment (eg, bandages, dressings, tape, blanket and pillow, upper and lower extremity splint sets). Oxygen equipment and a self-refilling bag-valve-mask combination (eg, Ambu bag) are optional. First responders also carry basic

Table 43–1. Training and procedures for emergency medical personnel.

Emergency Personnel Type	Hours of Training	Curriculum[1]	Skills and Procedures

First Responder	~ 40	Patient assessment
		Basic life support
		  Cardiopulmonary resuscitation
		  Bleeding and shock
		Wounds and fractures
		Medical emergencies
		  Poisoning, drug and alcohol emergencies, heart attack, stroke, epilepsy, asthma, emergency childbirth
		Environmental emergencies
		  Burns
		Psychiatric emergencies
		Stabilization and transfer
			Patient assessment
			Cardiopulmonary resuscitation
			Control of bleeding
			Bandaging and limited splinting
			Limited extrication

EMT-A (Basic)	81–140	Orientation and legal responsibilities
		Patient assessment
		Cardiopulmonary resuscitation
		Bleeding and shock
		Injuries
		Medical emergencies
		  Heart disease, stroke, substance abuse, pediatric emergencies
		Childbirth
		Environmental emergencies
		  Burns, hazardous materials, water hazards
		Psychologic aspects of emergency care
		Patient handling and extrication
		Ambulance operations and vehicle maintenance
		  Emergency driving, communications, report writing
		Optional skills
		  Intravenous therapy, advanced airway management, defibrillation by EMTs
			Patient assessment
			Airway management and oxygen therapy
			Control of bleeding
			Management of shock (including Military Anti-shock Trousers [MAST])
			Dressing and bandaging wounds
			Splinting (including traction splints)
			Spinal immobilization
			Extrication and triage

EMT-I (Intermediate)	110–1000	All EMT-A skills plus various advanced life support skills	All EMT-A skills plus specialized training in one or more life support skills, usually including
			  Manual or automatic defibrillation
			  Intravenous therapy
			  Selected emergency medications
			  Advanced (noninvasive) airway management

EMT-P (Advanced or Paramedic)	>1000	Role of the paramedic
		Human systems and patient assessment
		Fluids and shock
		General pharmacology
		Respiratory system
		Cardiovascular system
		Central nervous system
		Soft tissue injuries
		Musculoskeletal system
		Medical emergencies
		Obstetric and gynecologic emergencies
		Pediatric emergencies
		Management of the emotionally disturbed
		Communications and telemetry
		Multiple injuries, multiple casualties, and triage
			All EMT-A skills plus specialized training in advanced life support skills, including[2]
			  Intravenous cannulation
			  Invasive airway management including endotracheal intubation
			  Cardiac dysrhythmia recognition
			  Defibrillation
			  Emergency medications

[1]First responder curriculum adapted and reproduced, with permission, from Karren KJ, Hafen BQ: *First Responder: A Skills Approach,* 2nd ed. Morton, 1986. EMT-P curriculum reproduced, with permission, from Caroline NL: *Emergency Care in the Streets,* 2nd ed. Little Brown, 1983.

[2]Advanced procedures vary widely among communities and may include procedures not listed here.

tools to help them reach and extricate persons who are trapped. Increasingly, first responders are being trained and equipped to perform defibrillation using semiautomated defibrillators.

B. Emergency Medical Technicians (EMTs): The National Registry of Emergency Medical Technicians currently recognizes 3 formal grades of EMTs according to the typical number of hours of training given, the breadth of skills covered, and the range of procedures authorized: EMT-A (basic), EMT-I (intermediate), and EMT-P (advanced, paramedic). An EMT-D is a basic EMT trained in manual or automatic defibrillation but not authorized to perform any other advanced skill.

1. EMT-A–Basic EMTs constitute the essential work force of EMS systems throughout the USA. Most state laws require at least one certified EMT on board ambulance vehicles that transport patients.

The basic EMT course requires at least 81 hours of training standardized by the Department of Transportation. Basic classes frequently exceed this minimum by up to 140 hours. Students learn basic principles of patient care, how to identify signs and symptoms central to patient assessment and diagnosis, and how to treat patients in specific emergencies. Optional training in the use of military antishock trousers (MAST) lengthens the basic class.

2. EMT-I–Intermediate EMTs commonly have completed the basic EMT course as well as some advanced life support skills such as inserting intravenous catheters, administering selected emergency medications, or using automatic or manual defibrillators or advanced noninvasive airway management devices (eg, Ambu bag).

3. EMT-P–Advanced EMTs (paramedics) receive over 1000 hours of training in advanced life support techniques. Their skills include the basic EMT procedures as well as intravenous cannulation, invasive airway management (including endotracheal intubation), recognition of cardiac dysrhythmias, defibrillation, and the use of specific emergency medications. In addition to extensive classroom training, EMT-P personnel also complete clinical training and a field internship with experienced paramedic teams.

Paramedics operate under standing orders and treatment protocols developed by a physician medical director that are usually broader and more advanced than those guiding basic EMTs. These determine the type and level of care administered at the emergency site. Physicians who provide on-line medical supervision of paramedics (by radio and telemetry) from base hospitals may permit paramedics to deviate from established protocols or to provide treatment not specifically covered in standing orders.

Types of EMS Systems

EMS personnel can be organized in various ways. Some systems may include several different grades of personnel operating in a coordinated fashion. There are 2 basic forms of EMS response: a single-response system and a layered- (or tiered-) response system. In a single-response system, there is only one grade of EMS unit, and any available unit may be dispatched to any nearby emergency. In a layered-response system, 2 or more grades of EMS personnel respond hierarchically (eg, first responder, then EMT-A, then EMT-P) as needed. Layered-response systems usually provide for an EMT-A response for all less severe reported medical emergencies, reserving an EMT-P response for severe or life-threatening incidents (Table 43–2).

Communications Network

The communications network is important in tying together the components of an EMS system. It usually consists of a radio system with telemetric capability for transmission of electrocardiographic traces. A dispatcher at a communications center receives a telephone request from a caller at the site of the emergency and dispatches mobile EMS personnel via the radio network. Prehospital treatment by the EMS unit at the scene is guided by radio network communication with an on-line supervising physician at the hospital. In many areas of the USA, an easily remembered emergency telephone number (9–1–1) provides the public with rapid access to the communications center. Some systems offer an "enhanced 9–1–1" ser-

Table 43–2. Alternative EMS system designs.[1]

System Type	Response		Transport	
	Emergency	Nonemergency	Emergency	Nonemergency
Single-tier BLS	BLS		BLS	
Single-tier ALS	ALS		ALS	
Single-tier ALS with first responder	First responder + ALS	ALS	ALS	
Multitier (transport) with first responder	First responder + ALS	ALS	ALS	BLS
Multitier (response and transport) with first responder	First responder + ALS	BLS	ALS	BLS

[1]BLS = EMT-A ambulance; ALS = EMT-P ambulance; First responder = first aid or semiautomated defibrillation.

vice that provides immediate callback and location information to the dispatcher.

Hospital Facilities & Staffing

EMS systems typically include hospitals with a variety of treatment capabilities, ranging from local community hospitals with limited emergency department staffing to large teaching hospitals in urban areas with emergency physicians, surgeons, anesthesiologists, and surgical teams available 24 hours a day. Hospital facilities are frequently classified according to their relationship to EMS mobile units and their ability to provide definitive care.

A. Base Station Hospitals: Physicians or specially trained nurses with physician backup in the emergency department of the base station hospital provide EMS units with ongoing medical supervision and direction during patient treatment. EMS units may be housed at the base station hospital, but this is not always necessary or feasible since the units are usually strategically deployed in the hospital's service area. In many EMS systems, the base station hospital may also be the one most capable of providing definitive follow-up care.

B. Receiving Hospitals: Receiving hospitals are facilities to which patients may be transported. For each patient the receiving hospital is selected according to its proximity, its capability to provide definitive care, and the preference of the patient, family members, or family physician, as long as transport to the hospital does not draw the EMS unit away from its primary service area.

C. Hospitals Categorized by Capability: Hospitals may be categorized by their ability to provide acute care as determined by the availability of physicians, nurses, allied health personnel, and other hospital resources (operating rooms, laboratory, blood bank, etc). Many categorization schemes exist, both nationally and locally. The Joint Commission on Accreditation of Hospitals has established the following 4 levels of emergency service:

1. Level I–This service offers emergency care 24 hours a day with at least one physician experienced in emergency care on duty in the emergency care area. In addition, there must be in-house physician coverage by residents at the senior level or higher for the medical, surgical, orthopedic, obstetric/gynecologic, pediatric, and anesthesiologic services.

2. Level II–This service offers emergency care 24 hours a day with at least one physician experienced in emergency care on duty in the emergency care area. Specialty consultation should be available within 30 minutes.

3. Level III–This service offers emergency care 24 hours a day with at least one physician on duty in the emergency care area available within 30 minutes through a medical staff call roster.

4. Level IV–This service is capable of performing a triage function and can administer lifesaving

first aid until transportation to the nearest appropriate facility is available.

D. Hospitals Categorized by Areas of Care: Hospitals can also be categorized by special areas of care (eg, trauma, burns, neonatal intensive care), especially where regionalization of services in these areas is practiced. The American College of Surgeons, for example, has established the following categorization of trauma facilities:

1. Level I–This designates a full-service trauma center that can provide optimal care of the trauma patient. One or more experienced emergency physicians, a general surgeon, anesthesiology services, laboratory, blood bank, and an operating room team must be available in-house 24 hours a day. All surgical subspecialty services should be immediately available on call. A commitment to education and research in trauma must also be demonstrated.

2. Level II–This trauma center is similar to a level I center but does not necessarily include a commitment to education or research. Occasionally, the most severe injuries or those needing highly specialized care may be transferred from a level II center to a level I center.

3. Level III–This trauma center does not have all of the resources available at a level I or level II center but may represent the highest level available in a given community. Usually, initial stabilization and lifesaving procedures are performed and the patient is then transferred to a level I or level II center.

EMS Administration

EMS systems may be administered through a variety of organizations, including local health departments, public safety agencies such as police or fire departments, hospitals, or privately owned provider agencies. Often several of these agencies operate EMS systems in the same area, and these are coordinated through an EMS regional council, which interacts with hospitals, public agencies, and physician medical directors, sets operational standards, and monitors performance (quality assurance).

Operation of the EMS System

One way to visualize the interplay between various components of the EMS system is to review the sequence of events surrounding a typical emergency medical incident. There are 4 major phases: (**1**) report of the emergency and activation of the EMS system; (**2**) dispatch of appropriate prehospital units; (**3**) medical evaluation and field treatment by EMS personnel; and (**4**) transport of the patient to the appropriate hospital.

A. Report of the Emergency: In many areas of the USA, a single, easily remembered telephone number (9–1–1) can now be used to request emergency help from the police and fire departments and to activate the EMS system.

B. Dispatch: Dispatchers receive the emergency

call, interrogate the caller to determine the type and severity of the emergency, and dispatch the appropriate type of emergency medical response. In systems with heavy call volumes, calls may be priority ranked and then dispatched in order of urgency of need and resource availability. In some systems, dispatchers are also trained EMTs or EMT paramedics who can offer advice to callers concerning how to assist patients pending the arrival of the emergency units (pre-arrival instructions). Algorithms may be employed to guide the dispatcher in decision making (Fig 43–1). Dispatchers in layered-response emergency medical systems frequently follow specific protocols in determining which type of EMS unit to dispatch (ie, ALS, BLS, first responder; see Table 43–2). Dispatchers

may also be trained to provide effective CPR instructions by telephone to callers reporting cardiac or respiratory arrest. Dispatch centers may also monitor hospital availability, manage the status and geographic deployment of EMS vehicles, and through computer-aided dispatch perform EMS management information and quality assurance functions.

C. Medical Evaluation and Treatment: Most EMS systems in urban and suburban areas are capable of responding within a few minutes of receiving an emergency call. First responders can frequently arrive at the scene within 3–6 minutes, and paramedics within 5–10 minutes of receiving the call. Survival following time-sensitive medical emergencies such as cardiac arrest is closely correlated with unit re-

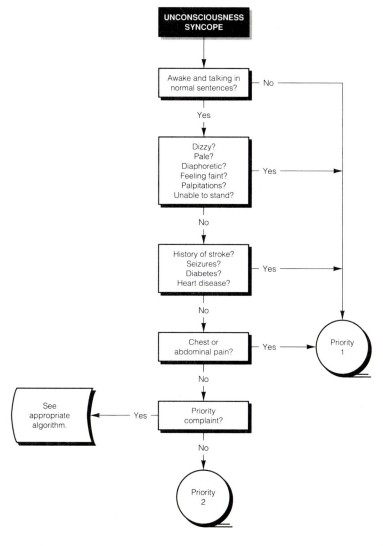

Figure 43–1. Sample algorithm to guide medical dispatchers when the subject's principal complaint or problem is unconsciousness or syncope.

sponse time, especially when basic EMTs have been trained in defibrillation. In layered-response systems, paramedics are held in reserve for such critical or life-threatening incidents, where their advanced skills may provide definitive or stabilizing care to patients. In some EMS systems, basic or intermediate EMT units are able to initiate advanced forms of treatment (eg, MAST garment application, defibrillation) before paramedic units arrive.

Upon arrival at the emergency scene, EMS personnel undertake patient assessment and examination (see below). EMT-paramedics may be authorized by standing orders to proceed with immediate patient care in cases of cardiac arrest or other life-threatening emergencies where quick action is critical. Following patient evaluation and, when needed, emergency stabilization and treatment, the EMS unit contacts the supervising emergency medical physician (or, in some states, a nurse) at the base station hospital by radio or telephone to describe the patient's condition and any treatment undertaken. The physician may give specific instructions for treatment at the scene or request immediate transport to the hospital for definitive care.

D. Transport: Transport of the patient to a nearby hospital is necessary in many EMS responses. The mode of transport (ground or air, with or without sirens or lights) depends on availability, stability of the patient's condition, transport time and distance, risks, etc. Hospital destination decisions are often guided by local protocols, with critically ill patients directed to the closest, most appropriate facility (special-care categories may apply). Noncritical cases may be transported to the hospital of the patient's choice.

1. Ground transport–Most patients are transported in surface ambulances. These vehicles vary slightly from state to state in their configuration and on-board equipment, but all follow guidelines set by the Department of Transportation. Ambulance drivers usually are allowed by local and state laws to violate certain traffic laws while carrying a patient in a life-threatening emergency if doing so does not jeopardize the lives of others. In the vast majority of cases, however, the patient's life is not in danger and posted speeds and traffic laws should be obeyed.

In some EMS systems, the responding unit is also the transporting unit. In others, especially layered-response systems, the responding unit may primarily evaluate and stabilize the patient and may summon another, lower-level unit or private ambulance to provide transport.

2. Air transport–Some EMS systems and regional trauma hospitals, particularly those serving large outlying rural areas, use helicopters or fixed-wing aircraft with trained medical teams on boards as additional resources for prehospital care and transportation. The majority are hospital-based, but some are operated by municipal or state governmental agencies. Where these services are unavailable, or when search and rescue missions are required, aircraft equipped for medical evacuation may be sent from local military bases, operating within the Military Assistance to Safety and Traffic (MAST) program.

Air ambulances are usually integrated into the EMS system and are activated according to certain locally established criteria. The decision to transport a patient by air requires careful consideration of the risks and benefits of air versus ground transport (see below).

Medical Supervision

A. On-Line Medical Direction: On-line medical direction is the direction given by radio to EMS personnel at the scene while prehospital care is being provided. It is usually given by emergency physicians or nurses at the base station hospital or receiving hospital. In many systems, there is a trend toward the use of standing orders, or written authorization to administer certain treatments under specific circumstances, *without* prior attempt at base contact by radio (Fig 43–2). This has the advantage of allowing treatment to begin as soon as possible when time is of the essence. However, systems that employ standing orders require effective monitoring, training, and quality assurance mechanisms.

B. Off-Line Medical Direction: Off-line medical direction is the overall direction of the activities of EMS personnel. It includes establishing protocols and standing orders, ensuring adequate training and skills, reviewing patient care records and voice tapes retrospectively, and reviewing performance and outcome data. Off-line medical direction is usually provided by a physician experienced in emergency services or by an agency in which physicians play an active role.

Performance Evaluation

System performance evaluation has many aspects, including the evaluation of input resources and operating guidelines (eg, protocol validation, personnel review, training assessment), evaluation of the process of delivering care in the field (eg, response times, service volume, treatment audits for adherence to protocols), and evaluation of the outcome of prehospital care (eg, complications, complaints, success in the performance of procedures, and patient survival). Outcome data are the most difficult to obtain.

PREHOSPITAL SKILLS & TECHNIQUES

Field Assessment

EMTs responding to a call usually have certain dispatch information, including the location, the nature of the complaint, and the number of patients. Upon

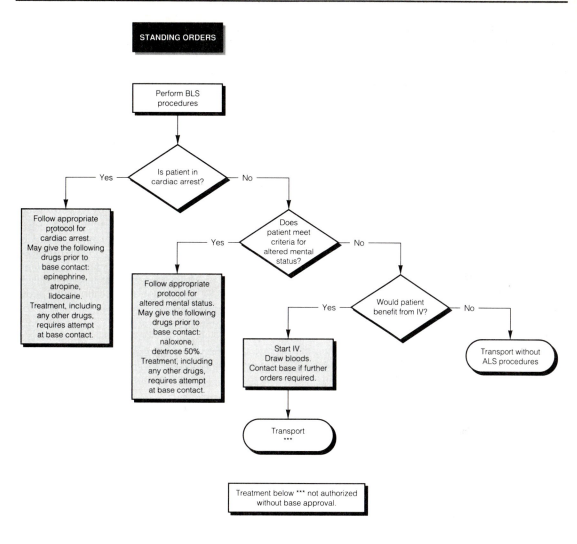

Figure 43–2. Standing orders for treatments and procedures that may be performed without prior attempt at base station contact by radio. BLS = EMT-A ambulance; ALS = EMT-P ambulance.

arrival, they must quickly determine the presence of hazards to themselves and the patient, ascertain the probable mechanism of injury, and identify other patients, if any. Support can be summoned for hazard suppression or additional medical assistance. Patients who are conscious and in minimal distress may be able to provide historical information. Information may also be obtained from witnesses or family members. Patients who are very ill, however, require an immediate survey assessment. This is brief, particularly in victims of trauma, and follows established priorities.

A. Primary Survey: The primary survey as-

sesses *responsiveness, airway patency, adequacy of breathing and circulation, and presence of profuse bleeding.* The purpose is to identify patients in need of immediate resuscitative measures, such as cardiopulmonary resuscitation or emergency intervention (eg, airway control, chest decompression).

B. Secondary Survey: The secondary survey consists of a comprehensive head-to-toe survey, including assessment of vital signs, and an interview of the patient and any witnesses or family members to obtain a history. The purpose is to detect any problem that may not be life-threatening but will need further evaluation or field treatment.

Field Treatment

A. Airway Control: Methods of airway control (p 855) depend on the level of skill and certification of the EMT. Initial steps to provide an airway include positioning the jaw and suctioning secretions (taking care in the trauma victim not to hyperextend the neck). Should this fail to achieve and maintain airway patency, and the basic EMT can insert an oral or nasal airway. Ventilation may be assisted by an Ambu bag.

In many states, basic EMTs are also trained to control the airway by inserting the esophageal obturator airway (EOA) or the esophageal gastric tube airway (EGTA). However, these devices are not universally accepted by physicians, most of whom are not experienced with their use or proper removal. Also, alveolar ventilation may, at times, be inadequate with these devices, and cases of esophageal rupture have been reported. Recently, the pharyngotracheal lumen airway has been introduced as a safer and more effective method of airway control in the hands of EMTs (Chapter 1). Experience is not yet widespread.

Endotracheal intubation is the preferred method of airway control in patients with inadequate ventilation. This skill is typically learned at the paramedic level and performed either by the oral route with direct visualization or by the blind nasotracheal route. Studies have shown that paramedics trained to perform endotracheal intubations have a nearly 90% success rate in the field.

B. Emergency Cardiac Care (ECC):

1. Cardiopulmonary resuscitation (CPR)– The probability of survival for victims of sudden cardiac arrest is inversely related to the elapsed time before an effective cardiac rhythm is reestablished. CPR is a temporizing measure which, when initiated within 4–6 minutes, increases the chances of survival. In most systems, a paramedic unit cannot routinely reach the scene within this period. In some systems, fire fighters trained as EMTs and police officers trained in CPR can provide basic life support as first responders within this time period until EMS units arrive.

2. Defibrillation– Ventricular fibrillation is the initial rhythm encountered in many victims of sudden death. The sooner defibrillation is performed, the higher the survival rate. Automatic defibrillators (Laerdal Heartstart 2000, others) can recognize ventricular fibrillation (or tachycardia) and deliver a countershock. The rescuer need not be able to recognize dysrhythmias but must be able to recognize cardiac arrest and operate the device. Automatic defibrillators have enabled nonparamedic first responders to provide rapid defibrillation and have consequently improved survival rates. An EMT who has passed the 4- to 8-hour EMT automatic defibrillation training course is certified as an EMT-D. Paramedics may perform manual defibrillation, a method that allows greater flexibility but requires more skill.

3. External pacing– External pacing devices (Zoll, others) deliver an electrical pacing spike through electrodes placed on the anterior and posterior surfaces of the thorax. They are easy to apply and operate and have been used by EMTs in prehospital treatment. While useful for patients in complete heart block, these devices have not, unfortunately, been shown to improve survival rates in victims of asystolic (agonal bradycardia) cardiac arrest. This may be due to the extensive myocardial damage present in this type of cardiac arrest.

C. Specialized Support Equipment:

1. Pneumatic antishock garment–(See also Fig 46–40.) The pneumatic antishock garment known as military antishock trousers (MAST) is an inflatable device that increases peripheral resistance below the level of the diaphragm. In the patient with shock it may increase systolic blood pressure and improve blood flow to the brain and myocardium. Most EMS systems are equipped with MAST garments, which are supplied by EMTs and paramedics under protocol, mainly for patients with hypovolemic shock. The MAST garment should be removed *only* after the patient is hemodynamically stable. It should be deflated gradually, abdominal compartment first, with ongoing monitoring of vital signs. Despite widespread use, the MAST garment has not been demonstrated to improve survival statistics, and its value is not universally accepted.

2. Mechanical resuscitators– Mechanical resuscitators (Thumper, others) are devices that perform mechanical chest compressions by means of a gas-powered piston positioned over the patient's sternum. A ventilator feature can also be used to inflate the lungs. They may be of value in preventing rescuer fatigue when resuscitation is prolonged, when it must be provided in a confined space, or when it must continue while the patient is moved (eg, down stairways). The device must be carefully monitored, however, to ensure proper functioning and piston position.

3. Mechanical ventilators– Compact gas-powered ventilators are often available for long-distance transport but are seldom used in urban prehospital care. Manually controlled positive pressure ventilators connected to a face mask or endotracheal tube are sometimes used to ventilate in tight spaces, during extrication, etc. However, routine use should be avoided, since they provide the rescuer no tactile feedback about airway resistance and may easily exceed the lower esophageal sphincter pressure and force part of the delivered air volume into the stomach.

D. Invasive Procedures:

1. Venous catheterization–(See Chapter 46.) The use of intravenous techniques by EMS field personnel is usually limited to cannulation of peripheral veins of the upper extremities. In most EMS systems, the procedure can be initiated under standing orders, when certain criteria are met, by intermediate or paramedic EMTs or basic EMTs who have had special training in intravenous techniques and fluid therapy. Studies have demonstrated that skilled paramedics in the field are able to start an intravenous line in approximately 3 minutes and achieve a success rate greater than 90%. However, when transport times are short (ie, 10 minutes or less), venous catheterization is usually unnecessary since it is unlikely that the volume of fluid infused or the medications administered during such a short period will be lifesaving. In addition, field placement of intravenous lines may increase the chances of infection. Needlestick injuries, which may occur during venous cannulation under adverse circumstances, such as in the back of a moving ambulance, are an increasing concern.

2. Needle thoracostomy–Chest decompression for suspected tension pneumothorax may occasionally be lifesaving and is performed by paramedics in some systems, usually after approval by the base physician via radio. A 14- or 16-gauge catheter-clad needle is inserted into the fourth intercostal space along the anterior axillary line immediately above the subjacent rib using sterile technique. The catheter is sealed with a Heimlich valve or a latex glove with the fingertip removed. (The open fingertip of the glove is secured around the catheter, allowing air to escape but preventing its reentry.)

3. Cricothyrotomy–(See Chapter 46.) Emergency surgical entry to the airway may be lifesaving in cases of supraglottic airway obstruction or laryngeal trauma. Cricothyrotomy may be performed by paramedics in some EMS systems, usually after approval by the base physician via radio. Because the procedure can be unexpectedly difficult, it should be performed as a last resort and only by properly trained personnel.

E. Extrication: Extrication is the process of removing a patient from a condition of entrapment, usually from a motor vehicle. It requires considerable skill and experience. Often, special tools are necessary, such as heavy bolt and metal cutters or large, powered spreading devices ("Jaws of Life," Hurst Tool, etc). In most EMS systems, when there is a report of a trapped victim, a fire rescue team is dispatched in addition to the EMS unit to clear fire hazards, wash away spilled gasoline, and provide additional heavy equipment and personnel.

As soon as the patient is accessible with minimal risk to emergency workers, the primary survey should be initiated while further efforts to free the patient continue. Once the patient is immobilized in place, emergency resuscitation can begin.

F. Immobilization and Splinting:

1. Immobilization–Victims of trauma may have injuries to the spine or extremities which, if manipulated, can lead to spinal cord or limb damage. Upon reaching a trauma victim, the rescue team must stabilize the cervical spine. If the patient is in the front seat of a motor vehicle, this can be accomplished by one rescuer in the rear seat grasping the patient's head and neck from behind and applying gentle axial traction while coworkers apply a rigid cervical collar and place a long spine board alongside the patient. The patient is then lifted (or logrolled) onto the spine board, with manual cervical spine traction maintained throughout. Spine boards are sometimes difficult to maneuver in closed spaces, but alternative devices are available, including the short spine board and flexible devices such as the Kendrick Extrication Device (KED) and the XP1. Immobilization is not considered complete until the patient is secured to the spine board with straps, the patient's head is secured to the spine board with tape across the forehead and beneath the chin, and a cervical collar and lateral neck rolls or sandbags are in place.

If endotracheal control intubation is necessary, the cervical spine should remain immobilized while it is performed. Should vomiting occur, the patient may be logrolled to face sideways while one rescuer maintains cervical spine traction.

2. Splinting–(See Chapters 22 and 23.) In general, extremities should be placed in an anatomic position, especially if pulses cannot be felt below a suspected fracture. If the patient protests or if resistance is felt, extremities should remain in a position of comfort. Reduction of fracture dislocations at a joint should be attempted only if there is impending vascular compromise, the duration of transport is long, and the rescuer is experienced in the technique. This usually requires approval by the base physician.

A pillow, rolled-up blanket, or other material may often serve as a simple splint. Specific splinting devices include cardboard splints, inflatable air splints, the MAST garment, and traction splints. Care must be taken with inflatable devices to monitor distal perfusion, since a compartment syndrome may occur with swelling of the extremity or changes in atmospheric pressure (eg, during air transport). Traction splints are used primarily with fractures of the femur.

G. Protocols and Standing Orders: Protocols are guidelines designed to assist the EMT in performing tasks in a complete and orderly fashion (Fig 43–3). Since actual situations vary widely and protocols cannot anticipate every variable, they are not meant to be absolute and must be accompanied by training, judgment, and experience. Each EMS system tailors its protocols to the training and skill of its EMTs and the needs of the local medical community.

Standing orders are express authorizations for the performance of a specific task or procedure. Under the standing order, an EMT may be authorized directly (or by applicable state regulations) to perform a task or procedure without first obtaining verbal authorization by radio. Standing orders are useful when radio contact is impractical or would delay lifesaving intervention (eg, CPR, defibrillation). Standing orders usually contain a clear list of circumstances under which the authorization applies (indications)

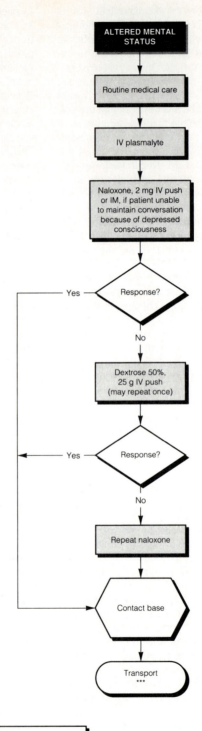

Figure 43–3. Sample protocol (in algorithmic form) for altered mental status. ***Note:*** The sequence for administering naloxone or glucose should be based on history and physical examination at the scene.

Treatment below *** not authorized without base approval.

***
Base hospital MD order only: Glucagon, 1 mg IM, if unable to establish IV.

Legend: Sample protocol (in algorithmic form) for altered mental status.

and detailed instructions on the manner in which the procedure should be performed. They are signed by the physician medical director, who shares legal responsibility for the outcome.

H. Communications:

1. Equipment and frequencies–EMS units communicate with receiving hospitals by various methods. In large cities, the field unit usually first contacts a medical communications center or relay station on a designated UHF or VHF radio frequency. The communications center may then assign the call to a different medical frequency ("channel") and "patch" the transmission into dedicated ground lines to the appropriate hospital. Communication is simplex; ie, signals pass in only one direction at a time, and neither party can simultaneously speak and be heard. In rural areas, communication may be direct, via radio, without a relay station or ground lines.

2. Communication technique–Radio communication must provide information in a concise, precise, and easily understood manner. To facilitate speed and understanding, a common format is followed, with slight variations depending on the community. However, no one should hesitate to ask for clarification, as misunderstandings may prove fatal.

a. The initial contact–The caller always names the party being called first, followed by the caller's own identification:

"Central Hospital, this is medic 19, how do you copy?"

b. The initial response–The initial response confirms the contact in the same manner:

"Medic 19, Central Hospital, receiving you loud and clear, over."

c. The report–The caller gives a concise, orderly report containing pertinent history, physical findings, destination, estimated time of arrival (ETA), and any necessary request for instructions. It should be as brief as possible:

"Central Hospital, medic 19 en route to your location, ETA 8 minutes, with a 20-year-old male victim of multiple, small-caliber gunshot wounds to the left chest, right flank, and right thigh. Patient is lethargic; blood pressure 80, pulse 140, respirations 46. Breath sounds absent over the left chest, abdomen soft. We have an ET tube in place, 2 IVs with lactated Ringer's wide open, and MAST garment inflated. Requesting permission for needle decompression of the left chest."

d. The report acknowledgment–This acknowledgment is kept brief; only essential queries should be made:

"Medic 19, have you checked ET tube position?"

"That's affirmative. Withdrawn 3 centimeters without improvement."

"Okay, medic 19; needle thoracostomy, left chest, is approved. Will stand by for update."

e. The sign-off–After receiving an order, the field personnel should repeat it to demonstrate that it was received accurately before signing off:

"Central Hospital, understand needle thoracostomy, left chest, is approved. Stand by."

3. 10-Codes–Ten-codes are phrases represented by 2 numbers, the first being 10 (Table 43–3). In many areas, these are used to ensure precise communication and to add some measure of privacy to the conversation. Unfortunately, few EMS personnel have all the possible 10-codes memorized. The result is often more confusion rather than less. Since mistakes may be dangerous, the codes should not be used unless thoroughly understood by all parties.

4. Telemetry–Receiving hospitals and ambulances may have equipment designed for the transmission of electrocardiographic traces (telemetry). This equipment is seldom used, however, because well-trained paramedics have shown the ability to interpret unstable rhythms (eg, ventricular fibrillation, ventricular tachycardia, bradycardia, and asystole) with acceptable precision, and more complex rhythms (eg, supraventricular tachycardia) rarely require treatment that cannot be postponed until arrival at the hospital. Studies are currently under way to assess the use of 12-lead electrocardiographic traces transmitted from the field to the hospital via cellular telephone to enable hospital-based physicians to direct thrombolytic therapy in the prehospital setting.

I. Air Transport:

1. Indications–As noted above, the benefits to the patient must outweigh the risks inherent in this mode of transport. Aeromedical transport is most advantageous when great distances must be covered rapidly, when ground transport is unavailable or impeded by geographic obstacles or dense traffic, or when specialized care (eg, trauma resuscitation) is needed at the scene or en route. Emergency medical helicopters serving rural areas often provide a higher level of care and more skilled procedures (eg, intubation, needle thoracostomy, cricothyrotomy) than are provided by localized services using basic EMTs. However, air transport is hazardous and helicopters operating at night and in inclement weather have crashed.

2. Requesting service–Helicopters equipped for medical evacuation can be requested, through the EMS communications network, from an area hospital that offers such services or from a local military base

Table 43–3. Common 10-codes.

10–4	Acknowledged (OK)
10–6	Busy at this time
10–7	Out of service
10–8	Back in service
10–9	Repeat message
10–20	What is your location?
10–23	Stand by
10–24	Police assistance needed
10–96	En route to scene
10–97	Arrival at scene
10–98	Departing scene, en route to hospital

that participates in the Military Assistance to Safety and Traffic (MAST) program.

3. Patient preparation–Before departure the patient should be stabilized on a spine board and immobilized as clinically indicated. Airway tubes and intravenous catheters should be secured. In the trauma patient, a MAST garment should be in place (not necessarily inflated) and a nasogastric tube inserted, time permitting, to minimize aspiration of gastric contents.

4. Anticipated physiologic consequences of air transport–

a. Hypoxia–Atmospheric pressure decreases with increasing altitude, as does the partial pressure of oxygen. Patients with existing heart or lung disease may suffer adverse consequences. Supplemental oxygen is required.

b. Expansion of trapped gas–The volume of trapped gas increases with decreasing barometric pressure. Thus, as altitude increases, air may expand in endotracheal tube cuffs, air splints, MAST garments, the bowel lumen, the stomach, pneumothoraces, abscess cavities, and the bottles and tubing of intravenous infusion apparatus. These compartments must be monitored frequently and vented as necessary. Intravenous flow rates should be adjusted accordingly.

c. Motion, noise, and vibration–These may cause patient discomfort. Forward acceleration with the patient's head forward may cause transient hypotension. This may be prevented by positioning the patient with feet forward.

5. Helicopter safety–

a. Site selection and lighting–A helicopter landing site should be level, approximately 100 feet square, and free of obstacles (eg, trees, wires) to approach and departure. It should also be clear of loose debris. The site should be secure from bystanders. At night, the site should be well lighted (eg, with vehicle headlights) but lights should never be directed upward toward the approaching helicopter, because they might interfere with the pilot's vision.

b. Approaching a helicopter–While the rotor blades are turning, the aircraft should be approached only from the front and only after prompting by the pilot. The tail rotor should be carefully avoided. Approach in a crouched position. Do not run. Never approach from uphill.

Tall objects such as poles associated with intravenous infusion apparatus should be lowered. Sheets, hats, and loose clothing should be secured. All smoking material should be extinguished.

REFERENCES

Bickell WH et al: Randomized trial of pneumatic antishock garments in the prehospital management of penetrating abdominal injuries. Ann Emerg Med 1987;16:653.

Cales RH: Trauma mortality in Orange County: The effect of implementation of a regional trauma system. Ann Emerg Med 1984;13:1.

Caroline NL: *Emergency Care in the Streets,* 3rd ed. Little, Brown, 1987.

Champion HR et al: Trauma score. Crit Care Med 1981;9:672.

Copass MK, Eisenberg MS, Macdonald SC: *The Paramedic Manual,* 2nd ed. Saunders, 1987.

Cummins RO et al: Survival of out-of-hospital cardiac arrest with early initiation of cardiopulmonary resuscitation. Am J Emerg Med 1985;3:114.

Cwinn AA et al: Prehospital advanced trauma life support for critical blunt trauma victims. Ann Emerg Med 1987;16:399.

Eisenberg MS, Hearne T: Prehospital emergency care in the USA: Effectiveness of paramedic and emergency medical technicians units. In: *Acute Phase of Ischemic Heart Disease and Myocardial Infarction.* Adgey AJ (editor). Martinus Nijhoff, 1982.

Eisenberg MS et al: Treatment of out-of-hospital cardiac arrests with rapid defibrillation by emergency medical technicians. N Engl J Med 1980;302:1379.

Fortner GS et al: The effects of prehospital trauma care on survival from a 50-meter fall. J Trauma 1983;23:976.

Gervin AS, Fischer RP: The importance of prompt transport in salvage of patients with penetrating heart wounds. J Trauma 1982;22:443.

Heckman JD et al (editors): *Emergency Care and Transportation of the Sick and Injured,* 4th ed. American Academy of Orthopedic Surgeons, 1986.

Hedges JR, Sacco WJ, Champion HR: An analysis of prehospital care of blunt trauma. J Trauma 1982;22:989.

Hedges JR et al: Factors contributing to paramedic on-scene time during evaluation and management of blunt trauma. Am J Emerg Med 1988;6:443.

Honigman B et al: Prehospital advanced life support for penetrating cardiac wounds. Ann Emerg Med 1990;19:145.

Jacobs LM et al: Prehospital advanced life support: Benefits in trauma. J Trauma 1984;24:8.

Karren KJ, Hafen BQ: *First Responder: A Skills Approach,* 2nd ed. Morton, 1986.

Kuehl A (editor): *National Association of EMS Physicians EMS Medical Director's Handbook.* Mosby, 1989.

Lewis RP, Stang JM, Warren JV: The role of paramedics in resuscitation of patients with prehospital cardiac arrest from coronary artery disease. Am J Emerg Med 1984;2:200.

Peacock JB, Blackwell VH, Wainscott M: Medical reliability of advanced prehospital cardiac life support. Ann Emerg Med 1985;14:407.

Pointer JE et al: The impact of standing orders on medication and skill selection, paramedic assessment, and hospital outcome: A follow-up report. Prehospital and Disaster Medicine 1991;6:303.

Romano TL et al: Paramedic services: Nationwide distribution and management structure. JACEP 1978;7:99.

Roush WR (editor): *Principles of EMS Systems.* American College of Emergency Physicians, 1989.

Slovis CM et al: A priority dispatch system for emergency medical services. Ann Emerg Med 1985;14:1055.

Soper RG et al: *EMT Handbook.* Saunders, 1984.

Standards and guidelines for cardiopulmonary resuscitation (CPR) and emergency cardiac care (ECC). JAMA 1986;255:2905.

Stewart RD: Prehospital care of trauma. Trauma Q 1985; 1:1.

Stults KR et al: Prehospital defibrillation performed by emergency medical technicians in rural communities. N Engl J Med 1984;310:219.

Weaver WD et al: Use of the automatic external defibrillator in the management of out-of-hospital cardiac arrest. N Engl J Med 1988;319:661.

44

Multicasualty Incidents & Disasters

Charles E. Saunders, MD, FACEP, FACP

Multicasualty incidents and disasters share a common principle. Both situations suddenly and unexpectedly produce victims of sufficient number and severity that local emergency medical resources are overwhelmed and special organization and resources are required. Although exact terminology varies, a **multicasualty incident** usually refers to an isolated, geographically focused event which produces a limited number of casualties that are managed within a community. The term **disaster** implies a more destructive event which produces a large number of casualties and which damages the social and physical environment of a community or region. Management of the event requires resources and assistance from sources outside the community.

The American College of Emergency Physicians (ACEP) has suggested the following terminology to categorize such events.

Level 1: A localized multiple casualty emergency wherein local medical resources are available and adequate to provide for triage, field medical treatment, and stabilization, including triage. The patients will be transported to the appropriate local medical facility for further diagnosis and treatment.

Level 2: A multiple casualty emergency where the large number of casualties or lack of local medical care facilities are such as to require multijurisdictional (regional) medical mutual aid.

Level 3: A mass casualty emergency wherein local and regional medical resource capabilities are exceeded or overwhelmed. Deficiencies in medical supplies and personnel are such as to require assistance from state or federal agencies.

EPIDEMIOLOGY OF DISASTERS

Specific types of disasters produce different patterns and numbers of injuries and have different effects on the social and physical environment. By understanding them and anticipating their potential effects on a community, effective mitigation and preparedness may be possible.

NATURAL DISASTERS

Natural disasters are events caused by natural forces and geophysical events. With the exception of war, these are historically the most common types of large-scale events (Table 44–1).

Earthquakes

An earthquake is the most likely large-scale event in the USA. There have been 6 major earthquakes greater than 8.0 on the Richter scale in United States history (New Madrid, 1811; Fort Tejon, 1857; Owens Valley, 1872; Charleston, 1886; San Francisco, 1906; and Alaska, 1964). Although they most commonly occur along the margins of tectonic plates, other areas have experienced earthquakes as well (Fig 44–1). Worldwide, there are approximately one million earthquakes per year, although only a small number produce significant casualties. In the 20th century, 1.3 million people have died in earthquakes, with the

Table 44–1. Sudden natural disasters causing 10,000 or more deaths from 1946–1985.[1]

Year	Event	Location	Approximate Death Toll
1949	Floods	China	57,000
1954	Floods	China	40,000
1960	Earthquake	Morocco	12,000
1962	Earthquake	Iran	12,000
1963	Tropical cyclone	Bangladesh	22,000
1965	Tropical cyclone	Bangladesh	17,000
1965	Tropical cyclone	Bangladesh	30,000
1965	Tropical cyclone	Bangladesh	10,000
1968	Earthquake	Iran	12,000
1970	Earthquake/ avalanche	Peru	70,000
1970	Tropical cyclone	Bangladesh	250,000–500,000
1971	Tropical cyclone	India	10,000–25,000
1976	Earthquake	China	225,000–650,000
1976	Earthquake	Guatemala	24,000
1977	Tropical cyclone	India	20,000
1978	Earthquake	Iran	25,000
1985	Tropical cyclone	Bangladesh	10,000
1985	Earthquake	Mexico	10,000
1985	Volcanic eruption	Colombia	22,000

[1]Reproduced, with permission, from Bernstein AB, Thompson P: The natural history of natural hazards. In: *Management of Wilderness and Environmental Emergencies*. Auerbach PS, Geehr EC (editors). Mosby, 1989.

Table 44–2. The deadliest earthquakes worldwide from 1900 to 1988.[1]

No. Killed	Place	Date
242,500	Tangshan, China	1976
200,000	Kansu, China	1920
142,800	Kanto, Japan	1923
66,800	Ankash, Peru	1970
58,000	Mossina, Italy	1908
40,900	Tsinghai, China	1927
32,700	Erzincan, Turkey	1939
32,600	Avezzano, Italy	1915
28,000	Chillán, Chile	1939
25,000	Quetta, Pakistan	1935
24,900	Armenia, USSR	1988
23,000	Guatemala City	1976
382,800 (29%)	Others	
1,300,000 (Total)		

[1]Reproduced, with permission, from Smith GS: Research issues in the epidemiology of injuries following earthquakes. In: *International Workshop on Earthquake Injury Epidemiology from Mitigation and Response*. Johns Hopkins Univ, 1989.

disruption of existing community infrastructure (food supply, power, sanitation, ongoing support for persons with chronic disease, etc). Predictably, the patterns of injury seen among casualties include lacerations, contusions, fractures, head and spinal cord injuries, burns, effects of exposure, infection, and exacerbation of chronic medical problems. The speed of rescue efforts has an important bearing on the outcome (Fig 44–2).

Tropical Cyclones (Hurricanes, Typhoons, & Tropical Cyclones)

Tropical cyclones (hurricanes in the USA and Atlantic; typhoons in the eastern Pacific; tropical cyclones elsewhere) are a circulating mass of clouds, rain, and wind around a clear central area of extreme low-barometric pressure. They occur most commonly in the late summer months. The most destructive tend to occur in the Indian Ocean (eg, in 1970, a tropical cyclone stuck Bangladesh, killing over 250,000). The most significant hurricanes of the 20th century in the USA are shown in Table 44–4.

The intensity of tropical cyclones is rated on a 5-point scale (Table 44–5); for hurricanes approaching the USA, this information is available from the National Weather Service, which can also provide information about the storm's probable path. Damage is commonly due to high winds, which can be in excess of 150 mph, torrential rain, and high seas, which may produce flooding and soil instability (eg, landslides).

Casualties may be caused by several factors, including trauma from flying debris, structural collapse, and evacuation and repair activities, from drowning, from famine related to damaged agriculture and food distribution systems, from disease related to loss of power, water, and sanitation, and occasionally from violence related to loss of public

majority of deaths occurring in 12 single events (Table 44–2).

Earthquake intensity is commonly measured in one of 2 ways. The **Richter scale** is a logarithmic scale that measures the intensity of seismic waves based on seismographic measurements. An earthquake of 2.0 magnitude is barely felt, whereas an 8.0 magnitude event is greatly destructive. The **modified Mercalli intensity scale** measures earthquakes subjectively by amount of ground movement felt by eyewitnesses and destruction caused to ground structures (Table 44–3). An earthquake of a given magnitude may produce varying amounts of destruction, depending on a complex interaction of many factors, including the type of ground underlying a structure, the degree of ground failure (eg, landslide, soil failures), and the construction quality of overlying structures.

Casualties can be predicted for an earthquake of a given magnitude at a specified location using computer-based casualty prediction models. These models take into account seismic, geophysical, structural, and demographic factors to yield an estimate of the expected number of casualties. They are notoriously inaccurate. Injuries are most often due to structural collapse with crush injuries, being struck by falling debris, fire, and falls. Illness also occurs as a result of

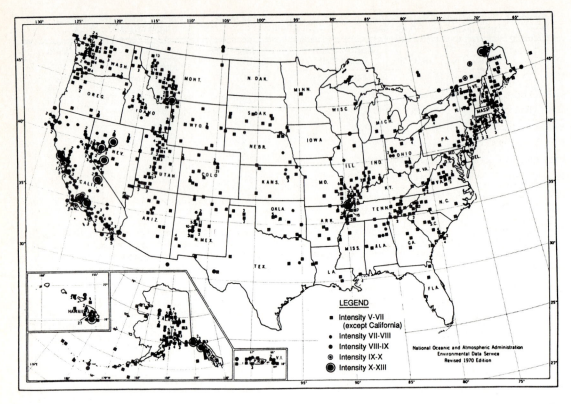

Figure 44–1. Epicenters of significant earthquakes in the USA, 1970. (Reproduced from: Centers for Disease Control: *The Public Health Consequences of Disasters*. United States Department of Health and Human Services Public Health Service, Centers for Disease Control, 1989.)

safety. Studies of emergency departments following a hurricane, however, show increased visits in a large variety of complaint categories, which trend may last days to months. Casualties may be reduced by effective early warning systems and evacuation efforts.

Tornadoes & Severe Storms

On an annual basis, tornadoes and severe thunderstorms are the most common cause of death due to natural disasters. In the USA, approximately 100,000 severe storms (eg, thunder, high winds, and hail) occur each year, including 1000 tornadoes. Most commonly affected are the midwestern and southern United States (Fig 44–3), usually during the summer months, and during late afternoons. The most deadly occurred in Missouri, Illinois, and Indiana, with 689 deaths. However, only about 3–4% of all tornadoes produce injury, with most deaths occurring in a small number of highly destructive events. Over the past 50 years, 9000 people have lost their lives to tornadoes.

Thunderstorms and tornadoes are caused by unstable air produced by convection currents associated with rapid heating of the earth's surface or by advancing low pressure cells. They may occur unpredictably on a hot summer afternoon, or along a squall line associated with an advancing front. Tornadoes

are characterized by a circulating funnel-shaped air mass with wind speeds up to 300 mph. They may be small, lasting only a few minutes over a path 1–2 miles long, or may less commonly last several hours and travel 100 miles or more. Destruction is caused by high winds lifting, tearing, or hurling structures and debris.

Casualties are related to trauma from structural collapse, flying debris, or being knocked to the ground or thrown. Head injuries, crush injuries, fractures, contusions, and lacerations are common. As with all disasters, secondary illness and injury may occur, although tornadoes most commonly tend to produce random, isolated groups of casualties wherever they touch down, rather than diffuse area-wide casualties and destruction to community infrastructure. Casualty mitigation through early warning and evacuation is hard to manage, since tornadoes are difficult to predict and the time frame for evacuation or protective cover is brief.

Floods

Floods are typically seasonal and result from one of several causes: (1) excessive rains or snow melts that lead to rivers overflowing their banks in a floodplain area, (2) tsunamis (tidal waves) or hurricanes in

Table 44–3. Modified Mercalli Earthquake Intensity scale, with associated relationship to the Richter magnitude.[1]

I. Not felt. Marginal and long-period effects of large earthquakes.

II. Felt by persons at rest, on upper floors, or favorably placed.

III. Felt indoors. Hanging objects swing. Vibration like passing of light trucks. Duration estimated. May not be recognized as an earthquake.

IV. Hanging objects swing. Vibration like passing of heavy trucks, or sensation of a jolt like a heavy ball striking the walls. Standing motor cars rock. Windows, dishes, doors rattle. Glasses clink. Crockery clashes. In the upper range of IV, wooden walls and frame creak.

V. Felt outdoors; direction estimated. Sleepers wakened. Liquids disturbed, some spilled. Small unstable objects displaced or upset. Doors swing, close, open. Shutters, pictures move. Pendulum clocks stop, start, change rate.

VI. Felt by all. Many frightened and run outdoors. Persons walk unsteadily. Windows, dishes, glassware broken. Knickknacks, books, etc., off shelves. Pictures off walls. Furniture moved or overturned. Weak plaster and masonry D cracked. Small bells ring (church, school). Trees, bushes shaken visibly or heard to rustle.

VII. Difficult to stand. Noticed by drivers of motor cars. Hanging objects quiver. Furniture broken. Damage to masonry D, including cracks. Weak chimney broken at roof line. Fall of plaster, loose bricks, stones, tiles, cornices, also unbraced parapets and architectural ornaments. Some cracks in masonry C. Waves on ponds; water turbid with mud. Small slides and caving in along sand or gravel banks. Large bells ring. Concrete irrigation ditches damaged.

VIII. Steering of motor cars affected. Damage to masonry C; partial collapse. Some damage to masonry B; none to masonry A. Fall of stucco and some masonry walls. Twisting, fall of chimneys, factory stacks, monuments, towers, elevated tanks. Frame houses moved on foundations if not bolted down; loose panel walls thrown out. Decayed piling broken off. Branches broken from trees. Changes in flow or temperature of springs and wells. Cracks in wet ground and on steep slopes.

IX. General panic. Masonry D destroyed; masonry C heavily damaged, sometimes with complete collapse; masonry B seriously damaged. General damage to foundations. Frame structures, if not bolted, shifted off foundations. Frames racked. Serious damage to reservoirs. Underground pipes broken. Conspicuous cracks in ground. In alluviated areas, sand and mud ejected, earthquake fountains, sand craters.

X. Most masonry and frame structures destroyed with their foundations. Some well-built wooden structures and bridges destroyed. Serious damage to dams, dikes, embankments. Large landslides. Water thrown on banks of canals, rivers, lakes, etc. Sand and mud shifted horizontally on beaches and flat land. Rails bent slightly.

XI. Rails bent greatly. Underground pipelines completely out of service.

XII. Damage nearly total. Large rock masses displaced. Lines of sight and level distorted. Objects thrown into the air.

	Approximate relationship between magnitude and intensity			
Richter Magnitude	**Energy Released (ergs)**	**Felt Area (sq mi)**	**Disturbance Felt**	**Maximum Modified Mercalli Intensity**
3.0–3.9	9.5×10^{15} – 4.0×10^{17}	750	15	II–III
4.0–4.9	6.0×10^{17} – 8.8×10^{18}	3,000	30	IV–V
5.0–5.9	9.5×10^{18} – 4.0×10^{20}	15,000	70	VI–VII
6.0–6.9	6.0×10^{20} – 8.8×10^{21}	50,000	125	VII–VIII
7.0–7.9	9.5×10^{22} – 4.0×10^{23}	200,000	250	IX–X
8.0–8.9	6.0×10^{23} – 8.8×10^{24}	800,000	450	XI–XII

[1]Reproduced, with permission, from Hammond DJ: A course in structural aspects of urban heavy rescue. In: *International Workshop on Earthquake Injury Epidemiology from Mitigation and Response.* Johns Hopkins Univ, 1989.

low-lying coastal areas, **(3)** flash floods in flat areas where rainfall produces surface water that exceeds the runoff or absorptive capacity of the soil, or failure of a dike or dam, usually due to heavy rains.

In the USA, the number of deaths each year from floods is small and sporadic. An exception was the 1976 Thompson Canyon flash flood in which 139 people died owing to inadequate early evacuation and the closed nature of the canyon. However, property damage can be considerable, as are secondary effects on crops, sanitation, and vector-borne infections. When casualties occur, they are usually due to drowning.

By contrast, developing countries with poor watershed management and rapid growth of agriculture and urban development on floodplains have seen large numbers of casualties in isolated events. Casu-alties from secondary effects, such as famine, have occasionally been large (eg, Bangladesh).

Mitigation (eg, through watershed engineering projects and limiting development on floodplains) and early warning are the most effective means of reducing deaths.

Tsunamis

Tsunamis are tidal waves due to sudden geologic events occurring at sea, such as earthquakes and volcanic eruptions. A resultant giant wave of water is produced that may travel from the epicenter at hundreds of miles per hour. The onset is often heralded by a sudden ebb of water that exposes the sea floor and is followed in minutes by a wall of water that may rise to 100 feet. Massive damage occurs to the shore and structures; casualties occur owing to

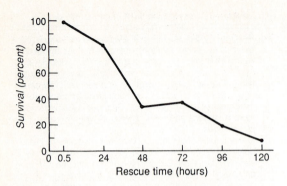

Figure 44–2. Survival rates versus rescue time for victims trapped in the Tangshan earthquake, 1976. (Adapted from Smith GS: Research issues in the epidemiology of injuries following earthquakes. In: *International Workshop on Earthquake Injury Epidemiology from Mitigation and Response.* Johns Hopkins Univ, 1989.)

Table 44–5. Saffir/Simpson rating scale for tropical cyclones.[1]

Scale	Winds (mph)	Surge (ft)	Damage Examples
1	74–95	4–5	Shrubberies, loose signs, unanchored mobile homes
2	96–100	6–8	Some trees down, roofs, windows, doors; small boats torn from moorings
3	111–130	9–12	Some flooding; small structures near coast destroyed
4	131–155	13–18	Roof failures, extensive flooding, beach erosion
5	>155	>18	Small buildings blown away, industrial building damage, extensive flooding

[1]Source: National Climatic Center, 1978.

Table 44–4. The deadliest hurricanes in the USA from 1900 to 1982.[1]

Hurricane	Year	Category	Deaths
1. Texas (Galveston)	1900	4	6,000
2. Florida (Lake Okeechobee)	1928	4	1,836
3. Florida (Keys/S. Texas)	1919	4	600–900[3]
4. New England	1938	3[2]	600
5. Florida (Keys)	1935	5	408
6. Audrey (Louisiana/Texas)	1957	4	390
7. Northeast USA	1944	3[2]	390[4]
8. Louisiana (Grand Isle)	1909	4	350
9. Louisiana (New Orleans)	1915	4	275
10. Texas (Galveston)	1915	4	275
11. Camille (Mississippi/Louisiana)	1969	5	256
12. Florida (Miami)	1926	4	243
13. Diane (Northeast USA)	1955	1	184
14. Southeast Florida	1906	2	164
15. Mississippi/Alabama/Pensacola	1906	3	134
16. Agnes (Northeast USA)	1972	1	122
17. Hazel (Carolinas)	1954	4[2]	95
18. Betsy (Florida/Louisiana)	1965	3	75
19. Carol (Northeast USA)	1954	3[2]	60
20. Southeast Florida/Louisiana-Mississippi	1947	4	51
21. Donna (Florida./Eastern USA)	1960	4	50
22. Georgia/Carolinas	1940	2	50
23. Carla (Texas)	1961	4	46
24. Texas (Velasco)	1909	3	41
25. Texas (Freeport)	1932	4	40
26. South Texas	1933	3	40
27. Hilda (Louisiana)	1964	3	38
28. Southwest Louisiana	1918	3	34
29. Southwest Florida	1910	3	30
30. Connie (North Carolina)	1955	3	25
31. Central Louisiana	1926	3	25

[1]Reproduced from Centers for Disease Control: *The Public Health Consequences of Disasters.* United States Department of Health and Human Services Public Health Service, Centers for Disease Control, 1989.
[2]Moving > 30 mph.
[3]Over 500 of these lost on ships at sea.
[4]344 of these lost on ships at sea.

drowning. The most deadly tsunami of modern times occurred in 1960 when an earthquake occurred off the coast of Chile. The resultant tsunami killed more than 2000 people across the Pacific.

Mitigation by building sea walls and locating structures on high ground and early warning are the only effective means of reducing casualties.

Volcanoes

Volcanoes are channels of molten rock (magma) from deep in the earth that vent to the surface in one of several forms. They may cause eruptions of molten rock (lava) or spew ash and debris. Volcanoes tend to be localized to the boundaries of tectonic plates (eg,

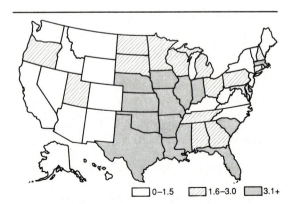

Figure 44–3. Total deaths from tornadoes in the USA per 10,000 square miles by state, 1952–1969. (Reproduced from: Centers for Disease Control: *The Public Health Consequences of Disasters.* United States Department of Health and Human Services Public Health Service, Centers for Disease Control, 1989.)

the Pacific rim). Six volcanic eruptions over the past 200 years have resulted in significant loss of life, the most recent of which, in Ruiz, Columbia, in 1985, killed 23,000 (Table 44–6). Injury is most commonly due to falling debris, collapse of structures under the weight of ash, being buried in mud slides or lava flows, or toxic effects of gases (CO_2, H_2S). Effects on agriculture and property can be extensive. In many cases, early warning, although imprecise, can allow evacuation and mitigate casualties.

NONNATURAL DISASTERS

Fires

Collectively, fires produce approximately 5000 deaths and 300,000 injuries each year in the USA, although the number has been on a steady decline over the past 50 years. Fire disasters have occurred in forests (some are natural disasters), cities, ships, hotels, theaters, hospitals, and schools (Table 44–7). Risk factors appear to include dry wood structures and winter months. Under the right conditions, hot gases can produce winds that collect in a rotating cyclone ("fire storm"). One which ignited in Dresden, Germany, in 1945 killed 135,000. Most deaths are due to asphyxia from carbon monoxide and other toxic gases and to burns.

Transportation Accidents

Transportation accidents are the most common incidents producing multiple casualties in the USA. Airplane crashes produce a high ratio of fatalities to total injuries and highway accidents the opposite. The worst aviation accident occurred in 1977, in Tenerife, Canary Islands, when two 747 jets collided on a

Table 44–7. Most serious fire disasters in the USA from 1871 to 1980.[1]

Category	Date	No. of Fatalities
Forests		
Michigan and Wisconsin	1871	1,000
Minnesota	1894	894
Minnesota and Wisconsin	1918	1,000
Cities		
Chicago	1871	766
Peshtigo, Wisconsin	1871	800
San Francisco	1906	1,188
Chelsea, Massachusetts	1908	18
Ships		
New York harbor	1904	1,000
Rhode Island coast	1954	103
Hotels		
Winecoff (Atlanta)	1946	119
LaSalle (Chicago)	1946	61
MGM Grand (Las Vegas)	1980	84
Hilton (Las Vegas)	1980	8
Stouffers Inn (New York)	1981	26
Places of entertainment		
Theater (Chicago)	1903	602
Dance Hall (Mississippi)	1940	207
Nightclub (Massachusetts)	1942	492
Circus (Connecticut)	1944	163
Supper Club (Kentucky)	1977	164
Health-Care Facilities		
Hospital (Oklahoma)	1918	38
Nursing home (Missouri)	1957	72
Hospital (Connecticut)	1961	16
Nursing home (Ohio)	1963	63
Nursing home (Ohio)	1970	31
Schools		
Collinwood, Ohio	1908	161
Chicago, Illnois	1958	93

[1]Reproduced from Centers for Disease Control: *The Public Health Consequences of Disasters.* United States Department of Health and Human Services Public Health Service, Centers for Disease Control, 1989.

Table 44–6. Most deadly volcanic eruptions world-wide from 1600 to 1985.[1]

Volcano	Date of Eruption	No. Killed	Lethal Agent
Laki, Iceland	1783	9,350	Ashfalls destroyed crops and animals, causing starvation.
Unzen, Japan	1792	14,300	70% killed by cone collapse; 30% by tsunami.
Tambora, Indonesia	1815	92,000	Most deaths due to starvation.
Krakatoa, Indonesia	1883	36,417	90% killed by tsunami.
Mt Pelee, Martinique	1902	29,025	Pyroclastic flows.
Ruiz, Colombia	1985	23,000	Mud flow.

[1]Reproduced from Centers for Disease Control: *The Public Health Consequences of Disasters.* United States Department of Health and Human Services Public Health Service, Centers for Disease Control, 1989.

runway, killing 577. Railway accidents may produce significant injuries if passengers are involved and also have resulted in release of hazardous materials.

Transportation accidents are the prototypical geographically localized multicasualty events that are practiced in most communities' disaster drills. They are realistically apt to occur, and they lend themselves to management within the jurisdiction and structure of local emergency medical services (EMS).

The patterns of injury are well known to most emergency workers and consist of fractures, contusions, lacerations, and head and thoracoabdominal blunt injury.

Industrial Accidents

Industrial accidents that cause large-scale disasters most commonly result in the release of a hazardous material (Table 44–8). The most notorious occurred in Bhopal, India, in 1984; a release of methyl isocyanate killed more than 2000 and injured up to 200,000.

Table 44–8. Deadliest industrial disasters worldwide from 1921 to 1984.[1]

Date	Place	Event	Result
9/21/21	Oppau, Germany	Explosion at a nitrate manufacturing plant destroyed plant and nearby village.	561 deaths; > 1500 persons injured.
4/16/47	Texas City, Texas	Explosion in freighter being loaded with ammonium nitrate.	561 deaths; much of city destroyed.
7/28/48	Ludwigshafen, Federal Democratic Republic of Germany	Vapor explosion from dimethyl ether.	209 deaths.
7/10/76	Seveso, Italy	Chemical reactor explosion released 2,3,7,8-TCDD.	100,000 animals killed; 760 people evacuated; 4450 acrees contaminated.
2/25/84	Cubatao, Sao Paulo, Brazil	Gasoline leak from a pipeline exploded and burned nearby shanty town.	> 500 deaths.
11/19/84	San Juan Ixtaheupec, Mexico City, Mexico	5 million liters of liquefied butane exploded at a storage facility.	> 400 deaths; 7231 persons injured; 700,000 evacuated.
12/3/84	Bhopal, India	Release of methyl isocyanate from pesticide plant.	> 2000 deaths; 100,000 persons injured.

[1]Reproduced from Centers for Disease Control: *The Public Health Consequences of Disasters.* United States Department of Health and Human Services Public Health Service, Centers for Disease Control, 1989.

Of the approximately 1300 releases of hazardous materials in the USA each year, 1–2 per day result in injury, death, or evacuation.

Injuries vary depending on the nature of the agent, but asphyxia, respiratory distress, skin and eye irritation, neurologic abnormalities, and teratogenic effects may occur.

Radiation & Nuclear Accidents

Aside from the atomic explosions in Japan in World War II, there have been few deaths due to nuclear disasters in the world, although several significant incidents have occurred (Table 44–9). The most deadly was the Chernobyl, Soviet Union, reactor explosion in 1986, in which 27 people died and 135,000 were evacuated, many of whom were exposed to high radiation levels.

Injuries are due to the immediate blast effects, to exposure to toxic chemicals used at reactor sites (eg, sulfuric acid, chlorine, ammonia), and to radiation exposure. (See Chapter 38.)

Structural Collapse & Explosions

Structural failure of a building or man-made structure can be precipitated by natural forces (eg, earthquake), or may occur unexpectedly (Hyatt skywalk collapse, Kansas City, 1981; 113 dead, 200 injured). However, most such events in the USA have been limited in scope and have not produced many casualties. Injuries are predictable and consist of head injuries, fractures, lacerations, and blunt thoracoabdominal injuries.

Acts of Violence

Unfortunately, acts of violence in the USA are not uncommon. Whereas in armed conflicts, casualties can be massive, in the civilian arena they are usually

Table 44–9. Major nuclear incidents worldwide from 1952 to 1986.[1]

Description of Incident	Site	Date	Adult Thyroid Dose (rem)
Minor core damage (no release of radiologic material)	Chalk River	1952	NA[2]
	Breeder Reactor, Idaho	1955	NA
	Westinghouse Test Reactor	1960	NA
	Detroit Edison Fermi	1966	NA
Major core damage (radioiodine released) Noncommercial	Windscale, England	1957	16
	Idaho Falls SL-1	1961	0.035
Commercial	Three Mile Island	1979	0.005
	Chernobyl, Soviet Union	1986	100[3]

[1]Reproduced from Centers for Disease Control: *The Public Health Consequences of Disasters.* United States Department of Health and Human Services Public Health Service, Centers for Disease Control, 1989.
[2]Not applicable.

limited to a small number (the difference primarily due to explosives). Injuries are penetrating trauma.

PREHOSPITAL MANAGEMENT OF MULTICASUALTY EVENTS & DISASTERS

Preparation for disaster is an important responsibility of any community's public safety agencies. A community should prepare actively for those events to which the area is vulnerable based on historical, geologic, demographic, transportation, and industrial sources. Many large cities practice an airplane crash scenario each year, despite the extremely low probability of such an event occurring, in part because the local airport is mandated by the FAA to conduct such drills. On occasion this has paid off. However, other realistic scenarios should not be neglected.

Organization of the Response
A. EMS versus "Civil Defense" Management: Most events are small level 1 events and are best managed by the local public safety or EMS jurisdiction as an extension of day-to-day operations under an organization or management system that can incorporate and coordinate outside assistance (see Incident Command System, below). At some point, large-scale events overwhelm local agencies and require the management and control to extend over a larger scale. Under the Civil Defense model, victims are collected and treated in supplementary casualty collection points or field hospitals that can stabilize them pending large-scale or distant evacuation. In many states (eg, California), plans exist for both such models although the EMS model is most commonly employed.

B. Incident Command System: The response by emergency personnel to a multicasualty event can be complex when multiple agencies are involved, jurisdictional boundaries are crossed, or the event occurs in multiple geographic locations. In order to devise a system to better coordinate events of varying size and complexity, federal, state, and local fire services joined together in 1982 in the FIRESCOPE project to devise the Incident Command System (ICS). ICS is a management system that allows incidents of varying size and complexity to be managed effectively, regardless of the diversity of agencies and resources involved.

The ICS has several functional components coordinated within an organizational framework (Fig 44–4). At the apex is the incident commander, who directs the Operations, Planning, Logistics, and Finance sections. Within the Operations section are various functional divisions, branches, and groups that carry out the actual line emergency response work. Various functional components or autonomous teams of individuals can maintain their "group" autonomy and fit into the organizational tree as a unit.

In complex incidents that have limited emergency medical needs, the EMS component may simply occupy a small division or group in the overall ICS structure. By contrast, a large, purely medical event may lead to the medical commander occupying the incident commander role.

C. Medical Management: The organization of medical resources to a disaster depends on the nature and level of the event. The easiest to illustrate is the geographically focused level 1 event. The medical response is directed by an on-scene medical commander who designates functional responsibilities to individuals or teams: triage, treatment, transport, communications, logistics, staging, and so on. The medical commander may, in fact, be a branch or division commander within a larger ICS structure or may be the event incident commander if the event is purely medical.

In typical smaller scale day-to-day incidents, the first-in ambulance remains out of service for the duration of the event and one paramedic assumes the role of medical commander, while the other begins triage or treatment responsibilities. As additional ambulances arrive, they report to the medical commander who assigns them roles or duties. Each crew then treats and transports patients in order of relative severity of injuries (as directed by a transport or loading officer).

If physicians or nurses are available, they are best used in treatment roles, since their expertise in assessing and treating patients may be considerable whereas their experience in working with other agencies in a command role in a fast-moving prehospital environment is usually limited.

A large-scale diffuse event, such as a major earthquake, is more difficult to manage. There may be no central focus of casualties. Instead, victims may be scattered or clustered over a large area, their existence made known by many hundreds of individual telephone requests (eg, via 9–1–1), provided that telephone services remain intact. This presents a coordinating problem if a limited number of ambulances are available or radio communications with ambulances are interrupted. Such loss of communications and central coordination capability may require decentralized management: ambulance resources disperse to individual neighborhoods to organize casualty collection and treatment at that level (eg, at each fire station).

Scene Organization
Geographic factors play an important role in disaster response. In remote areas, aeromedical services may be instrumental; at sea, rescue vessels are

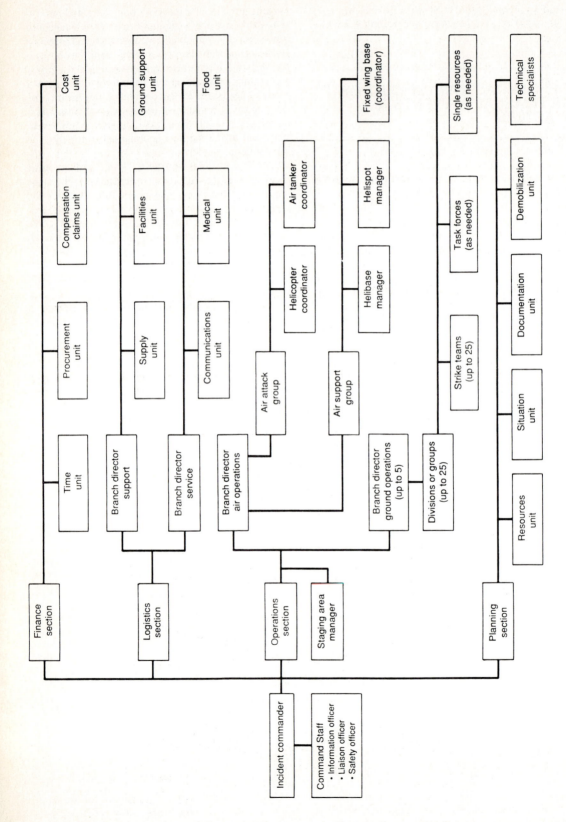

Figure 44-4. The Incident Command System (ICS) organizational diagram.

needed; in urban areas, crowd and traffic control may be important. If a hazard is present, the area must be isolated, and emergency vehicles positioned safely upwind. Fig 44–5 shows a typical ground schematic for a geographically focused multicasualty event.

Patients are most efficiently extricated and categorized (see Triage, below) if they are channeled to a single triage location and from there assigned to one of several treatment areas, depending on their level of treatment priority. From that point, patients depart the treatment areas through a single exit point. This arrangement ensures that the patients with the highest relative priority go first, no one is overlooked, and the total number of victims and their distribution are known.

Logistics

Logistics is a term applied to a support activity concerned with supplying and delivering resources to a rescue effort. Resources may be personnel, equipment, supplies, food and water, crew relief facilities, etc. In the first few minutes of the EMS response to a typical multicasualty event, the first-in paramedic (or the medical commander), provides an initial report by radio to the dispatch or communications center, relaying such information as type of incident, estimated number of victims and severity of injuries, presence of any hazard, number and type of additional resources needed, additional agencies requested (eg, police, fire), and recommended staging location of incoming vehicles. As soon as possible, and if per-

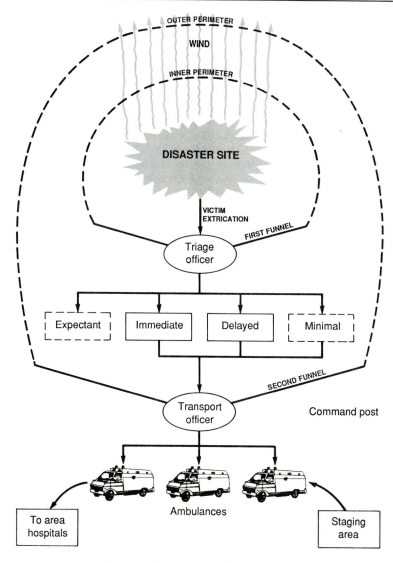

Figure 44–5. Scene diagram of a localized multicasualty incident.

sonnel are available, a logistics officer or team is designated by the medical commander.

Communications

Experience with modern multicasualty event management has shown communications to be the weak link in many incidents. Multiple jurisdictions and agencies may lack radios equipped with a common radio frequency, centralized radio relay equipment may be damaged, telephone services may be disabled, or simple frequency congestion may occur owing to heavy use. Lately, cellular telephones have added greatly to the ability to communicate during disasters from the field. In large-scale events, amateur radio operators have provided assistance. This is a particularly useful resource in remote areas.

In typical events, EMS units on scene should designate a radio frequency for communication between individuals at the scene and use a different one for communication with the central dispatch center to coordinate patient distribution and requests for additional resources. When disparate ambulance companies are involved that do not normally share a common frequency, they can still communicate with a central coordinating center if the federally designated UHF "Med Channels" (10 frequencies set aside for communications between ambulances and receiving hospitals) are temporarily used for this purpose.

Normal base hospital telemetry for on-line medical direction may need to be temporarily suspended owing to heavy traffic. Paramedics should then act on predesignated standing orders.

Triage

A. General Considerations: Triage is a process of sorting patients and classifying them by categories in terms of relative urgency. It ensures that those who need treatment sooner receive it and limited resources are not wasted on victims for whom care can be delayed with little chance of harm. Although triage systems are used in most busy emergency departments and are usually familiar to emergency workers, those used in disasters have an important difference: patients whose injuries are so severe that their survival is unlikely are given are given a *low* triage priority. This situation can be difficult for many emergency workers to accept, but it is important because diversion of precious limited resources to moribund victims makes them unavailable to others who could be saved. The objective of disaster triage is to categorize patients in a way that will do the most good for the largest number and to ensure that limited resources are efficiently utilized.

B. Triage Categories: The most effective triage systems are simple and require no complex scoring methodology. A 4-level triage system is commonly used in the USA:

1. Immediate (I)–Have life-threatening injuries that probably are survivable with immediate treat-

ment. Examples are tension pneumothorax, respiratory distress, major internal hemorrhage, and airway injuries.

2. Delayed (II)–Require definitive treatment but no immediate threat to life exists and can wait for treatment without jeopardy. Examples include minor extremity fractures, lacerations with hemorrhage controlled, and burns over less than 25% of body surface area.

3. Minimal (III)–Have minimal injuries, are ambulatory, and can self-treat or seek alternative medical attention independently. Examples include minor lacerations, contusions, and abrasions.

4. Expectant (0)–Have lethal injuries and will die despite treatment. Examples include devastating head injuries, major third-degree burns over most of the body, and destruction of vital organs.

The military system uses a 5-level triage system that adds a category for victims with no apparent injuries.

C. Assessment Methods: The method for rapidly assessing patients and deriving triage categories is based on evaluations that can be made quickly, easily, and by individuals with limited medical training. One such system employed in California is termed "START" (simple triage and rapid treatment; see Fig 44–6). Whatever system is used, the person with the greatest amount of experience, medical knowledge, and good judgment should be assigned this role.

D. Triage Tags: Detailed patient assessment information cannot practically be recorded in the field during a disaster, yet the need to communicate medical information about a patient to subsequent rescue workers still exists. Therefore, triage tags have been devised that can be attached to the patient and are simple and visual (Fig 44–7).

Treatment

In a disaster or multicasualty event, personnel and equipment may be in short supply. Hence, initially, treatment is limited to *austere* medical care, ie, only essential and urgently necessary treatments, such as endotracheal intubation, pressure dressings, and intravenous lines for volume or essential drug administration. "Prophylactic" intravenous lines, for example, are omitted.

Generally, a casualty collection point is designated in a convenient, safe, and sheltered location near the disaster site (Fig 44–5). The area is subdivided into sections for each triage category (ie, immediate, delayed, minimal, expectant), identifiable by colored tarps, tapes and cones, tents, etc. The areas should have controlled access and egress points to prevent violation of the triage and loading priority organization. Arriving EMS personnel and ancillary health care workers should be assigned by the medical commander to each area as needed. Victims, once directed to a treatment area by the triage officer, should be reassessed and treated according to need and the

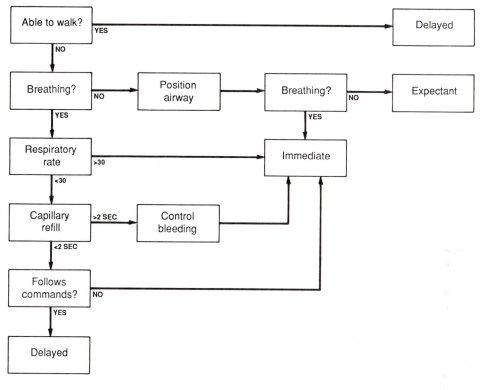

Figure 44–6. "START" triage algorithm.

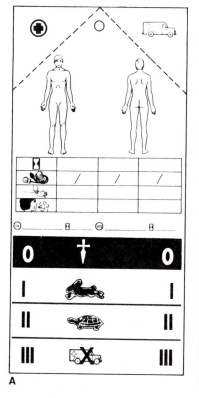

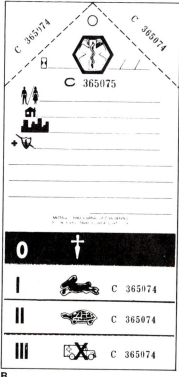

A   B

Figure 44–7. Example of triage tag, front and back. (Shown, with permission, from the Journal of Civil Defense.)

limitations of austere medical care. At any point, if a victim's condition changes, the victim may be moved to another area.

Victims in the "expectant" category are segregated and made comfortable. The dead are often not immediately extricated from the disaster site but are left for the medical examiner to remove at the conclusion of the event, unless public health reasons or security considerations require them to be moved to a temporary morgue.

Transport & Distribution of Patients

Ambulances or other transport vehicles (eg, bus or van) are directed to a specified loading location at a controlled egress point near the treatment areas. A Loading Officer (sometimes called Transport Officer) continually surveys the number of victims in each area and, when ambulances arrive, assigns victims for transport in order of relative priority based on the urgency of their condition. Generally, a typical ambulance can transport more than one victim (eg, one "immediate" plus one or 2 "delayed" victims) depending on the stretcher and seating capacity of the ambulance and the level of attention required by the victims en route.

Victim distribution to area hospitals differs significantly during a disaster compared with normal operations. Normally, destination may be determined by protocol factors, such as nature of problem, proximity to a given facility, or patient preference. Multicasualty events require victims to be *distributed* to area hospitals on a rotation protocol or according to each facility's capability to receive victims. This prevents the closest hospital from being inundated with large numbers of victims while more distant facilities remain idle.

Distribution can be accomplished by centrally coordinating destination assignments through the central dispatcher (if communications remain intact) or through the Loading (Transport) Officer, who maintains a log of each departing ambulance's destination. The advantage of central coordination is that individual hospital capacity information can be solicited by dispatch personnel more easily than by on-scene rescue workers. If feedback information is unavailable, a simple rotation protocol may be used.

Public Safety

Public safety involves protecting the public from hazards at the scene and allowing the rescue effort to unfold unimpeded by interference from the crowd. Most urban multicasualty events managed by EMS underutilize public safety personnel (police and fire fighters). While fire fighters have a prominent role when a hazard is present (eg, fire, explosion, collapse), an event that is predominantly medical presents a less clear role for them unless they are used to providing EMS care or participating actively in the medical response.

Most commonly, non-EMS fire fighters may be employed for hazard suppression, victim extrication and movement, and to the extent their training allows, initial triage. They should set up an inviolate perimeter barrier around the hazard area, position equipment and personnel in a safe, upwind position, and observe scene organization.

Similarly, police should enforce secure boundaries established by fire fighters and EMS and maintain the crowd at safe distance. Their assistance with traffic control and street closure may be necessary for the efficient ingress and egress of emergency vehicles.

Media Involvement

In some states, the press may have a statutory right of access to a disaster site and cannot be denied access unless they interfere with ongoing rescue efforts, even if they jeopardize their own safety in the process (eg, California Penal Code, Section 409). The objectives of rescue workers and members of the press may sometimes seem at odds and lead to conflict during a disaster. However, it is usually in the broadest public interest to communicate timely, accurate information about an event to the public, and rescue workers are often called upon to provide information to the press.

As a general rule, the following points are worth observing:

A. Allow the press access to the disaster site, but advise them about areas and activities which are dangerous to them or which may interfere with ongoing rescue efforts or victim treatment.

B. Actively provide the press with information that is as timely and as accurate as possible, and do so frequently. Appointing a press liaison or public relations officer is helpful.

C. Important information almost always involves the nature of the incident, number of victims, relative seriousness of injures (eg, number of deaths), and location where the victims were taken. A source of information (eg, telephone hotline) for relatives of victims to call is an important public service.

D. Do not speculate about facts that are not known to you.

Aeromedical Resources

Many communities and rural areas have access to aeromedical resources both for transport and for delivery of personnel and supplies. In remote areas, this may be the only form of disaster assistance. EMS helicopters may be utilized by designating a helicopter landing zone in a safe location upwind from the event. It should be distant enough that rotor noise and debris do not interfere with rescue activities, and it should be free of obstacles to landing and departing. In general, a relatively flat field (minimum of 100 feet square) with an unobstructed approach and departure path (into the wind) is ideal. An aircraft staging officer should be appointed who can coordinate the arrival of arriving helicopters on a mutual radio frequency.

However, not all disasters are amenable to aeromedical assistance, and at times, helicopters can be a nuisance. During the Loma Prieta earthquake in 1989, many structures in the San Francisco marina area were felt to be unstable and susceptible to collapse from helicopter rotor vibrations. As a result, access to the overlying airspace was restricted.

Local Accessory Resources

Accessory resources may be needed in certain circumstances. For example, structural collapse may require heavy equipment such as bulldozers provided and operated by the city's department of public works; utility loss or live power wires may require the assistance of the local power company. The ICS is a useful organizational structure for managing these resources.

Mutual Aid

Mutual aid refers to assistance provided by local EMS and public safety agencies from neighboring counties or towns. It is intended to provide mutual back-up resources for common events that temporarily overwhelm local capabilities. Ideally, prearranged operating agreements are helpful, as is the installation of a common radio frequency for mutual communications. Requests for mutual aid are normally made rapidly at the dispatch center, although in some cases, they may require authorization from some local authority, especially if an obligation for reimbursement occurs.

Special Considerations

A. Hazardous Materials: An incident involving a hazardous material ("hazmat") is a special type of situation that requires specialty management because a threat to rescue workers exits that may create additional casualties from among the rescuers or because contamination may spread to other areas in the community.

1. Priorities–The priorities in "hazmat" management are to

(a) Identify, isolate, and contain the hazard to prevent spread of the contamination.

(b) Decontaminate victims.

(c) Protect rescue workers and EMS personnel, who should not approach or receive victims unless they are properly decontaminated, or the rescuers have appropriate protective gear, or the contamination is "contained" in a protective wrap around the victim.

(d) Provide advance warning to receiving hospitals so that appropriate protective measures may be taken.

2. Special training and equipment–"Hazmat" incidents are best managed by a specially trained team of rescue workers who wear special protective

clothing and, when necessary, a respirator or self-contained breathing apparatus (Table 44–10). The appropriate training can be obtained from a variety of sources; one such is a 200-hour course provided by Federal Emergency Management Agency's National Fire Academy. "Hazmat" team individuals are familiar with methods of identifying hazardous substances, the nature of the substances and their effects, methods of hazard scene management, methods of hazard suppression, methods of decontamination, and operation of protective gear.

3. Specialty scene organization–The "hazmat" scene differs from the typical multicasualty event scene in that the immediate hazard area is isolated from entry by unprotected non-"hazmat" personnel ("hot zone"; see Fig 44–8). "Hazmat" team members in protective gear enter the hot zone and extricate the victims to an "intermediate zone" or area where victim decontamination occurs, performed by "hazmat" team members also in protective gear. Triage principles should be employed by "hazmat" team members to identify victims with the most immediate medical problems and the heaviest amounts of contamination. Decontamination often can be accomplished by removing the victim's clothing and dowsing the victim with copious quantities of water or some other irrigant solution, taking care to prevent hypothermia and to contain the effluent. Once decontaminated, victims are then transferred to awaiting EMS personnel, who perform triage and treatment as in a traditional multicasualty event.

Occasionally, victims with critical injuries require immediate lifesaving treatment before they can be decontaminated. Because this may happen, it is helpful to include individuals in the "hazmat" team who have medical training (eg, paramedics), are capable of performing triage of victims as they are extricated, and can perform limited lifesaving care before or during decontamination efforts. If decontamination is impossible, then the contamination should be contained in an occlusive wrap and the patient transferred to EMS personnel with adequate notification of the remaining contamination hazard.

B. Diffusely Distributed Victims: Multicasualty events or disasters that produce victims dispersed over a large geographic area, rather than a localized event, pose a special challenge. The method of response differs in approach and method of coordination and depends on the extent to which central

Table 44–10. Hazard exposure protective equipment.[1]

Level	Description
D	Work uniform, safety shoes, hard hat, gloves, eye protection
C	Add chemical-resistant suit, respirator
B	Add self-contained breathing apparatus (SCBA)
A	Total encapsulation with SCBA

[1]Source: Environmental Protection Agency.

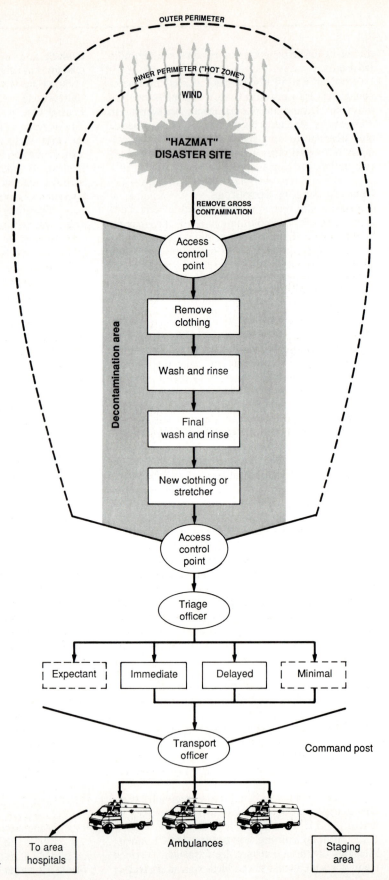

Figure 44–8. "Hazmat" scene organization diagram.

command, coordination, and communications remain functional.

1. The dispatch center remains intact and operational with functioning radio and telephone communications (eg, moderate earthquake or natural disaster). The number of incoming 9–1–1 calls may be markedly increased with patients distributed diffusely throughout the area. Steps in managing such an event are

(a) Obtain and deploy additional ambulance resources through reserve units, back-up arrangements, mutual aid, etc.

(b) Increase capacity for tracking deployed units by assigning additional dispatchers, reassigning radio frequencies, etc; it may be necessary to suspend telemetry transmission to decongest the airwaves and free the dispatchers from nonessential duties.

(c) Priority rank incoming calls and notify callers of anticipated delays; it may be necessary to temporarily suspend response to routine service requests.

2. The dispatch center or other elements of command and communications have been rendered ineffective, and there is no effective means of tracking resources, tracking incoming calls, or dispatching ambulances; a large number of victims are diffusely distributed in the area. This may occur with a major natural disaster and is the most difficult situation to manage.

(a) With loss of communication (or by declaration), centralized dispatch ceases and ambulances should disperse to predesignated station assignments in each neighborhood or area (eg, fire stations, hospitals, schools) that are natural locations for victims to self-report or around which neighborhood-level rescue efforts would be centered. Preestablished cache supplies at these sites should be utilized.

(b) EMS ambulance crews should assist the local neighborhoods at organizing casualty collection, triage, and treatment areas to the extent possible. It may not be practical for EMS crews to transport victims if they are the sole resource in a neighborhood with many casualties. Instead, they should concentrate on casualty collection and triage, use nonmedical transport, such as vans and buses, if available, and summon additional aid.

(c) The numbers of casualties at each location and need for additional resources should be communicated by hand-held radio or by runner to a central command post for the area.

(d) Efforts to reestablish radio communications should proceed immediately.

(e) Additional resources should be allocated to each area as they become available, and idle resources should be relocated.

(f) Outside aid should be requested, and victim evacuation from casualty collection points should proceed if needed.

Disaster Organizations & Assistance

In addition to local mutual aid from neighboring communities, several other sources of disaster assistance are available.

A. Military Assistance to Safety and Traffic (MAST): This program provides assistance from nearby military bases having a military medical mission in the form of aeromedical resources and medical support personnel in remote or rural areas. MAST can be requested directly by local public safety agencies. Usually, the response, which may consist of one or more aeromedical helicopter units, ranges from 30 to 90 minutes and consists of direct patient care and transport.

B. National Disaster Medical System (NDMS): The Federal Emergency Management Agency and the Department of Defense established the NDMS in 1984 as a cooperative program involving the Veteran's Administration hospital system and civilian hospitals. Its role is to provide for the distribution and care of large numbers of casualties from a major disaster or armed conflict in the USA. The principal component of the system is the network of civilian and Veteran's Administration hospitals spread throughout the USA that have pledged to provide a designated number of beds for disaster victims. The military would coordinate the collection, triage, and distribution of victims from the disaster site to these hospitals, using military airlift resources.

A second important component involves the on-scene management of casualties with disaster medical assistance teams (DMATs), which consist of volunteer health care and rescue workers who are willing to be deployed to a disaster area within the USA and serve a medical clearing and staging function or serve as part of a mobile Army surgical unit.

The NDMS system can be activated by request from a governor in the event of a major disaster, with Presidential approval, or by order of the Secretary of Defense during a military conflict.

C. Other Military Resources: Other agencies, such as the National Guard, Coast Guard, and local military bases may be available to respond with personnel, equipment, and medical resources upon request from local, regional, or state officials.

D. Disaster Relief Organizations: Various organizations, such as the American National or International Red Cross, Goodwill Industries, the Salvation Army, and various religious groups, are private or nonprofit organizations that provide assistance in the form of shelter, food, clothing, and services to victims of disasters. Internationally, the World Health Organization (WHO), while not directly participating in on-site disaster management, provides technical advice and assists with resources and finance. The United Nations Disaster Relief Office (UNDRO) acts as a direct coordinator of disaster relief. Other assistance may be provided by organizations such as the Organization of American States (OAS) and the regional arm of WHO, the Pan American Health Organization (PAHO).

E. Volunteerism: Volunteerism by both health care and lay individuals is common during a disaster. However well-intentioned, volunteerism is not without drawbacks. Many volunteers are not familiar with local policies, laws, equipment, or practices; the expertise and certification of volunteers is difficult for rescue workers to verify; and volunteers may place an additional burden on the local system by their own need for food, water, and medical assistance if they are injured during rescue activities. Volunteers who have traveled to foreign countries to lend assistance during disasters have occasionally found themselves without many basic necessities, including food, shelter, and transportation home. Emergency health care workers who contemplate lending such assistance should consider these factors.

EMERGENCY DEPARTMENT DISASTER MANAGEMENT

The term "disaster" may have a slightly different meaning to a hospital than to the prehospital community. Although a community multicasualty incident may overwhelm local EMS resources and require the activation of a community disaster plan, much of the response and resource requirement may relate to public safety needs, victim rescue, or hazard suppression, with relatively few casualties requiring hospitalization. In addition, the distribution of victims among several area hospitals may lessen the impact on a single institution, as will the existence of special destination criteria (eg, burns, trauma, pediatrics). On the other hand, internal problems at a hospital, such as utility failure, minor fires, and broken sewer lines may require the evacuation of the hospital or shut down critical services (eg, x-ray, laboratory), causing bottlenecks or patient flow problems. Even unexpected staffing problems coupled with a higher than normal emergency department census can be a minor "disaster" within a facility from time to time.

As a result, hospitals should have well-tested plans, worked out in advance, to provide special organization and management during such times.

Planning & Drilling

Community disasters large enough to require activation of a hospital's disaster plan are rare. Therefore, it is usually only through disaster drills that health care workers can gain experience with in-hospital disaster management. This is usually a committee or task force effort, and it should prominently involve input from emergency physicians and nurses in the hospital, as well as representatives from administration, plant services, security, etc. The Joint Committee on Accreditation of Hospital Organization (JCAHO) mandates that each member hospital have a disaster plan and conduct regular drills.

Disaster plans by be classified quantitatively in terms of the number of victims expected (eg, level 1, up to 20 victims; level 2, 20–50; level 3, over 50) or qualitatively in terms of the type of incident (eg, external trauma, radiation, fire, utility failure).

Notification & Activation

Notification of the hospital usually occurs via local emergency medical services with a telemetric call to the emergency department from incoming ambulances or from the community ambulance dispatch center to alert area hospitals of the potential for victims. This call should lead to a decision to activate the hospital's disaster plan, eg, by the emergency attending physician or by the hospital administrator or supervisor on duty. The decision may be protocol-driving by specific activation criteria, or it may be based on the judgment of a key individual who determines that special organization and resources are needed.

Notification should not only include in-hospital departments and personnel (Table 44–11) but also key individuals at their homes. An in-hospital overhead announcement or group paging capability is customary.

Mobilization of Disaster Resources

A. Personnel: Additional personnel resources, such as doctors, nurses, orderlies, and registration clerks, should be quickly mobilized and sent to the emergency department where incoming patients may soon arrive. Special support areas, such as radiology, blood bank, clinical laboratories, operating and recovery rooms, and central supply, may also need additional staff.

B. Supplies: Disaster cache medical supplies, registration packets, stretchers, blood products, etc, should be delivered immediately to the emergency department.

C. Space: The emergency department should be quickly surveyed and those patients with non–life-threatening complaints should be moved to another area to open up treatment rooms for incoming victims. The operating and recovery rooms should be placed on standby and elective cases postponed. The intensive care units should review existing patients to identify those who can be moved to the wards. Opening a separate clinic area for minor complaints may be helpful.

Triage for Incoming Victims

An experienced physician or nurse should perform triage for arriving casualties at the door and direct them to resuscitation (or operating) areas, treatment rooms, or waiting areas, using principles similar to those outlined above (ie, immediate, delayed, mini-

Table 44–11. Hospital disaster notification.[1]

Notify	Example of Typical Duties
ED: Attending physician	Prepare for arrivals, move minor patients out of the ED.
ED: Charge nurse	Prepare for arrivals, call in additional staff, set up triage.
Administrator in charge	Activate plan, notify chiefs of services, set up command post.
Hospital operator	Group page or call down list, announce plan in effect.
Trauma surgeon (one or more)	Report to ED; postpone elective cases.
Nursing supervisor	Obtain additional nursing staff, review nursing unit assignments.
Admitting and registration	Report to ED, mass admitting and registration, disaster tags.
Operating room (one or more)	Open idle rooms, obtain additional staff, postpone elective cases.
Radiology	Postpone elective studies, prepare for emergency radiography.
Blood bank	Inventory blood products available, order needed supplies.
Clinical laboratory	Call additional staff, suspend nonessential services.
Respiratory therapy	Report to ED, call additional staff.
Central supply	Disaster cache supplies to ED.
Pharmacy	Add staffing as needed.
Intensive care units	Inventory beds, triage patients to wards, call in added staffing.
Recovery room	Open if idle, call in staffing.
Medical and surgical wards	Inventory beds, identify patients for discharge, call in added staff.
Outpatient clinics	Open for ambulatory overflow from ED.
Security	Control pedestrian traffic and access.
Media relations	Report to command post, set up press area.
Plant services	Survey structural, utility, mechanical integrity.
Housekeeping	Report to ED for transport and cleaning assistance.
Dietary staff	Prepare for extended hours, obtain additional staff and supplies.

[1]ED = Emergency department.

mal, expectant levels). Use of the triage tags applied by field paramedics is important, not only to learn about the victim's prehospital course but to add information until a chart can be established.

Provision of Treatment

After emergency lifesaving treatment, such as airway control, has been provided, the emphasis is on providing definitive treatment rapidly for those who need it immediately and are likely to survive as a result. (Do the most good for the most people.) Unlike in the field, care need not be austere, but priority ranking is important and minor treatments may be delayed. Surgical resuscitation may be best handled in the operating room, since it tends to tie up personnel, space, and equipment in the emergency department.

Command & Communications Organization

It is important to establish early an administrative command center capable of communicating with each of the departments, coordinating logistics, and assessing resource and capacity needs. A link to the local EMS dispatch center is crucial to provide capacity information that will help the dispatchers equitably distribute patients to area hospitals.

Security Provisions

Enforcement of designated areas in the hospital and limitation of foot traffic by security personnel minimizes the stress and disorder accompanying any multicasualty event and makes the entire effort more effective.

Media Relations

A press area should be set aside and a media liaison and hospital spokesperson designated to keep the public informed of events. An accurate victim count as well as names of victims are of intense interest to concerned relatives.

Plant Services

An assessment of the structural integrity of the facility is critical in a damaging natural disaster. Problems should be communicated to the local ambulance dispatch center so that additional victims may be diverted elsewhere.

Specialty Management of Hazardous Materials & Radiation

Variations in the basic plan are required for different types of incidents and disasters. An important variation occurs when a hazardous or radioactive substance is involved. Although sizable casualties of this type are rare in the USA, they may occur, particularly along transportation routes.

A. Notify Team: Once it is known that there are incoming contaminated victims, the hospital's radiation safety or hazardous materials team should be notified immediately (if one exists). Immediate information about the nature of the agent (if its identity is known), its effects, and precautions can often be obtained from the local fire department "hazmat" team or from a regional poison center.

B. Designate Restricted Areas: Restricted areas in the emergency department should be designated and demarcated by a strictly enforced hazard boundary line ("hot zone"). The area should include an intake pathway from the ambulance loading bay up to a separate decontamination area. It should also include one or more treatment or resuscitation rooms in the event that immediate resuscitation is needed before adequate decontamination is possible. Equipment, air intake vents, and floors should be covered with paper or plastic depending on the nature of the contaminant.

C. Apply Protective Clothing: Emergency personnel who will be involved in the evaluation and treatment of the victims should wear protective gear.

Usually, a special "hazmat" suit, respirator, and self-contained breathing apparatus are not necessary. A surgical gown, scrubs, face shield, gloves, and shoe and head covering are usually adequate (the shoe covering should be removed when leaving the restricted area to prevent tracking contamination to other areas).

D. Decontaminate the Victim: The patient should receive a triage examination away from the emergency department treatment area. Unless already decontaminated in the field, the victim should be dowsed with water or other appropriate decontamination solution and, if necessary, scrubbed with soap and water (do not abrade the skin; pay attention to hair and nails) before entry into the treatment area. Rarely, if lifesaving care cannot be delayed for decontamination, then the victim should be contained in a plastic wrap and treated by individuals protected as described above until stabilized sufficiently for decontamination. Avoid washing cutaneous contamination into an open wound, where systemic absorption will be more rapid. Collect all clothing, dressings, and tissue specimens.

E. Monitor Contamination: In the case of ionizing radiation, the victim's level of contamination and also exposed areas of the emergency department should be assessed with a monitoring device.

F. Treat: Treatment varies considerably depending on the agent involved. In some cases, there are specific treatments, such as atropine for organophosphate toxicity and sodium nitrite for cyanide toxicity, but in most cases, treatment consists of providing airway and circulatory support and removing the offending agent. (See Chapters 38 and 39.)

G. Clean Up: The isolated area in the emergency department should be thoroughly decontaminated before access is granted. Depending on the agent involved, clean-up efforts should be directed by the hospital hazardous materials expert or radiation physicist.

STRESS MANAGEMENT & PSYCHOLOGICAL SUPPORT

Multicasualty incidents and disasters are not only stressful and fatiguing to emergency workers, but they may also produce extreme psychological reactions to witnessed trauma. These reactions may be immediate or delayed, and may be manifested as anxiety, fatigue, depression, guilt, sleep disorders, and nightmares. It is not uncommon for emergency workers who are used working with life-and-death situations to appear outwardly calm and unaffected owing to defense mechanisms, denial, and peer effects.

In addition to an operational debriefing or "postmortem" event analysis, a mandatory psychological debriefing should be performed by a team consisting of a psychologist or psychiatrist and others outside of the organization. In this session, individuals should be encouraged to express their feelings and emotions related to the event and to realize that such feelings are normal, that they are not alone in feeling them, and that support is available if needed.

REFERENCES

Abrams T: The feasibility of prehospital medical response teams for foreign disaster assistance. Prehosp Disast Med 1990;5:241.

Auf der Heide E: *Disaster Response: Principles of Preparation and Coordination.* Mosby, 1989.

Bern AI: Disaster medical services. In: *Principles of EMS Systems.* Roush WR et al (editors). American College of Emergency Physicians, 1989.

Bernstein AB, Thompson P: The natural history of natural hazards. In: *Management of Wilderness and Environmental Emergencies.* Auerbach PS, Geehr EC (editors). Mosby, 1989.

Centers for Disease Control: *The Public Health Consequences of Disasters.* United States Department of Health and Human Services Public Health Service, Centers for Disease Control, 1989.

Cowan ML, Cloutier MG: Medical simulation for disaster casualty management training. J Trauma 1988;28(1 Suppl):S178.

Cowley R, Edelstein S, Silverman M: *Mass Casualties: A Lessons Learned Approach.* United States Government Printing Office, Department of Transportation, No. (DOT) HS 806 302, 1982.

de Boer J: Definition and classification of disasters: Introduction of a disaster severity scale. J Emerg Med 1990;8:591.

Doyle CJ: Mass casualty incident: Integration with prehospital care. Emerg Med Clin North Am 1990;8:163.

Emergency Medical Services Authority, State of California: *Hazardous Materials Medical Management Protocols.* State of California, 1991.

Feldstein B: Disasters and disaster medicine: An introduction and overview. Top Emerg Med 1986;7:1.

Feldstein B et al: Disaster training for emergency physicians in the United States: A systems approach. Ann Emerg Med 1985;14:36.

Goodwin C: *Disaster Management.* Aspen Publishers, 1986.

Gunn SWA: The language of disasters. Prehosp Disast Med 1990;5:373.

Lilja PG, Madsen MA: Medical aspects of disaster management. In: *National Association of EMS Physicians EMS*

Medical Directors' Handbook. Kuehl A (editor). Mosby, 1989.

Mahoney LE, Lasek RW, Paris PM: Natural disaster management. In: *Management of Wilderness and Environmental Emergencies.* Auerbach PS, Geehr EC (editors). Mosby, 1989.

Mahoney LE et al: Disaster medical assistance teams. Ann Emerg Med 1987;16:354.

Morris G: Applying the incident command system to mass casualty incidents. Emerg Care Q 1986;2:15.

Plante DM, Walker JS: EMS response at a hazardous material incident: Some basic guidelines. J Emerg Med 1989;7:55.

Ratzan RM: Defining a rational back-up policy for emergency departments. J Emerg Med 1987;5:49.

Rutherford WH: An analysis of civil aircrash statistics 1977–86 for the purposes of planning disaster exercises. Injury 1988;19:384.

Waeckerle JE: Disaster planning and response. (Current Concepts.) N Engl J Med 1991;324:815.

45

Legal Aspects of Emergency Care

James E. George, MD, JD, FACEP

Medical malpractice lawsuits are a major concern for physicians and health care institutions. At least once in their careers, physicians may expect to become involved in some manner in litigation alleging physician negligence. The physician may not always be a target defendant. In some circumstances, physicians who have treated a patient suing another physician may be subpoenaed to testify in court. Physicians may also become involved in litigation by agreeing to present expert medical opinion on behalf of either party (plaintiff or defendant).

The filing of a malpractice action always generates a great deal of emotional stress for the defendant physician. This chapter discusses medicolegal problem areas in the emergency department and suggests ways in which the emergency department physician can avoid malpractice litigation.

The true extent of the emergency department malpractice problem is unknown, partly because emergency departments and emergency physicians are insured by many different professional liability insurance companies that have not pooled their claim information and partly because many claims involve events that occurred not only in the emergency department but also in other parts of the hospital.

Regardless of the magnitude of the malpractice problem, the net effect of malpractice suits has been to make emergency physicians, like physicians in general, practice "defensive medicine." Modern emergency departments provide mainly episodic care in a high-pressure environment that affords little time for leisurely contemplation and consultation when there is doubt about the diagnosis or the best course of treatment. These conditions mandate obtaining more supportive laboratory or radiologic studies than might be obtained under more ordered circumstances. Whether physicians like it or not, the public demands that defensive medicine be the standard of care.

This chapter is intended to provide the practitioner with an overview of relevant medicolegal aspects of emergency medicine. The reader should note that the outcome of a particular malpractice case depends on its particular facts and that changing a single fact in a case may result in an entirely different outcome. Furthermore, both statutory and case law may vary considerably in different jurisdictions. For these reasons, this chapter is not offered as legal advice.

GENERAL LEGAL PRINCIPLES

CRIMINAL VERSUS CIVIL LAW

There are 2 general categories of law in the USA: civil and criminal. Medical malpractice is one form of negligence, a specific tort action within civil law. Allegations of medical malpractice may encompass other torts, including (but not limited to) assault and battery, breach of confidentiality, and false imprisonment.

Criminal law involves a legal action filed by a state or the federal government against one or more defendants and deals with the definitions of crimes and their punishments. Civil law deals with legal actions that seek the redress of wrongs which are not criminal in nature. Contracts, torts, and domestic relations are a few of the areas within the category of civil law. Civil wrongs (other than breach of contract) committed by one individual against another are called torts. If a civil wrong is also classified as a criminal wrong, the offending individual could be subject to both civil and criminal penalties. Fraud and assault and battery are examples of wrongs potentially giving rise to both civil and criminal liability.

NEGLIGENCE

Negligence is defined as harmful conduct that deviates from accepted standards of duty and care. The law requires all persons to conduct their personal, business, and professional activities in a reasonably safe manner so as not to expose others to an unnecessary risk of harm. A physician who injures a patient by conduct that fails to meet the legal standard of due care may be liable for negligence in an action for malpractice. In order for a complaining party (plaintiff) to sustain an action for negligence against a defending party (defendant), 4 specific elements must be alleged and proved in a court of law: (1) the existence of a physician-patient relationship giving rise to a duty of due care, (2) breach of that duty, (3) proximate cause, and (4) damages. Failure to plead and prove any one of these items will prevent recovery for negligence.

Duty

To satisfy the first requirement for a negligence action, the existence of a legal relationship between the plaintiff and the defendant (a doctor-patient relationship) must be proved by the plaintiff. It is this legal relationship that imposes a duty of reasonable care on the physician. Usually, a physician who voluntarily undertakes to care for a patient establishes a legal relationship. A physician in a hospital emergency de-

partment, however, may have a legal duty to examine and treat all patients seeking emergency care. Such duty has been imposed by case law (court decisions) in some states in the USA and through statutes or regulations in others.

A federal law known as the Consolidated Omnibus Budget Reconciliation Act of 1985 and its 1989 amendment also require hospitals that provide emergency services and the emergency physicians who staff hospital emergency departments to follow specified procedures before refusing to examine or treat or before transferring any individual seeking a medical examination or treatment. The federal law was enacted to prevent the practice of "patient dumping" (the transfer of patients unable to pay for emergency services). Recent amendments to the law require an appropriate medical screening examination within the capabilities of the hospital's emergency facilities. The screening examination may not be delayed while inquiry is made about payment for services.

This law also set forth conditions that must be met before a person in active labor or other emergency condition may be transferred to another facility. Physicians and hospitals are subject to civil monetary and other penalties for a failure to comply with the law.

Private physicians practicing in their own offices have great latitude in choosing their patients and may refuse to provide care.

In undertaking the care of a patient, physicians assume a duty to conduct themselves according to the standard of care expected of a reasonably well trained, prudent physician in the same or similar circumstances. In the past, the scope and quality of this "reasonable man" duty were measured according to the standards prevailing in the geographic locality in which the physician practiced. This was known as the "locality rule," and in some cases rural practitioners were not held to the same high standard of care as urban practitioners. The development of electronic communication and rapid transportation and the wide availability of continuing medical education have led most courts to discard this rule in favor of a more uniform national standard of care.

Training in a specialty—or a claim to be a specialist even in the absence of training—will raise the standard of care and skill to which the physician is expected to conform.

Breach of Duty

Once a duty is established, the plaintiff must prove that the physician breached that duty by failing to exert a reasonable standard of care. Breach may consist of malfeasance or nonfeasance. Malfeasance is an affirmative act that does not comport with the accepted standard of care; nonfeasance is failure to do something that would be expected under the circumstances. For example, prescribing the wrong drug is malfeasance, whereas failure to prescribe any drug when one is clearly needed is nonfeasance.

Causation

The third element of negligence the plaintiff must prove is causation. Even if the plaintiff can prove that the defendant physician had a duty of care and that damages resulted after the physician breached the duty to conform to the accepted standard of care, the suit will not be successful unless the plaintiff can prove that the defendant's negligent conduct caused injury which would not otherwise have occurred.

For example, a patient who falls from a stretcher in the emergency department, sustains bruises, and 4 months later has a myocardial infarction is unlikely to be able to prove that the fall caused the myocardial infarction. If the myocardial infarction occurs moments after the fall, a causal relationship might be easier to prove.

In some jurisdictions, major changes in the traditional legal concept of causation have occurred in certain types of medical malpractice suits. In cases in which a plaintiff alleges that a delay in diagnosis or treatment of a preexisting condition reduced the chances of recovery, some courts may allow the plaintiff to prove his or her case based on a more relaxed standard of proof. For example, it may be alleged that a failure to timely diagnose and treat an abdominal aortic aneurysm deprived the plaintiff of a chance to survive. If the jury finds that the defendant physician was negligent, it may decide that the physician's negligence caused the plaintiff's death by increasing the risk of harm to the plaintiff and by becoming a substantial factor in increasing the risk of harm.

Damages

The plaintiff must prove that some injury has been sustained as a result of the physician's alleged negligence. This element is essential to the plaintiff's suit, because the purpose of legal redress is to obtain compensation for the damages suffered. A court will not entertain a suit for negligence in the absence of damages. A jury may award damages for medical expenses, physical pain, mental pain and suffering, lost wages, lost earning capacity, loss of services of a spouse, funeral expenses, and other items of damage. Some jurisdictions will also allow a jury to impose "punitive" damages in cases in which the defendant's conduct is proved to be done with malicious intent or with reckless indifference to the consequences of his or her action. In some states, the law prohibits the payment of punitive damages by professional liability insurance carriers.

STATUTE OF LIMITATIONS

The statute of limitations is a law that specifies how soon after an injury a plaintiff must file suit or be forever barred from doing so. The legislative purpose is both to prevent the threat of a lawsuit from hanging over a possible defendant's head forever and to force litigants to bring their actions before memories fade or witnesses die or leave the jurisdiction of the court where the matter must be tried. In the USA, the statutory interval is different in different states and depends on the type of complaint. The statute of limitations for negligence actions in most states is 2 years. There is some variation in the method used to determine when the limiting period actually begins to run. Some states provide that the statute of limitations begins when the negligent act occurred; in other states, the statute of limitations does not begin until the patient discovers or should reasonably discover that negligence has occurred and has caused damages. Furthermore, the statute of limitations does not usually begin in the case of a minor until the person is emancipated or reaches the age of majority. The age of majority varies from 18 to 21 years of age.

As a result, a malpractice suit may in some cases be filed many years after the event. A complete and accurate medical record is the physician's best defense in such cases, since the physician may have little recollection of the events in question.

RES IPSA LOQUITUR

In most medical malpractice cases, the plaintiff is required to prove negligence through the testimony of expert medical witnesses. An exception to this requirement is the doctrine of **res ipsa loquitur,** a Latin phrase meaning "the thing speaks for itself." This doctrine applies when the medical mishap could only be due to someone's negligence. For example, the presence of a surgical sponge or clamp in the internal cavities of a patient who has had surgery is a self-evident indication of negligent conduct by some member of the operating team.

The doctrine of res ipsa loquitur evolved as a means of assisting the plaintiff in recovering damages in circumstances in which it would be difficult or impossible to prove all of the elements of negligence. The application of the doctrine of res ipsa loquitur may relieve the plaintiff of the necessity of obtaining expert testimony. The plaintiff must prove 3 specific elements before the doctrine of res ipsa loquitur can be invoked: (1) the damages would not have occurred in the absence of someone's negligence; (2) the instrument or agency that caused the damage must have been under the exclusive control of the defendant at all times; and (3) the patient did nothing that could have contributed to the injury. The legal effect and benefit of successfully invoking the doctrine of res ipsa loquitur are to shift the burden of proof from the plaintiff to the defendant, who must now prove that there was no negligence (ie, the defendant is guilty until proved "innocent"). The doctrine of res ipsa loquitur has been broadly and at times improvidently applied in the area of medical malpractice, and this has been a cause of concern to both the medical and the legal professions.

LIABILITY FOR THE ACTS OF OTHERS (Vicarious Liability)

As a general rule, individuals are liable for their own acts of negligence. However, in medical malpractice actions, legal relationships between the various parties may determine the ultimate distribution of liability among the individuals involved. Another party may share the liability of the wrongdoer because of a preexisting legal relationship.

The hospital emergency department's cast of characters includes the hospital corporation, emergency physicians, other staff physicians, nurses, emergency department technicians, and other hospital employees. Various relationships may exist among these individuals, including employer-employee, independent contractor, and borrowed servant.

The doctrine of **respondeat superior** ("let the master answer" [for the servant]) imposes liability upon the employer for the torts of his or her employees committed within the scope of their employment. However, an employer is not usually liable for the torts of an independent contractor if the employer has no significant control or right of control over the actions of the independent contractor. Whether the hospital is liable for the negligence of emergency physicians who are independent contractors has been decided in different ways in different jurisdictions. The legal rules and exceptions in the area of vicarious liability are important when the hospital and physician are confronted with a negligence suit. Hospital attorneys will generally try to show that liability for negligence rests solely with the physician, while the physician's insurance company will argue that the insured's professional negligence should be shared by the hospital. It can safely be said that all emergency department personnel—as well as the hospital—will be joined as codefendants in a negligence suit to ensure that the plaintiff will recover money damages from somebody. In rendering a verdict for the plaintiff, the court will usually leave it to the defendants to sort out among themselves who will pay all or part of the damage judgment for negligence, and suits may therefore be filed by the defendants against one another to determine the distribution of damages.

DUTY TO PROVIDE EMERGENCY CARE

At one time, United States common law did not require a physician or hospital to provide medical treatment to all who sought it. Thus, private hospitals and some public hospitals could refuse to admit a patient needing emergency care if the treatment would result in no compensation to the hospital.

A series of abuses of the privilege not to provide emergency care and some landmark legal decisions reversed this doctrine in some jurisdictions. In some areas of the USA, no state law addressed the increasing problem of denial of emergency care or the transfers of patients to hospitals that would accept those persons unable to pay. Mounting concern over the practice of "patient dumping" resulted in the passage of the Consolidated Omnibus Budget Reconciliation Act of 1985, amended by the Omnibus Budget Reconciliation Act of 1989.

The goal of the federal legislation is to ensure access to emergency care for all who need it, regardless of ability to pay. The law requires that any hospital that receives Medicare funds provide a screening examination for all patients to determine whether an emergency condition exists. If so, the hospital must provide immediate and stabilizing care to all emergency patients and obstetric patients in active labor before transfers are considered. The 1989 amendments preclude transfer of obstetric patients under certain specified conditions. The law provides for civil monetary penalties for violations. In addition, civil suits may be filed in state or federal court, bypassing any peer review or arbitration system established in some states as part of tort reform. This new law change places an additional burden on emergency physicians as well as hospitals that transfer and receive transferred patients.

Hospitals have found that one of the best means of assuming these increased responsibilities is to staff their emergency departments with practitioners who specialize in emergency medicine. The responsibilities of emergency care are so important that any hospital which does not have a qualified emergency physician on duty in the emergency department might find itself unable to discharge its full legal duty to the public under the law.

GOOD SAMARITAN LAWS

Good Samaritan laws have been enacted in every state in the USA to encourage health professionals and others to render emergency care at the scene of accidents and emergencies. Good Samaritan laws generally provide immunity from civil liability to persons who in good faith render emergency aid to victims. The class of person granted immunity by Good Samaritan statutes depends on the particular wording of the statute. Some states grant immunity to "any person," while others grant such immunity only to licensed physicians or nurses. Application of these laws generally assumes that the aid has been rendered without expectation of payment. Good Samaritan statutes generally do not provide immunity from acts that amount to willful, wanton, or grossly negligent conduct in the rendering of emergency care. Also, a physician or nurse working in an emergency department may not receive Good Samaritan status for care provided there unless such immunity is clearly set forth in the applicable statute.

Physicians, nurses, and other health professionals are generally not required to stop and provide aid at the scene of accidents and emergencies. There are some exceptions, however. For example, most state motor vehicle codes require persons involved in motor vehicle accidents to stay at the scene of the accident and render appropriate emergency care to the victims. Vermont's "Duty to Aid the Endangered" act requires an individual who knows that another individual is exposed to grave physical harm to render appropriate assistance if to do so incurs no personal danger or peril. Failure to comply with this statute is punishable by a fine.

A physician who decides to render emergency aid to a victim at the scene must follow through with that decision. If it appears to others that a doctor has undertaken to render aid, it is reasonable to expect that other potential Good Samaritans may believe that their assistance is no longer required and so leave the scene. Should the physician later reverse the decision to help and instead provide no aid, and if the victim suffers harm as a result, the physician risks liability on grounds of abandonment.

It is important for health professionals to be aware that Good Samaritan statutes may not make the health professional completely immune from an action for malpractice. If the court finds that as a matter of law the protection of the Good Samaritan statute should be applied, the plaintiff's suit will be summarily dismissed. However, if the court finds on the evidence before it that disputed factual issues, if proved by the plaintiff, would remove the protection of the Good Samaritan statute (eg, conduct that a jury could conclude was grossly negligent), the plaintiff's case will be permitted to go forward.

If health professionals are sued, they must still retain defense counsel and affirmatively plead the protection of the Good Samaritan statute. Thus, Good Samaritan statutes do not make health professionals immune from suit but do make them immune from liability if they are sued.

COMMON LEGAL PROBLEMS IN THE EMERGENCY DEPARTMENT

CONSENT

General Principles Relating to Consent

It is a fundamental principle of the legal system of the USA that all adult competent persons have the right to make decisions involving their bodies. A physician who fails to obtain consent for treatment or who provides treatment beyond or contrary to what the patient has consented to is liable under the tort doctrine of **battery,** which is defined as "an unpermitted contact with the plaintiff's person." A threatening approach or gesture that makes a person apprehensive of imminent battery is an assault. Although distinct torts, these terms are often used interchangeably, or both together in the phrase "assault and battery."

Any physical examination or treatment must be with the consent of the patient. Consent may be *express,* either orally or in writing, or *implied* by the circumstances. A clear example of implied consent is voluntary submission to examination or treatment by a patient who has sought the physician's services. Although implied consent is legally sufficient under appropriate circumstances, the emergency physician may do well to eliminate any possible later claim of "battery" by securing a more definite express consent, preferably in writing.

Doctrine of Informed Consent

Consent cases today usually focus on the quality of the consent given, and the basis for the action is not battery but rather the physician's negligence in failing to obtain full and informed consent. Informed consent generally requires that the patient (1) be competent to consent and (2) understand the risks and benefits inherent in the proposed procedure as well as the consequences of alternative methods of treatment or of no treatment at all.

Court decisions in various states in the USA have set different legal standards regarding the extent of a physician's duty of disclosure. Under what is commonly referred to as a "professional community– or physician–oriented" standard, the duty to obtain informed consent is measured by the custom and practice within the medical community. This standard calls for the same degree of disclosure that a reasonable health practitioner would make under the same or similar circumstances. In other states, including Pennsylvania and New Jersey, a patient's standard of informed consent has evolved. Under this standard, the patient must be provided with information that would be regarded as material by an average, reasonable patient making a decision about whether to accept or refuse treatment or choose between different treatment options. At a minimum, disclosure is required of any material risks associated with the procedure.

The physician charged with the duty to disclose necessary information to the patient may be the emergency physician or the consulting physician who will provide appropriate inpatient or outpatient follow-up care. After the physician has spoken with the patient, it is appropriate to give a nurse the responsibility for obtaining the patient's written consent to treatment. Written consent may be obtained through the use of a consent form that the patient should read and sign. It is also appropriate for the patient to sign in the presence of a nurse or other individual who witnesses the act of signing.

Exceptions to Consent Requirements

Generally, a patient's consent must be obtained prior to medical and diagnostic procedures and surgical treatment. The **emergency doctrine** provides an exception to this rule in the event of an emergency requiring immediate action for the preservation of the life or health of the patient in circumstances that make it impractical to obtain the patient's consent. The emergency doctrine is based on the premise that if able to do so, anyone would authorize treatment to save his or her own life or prevent serious personal harm. The doctrine implies consent only for the treatment necessary to rescue the patient from the emergency situation. As in all implied consent cases, the emergency physician should make every effort to secure an express consent from the patient or someone authorized to consent on the patient's behalf. Attempts to secure consent should be noted in the patient's medical record.

The **extension doctrine** provides an exception to the general rule that a patient's consent is limited to those procedures contemplated when consent is given. If in the course of authorized medical treatment a physician discovers a life-threatening condition that requires immediate treatment and the patient is unable to consent (eg, the patient is under anesthesia), the physician may extend the operation or treatment without the patient's express consent.

Finally, in situations where full disclosure to the patient might be *harmful* and therefore contraindicated, a physician may have a **therapeutic privilege** to withhold information. This privilege avails only when the patient's distress and apprehension are so great that full disclosure of all the risks might cause emotional harm or induce the patient to refuse treatment, fail to cooperate with treatment, or make an irrational choice of treatment alternatives. The privilege is justified only in rare circumstances, and full documentation of the need for it must always be entered into the medical record.

Authority to Give Consent

All *competent adults* have the legal capacity to consent to treatment. A patient who is competent has the ability to understand his or her medical condition and the treatment offered in a general way and can appreciate the possible consequences of accepting or refusing a specific type of treatment. If the patient is an incompetent adult, the law requires that some other qualified person (parent, spouse, or guardian) consent to treatment on the patient's behalf. Incompetence may be caused by mental or physical incapacities such as mental illness, senility, alcohol or other drugs, or unconsciousness from trauma or other causes. Physicians may be presented with documents that purport to grant to a third person the authority to consent to care for an incompetent adult. Commonly known as powers of attorney, these instruments may be used as evidence of consent to treat when an effort to reach the next of kin would be futile or when reasonable efforts to reach the appropriate individual have failed.

Intoxicated Patients

Patients intoxicated with alcohol or drugs are frequent visitors to the emergency department and present special problems in consent. Intoxicated patients have a diminished capacity to give or withhold consent. Thus, the emergency department staff should make every effort to treat an intoxicated patient and ensure that not only the patient but also any family members or friends understand the seriousness of the injuries. It is far better to observe an extremely uncooperative patient than to refuse treatment and eject the person from the emergency department. The emergency department staff could be liable for failure to treat an intoxicated patient if the staff did not make every reasonable attempt to quiet the patient, impress upon the patient the seriousness of the injury, and obtain consent for treatment.

Police Custody

Patients who have been arrested and are on their way to jail—or persons already in jail—are often brought to the emergency department for treatment. These patients still have the same rights regarding consent to medical treatment as other people, so that consent for examination and treatment must be obtained.

Minors

The law requires that the consent of a minor's parents or legal guardian be obtained before treatment can be given. If the parent is not present in the emergency department, informed oral consent can be obtained over the telephone and "witnessed" by someone else listening on an extension, and the parent's consent can then be documented in the emergency department record.

A minor is any person under the legally recognized

age of majority. An emancipated minor may give consent for treatment. The minor's age, maturity, marital status, economic independence, and general ability to understand the nature of the proposed treatment are factors to be considered in determining whether a minor is emancipated. In the USA, some state statutes define the circumstances under which a minor may consent to medical treatment. For example, a New Jersey statute provides that a minor girl who is married or pregnant may consent to medical treatment for herself or any children she may have.

The emergency doctrine of implied consent also applies to minor patients. In the absence of a serious emergency, the physician who treats a minor without the consent of the minor's parents or legal guardian is at risk of liability for battery. This risk may be minimal, since parents rarely sue physicians for providing appropriate care to a child. When a minor's non–life-threatening condition requires treatment without undue delay, the physician should try to contact the responsible adult before rendering care and note in the patient's record that such an attempt has been made. If a responsible adult is unavailable, it is prudent to treat the minor who requires care rather than risk increased injury attributable to delay in obtaining consent.

Patient Refusal to Consent

A physician cannot force a competent adult patient to accept treatment even in the face of a life-threatening emergency. All competent patients have the right to decide what will be done to their bodies.

Thus, competent patients can sign out of the emergency department without treatment and against medical advice. If this occurs, the risks should be explained and the patient asked to sign a form releasing the hospital and emergency department staff from liability. If the patient or family members refuse to sign, this fact should be documented and witnessed by the emergency department staff. Efforts by the staff to make certain the patient understands his or her condition and the consequences of refusing treatment also should be noted in the record.

Members of Jehovah's Witnesses and other religious groups who refuse blood or blood product transfusions present a serious problem for the emergency department staff. In the USA, courts in some states have ordered lifesaving treatment despite the patient's objection when the patient is a minor. Other courts have reaffirmed the right of a competent individual to refuse treatment even when that individual's decision may result in the death of a parent of a minor. The hospital's counsel should be contacted immediately in the event of a conflict between the patient and his or her needs as perceived by the emergency physician.

Consent for Blood
Alcohol Samples

In the USA, many states have enacted stringent "DUI" (driving under the influence) laws that define intoxication on the basis of blood alcohol concentration. Most of the new laws have provisions under which motorists are deemed to have given their consent to the performance of certain chemical tests to determine the level of alcohol in the blood if the arresting officer has reasonable cause to suspect that the driver is impaired. In some states, this "implied consent" extends only to the testing of urine and breath samples and not to blood samples.

Emergency physicians should familiarize themselves with the provisions of the "DUI" (driving under the influence) laws in the states in which they practice. Physicians who practice emergency medicine in those states where implied consent laws do not apply to the taking of blood samples should exercise extra care to ensure that blood samples are obtained in a medically acceptable manner.

Emergency physicians who are confronted with an unconscious patient may obtain a clinically indicated blood sample for chemical testing. In the event that the test results are required for legal proceedings, the prosecutor may obtain a court order to obtain the test results if the state has no "implied consent" law.

When blood is drawn from a patient, the skin should be cleansed with a nonalcohol substance and all specimen tubes should be clearly labeled. The blood should be drawn and handed over directly to the witnessing police officer (when it is legally appropriate to do so), who should acknowledge receipt by signing the emergency department record. This procedure, as well as the patient's consent, should be witnessed by another emergency department staff member. The circumstances surrounding the taking of the specimen and the physical examination of the patient should be well documented in the emergency department record.

PSYCHIATRIC EMERGENCIES
(See also Chapter 41.)

Patients with psychiatric disorders are often unable to test and evaluate external reality and may experience delusions, hallucinations, and apparent personality disintegration. Such patients present special problems with regard to the legal principles of assault and battery as well as false imprisonment. The key question in deciding when and to what degree physical restraint can be used on a patient with mental illness is whether the patient is likely to cause self-inflicted harm or injure others. As a general rule, the emergency department staff may use appropriate and reasonable efforts, including the use of restraints, to protect the patient from self-injury and keep the patient from harming others. If the staff fails to use necessary, reasonable restraints, it risks incurring liability to innocent third parties injured by the patient and may even incur liability to the patient if the latter's unrestrained combativeness results in self-injury. On the other hand, unnecessary or excessive force may result in liability for injuries sustained by the patient. What constitutes excessive force depends on the facts and circumstances of each case. For this reason, the emergency department record should contain an objective and thorough documentation of the patient's behavior, the physician's conclusions with regard to the patient's mental status, and the efforts used to restrain the patient.

The problem may be complicated when an alert and apparently competent psychiatric patient protests against being held in the emergency department for further assessment. The emergency department staff may be exposed to liability for false imprisonment if such a patient is later determined not to be dangerous, either to himself or herself or to others. Actions for false imprisonment may arise when a person is unlawfully deprived of personal liberty by another person for any length of time without giving consent and is aware of such deprivation, and where no defense of privilege applies, as it does in the case of parents, schoolteachers, etc. Although the emergency department staff may be apprehensive about liability for false imprisonment, failure to hold and further assess a mentally unstable person may result in liability if the patient is released and subsequent self-injury or harm to others occurs. Physicians who have discharged psychiatric patients who subsequently committed suicide have been found liable for wrongful death of these patients in lawsuits brought by the patients' survivors. In these cases, juries have concluded that the physician's decisions to discharge their patients were made in a negligent manner.

Maintaining the patient in the emergency department for a reasonable period of time for examination and evaluation by a psychiatric health professional may be the most prudent course of action. If a psychiatrist or other mental health professional is not available, the emergency physician must decide whether to discharge the patient or start procedures for involuntary commitment to a mental institution. Laws vary greatly with regard to emergency involuntary commitments. The emergency department staff should be familiar with the details of these laws in the local jurisdiction.

ABANDONMENT

Abandonment is the unilateral termination of the physician-patient relationship by the physician without the patient's consent and without giving the patient sufficient opportunity to secure the services of another competent physician. While much emergency department care is episodic in nature and does not involve follow-up treatment, the emergency department physician and staff still have a responsibility to instruct the patient about the details of follow-up care.

Emergency department physicians are obligated under all circumstances to conduct themselves as any reasonable physician would in treating the same patient under the same or similar circumstances. This means that physicians may be liable for negligent disposition of the patient if they do not give follow-up care instructions appropriate for the patient's condition. In the USA, this principle also requires the translation of follow-up instructions for patients who do not read English if the emergency department is in an area where it would be reasonable to require the presence of translating personnel in the hospital or emergency department. The area of follow-up instructions is also one of concern for the Joint Commission on Accreditation of Health Care Organizations. When frequently required in an emergency care area, a means of communication should be available in the language of the predominant population groups served by the hospital emergency department.

Instruction Sheets

Many emergency departments have attempted to discharge their responsibilities to provide follow-up instructions by using emergency department instruction sheets to be signed by the patient. Instruction sheets are helpful but do not fully solve the problem of follow-up care. The patient can always allege in court that nobody explained what was written on the instruction sheet when it was handed out. Such explanations should be documented in the medical record. Translation of instruction sheets into the patient's native language may be required in some cases. The patient's signature on the instruction sheet should certify that he or she has received the form and has been given oral instructions as indicated on the sheet. A copy of the signed instruction sheet should be retained in the patient's medical record.

Telephone Consultation

Patients may also allege abandonment via telephone consultation. An example is the patient who is discharged from the emergency department, experiences a recurrence of symptoms, calls the emergency department, and is told not to worry about it until morning. If the patient's condition worsens, the emergency department staff may be liable for negligence and abandonment. As a general rule, emergency department staff should not diagnose or treat patients over the telephone. It may be a tempting convenience, but the medicolegal risks and hazards are many.

REPORTABLE EVENTS

All governments have statutes and administrative regulations that require reporting of certain events by emergency physicians and emergency department staff members. Among these reportable events are child abuse, rape, gunshot and stab wounds, certain communicable diseases (including most sexually transmitted diseases), HIV infection or AIDS, animal bites, and the receipt of patients who are dead on arrival. Emergency physicians should know which events are reportable and the procedure for reporting them in the area in which they practice, since these rules vary by state and county.

Child Abuse

All United States jurisdictions and many other countries have regulations or statutes requiring the reporting of actual or suspected cases of child abuse. Some of these statutes are permissive and allow the reporter to exercise discretion in deciding whether or not to report, while others require reporting of all cases under penalty of fine or imprisonment.

Many state reporting statutes grant immunity from civil liability (immunity from charges of slander, etc) to the reporting party. These immunity provisions were intended to make the public (including physicians and nurses) more inclined to report suspected child abuse cases by eliminating the fear of being sued by the parents. In some states, immunity for reporting and for participating in subsequent judicial proceedings is provided without any express qualification. Other states provide immunity for action taken "in good faith" or "without malice." Generally, no immunity provision will protect emergency department staff members who broadcast to third parties with no official status or right to know that the parents are child abusers.

In states lacking statutes granting immunity, the emergency physician and, more importantly, the child victim will be much better off if suspicion of child abuse is reported to the appropriate agency. Failure to report a reasonably suspected case of child abuse may result in criminal penalties for failure to report according to state law and may also result in civil liability for negligence in failing to report. A California case, which was settled before trial for damages in excess of $600,000, illustrates this problem. This case turned on whether failure to report a suspected case of battery on a child would be grounds for a civil suit for negligence. The case was settled before trial because the failure to report was so blatant and because the brain-damaged child would have gained the jury's sympathy, suggesting that the verdict would likely have been for the plaintiff.

Procedures for management of suspected child abuse are given in Chapter 42.

Rape

Rape has traditionally been defined as unlawful carnal knowledge of a woman by a man, not her husband, against her will or with deception, and with penetration, however slight, of the vagina by the penis. Many states in the USA have enacted modern criminal laws that redefine sexual offenses. Implicit in these new laws is the recognition that a victim of a sexual crime may be either male or female. An even more significant departure from the traditional legal definition is that under certain circumstances, marriage may not be a defense to a charge of rape. In some jurisdictions, sexual penetration of the vagina or other orifices is not a necessary element of the offense. A second category of rape is statutory rape, which is defined generally as proscribed sexual conduct with a victim under the statutory age, with or without consent.

Emergency department staff must recognize that rape is a legal conclusion and not a medical diagnosis. The legal conclusion of rape is customarily arrived at after a trial by jury. The medical diagnosis of the rape victim should be limited to the actual clinical findings at the time of examination.

Protocols for management of both male and female rape victims are given in Chapter 30.

Gunshot & Stab Wounds

Most jurisdictions require that injuries from acts of violence, such as gunshot and stab wounds, be reported to the appropriate reporting agency. Reports of these violent wounds are usually made to the local police, although this may be unnecessary if the police accompany the patient to the emergency department or are already investigating the incident.

Communicable Diseases

Public health laws may require the reporting of certain communicable diseases, including sexually transmitted infections, HIV infection or AIDS, acute infectious encephalitis, food poisoning, hepatitis, meningococcal infections, plague, and many others. Both documented and suspected cases should be reported. Lists of reportable diseases vary by locale and should be reviewed by the emergency physician, although the World Health Organization list of reportable diseases is widely regarded as a satisfactory minimum.

In general, all medical personnel who are aware of the patient's diagnosis (including the attending physician, nurses, and laboratory personnel) are obligated to report cases of communicable disease. Reporting in the USA is generally accomplished by means of a short written form (the Confidential Morbidity Reporting [CMR] card, but with certain diseases (eg, plague, botulism), reporting by telephone or telegraph may be required, for obvious reasons. It may be advisable for the physician to telephone in reports of other highly communicable and serious conditions (eg, HIV infection or AIDS), particularly if there is uncertainty about the health department's response to implementing contact tracing or other disease control measures. Although in most states, failure to report is a misdemeanor punishable by fines or brief imprisonment, punishment is seldom exacted. However, the physician who fails to notify the health department when he or she diagnoses a reportable communicable disease faces a risk of license revocation or civil suit if secondary cases result from the failure to report. Contrariwise, the need of the health department to know of these conditions transcends the usual absolute confidentiality of the doctor-patient relationship. The physician should discuss the need for reporting with the patient to preserve (if possible) the therapeutic relationship with the patient.

Individuals other than the health department may be notified of the patient's diagnosis directly by the physician if there is an immediate risk to the patient's health (eg, the spouse of a patient with syphilis). This notification may also be made by the health department. However, individuals not at immediate risk of contracting infection from the patient (this usually includes employers, fellow employees, landlords, and casual acquaintances) should not be informed of the patient's diagnosis by the physician. To do so would leave the physician at risk of civil liability for breach of confidentiality. The patient about whom such information is disclosed may bring a lawsuit alleging wrongful disclosure of private information. Also, the physician risks liability for defamation, which is defined broadly as that which tends to injure the plaintiff's reputation or to diminish the esteem or respect in which the plaintiff is held.

Animal Bites

Reporting laws in the USA usually require that the emergency physician and staff report an animal bite to the appropriate local health official within a specified number of hours after the bite has occurred. Such reporting is an obvious safeguard to protect the public from vicious animals and from the spread of animal-borne infections, especially rabies.

See Chapter 24 for management of bites.

Epilepsy

Epilepsy and other neurologic impairments, especially those resulting in episodic loss of consciousness, are reportable to the agency responsible for motor vehicle licensing in many states in the USA.

Dead on Arrival (DOA)

All states in the USA require that receipt of a body dead on arrival at the emergency department be reported to the coroner or medical examiner for possible investigation and for assessment of the need for postmortem examination. In such cases, the emergency physician and staff should do nothing to the corpse that would interfere with the gathering of evidence by the coroner or medical examiner. For example, the emergency department staff should not attempt to obtain blood and tissue for laboratory studies; all specimens in such cases should be obtained by the coroner or medical examiner. Similarly, the corpse should not be used to practice CPR, endotracheal intubation, or other procedures.

THE MEDICAL RECORD

The importance of medical records and good record keeping cannot be overstated. Medical records are the most constantly reviewed documents in the hospital, and they are seen by representatives of hospital administration, the medical staff, and the many state and national accreditation agencies that periodically review the hospital for certification purposes. When a lawsuit is filed against a physician or hospital, the outcome almost invariably depends on what is written or not written in the medical record. Where crucial facts such as vital signs or the results of neurologic examinations were not recorded in the patient's medical record, courts have permitted juries to conclude that the vital signs were not taken or that the neurologic examination was not performed. Thus, the medical record is both a legal document and a means of recording the course of the patient's illness.

The Joint Commission on Accreditation of Health Care Organizations has established standards for the emergency department medical record, which require that a medical record be maintained on every patient seeking emergency care and be incorporated into the patient's permanent hospital record. A control register should be continuously maintained that includes the following information for each individual seeking care: name, age, sex, date, time of arrival, means of arrival, nature of the complaint, disposition, and time of departure. In explaining this standard, the Joint Commission identifies 10 areas where emergency department documentation is of special importance:

1. Patient identification or documentation of the reason for the absence of such identification when it is not obtainable.

2. Time and means of arrival.

3. Pertinent history of the illness or injury and physical findings, including vital signs.

4. Emergency care given to the patient prior to arrival.

5. Diagnostic and therapeutic orders.

6. Clinical observations, including results of treatment.

7. Reports of procedures and tests and results.

8. Diagnostic impression.

9. Final disposition, condition on discharge or transfer, and follow-up care instructions given to the patient or family.

10. A patient leaving against medical advice.

The emergency department medical record should cover each of these essential areas to some extent. A medical form is designed to remind the emergency department staff about each of these areas. One of the most serious common errors by emergency department staffs is the failure to record a patient's complete vital signs. Another common error is failure to describe the follow-up treatment required and the indications for returning for care prior to that date.

The emergency physician should be aware that the information contained in the patient's medical record is confidential and should not be disclosed to the police, press, or other parties unless the patient has consented in writing to its disclosure. Exceptions to the general rule arise when the patient's medical record is sought by means of a valid subpoena or court order.

The emergency department physician can be forced to release confidential information by a court order requiring such release. Failure to obey such a court order may result in imprisonment or monetary penalties for contempt of court.

Medical records of patients seen in the emergency department because of drug or alcohol abuse must be handled with particular attention to confidentiality to avoid litigation for defamation. In the USA, federal regulations also govern the confidentiality of information concerning patients treated or referred for treatment for alcoholism or drug abuse by any facility that receives federal funds for any purpose.

All descriptions of the patient's clinical condition must be stated in an objective manner. The primary purpose of recording all relevant clinical information is diagnosis and treatment, both for the present condition and future care of the patient. Extraneous subjective remarks betraying the physician's or nurse's attitudes about the patient have no place in the medical record.

EMERGENCY PHYSICIAN & MEDICAL STAFF INTERACTION

The practice of hospital-based emergency medicine involves constant interaction of the emergency department staff with many members of the medical staff as well as the hospital administration and governing body. The clinical skills of the emergency physician are under constant prospective and retrospective scrutiny by the entire medical staff. As a result, the emergency department physicians and other staff must work in a highly charged professional environment.

A potential problem for the emergency department is created when a patient is instructed by a medical staff physician to go to the emergency department for treatment, and the physician then either fails to meet the patient and keep the appointment or fails to notify the emergency department staff of the patient's imminent arrival. The emergency physician must decide whether to exercise clinical control over the patient and institute diagnosis and treatment. If the patient is a nonemergency patient and wishes to be seen only by the private physician, there is no difficulty for the emergency department staff. However, when the patient's clinical problem requires immediate attention, the emergency physician may be sued for negligence if necessary emergency care is not given despite the wishes of the private physician. As a general rule, when in doubt, it is better to err on the side of treatment, assuming that the patient has consented to treatment in the first place. An effort should be made to contact the private physician under these circumstances, but administrative considerations should never interfere with appropriate patient care.

Another difficulty for the emergency physician is dealing with medical staff physicians' requests that the emergency physician write admission orders for patients admitted through the emergency department. The responsibility for writing admission orders rests with the medical staff physician to whose service the patient has been admitted. Having the emergency department physician write admission orders as a convenience for the medical staff only exposes the patient admitted through the emergency department to the added danger of not being promptly examined by the admitting physician.

Once a patient has been admitted through the emergency department, how soon should the patient be seen by the medical staff physician to whose service the patient has been admitted? If the patient's condition is serious, the patient should be seen as soon as possible after admission. Patients admitted to critical care units should be seen within a reasonable period of time, depending on the clinical conditions of each patient.

Another area of potential conflict between the hospital staff and the emergency physician is the area of on-call specialty consultation. Recent amendments to federal law require most hospitals to provide a list of on-call physicians who will respond to requests from emergency physicians to provide follow-up care. If emergency specialty consultation is requested and the on-call specialist fails to respond, the emergency physician may transfer the patient by certifying that the benefits of transfer outweigh the risks. Care must be taken to document requests for on-call consultation in a timely, accurate, and objective manner.

Problems such as these involving the emergency department and medical staff are of a delicate political nature and a source of much anxiety for both parties. It is important that the emergency department and medical staff keep lines of communication open so that these difficult areas can be discussed dispassionately. If this open communication does not exist, the inevitable result is strained personal and professional relations, which in turn cause a lowered standard of patient care and create a climate of confusion that engenders litigation.

HARVESTING OF ORGANS FOR TRANSPLANTATION

Emergency physicians can expect to be confronted with the issue of harvesting organs for transplantation. A possible scenario is as follows: An otherwise healthy young person is brought to the emergency department with intact cardiopulmonary function but obviously brain-dead as the result of a gunshot to the head. The emergency physician asks whether the parents would consent to organ donation. While the parents consider the request, the victim remains on a life-support system.

Legal and ethical problems may arise in securing organ donations, whether potential donors be alive or dead. The issue of informed consent must be fully explored with a potential competent adult donor. When the donor is deceased, consent may be obtained from the next of kin.

Deceased donors are most likely to be the source of donated organs in the emergency department setting. The primary legal question in such a situation appears to be the definition of death. Brain death legislation has been enacted in many states in the USA. Where brain death is recognized by statute, the express criteria set forth in the statute must be met. Where no statutory criteria exist, standards such as those accepted and recognized in the medical community must be applied (Chapter 10). The clinical indications of death should be documented in the medical record.

REFERENCES

Areen J: The legal status of consent obtained from families of adult patients to withhold or withdraw treatment. JAMA 1987;258:229.

Baker MT, Taub HA: Readability of informed consent forms for research in a Veterans Administration medical center. JAMA 1983;250:2646.

Curran WJ: Economic and legal considerations in emergency care. N Engl J Med 1985;312:374.

Fiscina SF: *Medical Law for the Attending Physician.* Southern Illinois Univ Press, 1982.

George JE: *Law and Emergency Care.* Mosby, 1980.

Goldberg RJ et al: A review of prehospital care litigation in a large metropolitan EMS system. Ann Emerg Med 1990;19:557.

Hirsch CS: *Handbook of Legal Medicine.* Mosby, 1979.

Hogue LL: *Public Health and the Law.* Aspen Systems, 1980.

Holder AR: *Medical Malpractice Law,* 2nd ed. Wiley, 1978.

Hospital Law Manual. Aspen Systems, 1980.

Kellerman AL, Hackman BB: Emergency department patient "dumping": An analysis of interhospital transfer to the Regional Medical Center at Memphis, Tennessee. Am J Public Health 1988;78:1287.

Ludlam J: *Informed Consent.* American Hospital Association, 1978.

Mancini MR, Gale ET: *Emergency Care and the Law.* Aspen Systems, 1981.

Mills M, Mills J: Legal aspects of infectious disease practice. Resident Staff Physician (Sept) 1983;29:85.

Rogers J: *Risk Management in Emergency Medicine.* American College of Emergency Physicians, 1985.

Rosoff AJ: *Informed Consent.* Aspen Systems, 1981.

46

Emergency Procedures

David Knighton, MD, FACS, Richard M. Locksley, MD, & John Mills, MD

GENERAL INSTRUCTIONS FOR SKIN PREPARATION & STERILE TECHNIQUE

Skin Preparation

A. There are 2 types of skin preparation: skin cleansing and skin sterilization.

1. Skin cleansing–Cleansing of the skin is sufficient for routine injections (subcutaneous, intramuscular, intravenous) and for simple venipuncture but *not* for venipuncture performed to draw blood for culture or to permit insertion of an indwelling device. In many countries, no skin preparation is used for routine venipuncture, and no complications are reported; however, in the USA, custom dictates skin cleansing before venipuncture or injection.

Skin cleansing is generally performed by swabbing the skin for a few seconds with a swab saturated with alcohol (70%) or organic iodine (eg, povidone-iodine or equivalent). To reduce the pain of venipuncture, the disinfectant should be allowed to dry on the skin before the skin is punctured: *Note: This procedure merely cleans the skin; it does not sterilize it.*

2. Skin sterilization–Skin sterilization should be performed before all procedures that involve puncturing or cutting the skin, with the exception of routine venipuncture and simple injections. This procedure eliminates superficial skin bacteria, leaving only a few organisms deep in hair follicles or sweat glands. Skin sterilization may be omitted if the delay involved would jeopardize the patient's life (eg, thoracostomy for tension pneumothorax).

B. A variety of techniques can be used to achieve skin sterilization:

1. Scrub the skin vigorously with copious amounts of 70% alcohol for 2 minutes. Or,

2. Using a sterile 10- × 10-cm (4- × 4-in) gauze pad, apply 2% iodine tincture to the area, and allow the iodine to dry. Then remove it, using 70% alcohol on a sterile pad, because iodine may cause skin burns. Or,

3. Apply an organic iodine disinfectant (eg, povidone-iodine or poloxamer-iodine) twice, allowing each application to dry. These particular disinfectants need not be removed before the procedure is started.

C. The following guidelines should be observed in all cases:

1. Sterilize a much larger area of skin than is required for the procedure.

2. Apply the disinfectant starting near the center of the area, and work outward toward the periphery.

3. Use sterile gloves to apply the disinfectant.

Sterile Technique

It is virtually impossible to achieve sterile technique at the bedside in the emergency department comparable to that obtainable in an operating room; however, following the guidelines outlined below decreases the risk of infection. Good lighting is helpful for maintaining sterile technique and is essential for performing procedures successfully.

1. Wash hands thoroughly, preferably with antiseptic soap, before performing any procedure.

2. Have all necessary equipment assembled and opened at the bedside, so that once sterile gloves have been donned, only sterile instruments and equipment will be touched. Alternatively, an assistant can open packaged sterile supplies.

3. Don sterile gloves.

4. Sterilize the skin, as described above.

5. Enlarge the sterile field by surrounding the sterile skin with sterile drapes made of cloth or paper. These may come with a window in them that is used to isolate the area of sterile skin selected for the procedure.

6. Make sure that catheters, needles, stopcocks, etc, are securely placed on the sterile field so that they cannot roll off the drape onto the floor, perhaps at a critical moment.

7. When performing complicated procedures that require stricter sterile conditions (eg, insertion of a catheter for total parenteral nutrition), wear a surgical cap, mask, and gown in addition to the sterile gloves.

UPPER EXTREMITY VENIPUNCTURE

Indications

Venipuncture is performed to obtain a sample of venous blood for laboratory testing.

Contraindications

Contraindications to venipuncture are as follows:

1. Cellulitis over the proposed site.

2. Phlebitis.

3. Venous obstruction.

4. Lymphangitis of the extremity.

5. Administration of intravenous fluid distal to the proposed site.

Personnel Required

One person can perform venipuncture unaided.

Equipment & Supplies Required

1. Materials for skin cleansing (or skin sterilization, if blood culture is to be performed).

2. Syringe of adequate size (10–50 mL) for the amount of blood needed, or Vacutainer tubes and appropriate Vacutainer syringe hub (Vacutainer equipment consists of a needle with a point at each end, evacuated glass tubes with rubber stoppers, and a plastic barrel. Blood is forced into the evacuated tube when the needle connects the tube with the vein).

3. Needle (21-gauge) for the syringe, or a Vacutainer needle with an automatic valve or rubber cuff to stop blood flow while tubes are being changed. If a large amount of blood is to be drawn, it is advisable to use an 18-gauge needle. Use smaller-gauge needles or scalp vein needles for infants and children.

4. Tourniquet.

5. Receptacle tubes for blood for the desired laboratory tests.

6. Gauze squares, 5×5 cm (2×2 in).

7. Adhesive dressing.

Positioning of the Patient

The upper extremity is the site most commonly used to draw venous blood. The patient should be in a comfortable position, with the upper extremity resting on a solid object. If the patient is in bed, the supine position is best, with the arm resting on the mattress close to the patient's side. The ambulatory patient should be sitting with the arm on a table or support at a comfortable height for the operator.

Procedure

1. Assemble all necessary equipment, and position the patient as described above.

2. Apply the tourniquet above the antecubital fossa in a manner that will allow quick removal with one hand. The tourniquet should be tight enough to occlude venous return but not so tight as to cause arterial obstruction or patient discomfort. It should be removed before the extremity turns purple.

3. Locate an appropriate vein. Have the patient open and close the fist of the selected arm to help pump blood from the muscle compartment of the arm into the superficial venous circulation.

a. Antecubital veins–The superficial basilic and cephalic veins course just under the skin on the volar side of the forearm. They run along the medial and lateral edge of the antecubital fossa at the elbow crease. In slender or muscular people, these veins often stand out and are easy to enter. If one of these veins is accessible, use it. In obese people, those who have had multiple venipunctures, and intravenous drug abusers, finding a patent antecubital vein (or any other vein) may be difficult.

Palpate the antecubital fossa with the tip of the index finger, and feel for the buoyant resilience of a distended vein. Be careful to differentiate the firm cord of a thrombosed vein from the resiliency of a patent vessel. When the veins are not visible, they must be located by feel. Even a small vein deep in the subcutaneous tissue may be detected on the basis of its resilient feel.

b. Arm veins–If a patient antecubital vein cannot be found, examine the forearm on both the volar and the dorsal surfaces. Look for the faint bluish color of a vein under the skin, or better yet, feel for a vein with the tip of the index finger.

c. Hand veins–If no vein is found on the forearm, proceed to the dorsal surface of the hand, and use one of the superficial veins on the hand. These veins are small, collapse easily, and are usually inadequate for drawing a large amount of blood. If large amounts of blood are needed, it is often better to go to another anatomic site such as the femoral vein rather than to persist in trying to draw large quantities of blood from a small hand vein. By the time an adequate amount has been obtained, it usually clots in the syringe, and another venipuncture then becomes necessary.

d. Repeated search–Do not give up after one examination of the arm. Carefully palpate the arm 2 or 3 times if necessary. A vein suitable for venipuncture may be obscured (eg, by hair) and may therefore be missed on initial examination. Occasionally, slapping repeatedly over the vein with the pads of the first and second fingers will help to distend a faint vein, or the patient can dangle the arm over the side of the bed to achieve the same result. Do not thrust blindly at a bluish mark on the patient's arm without first palpating the area to confirm that there is a patent vein underneath.

4. Prepare the skin. Skin cleansing is adequate unless blood is being obtained for culture, in which case the skin must be sterilized (see Skin Preparation, above).

5. Grasp the syringe or Vacutainer in the dominant hand while palpating the vein with the index finger of the other hand. Exert traction on the vein by pulling distally (toward the operator) on the skin next to the puncture site. Align the needle with the course of the vein, and make sure that the bevel is facing up. With a quick but smooth motion, push the needle through the skin at an angle of about 10–20 degrees (Fig 46–1). Then carefully advance the needle into the lumen of the vein with a smooth motion.

6. When the vein has been properly penetrated, blood will flow back into the needle when the plunger is pulled away from the needle or when the Vacutainer tube is pushed onto the needle.

7. If venous blood is not obtained on the first attempt, reassess the course of the vein. Try palpating the vein proximal to the needle site. Withdraw the needle to just below the skin, and attempt a second venipuncture.

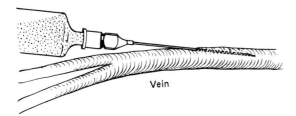

Figure 46–1. Technique of percutaneous venipuncture. The needle should be inserted into the lumen of the vein at an angle of about 10–20 degrees, and the bevel should be facing up. (Reproduced, with permission, from Krupp MA et al: *Physician's Handbook,* 21st ed. Lange, 1985.)

8. Once the needle is in the lumen of the vein, withdraw the required amount of blood with a steady, even pull on the plunger of the syringe. If too much force is applied and blood flow in the vein is less than the amount being drawn into the syringe, the vein will collapse, occluding the lumen of the needle. If this occurs, stop and allow the vein to fill, and then resume at a slower pace. If a large volume of blood is required, it may be necessary to select another, larger vein.

If a Vacutainer system is being used, simply fill all of the tubes required.

9. Draw enough blood to give accurate laboratory test results; clotted or hemolyzed specimens will give misleading information.

10. When enough blood has been obtained, remove the tourniquet, and then withdraw the needle quickly and smoothly. Have the patient immediately apply firm direct pressure on a 5- × 5-cm (2- × 2-in) piece of gauze over the site for 3–5 minutes. If the site is antecubital, flex the arm to stop the bleeding. Elevating the arm will speed hemostasis.

11. Quickly fill the blood receptacle tubes with the appropriate amount of blood, and mix each tube thoroughly if anticoagulant or preservative is present in the tube. Label the tubes with the patient's name, date of birth, and date of sample, and place any specimens on ice as required.

12. It is often helpful to put an adhesive dressing on the venipuncture site to absorb any blood that might ooze out.

EMERGENCY ANTECUBITAL FOSSA VENOUS CUTDOWN

Antecubital fossa cutdown provides a secure large-bore conduit for fluid resuscitation and central venous pressure measurement without the risks associated with placement of a subclavian or internal jugular vein catheter.

Indications
Emergency antecubital fossa cutdown is performed to gain immediate large-bore access to central veins for resuscitation and venous pressure measurements.

Contraindications
Contraindications to emergency antecubital fossa cutdown are as follows:

1. Previous antecubital fossa cutdown at the proposed insertion site (use the other arm or another site).

2. Trauma to the extremity proximal to the proposed cutdown site.

3. Known or suspected major vascular injury to the axillary or subclavian arterial or venous system on the side of the proposed cutdown.

Personnel Required
The operator may require an assistant to provide exposure and assist in insertion of the catheter.

Equipment & Supplies Required
A. Materials:

1. Materials for skin sterilization.

2. Lidocaine, 1%, with 10-mL syringe and 25-gauge needle.

3. Tourniquet.

4. Topical antibacterial ointment.

5. Expanded gauze roll and tape.

6. Padded armboard that fits under the mattress of the patient's gurney and extends (parallel to the floor) about 15 cm (6 in) beyond the patient's outstretched arm.

7. Tape to secure the patient's arm to the armboard.

8. Intravenous fluid in a container with a Y type blood infusion set and an in-line blood pump. The equipment should be flushed and fully assembled, ready for use.

B. Prepackaged sterile cutdown trays are commercially available. The following items are required:

1. Drapes

2. Gauze sponges (10 × 10 cm [4 × 4 in]).

3. Silk ligatures (size 3-0) (2).

4. Nylon or polypropylene skin suture (size 4-0) on a cutting needle.

5. Needle holder.

6. No. 15 and No. 11 scalpel blades, both mounted.

7. Curved Kelly clamps (3).

8. Mosquito clamps (2) (useful for small patients).

9. Tissue dissection scissors and straight suture scissors.

10. Self-retaining retractor or 2 right-angle retractors.

11. Pediatric feeding tubes, sizes 5F and 10F (1 each). (Use the largest one that fits the vein.)

12. Toothed and smooth forceps.

13. Plastic-coated absorbent pad to place beneath the patient's arm.

Positioning of the Patient

The patient should be supine, with the arm selected for cutdown insertion extended on an armboard that has been wrapped in an absorbent pad. Tape the arm in place at the wrist.

Anatomy Review

The deep basilic vein is found medial to the brachial artery beneath the superficial fascia. Accurate identification of the basilic vein is crucial. It is usually thin-walled when compared to the brachial artery, and it has a bluish tinge. The median nerve is fibrous and relatively avascular. However, the vein may be thick-walled in an elderly person or an intravenous drug abuser, or the artery may carry desaturated blood, which may also give it a bluish tinge.

Procedure

1. Apply the tourniquet proximal to the antecubital fossa.

2. Sterilize a wide area of skin around the antecubital fossa.

3. Drape the arm.

4. Measure the catheter (pediatric feeding tube), and cut it to the required length as follows: Place the hub end of the feeding tube at the antecubital fossa of the patient's outstretched arm, and extend the catheter to the suprasternal notch. This length ensures that the catheter will then be long enough to reach the central venous system (superior vena cava) without entering the right ventricle of the heart (which can cause serious ventricular arrhythmias). Cut the catheter at an angle, and trim off the sharp tip to avoid puncturing the vein distal to the insertion site.

5. Using the 1% lidocaine with the 10-mL syringe and 25-gauge needle, anesthetize the antecubital fossa over the medial aspect of the forearm at the level of the elbow crease, taking care not to puncture a superficial basilic vein. Omit this step if the patient is comatose.

6. With the No. 15 scalpel blade, make a 2.5- to 4-cm (1- to 1½-in) transverse incision on the median half of the antecubital fossa at the elbow crease. The incision should be at a right angle to the long axis of the arm and should extend down to the subcutaneous tissue. It may be helpful to palpate the brachial artery as a landmark, since the basilic vein lies medial to it. Be careful not to lacerate any large superficial veins that lie just under the skin.

7. If the patient has a large superficial basilic

vein, proceed with isolation and cannulation, as described in steps 8–11. If no superficial vein is present, continue to dissect deep to isolate the basilic vein (step 8). Be sure to differentiate the vein from the brachial artery and the median nerve. (See Anatomy Review, above.)

8. Using a curved Kelly clamp with the points aimed downward, dissect the subcutaneous tissue parallel to the long axis of the arm to isolate the basilic vein. Dissect the tissue on either side and then on top of the vein. Pass the clamp under the vein and dissect the tissue there. This maneuver should separate the vein from the surrounding structures and connective tissues. Small veins may be encountered in the subcutaneous tissue. *Do not* attempt to cannulate these veins. They have many valves and will not allow central passage of the catheter. Use the retractors to maintain exposure of the vein.

9. Leave the Kelly clamp in the open position under the vein for support. Using the smooth forceps as a clamp, pass the 2 silk ties under the vein, one proximal and one distal to the intended venotomy site. Ligate or loosely tie the distal portion of the vein while exerting traction on the distal silk tie. Perform a venotomy with the No. 11 scalpel blade (Fig 46–2):

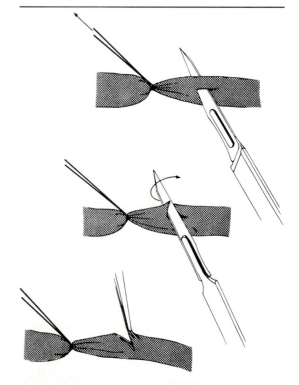

Figure 46–2. Venotomy technique. Exerting distal traction on the distal vein ligature, insert a No. 11 scalpel blade through the vein, and cut laterally. Open the venotomy incision with a mosquito clamp. (Reproduced, with permission, from Dunphy JE, Way LW [editors]: *Current Surgical Diagnosis & Treatment,* 5th ed. Lange, 1981.)

Hold the scalpel parallel to the long axis of the vein with the blade in a horizontal position, and pass it through the midportion of the superficial (or anterior) wall of the vein. Then turn the cutting edge of the blade upward, and open the top of the vein. Be careful not to transect the vein or puncture its outer wall.

10. Insert a closed mosquito clamp into the venotomy, and gently spread the clamp to dilate the vein.

11. With the bevel up, gently insert the catheter into the vein, and advance it until the hub reaches the incision. Remove the mosquito clamp.

12. Occasionally, the catheter fails to traverse the axilla and pass into the intrathoracic venous system. In this situation, abduct the arm, and slowly advance the catheter. This maneuver straightens the course of the vein and usually facilitates passage. If the catheter meets an obstruction at a valve, move the catheter gently backward and forward while rotating it, or attempt to open the valve by infusing fluid through the catheter. If the catheter does not pass easily into the central venous system, *stop*. Do not push so vigorously that the vein is perforated.

The most common problem is that the catheter has not entered the basilic vein. Withdraw the catheter, and tie off the proximal portion of the vein. Continue dissection, looking for the basilic vein. Occasionally, a basilic system vein of adequate diameter is not present, in which case an alternative method of central venous access must be found.

13. Allow blood to fill the catheter, and then remove the tourniquet. Insert the intravenous tubing in the catheter, and start the intravenous fluid drip. Ligate the distal portion of the vein with the distal silk tie, and using the same tie, secure the catheter to the ligated distal vein. Secure the catheter in the vein with a strong tie proximal to the venotomy site. Make sure that the ligatures are not so tight that they occlude the catheter (Fig 46–3).

14. Close the skin with a simple running skin stitch using the nylon or polypropylene skin suture.

15. Secure the catheter to the skin with a stitch, and tape all connections.

16. Dress the incision with the antibacterial ointment and a 10- × 10-cm (4- × 4-in) gauze sponge, and wrap the incision site with an expanded gauze roll.

17. Obtain a chest x-ray immediately to check the position of the catheter.

PERIPHERAL VENOUS CATHETERIZATION WITH A CATHETER-CLAD NEEDLE

Catheter-clad needles (eg, Angiocath) are generally preferred over needle-clad catheters (eg, Intracath) for peripheral intravenous access because they provide the largest-diameter catheter lumen possible for a given size of venipuncture. Their flexibility gives them an advantage over rigid needles for long-term use.

Indications

Peripheral venous catheterization with a catheter-clad needle is performed to gain peripheral venous access.

Contraindications

Contraindications to peripheral venous catheterization with a catheter-clad needle are as follows:

1. Phlebitis of the extremity.

2. Cellulitis over the projected site of insertion.

3. Potential or existing lymphedema or venous occlusive edema of the extremity.

4. Anticipated insertion of a Scribner shunt in the extremity.

Personnel Required

One person can insert a catheter-clad needle unaided.

Equipment & Supplies Required

1. Materials for skin sterilization.

2. Tourniquet.

3. Precut tape to secure the catheter in place.

4. Plastic-coated absorbent pad to place under the patient's arm.

5. Catheter-clad needle (eg, Angiocath) of sufficient size for the rate and type of fluid to be infused, but smaller than the cannulated vein. For administration of electrolyte or glucose solutions at rates of less than 200 mL/h, a 20-gauge catheter is usually sufficient. For infusion of blood or colloid solutions or rapid infusion of electrolyte solutions (200–1000 mL/h), an 18-gauge catheter is mandatory and a 16-gauge is preferred. In patients with multiple trauma, who may require large volumes of blood and electrolyte solutions, a 14-gauge catheter is preferable.

6. Container of fluid for intravenous administration, with proper connecting tubing. The equipment should be flushed and fully assembled ready for use.

Positioning of the Patient

Place peripheral intravenous catheters in the upper extremity if possible. Occasionally, a lower extremity intravenous catheter is necessary when all veins in the upper extremity are inaccessible and insertion of a central venous catheter is not practical. Intravenous

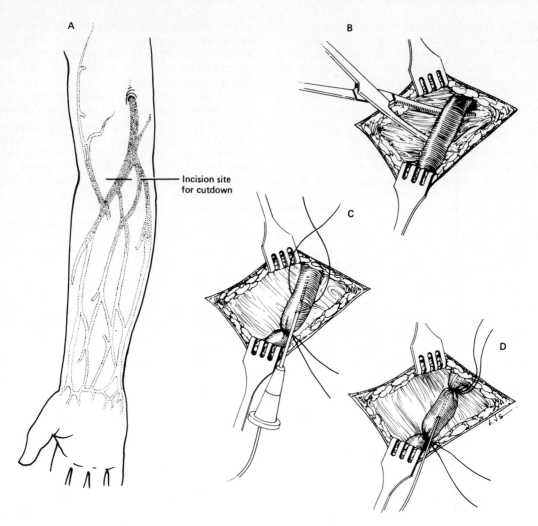

A

B

C

D

Incision site
for cutdown

Figure 46–3. Technique of cutdown insertion. After exposing the vein and making the venotomy incision (Fig 46–2), elevate and stabilize the vein with a straight clamp while inserting the tip of the catheter in the venotomy incision. As soon as the tip of the catheter is within the lumen of the vein, remove the clamp, slide the catheter the required distance up the vein, and tie the vein proximally and distally.

catheters in the lower extremity are associated with a much higher incidence of infection and thrombosis than are those inserted in the upper extremity.

The patient should be in a comfortable supine or sitting position, with the extremity to be used resting on a firm surface.

Procedure

1. Connect the container of fluid with the tubing, fill the connecting tubing with intravenous fluid, and make sure that all air is flushed from the tubing.

2. Apply the tourniquet above the antecubital fossa, and secure it so that it can be quickly removed with one hand.

3. Have the patient open and close the fist to help distend the superficial veins with blood. If veins are difficult to identify, having the patient hang the arm

below the level of the heart or wrapping the arm in a warm moist towel may be helpful.

4. Select an appropriate vein. The site at which 2 veins join is an excellent choice, since the vein is immobilized best in such a location. Possible sites include the radial aspect of the forearm just proximal to the wrist ("intern's vein"), the volar aspect of the forearm distal to the antecubital fossa on the ulnar side, and the dorsum of the hand. In slender people, these veins usually distend without difficulty; however, some individuals have deeply buried veins that can only be found by careful palpation. Remember that a vein does not have to be visualized in order to be successfully catheterized. Gentle tapping over the vein may help to distend it and make identification and catheterization easier. If it lies deep in the subcutaneous tissue, make a mental picture of its course and branches by means of systematic palpation up and down the vein.

5. Inspect the catheter to make sure that it slides easily off the needle and that both the catheter and the needle are smooth.

6. Place the plastic-coated drape under the arm selected for insertion.

7. Sterilize the skin around the insertion site.

8. Either grasp the needle directly with the dominant hand or place a syringe on the needle and grasp the syringe. Insert the needle through the skin at an angle of about 10–20 degrees, either on top of or next to the vein (Fig 46–1).

9. Pull the skin taut distal to the venipuncture site, and insert the needle and catheter into the vein. When the lumen of the vein is entered, blood flows back or can be withdrawn into the syringe.

10. Make sure that both the needle and the catheter are in the lumen of the vein. Blood may flow back when only the needle is in the vein and the catheter tip is against the wall of the vessel and has not actually entered the vessel lumen. In this position, the catheter cannot be advanced over the needle into the vein. To avoid this complication, advance the needle and catheter into the vein about 4–6 mm (⅛–¼ in) after blood initially returns. Check to be sure that blood continues to return when the needle and catheter are in this position.

11. Slide the catheter off the needle (Fig 46–4). Hold the needle steady by its hub in one hand at an angle of 10–20 degrees to the vein while gripping the hub of the catheter with the other hand, and gently push the catheter forward off the needle. Advance the catheter up to its hub while keeping the needle firmly in place. With practice, advancing the catheter and withdrawing the needle can be accomplished in one smooth motion. Be sure not to pull out both the catheter and needle at the same time. To avoid uncontrolled blood loss from the open catheter, occlude the vein proximal to the end of the catheter by applying direct pressure before pulling the needle out of the catheter.

12. *Note:* Occasionally, the catheter will encounter a valve in the vein that prevents complete advancement of the catheter. If this occurs, hold the catheter hub in place, remove the tourniquet, and connect the intravenous tubing to the catheter. Running intravenous fluid into the vein often opens the valve and allows complete insertion of the catheter.

13. Remove the tourniquet.

14. Attach the intravenous tubing to the catheter, and check the flow. A properly located catheter

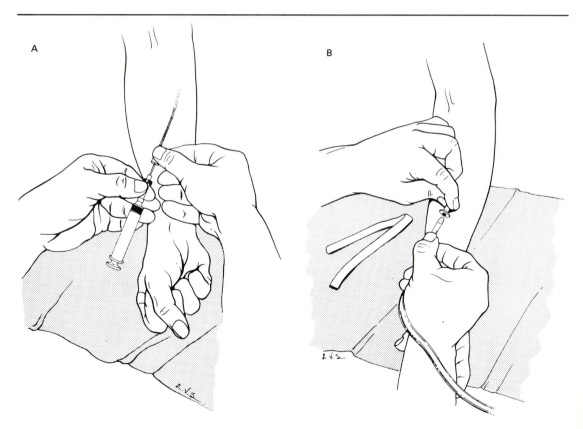

Figure 46–4. A: Technique of removing the needle from a catheter-clad needle. **B:** Connecting the intravenous tubing.

should allow rapid influx of fluid. If flow is slow or there is no flow at all, withdraw the catheter a few millimeters, and watch for change in the rate of flow. Occasionally, a branch vein or valve obstructs flow, and moving the catheter will be all that is required to achieve good flow.

15. Occasionally, the catheter is pushed through the opposite wall of the vein, causing swelling and pain at the insertion site as the intravenous fluid dissects the subcutaneous tissues. In this case, withdraw the catheter and needle completely, and try a second venipuncture in another vein or in the same vein proximal to the first insertion site. (Allow enough time for the first venipuncture to clot, or leave the catheter in place to occlude the venipuncture site until the more proximal catheter is inserted, and then withdraw the unused catheter.)

16. Secure the catheter in place with tape as shown in Fig 46–5. Tape all connections. Do not apply tape completely around the arm; it can act as a tourniquet and lead to distal edema. It is helpful to write the catheter gauge and date of insertion on the tape.

PERIPHERAL VENOUS CATHETERIZATION WITH A SCALP VEIN (BUTTERFLY) NEEDLE

Scalp vein needles are useful for short-term intravenous infusions in adults and for both long- and short-term use in children. They are also useful for phlebotomy in uncooperative patients, especially children, since the flexible connecting tubing prevents dislodgment of the needle when the patient moves.

Indications
Indications for peripheral venous catheterization with a scalp vein needle are as follows:

1. Need to gain peripheral venous access.

2. Need to perform phlebotomy in an uncooperative patient (the needle might otherwise become dislodged from the vein).

Contraindications
Contraindications to the use of scalp vein needles for peripheral venous catheterization are the same as those for catheter-clad needles.

Personnel Required
One person can perform venous catheterization with a scalp vein needle unaided if the patient is cooperative.

Equipment & Supplies Required
1. Materials for skin sterilization.

2. Tourniquet.

3. Precut tape to secure the catheter in place.

4. Plastic-coated absorbent pad to place beneath the patient's arm.

5. Scalp vein needle of appropriate size.

6. Container of intravenous fluid with connecting tubing. All equipment should be flushed and fully assembled ready for use.

Positioning of the Patient
If venipuncture in the upper extremity is planned, have the patient supine, with the arm extended volar side up. In infants, the veins of the scalp and the fist are also useful for catheterization (Fig 46–6A).

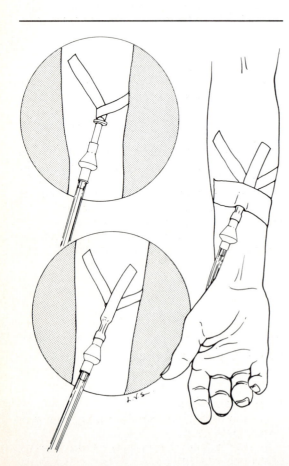

Figure 46–5. Technique of securing an intravenous catheter to the skin with tape after insertion.

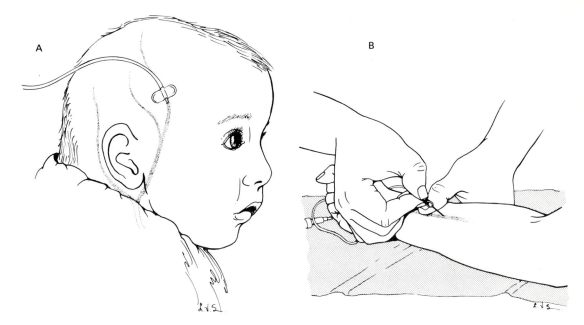

Figure 46–6. **A:** Scalp vein needle in an infant. **B:** Technique of inserting a butterfly needle. With the bevel of the needle facing up, oppose the 2 plastic "wings," and grip them between the thumb and forefinger while performing venipuncture.

Procedure

1. Connect the container of intravenous fluid with the tubing, and fill the connecting tubing with intravenous fluid. Make sure that all air is flushed from the tubing.

2. The short tubing connected to the scalp vein needle should be filled with fluid before the infusion begins. This can be accomplished either by letting the blood flow back into the tubing from the vein or by filling the tubing with infusion fluid before inserting the needle. Letting blood fill the tubing can lead to clotting if the flow of intravenous fluid is not established quickly.

3. Place the plastic-coated absorbent pad under the site chosen for catheterization.

4. If an extremity is to be catheterized, apply the tourniquet above the site.

5. Sterilize the skin around the insertion site.

6. Keeping the bevel of the needle facing up, grasp the plastic wings attached to the needle between the thumb and index finger of the dominant hand, and insert the needle into the vein at a 30-degree angle (Fig 46–6B).

7. Once the needle has entered the vein (blood appears in the tubing), decrease the angle between the needle and the vein to 10–20 degrees. Then carefully thread the needle into the lumen of the vein until the entire needle is in the vein. Failure to insert the needle completely makes securing it more difficult.

8. Secure the needle to the arm with tape, as shown in Fig 46–7, and tape all connections.

EXTERNAL JUGULAR VEIN CATHETERIZATION

Indications

External jugular vein catheterization is performed to gain peripheral or central venous access when sites other than the external jugular vein (eg, internal jugular or subclavian vein) are inaccessible or if catheterization of those sites is contraindicated (eg, coagulopathy).

Contraindications

Contraindications to external jugular vein catheterization are as follows:

1. Agitated, uncooperative patient (this is only a relative contraindication).

2. Cellulitis at the insertion site.

3. Previous neck surgery (the position of the vein

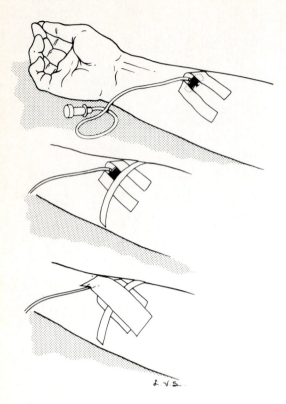

Figure 46–7. Technique of securing a butterfly needle to the skin with tape after insertion.

may be distorted, or it may have been ligated or removed).

Personnel Required

One person can perform simple external jugular vein catheterization unaided, although an assistant is helpful. Insertion of a central venous catheter through the external jugular vein by means of a J wire requires an assistant.

Equipment & Supplies Required

A. Peripheral Venous Access:

1. Materials for skin sterilization.

2. Catheter-clad needle (eg, Angiocath), 16- to 18-gauge.

3. Container of intravenous solution and connecting tubing.

4. Precut tape for securing the catheter.

5. Plastic-coated absorbent pad to place under the patient's head and neck.

6. Tincture of benzoin, 5 mL.

B. Central Venous Access:

1. Materials for skin sterilization.

2. Materials for sterile technique (cap, mask, gloves, and gown).

3. Lidocaine, 1%, with 10-mL syringe and 25-gauge needle.

4. Sterile medicine cup with normal saline for flushing intravenous catheters and tubing.

5. Needle-clad catheter (eg, Intracath) or 12.5- to 20-cm (5- to 8-in) catheter-clad needle (eg, Angiocath) of appropriate gauge for the patient. Most adults will need a 16- to 18-gauge catheter-clad needle or a 14-gauge needle-clad catheter. Make sure the needles and catheters are of the proper size and construction to accept and slip over the J wire.

6. J wire (flexible angiography wire) 35.5 cm (14 in) long, about 0.089 cm ($\frac{1}{32}$ in) in diameter, and with a curvature that has a radius of about 3 mm ($\frac{1}{8}$ in).

7. Silk skin suture (size 3-0) on a cutting needle.

8. Needle holder.

9. Straight scissors.

10. Container of intravenous fluid and connecting tubing. All equipment must be flushed and fully assembled ready for use.

11. Gauze squares, 10×10 cm (4×4 in).

12. Plastic-coated absorbent pad to place under the patient's head and neck.

13. Sterile drapes.

14. Antibacterial ointment.

15. Tincture of benzoin, 5 mL.

Positioning of the Patient

The patient should be placed in the Trendelenburg position (20–30 degrees), with the head turned 90 degrees away from the side of insertion. Place the plastic-coated absorbent pad under the patient's head and neck.

Anatomy Review

The external jugular vein courses from behind the angle of the jaw across to the sternocleidomastoid muscle and superficial to it to join the subclavian vein (Fig 46–8). The internal jugular vein and carotid artery lie deep to the external jugular vein and are separated from it by the sternocleidomastoid muscle.

Procedure

A. Peripheral Venous Access:

1. Assemble all necessary equipment, including the container of intravenous fluid and tubing, and make sure the tubing has been flushed to remove all air.

2. Position the patient.

3. Sterilize the skin around the area of insertion from the clavicle to the ear.

4. Have the patient take a deep breath and forcibly exhale against a closed glottis (Valsalva maneuver) to increase intrathoracic pressure and distend the external jugular vein with blood. It is sometimes helpful to have the patient put a thumb in his or her mouth and blow against it. If the patient is unable to cooperate, the vein may be distended by obstructing its outflow with a finger placed on the neck above the clavicle.

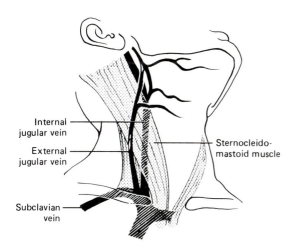

Figure 46–8. Anatomic relationships of the external jugular vein. The external jugular vein originates at the level of the angle of the mandible in the parotid gland, and it courses caudally and anteriorly across the sternocleidomastoid muscle. It enters the subclavian vein near the subclavian triangle.

5. Make a mental note of the position and size of the vein.

6. Have the patient resume normal breathing as soon as the size and position of the vein have been determined.

7. Insert the catheter-clad needle into the vein halfway between the angle of the jaw and the clavicle. While the patient performs the Valsalva maneuver, apply traction cephalad on the vein, and insert the catheter-clad needle into the vein lumen. Withdraw the needle, leaving the catheter in place. (See p 905 for technique of catheterization using a catheter-clad needle.)

8. Connect the intravenous tubing to the catheter, and start the intravenous infusion. To avoid air embolism, make sure either that intrathoracic pressure is elevated (eg, by the Valsalva maneuver) or that the hub of the needle is occluded with a thumb or finger.

9. Tape the tubing in place. When taping an intravenous line to the neck, it is helpful to use tincture of benzoin on both the patient's skin and the tubing. Tape the tubing up the side of the patient's neck and face superior to the ear, securing the line in several places with tape (Fig 46–9). Tape all connections.

10. Short catheters inserted in the external jugular vein are difficult to secure because of the constant motion of the patient's neck. The catheter may become dislodged from the vein and cause infiltration of intravenous fluid into the soft tissues of the neck. Before administering blood or drugs through an external jugular catheter, check to see that there is free flow of fluid into the line, that the neck is not swollen, and that blood can reflux freely into the in-

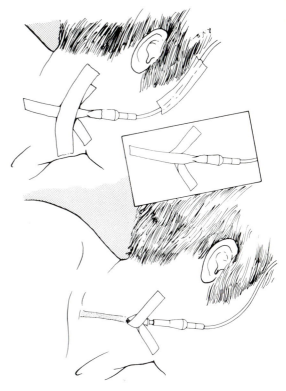

Figure 46–9. Technique of securing an external or internal jugular vein catheter to the skin with tape after insertion.

travenous tube when the intravenous bag or bottle is lowered below the level of the patient.

B. Central Venous Access:
1. Assemble all necessary equipment, including the container of intravenous fluid and tubing, and make sure the tubing has been flushed to remove all air.

2. Position the patient.

3. Sterilize the skin around the area of insertion from the clavicle to the ear.

4. Drape the area, and observe sterile technique (don cap, mask, gloves, and gown).

5. Have the patient take a deep breath and forcibly exhale against a closed glottis (Valsalva maneuver).

6. Note the course of the vein, and then have the patient resume normal breathing.

7. Select an insertion point about 4 cm (1⅝ in) above the clavicle, and infiltrate the area with the 1% lidocaine with the 10-mL syringe and 25-gauge needle.

8. While keeping the vein distended (by Valsalva maneuver or occlusion of outflow with finger compression), insert the catheter-clad needle or the needle from a needle-clad catheter into the external jugular vein. If a catheter-clad needle is being used, remove the central needle at this point, and cover the end of the catheter hub with a thumb to prevent aspiration of air.

9. Make sure the needle or catheter is properly placed in the vein by observing the return of blood through the catheter. Inject 5 mL of sterile saline, or run intravenous fluid through the line to establish its patency.

10. Insert the J wire through the needle or catheter, curved end first; guide the wire around the bends in the course of the external jugular vein-subclavian vein junction into the intrathoracic portion of the subclavian vein-superior vena cava system.

11. Secure the wire at the skin with a clamp or a finger. Do not allow the wire to slip all the way into the vein.

a. If a catheter-clad needle is being used, slide the catheter over the wire and into position in the intrathoracic portion of the venous system.

b. If a needle-clad catheter is being used, remove the insertion needle, taking care to grasp the J wire firmly to keep it from slipping forward all the way

into the vein. Slip the catheter over the J wire, and be careful not to let the J wire slip all the way into the vein as the catheter is being advanced.

12. Holding the catheter in place, remove the J wire, and cover the end of the catheter hub with a thumb until the setup can be tested for return of blood. Then start the intravenous infusion.

13. Secure the catheter in place with the silk suture run first through the skin and then wrapped around the catheter.

14. Take the patient out of the Trendelenburg position.

15. Obtain a portable chest x-ray immediately to confirm placement of the catheter.

16. Dress the insertion site with antibacterial ointment, cover it with a folded sterile 10- × 10-cm (4- × 4-in) gauze pad, and tape the pad in place.

17. Remember to tape all connections to prevent air embolism.

INTERNAL JUGULAR VEIN CATHETERIZATION

The internal jugular vein is used for insertion of central venous catheters. Pulmonary complications (hemothorax, pneumothorax) occur less commonly than with subclavian vein catheterization, but arterial injury (eg, to the carotid artery) is more common.

Indications

Internal jugular vein catheterization is performed to gain access to the central venous system for administration of fluids and measurement of central venous pressure.

Contraindications

Contraindications to internal jugular vein catheterization are as follows:

1. Previous neck injury that might have ligated or scarred the internal jugular vein and thereby altered its anatomy.

2. Superior vena cava occlusion.

3. Acquired or iatrogenic bleeding disorder.

4. Cellulitis over the proposed insertion site.

5. Agitated, uncooperative patient (this is only a relative contraindication).

6. Patient receiving CPR.

Personnel Required

The operator performing internal jugular vein catheterization requires an assistant to help handle sterile materials and position the patient.

Equipment & Supplies Required

A. Materials:

1. Materials for skin sterilization.

2. Materials for sterile technique (cap, mask, gloves, and gown).

3. Lidocaine, 1%, with 10-mL syringe and 25- and 22-gauge needles.

4. Topical antibacterial ointment.

5. Tape.

6. Container of intravenous fluid with all necessary tubing. All equipment should be flushed and fully assembled ready for use.

B. Prepackaged sterile cutdown trays are commercially available. The following are required:

1. Drapes.

2. Gauze sponges, 10 × 10 cm (4 × 4 in).

3. Nylon or silk skin suture (size 3-0 or 4-0) on a cutting needle.

4. Needle holder.

5. Straight scissors.

6. Plastic-coated absorbent pad to place beneath the patient's arm.

7. Syringe, 3-mL, with 22-gauge, 6.5-cm (2½-in) needle (for use as a probe).

8. Central venous catheter and insertion set. Many kinds are commercially available; most consist of an introducing needle and radiopaque catheter, usually 30.5 cm (12 in) long.

Positioning of the Patient

Use a bed or gurney which can be placed in the Trendelenburg position and which has a removable headboard. The patient should be supine, with the head turned 90 degrees away from the side selected for insertion. Place the patient in as steep a Trendelenburg position as possible in order to fully distend the internal jugular vein and also to create increased pressure inside the vein, thus decreasing the chances of air embolism during insertion.

Anatomy Review

The internal jugular vein leaves the base of the skull and courses laterally and posteriorly to the carotid artery and the carotid sheath. It joins the subclavian vein at the thoracic outlet. The internal jugular vein runs medial to the upper portion of the sternocleidomastoid muscle, deep to the triangle formed by the 2 heads at the midportion of this muscle, and deep to its clavicular head (Fig 46–8).

Procedure

A. Anterior (Triangle) Approach: (Fig 46–10).

1. Assemble and arrange all necessary equipment, including the container of intravenous fluid and intravenous tubing, and make sure the tubing has been flushed to remove all air.

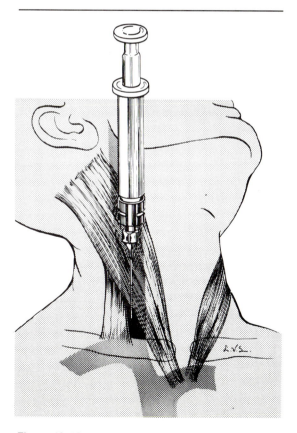

Figure 46–10. Internal jugular vein catheterization—anterior approach. (Reproduced, with permission, from Dunphy JE, Way LW [editors]: *Current Surgical Diagnosis & Treatment,* 5th ed. Lange, 1981.)

2. Position the patient, as described above.

3. Observe sterile technique (don cap, mask, gown, and gloves). Sterilize the skin around the area of insertion from the clavicle to the ear, and drape the patient.

4. The sternocleidomastoid muscle will be clearly outlined when the patient lifts the head slightly. Make a mental picture of the triangle formed by the 2 heads of the muscle, which has its apex pointed cephalad and its base formed by the clavicle.

5. Palpate the carotid artery, and make a mental note of the course of the internal jugular vein, which runs lateral and deep to the artery.

6. Choose a point near the apex of the triangle formed by the sternocleidomastoid, and anesthetize the skin with the 1% lidocaine with the 10-mL syringe and 25-gauge needle. Change to the 22-gauge needle, and infiltrate a path through the subcutaneous tissue toward the internal jugular vein, directing the needle downward at an angle of 45 degrees toward the ipsilateral nipple. Be careful when infiltrating the area to aspirate before injecting, so as to avoid injecting significant amounts of lidocaine into the vein. Omit this step if the patient is comatose.

7. Make a probe by placing the 22-gauge, 6.5-cm (2½-in) needle on the 3-mL syringe.

8. Use this small-gauge needle as a probe to locate the internal jugular vein. Pierce the skin near the apex of the triangle formed by the sternocleidomastoid, and direct the needle downward at a 30- to 45-degree angle toward the ipsilateral nipple. If the right hand is being used to guide the syringe and needle, palpate the carotid artery with the left hand to make sure that the needle is moving away from it. The needle should pierce the vein after advancing 2.5–4 cm (1–1½ in). If it does not, withdraw the needle until the point is just under the skin, reposition the needle in the subcutaneous tissue, and probe more medially, always keeping the left index finger on the carotid artery for reference. Once the needle has entered the internal jugular vein, dark venous blood should flow freely into the syringe. If the vein cannot be located after a few probing maneuvers, ask for assistance. *Caution: Do not use the larger catheter insertion needle or a catheter-clad needle (eg, Angiocath) if the vein cannot be located with the probing needle.* When the vein is located, withdraw the probing needle, and remove it from the syringe.

9. Now place the catheter insertion needle or catheter-clad needle on the syringe, and follow the course of the probing needle to enter the internal jugular vein. Always recheck the landmarks and position of the carotid artery while inserting this large needle.

10. Maintain a slight vacuum in the attached syringe while inserting the larger needle. Once the needle has entered the vein, dark venous blood will flow freely into the syringe. While aspirating, rotate the needle 360 degrees to make sure that the bevel of the needle is completely within the vein; cessation of blood flow at any point indicates that the needle should be slowly advanced or withdrawn, since it is near one wall of the vein.

11. When it is clear that the needle is properly positioned in the lumen of the vein, disconnect the syringe, and immediately occlude the orifice of the needle to prevent air embolization during inspiration. Pass the catheter through the needle into the vein, or slide the catheter off the needle, depending on the system being used. The catheter should meet no resistance. If it does, *do not* force it; withdraw the catheter and needle as a unit, apply pressure to the area for 5 minutes, and either try again on the same or opposite side (perhaps using a J wire to aid in passing the catheter [p 917]) or switch to the subclavian vein or some other method of central venous catheter placement. *Do not* withdraw only the catheter—especially with needle-clad catheters (eg, Intracath)—because this maneuver may cut off the catheter tip, which then may embolize distally.

12. When the catheter is fully inserted, check again to be sure there is good return, attach the intravenous tubing, and start the fluid infusion. If a needle-clad catheter is being used, withdraw the needle and catheter as a unit until the needle is fully exposed and the needle guard can be placed. Anchor the catheter in place with the nylon or silk size 3-0 or 4-0 skin suture. Make sure that the catheter is well secured, and tape it in place, using tincture of benzoin to help secure the tape to the skin and catheter. Tape all connections. Cover the insertion site with antibacterial ointment and a sterile 10- × 10-cm (4- × 4-in) gauze pad folded in half.

13. Take the patient out of the Trendelenburg position, and obtain a chest x-ray immediately to check placement of the catheter and to detect possible pneumothorax.

B. Posterior Approach: (Fig 46–11).

1–4. Steps 1–4 are the same as in the anterior approach.

5. Note the border where the posterior edge of the anterior belly of the sternocleidomastoid muscle meets the external jugular vein, and anesthetize with the 1% lidocaine. Use a 25-gauge needle for superficial infiltration and a 22-gauge needle for deeper anesthesia.

6. Using a 22-gauge, 6.5-cm (2½-in) needle attached to the 3-mL syringe as a probe, enter the skin just distal to the posterior edge of the sternocleidomastoid muscle, and direct the needle toward the suprasternal notch and under the sternocleidomastoid muscle. Pull back on the plunger as the needle is inserted. When the vein has been successfully entered,

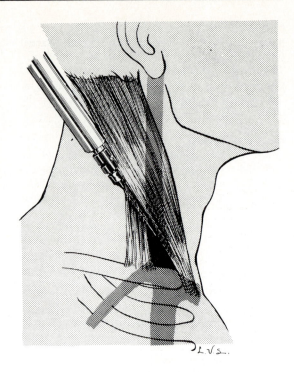

Figure 46–11. Internal jugular vein catheterization—posterior approach. (Reproduced, with permission, from Dunphy JE, Way LW [editors]: *Current Surgical Diagnosis & Treatment,* 5th ed. Lange, 1981.)

dark venous blood will flow back into the syringe. If the vein is not entered when the probing needle has been inserted its full length, withdraw the needle, and try again.

7. When the vein has been located with the probing needle, withdraw this needle, and insert the larger catheter insertion needle or catheter-needle combination. The needle should be attached to a syringe in which a slight vacuum is maintained.

8. When the vein has been successfully entered, dark venous blood will flow freely into the syringe.

9. Slip the catheter off the needle, or insert the catheter through the needle, depending on which system is being used. The catheter should pass easily without any resistance. If resistance is felt, stop, withdraw the catheter and needle together as a unit, apply pressure to the site for 5 minutes, and try again (perhaps using a J wire as a guide [p 910]), or use a different approach.

The remaining steps are the same as in the anterior approach.

SUBCLAVIAN VEIN CATHETERIZATION

Indications

Subclavian vein catheterization is performed to gain central venous access for monitoring of central venous pressure, insertion of a transvenous pacemaker, or administration of medications or intravenous fluids.

Contraindications

Contraindications to subclavian vein catheterization are as follows:

1. Edema or other manifestations of superior vena cava obstruction on the proposed side of insertion.

2. Previous surgery or irradiation to the subclavicular area.

3. Bleeding diathesis.

4. Infection or cellulitis over the proposed insertion site.

5. Pneumothorax on the contralateral site.

6. Uncooperative patient.

7. Patient receiving CPR.

Relative Contraindications

Relative contraindications to subclavian vein catheterization are as follows:

1. Assisted ventilation with high end expiratory pressures.

2. Mastectomy on the proposed side of insertion.

3. Severe hypovolemia (eg, hemorrhagic shock).

4. Recently discontinued subclavian line in the same area.

Personnel Required

Two people are usually required to perform percutaneous subclavian vein catheterization. The operator inserts the catheter, and an assistant opens sterile equipment and helps to position the patient.

Equipment & Supplies Required

A. Materials:

1. Materials for skin sterilization.

2. Materials for sterile technique (cap, mask, gloves, and gown).

3. Lidocaine, 1%, with 10-mL syringe and 22- and 25-gauge needles.

4. Topical antibacterial ointment.

5. Container of intravenous fluid with connector tubing.

6. Central venous catheter and insertion set. Many kinds are commercially available; most consist of an introducing needle and a radiopaque catheter, usually 30.5 cm (12 in) long.

7. Tape (including precut lengths).

8. Standard bath towel.

9. Tincture of benzoin.

B. Prepackaged sterile cutdown trays are commercially available. The following are required:

1. Drapes.

2. Gauze sponges, 10×10 cm (4×4 in).

3. Nylon or silk suture (size 3-0 or 4-0) on a cutting needle.

4. Needle holder.

5. Straight scissors.

6. Syringe, 3-mL, with 22-gauge, 6.5-cm ($2\frac{1}{2}$-in) needle for use as a probe (optional).

Positioning of the Patient

Proper positioning of the patient is crucial to successful subclavian vein catheterization.

1. Place the patient in the Trendelenburg position at an angle of 30 degrees, with the patient's head at a comfortable height for the operator. This position fully distends the subclavian vein and creates positive pressure inside the vein when the catheter is inserted, thus preventing air embolism.

2. Place the rolled bath towel between the patient's scapulas to allow the shoulders to fall backward and flatten the clavicles. Both arms should be at the patient's sides.

Anatomy Review

The subclavian vein courses under the clavicle near the subclavian artery and the apex of the lung (Fig 46–12). The artery is superior and deep to the vein. With a percutaneous approach, the vein is entered before the artery can be accidentally punctured. Laterally, the artery and vein drop caudally to enter the axilla.

Procedure

1. Make sure that all equipment is close at hand and ready for use. Assemble the container of intravenous fluid and tubing, and flush the tubing with fluid to remove all air.

2. Position the patient.

3. Sterilize the skin over the insertion site from the lateral aspect of the clavicle to the ear to the suprasternal notch.

4. The patient's head should be rotated away from the side of insertion, with the neck twisted as far as possible.

5. Observe sterile technique (don cap, mask, gloves, and gown).

6. Assemble the introducing needle and syringe, and make sure that the catheter is close by and quickly available.

7. Drape the infraclavicular area.

8. Using the index finger, palpate inferior to the

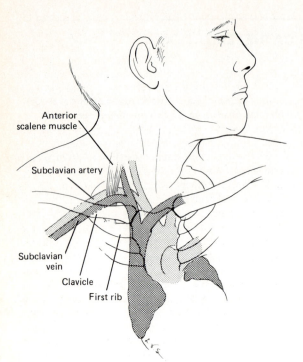

Figure 46–12. Anatomic relationships of the subclavian vein.

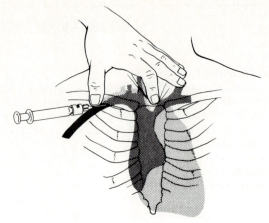

Figure 46–13. Technique of subclavian vein catheterization. With the index finger in the suprasternal notch and the thumb marking the costoclavicular ligament, insert the needle just medial to the thumb.

clavicle to find the costoclavicular ligament, which connects the clavicle and the first rib. This ligament lies where the clavicle bends posteriorly (about one-third the length of the clavicle from the suprasternal notch). Place the thumb between the clavicle and the first rib just lateral to this ligament, and place the index finger in the suprasternal notch. The subclavian vein traverses the imaginary line connecting these 2 fingers (Fig 46–13).

9. Anesthetize the skin with the 1% lidocaine using the 10-mL syringe and the 25-gauge needle; then use the 22-gauge needle to anesthetize the subcutaneous tissue and the periosteum of the clavicle along the expected route of insertion (ie, the inferior border of the clavicle). When anesthetizing, make sure that the needle is not in the vein (ie, that blood does not flow back when the plunger of the syringe is gently pulled back) before injecting lidocaine.

10. Reposition the index finger in the suprasternal notch and the thumb over the costoclavicular ligament. Place the catheter insertion needle or catheter-clad needle on the 3-mL syringe, and insert the needle under the skin 3 cm (1¹⁄₁₆ in) caudal to the clavicle just medial to the thumb (Fig 46–13). Insert the needle with the bevel facing up, so that its orientation can be maintained after it enters the vein. It may help to find the vein with a smaller needle (22-gauge, 6.5-cm [2½-in] needle attached to a 3-mL syringe) before using the introducing needle.

11. Advance the needle at a 10- to 20-degree angle until it contacts the clavicle. Decrease the angle of the needle until the needle shaft is parallel to the patient's back and close to the correct alignment (pointing to the finger in the suprasternal notch). Push the needle slowly inferiorly along the clavicle until it reaches the inferior surface. Always keep the tip in contact with the clavicle, and proceed slowly. When the inferior surface is reached, check the alignment of the needle with the suprasternal notch, and while pulling back on the plunger of the syringe, advance the needle toward the suprasternal notch, keeping the needle shaft parallel to the patient's back. When the needle enters the vein, venous blood will flow back into the syringe. If no blood flows out, slowly withdraw the needle while continuing to pull back on the plunger. Occasionally, blood will enter the syringe as the needle is being slowly pulled out.

12. If the first attempt fails, totally withdraw the needle, and flush it with air to clean out any tissue from the vein lumen. This maneuver is important, because a second attempt at catheterization with an obstructed needle will also fail. Occasionally, directing the needle a little cephalad or a little deeper will locate the vein, but do not make misguided attempts in all directions, because of the danger of penetrating nearby structures such as the lung or the subclavian artery. Seek assistance if 3 or 4 attempts to locate the vein fail. If assistance is not obtainable, attempt catheterization on the other side (obtain a chest x-ray first to rule out pneumothorax), or insert an internal jugular venous catheter instead.

13. After the vein has been entered, rotate the needle so that the bevel faces caudally (toward the patient's feet), and make sure that there is free flow of blood. Occasionally, if the tip of the needle lies against the wall of the vein, blood will flow if the bevel is facing cephalad but not when the bevel is rotated. If this is the case, advance or withdraw the needle a short distance, and check it again for blood flow.

14. When the needle is properly located in the lumen of the vein, hold it in place with the thumb and forefinger of one hand, remove the syringe, and *immediately* occlude the hub of the needle to prevent any air from entering the vein. (If a hypovolemic patient takes a deep breath just as the syringe is disconnected, air may be sucked into the vein, possibly causing air embolism.) If the needle is properly positioned, blood should flow freely from it.

15. While holding the needle in position with one hand, take the catheter with the other, and quickly pass the catheter through the introducing needle and into the vein. The catheter should pass smoothly and with relative ease; if resistance occurs, stop. Check for blood flow before advancing the catheter again.

If the catheter encounters an obstruction about a third of the way in, it may be at the junction of the subclavian and internal jugular veins. Pushing and twisting gently on the catheter will usually turn the tip past this junction into the superior vena cava. Leave the catheter positioned in the superior vena cava.

16. Remove the needle from the vein by withdrawing the needle and catheter together; be careful not to shear off the catheter on the needle.

17. Evacuate the insertion syringe of all blood clots, attach it to the catheter hub, and withdraw some blood to make sure that the catheter is in the vein. The blood should flow freely. Remove the syringe. An assistant should then insert the intravenous tubing into the catheter hub and check for rapid flow.

18. Take the patient out of the Trendelenburg position.

19. Secure the catheter at the insertion site by placing the skin suture through the skin, tying it, and then looping it around the catheter 3 times and tying it again. Make sure that the lumen of the catheter is not constricted by the tie.

20. Position the needle and the needle guard on the patient's chest, making sure there are no kinks in the tubing or catheter. Apply a small amount of antibacterial ointment to the insertion site, cover it and the needle with a folded 10- × 10-cm (4- × 4-in) sterile gauze sponge, and tape the sponge in place after applying tincture of benzoin to the skin to help secure the tape to the skin and the catheter.

21. Make sure that all connections are tight and patent, and tape all connections.

22. Obtain a chest x-ray immediately to check placement of the catheter and to detect possible pneumothorax.

FEMORAL VEIN PHLEBOTOMY OR CATHETERIZATION

Femoral vein catheterization is an easy way to gain rapid access to the central venous system, eg, during CPR. Because infection is common at this site, the femoral vein should not be used for procedures requiring elective long-term venous access (eg, parenteral nutrition). Femoral vein phlebotomy is useful in patients in whom peripheral veins of the extremities are not palpable (eg, intravenous drug abusers). However, this route should not be used to obtain blood for culture.

Indications
Femoral vein phlebotomy is used to obtain venous blood samples in patients in whom other sites cannot be used for venipuncture. Femoral vein catheterization is performed to gain central venous access.

Contraindications
Contraindications to femoral vein phlebotomy or catheterization are as follows:
1. Previous surgery in the groin.
2. Prosthetic graft placement in the groin.
3. Venous occlusive disease of the extremities.

4. Acquired or congenital bleeding disorder.
5. Cellulitis or burn over the proposed site of insertion.

Personnel Required
One operator can perform femoral vein phlebotomy or catheterization unaided if the patient is cooperative, but it is helpful to have an assistant.

Equipment & Supplies Required
A. Femoral Vein Phlebotomy:
1. Materials for skin cleansing.
2. Syringe (20- to 30-mL) with 18- or 20-gauge needle.
3. Gauze sponges, 5 × 5 cm (2 × 2 in).
4. Specimen tubes for blood.
5. Adhesive dressing.
B. Femoral Vein Catheterization:
1. Materials for skin sterilization.
2. Materials for sterile technique (cap, mask, gloves, and gown).
3. Lidocaine, 1%, with 10-mL syringe and 25-gauge needle.

4. Catheter-clad needle (eg, Angiocath), 16- to 18-gauge and 12.5–20.5 cm (5–8 in) long; or a 14-gauge needle-clad catheter (eg, Intracath), 30.5 cm (12 in) long.

5. Container of intravenous infusion fluid with connecting tubing. All equipment should be flushed and fully assembled ready for use.

6. Nylon or silk suture (size 3-0) on a cutting needle.

7. Needle holder.

8. Straight scissors.

9. Antibacterial ointment and dressings.

10. Drapes

11. Gauge sponges, 10 × 10 cm (4 × 4 in).

12. Tape.

Positioning of the Patient

The patient should be supine, with the leg externally rotated on the side selected for phlebotomy or catheterization.

Anatomy Review

The femoral vein normally lies 1–2 cm (⅜–¾ in) medial to the readily palpable femoral artery (Fig 46–14). In a patient without a palpable femoral pulse, the approximate position of the vein can be determined by dividing the distance from the anterior superior iliac spine to the pubic tubercle into 3 equal segments. The artery lies at the junction of the medial segment and the middle segment. The vein is about 1.5 cm (⅝ in) medial to this point and to the artery.

Procedure

A. Femoral Vein Phlebotomy:

1. Cleanse the skin.

2. Locate the femoral artery with the nondominant hand.

3. Using the 20- to 30-mL syringe and the 18- or 22-gauge needle in the dominant hand, hold the needle at an angle of 90 degrees to the long axis of the vein.

4. Insert the needle under the skin about 0.5 cm (³⁄₁₆ in) medial to the artery, and pull the plunger back gently to create a slight vacuum as the needle is advanced.

5. When the needle enters the vein, dark venous blood will flow back into the syringe. The blood should flow freely.

6. After obtaining the desired amount of blood, remove the needle quickly, and apply direct pressure over the puncture site.

7. Fill the specimen tubes as described under Upper Extremity Venipuncture, above.

B. Femoral Vein Catheterization:

1. Assemble all equipment, and make sure that it is readily at hand.

2. Shave the side of the groin chosen for insertion.

3. Observe sterile technique (don cap, mask, gloves, and gown).

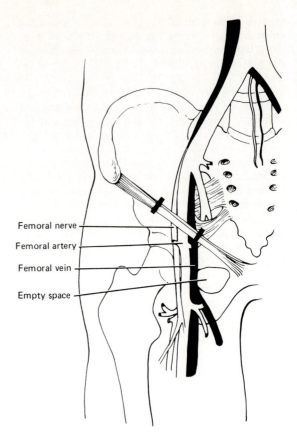

Femoral nerve
Femoral artery
Femoral vein
Empty space

Figure 46–14. Anatomic relationships of the femoral vein at the inguinal ligament.

4. Sterilize the skin around the groin, and drape the area.

5. Locate the femoral artery. Infiltrate the skin 1.5 cm (⅝ in) medial to the artery with the 1% lidocaine. Omit this step if the patient is comatose.

6. Using the catheter insertion needle attached to a syringe, insert the needle just under the skin, and pull the plunger back gently to create a slight vacuum. Then advance the needle at an angle of 45 degrees to the long axis of the vein; when the needle enters the vein, dark venous blood will flow back into the syringe. The blood should flow freely.

7. Advance the catheter into the vein. Once the catheter is in place, assemble any necessary needle guard, and check to make certain that the blood flows freely.

8. Obtain an x-ray immediately in order to check on the position of the catheter.

9. If the femoral artery instead of the femoral vein is entered, brighter red blood will flow into the syringe under systemic arterial pressure. A patient in shock or cardiac arrest may have desaturated blood, with little arterial pressure, so that differentiation between arterial and venous puncture may be difficult.

If the catheter is to be used solely for infusion of fluid or medication during emergency treatment (eg, CPR), temporary placement in the femoral artery is probably not harmful. If central venous access is re-quired, withdraw the needle and catheter from the ar-tery; maintain direct pressure over the area for 5 min-utes, and then either try again on the same side or attempt catheterization on the opposite side.

SAPHENOUS VEIN CUTDOWN

Indications

Saphenous vein cutdown is performed to gain emergency venous access when other sites are not available or when multiple intravenous lines are re-quired.

Contraindications

Contraindications to saphenous vein cutdown are as follows:

1. Previous use of the saphenous vein for a surgi-cal procedure (eg, cutdown, vein stripping, coronary artery bypass surgery).

2. Phlebitis.

3. Evidence of severe venous obstructive dis-ease.

4. Cellulitis over the proposed site of insertion.

5. Significant trauma to the legs.

Personnel Required

One person can perform saphenous vein cutdown unaided; however, an assistant is helpful.

Equipment & Supplies Required

A. Materials:

1. Materials for skin sterilization.

2. Lidocaine, 1%, with 10-mL syringe and 25-gauge needle.

3. Tourniquet.

4. Topical antibacterial ointment.

5. Expanded gauze roll and tape.

B. Prepackaged sterile cutdown trays are com-mercially available. The following are required:

1. Drapes.

2. Gauze sponges, 10×10 cm (4×4 in).

3. Silk ligatures (size 3-0) (2).

4. Nylon or polypropylene skin suture (size 3-0) on a cutting needle.

5. Needle holder.

6. No. 15 and No. 11 scalpel blades, both mounted.

7. Kelly clamps (2).

8. Mosquito clamps (2).

9. Dissection tissue scissors and straight scissors.

10. Self-retaining retractors or right-angle retrac-tors (2).

11. Pediatric feeding tubes, sizes 5F and 10F (1 each), cut to the proper length (sufficient to extend to the knee is usually satisfactory).

12. Toothed and smooth forceps.

13. Plastic-coated absorbent pad to place beneath the patient's leg.

C. Suitable intravenous infusion set (including blood pump and filter, if desired).

D. Container of intravenous fluid with connecting tubing.

Positioning of the Patient

The patient should be supine. The foot selected for the procedure should be externally rotated to expose the medial malleolus, and the plastic-coated absor-bent pad should be placed underneath the patient's leg.

Anatomy Review

The saphenous vein runs anterior to the medial malleolus, under the skin and subcutaneous tissue, but superficial to the malleolus (Fig 46–15). At this site, the vein is usually 4–5 mm ($\frac{1}{8}$–$\frac{3}{16}$ in) in diam-eter in adults.

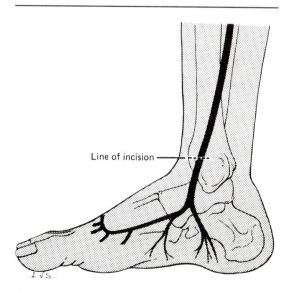

Line of incision

Figure 46–15. Anatomic relationships of the saphenous vein. (Reproduced, with permission, from Dunphy JE, Way LW [editors]: *Current Surgical Diagnosis & Treatment,* 5th ed. Lange, 1981.)

Procedure

1. Assemble all necessary equipment, including the container of intravenous fluid and connecting tubing, and make sure that the tubing has been flushed to remove all air.

2. Place a tourniquet around the lower extremity proximal to the venotomy site to occlude venous return and dilate the saphenous vein.

3. Sterilize the skin around the medial malleolus.

4. Drape the skin.

5. Anesthetize the area with the 1% lidocaine with the 10-mL syringe and 25-gauge needle. Omit this step if the patient is comatose.

6. With the No. 15 scalpel blade, make a 2-cm (¾-in) superficial transverse incision (the dotted line in Fig 46–15), just anterior to the medial malleolus, being careful not to cut through the vein.

7. Using a mosquito clamp, dissect the tissues in the long axis of the leg to isolate the vein. Pass the clamp under the vein and dissect the underlying tissue. Place a silk suture under the vein, and tie off the distal part of the vein. Maintain exposure with retractors.

8. Supporting the vein with an open Kelly clamp, perform a venotomy with the No. 11 scalpel blade: Hold the scalpel parallel to the long axis of the vein with the blade in a horizontal position, and pass it through the midportion of the superficial (or anterior) wall of the vein. Then turn the cutting edge of the blade upward, and open the top of the vein (Fig 46–2). Take care not to transect the vein or puncture its outer wall.

9. Dilate the vein with the closed point of the Kelly clamp.

10. Insert the catheter (Fig 46–3), and pass it 10–12.5 cm (4–5 in) proximally up the vein (it is unnecessary to pass it farther). Allow blood to fill the catheter, and then remove the tourniquet.

11. Connect the intravenous tubing to the catheter, and begin the infusion.

12. Now pass the second silk suture under and around the proximal portion of the vein (which now encloses the catheter). Tie this second suture around the vein and catheter proximal to the venotomy. Make it snug but not too tight, or it will cut through the vein, leaving the catheter loose.

13. Close the skin with the nylon or polypropylene suture using a simple running stitch. Secure the catheter to the skin with a skin stitch.

14. Apply antibacterial ointment to the wound, and wrap the ankle with an expanded gauze roll.

INTRAOSSEOUS INFUSION*

Indications

Intraosseous infusion is a *temporary* means of intravenous access in children to be replaced with conventional venous access as soon as possible. It is performed when other techniques of the venous cannulation have failed or would be too time-consuming (eg, in the presence of cardiac arrest, trauma, shock). Complications are infrequent (0.6%) and consist mostly of osteomyelitis and infection in adjacent tissues.

Site Selection

Several sites are suitable for infusion. In children under 3 years of age, the proximal tibia or distal femur is preferred, but these sites should not be used in patients beyond the age of 5 years, since the red marrow is replaced by fat beyond this age. The sternum is more suitable in older children, as it may be too thin and inadequately ossified in infants. The iliac crest is also acceptable.

Contraindications

Cutaneous infection or burn overlying the insertion site or major injury to the extremity proximal to the insertion site are contraindications.

Personnel Required

One person can perform the procedure. An assistant is helpful.

Equipment & Supplies Required

1. Materials for skin sterilization.

2. Lidocaine, 1%, with 5-mL syringe and 25-gauge needle.

3. Sterile drapes.

4. Sterile (latex) gloves.

5. Short, large-bore bone marrow needle or 18-gauge spinal needle. (Intraosseous infusion needles are commercially available.)

6. 10-mL syringe.

7. Intravenous infusion set, including sterile tubing and appropriate fluids for administration.

8. Gauze sponges (eg, 10×10 cm [4×4 in]).

9. Adhesive tape.

Positioning of the Patient

The patient should be supine. If the proximal tibia is selected, the leg should be rotated slightly externally.

---

*This section contributed by Charles E. Saunders, MD, FACEP, FACP.

Anatomy Review
The ideal insertion site on the tibia lies 1–2 cm distal to the tibial tuberosity on the anterior medial surface. On the femur it is 2–3 cm proximal to the lateral epicondyle in the midline.

Procedure
1. Sterilize the skin.
2. Drape the area.
3. Using sterile technique, locate the desired insertion site and infiltrate the skin with 1% lidocaine over a 2- to 3-cm area. Lidocaine should also be infiltrated along the anticipated course of insertion, down to and including the periosteum.
4. Using the bone marrow needle, spinal needle, or intraosseous infusion needle, penetrate the skin perpendicularly. Advance the needle toward the bone at a 60-degree angle (directed away from the growth plate; caudal at the tibia, and rostral at the femur).
5. Use firm pressure to penetrate the cortex, employing a rotating or twisting motion. Upon entry into the marrow space, a sudden "give" will be felt. *Cau-*

tion: Errant placement of the needle can cause injury to the growth place with resultant growth deformity.
6. Remove the trocar from the needle and attach a 10-mL syringe. Aspiration of blood and marrow contents confirms needle-tip placement in the marrow.
7. Connect fluid-filled intravenous tubing to the needle and observe free flow of fluid. Inability to infuse implies misplacement of the needle tip.
8. Apply gauze 10- × 10-cm (4- × 4-in) sponges (cut midway) against the skin at the entry site, surrounding the needle. Occasionally, deep penetration of the needle through the bone cortex on the opposite side can occur, with delivery of infusion into surrounding tissue spaces. This can also occur if the needle becomes dislodged and withdrawn from its intramedullary position; tape the needle firmly in place. (Commercially available intraosseous infusion needles may have a lip to which tape can be attached, securing the needle to the skin surface.) If a spinal needle is used, a styrofoam cup may be placed over the needle to protect it from being bumped.

RADIAL ARTERY PUNCTURE
(For Blood Gas & pH Analysis)

Indications
Indications for radial artery puncture are as follows:
1. Need to obtain arterial blood for blood gas and pH determinations.
2. Need to perform phlebotomy when other sites are inaccessible.

Contraindications
Contraindications to radial artery puncture are as follows:
1. Positive Allen test (see below), indicating that only one artery supplies the hand.
2. Absence of palpable radial artery pulse.
3. Cellulitis or other infection over the radial artery.
4. Coagulation defects (relative contraindication).

Personnel Required
One person can perform radial artery puncture unaided, but it is helpful to have an assistant to maintain pressure over the puncture site while the operator prepares the sample for transport to the laboratory.

Equipment & Supplies Required
1. Materials for skin cleansing.
2. Lidocaine, 1%, with 3- to 5-mL syringe and 23- to 25-gauge, 1.5-cm (½-in) needle.

3. Heparinized syringe, 3- to 5-mL, preferably of glass or of siliconized plastic made especially for arterial blood sampling. To heparinize the syringe, aspirate 0.5 mL of heparin (100–1000 units/mL) into the syringe, hold the syringe upright, pull the plunger all the way out to the end, and then return all of the heparin to the original container. This procedure ensures that there is a small amount of heparin in the tip of the syringe and needle hub that is adequate to heparinize the arterial blood gas sample but not enough to affect the accuracy of blood gas determinations.
4. Needle for arterial puncture, 23- to 25-gauge (depending on the size of the artery), 1.5-cm (½-in) long.
5. Ice for transport.

Positioning of the Patient
The patient should be in a comfortable position, either supine or sitting. If respiratory difficulties require that the patient sit upright, the upper extremity selected should be extended on a stable surface such as a bedside table or on the side of the bed. The arm should be positioned with the volar side up.

Anatomy Review
The radial artery runs along the lateral aspect of the volar forearm deep to the superficial fascia. The artery runs between the styloid process of the radius

and the flexor carpi radialis tendon. The point of maximum pulsation of the radial artery can usually be palpated just proximal to the wrist.

Allen Test

The Allen test should be performed to confirm the patency of the ulnar artery before any attempt is made to obtain a blood sample from the radial artery.

While the patient is elevating the arm and making a tight fist, occlude both radial and ulnar arterial flow with firm pressure over both the radial and the ulnar aspects of the volar forearm just proximal to the wrist. Allow a few minutes for the blood to drain from the hand, and then lower the arm to waist level and have the patient open the hand. Release the pressure on the ulnar artery while keeping the radial artery occluded. Normal skin color should return to the ulnar side of the palm in 1–2 seconds, followed by quick restoration of normal color to the entire palm. A hand that remains white indicates either absence or occlusion of the ulnar artery, in which case radial artery puncture is contraindicated. Failure to perform this test may result in a gangrenous finger or loss of the hand from spasm or clotting of the radial artery where there is no collateral flow through the ulnar artery.

Procedure

1. Palpate the radial artery just proximal to the wrist, and determine where the pulse is most prominent.

2. Locate the approximate position of the artery under the ball of the index finger by slowly rolling the finger from side to side. This maneuver causes the pulse to become alternately stronger and weaker and further helps to locate the relatively small radial artery.

3. Cleanse the skin over the proposed site of puncture.

4. Anesthetize the skin over the proposed site of puncture with the 1% lidocaine using the 3- to 5-mL syringe and 23- to 25-gauge needle.

5. Using the index and middle fingers of the nondominant hand, identify again the point of maximal pulsation of the radial artery (Fig 46–16).

6. Attach the 23- to 25-gauge needle to the heparinized syringe, and holding the needle perpendicular to the arm, insert the needle into the skin in the anesthetized area. The smaller the needle, the less the risk of injury to the artery and the less painful the procedure to the patient.

7. Guide the needle toward the point of maximum pulsation, and watch for a sudden gush of arterial blood into the hub of the needle or the lower part of the syringe. Once the needle has entered the lumen of the radial artery, the force of arterial pulsation should fill the syringe if it is specially designed for arterial puncture (glass or siliconized plastic). If an ordinary plastic syringe is used, a small amount of

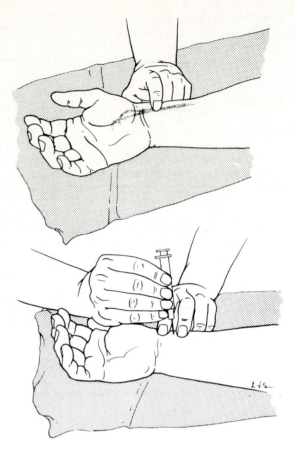

Figure 46–16. Technique of radial artery puncture. The index and middle fingers are used to identify the point of maximum pulsation.

suction may be required to obtain an adequate blood sample (only 1–2 mL of blood is required for blood gas and pH analysis).

8. If no blood is obtained with these maneuvers, it is possible that the needle has completely passed through the radial artery. Advance the needle until it meets the periosteum of the radius. Slowly withdraw the syringe and needle, and look for the gush of arterial blood into the hub of the needle.

9. If this attempt is still unsuccessful, withdraw the needle to a position just under the skin, move it 1 mm (1/16 in) to either side of the previous attempt, and try again. Make at least 3 attempts before giving up and trying another site or seeking assistance.

10. Remove the needle from the artery with a smooth, swift motion, and apply immediate direct pressure over the puncture site for 10 minutes. An assistant is helpful to apply pressure on the artery.

11. Evacuate all air bubbles from the sample by holding the syringe upright and allowing the bubbles to collect near the needle hub. Gently tapping the syringe with the end of a finger will help dislodge bubbles from the walls of the syringe. Once all of the air has been confined to the tip of the syringe, evacuate it by pushing on the plunger. Then, cap the needle with a rubber stopper, label the tube with the patient's name and number, and place the sample on ice for transport to the laboratory.

12. Return in 15 minutes, and check for adequate perfusion of the hand and for possible hematoma formation in the patient's wrist.

DIRECT LARYNGOSCOPY, OROTRACHEAL INTUBATION, & NASOTRACHEAL INTUBATION

Indications

A. Orotracheal Intubation: Indications for orotracheal intubation are as follows:

1. Inadequate oxygenation (decreased arterial PO_2, etc) that is not corrected by supplemental oxygen supplied by mask or nasal prongs.

2. Inadequate ventilation (increased arterial PCO_2).

3. Need to control and remove pulmonary secretions (bronchial toilet).

4. Need to provide airway protection in an obtunded patient or a patient with a depressed gag reflex.

B. Nasotracheal Intubation: Nasotracheal intubation is used for long-term intubation because it is more comfortable for the patient than orotracheal intubation. It is also used when access to the trachea through the oropharynx is difficult and emergency cricothyrotomy is not indicated. The advantages of nasotracheal intubation are **(1)** greater comfort for the patient; **(2)** greater ease in securing the tracheal tube; and **(3)** greater ease in communicating with the intubated patient through lip reading. Disadvantages include **(1)** need for a smaller airway, which results in increased airway resistance; **(2)** need for a more skilled operator, since the tube is usually inserted without direct vision; **(3)** possible bleeding caused by passage of the nasotracheal tube through the nasopharynx; and **(4)** sinusitis that may result owing to obstruction of the ostia of the sinuses.

Contraindications

The following are only relative contraindications to tracheal intubation.

1. Severe airway trauma or obstruction that does not permit safe passage of an endotracheal tube. Emergency cricothyrotomy is indicated in such cases.

2. Cervical spine injury, in which the need for complete immobilization of the cervical spine makes endotracheal intubation difficult (Chapter 21).

Personnel Required

One person can perform direct laryngoscopy or tra-

cheal intubation unaided. If an assistant is available, he or she should give 100% oxygen while equipment is being prepared.

Equipment & Supplies Required

1. Self-refilling bag-valve combination (eg, Ambu bag) or bag-valve unit (Ayres bag), connector, tubing, and oxygen source. Assemble all items before attempting intubation.

2. Laryngoscope with curved and straight blades of a size appropriate for the patient.

3. Endotracheal tubes of several different sizes (Table 46–1). Low-pressure, high-flow cuffed balloons are preferred. Tracheal tubes used in nasotracheal intubation should be smaller than those used for orotracheal intubation (Table 46–1).

4. Oral and nasal airways.

5. Tincture of benzoin and precut tape.

6. Introducer (stylets or Magill forceps).

7. Suction apparatus (tonsil tip and catheter suction).

8. Syringe, 10-mL, to inflate the cuff.

9. Mucosal anesthetics and astringents (eg, 4% cocaine).

10. Water-soluble sterile lubricant.

Positioning of the Patient

The sniffing position—patient supine, with the neck flexed, the occiput elevated, and the head tilted backward—permits visualization of the glottis and

Table 46–1. Guidelines for endotracheal tube selection.

Age	Orotracheal Tube[1]	Nasotracheal Tube
Premature	3.5–4	Not applicable
Term	4–5	Not applicable
3–18 months	5–6	Not applicable
1½–3 years	6–7	Not applicable
3–5 years	7–8	6–7
5–7 years	8–9	7–8
8–14 years	9–10	8–9
Over 14 years		
Female	10–12	8–10
Male	11–14	9–12

[1]Outside diameter in mm.

vocal cords and allows passage of the endotracheal tube. A towel rolled under the head usually makes it easier for the patient to maintain this position.

In infants under 1 month of age, the head and neck should be in a neutral position.

Procedure

A. Mask Ventilation: (Oxygen delivered with a face mask at a rate of 10–15 L/min.)

1. Select the proper-sized mask; it should cover the mouth and nose and fit snugly against the cheeks.

2. Place the patient in the sniffing position.

3. Place the mask over the patient's mouth and nose with the right hand.

4. With the left hand, place the small and ring fingers under the patient's mandible, and lift up to open the airway. Grasp the mask with the thumb and index finger, and press it to the patient's face while lifting the mandible with the ring and small fingers.

5. Compress the bag with the right hand.

6. The chest should rise with each breath, and airflow should be unimpeded. If not, reposition the mask, and try again. Occasionally, insertion of an oral or nasal airway facilitates ventilation by mask. Because of the lack of support for the lips, elderly edentulous patients may be especially hard to ventilate using a mask.

B. Topical Anesthesia: Anesthetize the mucosa of the nose, oropharynx, and upper airway with cocaine, 4%, or lidocaine, 2%, if time permits and the patient is awake.

C. Direct Laryngoscopy:

1. Place the patient in the sniffing position.

2. Check the laryngoscope and blade for proper fit, and make sure that the light works.

3. Make sure that all materials are assembled and close at hand.

4. Curved blade technique–

a. Open the patient's mouth with the right hand, and remove any dentures.

b. Grasp the laryngoscope in the left hand as shown (Fig 46–17).

c. Spread the patient's lips, and insert the blade between the teeth, being careful not to break a tooth.

d. Pass the blade to the right of the tongue, and advance the blade into the hypopharynx, pushing the tongue to the left.

e. Lift the laryngoscope upward and forward, without changing the angle of the blade, to expose the vocal cords.

5. Straight blade technique–Follow the steps outlined for curved blade technique, but advance the blade down the hypopharynx, and lift the epiglottis with the tip of the blade to expose the vocal cords. The tip of the laryngoscope blade fits below the epiglottis, which is no longer visible with the blade in position.

D. Orotracheal Intubation:

1. Select the proper-sized tube (Table 46–1).

a. Most adult men take an endotracheal tube that has an outside diameter of 12–13 mm (½ in).

b. Most adult women take an endotracheal tube that is 11–12 mm (⁷⁄₁₆ in) in diameter.

c. For children, a general rule is that the external diameter of the tube is equal to the diameter of the child's fifth finger.

2. With the 10-mL syringe, inflate the balloon with 5–8 mL of air. Make sure that the balloon is functional and intact.

3. Lubricate the end of the tube (optional).

4. Insert the stylet, and bend the tube and stylet gently into a crescent shape so that the tip of the stylet is at least 1 cm (³⁄₈ in) proximal to the end of the orotracheal tube.

5. Be sure that the syringe and the bag-valve combination are within easy reach.

6. Ventilate the patient with the bag-valve combination for 1–2 minutes with 100% oxygen.

7. Open the patient's mouth, remove dentures, and suction secretions or vomitus from the mouth.

8. Visualize the glottis and vocal cords and, by direct laryngoscopy, gently pass the tube through the vocal cords into the trachea. Occasionally, gently pressing posteriorly on the anterior neck at the level of the larynx will help to bring an anteriorly placed larynx into view and facilitate intubation.

9. Gently pass the tube next to the laryngoscope blade, through the vocal cords and far enough so that the balloon is just beyond the cords.

10. Withdraw the stylet.

11. Connect the bag-valve combination, and begin ventilation with 100% oxygen.

12. Confirm that the tube is properly positioned. First, listen over the stomach with a stethoscope while ventilating the patient. If sounds of airflow are heard or if distention of the stomach occurs, the tube is in the esophagus. If the esophagus has been intubated instead of the trachea, remove the tube, ventilate the patient with a mask, and try again.

Next, listen to each side of the chest, including the axilla, to be sure that breath sounds are equal. If the left chest has more distant breath sounds than the right chest, try withdrawing the tube 1–2 cm (³⁄₈–¾ in) and ventilating again. This maneuver helps to correct intubation of the right main stem bronchus as a cause of unequal ventilation. Airway anatomy makes intubation of the right main stem bronchus more likely than intubation of the left. When breath sounds are equal on both sides and the thorax rises equally on both sides with each inspiration, note the position of the tube (eg, mark the tube at the patient's mouth), and inflate the cuff with the 10-mL syringe until there is no air leak around the tube when positive pressure is applied.

13. Apply tincture of benzoin to the cheeks, upper lip, and endotracheal tube.

14. Wrap adhesive tape around the tube where it comes out of the mouth. Then carry the tape over the

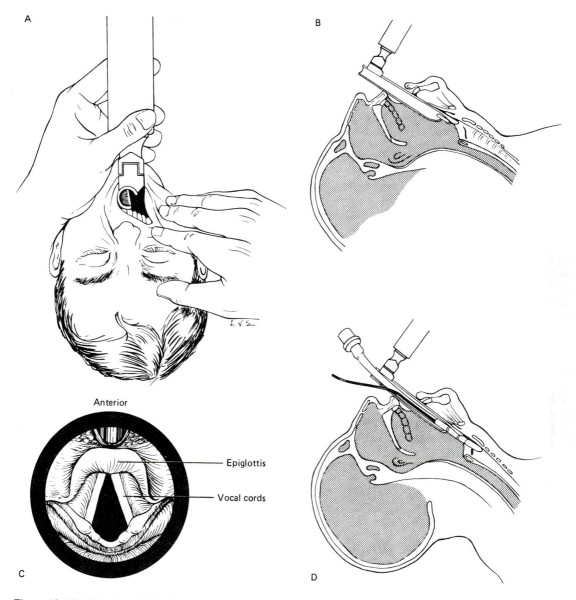

Figure 46–17. Technique of direct laryngoscopy and orotracheal intubation. *A:* The straight laryngoscope blade is passed behind the tongue and deep to the tip of the epiglottis. *B:* Lateral view showing straight laryngoscope blade deep to the tip of epiglottis exposing glottic opening. *C:* View of glottis as seen through a laryngoscope with a curved blade. *D:* Insertion of endotracheal tube (Parts A, B, and D reproduced, with permission, from Way LW [editor]: *Current Surgical Diagnosis & Treatment,* 3rd ed. Lange, 1977. Part C reproduced, with permission, from Kempe CH, Silver HK, O'Brien D: [editors]: *Current Pediatric Diagnosis & Treatment,* 4th ed. Lange, 1976.)

cheek and around the back of the head onto the other cheek. Fasten the end of the tape around the tube.

15. Obtain a chest x-ray immediately to check tube placement.

16. Obtain arterial blood gas measurements to assess the adequacy of ventilation.

E. Nasotracheal Intubation:

1–6. Steps 1–6 are the same as those for orotracheal intubation. The tube must be checked and lubricated, and all materials must be readily at hand.

7. Examine the patient's nose, and determine if one nasal passage is larger than the other. Insert the lubricated nasotracheal tube in the external naris, and pass it directly posteriorly until it meets the floor of the nasopharynx. The technique is similar to that used to pass a nasogastric tube (see Nasogastric Intubation, below).

8. Make sure that the natural bend in the tube (without the stylet in place) corresponds to the direction of passage, and with gentle, steady pressure, continue to advance the nasotracheal tube into the posterior pharynx. At this point, the tube may meet with obstruction. If the tube fails to pass into the posterior pharynx under gentle, steady pressure, withdraw the tube, and attempt insertion in the opposite nostril.

9. Once the nasotracheal tube is in the pharynx, flex the patient's head by lifting the occiput to help guide the tube through the vocal cords anteriorly into the larynx. The patient may start to cough when the tube passes through the vocal cords.

10. If the patient is breathing spontaneously, listen at the external end of the tube. If the tube is properly positioned over the larynx, air should be heard coming in and out of the tube. If no air is heard, the tube has slipped posteriorly and is in the esophagus. There is no quick way to determine the position of the tube during its insertion in an apneic patient. Insertion under direct vision is preferred (see below), and position must be confirmed after insertion (step 13).

11. When ventilation is heard, steady the patient's head in that position, and when inspiration begins, advance the tube into the trachea.

12. Once the tube is in the trachea, listen again to make sure that air is coming from the nasotracheal tube, and look at the tube to see the condensation of water vapor with exhalation.

13. Have an assistant steady the nasotracheal tube. Connect an air reservoir bag (eg, Ayers or Ambu bag) to the tube, ventilate the patient, and check for elevation of both sides of the chest on inspiration and the presence of breath sounds at each axilla. As with orotracheal intubation, inadvertent intubation of the right main stem bronchus (with poor ventilation of the left lung) occurs more commonly than intubation of the left bronchus.

14. When proper positioning of the tube in the trachea has been achieved, tape the tube to the patient's upper lip; make sure that there is no pressure on the external naris that might cause necrosis.

F.   Alternative Method of Insertion: In patients who are not breathing spontaneously, passage of a nasotracheal tube is difficult because of the absence of normal breath sounds that guide insertion into the larynx. If prolonged intubation is indicated and a nasotracheal tube is desired, passage can be done under direct vision, as follows:

1. Proceed as above (steps 1–8) until the tube is in the posterior pharynx.

2. Using a laryngoscope and direct laryngoscopy, identify the tracheal tube in the posterior pharynx, and manually guide the tube into the trachea using Magill forceps to grasp the tube. During this procedure, it is important to have an assistant gently push on the tube as it is being guided anteriorly into the trachea with the forceps. Be careful not to grasp the tube at the level of the balloon, since this commonly punctures the balloon and requires insertion of a new tube.

3. After the tube is inserted, check for proper placement as described above, and tape it in place.

G.   Removal of the Endotracheal Tube:

1. Ventilate the patient with a bag-valve combination for 1–2 minutes with 100% oxygen.

2. Suction the patient's trachea, mouth, and hypopharynx before removing the tube.

3. Deflate the cuff by withdrawing all air with the 10-mL syringe.

4. Have the patient take a deep breath, and remove the tube at the midpoint of expiration.

5. Suction the patient's mouth a second time to remove any remaining secretions.

6. Begin oxygen, 5 L/min, by mask. Obtain a sample of arterial blood to assess respiratory function.

NASOGASTRIC INTUBATION
(For Gastric Evacuation or Lavage)

Indications

Indications for nasogastric intubation are as follows:

1. Need to suppress vomiting caused by gastric distention or paralytic ileus.

2. Need to perform gastric lavage (therapeutic or diagnostic).

3. Need to perform gastric decompression.

4. Need to perform gastric evacuation.

Contraindications

A. Important contraindications to nasogastric intubation are as follows:

1. Choanal atresia.

2. Massive facial trauma or basilar skull fracture.

3. Esophageal atresia or stricture.

4. Ingestion of a caustic substance (eg, acid, lye)—unless nasogastric intubation can be performed under direct vision.

B. Relative contraindications to nasogastric intubation are as follows:

1. Recent gastric or esophageal surgery.

2. Recent oropharyngeal or nasal surgery.

3. Esophageal stricture.

4. Esophageal burn.

5. Zenker's diverticulum.

Personnel Required

One person can perform nasogastric intubation unaided, but an assistant is helpful.

Equipment & Supplies Required

1. Nasogastric tube of the proper diameter. There are 2 main types of tubes: straight suction tubes and sump suction tubes (with 2 lumens). The sump tube is less likely to be sucked against the stomach wall and become plugged. The only disadvantage is that because of the second air-inlet port, it has a slightly smaller lumen for suction than a similarly sized straight suction tube. Most adults require a 16–18F sump tube. The limiting factor is the size of the naris. Children usually require a 10F nasogastric tube and infants an 8F tube.

2. Lubricant.

3. Suction syringe with catheter tip.

4. Connector (usually supplied with the nasogastric tube).

5. Suction tube and suction device (wall suction, intermittent wall suction, or portable intermittent suction).

6. Glass of water and a straw.

7. Tape.

Positioning of the Patient

The patient should be in a comfortable, supported sitting position. Unconscious patients should either be supine and flat or supine with the head slightly elevated. Children or unusually overreactive adults may be asked to sit on their hands as a reminder to keep them away from the nose and the tube as it is being passed into the stomach.

Procedure

1. Explain exactly what the steps of the procedure will be, and explain the need for the patient's help at certain points.

2. Determine the length of tubing necessary by measuring the distance between the ear and the umbilicus.

3. Lubricate the end of the tube with lubricant.

4. Have the patient or an assistant hold the water and straw to the patient's mouth.

5. Insert the tube into the nostril at a 60- to 90-degree angle to the plane of the face, and advance it straight back until it meets resistance (the patient usually signals when this happens).

6. Using gentle pressure and pushing posteriorly and perpendicularly to the long axis of the head, advance the tip of the tube inferiorly and into the nasopharynx (Fig 46–18).

7. Have the patient take a small sip of water through the straw and hold it in the mouth without swallowing. Then have the patient swallow, and advance the tube into the esophagus simultaneously. If this maneuver is successful, the patient will gag. If it fails and the tube slips into the trachea, violent

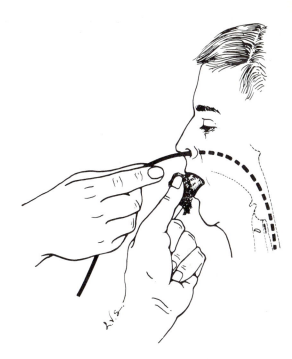

Figure 46–18. Technique of nasogastric intubation.

coughing will usually ensue. Withdraw the tube into the oropharynx, and try again. The most important step is timing the advancement of the tube to coincide with the swallow. Patients with an altered sensorium sometimes tolerate tracheal intubation without any reflex coughing. The tube is improperly positioned if air exchange is heard.

8. When the tube is in the esophagus, advance it into the stomach. In adults, the tube is usually in the stomach when it is advanced to the next-to-the-last mark on the sump tube.

9. Once the nasogastric tube is in the stomach, withdraw some gastric juice, and with a suction syringe inject air down the tube while listening over the left upper quadrant for the sound of air leaving the tube and bubbling in the stomach. If no sound is heard, reposition the tube, and inject more air. If several attempts fail, check to make sure that the tube is not in the trachea or curled in the patient's mouth. Obtain a chest x-ray to check the position of the tube. Injecting a small amount of water-soluble contrast medium down the tube and visualizing its position with fluoroscopy or standard x-ray is the definitive confirmatory procedure. *Never* assume that the tube is in the correct position without performing some confirming maneuver. Nasogastric tubes have been left in the peripheral lung, cranial vault, extraesophageal mediastinum, and peritoneal cavity.

10. Apply tincture of benzoin to the nose before securing the tube to the nose with tape, and make sure that the tube does not exert pressure on the external naris, which can result in pressure necrosis and sloughing of the naris.

Special Problems

A. Intubated Patients: Inserting a nasogastric tube in an intubated patient can be difficult. Follow the steps outlined above, and remember to deflate the cuff of the endotracheal tube if the nasogastric tube becomes stuck in the upper esophagus. In an unresponsive intubated patient, it may occasionally be necessary to use Magill forceps and a laryngoscope to advance the tube into the esophagus under direct vision.

B. Comatose Patients: A comatose or obtunded patient cannot swallow at the right time to facilitate passage of the tube. The natural bend of the tube as it passes into the pharynx from the naris is anterior; the tube therefore tends to enter the trachea. Any one of the following maneuvers may be helpful (they should be performed in the order given here).

1. Flex the patient's head when passing the tube. Make sure the patient does not have a cervical spine injury if this is attempted in the emergency department.

2. Before attempting intubation, put the tube in ice or in a freezer to stiffen it and give it more resistance to bending.

3. Pass the tube through the nostril and into the nasopharynx, and insert a finger into the patient's mouth to manually guide the tube posteriorly into the esophagus.

4. Use a laryngoscope and Magill forceps to pass the tube into the esophagus under direct vision.

INSERTION OF SENGSTAKEN-BLAKEMORE (SB) OR MINNESOTA TUBE

Minnesota and Sengstaken-Blakemore tubes (Fig 46–19) are used to control hemorrhage from esophageal varices and the esophagogastric junction. The Sengstaken-Blakemore tube is a triple-lumen rubber tube with 2 balloons: one that is inflated in the lumen of the stomach and pressed against the esophagogastric junction, and one that is inflated in the lumen of the esophagus to press directly against the varices. Two of the lumens are used to inflate the balloons; the third opens into a port on the distal tip of the tube and is used to irrigate and drain the stomach.

The Minnesota tube is currently preferable to the other tubes that are available. This tube has 4 lumens: 2 for filling the balloons, one that permits aspiration of gastric contents, and a fourth to aspirate the esophagus above the balloon. If a tube without an esophageal port is used (eg, a Sengstaken-Blakemore tube), a nasogastric tube must be tied to the Sengstaken-Blakemore tube just above the esophageal balloon in order to remove secretions collecting there.

Effective use of the Sengstaken-Blakemore or Minnesota tube requires close attention to the pressure in each balloon and monitoring for continued bleeding from the esophagogastric varices (blood aspirated through the gastric aspiration port of the Sengstaken-Blakemore tube or above the esophageal balloon through a nasogastric tube or the esophageal port of the Minnesota tube). Proper insertion will also ensure that the gastric balloon is not inflated in the esophagus, which may lead to esophageal rupture.

With either tube, patients may require orotracheal or nasotracheal intubation *first* to protect the airway before balloon tamponade is attempted. Intubation must *always* be done in comatose patients.

Indications

Indications for insertion of a Sengstaken-Blakemore tube are as follows:

1. Need to control massive upper gastrointestinal tract hemorrhage presumed to be from esophageal varices in a patient with hypovolemic shock.

2. Need to control documented esophagovariceal hemorrhage in a patient with or without hemodynamic compromise.

Contraindications

Insertion of a Sengstaken-Blakemore tube is contraindicated in patients who have undergone previous gastroesophageal surgery.

Personnel Required

The operator will require an assistant.

Equipment & Supplies Required

1. Sengstaken-Blakemore tube or Minnesota tube.

2. No. 18 Salem sump tube if Sengstaken-Blakemore tube is used.

3. Constant or intermittent wall or portable suction device.

4. Mercury manometer or aneroid pressure gauge.

5. Y connector.

6. Rubber-clad clamps (3).

7. Water-soluble lubricating jelly.

8. Cocaine spray, 4%.

9. Glass of water and a straw.

10. Manometer-grade rubber tubing, 0.6–1 m (2–3 ft).

11. Irrigating syringe, 50-mL; water, basin.

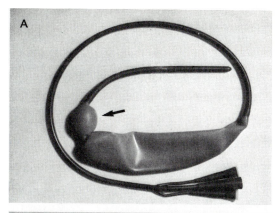

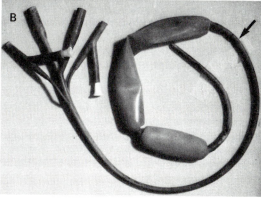

Figure 46–19. Balloon tamponade for bleeding varices. **A:** The Sengstaken-Blakemore tube has a small gastric balloon (arrow) that can be inflated to 250 mL with air. **B:** The 4-lumen Minnesota tube has a much larger gastric balloon that inflates to 450 mL and a series of aspirating ports (arrow) for removing secretions above the esophageal balloon.

12. Football helmet with a face mask.

13. Sponge rubber to act as cuff around the tube.

Positioning of the Patient

The patient should be supine, with the head of the bed elevated 30–45 degrees if possible. It is difficult to insert the tube with the patient in the Trendelenburg position.

Anatomy Review

Esophageal varices result from portal hypertension. When the distal esophageal veins become distended, they become susceptible to erosion, and the overlying mucosa becomes thinner. Mechanical or chemical (reflux of gastric acid) irritation may rupture the varices, causing hemorrhage.

Procedure

1. Protect the airway. In stuporous patients or those with a diminished gag reflex, endotracheal intu-

bation should be performed before passage of a Minnesota or Sengstaken-Blakemore tube.

2. Inflate the balloons to test for air leaks, and lubricate the distal end of the tube and balloons.

3. Make sure that all necessary equipment is readily at hand.

4. Deflate the balloons completely.

5. Anesthetize the patient's nasal passages, pharynx, and hypopharynx with the 4% cocaine spray, and wait 2–3 minutes.

6. Pass the tube through one nostril with steady pressure until the tip of the tube is in the posterior pharynx.

7. Have the patient sip some water through the straw and hold it in the mouth until told to swallow. Advance the tube into the esophagus as the patient swallows.

8. Advance the tube to at least the 50-cm mark. (In the typical adult, the tube should be in the stomach at this point.)

9. Fill the irrigating syringe with air, and listen over the patient's stomach with a stethoscope while injecting air through the gastric aspiration port. If the tube is properly positioned, a gurgling sound will be heard in the stomach as air escapes from the tube. If no air is heard, withdraw the tube, and insert it again. Do not inflate either balloon until the tube is known to be in the stomach.

10. When proper placement of the tube in the stomach has been confirmed, inflate the gastric balloon with air (250–275 mL for the Sengstaken-Blakemore tube; 450–500 mL for the Minnesota tube), and clamp the gastric balloon port with a rubber-clad clamp. If the patient develops substernal pain while the gastric balloon is being inflated, the balloon may be in the esophagus. Stop immediately, deflate the balloon, and push the tube farther into the stomach before attempting reinflation of the gastric balloon.

11. Pull back on the tube until resistance is felt, showing that tamponade of the gastroesophageal junction has been achieved. Secure the tube with a minimum of tension (about 0.45 kg [1 lb]) by taping a cuff of sponge rubber to the tube just distal to the patient's nostril.

12. Construct a pressure-reading mechanism by connecting the esophageal balloon port to a Y connector. Use part of the manometer-grade rubber tubing if needed. Connect the manometer or aneroid pressure gauge to one port of the Y connector and an inflating bulb or the 50-mL syringe to the other.

13. If inflation of the gastric balloon fails to stop the bleeding, inflate the esophageal balloon to 35–50 mm Hg of pressure, using manometer control. Use the lowest pressure possible that will control hemorrhage.

14. Aspirate through the gastric port of the tube, and evacuate the stomach of all blood and water. Irrigate and aspirate the stomach, if necessary, to completely evacuate all contents.

15. Continue gastric lavage for 30 minutes, and check for bright red blood. If bleeding continues, increase the esophageal balloon pressure by 5-mm Hg increments. Continue lavage to determine the exact pressure at which bleeding stops. Occlude the esophageal and gastric ports with a rubber-clad clamp proximal to the Y connector.

16. Record the pressures in the gastric and esophageal balloons, and transport the patient to an intensive care unit with one-on-one nursing.

17. Obtain a portable chest x-ray and abdominal film immediately to check for proper placement of the tube.

18. If a football helmet is available, secure the tube to the face mask instead of using pressure against the nostril to hold the tube in place.

19. If a Sengstaken-Blakemore tube is being used, pass a standard nasogastric Salem sump tube through the other nostril to evacuate all secretions that accumulate above the esophageal balloon. If a Minnesota tube is being used, attach the esophageal port to a suction device set to intermittent high suction.

20. Secure the tube as shown in Fig 46–20.

21. The pressure in both balloons should be checked every 30 minutes by releasing the rubber-clad clamps on the tube proximal to the Y connector while the tube used for inflation is occluded. This connects the balloon to the manometer for pressure measurement, and air leaks in the balloon can be quickly detected before bleeding recurs. Periodically irrigate and aspirate through the gastric port and through the esophageal port (Minnesota tube) or Salem sump tube (Sengstaken-Blakemore tube) to make sure that no gastric or esophageal bleeding goes undetected.

22. If the patient is comatose and the tube cannot

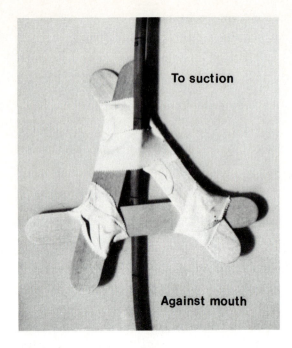

Figure 46–20. Securing tamponade tube using crossed tongue blades. The insertion tube is secured to the corner of the mouth as shown. Foam or gauze may be placed between the triangle and the patient's mouth to prevent damage to gingival mucosa.

be passed through the nose, insert it through the mouth, and guide it into the esophagus with a finger. An alternative is to use direct laryngoscopy and Magill forceps to guide the tube into the esophagus. Be careful not to puncture the balloon with the forceps.

CRICOTHYROTOMY*

Indications

Cricothyrotomy is performed when the airway must be secured or maintained and when attempts at orotracheal or nasotracheal intubation have failed.

Contraindications

Cricothyrotomy is contraindicated when any other less radical means of securing an airway is feasible.

Personnel Required

One person can perform cricothyrotomy unaided, but an assistant is helpful.

*This section contributed by Charles E. Saunders, MD, FACEP, FACP.

Equipment & Supplies Required

Because cricothyrotomy is almost always performed when speed is essential to save the patient's life, presterilized kits containing the required materials should be available in all hospital emergency departments.

1. Materials for skin sterilization.
2. Materials for sterile technique (cap, mask, gloves, and gown).
3. Lidocaine, 1%, with 10-mL syringe and 25-gauge needle.
4. Sponges, 10 × 10 cm (4 × 4 in).
5. Drapes and rolled bath towel.
6. No. 11 scalpel blade, mounted.
7. Mosquito clamps (2).

8. Kelly clamps (2).

9. Adhesive tape and tincture of benzoin.

10. Low-pressure, high-flow orotracheal tube sized to the patient (usually a small ⅛ in [3 to 4 mm] tube is used to fit the small opening) or, if available, low-pressure cuffed tracheostomy tubes of various sizes.

11. Syringe, 10-mL, to inflate the balloon on the orotracheal tube.

12. Self-refilling bag-valve-mask combination (eg, Ambu bag) or bag-valve unit (eg, Ayres bag), connector, tubing, and oxygen source.

Positioning of the Patient

The patient should be supine, with a rolled bath towel under the shoulders, and the neck hyperextended.

Anatomy Review

The cricothyroid membrane (conus elasticus and cricothyroid ligament) lies between the thyroid cartilage superiorly and the cricoid cartilage inferiorly (Fig 46–21). The membrane is a poorly vascularized ligamentous structure that lies under the subcutaneous tissue between the laterally placed cricothyroid muscles.

Procedure

1. Assemble all necessary equipment.

2. Position the patient.

3. Sterilize the skin of the neck from the chin to the sternal notch and laterally to the base of the neck, if time permits.

4. Observe sterile technique (don cap, mask, gloves, and gown) if time permits.

5. Check the endotracheal tube or tracheostomy tube for cuff leaks by inflating the tube with air from a syringe.

6. Identify the cricothyroid membrane. Using the 10-mL syringe with the 25-gauge needle, infiltrate the skin and underlying cricothyroid membrane with the 1% lidocaine in a line across the membrane while steadying the thyroid cartilage with the left hand. Omit this step if complete airway obstruction is present or if the patient is comatose.

7. Using the No. 11 blade, make a transverse incision of the skin over the membrane, and then continue the incision through the membrane.

8. Extend the incision in the subcutaneous tissue and membrane for approximately 1 cm (⅜ in) on each side of the midline.

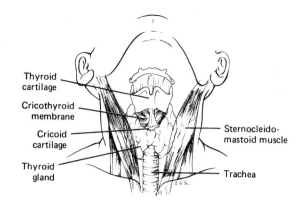

Figure 46–21. Anatomic relationships of the cricothyroid membrane. (Reproduced, with permission, from Dunphy JE, Way LW [editors]: *Current Surgical Diagnosis & Treatment,* 5th ed. Lange, 1981.)

9. Using a mosquito or Kelly clamp in the left hand (with the points downward), insert the clamp into the incision and spread it. This maneuver alone is sufficient to provide an airway for a patient with supraglottic airway obstruction.

10. Grasp the endotracheal tube or tracheostomy tube with the right hand, and insert the tube through the incision into the trachea, directing it caudally.

11. Connect the bag-valve unit to the tube, and immediately ventilate the patient with 100% oxygen. Check for respiratory movement of the chest and the presence of bilaterally symmetric breath sounds.

12. Inflate the balloon just enough to stop any audible air leak during the inspiratory phase of positive pressure ventilation.

13. Cut a 10- × 10-cm (4- × 4-in) gauze sponge halfway down the middle, and wrap it around the tube. If an orotracheal tube is being used, fashion a necklace of adhesive tape, apply tincture of benzoin to the tube, and tape it in place. If a tracheostomy tube is being used, secure the wings of the tube by tying the tapes around the patient's neck, leaving enough slack so that an index finger can easily slide under the tape. Tying the tape too tightly can cause erosion of the skin and venous congestion above the tie, while tying it too loosely invites dislodging of the tube.

14. Suction the trachea.

15. Obtain a chest x-ray immediately to check the position of the tube.

TRANSTRACHEAL JET VENTILATION*

Indications

Transtracheal jet ventilation (TTJV) is an alternative to cricothyrotomy in patients who require emergency assisted ventilation when conventional methods of endotracheal intubation are not possible.

Contraindications

TTJV is contraindicated if conventional methods of endotracheal intubation can be successfully employed or if the proper equipment for TTJV is not available.

Personnel Required

One person can perform the procedure unaided, although it is helpful to have an assistant to position the patient's head and handle equipment.

Equipment & Supplies Required

1. Materials for skin sterilization.
2. Sterile gloves.
3. Intravenous catheter, 12- or 14-gauge, or 13-gauge cannula designed specifically for TTJV that has lateral flanges to which tape may be attached.

*This section contributed by Charles E. Saunders, MD, FACEP, FACP.

4. Bag-valve mask set.
5. 50-psi oxygen source.
6. Demand valve device or Y adapter with connectors and tubing that connects to the 50-psi oxygen source.
7. Adapter (eg, Luer-Lok) for connecting the demand valve outflow tubing to the catheter (Fig 46–22).
8. Tape for securing catheter in place.
9. Syringe, 3-mL.

Positioning of the Patient

The patient is positioned supine with the head in the midline. It is helpful to have the neck slightly extended unless cervical spine injury is suspected.

Anatomy Review

The cricothyroid membrane is a 1- to 1.5-cm membrane that lies inferior to the thyroid cartilage and superior to the first tracheal ring. It can be located easily by palpating the protuberant midline portion of the thyroid cartilage ("Adam's apple") and then moving the fingertip inferiorly 1.5 cm until it rests in a soft, flat depression between the thyroid cartilage and the first tracheal ring. The examining fingertip will then be on the cricothyroid membrane.

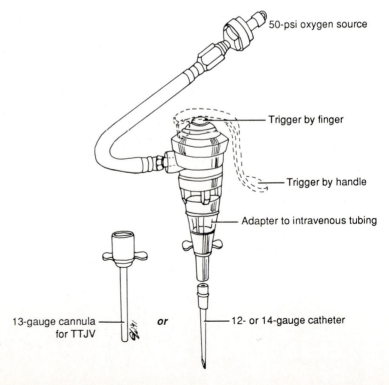

Figure 46–22. 50-psi Oxygen source is connected via a demand valve to the transtracheal jet ventilator.

Procedure

1. Position the head as described above. Have an assistant hold the patient's head or use tape across the forehead to prevent unexpected motion. If the patient requires assisted ventilation, provide it by a bag-valve-mask device.

2. Prepare the anterior surface of the neck with povidone-iodine.

3. Using sterile gloves, locate the cricothyroid membrane. It may be helpful to place the thumb and index finger of the nondominant hand on either side of the cricothyroid membrane to stabilize the trachea and anchor and stretch the skin slightly.

4. Connect the catheter or cannula to the 3-mL syringe. With the catheter or cannula and syringe in the dominant hand, pierce the skin and cricothyroid membrane at a 45-degree angle, directing the catheter tip inferiorly (Fig 46–23). When the catheter tip enters the tracheal lumen, a slight "give" will be felt. The patient may also cough when the catheter stimulates the tracheal wall. Traction in the syringe plunger during entry will confirm lumen entry when air is withdrawn freely.

5. Slide the catheter sheath forward until it is snug against the skin, and then withdraw the needle.

6. Connect the inflow tubing on the demand valve or Y adapter to the 50-psi oxygen source and the outflow tubing to the catheter via the adapter. (Note: 50 psi may be obtained from a step-down regulator that supplies oxygen to a demand valve, or from a venturi flow regulator opened wide to deliver 15 L/min.)

7. Begin ventilation at a rate of 20 breaths per minute, by pressing the button on the demand valve, or occluding the open port on the Y adapter, and inflating for 1 second, followed by a 2-second relaxation phase during which the patient will exhale passively through the oropharynx. Be prepared for secretions to be expelled during inflation as well as exhalation.

8. Tape the catheter firmly in place, with the hub of the catheter snug against the neck.

Emergency Alternative Method

If time is of the essence and a demand valve/50-psi oxygen source is not available, TTJV may be accomplished using a standard bag-valve-mask device and no special equipment other than a 12- or 14-gauge catheter. This method is not preferred, because oxygen flow rates achievable are not as high as those provided by the 50-psi oxygen source and hypercapnia may develop. However, the following may suffice temporarily until a definitive airway can be established, if the necessary equipment is not available, particularly in small children whose ventilatory requirements are less. Steps 1–5 are unchanged.

9. Leave the 3-mL syringe attached to the catheter, and remove the plunger. This converts it into a makeshift "adapter" into which the elbow joint of the bag-valve device will fit.

10. Connect the bag-valve device by inserting the elbow-joint opening into the end of the 3-mL syringe (Fig 46–24).

11. Ventilate the patient at 20 breaths per minute using a vigorous, 1-second compression, followed by a 2-second relaxation.

12. Tape the catheter firmly in place, with the hub snug against the skin.

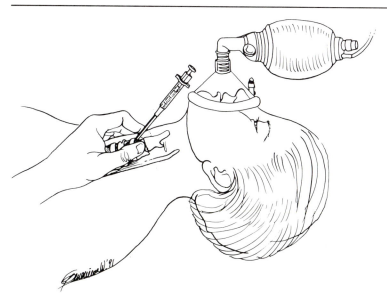

Figure 46–23. Proper orientation for introducing transtracheal catheter. The trachea is stabilized with the hand.

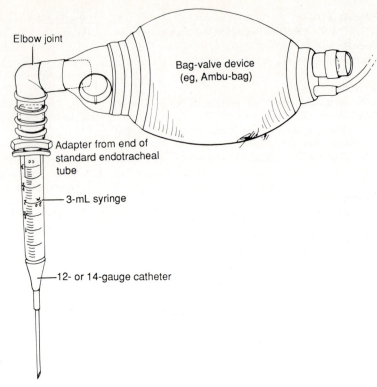

Figure 46–24. Makeshift "adapter" can be fashioned from a 3-mL syringe.

Labels in figure: Elbow joint; Bag-valve device (eg, Ambu-bag); Adapter from end of standard endotracheal tube; 3-mL syringe; 12- or 14-gauge catheter

THORACENTESIS

Indications

Indications for thoracentesis are as follows:

1. To relieve dyspnea or respiratory distress caused by accumulation of fluid in the pleural space.

2. To obtain pleural fluid for diagnostic tests.

Contraindications

Contraindications to thoracentesis are as follows:

1. Severe coagulopathy (should be corrected before thoracentesis, unless there is severe respiratory failure, as determined by arterial blood gas analysis).

2. Agitated, uncooperative patient (only a relative contraindication).

Personnel Required

One person can perform thoracentesis unaided.

Equipment & Supplies Required

1. Materials for skin sterilization.

2. Materials for sterile technique (cap, mask, gloves, and gown).

3. Lidocaine, 1%, with 5-ml syringe and 25- or 27-gauge needle.

4. Sterile towels (4) or sterile paper drapes.

5. Gauze sponges, 10 × 10 cm (4 × 4 in).

6. Catheter-clad needle (eg, Angiocath), 16- to 18-gauge, 30.5 cm (12 in) long; or needle-clad catheter (eg, Intracath) 14- to 16-gauge, with 30.5-cm (12-in) catheter; and 30-mL syringe to aid in insertion.

7. Three-way stopcock.

8. Luer-Lok syringe, 30-mL.

9. Sterile connecting tubing and empty intravenous bottle, or vacuum bottle specially designed for thoracentesis (if removal of more than a few hundred milliliters of fluid is anticipated). The connecting tube should not have a drip chamber.

10. Collection vessels and culture media for laboratory analysis.

Positioning of the Patient

Thoracentesis is usually performed with the operator positioned behind the seated patient. Occasionally, thoracentesis must be performed in the lateral position when the patient cannot sit.

For the posterior approach, the patient should be sitting on the edge of the bed or gurney with arms and trunk bent forward over a bedside stand and supported by the elbows or a pillow.

If the lateral approach must be used, have the patient lie at the edge of the bed on the affected side with the ipsilateral arm extended over the head. The midposterior line must be accessible for insertion of the needle. Elevating the head of the bed 30 degrees is sometimes helpful.

Anatomy Review

Access to the pleural space is gained through the intercostal spaces (Fig 46–25). Remember that nerves and blood vessels run on the underside of the rib, and that the domes of the diaphragm are highest posteriorly, occasionally as high as the seventh intercostal space.

Procedure

A. Position the patient, and prepare all equipment.

B. Initial Preparation:

1. If removing a large volume of fluid, assemble the connecting tubing and a collection vessel.

2. Observe sterile technique (don cap, mask, gloves, and gown) if time permits.

3. Arrange all of the equipment on a sterile field on a Mayo stand or bedside table.

4. Select the thoracentesis site by localizing the level of pleural fluid either by percussion (area of dullness) or ultrasonography. Insert the needle in the intercostal space below the level of fluid in the mid

posterior line (posterior insertion) or the midaxillary line (lateral insertion).

5. Sterilize a wide area of skin around the proposed insertion site.

6. Drape the patient (this may be impossible if the patient is sitting).

7. Anesthetize the skin over the insertion site with the 1% lidocaine with the 25- or 27-gauge needle and 5-mL syringe. Then anesthetize the superior surface of the rib and the parietal pleura.

C. Catheter-Clad Needle (eg, Angiocath) Insertion:

1. Attach a 30-mL syringe to the catheter-clad needle, and insert the needle through the skin over the rib selected. Advance the needle until its hits the rib.

2. Move the tip of the needle cephalad over the edge of the rib until it encounters the superior aspect of the rib.

3. Have the patient take a deep breath and hold it against a closed glottis.

4. Advance the needle over the superior surface of the rib and through the pleura into the pleural space. Maintain constant suction on the syringe so that the pleural fluid will enter the syringe instantly when the pleural space is entered. Apply controlled, gentle, steady pressure with both hands steadied on the patient's back to keep from suddenly spearing the

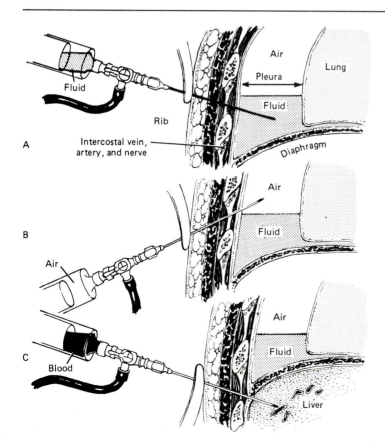

Figure 46–25. Technique of thoracentesis using a regular steel needle (not catheter-clad). **A:** Successful tap, with fluid obtained. Note the position of the needle with relation to the intercostal neurovascular bundle, and the use of the clamp to steady the needle at skin level (do not use a clamp with a catheter-clad needle). **B:** Air is obtained if the position of the needle tip is too high (lung is punctured, or preexisting pneumothorax is entered, as an illustration). **C:** A bloody tap may result from excessively low position of the needle with puncture of the liver. (Reproduced, with permission, from Wilson JL [editor]: *Handbook of Surgery*, 5th ed. Lange, 1973. Redrawn from GE Lindskog and AE Liebow.)

lung. Do not use a Kelly clamp to grip a catheter-clad needle.

5. When the catheter has entered the pleural space, angle the needle caudally, and push the catheter off the needle and into the base of the pleural space.

6. Occlude the lumen of the catheter, and have the patient exhale and breathe normally.

7. Have the patient take a deep breath again and hold it; insert the 3-way stopcock into the catheter hub. Make sure that the stopcock valve is set to occlude the catheter port. Have the patient resume normal breathing.

8. Connect the 30-mL Luer-Lok syringe to one port of the 3-way stopcock and (if needed) the intravenous tubing to the other.

9. Turn the stopcock valve to connect the syringe with the catheter, and withdraw fluid from the pleural space. Then turn the stopcock so as to connect the syringe to the intravenous tubing, and empty the syringe through the tubing into the intravenous bag or bottle. The first syringeful of fluid may be reserved for diagnostic tests.

10. Withdraw as much fluid as possible but no more than 1 L at one time. In order to completely evacuate the pleural space, the patient may have to be rocked from side to side while fluid is being withdrawn.

11. When no more fluid can be withdrawn, the patient should take a deep breath and hold it while the catheter is quickly withdrawn. Cover the insertion site with a sterile occlusive dressing.

12. Obtain an upright portable chest x-ray to check for possible pneumothorax and residual fluid.

D. Needle-Clad Catheter (eg, Intracath) Insertion: If a needle-clad catheter is used, the procedure is the same as described above, except for the following steps:

1. Insert the needle as described above (steps 1–4), and withdraw fluid to make sure that the needle is in the pleural space. (The fluid may be used for analysis.) A clamp may be used to grip the needle to prevent it from being inserted too far.

2. Instruct the patient to take a deep breath and hold it against a closed glottis, and then quickly insert the catheter through the needle so that it goes to the base of the pleural space. Withdraw the needle, leaving the catheter inside the pleural space.

3. Occlude the lumen of the catheter, and have the patient resume normal breathing.

4. Again have the patient take a deep breath and hold it, and insert the stopcock into the hub of the catheter. Follow the remaining steps (8–12) described above.

TUBE THORACOSTOMY
(Insertion of a Chest Tube)

Indications

Tube thoracostomy is performed in order to drain air or fluid from the pleural space.

Contraindications

There are no absolute contraindications to chest tube insertion. Usually, the patient is in distress, and any relative contraindication (eg, coagulopathy) is superseded by the need to reinflate a compressed lung or drain fluid from the lungs.

Personnel Required

One operator can insert a chest tube alone; however, an assistant is helpful.

Equipment & Supplies Required

Most hospitals have sterile thoracostomy trays ready for use. If a tray is not available, assemble the following instruments and materials:

A. Materials:
1. Materials for skin sterilization.
2. Materials for sterile technique (cap, mask, gloves, and gown).
3. Lidocaine, 1%, with 10-mL syringe and 25- and 22-gauge needles.

B. Equipment:
1. Sterile towels (4) or sterile paper drapes.
2. Chest tube of the appropriate size and style to suit the clinical situation (see below).
3. No. 11 surgical blade, mounted.
4. Mayo clamp.
5. Kelly clamp.
6. Surgical silk suture (size 0) with large curved cutting needle.
7. Needle holder.
8. Petrolatum-impregnated gauze.
9. Sterile gauze sponges, 10×10 cm (4×4 in).
10. Plastic adhesive tape, 5 cm (2 in) wide.
11. Suction apparatus, 3-bottle, with water-seal, collection, and water-column sections (Fig 46–26). In the USA, this device is usually supplied as a unit with tall connectors and tubes included (eg, Pleurevac).
12. Sterile Y connector (if 2 chest tubes are to be connected to the same suction apparatus).

Positioning of the Patient

Tubes are usually inserted laterally when fluid, pus, or blood is drained, irrespective of whether air is also being removed. The patient should lie with the affected side up, and the ipsilateral arm extended

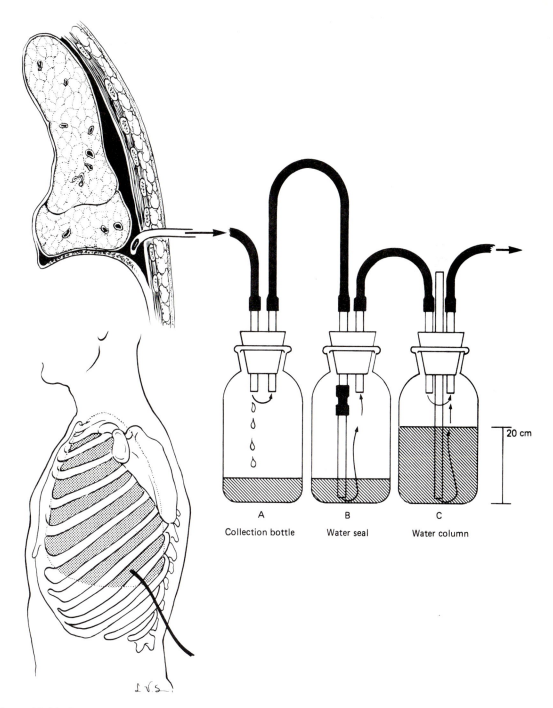

A
Collection bottle

B
Water seal

C
Water column

20 cm

Figure 46–26. Diagram of tube thoracostomy and 3-bottle suction apparatus. ***Bottle A*** is connected to the thoracostomy tube and collects pleural drainage for inspection and measurement of volume. ***Bottle B*** acts as a simple valve to prevent collapse of the lung if tubing distal to this point is opened to atmospheric pressure. Pulmonary air leak can be detected by the escape of bubbles from the submerged tube. ***Bottle C*** is a system for regulating the negative pressure delivered to the pleural space. Wall suction should be regulated to maintain continuous vigorous bubbling from the middle open tube in bottle C. The resulting negative pressure (in cm water) is equal to the difference in the height of the fluid levels in bottles B and C. (Reproduced, with permission, from Dunphy JE, Way LW [editors]: *Current Surgical Diagnosis & Treatment,* 3rd ed. Lange, 1977.)

over the head and grasping the top of the bed or the guardrail for security.

Rarely, chest tubes are inserted anteriorly to evacuate a pure pneumothorax. The patient should be supine, with the head raised about 10 degrees. Position the bed or gurney at a comfortable height to prevent back strain for the operator.

Anatomy Review

See Anatomy Review under Thoracentesis, above. Remember that the intercostal arteries and veins follow the inferior border of the rib.

Procedure

1. Prepare all necessary equipment, and arrange it on a sterile towel placed on a Mayo stand or bedside table.

2. Select the proper chest tube for insertion. In patients with trauma, insert the largest tube available (usually 36–40F), and consider using a 90-degree angled tube to ensure drainage at the base of the lung. In patients without trauma, use a 32–36F chest tube, either straight or curved. In a patient with pure pneumothorax, a smaller chest tube (12–20F) is usually sufficient. A general rule is that a large tube effectively drains any substance from the pleural space and thus is preferred in emergencies, when the diagnosis may be unclear.

3. Assemble the suction apparatus according to the manufacturer's directions.

4. Connect the suction apparatus to a wall suction outlet, and adjust the suction so that a steady stream of bubbles is produced in the water column.

5. Position the patient.

6. Determine the insertion site. Most tubes are inserted in the lateral thorax at the anterior axillary line, just lateral to the nipple. This places the tube in the fourth or fifth intercostal space, ensuring that it is above the dome of the diaphragm. Palpate the nearest rib, and double-check the position; liver or spleen laceration can occur if the patient is not properly positioned.

7. Observing sterile technique, open the sterile instrument tray, arrange all necessary instruments, and make sure that everything is present.

8. Sterilize the skin over the insertion site and a wide area around it.

9. Again locate the rib for the insertion site, and anesthetize the skin over the mid to inferior aspect of the rib with the 1% lidocaine with the 10-mL syringe and 25-gauge needle. Then anesthetize the surface of the rib and the tissue superior to it with the 22-gauge needle.

10. Drape the area around the insertion site.

11. Using the No. 11 blade, make a horizontal incision through the skin along the inferior aspect of the rib. The incision should be about 1½ times as wide as the tube selected. Incise the skin down to the subcutaneous tissue.

12. Use the Mayo clamp with the tips down as a dissector. Spread the tips to open tissue planes, and create a tunnel aiming toward the superior aspect of the rib. Make sure the clamp stays next to the rib.

13. When the Mayo clamp is just over the superior edge of the rib, close the clamp, and push it with steady pressure through the parietal pleura and into the chest. This maneuver requires more pressure than might be anticipated. Use steady, even, controlled pressure to provide control of the clamp after it has perforated the pleura. A lunging motion may cause a hole in the lung, liver, or spleen.

Once the clamp has penetrated the pleural space, air, fluid, blood, or pus may escape during expiration. Tension pneumothorax will whistle as air escapes under pressure, and the lung will collapse further during inspiration, because free air has access to the pleural space.

14. Widen the hole in the parietal pleura by spreading the Mayo clamp.

15. If a tube of large diameter is to be inserted, use the index finger to dilate the tract and hole in the pleura. This maneuver also ensures that entry has been made into the pleural space and not into a space inadvertently created between the parietal pleura and the chest wall.

16. Grasp the end of the chest tube with a Mayo or Kelly clamp (jaws parallel to the tube), and guide the tube down the tract into the pleural space, making sure that the last hole in the chest tube is within the pleural space. If a curved tube is being used, direct it inferiorly so that it lies along the base of the pleural space. A straight tube may be positioned inferiorly, laterally, or superiorly, depending on the clinical situation.

17. Connect the chest tube to the suction apparatus, and make sure that the level in the water column varies with respiration. Usually, fluid, blood, or pus drains from the tube, a sign that the tube is properly positioned in the pleural space (unless the tube was inserted for pure pneumothorax). *Note:* If the tube has been inadvertently inserted between the parietal pleura and the chest wall, no fluid will drain from the tube, and the level in the water column will not vary with respiration.

18. Sew the tube to the chest wall with the silk suture. Partially close the incision with a mattress stitch, and use one throw of a square knot to close the skin around the tube. Then, wind both ends of the suture around the tube, starting at the bottom and working toward the top (as if lacing up a shoe). Tie the ends of the suture snugly around the top of the tube.

19. Wrap Xeroform or petrolatum-impregnated gauze around the tube to seal it to the skin. Cover the tube with two 10- × 10-cm (4- × 4-in) sterile gauze sponges, cut so that they fit around the tube. Tape the sponges and the tube in place. Tape connections of the chest tube to the suction tube, and tape the chest tube to the patient's side below the insertion site.

20. Obtain a portable upright chest x-ray to check the position of the tube and to make sure that the lung is expanded and that all fluid has been evacuated.

EMERGENCY THORACOTOMY*

Emergency thoracotomy is performed to gain access to the heart and great vessels. It can occasionally be lifesaving, although controversy exists over the indications and the location where it should be performed. It should only be performed when the patient can be taken immediately afterwards to the operating room.

Indications

1. Traumatic cardiac arrest following penetrating chest trauma with signs of life in the prehospital setting (survival rate up to 40%).
2. Traumatic cardiac arrest following penetrating or blunt trauma with signs of life in the emergency department (low survival rate for blunt trauma victims).
3. Cardiac tamponade with profound shock; patient is unresponsive to rapid volume expansion, is deteriorating, and is unlikely to survive until operation.
4. Blunt or penetrating trauma to the chest or abdomen with profound shock; patient is unresponsive to rapid volume expansion, is deteriorating, and is unlikely to survive until operation.
5. Massive chest or abdominal bleeding with profound shock; patient is unresponsive to rapid volume expansion, is deteriorating, and is unlikely to survive until operation.

Contraindications

1. Traumatic cardiac arrest with no signs of life in the prehospital setting (survival rate virtually nil).
2. Appropriate operating facilities and personnel not immediately available.
3. Patient immediately responsive to volume expansion or decompression of tension pneumothorax.

Personnel Required

One individual experienced in the technique is required to perform the procedure, another to maintain an airway and assist ventilation, and, ideally, a third to prepare and hand equipment to the operator. In most cases, patients have multiple, concomitant needs that are best met by a team.

Equipment & Supplies Required

1. Materials for skin sterilization.
2. Sterile drapes.
3. Scalpel with No. 10 blades.
4. Rib spreaders.
5. Vascular clamps.

6. Nonvascular clamps.
7. Suture scissors.
8. Metzenbaum scissors (long).
9. Needle holder (long).
10. Suture (2-0 silk or comparable) on cutting needle.
11. 10-in DeBakey tangential occlusion clamp.
12. Suction catheter.
13. Tissue forceps.
14. Bone rongeur.
15. Rib approximator.

Positioning of the Patient

The patient should be supine. Place rolled sheet under the left scapula and lower ribs, and elevate the left arm above the head to expose the left chest and axilla. The patient should be intubated and ventilated with positive pressure (manual bag-valve method or mechanical ventilator).

Anatomy Review

The favored approach to the heart in an emergency setting is through a left thoracotomy. The incision follows the rib interspace, with care taken to avoid the intercostal vessels that run beneath each rib. The internal mammary artery runs parallel to the lateral margin of the sternum and must be ligated should hemorrhage from this vessel occur.

Procedure

1. Prepare the anterior thoracic surface generously on both sides with skin-sterilizing solution, and cover it with sterile drapes to the extent that time allows.
2. Using the No. 10 scalpel blade, make a horizontal incision in the left 4th–5th intercostal space, extending from the sternum to the posterior axillary line. It should be deep enough to expose the intercostal muscles and should follow the superior rib margin to avoid injury to the intercostal vascular bundle beneath the rib above. In women, make the incision beneath the breast.
3. With a scalpel or scissors, make a small opening through the intercostal muscles into the pleural space. Using Metzenbaum scissors, divide the intercostal muscles the entire length of the incision, remaining close to the superior margin of the rib. Ligate the internal mammary artery above and below. Using the scalpel or heavy scissors, cut through 2 sternocostal cartilages above the interspace.
4. Insert a rib spreader and spread the ribs as widely apart as possible. If necessary (eg, in penetrating trauma to the right chest), the incision may be ex-

*This section contributed by Charles E. Saunders, MD, FACEP, FACP.

tended across the sternum and into the right chest to increase exposure.

5. Inspect the heart. It will appear to be bluish if cardiac tamponade is present. To relieve tamponade or perform cardiac massage, open the pericardium. Pick up the pericardium with forceps and incise it from apex to base, using Metzenbaum scissors. Be careful to avoid the phrenic nerve, which courses longitudinally along the lateral heart margin. Remove any clotted blood; suction excess blood as needed.

6. If observable cardiac contractions are inadequate, or if cardiac arrest has occurred, perform internal cardiac massage by gently compressing the heart with both hands. If ventricular fibrillation is present, a quivering motion will be observed. Perform defibrillation using the internal paddles, at an energy level of 5–50 J. If a myocardial laceration is present, it can be temporarily controlled with a fingertip or with a 3-0 polypropylene suture. Horizontal mattress sutures through Teflon pledgets will help prevent further laceration of the myocardium. Place sutures through the epicardium and myocardium only. Avoid the coronary artery. Atrial wounds can be repaired with simple interrupted sutures.

7. Control massive bleeding from the lung or pulmonary vessels by cross-clamping the hilum of the involved lung.

8. If the patient fails to respond rapidly to volume administration, or if intra-abdominal bleeding is suspected, incise the overlying pleura and cross-clamp the aorta above the point where it enters the diaphragm. Be careful to avoid clamping the esophagus. As a temporary measure during internal cardiac massage, the aorta may be occluded with the index and long fingers placed behind the heart.

9. If resuscitation is successful, immediately transport the patient to the operating room for definitive care.

AUTOTRANSFUSION

Autotransfusion permits collection, anticoagulation, and reinfusion of a patient's blood. The Sorensen autotransfusion system is used most frequently in emergencies. This device removes blood from the patient into a collection bag and mixes it with an anticoagulant. The anticoagulated blood is then filtered through a 170-μm (about 0.0067-in) filter and infused back into the patient through a standard intravenous catheter. Emergency autotransfusion is performed almost exclusively in patients with traumatic hemothorax. Blood from the pleural space is ideal for autotransfusion because it rarely clots while in the chest, it is usually not contaminated with other body fluids or solid matter, and it can be easily removed by insertion of a chest tube.

Do not collect blood for autotransfusion from external hemorrhage.

Indications

Autotransfusion is performed to reduce the amount of blood needed from the blood bank for transfusion in patients with a large hemothorax due to penetrating or blunt chest trauma.

Contraindications

Contraindications to autotransfusion are as follows:

1. Infection in the pleural space.

2. Contamination of blood by fecal material, bacteria, or tumor cells.

3. Coagulation defects or significant liver or kidney dysfunction.

Personnel Required

Two people are required to perform autotransfusion. The operator inserts the chest tube, and an assistant sets up the suction and collection system.

Equipment & Supplies Required

1. Sorensen autotransfusion system (Fig 46–27) with a suction canister, sterile blood collection bag, and collection tubing to connect the chest tube to the collection bag.

2. Standard suction tubing and source of continuous suction (10–30 mm Hg).

3. Standard intravenous tubing for transferring anticoagulant to the collection container and for reinfusing the collected blood into the patient (2 sets).

4. Anticoagulant (citrate-phosphate-dextrose [CPD] anticoagulant is recommended). A 250-mL bottle of CPD is sufficient anticoagulant for 2500 mL of blood.

5. Blood filter, 170-μm (about 0.0067-in).

6. Thoracostomy tube and insertion set (see Tube Thoracostomy, above).

7. Kelly clamp.

Positioning of the Patient

Positioning of the patient is the same as that described for chest tube insertion. The patient should lie with the affected side up, with the ipsilateral arm extended over the head. The patient can grasp the top of the gurney or the guardrail for security.

Procedure

1. Assemble the autotransfusion unit as soon as a

A

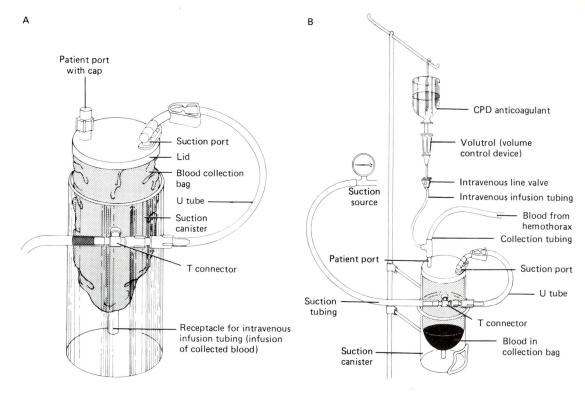

B

Figure 46–27. Sorensen autotransfusion system. **A:** Blood collection bag being inserted into suction canister. **B:** Completely assembled system.

diagnosis of hemothorax has been made and before a chest tube is inserted. Attach the suction canister to an intravenous administration pole. Hang the bottle of CPD anticoagulant and the attached infusion tubing above the suction canister.

2. Flush the infusion tubing with CPD anticoagulant so that the tubing is free of all air.

3. Extend the blood collection bag to its full length, and insert the bag into the suction canister. On top of the blood collection bag is a plastic lid that fits on top of the suction canister. On this lid are 2 ports, one marked "patient," and the other, with a U tube attached, marked "suction." Connect the distal end of the U tube to the adaptor on the T connector located on the upper side of the suction canister.

4. Using the suction tubing, connect the other side of the T connector to a source of continuous suction, and adjust the suction to 10–30 mm Hg.

5. Attach the yellow connector of the chest tube collection tubing to the port marked "patient" on the lid of the blood collection bag. Occlude the collection tubing with a clamp.

6. Attach the infusion tubing from the CPD bottle to the port marked "patient" on the top of the blood collection bag. The chest tube may now be inserted.

7. Attach the white connector (distal end) of the collection tubing to the chest tube draining the hemothorax.

8. Release the occluding clamp on the collection tubing, permitting blood to flow from the hemothorax into the blood collection bag. Simultaneously, start the flow of CPD anticoagulant into the collection bag by opening the infusion tubing.

9. As blood is evacuated from the pleural space, it is sucked into the blood collection bag. The ratio of CPD anticoagulant volume to blood volume should be 1:10 (eg, 100 mL of anticoagulant per liter of blood). As blood fills the bag in the canister, rotate the canister to make sure that blood is completely mixed with anticoagulant.

10. Observe the fluid level in the collection canister, and stop blood flow by clamping the collection tube when 1500 mL of blood has been collected.

11. Stop the infusion of CPD anticoagulant.

12. Disconnect the collection tubing and the CPD anticoagulant from the "patient" port on the lid of the blood collection bag.

13. Disconnect the CPD anticoagulant infusion tubing from the "patient" port on the lid of the blood collection bag.

14. Make sure the collection tubing is clamped before proceeding. If the vacuum is released with the collection tubing open, pneumothorax will result.

15. Disconnect the U tube that goes from the T connector to the lid of the blood collection bag, and remove the white spacer from the end of the line.

16. Place the male end of the white spacer into the open end of the collection tubing to maintain sterile conditions.

17. Connect the open end of the U tube to the "patient" port on the lid of the blood collection bag to close the receptacle system and maintain sterile conditions.

18. Remove the bag filled with anticoagulated blood from the canister, and hang it from the intravenous administration pole by the plastic hanger on top of the bag.

19. Insert a 170-μm (about 0.0067-in) blood filter into the bottom of the bag, and administer the blood to the patient through the infusion tubing.

20. Insert a new blood collection bag into the suction canister, attach the collection and suction tubing as described above, and continue collecting salvageable blood.

21. When blood return from the collecting tube stops because the hemothorax has been drained, clamp the thoracostomy tube, disconnect the collecting tube, and connect the thoracostomy tube to a standard water-seal suction apparatus (see Tube Thoracostomy, above).

PERICARDIOCENTESIS

Aspiration of pericardial fluid is both a diagnostic and a therapeutic procedure. Since noninvasive methods of detecting pericardial effusion (CT scan, echocardiography) are highly sensitive and pericardiocentesis is a dangerous procedure, the use of pericardiocentesis in the emergency department should be limited to relieving suspected decompensated cardiac tamponade in a desperately ill patient.

Indications

Pericardiocentesis is performed to relieve suspected decompensated cardiac tamponade (the diagnosis of pericardial effusion will be confirmed or ruled out at the same time).

Contraindications

In a patient who requires pericardiocentesis for decompensated or rapidly decompensating cardiac tamponade, there are no contraindications. In other patients, the following conditions are contraindications:

1. Infection along the proposed course of pericardiocentesis.

2. Bleeding diathesis (this is a relative contraindication only, especially if it can be corrected).

Personnel Required

Three people are required to perform pericardiocentesis: the operator, an assistant to monitor the electrocardiograph, and another physician besides the operator. A cardiothoracic surgeon should be available in case complications occur.

Equipment & Supplies Required

Many hospitals have prepackaged sterile pericardiocentesis trays that contain items 3–12. If these are not available, the following instruments and materials are required:

1. Materials for skin sterilization.

2. Materials for sterile technique (cap, mask, gloves, and gown).

3. Lidocaine, 1%, with 10-mL syringe and 25-gauge needle.

4. Pericardiocentesis needle: 17-gauge, 12.5-cm (5-in) thin-walled steel needle (usually a spinal needle) for aspiration. It is possible to use 16-gauge and even 14-gauge needles with plastic outer cannulas.

5. Syringes: assorted sizes, including 50-mL (2), 30-mL (2), 10-mL (2), 5-mL (1).

6. No. 11 scalpel blade, mounted.

7. Sterile conductive monitoring cable with alligator clamps at each end.

8. Three-way stopcock.

9. Silk suture (5-0) on a cutting needle.

10. Straight clamp and needle holder.

11. Needles: assorted sizes, including 25-gauge, 1.5-cm (⅝-in) (1); 22-gauge, 2.5-cm (1-in) (2); and 18-gauge, 4-cm (1½-in) (5), for transferring specimens.

12. Drapes.

13. Sterile, capped, 15-mL specimen tubes (10).

14. Heparin, to lightly heparinize cytologic specimen tubes.

15. Specimen tubes, 1 purple-topped and 3 red-topped.

16. Clean glass microscope slides.

17. Microhematocrit centrifuge tubes with occlusive sealant.

18.
Ice bucket to hold cytologic specimens.

19. Sterile dressing for entry and exit sites.

20. CPR cart and equipment and electrocardiograph.

Positioning of the Patient

The patient should be supine, and if time permits, the thorax should be elevated 30 degrees. Optimize bed height and lighting for the operator. A right-handed physician should stand on the patient's right side.

Procedure

A. Prepare the patient as follows (if time permits):

1. The patient should be in a bed where cardiac monitoring is available, preferably in a cardiac catheterization laboratory.

2. Position the patient, as described above.

3. Begin electrocardiographic monitoring with limb leads.

4. Gain secure intravenous access.

5. Give atropine, 0.6–1 mg intramuscularly or subcutaneously, before pericardiocentesis, since vagal responses during cardiac tamponade may be devastating.

6. Narcotics may be used as long as they do not depress consciousness or respiration.

7. Supplemental oxygen, 5–10 L/min, by mask or nasal prongs is advisable.

B. Observe sterile technique (don cap, mask, gloves, and gown).

1. Sterilize the skin in a wide area around the xiphoid process.

2. Drape the field widely with sterile towels if time permits.

C. Begin pericardiocentesis.

1. Locate the appropriate site to the left of and below the xiphoid process (Fig 46–28), and anesthetize the skin with the 1% lidocaine with the 10-mL syringe and 25-gauge needle. Switch to the 22-gauge needle, and anesthetize the tissue beneath the xiphoid process along the track of the pericardiocentesis needle. Omit this step if the patient is comatose.

2. Incise the skin with the No. 11 scalpel blade to facilitate entry of the pericardiocentesis needle.

3. With the help of an assistant, attach the conductive monitoring cable to the chest terminal lead of the electrocardiograph using one of the alligator clamps. Attach the other end to the hub of the pericardiocentesis needle. Operate the electrocardiograph on the V lead setting. The pericardiocentesis needle then becomes a probing electrocardiographic lead.

4. With the alligator clamp and conductive monitoring cable mounted, attach the pericardiocentesis needle to a 30-mL syringe.

5. Perform pericardiocentesis. If this procedure is being done during active CPR, make sure that everything is ready beforehand, work rapidly, and stop CPR for only as long as necessary. Enter the selected site, just caudal and to the left of the xiphoid process, and direct the needle at an angle of 30–45 degrees to the skin. Aim toward the patient's left shoulder. Advance the needle slowly, and aspirate the fluid continuously. There is usually a palpable feeling of resistance when the needle pierces the parietal pericardium.

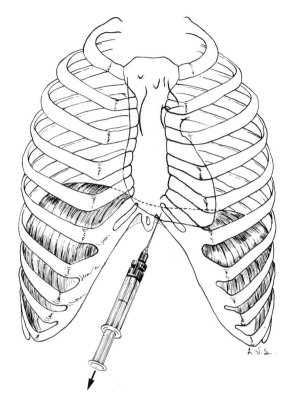

Figure 46–28. Diagram of pericardiocentesis showing position of needle and anatomic relationships. (Reproduced, with permission, from Way LW [editor]: *Current Surgical Diagnosis & Treatment,* 9th ed. Appleton & Lange, 1991.)

If the attempt to penetrate the pericardium is unsuccessful and no fluid is aspirated, bring the needle back to the subcutaneous tissue, and direct it more medially. Continue either until fluid is aspirated or until the needle hits the left side of the sternum, at which point it is safer to use fluoroscopic or echocardiographic guidance.

Pericardial aspiration by an anterior left intercostal approach (usually the fourth left intercostal space just left of the sternum) is less satisfactory because it penetrates the pleural space and has a potential for laceration of the left anterior descending coronary artery or a branch of the internal mammary artery. This approach may be used as a last resort in a dying patient.

6. Have an assistant continuously monitoring the electrocardiograph during the procedure. When fluid is aspirated and a flowing freely, the needle can be anchored at the chest wall with a surgical clamp to keep it from penetrating any farther. A myocardial current of injury or precipitation of arrhythmias on the ECG is a sign to slowly withdraw the needle until fluid is aspirated. In cardiac tamponade due to pericardial hemorrhage, the fact that pericardial blood does not clot (whereas intracardiac blood does) may be a helpful diagnostic clue.

7. Aspirate until the pericardium is dry by slowly withdrawing fluid under constant electrocardiographic monitoring. Secure any specimens that are required for diagnostic tests. In the presence of decompensated cardiac tamponade, removal of even a small amount of pericardial fluid should result in a dramatic improvement in the patient's hemodynamic status.

8. After aspiration is completed, withdraw the needle, and gain hemostasis with pressure. A single suture may be required.

9. Cover the entry site with a sterile dressing.

ABDOMINAL PARACENTESIS

Indications

Indications for abdominal paracentesis are as follows:

1. To determine the cause of ascites, including suspected intra-abdominal hemorrhage from trauma.

2. To lower intra-abdominal pressure in tense ascites (rarely indicated in the emergency department).

3. To obtain fluid for analysis and culture in patients with ascites who are thought to have an infection.

Contraindications

The following conditions are relative contraindications to abdominal paracentesis, and most can be corrected or circumvented if paracentesis must be performed:

1. Bleeding diathesis (coagulopathy or thrombocytopenia). Correct severe bleeding diathesis before performing paracentesis. Cautious paracentesis with a 22-gauge needle may be safely performed in patients with mild to moderate bleeding tendencies.

2. Previous abdominal surgery.

3. Severe bowel distention (correct with nasogastric suction and a rectal tube before performing paracentesis).

Personnel Required

One person can perform paracentesis unaided if the patient is cooperative. An assistant may be helpful if the patient is obese.

Equipment & Supplies Required

1. Materials for skin sterilization.

2. Materials for sterile technique (mask, gloves).

3. Lidocaine, 1%, with 10-mL syringe and 22- and 25-gauge needles.

4. Needles in various sizes, including a longer 20- or 22-gauge spinal needle and a 19-gauge catheter-clad needle (eg, Angiocath). Use a 22-gauge, 4-cm (1½-in) needle or spinal needle in patients with severe bleeding diathesis.

5. Syringe, 50-mL.

6. Drapes.

7. Specimen tubes, both with and without anticoagulant, and a blood culture bottle.

8. Ice bucket for cytology specimens.

9. Gauze sponges, 10×10 cm (4×4 in).

10. Topical antibacterial ointment.

11. Tape and dressing material.

12. Three-way stopcock, connector tubing, and 500-mL collection bottle (if therapeutic paracentesis is planned).

Positioning of the Patient

Have the patient supine at the edge of the bed nearest the operator (right side of the bed for a right-handed operator), with the trunk elevated 45 degrees. Allow 10 minutes for ascites to pool in the dependent portion of the abdomen and for air-filled bowel to float up away from the puncture site. Be sure the bladder has been emptied by voiding or catheterization.

The patient can be tipped 30 degrees to either side if paracentesis of the lower quadrants is necessary. Limited ascites can be aspirated successfully by having the patient bridge 2 beds or a bed and a chair on hands and knees. The approach in this case (a somewhat cramped one for the operator) is from below upward into the dependent abdomen.

Procedure

1. Observe sterile technique (don mask and gloves).

2. Sterilize the skin between the umbilicus and symphysis pubica and both lower quadrants.

3. Drape the field widely.

4. Using the 25-gauge needle, anesthetize the skin with the 1% lidocaine in the 10-mL syringe at the selected puncture site. The preferred site is on the poorly vascularized linea alba, about halfway between the symphysis pubica and the umbilicus (Fig 46–29). Change to the 22-gauge needle, and anesthetize down to and including the peritoneum.

5. Attach the 19-gauge catheter-clad needle to a 50-mL syringe. In patients with severe coagulopathy and thrombocytopenia, use a 22-gauge needle. In markedly obese patients, use a 20-gauge spinal needle.

6. Puncture the skin. Keeping the needle perpendicular to the abdominal wall, maintain continuous

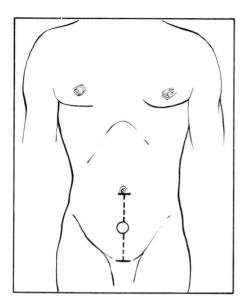

Figure 46–29. Insertion site for abdominal paracentesis. (Reproduced, with permission, from Dunphy JE, Way LW [editors]: *Current Surgical Diagnosis & Treatment,* 5th ed. Lange, 1981.)

negative suction in the syringe while slowly advancing the needle. In tense ascites, it may be useful to try Z-tracking the needle to minimize persistent leaking of ascitic fluid; ie, after penetrating the skin, move the needle and syringe 1–2 cm (3/8–3/4) in) before piercing the subcutaneous tissue, but maintain the perpendicular approach. Repeat this maneuver at the level of the peritoneum, thus describing an oblique Z

pattern through the various layers of tissue. In this manner, the track of the needle from the skin to the peritoneal space will not be a continuous line when the needle is removed.

7. The dense connective tissue of the peritoneum will yield noticeably ("pop") when pierced.

8. Fluid should flow freely into the syringe. To avoid bowel or visceral trauma, particularly in patients with bleeding tendencies, it is preferable to remove the steel needle, leaving the plastic catheter in place while specimens are collected. The patient can be safely moved into more dependent positions with the plastic catheter in place to facilitate drainage of sufficient fluid for analysis. In most cases of diagnostic paracentesis, a single collection of 50 mL is adequate. At a minimum, fluid should be sent to the laboratory for cell count, tests for protein, cultures, and staining with Gram's stain. For suspected neoplasia or for therapeutic relief of tense ascites, up to 1 L may be removed, although 750 mL is a more prudent upper limit in order to avoid adverse effects on intravascular volume. A 3-way stopcock can be used to minimize leakage while the operator is continually aspirating with a syringe. Alternatively, drainage can go directly into sterile 250- to 500-mL vacuum containers using connecting tubing.

9. After samples have been collected, remove the catheter or needle, and apply firm pressure to the site for 5 minutes.

10. Apply topical antibacterial ointment, and dress the site with a pressure dressing.

11. If leaking of ascitic fluid persists despite a pressure dressing, close the paracentesis tract with a mattress stitch.

PERITONEAL CATHETER INSERTION & PERITONEAL LAVAGE

Indications

Peritoneal lavage is performed to determine if intraperitoneal hemorrhage has occurred.

Contraindications

Contraindications to peritoneal lavage are as follows:

1. Previous intra-abdominal surgery of any kind.
2. Pregnancy.
3. Unstable patient who requires immediate surgery.

Personnel Required

1. Percutaneous approach–One operator and an assistant are required for peritoneal lavage using the percutaneous approach.

2. Operative approach–One operator and 2 assistants are required for peritoneal lavage using the operative approach.

Equipment & Supplies Required

Prepackaged trays with the necessary equipment are available commercially, or they can be made up by the hospital. Items required for peritoneal lavage are listed below.

1. Materials for skin sterilization.
2. Materials for sterile technique (cap, mask, gloves, and gown).
3. Sterile towels (4) or sterile paper drapes.
4. Lidocaine, 1%, with 5-mL syringe and 25-gauge needle.
5. No. 11 surgical blade, mounted.
6. Peritoneal lavage catheter (11–18F) and introducing stylet.

7. Sterile bottle containing 1 L of lactated Ringer's injection or normal saline, with intravenous connector tubing.

8. Nylon suture (size 4-0) on a cutting needle (percutaneous approach); chromic catgut (size 3-0) plus silk, nylon, or polypropylene sutures (size 3-0) (operative approach).

9. Needle holder and straight scissors.

10. Adhesive dressing.

11. For operative technique only: 2 Allis or Kocher clamps, 1 Kelly clamp, and 2 small right-angle retractors.

Positioning of the Patient

1. The patient should be supine on a level surface.

2. Examine the abdomen for scars; do not perform peritoneal lavage if abdominal surgery has been previously performed.

3. Take diagnostic abdominal x-rays before performing peritoneal lavage (the procedure may produce artifacts on the x-ray, eg, ileus or intraperitoneal air).

Procedure

A. Preparatory Measures:

1. Drain the bladder (by urination or catheterization, as required).

2. Position the patient, and check to see that all equipment is at hand.

3. Sterilize the skin of the anterior abdominal wall from the umbilicus to the symphysis pubica.

4. Drape the operative site.

5. Observe sterile technique (don cap, mask, gloves, and gown).

6. Using the 1% lidocaine with the 5-mL syringe and 25-gauge needle, anesthetize the skin about 2 cm (¾ in) caudal to the umbilicus in the midline. Then, directing the needle perpendicularly to the anterior abdominal wall, infiltrate the fascia (linea alba), preperitoneal space (between peritoneum and fascia), and parietal peritoneum. The needle will encounter resistance when it reaches the peritoneum.

B. Percutaneous Approach:

1. Using the No. 11 blade, make a 0.5-cm (¼-in) transverse incision through the skin and fascia to allow easy passage of the catheter and stylet.

2. Carefully insert the catheter and stylet into the anesthetized tract with gentle, steady, *controlled* pressure. (*Caution:* The abdominal aorta lies in the path of the catheter.) Control is best achieved by making sure that both hands are comfortably placed on the patient's abdomen and by advancing the catheter with steady pressure applied by the thumb and forefinger. Advance the catheter through the peritoneum and into the peritoneal cavity. There will be a definite give ("pop") as the catheter penetrates the peritoneum.

3. Once the catheter has penetrated the peritoneal cavity, slide it off the stylet and into the peritoneal cavity. The catheter should slide easily. If any resistance is encountered, withdraw the catheter and stylet together, and attempt insertion again. Difficulty in advancing the catheter may indicate that the stylet has not entered the peritoneal cavity and that the catheter is being inserted into the space between the peritoneum and the fascia; alternatively, there may be adhesions in the peritoneal cavity that have fixed the intraperitoneal structures. Failure to make this important distinction may result in false-positive or false-negative findings or perforation of intraperitoneal structures.

C. Operative Approach:
With this approach, a superficial laparotomy is performed to permit direct visualization of the peritoneum when the catheter is inserted. The advantage is that inadvertent insertion of the catheter into the preperitoneal space is unlikely to occur; however, more personnel are required to perform the procedure.

1. After the area has been anesthetized, use the No. 11 blade to make a 3-cm (1³⁄₁₆-in) vertical incision in the midline about 1 cm (⅜ in) inferior to the umbilicus.

2. Using the Kelly clamp, bluntly dissect through subcutaneous tissue to the fascia of the abdominal wall. Then incise the fascia for the length of the incision. Again using a Kelly clamp, spread the preperitoneal fat, and expose the parietal peritoneum.

3. Using 2 Allis or Kocher clamps, grasp the peritoneum, and lift it up to free it from any underlying visceral structures. (Grasp a bit of peritoneum with one clamp, grasp another bit with the second clamp about 1–2 cm [⅜–¾ in] away, and release the first clamp. Repeat as needed. This method of alternately grasping and releasing the peritoneum separates it from underlying structures.)

4. Holding the peritoneum up between 2 clamps (Allis or Kocher), make a small stab wound through the peritoneum with a No. 11 scalpel blade.

5. Insert the catheter into the peritoneal cavity under direct vision.

D. Results:
With either approach, gross blood may return after the catheter has been placed and the stylet has been removed. This finding signifies extensive intraperitoneal hemorrhage, and the patient should be prepared for surgery.

1. If blood does not return immediately, connect the intravenous tubing to the catheter, and instill 1 L of sterile Ringer's injection or normal saline (Fig 46–30). Gently massage the abdomen to spread the fluid, and roll the patient from side to side to make sure that the lavage fluid reaches all areas of the peritoneal cavity. Lower the intravenous bottle to the floor. The fluid in the peritoneal cavity should flow out of the cavity and back into the bottle. Again, roll the patient from side to side to return as much fluid as possible to the bottle.

2. After as much of the fluid as possible has been

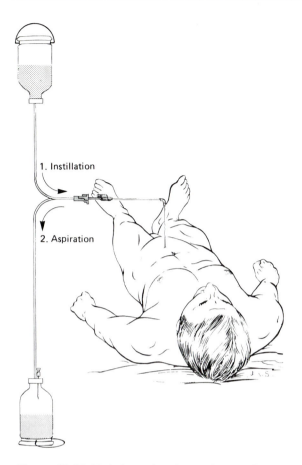

1. Instillation

2. Aspiration

Figure 46–30. Technique of peritoneal lavage. (Reproduced, with permission, from Dunphy JE, Way LW [editors]: *Current Surgical Diagnosis & Treatment,* 5th ed. Lange, 1981.)

removed from the peritoneal cavity (a reasonable return is 75–80% of the fluid instilled), remove the catheter, and close the incision. Use the size 4-0 nylon skin suture if the percutaneous approach was used, and cover it with an adhesive dressing. To close the incision made for the operative approach, close the peritoneum with chromic catgut sutures; close the anterior abdominal fascia with interrupted silk, polypropylene, or nylon sutures; approximate the subcutaneous tissue with absorbable sutures; and close the skin.

If immediate laparotomy is necessary, leave the incision open, and cover it with a sterile dressing that has been soaked in saline.

3. Make sure to record the amount of any excess fluid left in the patient's peritoneal cavity as fluid input on the fluid intake and output computation sheet.

Interpretation

Significant intraperitoneal hemorrhage is indicated by grossly bloody lavage fluid or gross blood coming from the catheter. Lavage fluid with a hematocrit of 1% or higher also indicates significant intraperitoneal hemorrhage and suggests the need for laparotomy. Completely clear fluid indicates lack of significant intraperitoneal bleeding.

INSERTION OF INDWELLING (FOLEY) URINARY CATHETER

Indications

Indications for insertion of an indwelling urinary catheter are as follows:

1. Diagnostic or therapeutic drainage of the urinary bladder.

2. Need for a reliable and frequent assessment of urine output (eg, for treatment of shock).

3. Need to perform retrograde cystography.

Contraindications

The following are only relative contraindications to insertion of an indwelling urinary catheter:

1. Previous urethral surgery.

2. Suspected or known urethral trauma (free-

floating prostate, blood issuing from urethral meatus). In this case, a urethrogram should be performed before urethral catheterization is attempted.

3. Inability to pass a catheter from the meatus up the urethra into the urinary bladder.

Personnel Required

One person can insert an indwelling urinary catheter unaided. An assistant is helpful if the patient is uncooperative.

Equipment & Supplies Required

Note: Most hospitals have disposable Foley insertion trays that contain most of the items listed below except for the catheter. It is important to check to see that the tray contains all of the needed materials and that the catheter, if it is supplied with the set, is of the proper size and desired material and has a balloon of the proper size.

1. Foley catheter of the appropriate size, material, and contour (different catheters are discussed below).

2. Urinary drainage bag and connecting tube.

3. Sterile lubricant.

4. Antiseptic solution and sterile cotton balls to sterilize the male urethral meatus and the female perineum.

5. Sterile syringe, 5- to 10-mL, filled with enough sterile water to inflate the balloon on the catheter. The size of the balloon is usually printed on the catheter (usually 5 mL).

6. Sterile gloves and drapes.

Selecting a Catheter

The Foley catheter is used in almost all cases when an indwelling urinary catheter is required. It consists of a double-lumen rubber tube with a terminal retaining balloon. The larger channel is for drainage of urine, and the smaller is for inflation of the balloon. Some indwelling catheters have a third lumen, for constant bladder irrigation. Foley catheters are of standard length 46 cm (18 in) but come in varying diameters that are numerically graded (French system), with the larger number indicating a larger diameter. Two sizes of balloon are commonly available: 5-mL balloons for routine catheterizations and 30-mL balloons for special situations. Most Foley catheters are made of rubber. Teflon or Silastic is sometimes used for long-term, indwelling catheters. (Specialized shapes and contours are not discussed here, because they should only be inserted by a urologist.)

1. For routine, short-term catheterization in males or females, a 14F or 18F rubber catheter with a 5-mL balloon is satisfactory. Smaller sizes are required for children.

2. Men with prostatic hypertrophy may require larger catheters, eg, 20–22F.

Positioning of the Patient

A. Females: The patient should be in the lithotomy position. If she is comatose or under anesthesia, flex her knees and hips, and allow the legs to abduct. If the soles of the feet are pressed together, this position can easily be held by the patient without assistance.

B. Males: The patient should be supine.

Anatomy Review

A. Females: The female urethra is short, and because there is no prostate gland, passage of a catheter is relatively easy. The only difficulty is locating the urethral meatus, which lies in the superior fornix of

the vulva, above the vaginal opening and below the clitoris. It appears as a small dimple or slit in the midline.

B. Males: The urethra leaves the bladder at the trigone, passes through the prostate, and then runs the length of the penis to exit at the meatus at the tip of the glans.

Procedure

A. Catheterization of Females:

1. Assemble all necessary equipment.

2. Open the catheter tray and selected catheter, and position them on a sterile field placed on a bedside table or stand so that all required materials are readily accessible.

3. Place a generous amount of lubricant on the sterile field.

4. Put on sterile gloves, and drape the perineal area.

5. Make sure that the catheter is open and the lubricating jelly is accessible.

6. Open the antiseptic packet, and moisten the cotton swabs provided with antiseptic.

7. Be sure that the syringe is filled with enough sterile water to inflate the balloon being used.

8. Using the left hand (standing on the patient's right side), spread the labia and identify the superior fornix with the clitoris at the apex. Thoroughly cleanse the entire area with 4–5 swabs soaked in antiseptic. Clean the labia with front to back strokes with 2 successive swabs; then cleanse the urethral meatus with another 2 successive swabs.

9. The left hand continues to hold the labia spread apart for the rest of the procedure.

10. Make a loop in the Foley catheter for easier handling. Grasp the catheter with the right hand, coat the tip and proximal portion with lubricating jelly, and insert the catheter into the urethral meatus, which lies just below the clitoris. Advance the catheter until urine returns. Then advance it 4–5 cm (1⅝–2 in) farther to make sure that the balloon is well within the bladder.

11. Inflate the balloon with the appropriate amount of sterile water (usually 5 mL; the balloon volume is usually printed on the catheter), and withdraw the catheter gently until the balloon is pulled snugly against the trigone (Fig 46–31).

12. Collect a small amount of urine in a sterile container for appropriate studies (urinalysis should be obtained routinely), and then connect the catheter to the urinary drainage bag.

13. Tape the Foley catheter and the urinary drainage tube to the upper thigh, leaving enough slack so that abduction of the legs will not put tension on the catheter.

14. *Note:* The most common mistake in catheterization of the female bladder is to miss the urethral meatus and inadvertently slip the catheter into the vagina. No urine will return. Leave the catheter in place

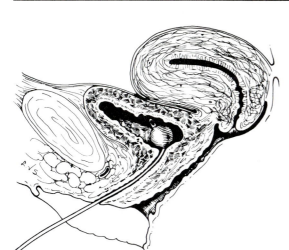

Figure 46–31. Sagittal section of female bladder showing balloon of Foley catheter fitting snugly against the trigone.

in the vagina as a marker. Obtain a new, sterile catheter, and try again. Remove the other catheter.

B. Catheterization of Males:

1–7. Steps 1–7 are the same as those described under Catheterization of Females, above.

8. Using the left hand (standing on the patient's right side), grasp the penis so that the shaft lies in the palm and the glans of the penis is free but secure. The penis should be held at a right angle to the abdomen. The left hand should remain in this position for the remainder of the procedure; it is no longer sterile.

9. Sterilize the glans and urethral meatus with 3–4 swabs dipped in antiseptic.

10. Put a single loop in the Foley catheter for easier handling, grasp the catheter in the right hand, and coat the tip of the catheter with lubricating jelly. It is often helpful to place some on the meatus as well.

11. Insert the catheter into the urethral meatus, and advance it down the penile urethra to the base of the penis with successive, steady movements.

12. Advance the catheter through the membranous and prostatic urethra into the bladder.

13. Advance the catheter to the hilt (even if urine is obtained earlier) to ensure that the balloon is not inflated in the urethra. As soon as the catheter has been advanced to the hilt, release the penis to free both hands for inflation of the balloon.

14. Inflate the balloon with the proper amount of sterile water for its size (usually 5 mL), and withdraw the catheter until the balloon is pulled snugly against the trigone.

15. Obtain a specimen for appropriate tests (at a minimum, routine urinalysis should be performed). Connect the urinary drainage system bag to the catheter, and tape the catheter to the upper thigh, leaving sufficient slack so that movement of the leg will not pull on the catheter.

16. Problem-solving–

a. Males with prostatic enlargement or false urethral passages–Conventional technique usually fails in patients with significant prostatic hypertrophy or false urethral passages. Listed below are a few techniques that have proved successful in catheterizing these patients. *Caution: Reasonable* persistence in attempting catheterization is acceptable; however, there comes a time when further manipulations may rupture the urethra or create new false passages. If attempts using the guidelines outlined below are still unsuccessful, consult a urologist, or insert a suprapubic catheter instead (see below).

(1) Increase the size of the catheter. Large catheters are stiffer and provide more forceful dilatation of the prostatic urethra. The larger, blunt tip tends to follow the true urethra rather than smaller false passages.

(2) Lubricate the urethra with sterile jelly by filling a 30- to 50-mL sterile catheter-tipped syringe with the jelly and injecting the jelly down the urethra with gentle pressure until no more can be injected. Then insert the catheter.

(3) Try injecting sterile lubricating jelly while the catheter is being passed. Fill the syringe as outlined above, insert the tip into the catheter, and fill the catheter with jelly. As the catheter is being passed, slowly inject more lubricant to ensure that the entire length of the catheter is lubricated and to help dilate the urethra just ahead of the catheter tip.

b. Traumatized patients–Most patients with major trauma have a Foley catheter inserted during resuscitation. A rectal examination must be performed before a catheter is inserted in a male patient with major blunt trauma. Feel for the prostrate and make sure that it is firmly attached to the surrounding tissues. A free-floating prostate or gross blood escaping from the urethra signifies urethral rupture until proved otherwise. In either case, Foley catheterization is contraindicated, and a suprapubic catheter should be inserted instead.

PERCUTANEOUS SUPRAPUBIC CYSTOSTOMY

Suprapubic bladder cystostomy is a means of bypassing the urethra to provide drainage of the urinary bladder.

Indications

Suprapubic bladder cystostomy is performed to provide bladder drainage when transurethral drainage is unsuccessful or contraindicated.

Contraindications

Contraindications to suprapubic cystostomy are as follows:
1. Nondistended, nonpalpable bladder.
2. Carcinoma of the bladder, because percutaneous catheterization of the bladder might lead to seeding of the cancer along the track of the catheter.
3. Gross hematuria, which would require a tube of large diameter to drain clots from the bladder.
4. Recent cystostomy (the percutaneous technique might disrupt suture lines).

Personnel Required

One person can perform percutaneous suprapubic cystostomy unaided, although an assistant may be helpful, particularly if the patient is uncooperative.

Equipment & Supplies Required

Many prepackaged commercial kits are available for percutaneous suprapubic cystostomy. The following items are required:
1. Materials for skin sterilization.
2. Materials for sterile technique (cap, mask, gloves, and gown).
3. Lidocaine, 1%, with 10-mL syringe and 25-gauge, 1-cm (½-in) and 22-gauge, 4-cm (1½-in) needles.
4. Sterile towels (4) or sterile paper drapes.
5. Razor.
6. No. 11 scalpel blade, mounted.
7. Catheter-clad needle (eg, Angiocath), 14-gauge, 30-cm (12-in); or needle-clad catheter (eg, Intracath), 14-gauge, 30-cm (12-in); or other commercially manufactured percutaneous suprapubic catheter set.
8. Syringe, 50-mL.
9. Closed urinary drainage system (sterile intravenous tubing and empty intravenous bag or bottle).
10. Silk suture (size 3-0) on a curved cutting needle.
11. Needle holder.
12. Suture scissors.
13. Antibacterial ointment.
14. Sterile gauze sponges, 5 × 5 cm (2 × 2 in), and tape.
15. Rolled bath towel for placement under the hips.

Positioning of the Patient

The patient should be supine, with a rolled-up towel placed under the hips.

Anatomy Review

The urinary bladder lies in the midline of the lower abdomen. When it is distended, its position can be detected by palpation or percussion.

Procedure

1. Locate the distended bladder by palpation, percussion, or ultrasonography. If the bladder cannot be located, percutaneous suprapubic cystostomy should not be performed. If the bladder is not distended, it can usually be filled by oral or intravenous hydration.
2. Prepare the area just above the symphysis pubica by shaving the pubic hair and sterilizing the skin. Extend the sterile field with drapes.
3. Assemble all necessary equipment.
4. Observe sterile technique (don cap, mask, gloves, and gown).
5. Determine the insertion point by measuring cephalad 1–2 cm (⅜–¾ in) from the superior edge of the symphysis pubica in the midline (Fig 46–32).
6. Using the 1% lidocaine with the 10-mL syringe and 25-gauge needle, anesthetize the skin at the point of insertion. Then switch to the 22-gauge needle to anesthetize the subcutaneous tissue and ante-

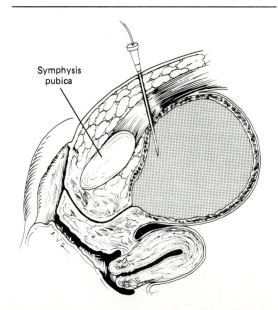

Figure 46–32. Suprapubic cystostomy. Sagittal cross section of distended bladder showing insertion site for catheter.

Symphysis pubica

rior wall of the bladder. If the position of the needle is correct, urine can be aspirated through the needle. Remove the needle.

7. Make a 0.5-cm ($\frac{3}{16}$-in) transverse incision in the skin over the anesthetized area with the No. 11 scalpel blade.

8. Actual placement of the catheter varies with the type of catheter used.

9. Catheter-clad needle–

a. Attach a 50-mL syringe to the 14-gauge, 30-cm (12-in) catheter-clad needle.

b. Insert the catheter unit through the skin incision.

c. Advance the catheter caudally at a 50- to 60-degree angle to the abdominal surface. Advance the catheter with a smooth, deliberate motion, and steady the guiding hands on the patient's abdomen as necessary. A "give" is felt as the catheter and needle penetrate each successive layer of the fascia and bladder wall. Maintaining gentle suction with the syringe will cause aspiration of urine as soon as the bladder cavity has been entered.

d. Once the bladder has been entered, slip the catheter tip off the needle by holding the hub of the needle in the left hand and advancing the catheter with the right.

e. Advance the catheter about 6–8 cm ($2\frac{3}{8}$–$3\frac{1}{8}$ in) to make sure that enough of it is within the bladder.

f. Attach the sterile intravenous tubing to the catheter hub. If no assistant is available, reattach the 50-mL syringe to the tubing to keep the system closed. Otherwise, have an assistant attach the end of the tubing to the empty intravenous bag or bottle that is to receive the urine.

g. Suture the catheter in place at the insertion site with the size 3-0 silk suture. Wind the ends of the suture around the catheter at least 3 times to make sure that it is secured to the abdominal wall.

h. Apply antibacterial ointment to the insertion site, cover it with sterile 5- × 5-cm (2- × 2-in) gauze sponges, and tape the sponges in place.

i. If not done earlier, attach the end of the tubing to the empty intravenous bag or bottle that is to receive the urine.

j. Tape all connections.

10. Needle-clad catheter–Steps **a–c** are the same as for the catheter-clad needle except that the introducing needle is used instead of a catheter-clad needle.

d. When the introducing needle is in the bladder, disconnect the syringe, and pass the catheter through the needle into the bladder. Pass it about 6–8 cm ($2\frac{3}{8}$–$3\frac{1}{8}$ in) through the needle to make sure that enough of the catheter is in the bladder.

e. Withdraw the needle, holding the catheter in place at the hub.

f. Seat the catheter in the hub of the introducing needle, and secure the guard to the end of the needle according to the directions provided with the set being used.

g. Attach the sterile intravenous tubing to the catheter hub, and reattach the 50-mL syringe to the tubing.

h. Secure the catheter, using the size 3-0 silk suture.

i. Apply antibacterial ointment to the insertion site, cover it with sterile 5- × 5-cm (2- ×-2 in) gauze sponges, and tape the sponges in place.

j. Attach the end of the intravenous tubing to the empty intravenous bag or bottle that is to receive the urine.

k. Tape all connections.

11. Percutaneous suprapubic catheter–Follow the manufacturer's instructions for use.

LUMBAR PUNCTURE

Indications

Indications for lumbar puncture are as follows:

1. Need to obtain cerebrospinal fluid for diagnostic tests (suspected meningitis, subarachnoid hemorrhage, etc).

2. Need to administer agents for diagnosis or treatment (eg, amphotericin B).

3. Need to lower cerebrospinal fluid pressure (rarely indicated).

Contraindications

Contraindications to lumbar puncture are as follows:

1. Local infection of the lumbar area. Cervical or cisternal puncture should be performed instead.

2. Suspected intracranial mass lesion (brain abscess, tumor, any posterior fossa lesion, subdural hematoma). Papilledema or focal cerebral defects (excluding ophthalmoplegia) suggest a mass lesion of the central nervous system. CT scan of the head, radionuclide brain scan, or angiography should precede lumbar puncture in these circumstances. However, suspected intracranial mass lesion is a *relative* contraindication only, and if meningitis is strongly suspected and there are only minimal signs suggestive of a mass lesion, lumbar puncture may be performed prior to radiographic procedures so that the need for antimicrobials can be assessed (see Meningitis in Chapter 13).

3. Bleeding diathesis. This is a relative contraindication and should be corrected if time permits.

4. Suspected spinal cord mass lesion, eg, epidural abscess, hematoma, or tumor. Myelography should be performed in consultation with a neurosurgeon to define the lower limit of the spinal block.

Personnel Required

One person can perform lumbar puncture unaided if the patient is cooperative. An assistant can help with positioning of the patient, lighting, handling of samples, etc, and is essential if the patient is uncooperative.

Equipment & Supplies Required

A. Prepackaged sterile disposable lumbar puncture trays are commercially available. If the tray is to be assembled at the hospital, the following items are required:

1. Spinal needles, 20- and 22-gauge (shorter, smaller-gauge needles are required for children).

2. Manometer.

3. Three-way stopcock.

4. Cerebrospinal fluid collection tubes (5).

5. Sponges, 10×10 cm (4×4 in).

6. Lidocaine, 1%, with 5-mL syringe and 22- and 25-gauge needles.

7. Sterile drapes.

8. Adhesive dressing.

9. Materials for skin sterilization.

10. Materials for sterile technique (gloves and mask; cap and gown are optional).

B. Ice bucket for specimens that must be put on ice immediately.

Positioning of the Patient

1. **Lateral decubitus**–Place the patient in the lateral decubitus position lying on the edge of the bed and facing away from the operator. The patient should flex the lumbar spine as much as possible by assuming the fetal position (forehead bent toward knees and knees drawn up to abdomen). The patient's head should rest on a pillow, so that the entire craniospinal axis is parallel to the bed. Positioning is the most crucial aspect of successful lumbar puncture, and the 3 key elements of proper positioning are achieving maximal lumbar flexion (to open the intervertebral spaces), keeping the patient's spine parallel to the bed, and having the line of the patient's shoulders and pelvis be perpendicular to the bed (to facilitate orientation of the needle track). Prevent pelvic rotation by keeping the patient's knees and ankles aligned. An assistant is useful to help the patient maintain the proper position.

2. **Sitting**–The patient sits facing away from the operator and bends over a bedside table to maximize lumbar flexion. This position is useful when cerebrospinal fluid pressure is low (eg, dehydration) or when the patient is obese. Cerebrospinal fluid pressure can be determined by having the patient lie in the decubitus position after the needle is in place.

After the patient has been properly positioned, raise the bed until the patient's lower lumbar spine is at the mid chest level of the operator, who should be seated. Adjust the lighting for optimal effect.

Anatomy Review

Lumbar puncture should enter the subarachnoid space below the level of the conus medullaris, which extends to L1–L2 in most adults and L2–L3 in children. The L3–L4 interspace, the most commonly used site for lumbar puncture, is at the level of the posterior iliac crests (Fig 46–33). The L4–L5 interspace may be preferable, however, since a traumatic spinal tap at this level may leave cerebrospinal fluid obtained at the higher interspace uncontaminated with red blood cells (because of the caudal direction of flow of cerebrospinal fluid).

With the patient properly positioned, find the posterior iliac crest, and palpate the spine at this level for the L3–L4 interspace. Other interspaces are counted

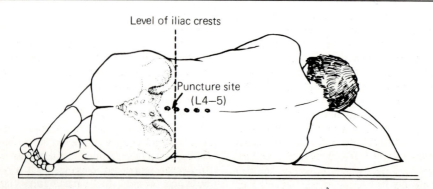

Figure 46–33. Decubitus position for lumbar puncture. (Reproduced, with permission, from Krupp MA et al: *Physician's Handbook,* 21st ed. Lange, 1985.)

from this landmark. The needle should enter the exact midpoint of the interspace between the spinous processes. Mark the point on the patient's skin with the end of a ballpoint pen or the indentation from a fingernail to facilitate locating the landmarks after the skin has been sterilized.

It may be difficult to palpate the spinous processes in obese patients. Using the gluteal cleft to mark the midline, locate the sacral promontory, which is palpable even in obese patients. Move cephalad until the promontory ends, indicating the L5–S1 interspace; the L4–L5 interspace is then easily identified.

Procedure

1. Observe sterile technique (don mask and gloves; cap and gown are optional).

2. Prepare all equipment. Assemble the manometer and stopcock (the channel from the spinal needle to the manometer should be open), open the specimen tubes, and draw up the 1% lidocaine into the 5-mL syringe with the 25-gauge needle.

3. Sterilize the skin in a wide field around the L2–L3 to L4–L5 interspaces.

4. Place a sterile drape under the patient that extends over the edge of the bed. Contamination of gloves may be avoided by folding the edge of the drape back over the gloves, pushing the edge beneath the patient's back, and carefully removing the gloved hands.

5. Place a second sterile drape over the top side of the patient, leaving only sterilized skin between the edges of the drapes. Although a drape with a center hole is preferred by some, it obscures the rest of the spine (a valuable landmark) and makes shifting to another interspace difficult.

6. Locate the puncture site, and anesthetize the skin using the 1% lidocaine in the 5-mL syringe with the 25-gauge needle. Change to the 22-gauge needle before anesthetizing between the spinous processes. Be sure to apply vacuum to the syringe to make sure that the needle has not entered a blood vessel (blood in the syringe).

7. Hold the spinal needle between the index and middle fingers, with the thumb over the stylet. It may be held with 2 hands, if necessary, for stability. Avoid touching the tip and shaft of the needle, since starch granules from the gloves may be introduced into the subarachnoid space and can cause sterile arachnoiditis. The 20-gauge needle is better for transmitting pressure changes in cerebrospinal fluid, but the 22-gauge needle is adequate in most cases; smaller needles should be used in children.

8. Introduce the needle in the midline perpendicular to a line connecting the iliac crests, aiming about 30 degrees rostrally toward the umbilicus. Be sure the long axis of the needle is parallel to the bed and that the plane of the patient's back is perpendicular to the bed. In infants, the entry angle is nearer to the perpendicular, whereas in elderly patients, the angle may approach 45 degrees rostrally to pass beneath the osteophytic lipping of the spinous processes. The bevel of the needle should be facing up (parallel to the spine) if the patient is in the lateral decubitus position, so that the fibers of the dura are split longitudinally.

9. Advance the needle slowly. There will be a "pop" as the needle passes through the ligamentum flavum and the spinal arachnoid membrane. Since the spinal venous plexus is *anterior* to the spinal canal, the chance of a traumatic spinal tap can be minimized by frequent checking of the position of the needle (withdraw the stylet).

10. If the needle hits bone deep in the penetration, withdraw to the ligamentum flavum, and redirect the tip in a more caudal direction. (The needle will follow the same course unless it is drawn back through the ligamentum flavum.) Pain radiating to the leg or buttock is an obvious indication to direct the needle toward the midline and away from the involved side.

11. When cerebrospinal fluid begins to flow from the needle, discard the first few drops. Establish free flow of cerebrospinal fluid—rotating the bevel of the needle may be helpful. Do not aspirate cerebrospinal fluid unless it cannot be obtained by other means, because a nerve root may be trapped against the needle and injured. Replace the stylet halfway in the shaft of the needle to prevent leakage. If the patient is in a seated position and if cerebrospinal fluid pressures are to be obtained, have an assistant help the patient into the decubitus position, taking care not to move the needle.

12. Remove the stylet, and attach the stopcock and the manometer to the needle.

13. If not already done, rotate the stopcock lever to open the channel between the needle and the manometer. Cerebrospinal fluid will rise into the manometer, and the opening cerebrospinal fluid pressure can be measured. Normal pressure is between 70 and 180 mm water. If pressure is elevated, make sure that the patient's position is not causing jugular or abdominal compression. Have the patient slowly relax and uncurl from the fetal position (if in the lateral decubitus position) and then inhale deeply. Cerebrospinal fluid pressure falls with inspiration and rises with expiration. Check pressure changes with the patient's head first flexed and then extended. To detect mass lesions in the spinal canal, look for a block to cerebrospinal fluid that is present only on either extension or flexion. Abnormally low pressures may be caused by dehydration.

14. Remove the manometer, and begin collecting samples of cerebrospinal fluid in the specimen tubes. This is most easily achieved by removing the 3-way stopcock and using the stylet to block flow between samples by replacing the stylet halfway in the shaft of the needle. Three tubes are routinely collected: tube 1 (0.5–1 mL); tube 2 (2–3 mL); and tube 3 (2–4 mL) in adults (smaller amounts are collected in children). Frequently, however, further information is desired, and more samples are collected in the extra tubes (see section on specimen collection, below). If in doubt, collect extra fluid in additional tubes.

15. If a diagnostic or therapeutic injection is necessary, inject the solution slowly over 30 seconds *after* having removed at least an equivalent volume of cerebrospinal fluid as a sample.

16. Replace the manometer, and obtain a closing pressure if spinal subarachnoid block is suspected.

17. Remove the needle, and place a small adhesive bandage over the puncture site.

18. Draw venous blood for determination of glucose concentration. The ratio of blood glucose to cerebrospinal fluid glucose is helpful in the diagnosis of inflammatory disease.

19. Have the patient lie *prone* for at least 2 hours following lumbar puncture in order to avoid lumbar puncture headache.

Special Problems Encountered in Lumbar Puncture

1. Massive obesity–If the patient is obese, landmarks are difficult to locate, and alternative methods for locating the L4–L5 interspace must be used (see Anatomy Review, above). Lumbar puncture with the patient sitting may be tried if attempts fail with the patient in the lateral decubitus position. The sitting position makes the midline easier to locate and increases lumbar flexion. A 12.5-cm (5-in) needle may be required. The patient must be cooperative. Cerebrospinal fluid pressures are not measured in this position, but the patient may be carefully repositioned in the lateral decubitus position after the needle is in place to record cerebrospinal fluid pressures. If lumbar puncture in the sitting position is unsuccessful, a neurosurgeon can use the cervical approach (done at the bedside), or a neuroradiologist can attempt a fluoroscopically guided approach (performed in the radiology department).

2. Osteoarthritis–As the body ages, desiccation of the nucleus pulposus of the intervertebral disk occurs, with subsequent narrowing of the disk space. This change, together with osteophytic "lipping" of the spinous process and calcification of the interspinous ligament and ligamentum flavum, combines to make lumbar puncture difficult. A larger-gauge needle (eg, 18- to 19-gauge) facilitates passage through calcified posterior ligaments. It may occasionally be necessary to resort to an oblique approach performed by a radiologist using fluoroscopy.

3. Previous lumbar surgery–Lumbosacral spine films assist in defining the extent of surgery and fusion. If all of the posterior approaches are unavailable for lumbar puncture, obtain neurologic or neurosurgical consultation.

4. Inadvertent arterial puncture–If arterial blood is obtained during lumbar puncture, completely withdraw the needle. Obtain a fresh spinal needle for the next attempt, since clotted blood makes replacement of the stylet difficult and also contaminates the sample. If the patient has an underlying coagulopathy, it should be corrected and the patient observed for signs of compressive spinal epidural or subdural hematoma (Chapter 10).

5. High opening pressure–If high cerebrospinal pressures are suspected before lumbar puncture is performed, use the smallest needle possible. Collect the *minimum* amount of fluid necessary (usually that in the manometer is sufficient), and withdraw the needle. Watch the patient carefully for signs of impending herniation, and treat accordingly (Chapter 10). Obtain a closing cerebrospinal fluid pressure; remove only as much fluid as causes the initial pressure to drop by one-half. A rapid drop in cerebrospinal fluid pressure to low levels with removal of only a small amount of fluid may be an ominous sign indicating impending herniation. Obtain urgent neurosurgical consultation.

6. Hypotension–Cerebrospinal fluid pressure is proportionate to venous pressure and PCO_2. Severe hypotension may decrease the volume of the subarachnoid space and make it difficult to penetrate. Slowly advance the needle, and each time the stylet is removed, attach a tuberculin syringe with a small air bubble in the hub, relying on the negative pressure in the epidural space to help define location (the bubble is sucked into the needle when the needle is in the epidural rather than the arachnoid space). Advancing the needle a few millimeters will place the tip within the subarachnoid space, permitting aspiration of cerebrospinal fluid.

The sitting position may be helpful in the patient with severe hypotension, provided that arterial blood pressure is sufficient to enable the patient to tolerate the upright position. The sitting position takes advantage of gravity to help raise cerebrospinal fluid pressure in the lumbar space.

7. Post—lumbar puncture headache–Headache following lumbar puncture can usually be avoided by using small-gauge needles and having the patient lie *prone* for at least 2 hours after the procedure. Post–lumbar puncture headache responds to nonnarcotic analgesics and bed rest. Some authorities recommend vigorous oral hydration, although supportive data are scant. Headache may rarely require potent analgesics.

8. Bloody cerebrospinal fluid–Features that point to a traumatic spinal tap rather than to subarachnoid hemorrhage include (**1**) normal cerebrospinal fluid pressure; (**2**) absence of xanthochromia after centrifugation; (**3**) bloody sample followed by clearer samples or bloodier samples; (**4**) white cell count proportionate to red cell count (700–1000 red blood cells per white blood cell; 1 mg/dL of protein per 1000 red blood cells); (**5**) changing red cell count in successive tubes; or (**6**) clot formation (rare). Repeat lumbar puncture at a higher interspace yields cerebrospinal fluid that is usually clear if the fluid was bloody owing to traumatic tap at a lower level. The presence or absence of crenated red cells is of no diagnostic value.

Specimens

At a minimum, collect 3 tubes: tube 1 (0.5–1 mL) for cell count, tube 2 (2–3 mL) for culture, and tube 3 for protein and glucose determinations and for chemistry studies (2–4 mL). Most authorities recommend another 0.5 mL for a VDRL study. There is no harm in collecting extra tubes, since a variety of other diagnostic tests may be indicated. If the specimen is bloody, perform comparison counts in tubes 1 and 3.

Cerebrospinal fluid should be clear and colorless. A tube containing at least 1 mL of cerebrospinal fluid should be examined down the long axis of the tube and compared to water in a similar tube. Turbidity of cerebrospinal fluid appears when there are about 400 cells/μL, but pleocytosis as low as 50 cells can be detected by making use of the Tyndall effect (the scattering of light by particles suspended in liquid). The tube is held in front of a dark background at right angles to a source of direct intense light (eg, the sun), and flicked at the bottom with a finger from the other hand. Appearance of a "snowy" flurry of sparkles indicates pleocytosis.

Table 46–2. Pigmentation of the cerebrospinal fluid following hemorrhage.

	Appearance	Maximum	Disappearance
Oxyhemoglo-bin (pink)	½–4 hours	24–35 hours	7–10 days
Bilirubin (yellow)	8–12 hours	2–4 days	2–3 weeks

In suspected subarachnoid hemorrhage, the supernatant in the tube should be examined for xanthochromia. Centrifuge 2–3 mL of cerebrospinal fluid at 1000 rpm for 5 minutes in a clinical centrifuge, and then examine the supernatant for the characteristic yellowish pigmentation of oxyhemoglobin and bilirubin. Xanthochromia does not appear until about 2–4 hours after hemorrhage, reaches a maximum around 36–48 hours, and may persist 2–4 weeks (Table 46–2). Jaundice, hypercarotenemia, and elevated cerebrospinal fluid protein (> 150 mg/dL) may also cause xanthochromic spinal fluid. Xanthochromia does not occur in the supernatant after a traumatic spinal tap, since the bloody cerebrospinal fluid is not exposed to the enzyme in the subarachnoid space that converts hemoglobin to bilirubin.

ANTERIOR & POSTERIOR NASAL PACKING FOR CONTROL OF EPISTAXIS

Bleeding from the anterior or posterior nasal passages is a commonly encountered emergency. The patient may present with bleeding ranging from mild epistaxis that is easily controlled by local pressure to exsanguinating hemorrhage causing hemorrhagic shock.

Successful treatment of epistaxis requires careful identification of the bleeding source. To accomplish this, proper positioning of the patient, proper instruments, and a bright, hand-directed light source are a necessity.

Bleeding in the anterior nares occurs most commonly in children and can be controlled by local measures such as direct pressure or cautery. Bleeding in adults usually occurs more posteriorly in the anterior nares and often requires anterior nasal packing; epistaxis in the elderly often requires both anterior and posterior nasal packing because the site of bleeding is in the posterior nares.

Indications

Nasal packing (Fig 46–34) is performed to control hemorrhage that cannot be controlled by local measures.

Contraindications

The patient's ability or inability to cooperate during the procedure is the only limiting factor in performing nasal packing. Occasionally, direct control of the bleeding site under general anesthesia in the operating room is required.

Personnel Required

One person can perform nasal packing unaided, although it is helpful to have an assistant to position the patient and handle instruments.

Equipment & Supplies Required
A. Anterior Packing:
1. Cocaine solution, 4% (10 mL).
2. Lidocaine, 1%, with epinephrine (10 mL).
3. Syringe, 5-mL, with 25-gauge needle.
4. Cotton-tipped swabs.
5. Silver nitrate–tipped sticks for coagulation.
6. Portable electrocautery device.
7. Nasal speculum.
8. Headlamp, or reflective eye mirror with suitable light source.
9. Continuous suction device with nasal suction tips.

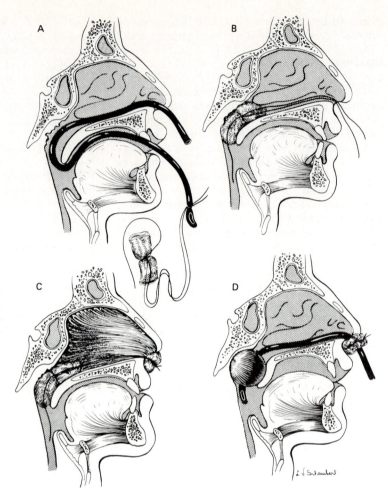

Figure 46–34. Packing to control bleeding from the posterior nose. **A:** Catheter inserted and pack attached. **B:** Pack drawn into position as catheter is removed. **C:** Strip tied over a bolster to hold pack in place with anterior pack installed "accordion pleating" style. **D:** Alternative method using balloon catheter instead of gauze pack. Anterior packing should follow placement of all posterior packs. (Reproduced, with permission, from Way LW [editor]: *Current Surgical Diagnosis & Treatment,* 9th ed. Appleton & Lange, 1991.)

10. Petrolatum-impregnated gauze packing (continuous strip).

11. Nasal packing forceps.

12. Cotton pledgets.

B. Posterior Nasal Packing: All of the equipment listed for anterior nasal packing is also required for posterior nasal packing. Additional equipment includes the following:

1. Occluding balloon catheters (specially designed for tamponade of the bleeding site) (2).

2. Absorbent cotton (4 × 5 cm [1⅝ × 2 in]), with 3 pieces of size 0 silk suture material tied around the middle (alternative to balloon catheterization).

3. No. 12 or No. 14 red rubber catheter.

4. Scissors.

5. Kelly clamp.

Positioning of the Patient

The patient should be either seated in an ENT chair or lying on a gurney with a backrest in the full upright position. The patient's head should also be supported.

Anatomy Review

Bleeding from the anterior nares most commonly occurs in Kiesselbach's area, located anteriorly along the nasal septum (see Fig 26–1). Bleeding that occurs more posteriorly in the anterior nares (a common occurrence in adults) may originate in the nasal turbinates. Posterior epistaxis usually occurs in elderly patients with calcified arteriosclerotic vessels which are refractory to the normal vasospastic control mechanism in response to bleeding and which may therefore bleed briskly. These posterior vessels are not accessible in a routine nasal examination, and control of epistaxis therefore requires tamponade with a balloon or pack.

Procedure

A. Anterior Nasal Pack:

1. Assemble and arrange all necessary equipment so that it is within easy reach.

2. Position the patient as described above, and make sure that the patient is comfortable but well supported and immobile.

3. Make sure that suction and adequate lighting are available.

4. While the operator is arranging equipment, an assistant can pinch the nose to stop bleeding from the septum.

5. Spread the patient's nostrils apart using the nasal speculum, and remove all blood with the suction device. Check the anterior septum for bleeding. Then examine the turbinates and the oropharynx to determine whether bleeding is occurring posteriorly.

6. If an anterior bleeding vessel is identified, eg, vessel in Kiesselbach's area, bleeding can be controlled in one of 3 ways.

a. Local vasoconstriction–Saturate cotton pledgets with the 4% cocaine, place one in each nostril, and have an assistant or the patient firmly pinch the nostrils together for 5 minutes. The cocaine will shrink the nasal mucosa and cause vasoconstriction, which, along with the pressure, often controls bleeding.

b. Silver nitrate—tipped sticks–After the bleeding site has been identified, cauterize the bleeding vessels using silver nitrate–tipped applicators. It is important to localize the site of cauterization precisely over the bleeding site. Overzealous cauterization of large areas of the nasal septum may cause septal necrosis with perforation.

c. Electrocautery–A single anterior bleeding vessel may also be cauterized using an electrocautery device. Exercise the same discretion that is required with chemical cautery.

7. Bleeding that is occurring more posteriorly in the anterior nasal passage, which cannot be controlled by local measures, requires anterior nasal packing. Using nasal forceps, pack the petrolatum-impregnated gauze in successive, tightly packed layers (accordion pleating), starting in the most posterior part of the accessible portion of the nose and working anteriorly. Insert only a small quantity of gauze at a time to ensure that the anterior naris is completely packed.

8. After the entire anterior nasal passage has been packed, check the oropharynx to see if bleeding is continuing posteriorly; if it is, insertion of a posterior pack is indicated (the anterior pack will have to be removed before this can be done). The anterior pack must then be replaced after posterior packing is completed.

B. Posterior Nasal Pack:

1. Sedate the patient (for adults, diazepam, 10 mg orally; or morphine, 5–10 mg intramuscularly).

2. Anesthetize the anterior nose with cocaine-saturated cotton pledgets before inserting the posterior nasal pack using either of the methods outlined below.

a. Balloon occlusion technique–

(1) Balloon catheters made specifically to pack the posterior nasopharynx are available commercially. They work on the same principle as a Foley catheter, with an air inflation port to inflate the balloon.

(2) The balloon-tipped distal end is inserted through the anterior naris into the posterior naris by guiding it directly posteriorly with gentle, steady pressure. After the catheter enters the posterior naris, inflate the balloon with the appropriate amount of air (the amount is printed on the balloon). Exert traction on the catheter to pull the balloon snugly up against the posterior nasal chamber, and secure the catheter at the external naris with gauze packing tied around the tube. Some nasal catheters have a small proximal balloon which, when inflated, will serve the same function as the gauze packing—to maintain tension on the distal intranasal balloon.

(3) After inserting the balloon catheter, check the anterior naris for coexisting anterior bleeding and the oropharynx to determine if posterior bleeding is continuing. If bleeding is occurring from both sides, a second balloon catheter may be placed. Insert an anterior nasal pack.

b. Gauze technique–

(1) If a balloon catheter is not available, posterior packing can be accomplished using a 4- × 5-cm (1⅝- × 2-in) piece of absorbent cotton or gauze. Tie the gauze around the middle with 3 strands of size 0 silk suture material. Two of the strands will be passed through the nasal passage and tied at the anterior naris. The third strand will be cut and allowed to hang down in the throat to facilitate removal of the pack after bleeding has been controlled.

(2) Pass the No. 12 rubber catheter through the external naris until the catheter is visible in the patient's throat.

(3) Using a Kelly clamp, grasp the end of the catheter in the throat, and bring it out through the patient's mouth (Fig 46–34A).

(4) Take the 2 ends of the size 0 silk suture material securing the gauze pack and tie them to the catheter.

(5) Pull the other end of the catheter through the patient's nose so that the sutures follow as the pack passes from the mouth to the posterior nasopharynx. This maneuver helps the pack fit snugly in the posterior nostril.

(6) Repeat the process for the other nostril. Tie the 4 silk strands (2 from each nostril) across a gauze sponge placed under the nose to prevent pressure on the nares from the septum.

(7) After the posterior packs are in place, pack the anterior nares, and check the oropharynx again to make sure that hemorrhage is controlled.

(8) In patients with preexisting cardiac or respiratory disease, draw blood for arterial blood gas determinations, since a significant fall in PO_2 may be seen.

All patients with posterior nasal packs should be hospitalized for monitoring of the airway. If the external gauze wrapping around the catheter slips, the balloon may be displaced posteriorly into the hypopharynx and may obstruct the airway. Antimicrobial prophylaxis (to prevent sinusitis) is recommended by many authorities, although its benefit is unproved. Give ampicillin, 150 mg/kg/d intravenously in 4–6 divided doses.

ARTHROCENTESIS
(Knee, Shoulder, Elbow, Ankle, Wrist, Hand, & Foot Joints)

The major peripheral joints can all be aspirated safely in the emergency department. Aspiration of the hip and other joints of the axial skeleton usually requires the aid of specialists (orthopedic surgeons or rheumatologists) and the use of ancillary techniques (fluoroscopy and radionuclide scans), and it will not be discussed here.

Indications

Indications for arthrocentesis are as follows:
1. Need to obtain synovial fluid for diagnosis.
2. Drainage of hemarthrosis when conservative management is unsuccessful.
3. Instillation of local analgesic and anti-inflammatory agents into a joint.

Contraindications

Contraindications to arthrocentesis are as follows:
1. Soft tissue infection overlying proposed site of aspiration.
2. Uncooperative patient (relative contraindication).
3. Severe bleeding diathesis or anticoagulant therapy.

Personnel Required

One person can perform arthrocentesis unaided if the patient is cooperative, although an assistant is helpful for handling samples and holding young children.

Equipment & Supplies Required

1. Materials for skin sterilization.
2. Materials for sterile technique (mask and gloves; cap and gown are optional).
3. Lidocaine, 1%, with 10-mL syringe and 22-gauge needle.
4. Needles: 25-gauge, 1.5-cm (⅝-in) (2); 22-gauge, 4-cm (1½-in) (2); 20-gauge, 4-cm (1½-in) (2); 27-gauge, 1.5-cm (½-in) (1). Select a needle size appropriate to the joint to be aspirated.
5. Syringes: 10-mL (2), 2-mL (2), 30-mL (1).
6. Sterile gloves.
7. Drapes.
8. Gauze pads, 10×10 cm (4×4 in) (2); 5×5 cm (2×2 in) (2).
9. Adhesive dressing.
10. Sterile capped specimen tubes (2–3).
11. Containers for synovial fluid: purple-topped or green-topped (EDTA or heparin anticoagulant, respectively, for cell count and differential and examination for crystals) (2); gray-topped (fluoride

inhibitor for glucose) (1); red-topped (no anticoagulant) (3).
12. Clean glass microscope slides and coverslips.

Positioning of the Patient

See Procedure for Specific Joints, below.

Procedure

1. Stabilize the joint to be aspirated. Identify landmarks, and mark the entry point with a scratch or indentation on the skin.
2. Sterilize the skin in a wide field around the puncture site.
3. Assemble all necessary equipment.
4. Observe sterile technique (don mask and gloves; cap and gown are optional).
5. Anesthetize the skin with the 1% lidocaine with the 10-mL syringe and 22- to 27-gauge needle; continue down to the joint capsule.
6. Select an appropriate needle (usually 20-gauge for knee, shoulder, elbow, ankle, or wrist; 25- or 27-gauge for small hand joints) and syringe (10-mL for knee, shoulder, elbow, ankle, or wrist; 2-mL for hand joints). A large-bore needle (eg, 18-gauge) may be required for aspiration of pus in larger joints. Use the 30-mL syringe for large effusions.
7. Penetrate the skin at the selected site, and cautiously advance the needle into the joint space; a "pop" will be felt when the needle passes through the synovium into the joint space. Aspirate continuously. Stop advancing the needle when joint fluid flows freely into the syringe.
8. Remove as much fluid as possible, but do not drain the joint dry if synovial biopsy is planned.
9. If joint fluid fails to flow freely, bring the needle all the way back to the subcutaneous tissue before redirecting it, in order to avoid joint trauma that might occur with deep probing.
10. After samples of fluid have been obtained, withdraw the needle, and apply firm pressure over the site for 1–2 minutes.
11. Cover the site with an adhesive dressing.

Procedure for Specific Joints

1. **Knee**—The joint space of the knee may be entered either medially or laterally (Fig 46–35). In either case, the leg should be fully extended, with the patient supine. Pressure on the opposite side of the joint will make the synovium bulge more prominently and assist in directing the needle.

From the lateral aspect, the entrance site is at the intersection of lines extended from the upper and lateral margins of the patella. A 22-gauge, 4-cm (1½-

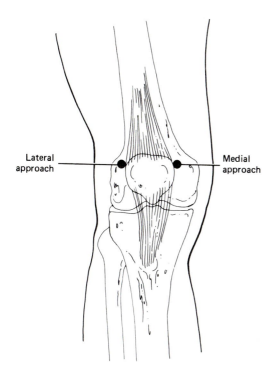

Figure 46–35. Aspiration of the knee joint.

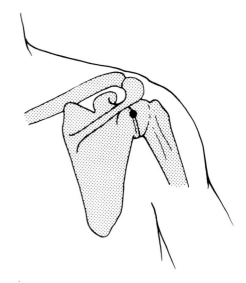

Figure 46–36. Posterior approach to shoulder joint aspiration.

in) needle held parallel to the bed is directed medially and just deep to the patella and into the suprapatellar space.

From the medial aspect, the needle is introduced anteromedially in the space between the patella and the medial condyle. The needle (held parallel to the bed) is advanced upward (toward the undersurface of the patella) and laterally, beneath the patella and into the joint space.

2. Shoulder–The shoulder joint can be aspirated from either an anterior or a posterior approach. The latter has the advantage of being out of the patient's line of vision.

For the posterior approach, the patient should sit in a chair and face backward (chest against the back of the chair). To open up the joint space and facilitate entry of the needle, the patient should put the arm of the side to be aspirated up against the chest and touch the opposite shoulder. This will adduct and internally rotate the arm. The head of the humerus is palpable posterolaterally. Use a 20- or 22-gauge, 4-cm (1½-in) needle, and keep it parallel to the floor. Direct it about 30 degrees medially into the joint space from a point just under the posterior inferior border of the acromion (Fig 46–36).

For the anterior approach, the patient should sit in a chair, facing forward, with the arm comfortably supported in the lap. Using a 20- or 22-gauge, 4-cm (1½-in) needle, enter the joint space at a spot medial to the head of the humerus and just below the palpa-

ble tip of the coracoid process (Fig 46–37). Direct the needle slightly laterally and superiorly into the scapulohumeral joint space.

3. Elbow–Be certain to differentiate olecranon bursitis that does not involve the elbow joint from bulging synovium.

Have the patient sit with the forearm supported from the elbow to the hand on a table, with the elbow joint in about 10–30 degrees of flexion. With significant effusion, the bulging synovium should be evi-

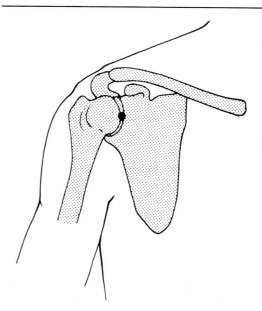

Figure 46–37. Anterior approach to shoulder joint aspiration.

dent laterally. Introduce the needle (usually a 20- or 22-gauge, 4-cm [1½-in] needle) just below the lateral epicondyle and proximal to the olecranon process of the radius (Fig 46–38). Advance the needle medially and slightly proximally into the joint space.

4. Ankle–Arthrocentesis of the ankle is more difficult than that of the other joints discussed here. The most common approach is anteromedial. Have the patient lie supine, with the knee extended and the foot slightly plantar-flexed. Identify the extensor hallucis longus tendon by having the patient extend the great toe. Just anterior (1 cm [≃⅜ in]) and inferior (1 cm [≃⅜ in]) to the medial malleolus and lateral to the extensor tendon is a small depression. Introduce the needle in this depression, and direct it toward the tibiotalar articulation (Fig 46–39). If swelling and pain are most severe on the *side* of the ankle, use a similar approach but from the anterolateral aspect of the joint. When subtalar disease is suspected (eg, pain on pronation and supination of the foot), the needle is introduced more distally, at the talonavicular articulation. Although fluid is seldom obtained at the talonavicular joint, injection of anti-inflammatory agents may be readily accomplished.

5. Wrist–A bulging, inflamed joint space at the wrist can be entered dorsally at prominent areas of swelling; such areas are invariably found on the radial or ulnar aspects. Use a 20- or 22-gauge, 4-cm (1½-in) needle.

For the radial (lateral) entry, position the hand with the palmar surface down, and flex it over a rolled towel at the wrist. Aspirate the joint at the midpoint of the distal articulation of the radius, just medial to the extensor tendon of the thumb. The needle should be perpendicular to the skin during aspiration.

The ulnar, or medial, approach is made in the middle of the palpable depression between the lateral as-

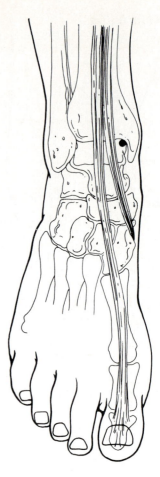

Figure 46–39. Determination of the needle entry site for ankle joint aspiration. A small depression can be palpated about 1 cm (½ in) anterior and inferior to the medial maleolus and lateral to the extensor hallucis longus.

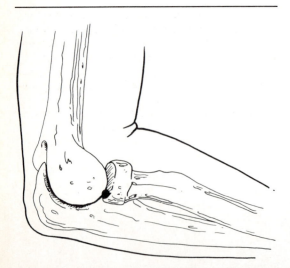

Figure 46–38. Aspiration of the elbow joint.

pect of the tip of the ulna and carpus. Position the hand as for a radial approach. Direct the needle ventrally toward the palmar surface and proximally into the joint space.

To administer corticosteroids into the carpal tunnel (to treat compression of the median nerve), place the needle between flexor creases of the wrist just lateral to the palmaris longus tendon (or medial to the flexor carpi radialis), and advance it distally until resistance to injection is minimal. (See Chapter 23 for details.)

6. Small joints of the hands and feet–Systemic arthritides frequently involve the proximal and distal interphalangeal joints and the first metatarsophalangeal joint. Enter the joint in the midline on the dorsolateral aspect, and gently work a 25- or 27-gauge needle into the joint space. A 2-mL syringe suffices for aspiration and is easier to handle than larger ones. Maintain a slight vacuum in the syringe, so that any trauma to digital vessels will be recognized immediately (blood will appear in the syringe).

Synovial Fluid Analysis

If minimal fluid is available, priorities must be established for processing the sample. If pyogenic arthritis is a diagnostic possibility, an appropriate approach would be to place one drop of fluid on a microscope slide for Gram's stain, another into a hemacytometer for cell count, and the remainder of the sample for culture. If 10–20 mL or more of synovial fluid is obtained, complete synovianalysis can be performed, as outlined below; partial analysis is possible on even as little as 1 mL of fluid.

A. Physical Characteristics:

1. Determine the total volume of fluid removed.

2. Assess color and clarity of fluid (normally a crystal-clear yellowish fluid through which print can be easily read).

3. Note viscosity by allowing a drop to fall from the needle. Normal joint fluid has high viscosity and easily forms a cord several inches long.

4. Perform the mucin clot test (Ropes test) by adding 1 mL of synovial fluid to diluted acetic acid (about 5%). Normally, the mucin in the fluid congeals within minutes, forming a gel (commonly called a clot) that remains firm for hours. In the case of infection or chronic inflammation, unstable gel forms that is easily broken up by gentle agitation. Examine the gel again at 1 hour for friability; normal mucin gel should be unchanged after 1 hour.

B. Laboratory Studies: The choice of studies is guided by clinical circumstances. Gram's stain and culture, cell count, and examination for crystal formation should always be performed when fluid from an acutely inflamed joint is being evaluated.

1. Cell count and differential–Place 2–10 mL of synovial fluid in a purple-topped (EDTA anticoagulant) or green-topped (heparin anticoagulant) tube for laboratory examination. If fluid is scanty, use 1–2 drops counterstained with methylene blue, and perform a cell count in the emergency department with a hemacytometer. Normal synovial fluid contains fewer than 200 white cells per microliter, of which less than 25% are PMNs.

2. Special stains–All joint fluid should be stained with Gram's stain and examined by microscopy. Special stains for fungi and acid-fast bacilli should also be performed when chronic monarticular arthritis is being evaluated. It should be noted, however, that these are specific but not sensitive for detection of fungal or mycobacterial arthritis.

3. Examination for crystals–Place a drop of synovial fluid on a clean glass microscope slide under a coverslip. Examine the specimen immediately; if this is impossible, slow the evaporation of joint fluid by sealing the edges of the coverslip with nail polish or petrolatum. Crystals can be detected using light microscopy and tentatively identified on the basis of morphologic characteristics seen at × 400 magnification. Urate crystals are needle-shaped; calcium pyrophosphate crystals are more rhomboid-shaped; and cholesterol crystals are flat, with notched corners. Polarized light microscopy demonstrates the negative birefringence of urate crystals and the positive birefringence of calcium pyrophosphate. The presence of crystals both free in fluid and within leukocytes is pathognomonic of crystal-induced arthropathy. If the laboratory is doing the examination, collect 1–2 mL of fluid in a purple-topped (EDTA anticoagulant) or green-topped (heparin anticoagulant) tube.

4. Culture–Sterile capped specimen tubes should be filled with 1–10 mL of fluid for bacterial cultures and, if indicated, mycobacterial and fungal cultures as well. In suspected gonococcal disease, chocolate agar should be inoculated with some of the fluid (in the emergency department if possible). When a potentially infected prosthetic joint is being evaluated, a jar of anaerobic transport media should also be inoculated.

5. Glucose determination–Place 0.5–1 mL of synovial fluid in a gray-topped (fluoride anticoagulant) tube. The sample must be compared with a simultaneously drawn blood sample. Blood glucose that is more than 40 mg/dL higher than synovial fluid glucose suggests infection.

6. Protein–Place 0.5–1 mL of synovial joint fluid in a red-topped (no anticoagulant) tube. Determine the total serum protein of a simultaneously drawn blood sample. Normal joint protein is about one-third that of serum.

Less commonly indicated studies include cytology studies in possible pigmented villonodular synovitis or metastatic disease (5–10 mL in a lightly heparinized specimen tube), pH determinations (1–2 mL in a sealed heparinized syringe), complement levels, and tests for rheumatoid factor, antinuclear antibody, immunoglobulins, and various enzymes.

The presence of fat globules (often with blood) is suggestive of intra-articular fracture.

INCISION & DRAINAGE OF SUPERFICIAL ABSCESS

Indications
A superficial abscess is incised in order to drain it.

Contraindications
There are no contraindications to incision and drainage of a superficial abscess.

Personnel Required
One person can usually incise and drain a superficial abscess unaided, although an assistant may be helpful to restrain an uncooperative patient.

Equipment & Supplies Required
Many incision and drainage kits are commercially available. The following items are required:
1. Materials for skin cleansing.
2. Protective gown or apron and gloves.
3. No. 11 surgical blade, mounted.
4. Drapes.
5. Curved Kelly and mosquito clamps.
6. Forceps.
7. Packing material, such as gauze strip packing.
8. Sterile gauze sponges, 10×10 cm (4×4 in), and tape.
9. Ethyl chloride skin-freezing solution (optional).
10. Lidocaine, 1%, with 25-gauge needle and 5-mL syringe.
11. Culture tube and slides.
12. Sterile saline for irrigation.
13. Irrigating syringe and basin.
14. Needle, 18-gauge, with 5-mL syringe.
15. Plastic-coated absorbent pad.

Positioning of the Patient
The patient should be lying on a firm surface in a comfortable position, with the area to be drained in full view and firmly supported.

Procedure
Anesthesia is the main difficulty in incision and drainage. Superficial abscesses suitable for drainage at the bedside are painful, and the patient should be assured that pain will decrease after the pressure is relieved and the pus is drained. Incising the skin and draining the pus are painful, however, and little relief can be obtained short of general or block anesthesia, both of which require an anesthesiologist and an operating room. Spraying the area with ethyl chloride to freeze the skin will prevent some but not all pain. Infiltrating the thin layer of skin over the pointing abscess with lidocaine is impossible, and injecting lidocaine into the abscess cavity is ineffective and may create more pain from increased pressure. Narcotic analgesics (eg, morphine, 2–10 mg intramuscularly or subcutaneously) may take the edge off the pain and relieve some of the patient's anxiety, but they will not provide total relief.

If an abscess is too large to be adequately drained at the bedside or if it appears that the patient may experience too much pain to be able to cooperate effectively, incision and drainage in the operating room is always an alternative.

A. Simple Abscess Not Involving a Vital Structure:
1. Assemble the necessary equipment, and arrange it on a table or bedside stand.
2. Position the patient. Place the plastic-coated absorbent pad under the body part with the abscess to be drained.
3. Don sterile gloves and put on a gown to protect clothing. Cleanse the skin over the area being drained. Drape the area, and have extra absorbent materials ready to catch any pus not absorbed by the drape.
4. If there is any doubt whether an abscess is actually present, take the 18-gauge needle and the 5-mL syringe, and aspirate the suspected abscess at the point of maximum fluctuance. If no pus is found, reassess the clinical situation, and proceed with incision and drainage if it is deemed appropriate.
5. If ethyl chloride or lidocaine is being used, it should be given at this time.
6. Using the No. 11 blade, open the abscess at the point of maximum fluctuance, and allow the pus to drain under its own pressure. Using a quick, decisive motion minimizes the patient's discomfort. Collect the first portion of pus for Gram's stain and culture and sensitivity testing.
7. After the pressure has been relieved, insert the Kelly or mosquito clamp and find the longest axis of the abscess. Point the curve of the clamp up at the farthest point from the central incision and determine the shortest possible length to be incised so that the abscess is completely drained. Incise the skin to that point, using one swift upward motion of the No. 11 blade. If it is necessary to make a long incision to completely drain the abscess, infiltrate the skin in the most lateral aspect with lidocaine. Repeat the procedure in the opposite direction. Allow any further pus to drain. *Note:* It is important to obtain an opening in the abscess wide enough to allow complete drainage of all pus. If the abscess is not opened completely, complete drainage cannot occur, and resolution of the abscess will be delayed.
8. Using the clamp, break up any loculated pus in the cavity.
9. Irrigate the abscess with saline until all pus is removed.

10. Pack the abscess cavity with iodoform or plain gauze packing. Fill the cavity tightly enough to cause hemostasis but not so tightly that it causes pain.

11. Dress the area with the sterile 10- × 10-cm (4- × 4-in) sponge and tape. On the extremities or in areas where there is movement, consider dressing the site with an expanded bandage around the extremity.

12. Begin antimicrobial therapy, if indicated (facial abscesses, cellulitis, etc). Dicloxacillin, 20 mg/kg/d orally in 4 divided doses, is usually satisfactory.

13. Schedule a follow-up appointment in 1–2 days.

B. Incision and Drainage of Abscesses Over Special Areas:

1. Face, head, and neck abscesses–The clinical situation in these anatomic areas must be carefully considered before incision and drainage is performed, because the large scar left by complete incision and drainage may be cosmetically unacceptable and because of the possibility of injuring vital structures beneath the skin. In small superficial abscesses on the face, drainage can be accomplished by making a small incision at the lower part of the abscess, removing all pus, and leaving a gauze wick in the incision to keep the wound from closing. Frequent irrigation will be needed during follow-up to keep the cavity clean and promote healing. Any abscess which is large or which might involve vital structures should be drained in the operating room by personnel experienced in this procedure.

2. Abscesses around joints–Make sure that the abscess does not involve the joint space. (Consult an orthopedic surgeon if there is any doubt.) If the abscess is superficial and does not involve the joint space, proceed with incision and drainage. Remember that splinting of the joint is necessary for adequate healing.

3. Abscesses around the anus–Differentiate pilonidal abscesses from perianal abscesses caused by anal fistulas. Both kinds of abscesses require surgical consultation and possibly drainage in the operating room.

4. Abscesses of the hands, wrists, ankles, and feet–The compact arrangement of many vital structures in the hand, wrist, ankle, and foot makes drainage of abscesses in these areas difficult to perform in the emergency department. It is recommended that any abscess around these structures be drained in the operating room by experienced personnel. Surgical consultation is advisable in all cases of abscesses in these areas.

TRANSCUTANEOUS CARDIAC PACING*

Transcutaneous cardiac pacing is a safe, rapid, noninvasive method of temporarily treating symptomatic bradyarrhythmias and asystole. Recent advances in technology have led to the development of several commercially available devices that are portable and easy to use. With these devices, transcutaneous pacing can be initiated in the prehospital setting or in the emergency department and is the procedure of choice in the treatment of asystole and bradycardic cardiac arrest.

Indications

1. Asystole.

2. Symptomatic bradycardia (< 40 beats/min) unresponsive to atropine.

3. Overdrive pacing for tachyarrhythmias (atrial, ventricular, torsade de pointes) unresponsive to medical and electrical cardioversion.

4. Transvenous pacing is difficult or contraindicated (eg, heart block in myocardial infarction patients treated with thrombolytic therapy).

Complications

The main complications to transcutaneous pacing are pain and local skin erythema due to first-degree burns. With the newer devices, pain from cutaneous nerve and muscle stimulation is now reported as tolerable. The energy levels used for pacing have not been shown to produce any significant myocardial damage. Other persons coming into contact with the pacing impulses may experience mild tingling. The risk of inducing ventricular fibrillation during transcutaneous pacing is negligible.

Personnel Required

One person can initiate transcutaneous pacing unaided.

Equipment Required

1. Transcutaneous pacing device, 2 pacing electrodes, and connecting cable.

2. Optional electrodes and connecting cable for electrocardiographic monitoring are available with some models.

Procedure

1. Place one pacing electrode over the left ante-

---

*This section contributed by Mary T. Ho, MD, MPH.

rior chest. Place the other electrode posteriorly in the interscapular area. Attach the connecting cables as indicated on the labels.

2. If the pacing device is equipped for electrocardiographic monitoring, attach monitor leads to both shoulders and left upper abdomen. *Note:* Standard electrocardiographic monitor results are usually uninterpretable owing to the strong pacing stimulus and movement artifact.

3. Set rate at 80 beats/min; select synchronous mode for bradycardia or asynchronous mode for asystole. (Depending on the model, rate and mode may be fixed and not operator-selected.) Turn on power; turn on pacing.

4. Begin at 70–80 mA current output.

5. Check for presence of a femoral pulse. Check the monitor for evidence of electrical capture (pacer spike before each QRS complex). If no pulse is de-

tected, gradually increase the current output until pulse appears or highest current setting is reached. *Caution:* The carotid pulse is usually difficult to detect owing to muscle contractions. A Doppler stethoscope may be needed to ascertain the presence or absence of a pulse.

6. Reduce current output to the lowest setting associated with a palpable pulse, and determine blood pressure.

7. If transcutaneous pacing is successful, interrupt pacing intermittently to check for return of spontaneous electrical activity. As soon as the patient is stable, if pacing is still needed, insert a transvenous pacemaker.

8. If transcutaneous pacing is unsuccessful and pacing is still required, attempt transvenous or transthoracic pacing.

APPLICATION & REMOVAL OF MAST GARMENT*
(Military Antishock Trousers; also Pneumatic Antishock Garment)

The MAST device is a garment that may be placed around a patient's legs and abdomen and inflated. Its primary use is as a temporizing measure in the treatment of shock until more definitive treatment (eg, transfusion, surgery) can be performed. Its predominant hemodynamic effect is to increase peripheral vascular resistance (afterload) by compressing vessels in regions of the patient's body enclosed by the garment. Autotransfusion from venous capacitance vessels in the abdomen and legs to the central circulation is minimal (< 300 mL). The MAST garment also reduces bleeding from the legs and abdomen by direct and indirect tamponade, respectively, and may also serve as a splint. The MAST garment is now widely accepted for use by emergency medical technicians, although its efficacy in prehospital treatment of shock remains controversial. Controlled studies of its use in this setting continue. The MAST garment should not be applied in a way that delays intravenous access and fluid administration.

Indications

1. Moderate to severe shock with supine systolic blood pressure less than 80 mm Hg or between 80 and 90 mm Hg with clinical evidence of hypoperfusion (eg, depressed or altered mental status, tachycardia > 100/min, prolonged [> 2 sec] capillary refill).

2. Splinting of pelvic and femoral fractures.

(MAST is the only effective emergency splint for combined fractures of the pelvis and femur.)

3. Tamponade of suspected intra-abdominal hemorrhage (eg, ruptured or leaking abdominal aortic aneurysm).

4. The MAST has been used as an adjunct to cardiopulmonary resuscitation for patients in cardiac arrest, but its efficacy is unknown.

Contraindications
A. Absolute:

1. Pulmonary edema, congestive heart failure, and cardiogenic shock due to pump failure. The MAST garment causes increased afterload.

2. Hypothermia (< 32 °C or 89.6 °F). Transfer of cold acidotic peripheral blood to the central circulation can precipitate cardiac arrest.

B. Relative: Burns involving areas that would be covered by the garment, which may exacerbate tissue ischemia. However, the need for cerebral and cardiac perfusion may override this consideration.

C. Relative Contraindications to Inflation of Abdominal Chamber: (These may be overruled if necessary to save life.)

1. Pregnancy.

2. Object impaling the abdomen (the object may be providing tamponade).

3. Evisceration.

4. Tension pneumothorax (the MAST garment may increase intrathoracic pressure).

5. Cardiac tamponade.

6. Bleeding above the diaphragm (bleeding may

---

*This section contributed by Mary T. Ho, MD, MPH.

be worsened by the MAST garment). However, this increase in bleeding may be more than compensated for by improved cerebral and cardiac perfusion.

Note: Head injury is *not* a contraindication. Increase in intracranial pressure is minimal and more than compensated for by improved cerebral and cardiac perfusion.

Personnel Required

One person can apply and deflate the MAST garment if the patient does not have a spine injury. However, 4 or more persons are usually needed if immobilization of the spine is required.

Equipment

The MAST garment is a commercially produced device containing an independently inflatable chamber for each leg and an inflatable abdominal chamber (Fig 46–40A). The garment fastens with Velcro straps, and airflow to each chamber is controlled by a stopcock. Two models are available, one equipped with a pop-off valve, the other with one or more pressure gauges. Depending on the manufacturer, the garment comes in one size that fits all or in 2 sizes (adult and child). A foot pump is also included.

Application

A. Spine Immobilization Required:

1. Place the MAST garment on a spine board, open it completely, and roll the inner leg flaps medially and the abdominal flap downward (Fig 46–40B).

2. Place the patient on the garment while maintaining spine immobilization. (Be sure the patient's crotch is over the crotch of the garment. If the patient is already on the spine board, lift the patient while maintaining spine immobilization and slip the opened garment between the patient and the spine board. (This requires at least 4 people—one to maintain neck traction, 2 or more to support the back and pelvis, and one to slip the garment underneath.)

3. Undress the patient as much as possible below the waist, and examine the abdomen, pelvis, and legs—*regions covered by the garment cannot be examined after the garment has been inflated.* If undressing the patient is not feasible, remove sharp or bulky objects from clothing and pockets.

4. Wrap the garment flaps snugly around the patient, and fasten the Velcro straps.

5. Connect the abdominal and leg chamber tubes on the foot pump to their respective tubes on the garment.

6. Open the stopcock corresponding to the chamber to be inflated. Be sure that stopcocks of chambers not to be inflated are closed.

7. Apply traction splints (eg, Hare), if needed, before inflating the garment.

8. Inflate chambers in the following sequence: (1) chamber of injured leg, (2) chamber of uninjured leg, and (3) abdominal chamber. *Never inflate the abdominal chamber before completely inflating both leg chambers.* (See contraindications to abdominal chamber inflation, above.)

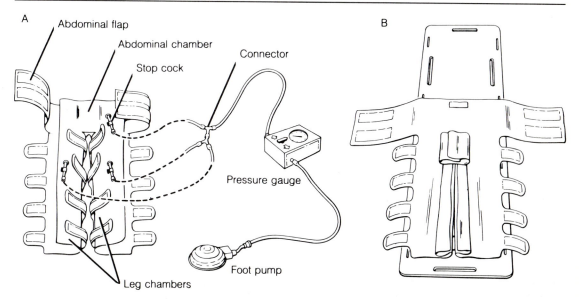

Figure 46–40. *A:* MAST garment and equipment to inflate the 3 separate compartments. *B:* MAST garment prepared for receiving patient—inner leg flaps rolled medially and abdominal flap rolled downward. If the patient requires immobilization, the MAST suit should be placed on the stretcher or spine board before the patient is positioned. (Reproduced, with permission, from Markovchick VJ: Mast suit. In: *Critical Decisions in Trauma.* Moore EE, Eiseman B, Van Way CW III [editors]. Mosby, 1984.)

9. Inflate until pop-off valve pops, Velcro straps crackle and begin to loosen, or pressure gauge records 100 mm Hg. Lower inflation pressures may be adequate if the MAST garment is applied for splinting only.

10. Close stopcock when chamber is fully inflated.

11. Check patient's blood pressure, pulse, and respiration. Monitor these signs every 5 minutes as long as the garment is inflated. Patients may occasionally require respiratory support if the inflated abdominal chamber compromises respiration by decreasing diaphragm excursion.

12. Monitor chamber pressures frequently, especially if changes in altitude or temperature occur during transport. Changes in altitude or temperature cause concomitant changes in chamber pressure (increases in altitude or temperature cause increased pressure). Pop-off valves automatically prevent hyperinflation, but with MAST garments that have only pressure gauges it may be necessary to release, or leak, air to reduce the pressure to 100 mm Hg. When partially deflating the garment, release air from abdominal chamber first, then from the chamber of the uninjured leg; release air from the chamber of the injured leg last. When reinflating the garment, follow the reverse order. The chamber pressure should be maintained at 100 mm Hg.

B. Spine Mobilization Not Required:

1. Raise the patient's legs and lower body.

2. Slip an opened MAST under the patient, and position the MAST so that the top of the abdominal flap reaches just below the patient's rib cage. Proceed with steps 3–12, above.

The following is an alternative procedure: (1) Undress the patient below the waist (or remove sharp or bulky objects from clothing) and examine the abdomen and legs. (2) Before fitting the MAST garment onto the patient, loosely fasten the Velcro straps on both leg chambers. Slide your arms up through the leg chambers, and bunch the garment so that your hands emerge at the top of the chambers. (3) Grasp the patient's feet and lift the patient's legs. Have an assistant slide the MAST garment off your arms and onto the patient's legs. (4) Wrap the garment snugly around the patient and refasten the Velcro. Proceed with steps 5–12, above.

Removal

A. *Caution: Never cut the MAST garment off or suddenly deflate all chambers.* Sudden decrease in afterload and release of lactic acid from ischemic extremities can cause irreversible shock or cardiac arrest. The garment should not be deflated until other resuscitative measures have restored effective intravascular volume. The abdominal chamber can be deflated just prior to abdominal surgery; leg chambers should remain inflated until deflation is indicated.

B. Removal Procedure:

1. When resuscitation is judged successful and the MAST garment is no longer needed, proceed with deflation.

2. Always deflate the abdominal chamber first. To do so, disconnect the foot pump from the garment. Turn the abdominal stopcock toward the open position and, while monitoring the patient's systolic pressure, allow a small amount of air to escape. Some MAST models have a control valve to regulate deflation.

3. After the abdominal chamber is fully deflated, deflate the uninjured leg chamber. Deflate the injured leg chamber last.

4. Stop deflation whenever systolic pressure declines by 5 mm Hg. Administer intravenous fluids until blood pressure is restored; then continue deflation.

5. Severe metabolic acidosis (pH < 7.2) may manifest as hypotension or arrhythmias and may need treatment with sodium bicarbonate (p 686). However, when deflation is performed slowly and correctly, severe acidosis is seldom a problem.

6. After deflation, open the garment to examine the patient, but leave it in place for reinflation until it is definitely no longer needed.

Index

Note: Page numbers in **bold face** type indicate a major discussion. A *t* following a page number indicates tabular material and an *i* following a page number indicates an illustration. Drugs are listed under their generic names. When a drug trade name is listed, the reader is referred to the generic name.

Basic Science Textbooks

Jawetz, Melnick & Adelberg's
Medical Microbiology, 19/e
Brooks, Butel & Ornston
1991, ISBN 0-8385-6241-8, A6241-2
Concise Pathology
Chandrasoma & Taylor
1991, ISBN 0-8385-1320-4, A1320-9
Correlative Neuroanatomy, 21/e
deGroot & Chusid
1991, ISBN 0-8385-1332-8, A1332-4
Review of Medical Physiology, 15/e
Ganong
1991, ISBN 0-8385-8418-7, A8418-4
Physiology: A Study Guide, 3/e
Ganong
1989, ISBN 0-8385-7875-6, A7875-6
Basic Histology, 7/e
Junqueira, Carniero & Kelly
1992, ISBN 0-8385-0576-7, A0576-7
Basic & Clinical Pharmacology, 5/e
Katzung
1992, ISBN 0-8385-0562-7, A0562-7
Pharmacology: Examination & Review, 3/e
Katzung & Trevor
1992, ISBN 0-8385-7807-1, A7807-9
Medical Microbiology & Immunology
Examination & Board Review, 2/e
Levinson & Jawetz
1991, ISBN 0-8385-6262-0, A6262-8
Harper's Biochemistry, 22/e
Murray, et al.
1991, ISBN 0-8385-3640-9, A3640-8
Basic Histology
Examination & Board Review, 2/e
Paulsen
1992, ISBN 0-8385-0569-4, A0569-2
Basic & Clinical Immunology, 7/e
Stites & Terr
1991, ISBN 0-8385-0544-9, A0544-5
Basic Human Immunology
Stites & Terr
1991, ISBN 0-8385-0543-0, A0543-7

Clinical Science Textbooks

Fluid & Electrolytes
Physiology & Pathophysiology
Cogan
1991, ISBN 0-8385-2546-6, A2546-8
Basic and Clinical Biostatistics
Dawson-Saunders & Trapp
1990, ISBN 0-8385-6200-0, A6200-8
Review of General Psychiatry, 3/e
Goldman
1992, ISBN 0-8385-8428-4, A8428-3
Principles of Clinical Electrocardiography, 13/e
Goldschlager & Goldman
1989, ISBN 0-8385-7951-5, A7951-5

Basic and Clinical Endocrinology, 3/e
Greenspan
1990, ISBN 0-8385-0545-7, A0545-2
Occupational Medicine
LaDou
1990, ISBN 0-8385-7207-3, A7207-2
Clinical Anatomy
Lindner
1989, ISBN 0-8385-1259-3, A1259-9
Clinical Anesthesiology
Morgan & Mikhail
1992, ISBN 0-8385-1324-7, A1324-1
Dermatology
Orkin, Maibach & Dahl
1991, ISBN 0-8385-1288-7, A1288-8
Clinical Neurology, 2/e
Simon, Aminoff & Greenberg
1992, ISBN 0-8385-1311-5, A1311-8
Clinical Cardiology, 5/e
Sokolow, McIlroy & Cheitlin
1990, ISBN 0-8385-1266-6, A1266-4
Clinical Thinking in Surgery
Sterns
1988, ISBN 0-8385-5686-8, A5686-9
Smith's General Urology, 13/e
Tanagho & McAninch
1992, ISBN 0-8385-8608-2, A8608-0
General Ophthalmology, 13/e
Vaughan, Asbury & Riordan-Eva
1992, ISBN 0-8385-3115-6, A3115-1

CURRENT Clinical References

CURRENT Pediatric Diagnosis & Treatment, 11/e
Hathaway, et al.
1992, ISBN 0-8385-1440-5, A1440-5
CURRENT Obstetric & Gynecologic Diagnosis & Treatment, 7/e
Pernoll
1991, ISBN 0-8385-1424-3, A1424-9
CURRENT Emergency Diagnosis & Treatment, 4/e
Saunders & Ho
1992, ISBN 0-8385-1347-6, A1347-2
CURRENT Medical Diagnosis & Treatment 1992, 31/e
Schroeder, et al.
1992, ISBN 0-8385-1438-3, A1438-9
CURRENT Surgical Diagnosis & Treatment, 9/e
Way
1991, ISBN 0-8385-1426-X, A1426-4

Order information on reverse.

LANGE Clinical Manuals

Dermatology
Diagnosis and Therapy
Bondi, Jegasothy & Lazarus
1990, ISBN 0-8385-1274-7, A1274-8
Office & Bedside Procedures
Chesnutt & Dewar
1992, ISBN 0-8385-1095-7, A1095-7
Psychiatry
Diagnosis & Treatment, 2/e
Flaherty, Davis & Janicak
1992, ISBN 0-8385-1267-4, A1267-2
Neonatology
Management, Procedures, On-Call Problems, Diseases, Drugs, 2/e
Gomella
1992, ISBN 0-8385-1284-4, A1284-7
Clinician's Pocket Reference, 6/e
Gomella
1989, ISBN 0-8385-1212-7, A1212-8
Drug Therapy, 2/e
Katzung
1991, ISBN 0-8385-1312-3, A1312-6
Poisoning and Drug Overdose
Olson
1990, ISBN 0-8385-1297-6, A1297-9
Ambulatory Medicine
Primary Care of Families
Schwiebert & Mengle
1992, ISBN 0-8385-1294-1, A1294-6
Internal Medicine
Diagnosis and Therapy, 2/e
Stein
1991, ISBN 0-8385-1299-2, A1299-5
Surgery
Diagnosis & Therapy
Stillman
1989, ISBN 0-8385-1283-6, A1283-9
Medical Perioperative Management
Wolfsthal
1989, ISBN 0-8385-1298-4, A1298-7

LANGE Handbooks

Handbook of Gynecology & Obstetrics
Brown & Crombleholme
1992, ISBN 0-8385-3608-5, A3608-5
Handbook of Clinical Endocrinology, 2/e
Fitzgerald
1991, ISBN 0-8385-3615-8, A3615-0
Silver, Kempe, Bruyn & Fulginiti's
Handbook of Pediatrics, 16/e
Merenstein, Kaplan & Rosenberg
1991, ISBN 0-8385-3639-5, A3639-0
Pocket Guide to Commonly Prescribed Drugs
Levine
1992, ISBN 0-8385-8023-8, A8023-2
Pocket Guide to Diagnostic Tests
Detmer, et al.
1992, ISBN 0-8385-8020-3, A8020-8

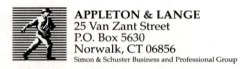